2012

the calorie carb and fat bible 2012

Juliette Kellow BSc RD, Lyndel Costain BSc RD & Laurence Beeken

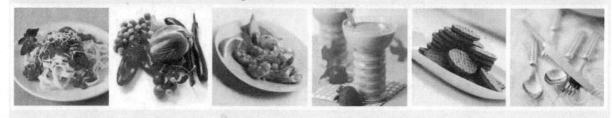

The UK's Most Comprehensive Calorie Counter

The Calorie, Carb & Fat Bible 2012

© Weight Loss Resources 2012
Lyndel Costain's contributions © Lyndel Costain 2007

Published by:
Weight Loss Resources Ltd
29 Metro Centre
Woodston,
Peterborough
PE2 7UH.

Tel: 01733 345592
www.weightlossresources.co.uk

Companies and other organisations wishing to make bulk purchases of the Calorie, Carb and Fat Bible should contact their local bookstore or Weight Loss Resources direct.

ISBN 978-1-904512-10-3

Authors: Lyndel Costain BSc RD
Juliette Kellow BSc RD
Laurence Beeken, Weight Loss Resources

Database Editor: Laurence Beeken

Design and Layout: Joanne Readshaw

Printed and bound by:
CPI Group (UK) Ltd, Croydon, CR0 4YY

Contents

Losing weight – the easy way

Juliette Kellow BSc RD

CHINESE TAKEAWAYS, curries, chocolate, chips and a glass of wine! Imagine being told the best diet to help you lose weight includes all these foods and more. It sounds too good to be true, doesn't it? But the truth is, these are exactly the types of foods you can still enjoy if you opt to lose weight by counting calories.

But you'd be forgiven for not knowing you can still eat all your favourite foods *and* lose weight. In recent years, endless trendy diets that cut carbs, boost protein intake or skip entire groups of foods, have helped to make dieting a complicated business. Added to this, an increasing number of celebrities and so-called nutrition experts have helped mislead us into thinking that dieting is all about restriction and denial. Is it any wonder then that most of us have been left feeling downright confused and miserable about what we should and shouldn't be eating to shift those pounds?

Dieting doesn't have to be complicated or an unhappy experience. In fact, there's really only one word you need to remember if you want to shift those pounds healthily and still eat all your favourite foods. And that's CALORIE!

It's calories that count

When it comes to losing weight, there's no getting away from the fact that it's calories that count. Ask any qualified nutrition expert or dietitian for advice on how to fight the flab and you'll receive the same reply: quite simply you need to create a calorie deficit or shortfall. In other words, you need to take in fewer calories than you use up so that your body has to draw on its fat stores to provide it with the energy it needs to function properly. The result: you start losing fat and the pounds start to drop off!

Fortunately, it couldn't be easier to create this calorie deficit. Regardless of your age, weight, sex, genetic make up, lifestyle or eating habits, losing weight is as simple as reducing your daily calorie intake slightly by modifying your diet and using up a few more calories by being slightly more active each day.

Better still, it's a complete myth that you need to change your eating and exercise habits dramatically. You'll notice I've said you need to reduce your calorie intake 'slightly' and be 'slightly' more active. It really is just LITTLE differences between the amount of calories we take in and the amount we use up that make BIG differences to our waistline over time. For example, you only need to consume one can of cola more than you need each day to gain a stone in a year. It's no wonder then that people say excess weight tends to 'creep up on them'.

10 simple food swaps you can make every day (and won't even notice!)

Make these simple swaps every day and in just 4 weeks you'll lose 7lb!

SWAP THIS...	FOR THIS...	SAVE...
300ml full-fat milk (195 calories)	300ml skimmed milk (100 calories)	95 calories
1tsp butter (35 calories)	1tsp low-fat spread (20 calories)	15 calories
1tbsp vegetable oil (100 calories)	10 sprays of a spray oil (10 calories)	90 calories
1tsp sugar (16 calories)	Artificial sweetener (2 calories)	14 calories
1tbsp mayonnaise (105 calories)	1tbsp fat-free dressing (10 calories)	95 calories
Regular sandwich (600 calories)	Low-fat sandwich (350 calories)	250 calories
Can of cola (135 calories)	Can of diet cola (1 calorie)	134 calories
Large (50g) packet of crisps (250 calories)	Small (25g) packet of crisps (125 calories)	125 calories
1 chocolate digestive (85 calories)	1 small chocolate chip cookie (55 calories)	30 calories
1 slice thick-cut wholemeal bread (95 calories)	1 slice medium-cut wholemeal bread (75 calories)	20 calories
	TOTAL CALORIE SAVING:	868 calories

The good news is the reverse is also true. You only need to swap that daily can of cola for the diet version or a glass of sparking water and you'll lose a stone in a year – it really is as easy as that!

Of course, most people don't want to wait a year to shift a stone. But there's more good news. To lose 1lb of fat each week you need to create a calorie deficit of just 500 calories a day. That might sound like a lot, but you can achieve this by simply swapping a croissant for a wholemeal fruit scone, a regular sandwich for a low-fat variety, a glass of dry white wine for a gin and slimline tonic and using low-fat spread on two slices of toast instead of butter. It is also important to become more active and increase your level of exercise. Losing 1lb a week, amounts to a stone in 14 weeks, or just under 4 stone in a year!

Taking control of calories

By now you've seen it really is calories that count when it comes to shifting those pounds. So it should be no surprise that a calorie-controlled diet is the only guaranteed way to help you shift those pounds – and that's a scientific fact! But better still, a calorie-controlled diet is one of the few that allows you to include anything, whether it's pizza, wine or chocolate. A healthy diet means including a wide range of foods *(see 'Healthy Eating Made Easy' page 32)*.

And that's where this book can really help. Gone are the days when it was virtually impossible to obtain information about the calorie contents of foods. This book provides calorie information for more than 22,000 different branded and unbranded foods so that counting calories has never been easier.

The benefits of counting calories
• *It's guaranteed to help you lose weight providing you stick to your daily calorie allowance*
• *You can include favourite foods*
• *No foods are banned*
• *It's a great way to lose weight slowly and steadily*
• *Nutrition experts agree that it's a proven way to lose weight*

Calorie counting made easy

Forget weird and wacky science, complicated diet rules and endless lists of foods to fill up on or avoid every day! Counting calories to lose weight couldn't be easier. Quite simply, you set yourself a daily calorie allowance to help you lose between ½-2lb (¼-1kg) a week and then add up the calories of everything you eat and drink each day, making sure you don't go over your limit.

To prevent hunger from kicking in, it's best to spread your daily calorie allowance evenly throughout the day, allowing a certain amount of calories for breakfast, lunch, dinner and one or two snacks. For example, if you are allowed 1,500 calories a day, you could have 300 calories for breakfast, 400 calories for lunch, 500 calories for dinner and two snacks or treats of 150 calories each. You'll find more detailed information on p26-31 (Your step-by-step guide to using this book and shifting those pounds).

QUESTION
What affects the calorie content of a food?

ANSWER:
Fat, protein, carbohydrate and alcohol all provide the body with calories, but in varying amounts:

- *1g fat provides 9 calories*

- *1g alcohol provides 7 calories*

- *1g protein provides 4 calories*

- *1g carbohydrate provides 3.75 calories*

The calorie content of a food depends on the amount of fat, protein and carbohydrate it contains. Because fat provides more than twice as many calories as an equal quantity of protein or carbohydrate, in general, foods that are high in fat tend to contain more calories. This explains why 100g of chips (189 calories) contains more than twice as many calories as 100g of boiled potato (72 calories).

DIET MYTH:
Food eaten late at night stops you losing weight

DIET FACT:
It's not eating in the evening that stops you losing weight. It's consuming too many calories throughout the day that will be your dieting downfall! Providing you stick to your daily calorie allowance you'll lose weight, regardless of when you consume those calories. Nevertheless, it's a good idea to spread your calorie allowance throughout the day to prevent hunger from kicking in, which leaves you reaching for high-calorie snack foods.

Eat for good health

While calories might be the buzz word when it comes to shifting those pounds, it's nevertheless important to make sure your diet is healthy, balanced and contains all the nutrients you need for good health. Yes, you can still lose weight by eating nothing but, for example, chocolate, crisps and biscuits providing you stick to your calorie allowance. But you'll never find a nutrition expert or dietitian recommending this. And there are plenty of good reasons why.

To start with, an unbalanced diet is likely to be lacking in essential nutrients such as protein, vitamins, minerals and fibre, in the long term putting you at risk of nutritional deficiencies. Secondly, research proves that filling up on foods that are high in fat and/or salt and sugar can lead to many different health problems. But most importantly, when it comes to losing weight, it's almost impossible to stick to a daily calorie allowance if you're only eating high-calorie foods.

Filling up on lower-calorie foods also means you'll be able to eat far more with the result that you're not constantly left feeling unsatisfied. For example, six chocolates from a selection box contain around 300 calories, a lot of fat and sugar, few nutrients – and are eaten in just six mouthfuls! For 300 calories, you could have a grilled skinless chicken breast (packed with protein and zinc), a large salad with fat-free dressing (a great source of fibre, vitamins and minerals), a slice of wholemeal bread with low-fat spread (rich in fibre and B vitamins) and a satsuma (an excellent source of vitamin C). That's a lot more food that will take you a lot more time to eat! Not convinced? Then put six chocolates on one plate, and the chicken, salad, bread and fruit on another!

Bottom line: while slightly reducing your calorie intake is the key to losing weight, you'll be healthier and far more likely to keep those pounds off if you do it by eating a healthy diet *(see 'Healthy Eating Made Easy' page 32).*

Eight steps to a healthy diet

1 *Base your meals on starchy foods.*

2 *Eat lots of fruit and vegetables.*

3 *Eat more fish.*

4 *Cut down on saturated fat and sugar.*

5 *Try to eat less salt - no more than 6g a day.*

6 *Get active and try to be a healthy weight.*

7 *Drink plenty of water.*

8 *Don't skip breakfast.*   SOURCE: FSA www.eatwell.gov.uk

Fat facts

Generally speaking, opting for foods that are low in fat can help slash your calorie intake considerably, for example, swapping full-fat milk for skimmed, switching from butter to a low-fat spread, not frying food in oil and chopping the fat off meat and poultry. But don't be fooled into believing that all foods described as 'low-fat' or 'fat-free' are automatically low in calories or calorie-free. In fact, some low-fat products may actually be higher in calories than standard products, thanks to them containing extra sugars and thickeners to boost the flavour and texture. The solution: always check the calorie content of low-fat foods, especially for things like cakes, biscuits, crisps, ice creams and ready meals. You might be surprised to find there's little difference in the calorie content when compared to the standard product.

Uncovering fat claims on food labels

Many products may lure you into believing they're a great choice if you're trying to cut fat, but you need to read between the lines on the labels if you want to be sure you're making the best choice. Here's the lowdown on what to look for:

LOW FAT	by law the food must contain less than 3g of fat per 100g for solids. These foods are generally a good choice if you're trying to lose weight.
REDUCED FAT	by law the food must contain 25 percent less fat than a similar standard product. This doesn't mean the product is low-fat (or low-calorie) though! For example, reduced-fat cheese may still contain 14g fat per 100g.
FAT FREE	the food must contain no more than 0.5g of fat per 100g or 100ml. Foods labelled as Virtually Fat Free must contain less than 0.3g fat per 100g. These foods are generally a good choice if you're trying to lose weight.
LESS THAN 8% FAT	this means the product contains less than 8g fat per 100g. It's only foods labelled 'less than 3% fat' that are a true low-fat choice.
X% FAT FREE	claims expressed as X% Fat Free shall be prohibited.
LIGHT OR LITE	claims stating a product is 'light' or 'lite' follows the same conditions as those set for the term 'reduced'.

10 easy ways to slash fat (and calories)

1 Eat fewer fried foods – grill, boil, bake, poach, steam, roast without added fat or microwave instead.

2 Don't add butter, lard, margarine or oil to food during preparation or cooking.

3 Use spreads sparingly. Butter and margarine contain the same amount of calories and fat – only low fat spreads contain less.

4 Choose boiled or jacket potatoes instead of chips or roast potatoes.

5 Cut off all visible fat from meat and remove the skin from chicken before cooking.

6 Don't eat too many fatty meat products such as sausages, burgers, pies and pastry products.

7 Use semi-skimmed or skimmed milk instead of full-fat milk.

8 Try low-fat or reduced-fat varieties of cheese such as reduced-fat Cheddar, low-fat soft cheese or cottage cheese.

9 Eat fewer high-fat foods such as crisps, chocolates, cakes, pastries and biscuits.

10 Don't add cream to puddings, sauces or coffee.

Getting Ready for Weight Loss Success

Lyndel Costain BSc RD

THIS BOOK not only provides tools to help you understand more about what you eat and how active you are, but guidance on how to use this information to develop a weight loss plan to suit your needs. Getting in the right frame of mind will also be a key part of your weight control journey, especially if you've lost weight before, only to watch the pounds pile back on.

The fact is that most people who want to lose weight know what to do. But often there is something that keeps stopping them from keeping up healthier habits. The same may be true for you. So what's going on? For many it's a lack of readiness. When the next diet comes along with its tempting promises it's so easy to just jump on board. But if you have struggled with your weight for a while, will that diet actually help you to recognise and change the thoughts and actions that have stopped you shifting the pounds for good?

Check out your attitude to weight loss programmes

Before starting any new weight loss programme, including the Weight Loss Resources approach, ask yourself:

Am I starting out thinking that I like myself as a person right now?	(YES or NO)
OR I feel I can only like myself once I lose weight?	(YES or NO)
Do I want to stop overeating, but at the same time find myself justifying it – in other words I want to be able to eat what I want, but with no consequences?	(YES or NO)
Do I believe that I need to take long-term responsibility for my weight?	(YES or NO)
OR Am I relying on 'it' (the diet) to do it for me?	(YES or NO)

Keep these questions, and your replies, in mind as you read through this chapter.

Next Steps

You may have already assessed the healthiness of your weight using the BMI guide on page 37. If not, why not do it now, remembering that the tools are a guide only. The important thing is to consider a weight at which you are healthy and comfortable – and which is realistic for the life you lead *(see opposite - What is a healthy weight?)*.

The next step is to have a long hard think about why you want to lose weight. Consider all the possible benefits, not just those related to how you look. Psychologists have found that if we focus only on appearance we are less likely to succeed in the long-term. This is because it so often reflects low self-esteem or self-worth – which can sabotage success – as it saps confidence and keeps us stuck in destructive thought patterns. Identifying key motivations other than simply how you look - such as health and other aspects of physical and emotional well being - is like saying that you're an OK person right now, and worth making changes for. Making healthy lifestyle choices also has the knock on effect of boosting self-esteem further.

Write down your reasons for wanting to lose weight in your Personal Plan *(see page 42)* – so you can refer back to them. This can be especially helpful when the going gets tough. It may help to think of it in terms of what your weight is stopping you from doing now. Here's some examples: to feel more confident; so I can play more comfortably with my kids; my healthier diet will give me more energy; to improve my fertility.

What is a Healthy Weight?

With all the 'thin is beautiful' messages in the media it can be easy to get a distorted view about whether your weight is healthy or not. However, as the BMI charts suggest, there is no single 'ideal' weight for anybody. Research also shows that modest amounts of weight loss can be very beneficial to health and are easier to keep off. Therefore, health professionals now encourage us to aim for a weight loss of 5-10%. The ideal rate of weight loss is no more than 1-2 pounds (0.5-1kg) per week – so averaging a pound a week is great, and realistic progress.

The health benefits of modest weight loss include:

- *Reduced risk of developing heart disease, stroke and certain cancers*

- *Reduced risk of developing diabetes and helping to manage diabetes*

- *Improvements in blood pressure*

- *Improvements in mobility, back pain and joint pain*

- *Improvements with fertility problems and polycystic ovarian syndrome*

- *Less breathlessness and sleep/snoring problems*

- *Increased self esteem and control over eating*

- *Feeling fitter and have more energy*

Are You Really Ready to Lose Weight?

When you think of losing weight, it's easy just to think of what weight you'd like to get to. But weight loss only happens as a result of making changes to your usual eating and activity patterns – which allow you to consume fewer calories than you burn *(see 'It's calories that count' page 5)*.

So here comes the next big question. Are you really ready to do it? Have you thought about the implications of your decision? If you have lost weight in the past, and put it all back on - have you thought about why that was? And how confident do you feel about being successful this time?

To help you answer these questions, try these short exercises.

Where would you place yourself on the following scales?

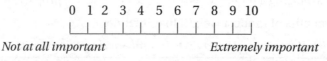

Importance

How important is it to you, to make the changes that will allow you to lose weight?

0 1 2 3 4 5 6 7 8 9 10

Not at all important   *Extremely important*

If you ranked yourself over half way along the scale then move on to the next question. If you were half way or less along the scale, you may not be mentally ready to make the required changes to lose weight. To further explore this, go to *'The Pros and Cons of Weight Loss' (page 17).*

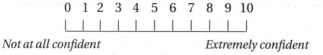

Confidence

How confident are you in your ability to make the changes that will allow you to lose weight?

0 1 2 3 4 5 6 7 8 9 10

Not at all confident   *Extremely confident*

Now ask yourself (regarding your confidence ratings):

1. Why did I place myself here?

2. What is stopping me moving further up the scale (if anything)?

3. What things, information, support would help me move further up the scale? (if not near 10)

If you aren't sure about answers to question 3, then keep reading for some pointers.

The Pros and Cons of Weight Loss

Making lifestyle changes to lose weight is simpler if there are lots of clear benefits or pros, for example, clothes fit again, more energy, helps back pain - but there will also be associated downsides or cons. For example, some may feel it interferes with their social life, or don't have the time to plan meals or check food labels. Or overeating can help, if only temporarily, as a way of coping with unwanted feelings. Being overweight allows some people to feel strong and assertive, or to control their partner's jealousy. So in these cases there are downsides to losing weight, even if the person says they are desperate to do it.

If you are aware of the possible downsides, as well as the pros, you will be better prepared to deal with potential conflicts. Understanding what could be (or were with past weight loss efforts) barriers to success gives you the chance to address them. This boosts confidence in your ability to succeed this time, which in turn maintains your motivation.

Have a go at weighing up the pros and cons using the charts below and on page 18. Some examples are included. If you decide that the pros outweigh the cons, then great. You can also use the cons as potential barriers to plan strategies for *(see page 42)*. If you find it's the other way around, this may not be the best time to actively lose weight. Try the exercise again in a month or so.

Making Lifestyle Changes to Lose Weight Now

CONS *e.g. Must limit eating out, take aways*	PROS *e.g. Feel more energetic, slimmer*

Not Making Changes Now – how would I feel in 6 months time?

PROS *e.g. Haven't had to worry about failing;* *Still able to eat take aways a lot*	CONS *e.g. Probably gained more weight;* *Back pain may be worse*

To change your weight, first change your mind

To lose weight you may already have a list of things to change, such as eating more fruit and veg, calculating your daily calorie intake, going for a walk each morning or buying low fat options. Others could also give you tips to try. But knowing what to do isn't the same as feeling motivated or able to do it. To be effective, you have to believe the changes are relevant, do-able and worth it.

What you think, affects how you feel, and in turn the actions you take.

Self-efficacy

In fact, research is telling us that one of the most important factors that influences weight loss success are your feelings of 'self-efficacy'. Self-efficacy is a term used in psychology to describe a person's belief that any action they take will have an effect on the outcome. It reflects our inner expectation that what we do will lead to the results we want. Not surprisingly, high levels of self-efficacy can enhance motivation, and allow us to deal better with uncertainty and conflict, and recovery from setbacks. But low levels, can reduce our motivation. We fear that whatever we do will not bring about our desired goal. This can lead self-defeating thoughts or 'self-talk', which make it hard to deal with set-backs, meaning we are more likely to give up. Here's some examples.

Examples: Low self-efficacy

'*No matter how carefully I diet, I don't lose weight . . .*'

'*I have eaten that chocolate and as usual blown my diet, so I may as well give up now.*'

'*I had a rich dessert – I have no willpower to say no. I can't stand not being able to eat what I want.*'

If you have a strong sense of self-efficacy, your mindset and 'self-talk' will be more like:

Examples: High self-efficacy

'*I know from previous weight loss programmes, that if I stay focussed on what I am doing I do lose weight. I have always expected to lose too much too quickly which frustrates me. I know that I will lose weight if I keep making the right changes, and this time it is important to me.*'

'*The chocolate bar won't ruin my diet, but if I think it has and keep on eating, then my negative self-talk will. So I will get back on track.*'

'*I don't like having to eat differently from others, but losing weight is very important to me, so I **can** stand it. After all, the world won't stop if I say no to dessert, and I will feel great afterwards. If I think about it, I am not hungry so would just feel bloated and guilty if I ate it.*'

Willpower is a Skill

Many people feel that they just need plenty of willpower or a good telling off to lose weight. But willpower isn't something you have or you don't have. Willpower is a skill. Like the dessert example on page 19, it's a sign that you've made a conscious choice to do something, because you believe the benefits outweigh any downsides. In reality everything we do is preceded by a thought. This includes everything we eat. It just may not seem like it because our actions often feel automatic *(see 'Look out for trigger eating' page 21).*

When it comes to weight loss, developing a range of skills – including choosing a lower calorie diet, coping with negative self-talk and managing things that don't go to plan - will boost your sense of self-efficacy to make the changes you want. This is especially important because we live in such a weight-promoting environment.

Our weight-promoting environment

We are constantly surrounded by tempting food, stresses that can trigger comfort eating and labour-saving devices that make it easy not to be physically active. In other words, the environment we live in makes it easy to gain weight, unless we stop and think about the food choices we make and how much exercise we do. In fact, to stay a healthy weight/maintain our weight, just about all of us need to make conscious lifestyle choices everyday. This isn't 'dieting' but just part of taking care of ourselves in the environment we live in.

It is also true that some people find it more of a challenge than others to manage their weight, thanks to genetic differences in factors such as appetite control, spontaneous activity level and emotional responses to food – rather than metabolic rate, as is often believed. The good news is that with a healthy diet and active lifestyle a healthier weight can still be achieved. But do talk to your doctor if you feel you need additional support.

Coping with Common Slimming Saboteurs

Lyndel Costain BSc RD

Look out for 'trigger' eating

Much of the overeating we do or cravings we have are actually down to unconscious, habitual, responses to a variety of triggers. These triggers can be external, such as the sight or smell of food, or internal and emotion-led, such as a response to stress, anger, boredom or emptiness. Your food diary (see page 43) helps you to recognise 'trigger' or 'non-hungry' eating which gives you the chance to think twice before you eat (see below).

Get some support

A big part of your success will be having someone to support you. It could be a friend, partner, health professional, health club or website. Let them know how they can help you most.

Make lapses your ally

Don't let a lapse throw you off course. You can't be, nor need to be perfect all the time. Doing well 80-90% of the time is great progress. Lapses are a normal part of change. Rather than feel you have failed and give up, look at what you can learn from a difficult day or week and use it to find helpful solutions for the future.

Understand why you eat

When I ask people what prompts them to eat, hunger usually comes down near the bottom of their list of reasons. Some people struggle to remember or appreciate what true hunger feels like. We are lucky that we have plenty of food to eat in our society. But its constant presence makes it harder to control what we eat, especially if it brings us comfort or joy.

If you ever find yourself in the fridge even though you've recently eaten, then you know hunger isn't the reason but some other trigger. The urge to eat can be so automatic that you feel you lack willpower or are out of control. But it is in fact a learned or conditioned response. A bit like Pavlov's dogs. He rang a bell every time he fed them, and from then on, whenever they heard the bell ring they were 'conditioned' to salivate in anticipation of food.

Because this 'non-hungry' eating is learned, you can reprogramme your response to the situations or feelings that trigger it. The first step is to identify when these urges strike. When you find yourself eating when you aren't hungry ask yourself 'why do I want to eat, what am I feeling?' If you aren't sure think back to what was happening before you ate. Then ask yourself if there is another way you can feel better without food. Or you could chat to your urge to eat in a friendly way, telling it that you don't want to give into it, you have a planned meal coming soon, and it's merely a learned response. Whatever strategy you choose, the more often you break into your urges to eat, the weaker their hold becomes.

Practise positive self-talk

Self-talk may be positive and constructive (like your guardian angel) or negative and irrational (like having a destructive devil on your shoulder).

If you've had on-off battles with your weight over the years, it's highly likely that the 'devil' is there more often. 'All or nothing' self-talk for example, 'I ate a "bad food" so have broken my diet', can make you feel like a failure which, can then trigger you into the action of overeating and/or totally giving up *(see 'Diet-binge cycle' page 23)*. One of the most powerful things about it is that the last thoughts we have are what stays in our mind. So if we think 'I still look fat' or 'I will never be slim', these feelings stay with us.

To change your self-talk for the better, the trick is to first recognise it's happening (keeping a diary really helps, *see Keep a Food Diary, page 29*). Then turn it around into a positive version of the same events *(see Self-efficacy, page 18)* where the resulting action was to feel good and stay on track. Reshaping negative self-talk helps you to boost your self-esteem and feelings of self-efficacy, and with it change your self-definition - from someone who can't 'lose weight' or 'do this or that', to someone 'who can'. And when you believe you can…

The Diet – Binge Cycle

If this cycle looks familiar, use positive self-talk, and a more flexible dietary approach, to help you break free.

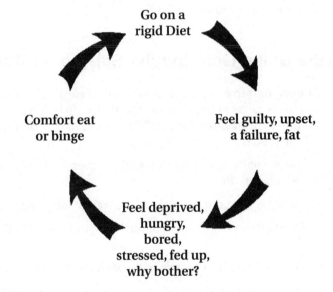

Go on a rigid Diet

Feel guilty, upset, a failure, fat

Feel deprived, hungry, bored, stressed, fed up, why bother?

Comfort eat or binge

Really choose what you want to eat

This skill is like your personal brake. It also helps you to manage 'trigger/non-hungry' eating and weaken its hold. It legalises food and stops you feeling deprived. It helps you to regularly remind yourself why you are making changes to your eating habits, which keeps motivation high. But it doesn't just happen. Like all skills it requires practise. Sometimes it will work well for you, other times it won't – but overall it will help. Basically, ask yourself if you really want to eat that food in front of you. This becomes the prompt for you to make a conscious choice, weighing up the pros and cons or consequences of making that choice, and feeling free to have it, reject it or just eat some. Remembering all the while that you can eat this food another time if you want to.

Action Planning

Successful people don't just wait for things to happen. They believe in themselves, plan ahead, take action and then refine their plan until it gets, and keeps on getting the results they want. Successful slimmers use a very similar approach. They don't rely on quick-fixes or magic formulas, but glean information from reliable sources to develop a plan or approach that suits their needs, tastes and lifestyle. Thinking of weight management as a lifelong project, which has a weight loss phase and a weight maintenance phase, is also a route to success.

When the Going Gets Tough - Staying on Track

If things start to go off track, don't panic. Learning new habits takes time. And life is never straightforward so there will be times when it all seems too much, or negative 'self- talk' creeps in to try and drag you back into old ways. So if the going gets tough:

- Value what you've achieved so far, rather than only focus on what you plan to do.

- Look back at your reasons to lose weight and refer to the list often.

- Don't expect to change too much, too quickly. Take things a step at a time.

- Accept difficulties as part of the learning and skill building process.

- Enjoy a non-food reward for achieving your goals (including maintaining your weight).

- Use recipes and meal ideas to keep things interesting.

- Talk to your supporters and get plenty of encouragement. This is really vital!

Strategies of Successful Slimmers

Thanks to research conducted by large studies such as the US National Weight Control Registry and the German Lean Habits Study, we now know more about what works best for people who have lost weight and successfully kept it off. So be inspired!

The key elements of success are to:

- Believe that you can control your weight and the changes involved are really worth it.
- Stay realistic and value what you have achieved rather than dwell on a weight you 'dream' of being.
- Be more active – plan ways to fit activity into your daily life – aim for 1 hour of walking daily.
- Plan ahead for regular meals and snacks, starting with breakfast.
- Choose a balanced, low-fat diet with plenty of fruit and vegetables (see *Healthy Eating Made Easy, page 32*).
- Watch portion size and limit fast food.
- Sit down to eat and take time over meals, paying attention to what you are eating.
- Have a flexible approach – plan in and enjoy some favourite foods without guilt.
- Recognise and address 'all or nothing' thinking and other negative 'self-talk'.
- Keep making conscious choices.
- Learn to confront problems rather than eat, drink, sleep or wish they would go away.
- Enlist ongoing help and support from family, friends, professionals or websites.
- Regularly (at least once a week but not more than once daily) check your weight.
- Take action before your weight increases by more than 4-5lb (2kg).
- Accept that your weight management skills need to be kept up long-term.
- Take heart from successful slimmers, who say that it gets easier over time.

Your step-by-step guide to using this book and shifting those pounds

Juliette Kellow BSc RD and Rebecca Walton

1. Find your healthy weight

Use the weight charts, body mass index table and information on pages 36-43 to determine the right weight for you. Then set yourself a weight to aim for. Research shows it really helps if you make losing 10% of your weight your first overall target. It also brings important health benefits too *(see 'What is a Healthy Weight?' page 15)*. You can break this down into smaller manageable steps, for example, 3kg/6.5lbs at a time. If 10% is too much, then go for a 5% loss – this has important health benefits too. In fact, just keeping your weight stable is a great achievement these days, because of our weight-promoting environment *(see page 20)*.

Waist Management

In addition to BMI, another important way to assess your weight is by measuring your waist just above belly button level. It is especially useful for men as they tend to carry more excess weight around their bellies, but women should test it out too. Having excess weight around your middle (known as being 'apple-shaped') increases your risk of heart disease and type 2 diabetes. A simple way to stay aware of your waist is according to how well, or otherwise, skirts and trousers fit. Talk to your doctor about any weight and health concerns.

WAIST MEASUREMENT

	Increased Health Risk	High Risk to Health
Women	32-35in (81-88cm)	more than 35in (88cm)
Men	37-40in (94-102cm)	more than 40in (102cm)

---

2. Set a realistic time scale

With today's hectic lifestyles, everything tends to happen at breakneck speed, so it's no wonder that when it comes to losing weight, most of us want to shift those pounds in an instant. But it's probably taken years to accumulate that extra weight, with the result that it's unrealistic to expect to lose the excess in just a few weeks! Instead, prepare yourself to lose weight slowly and steadily. It's far healthier to lose weight like this. But better still, research shows you'll be far more likely to maintain your new, lower weight.

If you only have a small amount of weight to lose, aim for a weight loss of around 1lb (½kg) a week. But if you have more than 2 stone (28kg) to lose, you may prefer to aim for 2lb (1kg) each week. Remember though, it's better to keep going at 1lb (½kg) a week than to give up because trying to lose 2lb (1kg) a week is making you miserable! The following words may help you to keep your goal in perspective:

'Never give up on a goal because of the time it will take to achieve it – the time will pass anyway.'

Weight Fluctuations

Weight typically fluctuates on a day to day basis. You know that shock/horror feeling when you weigh yourself in the morning then later in the day, or after a meal out, and it looks like youve gained pounds in hours! But this is due to fluid not fat changes. Real changes in body fat can only happen more gradually (remember, to gain 1lb you need to eat 3500 calories more than you usually do). Don't be confused either by seemingly very rapid weight loss in the first week or so.

When calorie intake is initially cut back, the body's carbohydrate stores in the liver and muscles (known as glycogen) are used up. Glycogen is stored with three times its weight in water, meaning that rapid losses of 4.5- 6.6lb (2 -3 kg) are possible. These stores can be just as rapidly refilled if normal eating is resumed. True weight loss happens more gradually and this book helps you to lose weight at the steady and healthy rate of no more than 1-2 lbs per week.

3. Calculate your calorie allowance

Use the calorie tables on pages 39-40 to find out how many calories you need each day to maintain your current weight. Then use the table below to discover the amount of calories you need to subtract from this amount every day to lose weight at your chosen rate. For example, a 35 year-old woman who is moderately active and weighs 12 stone (76kg) needs 2,188 calories a day to keep her weight steady. If she wants to lose ½lb (¼kg) a week, she needs 250 calories less each day, giving her a daily calorie allowance of 1,938 calories. If she wants to lose 1lb (½kg) a week, she needs 500 calories less each day, giving her a daily calorie allowance of 1,688 calories, and so on.

TO LOSE...	Cut your daily calorie intake by	In three months you could lose...	In six months you could lose...	In one year you could lose...
½lb a week	250	6.5lb	13lb	1st 12lb
1lb a week	500	13lb	1st 12lb	3st 10lb
1½lb a week	750	1st 5.5lb	2st 11lb	5st 8lb
2lb a week	1,000	1st 12lb	3st 10lb	7st 6lb

TO LOSE...	Cut your daily calorie intake by	In three months you could lose...	In six months you could lose...	In one year you could lose...
¼kg a week	250	3.25kg	6.5kg	13kg
½kg a week	500	6.5kg	13kg	26kg
¾kg a week	750	9.75kg	19.5kg	39kg
1kg a week	1,000	13kg	26kg	52kg

4. Keep a food diary

Writing down what you eat and drink and any thoughts linked to that eating helps you become more aware of your eating habits. Recognising what is going on helps you feel in control and is a powerful way to start planning change. Keeping a food diary before you start to change your eating habits will also help you identify opportunities for cutting calories by substituting one food for another, cutting portion sizes of high-calorie foods or eating certain foods less often. Simply write down every single item you eat or drink during the day and use this book to calculate the calories of each item. Then after a few days of eating normally, introduce some changes to your diet to achieve your daily calorie allowance. Remember to spread your daily calorie allowance fairly evenly throughout the day to prevent hunger. You'll find a template for a daily food and exercise diary on page 43. Try to use it as carefully as you can as research shows that people who do, do best.

Top Tip

If you only fill in your main food diary once a day, keep a pen and notepad with you to write down all those little extras you eat or drink during the day – that chocolate you ate in the office, the sliver of cheese you had while cooking dinner and the few chips you pinched from your husband's plate, for example! It's easy to forget the little things if they're not written down, but they can make the difference between success and failure.

QUESTION: Why are heavier people allowed more calories than those who have smaller amounts of weight to lose?

ANSWER: This confuses a lot of people but is easily explained. Someone who is 3 stone overweight, for example, is carrying the equivalent of 42 small packets of butter with them everywhere they go – up and down the stairs, to the local shops, into the kitchen. Obviously, it takes a lot more energy simply to move around when you're carrying that extra weight. As a consequence, the heavier you are, the more calories you need just to keep your weight steady. In turn, this means you'll lose weight on a higher calorie allowance. However, as you lose weight, you'll need to lower your calorie allowance slightly as you have less weight to carry around.

5. Control your portions

As well as making some smart food swaps to cut calories, it's likely you'll also need to reduce your serving sizes for some foods to help shift those pounds. Even 'healthy' foods such as brown rice, wholemeal bread, chicken, fish and low-fat dairy products contain calories so you may need to limit the amount you eat. When you first start out, weigh portions of foods like rice, pasta, cereal, cheese, butter, oil, meat, fish, and chicken rather than completing your food diary with a 'guesstimated' weight! That way you can calculate the calorie content accurately. Don't forget that drinks contain calories too, alcohol, milk, juices and sugary drinks all count.

6. Measure your success

Research has found that regular weight checks do help. Weighing yourself helps you assess how your eating and exercise habits affect your body weight. The important thing is to use the information in a positive way – to assess your progress - rather than as a stick to beat yourself up with. Remember that weight can fluctuate by a kilogram in a day, for example, due to fluid changes, premenstrually, after a big meal out, so weigh yourself at the same time of day and look at the trend over a week or two.

People who successfully lose weight and keep it off, also tend to continue weighing themselves at least once a week, and often daily (but not in an obsessive way), because they say it helps them stay 'on track'. Probably because they use it as an early warning system. People who weigh themselves regularly (or regularly try on a tight fitting item of clothing) will notice quickly if they have gained a couple of kilograms and can take action to stop gaining more. Checking your weight less often can mean that you might discover one day that you gained 6kg. That can be pretty discouraging, and it might trigger you to just give up.

Top Tip

Don't just focus on what the bathroom scales say either – keep a record of your vital statistics, too. Many people find it doubly encouraging to see the inches dropping off, as well as the pounds!

7. Stay motivated

Each time you lose half a stone, or reach your own small goal – celebrate! Treat yourself to a little luxury – something new to wear, a little pampering or some other (non-food) treat. It also helps replace the comfort you once got from food and allows you to take care of yourself in other ways. Trying on an item of clothing that used to be tight can also help to keep you feeling motivated. Make sure you keep in touch with your supporters, and if the going gets tough take another look at the 'Coping with Slimming Saboteurs' section. Once you've reviewed how well you've done, use this book to set yourself a new daily calorie allowance based on your new weight to help you lose the next half stone *(see point 3 - page 28 - Calculate your calorie allowance).*

8. Keep it off

What you do to stay slim is just as important as what you did to get slim. Quite simply, if you return to your old ways, you are likely to return to your old weight. The great thing about calorie counting is that you will learn so much about what you eat, and make so many important changes to your eating and drinking habits, that you'll probably find it difficult to go back to your old ways – and won't want to anyway. It's still a good idea to weigh yourself at least once a week to keep a check on your weight. The key is to deal with any extra pounds immediately, rather than waiting until you have a stone to lose *(see page 30).* Simply go back to counting calories for as long as it takes to shift those pounds and enjoy the new slim you. Page 25 has more information about how successful slimmers keep it off.

QUESTION: Do I need to stick to exactly the same number of calories each day or is it OK to have a lower calorie intake during the week and slightly more at the weekend?

ANSWER: The key to losing weight is to take in fewer calories than you need for as long as it takes to reach your target, aiming for a loss of no more than 2lb (1kg) a week. In general, most nutrition experts recommend a daily calorie allowance. However, it's just as valid to use other periods of time such as weeks. If you prefer, simply multiply your daily allowance by seven to work out a weekly calorie allowance and then allocate more calories to some days than others. For example, a daily allowance of 1,500 calories is equivalent to 10,500 calories a week. This means you could have 1,300 calories a day during the week and 2,000 calories a day on Saturday and Sunday.

Healthy Eating Made Easy

Juliette Kellow BSc RD

GONE ARE THE DAYS when a healthy diet meant surviving on bird seed, rabbit food and carrot juice! The new approach to eating healthily means we're positively encouraged to eat a wide range of foods, including some of our favourites – it's just a question of making sure we don't eat high fat, high sugar or highly processed foods too often.

Eating a healthy diet, together with taking regular exercise and not smoking, has huge benefits to our health, both in the short and long term. As well as helping us to lose or maintain our weight, a healthy diet can boost energy levels, keep our immune system strong and give us healthy skin, nails and hair. Meanwhile, eating well throughout life also means we're far less likely to suffer from health problems such as constipation, anaemia and tooth decay or set ourselves up for serious conditions in later life such as obesity, heart disease, stroke, diabetes, cancer or osteoporosis.

Fortunately, it couldn't be easier to eat a balanced diet. To start with, no single food provides all the calories and nutrients we need to stay healthy, so it's important to eat a variety of foods. Meanwhile, most nutrition experts also agree that mealtimes should be a pleasure rather than a penance. This means it's fine to eat small amounts of our favourite treats from time to time.

To help people eat healthily, the Food Standards Agency recommends eating plenty of different foods from four main groups of foods and limiting the amount we eat from a smaller fifth group. Ultimately, we should eat more fruit, vegetables, starchy, fibre-rich foods and fresh products, and fewer fatty, sugary, salty and processed foods.

The following guidelines are all based on the healthy eating guidelines recommended by the Food Standards Agency.

Bread, other cereals and potatoes

Eat these foods at each meal. They also make good snacks.

Foods in this group include bread, breakfast cereals, potatoes, rice, pasta, noodles, yams, oats and grains. Go for high-fibre varieties where available, such as wholegrain cereals, wholemeal bread and brown rice. These foods should fill roughly a third of your plate at mealtimes.

TYPICAL SERVING SIZES

- *2 slices bread in a sandwich or with a meal*
- *a tennis ball sized serving of pasta, potato, rice, noodles or couscous*
- *a bowl of porridge*
- *around 40g of breakfast cereal*

Fruit and vegetables

Eat at least five portions every day.

Foods in this group include all fruits and vegetables, including fresh, frozen, canned and dried products, and unsweetened fruit juice. Choose canned fruit in juice rather than syrup and go for veg canned in water without added salt or sugar.

TYPICAL PORTION SIZES

- *a piece of fruit eg: apple, banana, pear*
- *2 small fruits eg: satsumas, plums, apricots*
- *a bowl of fruit salad, canned or stewed fruit*
- *a small glass of unsweetened fruit juice*
- *a cereal bowl of salad*
- *3tbsp vegetables*

Milk and dairy foods

Eat two or three servings a day.

Foods in this group include milk, cheese, yoghurt and fromage frais. Choose low-fat varieties where available such as skimmed milk, reduced-fat cheese and fat-free yoghurt.

TYPICAL SERVING SIZES

• 200ml milk

• a small pot of yoghurt or fromage frais

• a small matchbox-sized piece of cheese

Meat, fish and alternatives

Eat two servings a day

Foods in this group include meat, poultry, fish, eggs, beans, nuts and seeds. Choose low-fat varieties where available such as extra-lean minced beef and skinless chicken and don't add extra fat or salt.

TYPICAL SERVING SIZES

• a piece of meat, chicken or fish the size of a deck of cards

• 1-2 eggs

• 3 heaped tablespoons of beans

• a small handful of nuts or seeds

Healthy Eating on a plate

A simple way to serve up both balance and healthy proportions is to fill one half of your plate with salad or vegetables and divide the other half between protein-rich meat, chicken, fish, eggs or beans, and healthy carbs (potatoes, rice, pasta, pulses, bread or noodles).

Fatty and sugary foods

Eat only small amounts of these foods

Foods in this group include oils, spreading fats, cream, mayonnaise, oily salad dressings, cakes, biscuits, puddings, crisps, savoury snacks, sugar, preserves, confectionery and sugary soft drinks.

TYPICAL SERVING SIZES:

- *a small packet of sweets or a small bar of chocolate*
- *a small slice of cake*
- *a couple of small biscuits*
- *1 level tbsp mayo, salad dressing or olive oil*
- *a small packet of crisps*

Useful Tools

Body Mass Index

The Body Mass Index (BMI) is the internationally accepted way of assessing how healthy our weight is. It is calculated using an individual's height and weight. Use the Body Mass Index Chart to look up your BMI, and use the table below to see what range you fall into.

BMI Under 18.5	*Underweight*
BMI 18.5-25	*Healthy*
BMI 25-30	*Overweight*
BMI 30-40	*Obese*
BMI Over 40	*Severely Obese*

This is what different BMI ranges mean.

- **Underweight:** you probably need to gain weight for your health's sake. Talk to your doctor if you have any concerns, or if you feel frightened about gaining weight.

- **Healthy weight:** you are a healthy weight, so aim to stay in this range (note that most people in this range tend to have a BMI between 20-25).

- **Overweight:** aim to lose some weight for your health's sake, or at least prevent further weight gain.

- **Obese:** your health is at risk and losing weight will benefit your health.

- **Severely obese:** your health is definitely at risk. You should visit your doctor for a health check. Losing weight will improve your health.

Please note that BMI is not as accurate for athletes or very muscular people (muscle weighs more than fat), as it can push them into a higher BMI category despite having a healthy level of body fat. It is also not accurate for women who are pregnant or breastfeeding, or people who are frail.

Body Mass Index Table

HEIGHT IN FEET / INCHES

WEIGHT IN STONES / LBS	4'6	4'8	4'10	5'0	5'2	5'4	5'6	5'8	5'10	6'0	6'2	6'4	6'6	6'8	6'10
6st 7	22.0	20.5	19.1	17.8	16.7	15.7	14.7	13.9	13.1	12.4	11.7	11.1	10.6	10.0	9.5
7st 0	23.7	22.1	20.6	19.2	18.0	16.9	15.9	15.0	14.1	13.3	12.6	12.0	11.4	10.8	10.3
7st 7	25.4	23.6	22.0	20.6	19.3	18.1	17.0	16.0	15.1	14.3	13.5	12.8	12.2	11.6	11.0
8st 0	27.1	25.2	23.5	22.0	20.6	19.3	18.1	17.1	16.1	15.2	14.4	13.7	13.0	12.3	11.8
8st 7	28.8	26.8	25.0	23.3	21.8	20.5	19.3	18.2	17.1	16.2	15.3	14.5	13.8	13.1	12.5
9st 0	30.5	28.4	26.4	24.7	23.1	21.7	20.4	19.2	18.1	17.2	16.2	15.4	14.6	13.9	13.2
9st 7	32.2	29.9	27.9	26.1	24.4	22.9	21.5	20.3	19.2	18.1	17.1	16.2	15.4	14.7	14.0
10st 0	33.9	31.5	29.4	27.4	25.7	24.1	22.7	21.4	20.2	19.1	18.0	17.1	16.2	15.4	14.7
10st 7	35.6	33.1	30.8	28.8	27.0	25.3	23.8	22.4	21.2	20.0	18.9	18.0	17.0	16.2	15.4
11st 0	37.3	34.7	32.3	30.2	28.3	26.5	24.9	23.5	22.2	21.0	19.8	18.8	17.9	17.0	16.2
11st 7	39.0	36.2	33.8	31.6	29.6	27.7	26.1	24.6	23.2	21.9	20.7	19.7	18.7	17.8	16.9
12st 0	40.7	37.8	35.2	32.9	30.8	28.9	27.2	25.6	24.2	22.9	21.6	20.5	19.5	18.5	17.6
12st 7	42.3	39.4	36.7	34.3	32.1	30.1	28.3	26.7	25.2	23.8	22.5	21.4	20.3	19.3	18.4
13st 0	44.0	41.0	38.2	35.7	33.4	31.4	29.5	27.8	26.2	24.8	23.5	22.2	21.1	20.1	19.1
13st 7	45.7	42.5	39.6	37.0	34.7	32.6	30.6	28.8	27.2	25.7	24.4	23.1	21.9	20.8	19.8
14st 0	47.4	44.1	41.1	38.4	36.0	33.8	31.7	29.9	28.2	26.7	25.3	23.9	22.7	21.6	20.6
14st 7	49.1	45.7	42.6	39.8	37.3	35.0	32.9	31.0	29.2	27.6	26.2	24.8	23.5	22.4	21.3
15st 0	50.8	47.3	44.0	41.2	38.5	36.2	34.0	32.0	30.2	28.6	27.1	25.7	24.4	23.2	22.0
15st 7	52.5	48.8	45.5	42.5	39.8	37.4	35.2	33.1	31.2	29.5	28.0	26.5	25.2	23.9	22.8
16st 0	54.2	50.4	47.0	43.9	41.1	38.6	36.3	34.2	32.3	30.5	28.9	27.4	26.0	24.7	23.5
16st 7	55.9	52.0	48.5	45.3	42.4	39.8	37.4	35.2	33.3	31.4	29.8	28.2	26.8	25.5	24.2
17st 0	57.6	53.6	49.9	46.6	43.7	41.0	38.6	36.3	34.3	32.4	30.7	29.1	27.6	26.2	25.0
17st 7	59.3	55.1	51.4	48.0	45.0	42.2	39.7	37.4	35.3	33.3	31.6	29.9	28.4	27.0	25.7
18st 0	61.0	56.7	52.9	49.4	46.3	43.4	40.8	38.5	36.3	34.3	32.5	30.8	29.2	27.8	26.4
18st 7	62.7	58.3	54.3	50.8	47.5	44.6	42.0	39.5	37.3	35.3	33.4	31.6	30.0	28.6	27.2
19st 0	64.4	59.9	55.8	52.1	48.8	45.8	43.1	40.6	38.3	36.2	34.3	32.5	30.8	29.3	27.9
19st 7	66.1	61.4	57.3	53.5	50.1	47.0	44.2	41.7	39.3	37.2	35.2	33.3	31.7	30.1	28.6
20st 0	67.8	63.0	58.7	54.9	51.4	48.2	45.4	42.7	40.3	38.1	36.1	34.2	32.5	30.9	29.4
20st 7	69.4	64.6	60.2	56.3	52.7	49.4	46.5	43.8	41.3	39.1	37.0	35.1	33.3	31.6	30.1
21st 0	71.1	66.2	61.7	57.6	54.0	50.6	47.6	44.9	42.3	40.0	37.9	35.9	34.1	32.4	30.9
21st 7	72.8	67.7	63.1	59.0	55.3	51.9	48.8	45.9	43.3	41.0	38.8	36.8	34.9	33.2	31.6
22st 0	74.5	69.3	64.6	60.4	56.5	53.1	49.9	47.0	44.4	41.9	39.7	37.6	35.7	34.0	32.3
22st 7	76.2	70.9	66.1	61.7	57.8	54.3	51.0	48.1	45.4	42.9	40.6	38.5	36.5	34.7	33.1
23st 0	77.9	72.5	67.5	63.1	59.1	55.5	52.2	49.1	46.4	43.8	41.5	39.3	37.3	35.5	33.8
23st 7	79.6	74.0	69.0	64.5	60.4	56.7	53.3	50.2	47.4	44.8	42.4	40.2	38.2	36.3	34.5
24st 0	81.3	75.6	70.5	65.9	61.7	57.9	54.4	51.3	48.4	45.7	43.3	41.0	39.0	37.0	35.3
24st 7	83.0	77.2	71.9	67.2	63.0	59.1	55.6	52.3	49.4	46.7	44.2	41.9	39.8	37.8	36.0
25st 0	84.7	78.8	73.4	68.6	64.2	60.3	56.7	53.4	50.4	47.6	45.1	42.8	40.6	38.6	36.7
25st 7	86.4	80.3	74.9	70.0	65.5	61.5	57.8	54.5	51.4	48.6	46.0	43.6	41.4	39.4	37.5
26st 0	88.1	81.9	76.3	71.3	66.8	62.7	59.0	55.5	52.4	49.5	46.9	44.5	42.2	40.1	38.2
26st 7	89.8	83.5	77.8	72.7	68.1	63.9	60.1	56.6	53.4	50.5	47.8	45.3	43.0	40.9	38.9
27st 0	91.5	85.1	79.3	74.1	69.4	65.1	61.2	57.7	54.4	51.5	48.7	46.2	43.8	41.7	39.7
27st 7	93.2	86.6	80.8	75.5	70.7	66.3	62.4	58.7	55.4	52.4	49.6	47.0	44.7	42.4	40.4
28st 0	94.9	88.2	82.2	76.8	72.0	67.5	63.5	59.8	56.4	53.4	50.5	47.9	45.5	43.2	41.1
28st 7	96.5	89.8	83.7	78.2	73.2	68.7	64.6	60.9	57.5	54.3	51.4	48.7	46.3	44.0	41.9
29st 0	98.2	91.4	85.2	79.6	74.5	69.9	65.8	62.0	58.5	55.3	52.3	49.6	47.1	44.8	42.6
29st 7	99.9	92.9	86.6	80.9	75.8	71.1	66.9	63.0	59.5	56.2	53.2	50.5	47.9	45.5	43.3

Weight Chart

Underweight
BMI less than 18.5

HEALTHY
WEIGHT
BMI 18.5-25

Overweight
BMI 25-30

Obese
BMI 30-40

Severely
Obese
BMI 40 or more

BMI: 10, 11, 12, 13, 14, 15, 16, 17, 18, 19, 20, 21, 22, 23, 24, 25, 26, 27, 28, 29, 30, 31, 32, 33, 34, 35, 36, 37, 38

Height: 6ft 6" / 197.5cm, 6ft 5" / 195cm, 6ft 4" / 192.5cm, 6ft 3" / 190cm, 6ft 2" / 187.5cm, 6ft 1" / 185cm, 6ft 0" / 182.5cm, 5ft 11" / 180cm, 5ft 10" / 177.5cm, 5ft 9" / 175cm, 5ft 8" / 172.5cm, 5ft 7" / 170cm, 5ft 6" / 167.5cm, 5ft 5" / 165cm, 5ft 4" / 162.5cm, 5ft 3" / 160cm, 5ft 2" / 157.5cm, 5ft 1" / 155cm, 5ft 0" / 152.5cm, 4ft 11" / 150cm, 4ft 10" / 147.5cm, 4ft 9" / 145cm, 4ft 8" / 142.5cm, 4ft 7" / 140cm, 4ft 6" / 137.5cm

Weight: 4st 7lb / 29kg, 5st 0lb / 32kg, 5st 7lb / 35kg, 6st 0lb / 38kg, 6st 7lb / 41kg, 7st 0lb / 45kg, 7st 7lb / 48kg, 8st 0lb / 51kg, 8st 7lb / 54kg, 9st 0lb / 57kg, 9st 7lb / 60kg, 10st 0lb / 64kg, 10st 7lb / 67kg, 11st 0lb / 70kg, 11st 7lb / 73kg, 12st 0lb / 76kg, 12st 7lb / 79kg, 13st 0lb / 83kg, 13st 7lb / 86kg, 14st 0lb / 89kg, 14st 7lb / 92kg, 15st 0lb / 95kg, 15st 7lb / 98kg, 16st 0lb / 102kg, 16st 7lb / 105kg, 17st 0lb / 108kg, 17st 7lb / 111kg, 18st 0lb / 114kg, 18st 7lb / 118kg, 19st 0lb / 121kg, 19st 7lb / 124kg, 20st 0lb / 127kg, 20st 7lb / 130kg, 21st 0lb / 133kg, 21st 7lb / 137kg, 22st 0lb / 140kg, 22st 7lb / 143kg, 23st 0lb / 146kg, 23st 7lb / 149kg

Calories Required to Maintain Weight
Adult Females

ACTIVITY LEVEL / AGE

WEIGHT IN STONES / LBS	VERY SEDENTARY			MODERATELY SEDENTARY			MODERATELY ACTIVE			VERY ACTIVE		
	<30	30-60	60+	<30	30-60	60+	<30	30-60	60+	<30	30-60	60+
7st 7	1425	1473	1304	1544	1596	1412	1781	1841	1630	2138	2210	1956
8st 0	1481	1504	1338	1605	1629	1450	1852	1880	1673	2222	2256	2008
8st 7	1537	1535	1373	1666	1663	1487	1922	1919	1716	2306	2302	2059
9st 0	1594	1566	1407	1726	1696	1524	1992	1957	1759	2391	2349	2111
9st 7	1650	1596	1442	1787	1729	1562	2062	1996	1802	2475	2395	2163
10st 0	1706	1627	1476	1848	1763	1599	2133	2034	1845	2559	2441	2214
10st 7	1762	1658	1511	1909	1796	1637	2203	2073	1888	2644	2487	2266
11st 0	1819	1689	1545	1970	1830	1674	2273	2111	1931	2728	2534	2318
11st 7	1875	1720	1580	2031	1863	1711	2344	2150	1975	2813	2580	2370
12st 0	1931	1751	1614	2092	1897	1749	2414	2188	2018	2897	2626	2421
12st 7	1987	1781	1648	2153	1930	1786	2484	2227	2061	2981	2672	2473
13st 0	2044	1812	1683	2214	1963	1823	2555	2266	2104	3066	2719	2525
13st 7	2100	1843	1717	2275	1997	1861	2625	2304	2147	3150	2765	2576
14st 0	2156	1874	1752	2336	2030	1898	2695	2343	2190	3234	2811	2628
14st 7	2212	1905	1786	2397	2064	1935	2766	2381	2233	3319	2858	2680
15st 0	2269	1936	1821	2458	2097	1973	2836	2420	2276	3403	2904	2732
15st 7	2325	1967	1855	2519	2130	2010	2906	2458	2319	3488	2950	2783
16st 0	2381	1997	1890	2580	2164	2047	2976	2497	2362	3572	2996	2835
16st 7	2437	2028	1924	2640	2197	2085	3047	2535	2405	3656	3043	2887
17st 0	2494	2059	1959	2701	2231	2122	3117	2574	2449	3741	3089	2938
17st 7	2550	2090	1993	2762	2264	2159	3187	2613	2492	3825	3135	2990
18st 0	2606	2121	2028	2823	2298	2197	3258	2651	2535	3909	3181	3042
18st 7	2662	2152	2062	2884	2331	2234	3328	2690	2578	3994	3228	3093
19st 0	2719	2182	2097	2945	2364	2271	3398	2728	2621	4078	3274	3145
19st 7	2775	2213	2131	3006	2398	2309	3469	2767	2664	4162	3320	3197
20st 0	2831	2244	2166	3067	2431	2346	3539	2805	2707	4247	3366	3249
20st 7	2887	2275	2200	3128	2465	2383	3609	2844	2750	4331	3413	3300
21st 0	2944	2306	2235	3189	2498	2421	3680	2882	2793	4416	3459	3352
21st 7	3000	2337	2269	3250	2531	2458	3750	2921	2836	4500	3505	3404
22st 0	3056	2368	2303	3311	2565	2495	3820	2960	2879	4584	3552	3455
22st 7	3112	2398	2338	3372	2598	2533	3890	2998	2923	4669	3598	3507
23st 0	3169	2429	2372	3433	2632	2570	3961	3037	2966	4753	3644	3559
23st 7	3225	2460	2407	3494	2665	2608	4031	3075	3009	4837	3690	3611
24st 0	3281	2491	2441	3554	2699	2645	4101	3114	3052	4922	3737	3662
24st 7	3337	2522	2476	3615	2732	2682	4172	3152	3095	5006	3783	3714
25st 0	3394	2553	2510	3676	2765	2720	4242	3191	3138	5091	3829	3766
25st 7	3450	2583	2545	3737	2799	2757	4312	3229	3181	5175	3875	3817
26st 0	3506	2614	2579	3798	2832	2794	4383	3268	3224	5259	3922	3869
26st 7	3562	2645	2614	3859	2866	2832	4453	3307	3267	5344	3968	3921
27st 0	3618	2676	2648	3920	2899	2869	4523	3345	3310	5428	4014	3973
27st 7	3675	2707	2683	3981	2932	2906	4594	3384	3353	5512	4060	4024
28st 0	3731	2738	2717	4042	2966	2944	4664	3422	3397	5597	4107	4076
28st 7	3787	2768	2752	4103	2999	2981	4734	3461	3440	5681	4153	4128

Calories Required to Maintain Weight
Adult Males

ACTIVITY LEVEL / AGE

WEIGHT IN STONES / LBS	VERY SEDENTARY			MODERATELY SEDENTARY			MODERATELY ACTIVE			VERY ACTIVE		
	<30	30-60	60+	<30	30-60	60+	<30	30-60	60+	<30	30-60	60+
9st 0	1856	1827	1502	2010	1979	1627	2320	2284	1878	2784	2741	2254
9st 7	1913	1871	1547	2072	2026	1676	2391	2338	1933	2870	2806	2320
10st 0	1970	1914	1591	2134	2074	1724	2463	2393	1989	2955	2871	2387
10st 7	2027	1958	1636	2196	2121	1772	2534	2447	2045	3041	2937	2454
11st 0	2084	2001	1680	2258	2168	1820	2605	2502	2100	3127	3002	2520
11st 7	2141	2045	1724	2320	2215	1868	2677	2556	2156	3212	3067	2587
12st 0	2199	2088	1769	2382	2262	1916	2748	2611	2211	3298	3133	2654
12st 7	2256	2132	1813	2444	2310	1965	2820	2665	2267	3384	3198	2720
13st 0	2313	2175	1858	2506	2357	2013	2891	2719	2322	3470	3263	2787
13st 7	2370	2219	1902	2568	2404	2061	2963	2774	2378	3555	3329	2854
14st 0	2427	2262	1947	2630	2451	2109	3034	2828	2434	3641	3394	2920
14st 7	2484	2306	1991	2691	2498	2157	3106	2883	2489	3727	3459	2987
15st 0	2542	2350	2036	2753	2545	2205	3177	2937	2545	3813	3525	3054
15st 7	2599	2393	2080	2815	2593	2253	3248	2992	2600	3898	3590	3120
16st 0	2656	2437	2125	2877	2640	2302	3320	3046	2656	3984	3655	3187
16st 7	2713	2480	2169	2939	2687	2350	3391	3100	2711	4070	3721	3254
17st 0	2770	2524	2213	3001	2734	2398	3463	3155	2767	4155	3786	3320
17st 7	2827	2567	2258	3063	2781	2446	3534	3209	2823	4241	3851	3387
18st 0	2884	2611	2302	3125	2828	2494	3606	3264	2878	4327	3917	3454
18st 7	2942	2654	2347	3187	2876	2542	3677	3318	2934	4413	3982	3520
19st 0	2999	2698	2391	3249	2923	2591	3749	3373	2989	4498	4047	3587
19st 7	3056	2741	2436	3311	2970	2639	3820	3427	3045	4584	4112	3654
20st 0	3113	2785	2480	3373	3017	2687	3891	3481	3100	4670	4178	3721
20st 7	3170	2829	2525	3434	3064	2735	3963	3536	3156	4756	4243	3787
21st 0	3227	2872	2569	3496	3112	2783	4034	3590	3211	4841	4308	3854
21st 7	3285	2916	2614	3558	3159	2831	4106	3645	3267	4927	4374	3921
22st 0	3342	2959	2658	3620	3206	2880	4177	3699	3323	5013	4439	3987
22st 7	3399	3003	2702	3682	3253	2928	4249	3754	3378	5098	4504	4054
23st 0	3456	3046	2747	3744	3300	2976	4320	3808	3434	5184	4570	4121
23st 7	3513	3090	2791	3806	3347	3024	4392	3862	3489	5270	4635	4187
24st 0	3570	3133	2836	3868	3395	3072	4463	3917	3545	5356	4700	4254
24st 7	3627	3177	2880	3930	3442	3120	4534	3971	3600	5441	4766	4321
25st 0	3685	3220	2925	3992	3489	3168	4606	4026	3656	5527	4831	4387
25st 7	3742	3264	2969	4054	3536	3217	4677	4080	3712	5613	4896	4454
26st 0	3799	3308	3014	4116	3583	3265	4749	4135	3767	5699	4962	4521
26st 7	3856	3351	3058	4177	3630	3313	4820	4189	3823	5784	5027	4587
27st 0	3913	3395	3103	4239	3678	3361	4892	4243	3878	5870	5092	4654
27st 7	3970	3438	3147	4301	3725	3409	4963	4298	3934	5956	5158	4721
28st 0	4028	3482	3191	4363	3772	3457	5035	4352	3989	6042	5223	4787
28st 7	4085	3525	3236	4425	3819	3506	5106	4407	4045	6127	5288	4854
29st 0	4142	3569	3280	4487	3866	3554	5177	4461	4101	6213	5354	4921
29st 7	4199	3612	3325	4549	3913	3602	5249	4516	4156	6299	5419	4987
30st 0	4256	3656	3369	4611	3961	3650	5320	4570	4212	6384	5484	5054

Calories Burned in Exercise

This table shows the approximate number of extra* calories that would be burned in a five minute period of exercise activity.

ACTIVITY	CALORIES BURNED IN 5 MINUTES	ACTIVITY	CALORIES BURNED IN 5 MINUTES
Aerobics, Low Impact	25	Situps, Continuous	17
Badminton, Recreational	17	Skiing, Moderate	30
Cross Trainer	30	Skipping, Moderate	30
Cycling, Recreational, 5mph	17	Squash Playing	39
Dancing, Modern, Moderate	13	Tennis Playing, Recreational	26
Fencing	24	Toning Exercises	17
Gardening, Weeding	19	Trampolining	17
Hill Walking, Up and Down, Recreational	22	Volleyball, Recreational	10
Jogging	30	Walking, Uphill, 15% Gradient, Moderate	43
Kick Boxing	30	Walking Up and Down Stairs, Moderate	34
Netball Playing	23	Walking, 4mph	24
Rebounding	18	Weight Training, Moderate	12
Roller Skating	30	Yoga	13
Rowing Machine, Moderate	30		
Running, 7.5mph	48		

*Extra calories are those in addition to your normal daily calorie needs.

My Personal Plan

Date: _____

Body Mass Index: _____

Weight: _____

Waist Measurement: _____

Height: _____

Body Fat % (if known) _____

10% Weight Loss Goal: _____

Current weight	16stone (224lb)	100kg
- 10% weight	1stone 8½lb (22½lb)	10kg
= 10% loss goal	14stone 5½lb (201½lb)	90kg

My smaller weight targets on the way to achieving my 10% goal will be:

_____ _____ _____

Reasons why I want to lose weight:

_____

Changes I will make to help me lose weight:

Diet:

_____

_____

Activity:

_____

_____

Potential saboteurs or barriers will be:

_____

_____

_____

Ways I will overcome these:

_____

_____

_____

My supporters will be:

_____

I will monitor my progress by:

_____

_____

I will reward my progress with:

In the short term:

_____

_____

In the long term:

_____

_____

Food and Exercise Diary

Date:

/ /

Daily Calorie Allowance: **A**

Food/Drink Consumed	Serving Size	Calories

Total calories consumed **B**

Exercise/Activity	No. mins	Calories

Calories used in exercise **C**

Calorie balance **D**

You are aiming for your Calorie Balance (Box D) to be as close to zero as possible - ie. you consume the number of calories you need.

Your Daily Calorie Allowance (Box A) should be set to lose ½-2lb (¼-1kg) a week, or maintain weight, depending on your goals.

Daily Calorie Allowance (A) *plus* Extra Calories used in Exercise (C) *minus* Total Calories Consumed (B) *equals* Calorie Balance (D)

$A + C - B = D$

You can also write down any comments or thoughts related to your eating if you want to.

Food Information

Nutritional Information

CALORIE AND FAT values are given per serving, plus calorie and nutrition values per 100g of product. This makes it easy to compare the proportions of fat, protein, carbohydrate and fibre in each food.

The values given are for uncooked, unprepared foods unless otherwise stated. Values are also for only the edible portion of the food unless otherwise stated. ie - weighed with bone.

Finding Foods

The Calorie, Carb & Fat Bible has an Eating Out section which is arranged alphabetically by brand. In the General Foods and Drinks A-Z most foods are grouped together by type, and then put in to alphabetical order. This makes it easy to compare different brands, and will help you to find lower calorie and/or fat alternatives where they are available.

This format also makes it easier to locate foods. Foods are categorised by their main characteristics so, for example, if it is bread, ciabatta or white sliced, you'll find it under "Bread".

Basic ingredients are highlighted to make them easier to find at a glance. You'll find all unbranded foods in bold - making the index easier to use, whether it's just an apple or all the components of a home cooked stew.

There are, however, some foods which are not so easy to categorise, especially combination foods like ready meals. The following pointers will help you to find your way around the book until you get to know it a little better.

FILLED ROLLS AND SANDWICHES - Bagels, baguettes, etc which are filled are listed as "Bagels (filled)" etc. Sandwiches are under "Sandwiches".

CURRIES - Popular types of curry, like Balti or Jalfrezi, are listed under their individual types. Unspecified or lesser known types are listed under their main ingredient.

BURGERS - All burgers, including chicken-type sandwiches from fast-food outlets, are listed under "Burgers". CHIPS & FRIES - Are listed separately, depending on the name of the particular brand. All other types of potato are listed under "Potatoes".

SWEETS & CHOCOLATES - Well-known brands, eg. Aero, Mars Bar, are listed under their brand names. Others are listed under "Chocolate" (for bars) and "Chocolates" (for individual sweets).

READY MEALS - Popular types of dishes are listed under their type, eg. "Chow Mein", "Casserole", "Hot Pot", etc. Others are listed by their main ingredient, eg. "Chicken With", "Chicken In", etc.

EATING OUT & FAST FOODS - By popular demand this edition has the major eating out and fast food brands listed separately, at the back of the book. They are alphabetised first by brand, then follow using the same format as the rest of the book.

Serving Sizes

Many ready-meal type foods are given with calories for the full pack size, so that an individual serving can be worked out by estimating the proportion of the pack that has been consumed. For example, if you have eaten a quarter of a packaged pasta dish, divide the calorie value given for the whole pack by 4 to determine the number of calories you have consumed. Where serving sizes are not appropriate, or unknown, values are given per 1oz/28g. Serving sizes vary greatly from person to person and, if you are trying to lose weight, it's very important to be accurate – especially with foods that are very high in calories such as those that contain a fair amount of fat, sugar, cream, cheese, alcohol etc.

Food Data

Nutrition information for basic average foods has been compiled by the Weight Loss Resources food data team using many sources of information to calculate the most accurate values possible. Some nutrition information for non-branded food records is from The Composition of Foods 6th Edition (2002). Reproduced under licence from The Controller of Her Majesty's Stationary Office. Where basic data is present for ordinary foodstuffs such as 'raw carrots'; branded records are not included.

Nutrition information for branded goods is from details supplied by retailers and manufacturers, and researched by Weight Loss Resources staff. The Calorie Carb & Fat Bible contains data for over 1400 UK brands, including major supermarkets and fast food outlets.

The publishers gratefully acknowledge all the manufacturers and retailers who have provided information on their products. All product names, trademarks or registered trademarks belong to their respective owners and are used only for the purpose of identifying products.

Calorie & nutrition data for all food and drink items are typical values.

Caution

The information in The Calorie, Carb and Fat Bible is intended as an aid to weight loss and weight maintenance, and is not medical advice. If you suffer from, or think you may suffer from a medical condition you should consult your doctor before starting a weight loss and/or exercise regime. If you start exercising after a period of relative inactivity, you should start slowly and consult your doctor if you experience pain, distress or other symptoms.

Weights, Measures
& Abbreviations

ABBREVIATIONS

kcal	kilocalories / calories
prot	protein
carb	carbohydrate
sm	small
med	medium
av	average
reg	regular
lge	large
tsp	teaspoon
tbsp	tablespoon
dtsp	dessertspoon

BRAND ABBREVIATIONS USED

ASDA

Good for You	GFY

MARKS & SPENCER — M & S

Count on Us	COU

MORRISONS

Better For You	BFY

SAINSBURY'S

Be Good to Yourself	BGTY
Way to Five	WTF
Taste the Difference	TTD

TESCO

Healthy Living	HL

WAITROSE

Perfectly Balanced	PB

	Measure INFO/WEIGHT	per Measure		Nutrition Values per 100g / 100ml				
		KCAL	FAT	KCAL	PROT	CARB	FAT	FIBRE
ABALONE								
Cooked, Fried, Weighed without Shells	1 Serving/100g	189	6.8	189	19.6	11.0	6.8	0.0
Raw, Weighed without Shells	1 Serving/100g	105	0.8	105	17.1	6.0	0.8	0.0
ABSINTHE								
Average	*1 Shot/35ml*	*127*	*0.0*	*363*	*0.0*	*38.8*	*0.0*	*0.0*
ACKEE								
Canned, Drained, Average	*1oz/28g*	*42*	*4.3*	*151*	*2.9*	*0.8*	*15.2*	*0.0*
ADVOCAAT								
Average	*1 Shot/35ml*	*91*	*2.2*	*260*	*4.7*	*28.4*	*6.3*	*0.0*
AERO								
Bar, Milk, Giant, Nestle*	1 Bar/125g	674	38.6	539	6.6	57.7	30.9	2.2
Bar, Milk, Standard, Nestle*	1 Bar/31g	165	9.6	531	6.3	56.9	30.9	0.8
Creamy White Centre, Nestle*	1 Bar/46g	244	13.8	530	7.6	57.4	30.0	0.0
Honeycomb, Nestle*	1 Serving/40g	199	10.0	497	5.9	62.2	25.0	0.0
Minis, Nestle*	1 Bar/11g	57	3.2	518	6.8	58.1	28.7	0.8
Mint, Nestle*	1 Bar/46g	245	13.7	533	4.9	61.2	29.8	0.4
ALFALFA SPROUTS								
Raw, Average	1 Serving/100g	27	0.9	27	4.5	1.1	0.9	1.3
ALLSPICE								
Ground, Schwartz*	1 Tsp/3g	11	0.1	358	6.1	74.3	4.0	0.0
ALMONDS								
Blanched, Average	*1oz/28g*	*171*	*15.0*	*610*	*24.9*	*7.1*	*53.5*	*8.5*
Flaked, Average	*1oz/28g*	*172*	*15.2*	*613*	*24.9*	*6.5*	*54.3*	*7.6*
Flaked, Toasted, Average	*1oz/28g*	*176*	*15.8*	*629*	*24.6*	*5.8*	*56.4*	*7.5*
Ground, Average	*1 Serving/10g*	*62*	*5.6*	*625*	*24.0*	*6.6*	*55.8*	*7.4*
Marcona, Average	*1 Serving/100g*	*608*	*53.7*	*608*	*22.1*	*13.0*	*53.7*	*9.7*
Toasted, Average	*1oz/28g*	*178*	*15.8*	*634*	*24.9*	*6.6*	*56.4*	*6.6*
Whole, Average	*1 Serving/20g*	*122*	*11.0*	*612*	*23.4*	*21.2*	*54.8*	*8.4*
ALOO TIKKI								
Indian Selection, Tesco*	1 Serving/23g	49	3.1	211	2.3	20.1	13.5	3.5
Mini, from Indian Snack Selection, Sainsbury's*	1 Piece/25g	44	1.9	175	4.8	22.1	7.5	3.9
ANCHOVIES								
Fillets, Flat, John West*	1 Can/50g	113	7.0	226	25.0	0.1	14.0	0.0
in Oil, Canned, Drained, Average	*1 Serving/30g*	*58*	*3.4*	*194*	*22.9*	*0.0*	*11.3*	*0.0*
Marinated, Sainsbury's*	¼ Pot/44g	78	4.0	177	22.0	2.0	9.0	0.1
Salted, Finest, Tesco*	1 Serving/10g	9	0.2	93	18.2	0.0	2.2	0.0
ANGEL DELIGHT								
Banana Flavour, Kraft*	1 Sachet/59g	289	12.4	490	2.5	72.0	21.0	0.0
Butterscotch Flavour, Kraft*	1 Sachet/59g	280	11.2	475	2.4	73.5	19.0	0.0
Butterscotch Flavour, No Added Sugar, Kraft*	1 Sachet/47g	226	11.3	480	4.5	61.0	24.0	0.0
Chocolate Flavour, Kraft*	1 Sachet/67g	305	12.1	455	3.7	69.5	18.0	0.4
Raspberry Flavour, Kraft*	1 Sachet/59g	289	12.4	490	2.5	72.0	21.0	0.0
Raspberry Flavour, No Added Sugar, Kraft*	1 Sachet/59g	292	15.3	495	4.8	59.5	26.0	0.0
Strawberry Flavour, Kraft*	1 Sachet/59g	286	12.4	485	2.5	71.0	21.0	0.0
Strawberry Flavour, No Added Sugar, Kraft*	1 Sachet/47g	230	12.5	490	4.8	59.0	26.5	0.0
ANGEL HAIR								
Pasta, Spaghetti, Sainsbury's*	1 Serving/100g	357	1.7	357	12.3	73.1	1.7	2.5
ANTIPASTO								
Artichoke, Sainsbury's*	1 Serving/50g	67	6.2	135	2.0	3.6	12.5	2.3
Coppa, from Selection Platter, TTD, Sainsbury's*	1 Serving/100g	255	17.1	255	25.2	0.1	17.1	0.0
Felino, from Selection Platter, TTD, Sainsbury's*	1 Serving/100g	349	24.9	349	31.1	0.1	24.9	0.0
Mixed, Misto Cotto, Arrosto Erbe, Waitrose*	1 Slice/9g	11	0.4	129	22.2	0.0	4.4	0.0
Parma, Salami Milano, Bresaola, Finest, Tesco*	¼ Pack/30g	118	8.2	395	36.0	0.5	27.3	0.0
Parma Ham, from Selection Platter, TTD, Sainsbury's*	1 Serving/100g	236	12.9	236	29.9	0.1	12.9	0.0

A

	Measure INFO/WEIGHT	per Measure KCAL	FAT	Nutrition Values per 100g / 100ml KCAL	PROT	CARB	FAT	FIBRE
ANTIPASTO								
Roasted Pepper, Drained, Tesco*	1 Jar /170g	127	9.3	75	0.9	5.5	5.5	4.1
Sun Dried Tomato, Sainsbury's*	¼ Jar/70g	275	25.0	393	4.5	13.4	35.7	6.2
APPLES								
Braeburn, Average	*1 Apple/165g*	*79*	*0.2*	*48*	*0.4*	*11.3*	*0.1*	*1.8*
Cooking, Baked with Sugar, Flesh Only, Average	*1 Serving/140g*	*109*	*0.1*	*78*	*0.5*	*20.1*	*0.1*	*1.7*
Cooking, Raw, Peeled, Average	*1oz/28g*	*10*	*0.0*	*35*	*0.3*	*8.9*	*0.1*	*1.6*
Cooking, Stewed with Sugar, Average	*1 Serving/140g*	*104*	*0.1*	*74*	*0.3*	*19.1*	*0.1*	*1.2*
Cooking, Stewed without Sugar, Average	*1 Serving/140g*	*46*	*0.1*	*33*	*0.3*	*8.1*	*0.1*	*1.5*
Cox, English, Average	*1 Apple/108g*	*53*	*0.1*	*49*	*0.4*	*11.6*	*0.1*	*2.2*
Discovery, Average	*1 Apple/182g*	*95*	*0.3*	*52*	*0.3*	*13.8*	*0.2*	*2.4*
Dried, Average	*1 Pack/250g*	*554*	*0.7*	*221*	*1.0*	*57.3*	*0.3*	*6.6*
Empire, Average	*1 Serving/100g*	*48*	*0.1*	*48*	*0.4*	*11.8*	*0.1*	*2.0*
Gala, Average	*1 Apple/152g*	*74*	*0.2*	*49*	*0.4*	*11.5*	*0.1*	*1.4*
Golden Delicious, Average	*1 Med/102g*	*49*	*0.1*	*48*	*0.4*	*11.5*	*0.1*	*1.7*
Granny Smith, Average	*1 Sm/125g*	*62*	*0.1*	*50*	*0.4*	*11.9*	*0.1*	*2.0*
Green, Raw, Average	*1 Med/182g*	*86*	*0.2*	*47*	*0.3*	*11.3*	*0.1*	*1.7*
Mackintosh, Red, Average	*1 Apple/165g*	*81*	*0.5*	*49*	*0.2*	*12.8*	*0.3*	*1.8*
Pink Lady, Average	*1 Apple/125g*	*62*	*0.1*	*49*	*0.4*	*11.7*	*0.1*	*1.8*
Sliced, Average	*1oz/28g*	*14*	*0.0*	*49*	*0.4*	*11.6*	*0.1*	*1.8*
APPLETISE								
Schweppes*	1 Bottle/275ml	129	0.0	47	0.0	11.0	0.0	0.4
APRICOTS								
Canned, in Syrup, Average	*1oz/28g*	*18*	*0.0*	*63*	*0.4*	*16.1*	*0.1*	*0.9*
Dried, Average	*1 Apricot/10g*	*17*	*0.1*	*171*	*3.6*	*37.4*	*0.5*	*6.3*
Dried, Soft, Average	*1 Serving/100g*	*208*	*0.5*	*208*	*3.2*	*47.7*	*0.5*	*6.6*
Halves, in Fruit Juice, Average	*1 Can/221g*	*87*	*0.1*	*40*	*0.5*	*9.2*	*0.1*	*1.0*
Raw, Flesh Only, Average	*1 Apricot/37g*	*19*	*0.2*	*52*	*1.5*	*12.0*	*0.4*	*2.1*
Raw, Weighed with Stone, Average	*1 Apricot/40g*	*19*	*0.2*	*48*	*1.4*	*11.1*	*0.4*	*2.0*
ARCHERS*								
Aqua, Peach, Archers*	1 Bottle/275ml	206	0.0	75	0.3	5.1	0.0	0.0
Peach, Calculated Estimate, Archers*	1 Shot/35ml	91	0.0	260	0.0	0.0	0.0	0.0
Vea, Wildberry, Schnapps, Archers*	1 Bottle/275ml	124	0.0	45	0.0	5.8	0.0	0.0
ARTICHOKE								
Chargrilled, in Olive Oil, Cooks Ingredients, Waitrose*	1 Serving/40g	52	4.9	129	1.7	2.7	12.3	2.7
Hearts, Canned, Drained, Average	*½ Can/117g*	*35*	*0.1*	*30*	*1.9*	*5.4*	*0.0*	*2.1*
Hearts, Marinated & Grilled, Waitrose*	1 Serving/50g	57	5.0	114	3.0	3.0	10.0	3.0
Hearts, Sliced, with Extra Virgin Olive Oil, Waitrose*	1 Serving/40g	24	1.6	59	1.3	4.4	4.0	7.0
Marinated, in Oil, with Parsley & Garlic, Drained, M & S*	1 Serving/100g	115	11.9	115	1.5	0.5	11.9	4.7
Marinated, Roasted, M & S*	1 Pack/200g	300	26.6	150	1.9	5.0	13.3	2.3
Raw, Fresh, Average	*1oz/28g*	*13*	*0.0*	*47*	*3.3*	*10.5*	*0.1*	*5.4*
ASPARAGUS								
Boiled, in Salted Water, Average	*5 Spears/125g*	*32*	*1.0*	*26*	*3.4*	*1.4*	*0.8*	*1.4*
British, with Butter, Tesco*	1 Serving/50g	26	2.0	52	2.6	1.6	4.0	2.0
Canned, Average	*1 Can/250g*	*47*	*0.5*	*19*	*2.3*	*2.0*	*0.2*	*1.6*
Raw, Trimmed, Average	*1 Serving/80g*	*20*	*0.5*	*25*	*2.9*	*2.0*	*0.6*	*1.7*
ASPIRE								
Cranberry Flavoured Soft Drink, Aspire*	1 Can/250ml	12	0.0	5	0.0	1.1	0.0	0.0
AUBERGINE								
Fried, Average	*1oz/28g*	*85*	*8.9*	*302*	*1.2*	*2.8*	*31.9*	*2.3*
Raw, Fresh, Average	*1 Sm/250g*	*37*	*1.0*	*15*	*0.9*	*2.2*	*0.4*	*2.0*
AVOCADO								
Flesh Only, Average	*1 Med/145g*	*275*	*28.3*	*190*	*1.9*	*1.9*	*19.5*	*3.4*

	Measure INFO/WEIGHT	per Measure KCAL	FAT	Nutrition Values per 100g / 100ml KCAL	PROT	CARB	FAT	FIBRE
BACARDI*								
*37.5% Volume, Bacardi**	*1 Shot/35ml*	72	0.0	207	0.0	0.0	0.0	0.0
*40% Volume, Bacardi**	*1 Shot/35ml*	78	0.0	222	0.0	0.0	0.0	0.0
Breezer, Cranberry, Bacardi*	1 Bottle/275ml	154	0.0	56	0.0	7.1	0.0	0.0
Breezer, Half Sugar, Bacardi*	1 Bottle/275ml	122	0.0	44	0.0	0.0	0.0	0.0
Breezer, Lemon, Diet, Bacardi*	1 Bottle/275ml	96	0.0	35	0.0	1.2	0.0	0.0
Breezer, Lime, Bacardi*	1 Bottle/275ml	181	0.0	66	0.0	9.1	0.0	0.0
Breezer, Orange, Bacardi*	1 Bottle/275ml	179	0.0	65	0.0	8.2	0.0	0.0
Breezer, Orange, Diet, Bacardi*	1 Bottle/275ml	80	0.0	29	0.0	0.0	0.0	0.0
Breezer, Pineapple, Bacardi*	1 Bottle/275ml	102	0.0	37	0.0	3.1	0.0	0.0
Breezer, Watermelon, Bacardi*	1 Bottle/275ml	100	0.0	36	0.0	3.2	0.0	0.0
BACON								
Back, Dry Cured, Average	*1 Rasher/31g*	77	4.7	250	28.1	0.3	15.1	0.3
Back, Dry Fried Or Grilled, Average	*1 Rasher/25g*	76	5.5	304	26.5	0.1	21.9	0.0
Back, Lean, Average	*1 Rasher/33g*	57	4.0	173	16.3	0.1	12.0	0.5
Back, Smoked, Average	*1 Rasher/25g*	66	5.0	265	20.9	0.0	19.9	0.0
Back, Smoked, Lean, Average	*1 Rasher/25g*	41	1.2	163	28.2	1.1	5.0	0.2
Back, Smoked, Rindless, Average	*1 Rasher/25g*	60	4.3	241	21.0	0.1	17.4	0.0
Back, Tendersweet, Average	*1 Rasher/25g*	63	3.6	250	29.8	0.4	14.3	0.0
Back, Unsmoked, Average	*1 Rasher/32g*	78	5.5	243	21.3	0.4	17.3	0.0
Back, Unsmoked, Rindless, Average	*1 Rasher/23g*	56	3.9	241	22.5	0.0	16.9	0.0
Chops, Average	*1oz/28g*	62	4.2	222	22.3	0.0	14.8	0.0
Collar Joint, Lean & Fat, Boiled	*1oz/28g*	91	7.6	325	20.4	0.0	27.0	0.0
Collar Joint, Lean & Fat, Raw	*1oz/28g*	89	8.1	319	14.6	0.0	28.9	0.0
Collar Joint, Lean Only, Boiled	*1oz/28g*	53	2.7	191	26.0	0.0	9.7	0.0
Fat Only, Cooked, Average	*1oz/28g*	194	20.4	692	9.3	0.0	72.8	0.0
Fat Only, Raw, Average	*1oz/28g*	209	22.7	747	4.8	0.0	80.9	0.0
Gammon Rasher, Lean Only, Grilled	*1oz/28g*	48	1.5	172	31.4	0.0	5.2	0.0
Lean, Average	*1oz/28g*	40	1.9	142	19.6	0.9	6.7	0.2
Lean Only, Fried, Average	*1 Rasher/25g*	83	5.6	332	32.8	0.0	22.3	0.0
Lean Only, Grilled, Average	*1 Rasher/25g*	73	4.7	292	30.5	0.0	18.9	0.0
Loin Steaks, Grilled, Average	*1 Portion/120g*	229	11.6	191	25.9	0.0	9.7	0.0
Medallions, Average	*1 Rasher/18g*	27	0.6	151	29.3	0.9	3.3	0.1
Middle, Fried	*1 Rasher/40g*	140	11.4	350	23.4	0.0	28.5	0.0
Middle, Grilled	*1 Rasher/40g*	123	9.2	307	24.8	0.0	23.1	0.0
Middle, Raw	*1 Rasher/43g*	104	8.6	241	15.2	0.0	20.0	0.0
Rindless, Average	*1 Rasher/20g*	30	1.7	150	18.5	0.0	8.5	0.0
Smoked, Average	*1 Rasher/28g*	46	2.1	166	24.7	0.2	7.3	0.0
Smoked, Crispy, Cooked, Average	*1 Serving/10g*	46	2.7	460	53.0	2.1	26.9	0.0
Smoked, Rindless, Average	*1 Rasher/20g*	21	0.6	106	19.8	0.0	3.0	0.0
Streaky, Average	*1oz/28g*	76	5.9	270	20.0	0.0	21.0	0.0
Streaky, Cooked, Average	*1 Rasher/20g*	68	5.6	342	22.4	0.3	27.8	0.0
BACON BITS								
Average	*1oz/28g*	66	4.9	235	19.6	0.0	17.4	0.0
BACON VEGETARIAN								
Rashers, Cheatin', The Redwood Co*	1 Rasher/16g	32	1.2	196	25.9	7.3	7.3	0.5
Realeat*	1 Rasher/19g	49	1.1	260	27.0	25.0	5.8	1.6
BAGEL								
Bacon, & Soft Cheese, Boots*	1 Serving/148g	481	25.2	325	12.0	31.0	17.0	2.2
Ham, & Pesto, COU, M & S*	1 Serving/173g	259	2.4	150	11.1	23.5	1.4	1.7
Soft Cheese, & Salmon, Smoked, Finest, Tesco*	1 Pack/173g	396	10.0	229	13.1	31.2	5.8	1.7
Tuna, & Salad, BGTY, Sainsbury's*	1 Bagel/170g	325	7.1	191	10.4	26.0	4.2	1.0
Turkey, & Cranberry, Bagelmania*	1 Pack/198g	325	7.3	164	9.0	24.5	3.7	1.1
Turkey, Pastrami & American Mustard, Shapers, Boots*	1 Bagel/146g	296	5.0	203	11.0	32.0	3.4	1.4

B

	Measure INFO/WEIGHT	per Measure KCAL	FAT	Nutrition Values per 100g / 100ml KCAL	PROT	CARB	FAT	FIBRE
BAGUETTE								
All Day Breakfast, Darwins Deli*	1 Serving/184g	498	21.5	271	13.4	31.9	11.7	0.0
Beef & Horseradish, Fresh, M & S*	1 Serving/274g	795	31.0	290	12.1	37.2	11.3	2.0
Brie, Tomato & Rocket, Freshly Prepared, M & S*	1 Serving/219g	570	21.7	260	10.3	33.2	9.9	1.9
Cheese, & Ham, Snack 'n' Go, Sainsbury's*	1 Serving/178g	383	9.1	215	12.6	29.6	5.1	1.9
Cheese, & Tomato, Tesco*	1 Serving/108g	243	8.3	225	9.7	29.3	7.7	1.8
Cheese, Mixed, & Spring Onion, Asda*	1 Pack/190g	629	34.8	331	9.5	32.1	18.3	1.3
Chicken, & Mayonnaise, Asda*	1 Pack/190g	407	16.5	214	9.7	30.5	8.7	1.3
Chicken, & Salad, Shapers, Boots*	1 Serving/132g	222	2.6	168	11.0	27.0	2.0	1.5
Chicken, & Spicy Tomato, Snack, Sainsbury's*	1 Serving/160g	344	5.9	215	14.1	31.2	3.7	2.2
Chicken, & Stuffing, Hot, Sainsbury's*	1 Serving/227g	543	16.3	239	13.7	29.6	7.2	0.0
Chicken, Honey & Mustard, BGTY, Sainsbury's*	1 Pack/187g	340	3.7	182	11.0	30.0	2.0	0.0
Chicken, Tikka, Hot, Sainsbury's*	1 Pack/190g	386	11.6	203	8.5	28.4	6.1	0.0
Egg, & Tomato, Oldfields*	1 Pack/198g	416	15.0	210	8.7	27.0	7.6	0.0
Egg, Bacon & Tomato, Freshly Prepared, M & S*	1 Serving/182g	455	17.3	250	12.9	28.0	9.5	1.7
Egg Mayonnaise, & Cress, Cafe, Sainsbury's*	1 Pack/100g	480	20.4	480	13.8	60.2	20.4	0.0
Ham, & Turkey, Asda*	1 Serving/360g	774	18.4	215	11.6	30.7	5.1	1.3
Ham & Cheese, Freshly Prepared, M & S*	1 Serving/231g	555	11.3	240	13.4	35.9	4.9	2.4
Mozzarella, Tomato, & Pesto, Darwins Deli*	1 Serving/210g	531	20.4	253	11.7	29.7	9.7	0.0
Oakham Chicken, Fresh, M & S*	1 Serving/225g	450	10.8	200	12.4	26.7	4.8	1.5
Prawn Mayonnaise, Asda*	1 Pack/190g	399	9.3	210	9.1	32.5	4.9	1.3
Smoked Salmon & Egg, Freshly Prepared	1 Serving/178g	455	17.3	255	13.7	28.4	9.7	1.6
Steak, & Onion, Snack 'n' Go, Sainsbury's*	1 Serving/177g	398	8.8	225	14.3	30.6	5.0	2.2
Tuna, Melt, Sainsbury's*	1 Serving/204g	373	8.0	183	11.3	25.8	3.9	0.0
BAILEYS*								
Glide, Baileys*	1 Glass/200ml	212	2.4	106	0.0	18.0	1.2	0.0
Irish Cream, Original, Baileys*	**1 Glass/37ml**	**121**	**4.8**	**327**	**3.0**	**25.0**	**13.0**	**0.0**
BAKE								
Aubergine & Mozzarella, Finest, Tesco*	1 Pack/400g	288	13.6	72	3.6	6.7	3.4	2.6
Bean & Pasta, Asda*	1 Pack/450g	598	22.5	133	5.0	17.0	5.0	1.7
Broccoli & Cheese, M & S*	1 Pack/400g	380	22.8	95	4.8	5.6	5.7	1.1
Cauliflower & Broccoli Bake, Tesco*	½ Pack/250g	177	10.2	71	2.8	5.8	4.1	1.0
Cheese & Spinach, Tesco*	1 Bake/140g	269	10.9	192	4.5	26.0	7.8	1.4
Cheesy Broccoli, Asda*	1 Pack/400g	400	17.6	100	4.5	10.6	4.4	1.4
Chicken, Bacon & Potato, British Classics, Tesco*	½ Pack/375g	435	16.5	116	7.0	12.2	4.4	1.4
Chicken, Tomato, & Mascarpone, HL, Tesco*	1 Serving/400g	468	10.8	117	7.6	15.5	2.7	0.8
Chicken, Tomato & Mozzarella, Birds Eye*	1 Pack/285g	370	5.4	130	7.1	14.3	1.9	0.3
Chicken & Mushroom, COU, M & S*	1 Serving/360g	324	8.3	90	7.3	10.3	2.3	1.1
Chicken & Pasta, BGTY, Sainsbury's*	1 Pack/400g	394	10.0	98	9.0	10.0	2.5	2.5
Chicken Pasta, Frozen, Light Choices, Tesco*	1 Pack/369g	351	5.2	95	6.8	13.1	1.4	1.0
Chicken Spiralli, M & S*	1 Serving/400g	400	15.2	100	7.9	9.1	3.8	1.1
Cod & Prawn, COU, M & S*	1 Pack/400g	320	8.0	80	6.5	8.8	2.0	1.0
Creamy Peppercorn, Vegetarian, Tesco*	1 Serving/140g	322	16.8	230	3.6	27.0	12.0	1.2
Fish, Broccoli & Sweetcorn, Light & Easy, Youngs*	1 Pack/240g	187	5.5	78	8.6	5.7	2.3	0.6
Fish, Haddock, Smoked, Light & Easy, Youngs*	1 Pack/310g	242	7.1	78	6.4	8.0	2.3	0.9
Fish Dinner, Light & Easy, Youngs*	1 Pack/385g	370	13.5	96	6.4	9.7	3.5	1.6
Haddock, Smoked, Light & Easy, Youngs*	1 Pack/300g	234	6.9	78	6.4	8.0	2.3	0.9
Haddock, Smoked, Luxury, Light & Easy, Youngs*	1 Pack/355g	390	17.0	110	7.5	9.2	4.8	0.6
Minced Beef & Root Vegetable, COU, M & S*	1 Pack/400g	320	11.6	80	6.6	6.0	2.9	3.0
Mushroom, Leek & Cheddar, Chosen By You, Asda*	½ Pack/199g	181	8.8	91	3.7	8.1	4.4	1.9
Mushroom, Leek & Spinach, Cumberland, Sainsbury's*	1 Pack/450g	518	24.3	115	3.6	12.9	5.4	1.2
Penne Bolognese, Sainsbury's*	1 Pack/397g	603	27.8	152	7.6	14.8	7.0	2.0
Potato, Cheese, & Bacon, Homepride*	1 Serving/210g	277	26.2	132	1.6	3.2	12.5	0.0
Potato, Cheese, & Onion, Tesco*	1 Pack/400g	376	19.6	94	2.4	10.0	4.9	1.0

	Measure INFO/WEIGHT	per Measure KCAL	FAT	Nutrition Values per 100g / 100ml KCAL	PROT	CARB	FAT	FIBRE
BAKE								
Potato, Mushroom & Leek, M & S*	1 Serving/225g	225	13.3	100	3.5	10.0	5.9	2.0
Potatoes, Cherry Tomatoes & Mozzarella, M & S*	½ Pack/165g	140	5.6	85	2.2	11.5	3.4	2.6
Roast Onion & Potato, COU, M & S*	1 Pack/450g	337	5.8	75	1.9	13.6	1.3	1.5
Roast Potato, Cheese & Onion, Asda*	½ Pack/200g	288	16.0	144	4.2	14.0	8.0	1.1
Salmon & Prawn, M & S*	1 Bake/329g	460	31.2	140	7.4	6.6	9.5	0.7
Smoked Haddock & Prawn, BGTY, Sainsbury's*	1 Pack/350g	318	2.4	91	7.5	13.6	0.7	1.1
Vegetable, M & S*	½ Pack/225g	157	6.1	70	1.9	8.9	2.7	1.6
BAKING POWDER								
Average	*1 Tsp/2g*	*3*	*0.0*	*163*	*5.2*	*37.8*	*0.0*	*0.0*
BAKLAVA								
Average	1 Serving/100g	393	21.0	393	5.0	46.0	21.0	0.0
BALTI								
Chicken, & Rice, M & S*	1 Pack/400g	380	6.0	95	6.9	14.1	1.5	1.2
Chicken, Asda*	1 Pack/450g	324	9.9	72	8.0	5.0	2.2	0.0
Chicken, M & S*	½ Pack/175g	245	15.2	140	13.0	2.0	8.7	1.7
Chicken, Morrisons*	1 Pack/350g	441	26.6	126	12.1	2.3	7.6	1.5
Chicken, Sainsbury's*	½ Pack/200g	222	11.2	111	11.6	3.6	5.6	1.3
Chicken, Take Away, Tesco*	½ Pack/200g	170	7.6	85	8.1	4.6	3.8	1.9
Chicken, Takeaway, Sainsbury's*	1 Pack/400g	404	18.0	101	10.4	4.8	4.5	1.4
Chicken, Tesco*	1 Pack/460g	662	25.8	144	6.1	17.4	5.6	1.6
Chicken, with Naan Bread, Sharwood's*	1 Pack/375g	529	23.2	141	7.3	14.1	6.2	2.2
Chicken, with Pilau Rice, Asda*	1 Pack/504g	625	24.7	124	5.0	15.0	4.9	1.3
Chicken, with Pilau Rice, Light Choices, Tesco*	1 Pack/400g	440	5.2	110	6.3	17.4	1.3	1.8
Chicken, with Pilau Rice, Weight Watchers*	1 Pack/329g	306	4.3	93	6.9	13.4	1.3	1.2
Chicken, with Pilau Rice & Naan Bread, Tesco*	1 Meal/550g	660	19.8	120	6.1	15.5	3.6	1.4
Chicken, with Potato Wedges, HL, Tesco*	1 Pack/450g	387	9.4	86	6.0	10.8	2.1	1.1
Chicken, with Rice, Curry Break, Patak's*	1 Pack/220g	198	6.2	90	4.7	11.6	2.8	0.0
Chicken, with Rice, Patak's*	1 Pack/370g	440	12.9	119	6.1	16.7	3.5	1.7
Lamb, Bhuna, Tesco*	1 Pack/400g	360	14.8	90	9.2	4.8	3.7	1.1
Vegetable, Asda*	½ Can/200g	206	12.0	103	2.2	10.0	6.0	2.5
Vegetable, Chosen By You, Asda*	1 Pack/200g	190	11.6	95	2.0	7.7	5.8	2.0
Vegetable & Rice, Tesco*	1 Pack/450g	378	7.2	84	2.0	15.6	1.6	1.3
BAMBOO SHOOTS								
Canned, Average	*1 Can/120g*	*11*	*0.2*	*9*	*1.1*	*0.9*	*0.1*	*0.9*
BANANA								
Raw, Flesh Only, Average	*1 Sm/95g*	*90*	*0.3*	*95*	*1.2*	*20.9*	*0.3*	*4.2*
Raw, Weighed with Skin, Average	*1 Lge/185g*	*176*	*0.6*	*95*	*1.2*	*20.9*	*0.3*	*4.2*
Slices, Dried, Love Life, Waitrose*	1 Serving/25g	74	0.1	295	4.8	66.5	0.6	5.2
BANANA CHIPS								
Average	*1oz/28g*	*143*	*8.8*	*511*	*1.0*	*59.9*	*31.4*	*1.7*
BANANA SPLIT								
Fresh Cream, Tesco*	1 Serving/240g	463	31.2	193	1.7	17.2	13.0	0.3
BANGERS & MASH								
Asda*	1 Pack/400g	636	28.0	159	9.0	15.0	7.0	1.6
Meal for One, M & S*	1 Pack/431g	560	34.0	130	4.7	9.5	7.9	1.1
BARS								
All Bran, Apple, Kellogg's*	1 Bar/40g	158	7.6	395	8.0	48.0	19.0	5.0
All Bran, Honey & Oat, Kellogg's*	1 Bar/27g	99	2.2	366	6.0	67.0	8.0	12.0
All Fruit, Frusli, Passion Fruit, Jordans*	1 Bar/30g	92	0.2	307	1.3	74.0	0.7	5.0
All Fruit, Frusli, Strawberry, Jordans*	1 Bar/30g	94	0.1	313	2.3	81.3	0.3	5.0
Almond, Apricot, & Mango, M & S*	1 Bar/50g	205	7.4	410	9.0	60.2	14.8	5.0
Almond & Apricot, Weight Watchers*	1 Bar/34g	151	6.6	443	8.6	55.9	19.4	5.2
Almond & Cranberry, Day Break, Atkins*	1 Bar/37g	137	5.7	370	37.8	22.7	15.4	15.1

BARS

	Measure INFO/WEIGHT	per Measure KCAL	FAT	Nutrition Values per 100g / 100ml KCAL	PROT	CARB	FAT	FIBRE
Am, Cereal, Apple, McVitie's*	1 Bar/40g	160	5.4	400	4.3	65.4	13.5	3.1
Am, Cereal, Apricot, McVitie's*	1 Bar/30g	146	6.1	486	6.5	68.8	20.5	0.5
Am, Cereal, Berry, McVitie's*	1 Bar/30g	146	6.1	486	6.5	68.8	20.5	0.5
Am, Cereal, Fruit & Nut, McVitie's*	1 Bar/35g	167	7.5	477	6.6	64.9	21.4	3.4
Am, Cereal, Grapefruit, McVitie's*	1 Bar/35g	136	3.3	389	5.1	70.9	9.4	3.1
Am, Cereal, Raisin & Nut, McVitie's*	1 Bar/35g	148	5.8	422	6.4	62.1	16.4	2.4
Am, Cereal, Strawberry, McVitie's*	1 Bar/35g	138	3.5	395	5.7	70.5	10.1	2.7
Am, Muesli Fingers, McVitie's*	1 Bar/35g	154	6.9	440	6.0	59.8	19.6	3.1
Apple, Fruit Bake, Go Ahead, McVitie's*	1 Bar/35g	124	2.5	354	2.7	73.8	7.2	1.2
Apple, Geobar, Traidcraft*	1 Bar/35g	132	3.1	376	5.3	69.0	8.8	3.5
Apple, Granola, McVitie's*	1 Bar/35g	128	3.4	366	6.6	63.1	9.7	4.3
Apple & Blackberry, Fruit Bake, McVitie's*	1 Bar/35g	124	2.5	354	2.7	73.8	7.2	1.2
Apple & Cinnamon, Breakfast Snack, Tesco*	1 Bar/38g	137	4.7	365	4.3	58.8	12.5	2.0
Apple & Cinnamon, Chewy, GFY, Asda*	1 Bar/27g	95	0.7	351	6.0	76.0	2.6	3.5
Apple & Cinnamon, Solo Slim, Rosemary Conley*	1 Bar/35g	114	1.3	327	26.7	46.6	3.8	8.3
Apple Pie, Nak'd*	1 Bar/68g	221	5.9	325	6.8	57.2	8.7	7.3
Apricot, Dried Fruit, Sunsweet*	1 Bar/33g	96	0.0	292	3.6	72.5	0.1	0.0
Apricot, Fruity Grain, Tesco*	1 Bar/37g	135	2.6	366	6.5	65.0	7.0	2.5
Apricot & Almond, Yoghurt Coated, Eat Natural*	1 Bar/50g	228	12.3	456	5.7	52.8	24.7	5.7
Apricot & Orange, Diet Chef Ltd*	1 Bar/25g	97	1.7	388	4.3	75.2	7.0	2.4
Apricot & Peach, Multigrain, BGTY, Sainsbury's*	1 Bar/25g	70	0.6	282	6.6	58.2	2.5	23.1
Baked Apple Pie, Weight Watchers*	1 Bar/27g	76	0.4	283	4.4	55.7	1.5	14.7
Banana, Apricot, & Milk Chocolate, Eat Natural*	1 Bar/30g	108	2.0	362	3.7	71.8	6.7	4.0
Banana Break, Breakfast in a Bar, Jordans*	1 Bar/40g	152	3.6	381	5.7	69.1	9.1	5.0
Banoffee, Weight Watchers*	1 Bar/18g	68	0.9	379	6.3	77.0	5.1	3.0
Berry Delight, Gluten Free, Nak'd*	1 Bar/35g	135	5.2	385	9.0	52.0	15.0	6.0
Berry Snack, Diet Chef Ltd*	1 Bar/27g	96	2.2	356	7.2	64.0	8.2	5.5
Biscuit, Chocolate, Penguin, McVitie's*	1 Bar/25g	130	6.9	520	5.2	62.4	27.7	2.4
Biscuit, Chocolate Mint, Penguin, McVitie's*	1 Bar/25g	133	6.9	531	5.4	65.0	27.7	1.5
Biscuit, Chocolate Orange, Penguin, McVitie's*	1 Bar/25g	133	6.9	531	5.4	65.0	27.7	1.5
Black Forest, Weight Watchers*	1 Bar/23g	94	2.0	408	3.9	78.4	8.8	1.4
Blackcurrant & Raspberry, Diet Chef Ltd*	1 Bar/25g	98	1.8	392	3.7	75.5	7.4	3.3
Blue Riband, 99 Calories, Nestle*	1 Bar/19g	99	4.9	513	4.8	66.4	25.3	0.0
Blue Riband, Double Choc, Nestle*	1 Bar/22g	113	5.6	513	4.8	66.4	25.3	1.1
Blue Riband, Nestle*	1 Bar/21g	104	5.2	495	4.5	64.5	24.5	1.0
Blueberry, Fruit & Grain, Asda*	1 Bar/37g	124	2.6	335	4.1	64.0	7.0	3.9
Blueberry, Weight Watchers*	1 Bar/25g	91	1.8	365	4.5	74.9	7.4	2.2
Blueberry, Yoghurt & Honey, Altu*	1 Bar/40g	129	4.7	323	12.9	45.5	11.7	12.0
Blueberry & Yoghurt Nougat, Shapers, Boots*	1 Bar/23g	89	3.7	385	1.7	58.0	16.0	0.7
Brazils, Sultanas, Almonds & Hazelnuts, Eat Natural*	1 Bar/50g	234	14.3	469	12.1	40.5	28.7	5.8
Breakfast, Apple Crisp, Morning Start, Atkins*	1 Bar/37g	145	7.9	392	29.2	25.4	21.4	13.8
Breakfast, Blueberry, Free From, Sainsbury's*	1 Bar/35g	163	7.8	467	3.8	62.6	22.4	0.2
Breakfast, Cherry, Oats & More, Nestle*	1 Bar/30g	109	1.9	363	6.0	70.2	6.5	3.6
Breakfast, Chocolate Chip Crisp, Morning Start, Atkins*	1 Bar/37g	137	7.0	370	31.8	22.5	18.8	15.0
Breakfast, Muesli, Country Garden Cakes*	1 Bar/25g	94	2.3	376	5.6	67.6	9.2	3.6
Caramel, Chocolate Nut Roll, Advantage, Atkins*	1 Bar/44g	170	12.0	386	18.2	43.2	27.3	18.2
Caramel, Double, Chocolate, Crunch, Atkins*	1 Bar/44g	160	9.0	364	22.7	50.0	20.4	25.0
Caramel, Endulge, Atkins*	1 Bar/24g	89	3.0	369	7.8	54.4	12.6	8.6
Caramel Chocolate Peanut Nougat, Advantage, Atkins*	1 Bar/44g	180	11.0	409	22.7	40.9	25.0	25.0
Caramel Crisp, Go Ahead, McVitie's*	1 Bar/33g	141	4.0	428	4.8	75.1	12.0	0.8
Caramel Crunch, Go Ahead, McVitie's*	1 Bar/24g	106	3.3	440	4.7	76.6	13.8	0.8
Caramel Nougat, Soft, Shapers, Boots*	1 Bar/25g	86	2.5	343	2.9	60.4	10.0	0.6
Caramel Wafer, Weight Watchers*	1 Bar/18g	78	3.7	427	5.7	64.7	20.2	1.9

	Measure	per Measure		Nutrition Values per 100g / 100ml				
	INFO/WEIGHT	KCAL	FAT	KCAL	PROT	CARB	FAT	FIBRE

BARS

	Measure INFO/WEIGHT	KCAL	FAT	KCAL	PROT	CARB	FAT	FIBRE
Cashew Cookie, Gluten Free, Nak'd*	1 Bar/35g	143	8.0	410	10.0	46.0	23.0	0.0
Cereal, Apple, Chewy, BGTY, Sainsbury's*	1 Bar/25g	85	0.5	340	4.8	76.0	2.0	2.0
Cereal, Apple & Blackberry, with Yoghurt, Alpen*	1 Bar/29g	117	3.1	404	5.4	71.8	10.6	5.0
Cereal, Apple & Raspberry, Waitrose*	1 Bar/25g	90	0.8	359	5.0	77.1	3.4	4.6
Cereal, Apple & Sultana, Light, Alpen*	1 Bar/21g	59	0.8	283	5.7	66.6	4.0	23.7
Cereal, Apricot & Yoghurt, COU, M & S*	1 Bar/21g	75	0.5	360	5.3	79.6	2.4	3.8
Cereal, Banoffee, COU, M & S*	1 Bar/20g	75	0.4	375	4.5	82.5	2.0	2.5
Cereal, Berry & Cream, COU, M & S*	1 Bar/20g	72	0.5	360	5.3	79.7	2.3	3.1
Cereal, Brownie, COU, M & S*	1 Bar/21g	75	0.5	365	5.5	79.7	2.6	4.6
Cereal, Cheerios & Milk Bar, Nestle*	1 Bar/22g	92	3.0	416	7.6	66.1	13.5	2.0
Cereal, Chewy & Crisp with Choc Chips, Tesco*	1 Bar/27g	125	6.3	463	9.2	54.0	23.4	3.8
Cereal, Chewy & Crisp with Roasted Nuts, Tesco*	1 Bar/27g	127	6.2	471	9.3	57.0	22.9	2.5
Cereal, Chewy Apple, Fruitus, Lyme Regis Foods*	1 Bar/35g	132	3.8	378	5.4	64.8	10.8	5.4
Cereal, Chewy Pomegranate, Vitality, Asda*	1 Bar/22g	76	0.6	346	4.1	69.3	2.8	13.4
Cereal, Choc Chip & Nut, Chewy & Crisp, Sainsbury's*	1 Bar/27g	129	7.0	476	8.8	51.8	26.0	4.4
Cereal, Chocolate, Geobar, Traidcraft*	1 Bar/32g	130	2.7	407	4.3	78.5	8.4	0.0
Cereal, Chocolate & Fudge, Light, Alpen*	1 Bar/21g	62	1.3	296	5.9	54.5	6.0	25.1
Cereal, Chocolate & Orange, Light, Alpen*	1 Bar/21g	62	1.1	295	6.0	56.0	5.2	22.2
Cereal, Chocolate & Pear, Fitnesse, Nestle*	1 Bar/24g	88	1.3	374	4.7	76.3	5.5	3.2
Cereal, Chocolate Chip, Special K, Kellogg's*	1 Bar/21g	84	1.5	401	9.0	76.0	7.0	1.5
Cereal, Citrus Fruits, Light, Alpen*	1 Bar/21g	59	0.9	283	5.6	55.9	4.1	22.4
Cereal, Coconut, Original Crunchy, Jordans*	1 Bar/30g	141	6.8	470	6.5	60.0	22.7	6.2
Cereal, Cranberry & Blackcurrant, HL, Tesco*	1 Bar/25g	121	7.0	485	7.2	50.3	27.9	3.8
Cereal, Cranberry & Orange, BGTY, Sainsbury's*	1 Bar/26g	93	1.3	358	2.7	75.8	4.9	2.3
Cereal, Cranberry & Orange, Weight Watchers*	1 Bar/28g	102	1.1	365	4.5	77.6	4.1	2.3
Cereal, Crunchy Granola, Apple Crunch, Nature Valley*	1 Bar/21g	92	3.1	440	7.3	69.0	15.0	5.7
Cereal, Crunchy Granola, Ginger Nut, Nature Valley*	1 Bar/42g	189	7.1	451	7.9	64.2	16.9	2.3
Cereal, Dark Chocolate, Le Noir, Orco*	1 Bar/21g	95	3.3	451	7.3	69.9	15.8	0.0
Cereal, Double Milk Chocolate, Special K, Kellogg's*	1 Bar/20g	80	1.8	398	9.0	66.0	9.0	10.0
Cereal, Fruit & Fibre, Asda*	1 Bar/29g	111	2.8	390	6.0	69.0	10.0	4.1
Cereal, Fruit & Nut, Ainsley Harriott*	1 Bar/35g	151	6.1	431	5.4	63.2	17.4	3.8
Cereal, Fruit & Nut, Alpen*	1 Bar/28g	110	2.8	394	6.6	69.6	9.9	5.0
Cereal, Fruit & Nut, Chewy Trail Mix, Nature Valley*	1 Bar/30g	114	3.2	379	7.7	63.2	10.6	7.3
Cereal, Fruit & Nut Break, Jordans*	1 Bar/37g	138	3.8	374	7.0	63.2	10.4	8.1
Cereal, Fruit & Nut with Milk Chocolate, Alpen*	1 Bar/29g	124	4.1	427	7.1	67.8	14.1	4.0
Cereal, Frusli, Blueberry Burst, Jordans*	1 Bar/30g	118	2.9	392	5.8	70.1	9.8	5.1
Cereal, Frusli, Cranberry & Apple, Jordans*	1 Bar/30g	118	3.0	393	5.7	70.0	10.0	5.3
Cereal, Frusli, Raisin & Hazelnut, Jordans*	1 Bar/30g	117	3.7	390	5.8	64.3	12.2	4.5
Cereal, Frusli, Red Berries, Jordans*	1 Bar/30g	113	2.4	378	5.1	71.7	7.9	4.5
Cereal, Frusli, Tangy Citrus, Jordans*	1 Bar/33g	124	3.2	376	4.4	67.7	9.8	4.8
Cereal, Frusli, Wild Berries, Jordans*	1 Bar/30g	118	2.9	392	5.7	70.0	9.8	5.0
Cereal, Ginger, Essential, Waitrose*	1 Bar/23g	81	0.6	353	4.9	77.7	2.5	3.2
Cereal, Ginger & Dark Chocolate, Weight Watchers*	1 Bar/22g	82	1.5	371	4.5	67.1	6.8	11.9
Cereal, Ginger & Raisin, BGTY, Sainsbury's*	1 Bar/40g	91	1.1	227	2.0	48.5	2.7	0.0
Cereal, Hazelnut & Pistachio, Go Ahead, McVitie's*	1 Bar/30g	117	3.4	389	4.8	66.5	11.5	2.5
Cereal, Hazelnut & Sultana, Organic, Seeds of Change*	1 Bar/29g	116	3.7	399	5.9	65.5	12.6	5.1
Cereal, Marmite*	1 Bar/25g	93	2.0	372	18.5	56.2	8.1	6.0
Cereal, Milk Chocolate, Weetos, Weetabix*	1 Bar/20g	88	2.9	440	5.9	70.9	14.7	1.6
Cereal, Mint Chocolate, Kellogg's*	1 Bar/22g	88	2.2	401	4.5	74.0	10.0	3.5
Cereal, Mixed Berry, Go Ahead, McVitie's*	1 Bar/35g	134	2.2	383	4.6	77.1	6.3	3.1
Cereal, Muesli Break, Breakfast in a Bar, Jordans*	1 Bar/46g	178	5.0	387	5.9	66.6	10.8	4.3
Cereal, Multigrain Balance, Maple, BGTY, Sainsbury's*	1 Bar/27g	75	0.8	276	6.4	56.2	2.8	25.5
Cereal, Nut & Seed, Organic, Green & Black's*	1 Bar/50g	258	16.3	516	8.4	47.2	32.6	10.0

B

BARS

	Measure INFO/WEIGHT	per Measure KCAL	FAT	Nutrition Values per 100g / 100ml KCAL	PROT	CARB	FAT	FIBRE
Cereal, Nutty, Free From, Sainsbury's*	1 Bar/25g	114	5.0	454	6.8	61.8	20.0	2.3
Cereal, Oats & More, Chocolate, Nestle*	1 Bar/30g	118	3.1	395	6.8	68.3	10.5	3.4
Cereal, Oats & More, Strawberry, Nestle*	1 Bar/30g	109	1.9	363	6.1	69.9	6.5	4.1
Cereal, Oaty, Milk Chocolate, Weetabix*	1 Bar/23g	80	1.5	342	6.9	51.7	6.5	24.3
Cereal, Oaty, Strawberry, Weetabix*	1 Bar/23g	69	1.4	299	6.2	54.7	6.1	24.5
Cereal, Oaty, Toffee Dazzler, Weetabix*	1 Bar/23g	80	1.5	348	6.2	54.9	6.7	21.5
Cereal, Oaty, White Chocolate Flavour, Weetabix*	1 Bar/23g	67	1.4	290	6.5	51.9	6.3	26.9
Cereal, Peanut Butter & Oat, Organic, Meridian Foods*	1 Bar/50g	203	9.2	407	12.6	50.9	18.4	5.0
Cereal, Pink Grapefruit, Chewy, BGTY, Sainsbury's*	1 Bar/25g	86	0.5	345	5.0	76.5	2.1	2.4
Cereal, Pomegranate, with Prebiotic, GFY, Asda*	1 Bar/22g	76	0.6	345	6.2	69.3	2.8	13.4
Cereal, Raisin & Apricot, Weight Watchers*	1 Bar/28g	100	1.3	358	6.8	72.2	4.6	3.2
Cereal, Raisin & Chocolate Chip, Fairtrade, Co-Op*	1 Bar/49g	185	4.6	378	5.3	69.2	9.4	3.7
Cereal, Raisin & Nut Snack Bar, Benecol*	1 Bar/25g	97	2.8	390	3.9	68.5	11.1	2.0
Cereal, Redberry & Chocolate, Sveltesse, Nestle*	1 Bar/25g	97	2.5	389	5.4	69.2	9.9	6.8
Cereal, Roast Hazelnut, Organic, Jordans*	1 Bar/33g	150	7.2	455	8.0	56.7	21.8	7.8
Cereal, Strawberry, Fitness, Nestle*	1 Bar/24g	89	1.6	378	4.9	73.8	7.0	4.1
Cereal, Strawberry with Yoghurt, Alpen*	1 Bar/29g	119	3.1	409	5.7	72.6	10.6	0.0
Cereal, Sultana & Apple, Sainsbury's*	1 Bar/27g	101	1.4	374	6.7	75.3	5.1	4.3
Cereal, Sultana & Honey, Jordans*	1 Bar/36g	130	3.0	361	6.0	65.9	8.2	9.2
Cereal, Summer Fruits, Light, Alpen*	1 Bar/21g	61	0.8	289	5.6	68.0	4.0	22.4
Cereal, Super High Fibre, Dorset Cereals*	1 Bar/35g	149	5.6	425	9.6	60.8	16.0	7.1
Cereal, Tropical Fruit & Nut, Organic, Dove's Farm*	1 Bar/40g	196	4.6	490	6.5	63.3	11.5	5.3
Cereal, Tropical Fruit & Nut Bar, Delicious, Boots*	1 Bar/40g	201	12.0	502	7.5	52.5	30.0	2.2
Cereal & Milk, Nesquik, Nestle*	1 Bar/25g	108	3.7	433	6.2	68.5	14.9	1.0
Chocolate, Caramel, & Biscuit, Asda*	1 Bar/30g	150	8.3	508	8.0	56.0	28.0	2.5
Chocolate, Crisp, Weight Watchers*	1 Bar/25g	92	2.5	369	5.4	75.1	10.2	0.8
Chocolate, Fruit & Nut, M & S*	1 Bar/50g	235	12.0	470	6.5	57.1	24.1	2.5
Chocolate, Healthy Meal, Herbalife*	1 Bar/56g	207	5.9	370	23.9	37.5	10.6	14.5
Chocolate, Milk, Belgian, Sugar Free, Sweet' N Low*	1 Bar/42g	202	14.3	480	7.1	52.7	34.1	1.8
Chocolate, Milk, Crispy, Endulge, Atkins*	1 Bar/30g	140	9.6	467	14.0	30.7	32.0	2.0
Chocolate, Milkshake, Crisp, Weight Watchers*	1 Bar/21g	82	2.1	391	4.4	59.6	10.0	13.4
Chocolate, Slim Fast*	1 Bar/39g	107	3.5	274	20.6	35.3	9.0	5.5
Chocolate, Toffee Pecan, M & S*	1 Bar/36g	179	9.8	498	4.9	58.3	27.3	0.7
Chocolate & Caramel, Lo Carb, Boots*	1 Bar/28g	101	3.1	359	2.8	82.0	11.0	1.8
Chocolate & Crispy Rice, Organic, Dove's Farm*	1 Bar/35g	147	5.3	421	4.4	66.9	15.1	3.0
Chocolate & Mint, Bliss, Special K, Kellogg's*	1 Bar/22g	90	2.2	403	5.0	74.0	10.0	3.5
Chocolate & Orange, Crispy, Free From, Sainsbury's*	1 Bar/30g	132	4.9	440	4.8	68.2	16.2	1.2
Chocolate & Orange, Crispy, Shapers, Boots*	1 Bar/22g	93	2.6	425	3.6	77.0	12.0	0.8
Chocolate & Peanut Butter, Atkins*	1 Bar/60g	240	12.0	400	31.7	36.7	20.0	16.7
Chocolate & Raisin, Shapers, Boots*	1 Bar/30g	99	2.0	331	5.4	55.0	6.8	5.0
Chocolate & Raspberry, COU, M & S*	1 Bar/25g	90	0.7	360	5.4	78.2	2.7	3.2
Chocolate Almond Fudge	1 Bar/68g	230	4.5	338	14.7	55.9	6.6	7.3
Chocolate Brownie	1 Bar/68g	240	4.0	353	14.7	60.3	5.9	8.8
Chocolate Caramel, Slim Fast*	1 Bar/26g	95	2.5	365	3.5	61.5	9.6	1.5
Chocolate Caramel, Weight Watchers*	1 Bar/20g	80	2.5	400	5.0	70.0	12.5	0.0
Chocolate Caramel Whip, Weight Watchers*	1 Bar/25g	88	2.7	353	2.7	72.4	10.8	1.0
Chocolate Chip, Slim Fast*	1 Bar/26g	98	3.0	378	4.9	70.4	11.4	1.8
Chocolate Chip, Snack, Slim Fast*	1 Bar/26g	99	3.0	382	4.9	70.4	11.4	1.8
Chocolate Chip Granola, Advantage, Atkins*	1 Bar/48g	200	8.0	417	35.4	37.5	16.7	12.5
Chocolate Chip Muesli, Diet Chef Ltd*	1 Bar/50g	191	5.9	382	5.8	59.8	11.9	6.1
Chocolate Cookie Dough, Meal, Slim Fast*	1 Bar/56g	220	5.0	393	14.3	64.3	8.9	3.6
Chocolate Creme, Endulge, Atkins*	1 Bar/14g	70	4.8	504	12.5	38.6	34.3	2.5
Chocolate Crisp, Weight Watchers*	1 Bar/25g	94	2.5	378	4.8	66.8	10.2	1.6

	Measure INFO/WEIGHT	per Measure KCAL	FAT	Nutrition Values per 100g / 100ml KCAL	PROT	CARB	FAT	FIBRE
BARS								
Chocolate Crunch, Slim Fast*	1 Bar/60g	210	5.0	350	23.3	51.7	8.3	6.7
Chocolate Decadence, Atkins*	1 Bar/60g	227	12.2	378	27.1	30.7	20.4	11.6
Chocolate Heaven, Ainsley Harriott*	1 Bar/26g	141	7.8	541	7.0	60.0	30.0	2.0
Chocolate Mint, The Cambridge Diet*	1 Bar/50g	174	5.8	348	24.8	30.2	11.6	14.4
Chocolate Muesli, Slim Fast*	1 Bar/26g	97	3.7	373	4.6	53.8	14.2	6.5
Chocolate Muesli, Snack, Slim Fast*	1 Bar/26g	99	3.5	379	4.7	64.5	13.3	6.5
Chocolate Peanut, Slim Fast*	1 Bar/26g	99	3.3	382	5.4	67.8	12.6	1.1
Chocolate Truffle, M & S*	1 Bar/35g	168	11.4	480	5.9	41.7	32.5	8.3
Club, Fruit, Jacob's*	1 Bar/25g	124	6.2	496	5.6	62.2	25.0	2.3
Club, Milk Chocolate, Jacob's*	1 Bar/24g	123	6.3	511	5.8	62.6	26.4	2.0
Club, Mint, Jacob's*	1 Bar/24g	124	6.5	517	5.6	62.5	27.2	1.7
Club, Orange, Jacob's*	1 Bar/23g	117	6.1	509	5.7	61.8	26.5	2.3
Coco Pops, & Milk, Kellogg's*	1 Bar/20g	85	2.6	423	7.0	70.0	13.0	1.0
Cocoa Loco, Nak'd*	1 Bar/30g	100	3.0	332	8.0	55.0	10.0	7.0
Cocoa Orange, Gluten Free, Nak'd*	1 Bar/35g	131	7.0	373	9.0	48.0	20.0	0.0
Coconut Chocolate Crisp, Weight Watchers*	1 Bar/25g	89	2.6	356	3.6	71.2	10.4	3.2
Coconut Cream Pie, Larabar*	1 Bar/48g	200	10.0	417	6.2	56.2	20.8	10.4
Coconut Whip, Weight Watchers*	1 Bar/20g	81	2.8	404	2.4	70.6	14.1	1.5
Corn Flakes, & Chocolate Milk, Kellogg's*	1 Bar/40g	176	6.4	440	9.0	66.0	16.0	2.0
Cranberry, Crunch, The Cambridge Diet*	1 Bar/50g	152	5.3	305	23.7	28.7	10.6	17.9
Cranberry & Macadamia Porridge Oat, Stoats*	1 Bar/85g	385	22.9	453	6.9	71.8	26.9	5.9
Cranberry & Raisin, Geobar, Traidcraft*	1 Bar/35g	131	2.8	374	3.7	72.6	8.0	2.3
Crazy Caramel, Tesco*	1 Bar/40g	192	9.2	480	3.9	64.0	23.0	1.0
Creme Brulee Chocolate, M & S*	1 Bar/36g	178	10.5	495	4.4	54.0	29.2	0.4
Crunchy Caramel, Tesco*	1 Bar/21g	98	5.2	467	4.6	56.0	25.0	1.4
Crunchy Granola, Oats 'n Honey, Nature Valley*	1 Bar/21g	97	3.4	460	8.3	70.4	16.1	6.2
Crunchy Nut, Chocolate Peanut Crisp, Kellogg's*	1 Bar/35g	169	8.7	483	12.0	53.0	25.0	3.5
Crunchy Nut, Kellogg's*	1 Bar/30g	119	1.5	397	6.0	82.0	5.0	2.5
Date & Fig, Lyme Regis Foods*	1 Bar/42g	143	4.9	341	7.0	52.0	11.7	9.3
Date & Fruit, Lyme Regis Foods*	1 Bar/42g	169	6.5	402	7.3	58.2	15.5	8.9
Date & Walnut, Eat Natural*	1 Bar/50g	220	10.0	441	8.0	57.1	20.1	3.3
Digestive, Milk Chocolate, McVitie's*	1 Bar/23g	118	5.8	511	6.6	64.6	25.1	1.9
Fig & Mango, The Food Doctor*	1 Bar/35g	103	0.9	293	8.6	58.6	2.7	10.3
Food Bar, Apple & Walnut, The Food Doctor*	1 Bar/35g	117	4.0	333	10.8	46.8	11.4	15.3
Forest Fruit & Raisin, Light Choices, Tesco*	1 Bar/27g	95	0.7	350	4.5	76.8	2.7	3.6
Frosties, & Milk, Kellogg's*	1 Bar/25g	102	2.7	408	7.0	71.0	11.0	1.0
Frosties, Chocolate, Kellogg's*	1 Bar/25g	103	3.0	412	6.0	72.0	12.0	1.6
Fruit, Apple, Trimlyne*	1 Bar/27g	88	0.7	326	4.5	69.6	2.7	3.8
Fruit, Fig, Castus*	1 Bar/27g	80	1.3	300	3.0	60.0	5.0	0.0
Fruit, Raisin & Apple, Light Choices, Tesco*	1 Bar/27g	95	0.7	350	4.5	76.8	2.7	3.6
Fruit, Strawberry, Fruitina*	1 Bar/15g	43	0.2	289	1.9	61.9	1.1	12.2
Fruit & Fibre, Whole Grain, Sainsbury's*	1 Bar/27g	109	3.0	405	6.2	70.1	11.1	3.8
Fruit & Nut, Breakfast, Replacement, The Biggest Loser*	1 Bar/55g	220	7.1	400	23.1	48.1	12.9	5.5
Fruit & Nut, Eat Natural*	1 Bar/50g	223	11.1	446	11.6	49.8	22.3	5.3
Fruit & Nut, Ginger Snap, Larabar*	1 Bar/51g	220	14.0	431	9.8	47.1	27.4	9.8
Fruit & Nut, Multigrain, Jordans*	1 Bar/40g	164	6.5	410	7.0	59.1	16.2	5.7
Fruit 'n' Fibre, Kellogg's*	1 Bar/25g	95	2.2	380	5.0	71.0	9.0	5.0
Fruit 'n' Fibre Bakes, with Sultanas, Kellogg's*	1 Bar/40g	146	5.2	365	4.5	58.0	13.0	9.0
Fruity, Oat, Low Fat, Organic, Dove's Farm*	1 Bar/40g	142	1.1	354	5.0	71.5	2.7	2.4
Fruity Cereal, Go, Soreen*	1 Bar/40g	143	1.8	358	6.8	72.6	4.5	0.0
Fudge Mallow Delight, Whipple Scrumptious, Wonka*	1 Bar/38g	205	12.0	537	4.6	59.2	31.3	0.6
Ginger, Solo Slim, Rosemary Conley*	1 Bar/35g	117	1.3	335	27.2	48.1	3.8	8.5
Ginger & Oat, Chocolate Covered, Snack, Waitrose*	1 Bar/27g	120	5.0	444	4.2	65.0	18.6	2.1

BARS

Measure INFO/WEIGHT	per Measure KCAL	FAT	Nutrition Values per 100g / 100ml KCAL	PROT	CARB	FAT	FIBRE
Goji Berries & Fax Seeds, Porridge Oat, Stoats*	1 Bar/85g	374	24.4	440	10.9	62.3	28.7	8.2
Granola, Crunchy, Roasted Almond, Nature Valley*	1 Bar/42g	193	7.6	459	8.1	65.6	18.2	3.7
Granola, Peanut Butter, Advantage, Atkins*	1 Bar/48g	210	11.0	437	29.2	39.6	22.9	10.4
Granola, Peanut Butter, Quaker Oats*	1 Bar/28g	110	3.5	393	7.1	64.3	12.5	3.6
Granola, with Peanut Butter, Natco*	1 Bar/29g	129	4.1	445	10.0	69.0	14.1	5.5
Hi-Fi, Luscious Lemon, Slimming World*	1 Bar/32g	106	3.1	332	4.4	54.2	9.7	12.4
Hi-Fi, Ravishing Ruby, Slimming World*	1 Bar/32g	117	2.7	365	5.2	65.4	8.5	9.3
Hi-Fi Cheeky Chocolate & Orange, Slimming World*	1 Bar/32g	119	2.8	373	4.4	66.6	8.8	10.6
Hi-Fi Deluxe Chocolate Bliss, Slimming World*	1 Bar/31g	121	3.6	390	6.8	52.9	11.6	21.0
Honey, Natural, Trail Mix, Kallo*	1 Bar/40g	196	13.3	490	15.7	40.9	33.2	5.7
Honey Nut, Special K, Special K, Kellogg's*	1 Bar/22g	90	2.0	409	9.1	72.7	9.1	13.6
Honey Rice Crisp, Lower Fat, Go Ahead, McVitie's*	1 Bar/22g	90	2.2	411	3.9	75.8	10.2	1.1
Macadamia & Fruit, Eat Natural*	1 Bar/50g	242	15.4	485	7.3	44.6	30.8	0.0
Macaroon, Lees*	1 Bar/70g	276	4.7	395	1.2	82.5	6.7	0.0
Mango & Brazil, Tropical Whole Foods*	1 Bar/40g	172	7.6	429	4.7	61.4	19.1	4.2
Maple & Pecan, Crunchy, Jordans*	1 Bar/33g	153	7.6	464	7.7	56.8	22.9	6.5
Maple & Pecan, Organic, Jordans*	1 Bar/25g	101	3.3	405	5.5	66.2	13.1	3.2
Mars, Minis, Mars*	1 Bar/18g	80	11.6	444	3.3	0.0	64.4	1.1
Marshmallow, Chewy, Rice Krispies Sqr, Kellogg's*	1 Bar/28g	119	3.4	424	3.0	76.0	12.0	0.9
Marshmallow Mudslide, Advantage, Atkins*	1 Bar/48g	210	10.0	437	31.2	39.6	20.8	10.4
Mint, Double Take, Sainsbury's*	1 Bar/20g	107	6.2	534	7.2	56.9	30.8	1.3
Mint Chocolate Whip, Weight Watchers*	1 Bar/20g	80	2.0	402	3.6	74.0	9.9	0.7
Mixed Berry, Trek, Natural Balance Foods*	1 Bar/68g	204	1.5	300	15.6	56.5	2.2	6.0
Mixed Nut Feast, Eat Natural*	1 Bar/50g	278	20.5	556	18.8	28.0	41.0	0.0
Muesli, Apricot & Almond, Carmen's*	1 Bar/45g	190	8.2	423	10.4	50.6	18.2	7.4
Muesli, Cherry & Milk, Sirius*	1 Bar/25g	104	2.8	417	7.2	71.3	11.4	3.9
Multigrain, Apple & Sultana, Jordans*	1 Bar/40g	141	2.5	353	4.4	70.0	6.2	4.8
Multigrain, Cranberry & Raspberry, Jordans*	1 Bar/37g	135	2.4	364	4.8	71.3	6.6	4.8
Multigrain, Fruit & Nut, Jordans*	1 Bar/40g	164	6.5	410	7.0	59.1	16.2	5.7
Nougat, Summer Strawberry, Shapers, Boots*	1 Bar/23g	83	3.0	361	2.7	73.0	13.0	0.6
Nutri-Grain, Apple, Kellogg's*	1 Bar/37g	131	3.3	355	4.0	67.0	9.0	4.0
Nutri-Grain, Blackberry & Apple, Kellogg's*	1 Bar/37g	131	3.3	355	4.0	67.0	9.0	4.0
Nutri-Grain, Blueberry, Kellogg's*	1 Bar/37g	130	3.3	351	4.0	66.0	9.0	4.0
Nutri-Grain, Cherry, Kellogg's*	1 Bar/37g	129	3.0	348	4.0	67.0	8.0	4.0
Nutri-Grain, Chocolate, Kellogg's*	1 Bar/37g	136	3.7	367	4.5	66.0	10.0	4.0
Nutri-Grain, Chocolate Chip, Chewy, Kellogg's*	1 Bar/25g	103	3.0	413	4.5	73.0	12.0	2.5
Nutri-Grain, Elevenses, Choc Chip, Kellogg's*	1 Bar/45g	179	5.8	397	4.0	66.0	13.0	2.0
Nutri-Grain, Elevenses, Ginger, Kellogg's*	1 Bar/45g	168	4.0	373	5.0	68.0	9.0	3.0
Nutri-Grain, Elevenses, Raisin, Kellogg's*	1 Bar/45g	164	4.0	364	5.0	66.0	9.0	3.5
Nutri-Grain, Honey Oat & Raisin, Chewy, Kellogg's*	1 Bar/25g	98	2.0	393	3.5	78.0	8.0	2.5
Nutri-Grain, Oat Bakes, Totally Oaty, Kellogg's*	1 Bar/50g	205	7.5	411	5.0	64.0	15.0	3.0
Nutri-Grain, Raspberry, Kellogg's*	1 Bar/37g	131	3.3	355	4.0	67.0	9.0	4.0
Nutri-Grain, Strawberry, Kellogg's*	1 Bar/37g	133	3.0	359	3.5	69.0	8.0	3.5
Oat, Mixed Berry, Quaker Oats*	1 Bar/38g	137	3.3	360	6.8	64.5	8.8	8.0
Oat, Original with Golden Syrup, Quaker Oats*	1 Bar/38g	139	3.6	366	7.1	64.5	9.5	7.9
Oat, Quaker Oats*	1 Bar/38g	137	3.4	360	6.8	64.5	8.8	8.0
Oats, Raisins, Honey & Apricots, Geobar, Traidcraft*	1 Bar/35g	132	3.1	376	5.3	69.0	8.8	3.5
Oaty, Strawberry Crusher, Weetabix*	1 Bar/23g	79	1.4	345	6.1	55.2	6.1	22.2
Oaty with Cranberry & Blueberry, Tesco*	1 Bar/38g	141	2.8	370	5.5	69.0	7.5	6.2
Optivita, Berry Oat, Kellogg's*	1 Bar/28g	101	2.0	360	7.0	68.0	7.0	9.0
Orange Crunch, Go Ahead, McVitie's*	1 Bar/23g	99	2.9	430	4.1	78.0	12.8	0.8
Orange Truffle, M & S*	1 Bar/33g	177	10.5	535	6.6	55.6	31.9	1.4
Orchard Fruits & Yoghurt, Fruit & Fibre, Sainsbury's*	1 Bar/27g	102	1.6	379	5.9	75.3	6.0	4.1

BARS

Measure INFO/WEIGHT	per Measure KCAL	FAT	Nutrition Values per 100g / 100ml KCAL	PROT	CARB	FAT	FIBRE
BARS							
Original, Crunchy, Honey & Almond, Jordans*	1 Bar/30g	139	6.8	463	8.3	56.7	22.7	6.7
Original, Nut Free, Get Buzzing*	1 Bar/62g	248	12.0	400	6.8	51.6	19.3	3.7
Original Muesli, Diet Chef Ltd*	1 Bar/50g	199	6.9	398	6.1	59.0	13.8	6.4
Peach, Apricot & Almond, Altu*	1 Bar/40g	158	4.6	395	7.9	65.2	11.4	4.3
Peach & Raspberry, Solo Slim, Rosemary Conley*	1 Bar/35g	115	1.4	329	26.9	46.7	4.0	9.4
Peanut, Cashew & Thai Sweet Chilli, Altu*	1 Bar/40g	172	8.1	430	14.7	47.0	20.3	3.1
Peanut, Raisin & Chocolate, Weight Watchers*	1 Bar/25g	97	2.8	388	7.6	60.0	11.2	12.8
Peanut & Caramel Whip, Weight Watchers*	1 Bar/20g	76	2.7	381	4.4	73.7	13.7	1.2
Peanut Butter, Chewy, Granola, Slim Fast*	1 Bar/56g	123	3.4	220	8.0	35.0	6.0	0.0
Peanut Fudge Granola, Advantage, Atkins*	1 Bar/48g	210	10.0	437	33.3	35.4	20.8	18.7
Pear & Ginger, Fruit Break, Lyme Regis Foods*	1 Bar/42g	160	8.8	381	2.7	45.4	20.9	9.9
Pecan Apricot & Peach, M & S*	1 Bar/50g	255	17.7	510	9.3	38.2	35.5	4.9
Pecan Pie, Larabar*	1 Bar/45g	200	14.0	444	6.7	48.9	31.1	8.9
Raisin & Apricot, Geobar, Traidcraft*	1 Bar/35g	132	3.1	376	5.3	69.0	8.8	3.5
Raisin & Hazelnut, Weight Watchers*	1 Bar/24g	95	2.4	396	5.0	71.2	10.0	2.9
Raisin & Oatmeal, Breakfast Snack, Tesco*	1 Bar/38g	133	4.4	355	5.6	56.8	11.7	2.8
Raspberry, Baked, Asda*	1 Bar/27g	104	2.1	385	3.4	74.2	7.6	1.8
Raspberry, Fruit Bake, Go Ahead, McVitie's*	1 Bar/35g	124	2.5	354	2.7	73.8	7.2	1.2
Raspberry & White Chocolate Crispie, Shapers, Boots*	1 Bar/24g	93	2.0	387	3.8	68.0	8.5	11.0
Replacement, Bar, Peanut Crunch, The Cambridge Diet*	1 Bar/50g	173	7.3	346	26.7	27.0	14.6	14.8
Rice Krispies, Snack, Kellogg's*	1 Bar/20g	83	2.0	415	7.0	70.0	10.0	0.5
Rice Krispies & Milk, Kellogg's*	1 Bar/20g	83	2.4	416	7.0	71.0	12.0	0.3
Rich Toffee, Weight Watchers*	1 Bar/26g	83	2.8	319	3.6	52.3	10.6	0.8
Roasted Nut, Chewy & Crisp, Sainsbury's*	1 Bar/27g	120	6.6	446	10.1	46.6	24.3	3.9
Roasted Peanut, Weight Watchers*	1 Bar/25g	104	3.2	415	9.6	65.3	12.8	3.7
Smarties, Nestle*	1 Bar/45g	238	13.5	528	6.2	58.2	30.0	0.9
Snack, Ginger, Diet Chef Ltd*	1 Bar/27g	94	1.9	348	5.5	65.6	7.1	4.4
Special Fruit Muesli, Jordans*	1 Bar/40g	140	2.4	349	5.0	68.8	6.0	5.0
Special K, Apple & Pear, Kellogg's*	1 Bar/23g	92	1.8	400	8.0	73.0	8.0	2.0
Special K, Bliss Bar, Raspberry & Chocolate, Kellogg's*	1 Bar/22g	88	2.2	399	4.0	74.0	10.0	4.0
Special K, Cereal with Chocolate Chip, Kellogg's*	1 Bar/21g	83	1.3	396	9.0	77.0	6.0	1.5
Special K, Chocolate Chip, Kellogg's*	1 Bar/22g	90	1.6	401	9.0	76.0	7.0	1.5
Special K, Fruits of the Forest, Kellogg's*	1 Bar/22g	87	1.8	397	8.0	74.0	8.0	2.5
Special K, Peach & Apricot, Kellogg's*	1 Bar/21g	84	1.9	400	8.0	73.0	9.0	2.5
Special K, Red Berry, Kellogg's*	1 Bar/23g	88	1.1	383	8.0	77.0	5.0	2.0
Special Muesli, Jordans*	1 Bar/40g	152	4.8	379	6.0	61.6	12.1	5.8
Strawberry, Fruit Bakes, Go Ahead, McVitie's*	1 Bar/35g	124	2.5	355	2.7	74.0	7.2	1.2
Strawberry, Morning Shine, Atkins*	1 Bar/37g	145	8.0	392	28.9	24.9	21.6	14.1
Sultana, Apple & Yoghurt, Balance, Sainsbury's*	1 Bar/27g	104	1.6	387	6.1	77.4	5.9	2.3
Summer Berry, Meal, Slim Fast*	1 Bar/60g	210	5.0	350	23.3	51.7	8.3	5.8
Sweet & Salty, Almond Crunch, Advantage, Atkins*	1 Bar/40g	200	15.0	500	17.5	35.0	37.5	12.5
Toffee, Slim Fast*	1 Bar/39g	122	3.3	314	19.7	47.1	8.5	5.6
Toffee & Banana, Weight Watchers*	1 Bar/18g	67	0.7	372	6.1	77.2	3.9	1.7
Totally Chocolate Orange, Rice Krispies Sqr, Kellogg's*	1 Bar/34g	149	4.8	437	4.5	73.0	14.0	1.5
Totally Chocolatey, Rice Krispies Squares, Kellogg's*	1 Bar/36g	156	4.7	432	4.5	74.0	13.0	1.5
Tracker, Breakfast, Banana, Mars*	1 Bar/37g	176	8.4	476	4.7	63.3	22.6	9.4
Tracker, Breakfast, Lemon, Mars*	1 Bar/26g	124	5.8	477	4.6	64.3	22.4	0.0
Tracker, Chocolate Chip, Mars*	1 Bar/37g	178	8.7	480	6.8	58.0	23.6	3.8
Tracker, Forest Fruits, Mars*	1 Bar/26g	123	5.8	474	4.6	64.1	22.2	0.0
Tracker, Roasted Nut, Mars*	1 Bar/26g	127	6.6	489	8.1	55.0	25.3	4.9
Tracker, Yoghurt, Mars*	1 Bar/27g	133	6.3	491	6.3	64.2	23.2	0.0
BASIL							
Dried, Ground	1 Tsp/1.4g	4	0.1	251	14.4	43.2	4.0	0.0

	Measure INFO/WEIGHT	per Measure KCAL	FAT	Nutrition Values per 100g / 100ml KCAL	PROT	CARB	FAT	FIBRE
BASIL								
Fresh, Average	*1 Tbsp/5g*	*2*	*0.0*	*40*	*3.1*	*5.1*	*0.8*	*0.0*
BATTER MIX								
for Yorkshire Puddings & Pancakes, Morrisons*	1 Pudding/30g	43	0.8	143	6.4	23.1	2.8	4.1
for Yorkshire Puddings & Pancakes, Tesco*	1 Serving/17g	34	0.3	200	2.3	43.3	1.5	2.5
Green's*	1 Bag/125g	296	9.0	237	8.7	34.3	7.2	0.0
Pancake, Sainsbury's*	1 Pancake/63g	96	1.1	152	6.5	27.4	1.8	3.1
BAY LEAVES								
Dried, Average	*1 Tsp/0.6g*	*2*	*0.1*	*313*	*7.6*	*48.6*	*8.4*	*0.0*
BEAN SPROUTS								
Mung, Canned, Drained, Average	*1 Serving/90g*	*9*	*0.1*	*10*	*1.6*	*0.8*	*0.1*	*0.7*
Mung, Raw, Average	*1oz/28g*	*9*	*0.1*	*31*	*2.9*	*4.0*	*0.5*	*1.5*
Mung, Stir-Fried in Blended Oil, Average	*1 Serving/90g*	*65*	*5.5*	*72*	*1.9*	*2.5*	*6.1*	*0.9*
Raw, Average	*1 Serving/150g*	*45*	*0.3*	*30*	*3.0*	*5.9*	*0.2*	*1.8*
BEANFEAST								
Bolognese Style, Dry, Batchelors*	1 Pack/120g	362	6.7	302	23.9	39.0	5.6	13.5
Mexican Chilli, Batchelors*	1 Serving/65g	203	3.2	312	24.3	42.7	4.9	13.6
BEANS								
Aduki, Cooked in Unsalted Water, Average	*1 Tbsp/30g*	*37*	*0.1*	*123*	*9.3*	*22.5*	*0.2*	*5.5*
Aduki, Dried, Raw	*1 Tbsp/30g*	*82*	*0.1*	*272*	*19.9*	*50.1*	*0.5*	*11.1*
Adzuki, Dry, Love Life, Waitrose*	1 Serving/100g	340	0.5	340	19.9	62.9	0.5	12.7
Adzuki, in Water, Drained, Tesco*	1 Can/236g	201	0.9	85	6.5	13.6	0.4	6.5
Baked, & Jumbo Sausages, Asda*	1 Serving/210g	317	14.7	151	7.0	15.0	7.0	2.6
Baked, & Pork Sausages, Sainsbury's*	1 Serving/210g	248	9.2	118	5.7	13.9	4.4	3.4
Baked, & Sausages, GFY, Asda*	1 Serving/217g	178	5.6	82	4.7	10.0	2.6	1.8
Baked, & Sausages, Meatfree, Sainsbury's*	1 Can/420g	500	16.8	119	8.0	12.6	4.0	2.7
Baked, Barbecue, Smokey, Beanz, Heinz*	1 Can/420g	332	0.8	79	4.9	14.3	0.2	3.8
Baked, Cheezy, Heinz*	1oz/28g	53	1.4	189	11.6	24.5	4.9	6.2
Baked, Curried, Average	*½ Can/210g*	*203*	*1.9*	*96*	*4.8*	*17.2*	*0.9*	*3.6*
Baked, in Tomato Sauce, Average	*1 Can/400g*	*346*	*1.8*	*86*	*4.8*	*15.9*	*0.5*	*3.3*
Baked, in Tomato Sauce, Beanz, Heinz*	½ Can/208g	164	0.4	79	4.7	12.9	0.2	3.7
Baked, in Tomato Sauce, Beanz, Snap Pot, Heinz*	1 Pot/200g	160	0.4	80	4.7	12.9	0.2	3.7
Baked, in Tomato Sauce, Healthy Range, Average	*½ Can/210g*	*143*	*0.5*	*68*	*3.9*	*12.8*	*0.2*	*2.8*
Baked, in Tomato Sauce, Reduced Sugar & Salt	*½ Can/210g*	*159*	*0.7*	*75*	*4.5*	*13.6*	*0.3*	*3.8*
Baked, Jalfrezi, Mean, Beanz, Heinz*	1 Serving/195g	135	2.5	69	4.5	9.8	1.3	3.6
Baked, Mexican, Mean, Beanz, Heinz*	½ Can/208g	158	1.0	76	5.0	12.9	0.5	4.0
Baked, Sweet Chilli, Mean, Beanz, Heinz*	½ Can/195g	142	0.6	73	4.5	13.0	0.3	3.6
Baked, Tikka, Mean, Beanz, Heinz*	1 Serving/195g	172	5.9	88	4.8	10.6	3.0	3.5
Baked, Virtually Fat Free, Heinz*	1 Serving/100g	79	0.2	79	4.7	12.9	0.2	3.7
Baked, with Chicken Nuggets, Beanz, Heinz*	1 Can/200g	210	6.3	105	6.7	12.4	3.1	3.2
Baked, with Hidden Veg, Beanz, Heinz*	½ Can/208g	156	0.6	75	4.7	13.5	0.3	4.1
Baked, with HP Sauce, Beanz, Heinz*	½ Can/208g	158	0.6	76	4.8	13.7	0.3	3.9
Baked, with Lea & Perrins Sauce, Beanz, Heinz*	1 Can/415g	303	0.8	73	4.8	13.1	0.2	3.8
Baked, with Sausages, Branston, Crosse & Blackwell*	½ Can/202g	233	6.5	115	6.9	12.2	3.2	5.0
Baked, with Spicy Meatballs, Beanz, Heinz*	1 Can/400g	372	9.6	93	5.8	12.0	2.4	2.9
Baked, with Steak Chunks, Beanz, Heinz*	1 Can/415g	340	2.9	82	6.9	12.1	0.7	3.5
Black, Cooked, Average	*1 Cup/172g*	*227*	*0.9*	*132*	*8.8*	*23.7*	*0.5*	*8.7*
Black, Dried, Average	*1 Serving/100g*	*341*	*1.4*	*341*	*21.6*	*62.4*	*1.4*	*15.2*
Blackeye, Canned, Average	*1 Can/172g*	*206*	*1.3*	*119*	*8.4*	*19.7*	*0.7*	*3.3*
Blackeye, Dried, Raw	*1oz/28g*	*87*	*0.4*	*311*	*23.5*	*54.1*	*1.6*	*8.2*
Borlotti, Canned, Average	*1oz/28g*	*29*	*0.1*	*103*	*7.6*	*16.9*	*0.5*	*4.7*
Borlotti, Dried, Raw, Average	*1 Serving/100g*	*335*	*1.2*	*335*	*23.0*	*60.0*	*1.2*	*24.7*
Broad, Canned, Drained, Average	*1 Can/195g*	*136*	*1.1*	*70*	*6.9*	*9.2*	*0.6*	*6.8*
Broad, Dried, Raw, Average	*1oz/28g*	*69*	*0.6*	*245*	*26.1*	*32.5*	*2.1*	*27.6*

	Measure INFO/WEIGHT	per Measure		Nutrition Values per 100g / 100ml				
		KCAL	FAT	KCAL	PROT	CARB	FAT	FIBRE
BEANS								
Broad, Weighed with Pod, Raw, Average	1oz/28g	17	0.3	59	5.7	7.2	1.0	6.1
Butter, Canned, Average	1oz/28g	22	0.1	79	5.9	12.9	0.5	4.0
Butter, Dried, Boiled, Average	1oz/28g	30	0.2	106	7.2	18.6	0.6	5.2
Butter, Dried, Raw, Average	1oz/28g	81	0.5	290	19.1	52.9	1.7	16.0
Cannellini, Canned, Average	1oz/28g	26	0.1	94	7.2	15.0	0.5	5.7
Chilli, Canned, Average	1 Can/420g	381	3.1	91	5.2	15.8	0.7	4.3
Edamame, Shelled, Frozen, Raw, Average	1 Serving/80g	88	3.8	110	10.2	8.6	4.7	4.8
Flageolet, Canned, Average	1 Can/265g	235	1.6	89	6.7	14.0	0.6	3.5
French, Boiled, Average	1 Serving/150g	37	0.0	25	2.3	3.8	0.0	3.7
French, Canned, Average	1oz/28g	6	0.1	22	1.6	3.5	0.3	2.5
French, Raw	1oz/28g	7	0.1	24	1.9	3.2	0.5	2.2
Green, Cut, Average	1oz/28g	6	0.1	22	1.7	3.7	0.2	2.1
Green, Fine, Average	1 Serving/75g	18	0.3	24	1.8	3.4	0.4	2.6
Green, Sliced, Average	1oz/28g	6	0.1	23	1.9	3.5	0.2	2.1
Green, Sliced, Frozen, Average	1 Serving/50g	13	0.0	26	1.8	4.4	0.1	4.1
Green, Whole, Average	1oz/28g	6	0.1	22	1.6	3.0	0.4	1.7
Haricot, Dried, Boiled in Unsalted Water	1oz/28g	27	0.1	95	6.6	17.2	0.5	6.1
Haricot, Dried, Raw	1oz/28g	80	0.4	286	21.4	49.7	1.6	17.0
Kidney, Red, Canned, Average	½ Can/90g	92	0.5	102	7.8	16.7	0.6	5.6
Kidney, Red, Dried, Boiled in Unsalted Water	1oz/28g	29	0.1	103	8.4	17.4	0.5	6.7
Kidney, Red, Dried, Raw	1oz/28g	74	0.4	266	22.1	44.1	1.4	15.7
Mixed, Canned, Average	1 Can/300g	300	3.5	100	6.7	15.6	1.2	4.1
Mixed, Spicy, Average	1 Serving/140g	108	0.7	77	4.8	13.4	0.5	3.9
Mixed, with Lentils, Waitrose*	1 Pack/300g	399	21.9	133	5.1	11.6	7.3	3.1
Mung, Whole, Dried, Boiled in Unsalted Water	1oz/28g	25	0.1	91	7.6	15.3	0.4	3.0
Mung, Whole, Dried, Raw	1oz/28g	78	0.3	279	23.9	46.3	1.1	10.0
Pinto, Dried, Boiled in Unsalted Water	1oz/28g	38	0.2	137	8.9	23.9	0.7	0.0
Pinto, Dried, Raw	1oz/28g	92	0.4	327	21.1	57.1	1.6	14.0
Refried, Average	1 Serving/215g	162	1.5	75	4.6	12.7	0.7	1.7
Runner, Average	1 Serving/80g	16	0.3	20	1.4	2.8	0.4	2.2
Soya, Dried, Average	1oz/28g	104	5.1	370	34.2	15.4	18.3	19.6
Soya, Dried, Boiled in Unsalted Water	1oz/28g	39	2.0	141	14.0	5.1	7.3	6.1
Soya, Frozen, Birds Eye*	1 Serving/80g	98	5.1	123	12.4	4.0	6.4	4.2
Soya, in Water, Salt Added, Sainsbury's*	1 Serving/100g	102	7.3	102	4.0	5.1	7.3	6.1
White, Campo Largo*	½ Jar/200g	180	1.0	90	7.1	11.2	0.5	0.0
BEEF								
Brisket, Boiled, Lean	1 Serving/100g	225	11.0	225	31.4	0.0	11.0	0.0
Brisket, Boiled, Lean & Fat	1 Serving/100g	268	17.4	268	27.8	0.0	17.4	0.0
Brisket, Braised, Lean	1 Serving/100g	280	17.4	280	29.0	0.0	17.4	0.0
Brisket, Raw, Lean	1oz/28g	39	1.7	139	21.1	0.0	6.1	0.0
Brisket, Raw, Lean & Fat	1oz/28g	61	4.5	218	18.4	0.0	16.0	0.0
Cooked, Sliced, From Supermarket, Average	1 Slice/35g	35	0.8	101	17.4	2.6	2.4	0.4
Escalope, Healthy Range, Average	1 Serving/170g	233	6.7	137	24.2	1.2	4.0	0.4
Flank, Pot-Roasted, Lean	1oz/28g	71	3.9	253	31.8	0.0	14.0	0.0
Flank, Pot-Roasted, Lean & Fat	1oz/28g	87	6.2	309	27.1	0.0	22.3	0.0
Flank, Raw, Lean	1oz/28g	49	2.6	175	22.7	0.0	9.3	0.0
Flank, Raw, Lean & Fat	1oz/28g	74	5.8	266	19.7	0.0	20.8	0.0
for Casserole, Lean, Diced, Average	1oz/28g	35	1.1	126	23.0	0.0	3.8	0.0
Fore Rib, Lean & Fat, Average	1oz/28g	40	1.7	143	21.7	0.0	6.2	0.2
Fore Rib, Raw, Lean	1oz/28g	41	1.8	145	21.5	0.0	6.5	0.0
Fore Rib, Roasted, Lean	1oz/28g	66	3.2	236	33.3	0.0	11.4	0.0
Fore Rib, Roasted, Lean & Fat	1oz/28g	84	5.7	300	29.1	0.0	20.4	0.0
Grill Steak, Average	1 Steak/170g	501	39.5	295	19.3	2.1	23.2	0.1

B

BEEF

	Measure INFO/WEIGHT	per Measure KCAL	per Measure FAT	Nutrition Values per 100g / 100ml KCAL	PROT	CARB	FAT	FIBRE
Grill Steak, Peppered, Average	1 Serving/172g	419	24.4	243	23.6	5.2	14.2	0.3
Joint, for Roasting, Average	1oz/28g	38	1.0	134	24.5	1.4	3.4	0.2
Joint, Sirloin, Roasted, Lean	1oz/28g	53	1.8	188	32.4	0.0	6.5	0.0
Joint, Sirloin, Roasted, Lean & Fat	1oz/28g	65	3.5	233	29.8	0.0	12.6	0.0
Mince, Cooked, Average	1 Serving/75g	214	15.3	286	23.9	0.0	20.3	0.0
Mince, Extra Lean, Raw, Average	1 Serving/100g	131	5.3	131	21.0	0.0	5.3	0.0
Mince, Extra Lean, Stewed	1oz/28g	50	2.4	177	24.7	0.0	8.7	0.0
Mince, Lean, Raw, Average	1oz/28g	49	2.7	175	22.0	0.0	9.7	0.0
Mince, Raw, Average	1oz/28g	67	5.0	239	18.7	0.2	18.0	0.1
Mince, Steak, Extra Lean, Average	1oz/28g	37	1.6	131	20.5	0.4	5.6	0.0
Mince, Steak, Raw, Average	1 Serving/125g	317	25.0	254	17.2	0.0	20.0	0.0
Mince, Stewed	1oz/28g	59	3.8	209	21.8	0.0	13.5	0.0
Peppered, Sliced, Average	1 Slice/20g	26	1.1	129	18.2	1.3	5.6	1.0
Roast, Sliced, Average	1 Slice/35g	48	1.3	136	26.1	0.4	3.6	0.2
Salt, Average	1 Serving/70g	80	1.7	114	21.7	1.0	2.5	0.1
Salted, Dried, Raw	1oz/28g	70	0.4	250	55.4	0.0	1.5	0.0
Silverside, Pot-Roasted, Lean	1oz/28g	54	1.8	193	34.0	0.0	6.3	0.0
Silverside, Pot-Roasted, Lean & Fat	1oz/28g	69	3.8	247	31.0	0.0	13.7	0.0
Silverside, Raw, Lean	1oz/28g	38	1.2	134	23.8	0.0	4.3	0.0
Silverside, Raw, Lean & Fat	1oz/28g	60	4.1	215	20.4	0.0	14.8	0.0
Silverside, Salted, Boiled, Lean	1oz/28g	52	1.9	184	30.4	0.0	6.9	0.0
Silverside, Salted, Boiled, Lean & Fat	1oz/28g	63	3.5	224	27.9	0.0	12.5	0.0
Silverside, Salted, Raw, Lean	1oz/28g	39	2.0	140	19.2	0.0	7.0	0.0
Silverside, Salted, Raw, Lean & Fat	1oz/28g	64	5.0	227	16.3	0.0	18.0	0.0
Steak, Braising, Braised, Lean	1oz/28g	63	2.7	225	34.4	0.0	9.7	0.0
Steak, Braising, Braised, Lean & Fat	1oz/28g	69	3.6	246	32.9	0.0	12.7	0.0
Steak, Braising, Lean, Raw, Average	1oz/28g	40	1.4	144	24.8	0.0	5.0	0.0
Steak, Braising, Raw, Lean & Fat	1oz/28g	45	2.4	160	20.7	0.0	8.6	0.0
Steak, Economy, Average	1oz/28g	53	2.4	190	26.9	1.2	8.7	0.4
Steak, Fillet, Cooked, Average	1oz/28g	54	2.4	191	28.6	0.0	8.5	0.0
Steak, Fillet, Lean, Average	1oz/28g	42	2.0	150	21.0	0.0	7.3	0.0
Steak, Fillet, Lean, Cooked, Average	1oz/28g	52	2.2	186	28.6	0.0	7.9	0.0
Steak, Frying, Average	1 Steak/110g	128	2.7	116	23.7	0.0	2.5	0.0
Steak, Rump, Cooked, Average	1oz/28g	69	4.0	245	29.1	0.5	14.1	0.0
Steak, Rump, Grilled, Rare, Lean	1 Steak/227g	381	15.6	168	26.5	0.0	6.9	0.0
Steak, Rump, Lean, Cooked, Average	1oz/28g	50	1.7	179	31.0	0.0	6.1	0.0
Steak, Rump, Raw, Lean	1oz/28g	35	1.1	125	22.0	0.0	4.1	0.0
Steak, Rump, Raw, Lean & Fat	1oz/28g	49	2.8	174	20.7	0.0	10.1	0.0
Steak, Sirloin, Fried, Rare, Lean	1oz/28g	53	2.3	189	28.8	0.0	8.2	0.0
Steak, Sirloin, Fried, Rare, Lean & Fat	1oz/28g	65	3.9	233	26.8	0.0	14.0	0.0
Steak, Sirloin, Grilled, Medium-Rare, Lean	1oz/28g	49	2.2	176	26.6	0.0	7.7	0.0
Steak, Sirloin, Grilled, Medium-Rare, Lean & Fat	1oz/28g	60	3.5	213	24.8	0.0	12.6	0.0
Steak, Sirloin, Grilled, Rare, Lean	1oz/28g	46	1.9	166	26.4	0.0	6.7	0.0
Steak, Sirloin, Grilled, Rare, Lean & Fat	1oz/28g	60	3.6	216	25.1	0.0	12.8	0.0
Steak, Sirloin, Grilled, Well-Done, Lean	1oz/28g	63	2.8	225	33.9	0.0	9.9	0.0
Steak, Sirloin, Grilled, Well-Done, Lean & Fat	1oz/28g	72	4.0	257	31.8	0.0	14.4	0.0
Steak, Sirloin, Raw, Lean	1oz/28g	38	1.3	135	23.5	0.0	4.5	0.0
Steak, Sirloin, Raw, Lean & Fat	1oz/28g	56	3.6	201	21.6	0.0	12.7	0.0
Stewed Steak, Average	1 Serving/220g	258	10.1	117	15.8	3.3	4.6	0.0
Stewing Steak, Lean & Fat, Raw, Average	1oz/28g	41	1.8	146	22.1	0.0	6.4	0.0
Stewing Steak, Raw, Lean	1oz/28g	34	1.0	122	22.6	0.0	3.5	0.0
Stewing Steak, Stewed, Lean	1oz/28g	52	1.8	185	32.0	0.0	6.3	0.0
Stewing Steak, Stewed, Lean & Fat	1oz/28g	57	2.7	203	29.2	0.0	9.6	0.0

B

	Measure INFO/WEIGHT	per Measure KCAL	FAT	Nutrition Values per 100g / 100ml KCAL	PROT	CARB	FAT	FIBRE
BEEF								
Stir Fry Strips, Raw, Average	1 Serving/125g	146	3.1	116	23.5	0.0	2.5	0.3
Topside, Lean & Fat, Average	1oz/28g	61	3.4	219	27.5	0.0	12.2	0.0
Topside, Raw, Lean	1oz/28g	32	0.8	116	23.0	0.0	2.7	0.0
Wafer Thin Sliced, Cooked, Average	1 Slice/10g	13	0.3	129	24.5	0.5	3.2	0.1
BEEF &								
Beer, Princes*	½ Can/205g	215	6.1	105	14.0	5.5	3.0	0.0
Black Bean, Sizzling, Oriental Express*	1 Pack/400g	420	8.4	105	7.2	14.0	2.1	2.1
Black Bean, with Rice, Weight Watchers*	1 Pack/320g	288	4.2	90	5.0	14.6	1.3	0.1
Mashed Potato, Braised, Sainsbury's*	1 Pack/434g	425	14.3	98	7.6	9.4	3.3	0.8
Onions, Minced, Asda*	½ Can/196g	314	19.6	160	13.0	4.6	10.0	0.1
Onions, with Gravy, Minced, Lean, Sainsbury's*	1 Can/198g	285	13.9	144	17.0	3.1	7.0	0.2
BEEF BORDELAISE								
Sainsbury's*	1 Pack/401g	525	25.7	131	8.7	9.7	6.4	1.0
BEEF BOURGUIGNON								
Extra Special, Asda*	1 Serving/300g	279	11.0	93	9.3	5.7	3.7	0.7
Finest, Tesco*	½ Pack/300g	247	7.8	82	9.9	4.8	2.6	0.5
BEEF BRAISED								
Steak, & Cabbage, COU, M & S*	1 Pack/380g	323	9.9	85	8.3	6.7	2.6	1.9
Steak, & Carrots, Mini Favourites, M & S*	1 Serving/200g	140	5.0	70	8.0	4.2	2.5	1.3
Steak, & Mash, GFY, Asda*	1 Pack/400g	260	3.2	65	3.4	11.0	0.8	0.7
Steak, & Mash, HL, Tesco*	1 Pack/450g	418	12.1	93	7.0	10.2	2.7	0.7
Steak, & Red Wine, Veg Mash, HL, Tesco*	1 Pack/500g	360	13.5	72	5.1	6.9	2.7	1.2
Steak, with Colcannon Mash, Tesco*	1 Pack/450g	477	15.7	106	9.5	9.0	3.5	0.9
Tender, Pub Specials, Birds Eye*	1 Pack/450g	243	3.6	54	5.5	6.1	0.8	1.8
BEEF CHASSEUR								
& Potato Mash, BGTY, Sainsbury's*	1 Pack/450g	387	10.8	86	7.8	8.4	2.4	1.3
BEEF CHILLI								
Crispy, Cantonese, Chilled, Sainsbury's*	1 Pack/250g	682	38.7	273	11.4	22.1	15.5	1.9
Crispy, Tesco*	1 Pack/250g	472	17.2	189	10.8	21.0	6.9	0.5
Sweet, Asda*	1 Pack/400g	356	3.6	89	7.8	12.3	0.9	1.9
BEEF DINNER								
Roast, Sainsbury's*	1 Pack/400g	356	6.8	89	6.5	12.0	1.7	1.9
Roast with Trimmings	1 Dinner/840g	1310	63.0	156	6.1	17.7	7.5	2.3
BEEF HOT & SOUR								
Chef's Selection, M & S*	1 Pack/329g	395	17.4	120	9.2	8.4	5.3	1.3
with Garlic Rice, BGTY, Sainsbury's*	1 Pack/400g	428	6.8	107	5.9	17.0	1.7	0.6
with Vegetable Rice, COU, M & S*	1 Pack/400g	360	5.6	90	5.5	14.4	1.4	0.6
BEEF IN								
Ale Gravy, Chunky, Birds Eye*	1 Pack/340g	272	6.8	80	7.4	8.3	2.0	1.5
Ale with Mushrooms, BGTY, Sainsbury's*	1 Pack/251g	193	3.8	77	10.2	5.6	1.5	0.4
Black Bean, with Egg Noodles, M & S*	1 Pack/400g	460	6.0	115	8.6	16.7	1.5	1.8
Black Bean Sauce, M & S*	1 Pack/350g	402	22.4	115	8.9	5.7	6.4	1.1
Black Pepper Sauce & Egg Fried Rice, Tesco*	1 Pack/451g	622	24.8	138	7.0	15.2	5.5	1.2
Black Velvet Porter, Diet Chef Ltd*	1 Meal/300g	201	3.6	67	8.2	6.0	1.2	2.1
Burgundy Red Wine, GFY, Asda*	1 Pack/405g	348	8.1	86	8.0	9.0	2.0	1.1
Chilli Sauce, Strips, Tesco*	1 Pack/166g	290	7.8	175	23.2	9.6	4.7	0.0
Creamy Peppercorn Sauce, Steak, Tesco*	1 Steak/150g	189	8.2	126	16.5	2.6	5.5	0.1
Gravy, Sliced, Sainsbury's*	1 Serving/125g	100	2.2	80	13.5	2.6	1.8	0.2
Madeira & Mushroom Gravy, Sliced, Finest, Tesco*	1 Pack/400g	536	24.8	134	15.2	4.3	6.2	1.0
Oriental Sauce, Lean Cuisine, Findus*	1 Pack/350g	420	8.7	120	4.5	20.0	2.5	1.5
Oyster Sauce, Asda*	1 Serving/100g	82	4.0	82	7.0	4.4	4.0	1.7
Peppercorn Sauce, & Mash Potato, Weight Watchers*	1 Pack/400g	312	8.0	78	5.0	10.0	2.0	1.0

	Measure INFO/WEIGHT	per Measure KCAL	FAT	Nutrition Values per 100g / 100ml KCAL	PROT	CARB	FAT	FIBRE
BEEF SZECHUAN								
Sizzling Hot Spicy, Oriental Express*	1 Pack/400g	380	7.6	95	6.4	13.2	1.9	2.0
BEEF TERIYAKI								
Incredibly Tender, Charlie Bigham's*	½ Pack/300g	477	26.7	159	5.0	10.9	8.9	0.9
with Noodles, BGTY, Sainsbury's*	1 Pack/400g	320	4.0	80	7.7	10.1	1.0	1.0
BEEF WELLINGTON								
Average	1 Serving/200g	530	33.3	265	12.3	16.9	16.6	1.0
BEEF WITH								
Black Bean Sauce, Chilli, Sainsbury's*	1 Pack/300g	336	14.4	112	8.7	8.6	4.8	1.0
Horseradish & Mustard Crust, Joint, Easy, Waitrose*	1/5 Pack/110g	153	5.6	139	20.9	2.5	5.1	0.7
Onion & Gravy, Minced, Princes*	1 Serving/200g	342	24.4	171	9.9	5.5	12.2	0.0
Oyster Sauce, Ooodles of Noodles, Oriental Express*	1 Pack/425g	378	5.5	89	4.9	14.2	1.3	1.5
Peppercorn Sauce, Steak, Just Cook, Sainsbury's*	½ Pack/128g	174	7.3	136	17.7	3.4	5.7	1.2
Red Wine Sauce, Steaks, Just Cook, Sainsbury's*	½ Pack/70g	83	2.3	118	20.0	2.0	3.3	0.2
Vegetables, Tesco*	1 Pot/300g	102	3.0	34	2.9	3.3	1.0	1.1
Vegetables & Gravy, Minced, Birds Eye*	1 Pack/178g	155	6.1	87	9.1	5.1	3.4	0.6
BEER								
Ale, Bottled, Old Speckled Hen*	1 Bottle/330ml	148	0.0	45	0.0	0.0	0.0	0.0
Ale, Ruby, Hobgoblin*	1 Bottle/500ml	255	0.0	51	0.2	5.0	0.0	0.0
Bitter, Canned, Average	*1 Can/440ml*	*141*	*0.0*	*32*	*0.3*	*2.3*	*0.0*	*0.0*
Bitter, Draught, Average	*1 Pint/568ml*	*182*	*0.0*	*32*	*0.3*	*2.3*	*0.0*	*0.0*
Bitter, Keg, Average	*1 Pint/568ml*	*176*	*0.0*	*31*	*0.3*	*2.3*	*0.0*	*0.0*
Bitter, Low Alcohol, Average	*1 Pint/568ml*	*74*	*0.0*	*13*	*0.2*	*2.1*	*0.0*	*0.0*
Brown Ale, Bottled, Average	*1 Bottle/330ml*	*99*	*0.0*	*30*	*0.3*	*3.0*	*0.0*	*0.0*
Guinness, Draught*	*1 Pint/568ml*	*210*	*0.3*	*37*	*0.3*	*3.2*	*0.0*	*0.0*
Guinness, Stout*	*1 Pint/568ml*	*170*	*0.0*	*30*	*0.4*	*3.0*	*0.0*	*0.0*
Guinness Extra Stout, Bottled*	*1 Bottle/500ml*	*215*	*0.0*	*43*	*4.0*	*0.0*	*0.0*	*0.0*
Mild, Draught, Average	*1 Pint/568ml*	*136*	*0.0*	*24*	*0.2*	*1.6*	*0.0*	*0.0*
Non Alcoholic, Cobra*	1 Bottle/330ml	79	0.0	24	0.8	2.0	0.0	0.0
Premium, Lager, San Miguel*	1 Bottle/330ml	148	0.0	45	0.3	3.7	0.0	0.0
Raspberry, Framboise, Lindemans*	1 Glass/355ml	185	0.0	52	0.0	8.8	0.0	0.0
BEETROOT								
Baby, Pickled, Average	*1oz/28g*	*10*	*0.0*	*37*	*1.7*	*7.2*	*0.1*	*1.2*
Cooked, Boiled, Drained, Average	*1 Serving/100g*	*44*	*0.2*	*44*	*1.7*	*10.0*	*0.2*	*2.0*
Crinkle Cut, Drained, Baxters*	1 Slice/10g	3	0.0	26	1.2	5.1	0.1	1.2
Pickled, in Sweet Vinegar, Average	*1oz/28g*	*16*	*0.0*	*57*	*1.2*	*12.8*	*0.1*	*1.5*
Pickled, in Vinegar, Average	*1 Serving/50g*	*19*	*0.0*	*37*	*1.6*	*7.5*	*0.1*	*1.2*
Raw, Average	*1oz/28g*	*9*	*0.0*	*32*	*1.5*	*6.0*	*0.1*	*1.8*
BHAJI								
Aubergine & Potato, Fried in Vegetable Oil, Average	1oz/28g	36	2.5	130	2.0	12.0	8.8	1.7
Cabbage & Pea, Fried in Vegetable Oil, Average	1oz/28g	50	4.1	178	3.3	9.2	14.7	3.4
Cauliflower, Fried in Vegetable Oil, Average	1oz/28g	60	5.7	214	4.0	4.0	20.5	2.0
Mushroom, Fried in Vegetable Oil, Average	1oz/28g	46	4.5	166	1.7	4.4	16.1	1.3
Okra, Bangladeshi, Fried in Butter Ghee, Average	1oz/28g	27	1.8	95	2.5	7.6	6.4	3.2
Onion, Indian Starter Selection, M & S*	1 Bhaji/22g	65	5.1	295	5.7	15.8	23.3	2.8
Onion, Mini, Snack Selection, Sainsbury's*	1 Bhaji/22g	49	3.4	226	4.1	17.4	15.5	3.5
Onion, Waitrose*	1 Bhaji/45g	124	9.4	276	4.7	17.5	20.8	2.5
Onion, with Tomato & Chilli Dip, M & S*	1 Bhaji/54g	111	6.3	205	4.1	21.1	11.7	3.6
Potato, Onion & Mushroom, Fried, Average	1oz/28g	58	4.9	208	2.0	12.0	17.5	1.5
Potato, Spinach & Cauliflower, Fried, Average	1oz/28g	47	4.2	169	2.2	7.1	15.1	1.4
Potato & Onion, Fried in Vegetable Oil, Average	1oz/28g	45	2.8	160	2.1	16.6	10.1	1.6
Spinach, Fried in Vegetable Oil, Average	1oz/28g	23	1.9	83	3.3	2.6	6.8	2.4
Spinach & Potato, Fried in Vegetable Oil, Average	1oz/28g	53	3.9	191	3.7	13.4	14.1	2.3
Turnip & Onion, Fried in Vegetable Oil, Average	1oz/28g	36	3.1	128	1.3	7.1	10.9	2.2

	Measure INFO/WEIGHT	per Measure KCAL	FAT	Nutrition Values per 100g / 100ml KCAL	PROT	CARB	FAT	FIBRE
BHAJI								
Vegetable, Fried in Vegetable Oil, Average	1oz/28g	59	5.2	212	2.1	10.1	18.5	2.4
BHUNA								
Chicken, Indian Takeaway, Tesco*	1 Pack/350g	437	27.6	125	8.3	4.6	7.9	2.2
Chicken, with Naan Bread, Sharwood's*	1 Pack/375g	465	19.1	124	6.8	12.8	5.1	2.8
Chicken Tikka, Tesco*	1 Pack/350g	437	23.4	125	11.3	5.0	6.7	0.9
King Prawn, M & S*	1 Pack /350g	262	13.3	75	6.7	3.3	3.8	1.5
King Prawn, Morrisons*	1 Pack/350g	301	20.6	86	6.5	1.8	5.9	0.5
Lamb, & Rice, Sainsbury's*	1 Pack/500g	619	26.5	124	7.4	11.6	5.3	2.0
BIERWURST								
Average	*1 Slice/10g*	*25*	*2.1*	*252*	*14.4*	*0.9*	*21.2*	*0.0*
BILBERRIES								
Fresh, Raw	*1oz/28g*	*8*	*0.1*	*30*	*0.6*	*6.9*	*0.2*	*1.8*
BILTONG								
Average	*1 Serving/25g*	*64*	*1.0*	*256*	*50.0*	*0.0*	*4.0*	*0.0*
BIRYANI								
Chicken, COU, M & S*	1 Pack/400g	360	8.4	90	6.9	10.8	2.1	1.9
Chicken, Light Choices, Tesco*	1 Serving/450g	495	10.3	110	7.0	15.0	2.3	3.4
Chicken, Weight Watchers*	1 Pack/330g	308	3.7	93	6.2	14.6	1.1	0.6
Chicken Tikka, Northern Indian, Sainsbury's*	1 Pack/450g	697	25.6	155	9.4	16.5	5.7	1.2
Chicken Tikka, with Basmati Rice, Sharwood's*	1 Pack/373g	481	16.0	129	6.3	16.2	4.3	0.9
Lamb, HL, Tesco*	1 Pack/400g	560	17.6	140	5.1	19.0	4.4	3.1
Seafood, M & S*	1 Pack/450g	619	25.7	138	7.1	14.4	5.7	1.7
Vegetable, Perfectly Balanced, Waitrose*	1 Serving/350g	238	0.7	68	2.6	14.0	0.2	2.7
Vegetable, Waitrose*	1 Pack/450g	486	18.0	108	2.8	15.2	4.0	2.2
Vegetable, with Rice, Patak's*	½ Pack/125g	194	1.9	155	3.6	32.9	1.5	1.2
BISCOTTI								
Almond, Kate's Cakes Ltd*	1 Serving/100g	381	15.4	381	8.8	51.7	15.4	3.1
Almond, Pan Ducale*	1 Serving/30g	130	5.0	433	10.0	60.0	16.7	3.3
Chocolate, Heinz*	1 Biscuit/20g	80	1.7	398	8.5	72.0	8.7	5.8
Chocolate Chip, Kate's Cakes Ltd*	1 Serving/100g	372	12.7	372	6.5	57.9	12.7	2.7
BISCUITS								
Abbey Crunch, McVitie's*	1 Biscuit/9g	43	1.6	477	6.0	72.8	17.9	2.5
Ace Milk Chocolate, McVitie's*	1 Biscuit/24g	122	5.9	510	6.1	66.2	24.5	1.6
After Eight, Nestle*	1 Biscuit/5g	26	1.4	525	6.5	62.6	27.7	1.5
All Butter, Tesco*	1 Biscuit/9g	44	2.1	486	6.3	63.5	23.0	1.9
Almond & Chocolate, Biscotti, TTD, Sainsbury's*	1 Biscuit/30g	132	4.8	440	8.4	65.6	16.0	3.1
Almond Butter Thins, Extra Special, Asda*	1 Biscuit/4g	15	0.5	375	5.0	60.0	12.5	2.5
Almond Fingers, Tesco*	1 Finger/46g	180	6.8	391	6.2	58.4	14.7	1.0
Almond Thins, Continental, Tesco*	1 Biscuit/3g	15	0.5	450	6.7	72.8	14.7	3.1
Almond Thins, Sainsbury's*	1 Biscuit/3g	13	0.3	430	7.0	80.3	9.0	1.0
Amaretti, M & S*	1 Biscuit/6g	30	1.1	480	9.6	71.3	17.2	3.8
Animals, Milk Chocolate, Cadbury*	1 Biscuit/19g	94	4.0	493	6.6	69.8	20.9	0.0
Apple & Cinnamon Thins, Finest, Tesco*	1 Biscuit/5g	22	0.8	470	5.9	71.7	17.5	1.5
Apple Strudel, Big Softies, Fox's*	1 Biscuit/23g	80	0.4	348	5.3	77.0	1.6	2.8
Apricot, Low Fat, M & S*	1 Biscuit/23g	79	1.0	343	6.1	69.6	4.4	7.8
Arrowroot, Thin, Crawfords*	1 Biscuit/7g	35	1.1	473	7.4	76.7	15.2	2.2
Berry GI, Diet Chef Ltd*	1 Serving/20g	87	3.2	435	7.0	65.2	16.1	7.2
Blackcurrant with Wheat Bran, Bisca*	1 Biscuit/8g	31	0.9	420	6.0	72.0	12.0	5.5
Blueberry & Vanilla, Oaty, Weight Watchers*	1 Biscuit/22g	101	4.1	460	7.1	65.6	18.8	4.2
BN, Chocolate Flavour, McVitie's*	1 Biscuit/18g	83	3.0	460	6.6	71.0	16.7	2.6
BN, Strawberry Flavour, McVitie's*	1 Biscuit/18g	71	1.2	395	5.6	78.0	6.8	0.0
BN, Vanilla Flavour, McVitie's*	1 Biscuit/18g	85	3.0	470	5.9	74.0	16.6	1.2
Boasters, Hazelnut & Choc Chip, McVitie's*	1 Biscuit/16g	88	5.3	549	7.0	55.5	33.3	2.4

BISCUITS

	Measure INFO/WEIGHT	per Measure KCAL	FAT	Nutrition Values per 100g / 100ml KCAL	PROT	CARB	FAT	FIBRE
Bourbon, Gluten & Wheat Free, Lovemore*	1 Biscuit/15g	70	2.9	469	4.1	67.9	19.1	4.7
Bourbon Creams, Sainsbury's*	1 Biscuit/13g	60	2.4	476	5.7	70.4	19.1	1.7
Brandy Snaps	1oz/28g	122	5.7	437	2.5	64.0	20.3	0.8
Breakfast, Honey & Nuts Belvita, Belvita, Kraft*	1 Biscuit/13g	60	2.2	465	7.9	68.0	17.0	3.3
Breakfast, Yogurt Crunch, Belvita*	2 Biscuits/50g	238	9.1	470	7.7	67.0	18.0	3.9
Butter, Crinkle Crunch, Fox's*	1 Biscuit/11g	50	1.9	460	5.8	69.8	17.5	2.4
Cantuccini, with Almonds, Average	1 Biscotti/30g	130	5.0	433	10.0	60.0	16.7	3.3
Caramels, Milk Chocolate, McVitie's*	1 Serving/17g	81	3.6	478	5.6	65.8	21.4	1.8
Cheddars, Real Cheddar Cheese, Jacob's*	1 Biscuit/4g	20	1.2	526	11.0	48.6	32.1	3.0
Cheese, & Chutney, Delicious, Boots*	1 Pack/133g	290	14.7	217	9.0	19.0	11.0	2.3
Cheese Melts, Carr's*	1 Biscuit/5g	22	1.0	479	11.9	58.2	22.0	2.2
Cheese Sandwich, Ritz*	1 Biscuit/9g	50	2.8	530	9.5	55.0	30.2	2.0
Choc Chip, Paterson's*	1 Biscuit/17g	79	3.6	474	5.6	64.0	21.6	3.1
Chocahoops, Cadbury*	1 Biscuit/13g	65	3.4	510	5.8	62.7	26.4	0.0
Choco Leibniz, Dark Chocolate, Bahlsen*	1 Biscuit/14g	69	3.6	493	6.8	59.0	26.0	5.1
Choco Leibniz, Milk, Bahlsen*	1 Biscuit/10g	51	2.5	515	7.9	63.4	25.5	0.0
Choco Leibniz, Orange Flavour, Bahlsen*	1 Biscuit/14g	70	3.7	504	7.9	58.5	26.4	0.0
Chocolate, Belgian Chocolate, Weight Watchers*	1 Biscuit/18g	87	4.1	481	7.1	61.8	22.8	4.5
Chocolate, Quirks, McVitie's*	1 Biscuit/13g	66	3.6	509	5.0	58.7	27.7	2.5
Chocolate & Coconut, Duchy Originals*	1 Biscuit/13g	68	4.3	543	6.3	52.1	34.4	2.6
Chocolate & Hazelnut, Quirks, McVitie's*	1 Biscuit/13g	66	3.6	511	5.0	58.4	28.0	2.6
Chocolate Chip & Peanut, Trufree*	1 Biscuit/11g	55	2.6	496	4.0	66.0	24.0	2.0
Chocolate Chip GI, Diet Chef Ltd*	1 Pack/20g	90	3.6	450	7.4	64.4	17.9	6.4
Chocolate Fingers, Caramel, Cadbury*	1 Finger/8g	39	1.9	490	5.8	63.2	23.8	0.0
Chocolate Fingers, Milk, Cadbury*	1 Biscuit/6g	31	1.6	515	6.8	60.8	27.1	1.7
Chocolate Fingers, Milk, Extra Crunchy, Cadbury*	1 Biscuit/5g	25	1.2	505	6.6	66.2	23.6	0.0
Chocolate Fingers, Plain, Cadbury*	1 Biscuit/6g	30	1.6	508	6.2	60.6	26.8	0.0
Chocolate Florentine, M & S*	1 Serving/39g	195	9.7	500	7.4	64.5	24.9	1.7
Chocolate Ginger, Thorntons*	1 Biscuit/19g	96	5.3	512	5.9	58.2	28.4	0.0
Chocolate Kimberley, Jacob's*	1 Biscuit/20g	86	3.4	428	3.9	64.4	17.2	1.1
Chocolate Mini Shorties, McVitie's*	1 Pack/25g	131	7.1	524	6.0	61.2	28.3	2.0
Chocolate Nibbles, High Lights, Cadbury*	1 Pack/16g	75	2.6	465	6.2	73.4	16.1	1.7
Chocolate Toffee, Crunch, Moments, McVitie's*	1 Biscuit/17g	89	4.7	520	5.6	62.3	27.6	1.7
Chocolate Viennese, Fox's*	1 Biscuit/16g	85	4.9	530	6.7	56.6	30.7	1.7
Chocolinis, Milk Chocolate, Go Ahead, McVitie's*	1 Biscuit/12g	56	1.7	466	7.7	77.2	14.0	2.0
Chocolinis, Plain Chocolate, McVitie's*	1 Biscuit/12g	56	1.8	468	6.9	77.0	14.7	2.6
Christmas Shapes, Assorted, Sainsbury's*	1 Biscuit/15g	77	4.3	525	5.2	59.0	29.8	1.7
Classic, Creams, Fox's*	1 Biscuit/14g	72	3.6	516	4.4	65.2	25.8	1.7
Classic, Milk Chocolate, Fox's*	1 Biscuit/13g	67	3.1	517	6.1	64.9	24.0	1.6
Coconut Crinkle, Sainsbury's*	1 Biscuit/11g	54	2.8	500	6.4	59.6	26.2	3.7
Coconut Ring, Asda*	1 Biscuit/8g	37	1.7	486	6.0	66.0	22.0	2.6
Cranberry, Crispy Slices, Light Choices, Tesco*	1 Biscuit/14g	54	0.6	370	6.0	76.0	3.9	5.5
Cranberry & Pumpkin Seed, BGTY, Sainsbury's*	1 Biscuit/17g	68	2.8	410	7.2	56.6	17.1	13.9
Cranberry & Sunflower Seed, Oaty, Weight Watchers*	1 Biscuit/22g	103	4.6	469	7.5	62.4	21.0	5.3
Crinkles, Classics, Milk Chocolate, Fox's*	1 Biscuit/13g	67	3.1	487	5.7	65.2	22.7	2.7
Crispy Fruit Slice, Apple, Sultana, Go Ahead, McVitie's*	1 Slice/13g	49	0.8	379	5.2	73.7	6.4	3.0
Crispy Fruit Slices, Forest Fruit, Go Ahead, McVitie's*	1 Biscuit/14g	56	0.9	395	5.5	75.4	6.4	2.4
Crispy Slices, Raspberry, Go Ahead, McVitie's*	1 Slice/14g	54	1.0	389	5.9	75.9	6.9	3.0
Crispy Slices, Red Cherry, Go Ahead, McVitie's*	1 Slice/15g	58	1.0	390	6.0	76.0	6.9	2.9
Crunchy Oats, Breakfast, Belvita, Nabisco*	1 Biscuit/13g	59	2.1	455	8.0	67.0	16.0	5.5
Custard Creams, 25% Less Fat, Sainsbury's*	1 Biscuit/13g	59	2.2	469	5.8	72.7	17.3	1.3
Custard Creams, Crawfords*	1 Biscuit/11g	57	2.7	517	5.9	69.2	24.1	1.5
Custard Creams, Jacob's*	1 Biscuit/16g	77	3.3	481	5.3	68.0	20.9	1.6

INFO/WEIGHT	Measure	per Measure KCAL	FAT	Nutrition Values per 100g / 100ml KCAL	PROT	CARB	FAT	FIBRE

BISCUITS

	Measure INFO/WEIGHT	per Measure KCAL	FAT	KCAL	PROT	CARB	FAT	FIBRE
Custard Creams, Trufree*	1 Biscuit/12g	60	2.8	504	8.7	65.0	23.0	1.0
Digestive, 25% Less Fat, Asda*	1 Biscuit/16g	73	2.6	455	7.3	69.8	16.3	2.6
Digestive, Caramels, Milk Chocolate, McVitie's*	1 Biscuit/17g	81	3.7	478	5.6	65.1	21.7	2.3
Digestive, Caramels, Plain Chocolate, McVitie's*	1 Biscuit/17g	82	3.8	481	5.7	65.5	22.1	2.1
Digestive, Chocolate	1 Biscuit/ 17g	84	4.1	493	6.8	66.5	24.1	2.2
Digestive, Dark Chocolate, McVitie's*	1 Biscuit/17g	82	4.0	487	6.0	61.6	24.0	4.0
Digestive, Gluten & Wheat Free, Lovemore*	1 Biscuit/15g	55	2.7	378	3.4	49.3	18.5	18.4
Digestive, High Fibre, Reduced Sugar, M & S*	1 Biscuit/13g	60	2.8	460	6.5	59.3	21.7	9.4
Digestive, Lemon & Ginger, McVitie's*	1 Biscuit/15g	72	3.1	480	6.7	66.7	20.7	2.7
Digestive, Milk Chocolate, Homewheat, McVitie's*	1 Biscuit/17g	83	4.1	486	6.0	61.5	24.0	4.0
Digestive, Milk Chocolate, M & S*	1 Biscuit/17g	85	4.4	505	6.1	62.2	26.0	2.6
Digestive, Milk Chocolate Mint, McVitie's*	1 Biscuit/17g	81	3.9	487	6.7	62.6	23.4	2.9
Digestive, Oat, Weight Watchers*	1 Biscuit/11g	50	2.1	457	6.0	66.3	18.6	6.9
Digestive, Plain	1 Biscuit/14g	66	2.9	471	6.3	68.6	20.9	2.2
Fig Roll, Tesco*	1 Biscuit/18g	70	1.6	375	4.0	69.3	8.8	3.1
for Cheese, Bran Cracker, Christmas, Tesco*	1oz/28g	127	5.1	454	9.7	62.8	18.2	3.2
for Cheese, Chive Cracker, Christmas, Tesco*	1oz/28g	125	4.5	448	9.3	66.6	16.0	2.4
for Cheese, Cornish Wafer, Christmas, Tesco*	1oz/28g	148	8.7	530	8.0	56.8	31.2	2.4
for Cheese, Cream Cracker, Christmas, Tesco*	1oz/28g	118	3.6	421	9.9	71.9	12.7	5.1
for Cheese, Digestive, Hovis, Christmas, Tesco*	1oz/28g	127	5.1	453	4.2	74.6	18.2	7.0
for Cheese, Poppy Snack, Christmas, Tesco*	1oz/28g	129	5.1	461	10.0	64.4	18.2	3.1
for Cheese, Sesame Carlton, Christmas, Tesco*	1oz/28g	133	6.0	476	9.1	61.5	21.5	2.7
for Cheese, Whole Grain, Christmas, Tesco*	1oz/28g	128	5.2	458	9.0	63.9	18.5	4.1
Fruit, All Butter, Sainsbury's*	1 Biscuit/9g	45	2.0	477	5.6	66.0	21.2	1.9
Fruit, Oat, GI, Diet Chef Ltd*	1 Serving/20g	85	2.9	425	7.8	65.3	14.7	7.6
Fruit & Fibre, Breakfast, Belvita, Nabisco*	1 Biscuit/13g	56	2.1	430	7.5	64.0	16.0	7.8
Fruit Bake, Organic, Tesco*	1 Biscuit/12g	53	2.1	453	7.5	65.1	18.1	5.6
Fruit Jambos, Rowntree's*	1 Biscuit/11g	47	1.4	435	4.7	73.6	13.4	1.7
Fruit Shortcake, McVitie's*	1 Biscuit/8g	37	1.6	464	5.7	65.1	20.1	2.7
Fruit Shrewsbury, Mini Pack, Paterson's*	1 Biscuit/17g	81	3.8	483	4.9	64.9	22.7	1.9
Fruity Oat, Organic, Dove's Farm*	1 Biscuit/12g	53	2.1	453	7.5	65.1	18.1	5.6
Galettes, Bonne Maman*	1 Serving/90g	460	22.5	511	6.0	65.7	25.0	0.0
Garibaldi, Waitrose*	1oz/28g	109	3.1	389	5.7	67.1	10.9	1.3
Ginger, Traditional, Fox's*	1 Biscuit/8g	33	1.0	404	4.4	70.1	11.7	1.4
Ginger Crinkle Crunch, Fox's*	1 Biscuit/12g	50	1.4	435	4.7	75.3	12.5	1.6
Ginger Crunch Creams, Fox's*	1 Biscuit/14g	73	3.7	518	4.6	64.8	26.7	0.0
Ginger Snap, Fox's*	1 Biscuit/8g	35	1.0	443	4.6	77.1	12.8	1.5
Ginger Thins, Anna's*	1 Biscuit/2g	10	0.4	480	6.0	67.0	20.0	0.4
Gingerbread Man, Gluten & Wheat Free, Lovemore*	1 Biscuit/37g	179	7.6	485	4.7	70.1	20.5	1.7
Gingernut	1 Biscuit/11g	50	1.7	456	5.6	79.1	15.2	1.4
Golden Crunch Creams, Fox's*	1 Biscuit/15g	75	3.8	515	4.7	64.8	26.3	1.2
Golden Shortie, Jacob's*	1 Biscuit/11g	54	2.6	492	6.0	64.9	23.2	0.0
Golden Syrup, McVitie's*	1 Biscuit/12g	63	3.0	508	5.1	67.3	24.2	2.2
Happy Faces, Jacob's*	1 Biscuit/16g	78	3.6	485	4.8	66.1	22.3	1.6
Hob Nobs, Chocolate Creams, McVitie's*	1 Biscuit/12g	60	3.1	503	6.7	60.3	26.1	4.0
Hob Nobs, Light, 25% Reduced Fat, McVitie's*	1 Biscuit/14g	62	2.3	435	8.1	64.6	16.1	6.2
Hob Nobs, McVitie's*	1 Biscuit/14g	67	3.1	466	7.1	60.8	21.7	5.5
Hob Nobs, Milk Chocolate, McVitie's*	1 Biscuit/19g	92	4.5	479	6.8	60.7	23.3	4.5
Hob Nobs, Milk Chocolate, Mini, McVitie's*	1 Pack/25g	121	5.9	483	6.6	61.3	23.5	4.4
Hob Nobs, Plain Chocolate, McVitie's*	1 Biscuit/16g	81	3.9	498	6.7	63.3	24.3	4.2
Hob Nobs, Vanilla Creams, McVitie's*	1 Biscuit/12g	60	3.0	501	6.1	62.3	25.2	3.6
Honeycomb Nibbles, High Lights, Cadbury*	1 Bag/16g	75	2.6	465	6.2	73.4	16.2	1.8
Iced Gems, Jacob's*	1 Portion/30g	116	0.9	388	5.0	85.5	2.9	1.5

BISCUITS

	Measure INFO/WEIGHT	per Measure KCAL	FAT	Nutrition Values per 100g / 100ml KCAL	PROT	CARB	FAT	FIBRE
Jaffa Cakes, Blackcurrant, McVitie's*	1 Cake/12g	45	1.0	371	4.8	69.7	8.1	2.3
Jaffa Cakes, Dark Chocolate, M & S*	1 Cake/11g	45	1.5	395	3.7	64.9	13.2	2.8
Jaffa Cakes, Free From, Asda*	1 Cake/12g	42	0.9	340	5.8	62.6	7.4	8.0
Jaffa Cakes, Lemon & Lime, McVitie's*	1 Cake/12g	45	1.0	370	4.7	69.5	8.1	2.1
Jaffa Cakes, Lunch Box, McVitie's*	1 Cake/7g	26	0.6	395	4.2	74.3	9.0	1.4
Jaffa Cakes, McVitie's*	1 Cake/12g	45	1.0	374	4.8	70.6	8.0	2.1
Jam Creams, Jacob's*	1 Biscuit/15g	75	3.4	486	5.0	67.4	21.8	1.6
Jam Rings, Crawfords*	1 Biscuit/12g	56	2.1	470	5.5	73.0	17.2	1.9
Jammie Dodgers, Minis. Lunchbox, Burton's*	1 Pack/20g	90	2.9	452	5.5	72.7	14.7	2.5
Jammie Dodgers, Original, Burton's*	1 Biscuit/19g	83	3.0	437	5.1	69.5	15.9	1.9
Jestives, Milk Chocolate, Cadbury*	1 Biscuit/17g	86	4.2	506	6.4	64.4	24.8	0.0
Lebkuchen, Sainsbury's*	1 Biscuit/10g	39	0.8	400	5.7	76.1	8.0	1.3
Lemon Butter, Thins, Sainsbury's*	1 Biscuit/13g	65	3.5	515	5.3	60.7	27.9	2.2
Lemon Curd Sandwich, Fox's*	1 Biscuit/14g	69	3.3	494	4.7	66.2	23.4	1.3
Lemon Puff, Jacob's*	1 Biscuit/13g	69	4.1	533	4.3	58.8	31.2	2.8
Lincoln, McVitie's*	1 Biscuit/8g	41	1.9	514	6.3	69.0	23.6	2.0
Malted Milk, Milk Chocolate, Asda*	1 Biscuit/11g	56	2.7	509	7.0	64.0	25.0	1.7
Malted Milk, Sainsbury's*	1 Biscuit/8g	40	1.8	488	7.1	65.5	21.9	2.0
Maple Leaf, M & S*	1 Biscuit/13g	50	1.9	395	5.1	59.8	14.8	2.0
Marie, Crawfords*	1 Biscuit/7g	33	1.1	475	7.5	76.3	15.5	2.3
Melts, Carr's*	1 Biscuit/4g	20	0.9	468	11.0	58.3	21.2	4.9
Mikado, Jacob's*	1 Biscuit/13g	53	1.6	397	4.2	67.7	12.1	2.5
Milk & Cereals, Breakfast, Belvita, Nabisco*	1 Biscuit/13g	58	1.9	448	8.7	69.0	15.0	3.6
Mini Assortment, M & S*	1 Biscuit/3g	12	0.6	480	6.1	63.9	22.5	2.8
Mint, Viscount*	1 Biscuit/13g	73	3.8	552	5.1	60.6	28.8	1.3
Morning Coffee, Asda*	1 Biscuit/5g	22	0.7	455	8.0	72.0	15.0	2.4
Nice, Cream, Tesco*	1 Serving/10g	50	2.4	503	5.3	66.2	24.1	1.9
Nice, Fox's*	1 Biscuit/9g	39	1.7	450	6.3	62.4	19.4	5.0
Nice, Jacob's*	1 Biscuit/7g	33	1.3	471	6.1	68.5	19.2	1.8
Oat, Fruit & Spice, Nairn's*	1 Biscuit/10g	43	1.5	425	7.8	65.3	14.7	7.6
Oat, Mixed Berries, Nairn's*	1 Biscuit/10g	43	1.5	430	7.7	67.0	14.6	5.9
Oat, Santiveri*	1 Biscuit/5g	23	0.9	428	10.0	58.8	17.0	7.0
Oat, Stem Ginger, Nairn's*	1 Biscuit/10g	43	1.5	434	8.8	65.6	15.2	6.1
Oat & Wholemeal, Crawfords*	1 Biscuit/14g	67	3.0	482	7.7	64.2	21.6	4.8
Oat Bites, Caramelised Onion, Diet Chef Ltd*	1 Pack/23g	99	3.9	430	7.5	64.2	16.8	6.0
Oat Bites, Cheese, Diet Chef Ltd*	1 Pack/23g	99	3.6	430	15.0	57.4	15.8	4.9
Oat Bites, Chilli, Diet Chef Ltd*	1 Serving/23g	128	3.1	556	8.1	68.4	13.3	7.2
Oat Crunch, M & S*	1 Biscuit/14g	65	2.7	450	7.8	62.0	18.7	6.1
Oat Crunch, Weight Watchers*	1 Biscuit/12g	52	2.1	448	7.4	65.2	17.8	6.1
Oatmeal Crunch, Jacob's*	1 Biscuit/8g	37	1.5	458	6.8	65.9	18.6	3.6
Oaty Thins, Rude Health*	1 Thin/6g	23	0.3	380	11.5	68.5	4.7	8.7
Parmesan Cheese, Sainsbury's*	1 Biscuit/3g	18	1.0	553	14.7	56.4	29.9	1.8
Party Rings, Iced, Fox's*	1 Biscuit/6g	29	0.9	459	5.1	75.8	15.0	0.0
Peanut Butter, American Style, Sainsbury's*	1 Biscuit/13g	63	2.9	504	5.2	68.7	23.1	2.2
Redcurrant Puffs, Eat Well, M & S*	1 Biscuit/7g	32	1.4	470	5.6	67.7	19.8	2.0
Rich Shorties, Asda*	1 Biscuit/10g	50	2.3	486	6.0	66.0	22.0	2.0
Rich Tea, Classic, McVitie's*	1 Biscuit/8g	38	1.3	453	7.1	71.2	15.5	2.9
Rich Tea, Essential, Waitrose*	1 Biscuit/8g	36	1.2	452	7.1	71.1	15.2	2.9
Rich Tea, Light, McVitie's*	1 Biscuit/8g	36	0.9	431	7.5	75.0	11.3	3.1
Rich Tea, Low Fat, M & S*	1 Biscuit/9g	40	1.0	435	8.3	76.7	10.5	2.4
Rich Tea, Milk Chocolate Covered, Cadbury*	1 Biscuit/12g	60	2.6	490	6.6	67.6	21.4	0.0
Rich Tea, Plain Chocolate, Sainsbury's*	1 Biscuit/13g	65	3.0	497	6.6	66.0	23.0	2.6
Rich Tea Creams, Fox's*	1 Biscuit/11g	52	2.3	456	5.3	62.7	20.4	1.4

	Measure INFO/WEIGHT	per Measure KCAL	FAT	Nutrition Values per 100g / 100ml KCAL	PROT	CARB	FAT	FIBRE
BISCUITS								
Rich Tea Finger, Tesco*	1 Finger/5g	23	0.7	451	7.4	72.9	14.4	2.3
Riva Milk, McVitie's*	1 Biscuit/25g	136	7.9	540	6.4	57.7	31.5	1.6
Rocky, Chocolate, Fox's*	1 Biscuit/21g	106	5.4	505	5.7	62.4	25.7	2.4
Rocky, Chocolate & Caramel, Fox's*	1 Biscuit/21g	107	4.1	507	6.9	60.3	19.3	15.5
Rocky, Funki Fudge, Fox's*	1 Biscuit/24g	125	6.6	520	6.9	60.3	27.7	1.1
Rocky Rounds, Caramel, Fox's*	1 Biscuit/15g	72	3.4	480	6.2	62.3	22.9	1.1
Rolo, Nestle*	1 Biscuit/22g	110	5.6	498	5.4	62.0	25.4	0.6
Rosemary & Raisin, M & S*	1 Biscuit/7g	35	1.7	490	5.1	62.5	24.1	1.8
Rosemary & Thyme, Savoury, Weight Watchers*	1 Biscuit/8g	33	1.5	419	8.1	55.0	18.7	13.1
Savoury, Gluten, Wheat & Dairy Free, Sainsbury's*	1 Biscuit/17g	77	2.9	467	11.7	65.1	17.7	2.4
Savoury, Organic, M & S*	1 Biscuit/7g	28	1.0	395	7.0	58.4	14.6	8.7
Savoury Oat, with Thyme, Rick Stein*	1 Biscuit/10g	46	2.1	460	9.8	66.9	21.4	10.4
Savoury Seed, Organic, The Village Bakery*	1 Biscuit/14g	63	3.8	438	12.6	42.5	26.5	7.0
Shortbread Fingers, Kate's Cakes Ltd*	2 Fingers/30g	141	8.0	471	4.6	52.8	26.8	1.6
Shortcake, Asda*	1 Biscuit/14g	73	3.6	518	5.0	66.0	26.0	2.0
Shortcake, Caramel, Mr Kipling*	1 Biscuit/36g	182	10.4	506	4.2	57.6	28.8	1.3
Shortcake, Caramel, Squares, M & S*	1 Square/40g	190	9.6	475	5.5	59.7	23.9	1.0
Shortcake, Crawfords*	1 Biscuit/10g	53	2.5	518	6.4	68.1	24.4	2.0
Shortcake, Dairy Milk Chocolate, Cadbury*	1 Bar/49g	252	13.5	515	7.5	59.2	27.5	0.0
Shortcake, Dutch, M & S*	1 Biscuit/17g	90	5.2	530	5.7	58.2	30.6	0.9
Shortcake, Fruit Biscuits, Crawfords*	1 Biscuit/8g	34	1.5	419	5.4	55.9	19.3	2.4
Shortcake, Jacob's*	1 Biscuit/10g	48	2.2	485	6.7	65.6	21.8	2.0
Shortcake, Organic, Waitrose*	1 Biscuit/13g	64	3.2	495	5.8	63.0	24.4	1.8
Shortcake, Snack, Cadbury*	1 Biscuit/7g	35	1.8	515	7.2	61.0	26.7	1.8
Shortcake, with Real Milk Chocolate, Cadbury*	1 Biscuit/15g	75	3.5	500	6.3	65.8	23.5	0.0
Shortcake Ring, Creations, Fox's*	1 Biscuit/20g	105	5.6	515	7.8	59.1	27.4	1.0
Shorties, Cadbury*	1 Biscuit/15g	77	3.6	511	6.5	67.3	24.0	0.0
Shorties, Sainsbury's*	1 Biscuit/10g	50	2.2	500	6.4	69.8	21.8	2.0
Taxi, McVitie's*	1 Biscuit/27g	134	6.9	504	4.2	63.3	26.0	0.7
Twix, Caramel Slice, McVitie's*	1 Slice/29g	142	7.8	491	4.5	57.3	26.8	1.4
Vanilla, Ser*	1 Biscuit/4g	14	0.3	408	8.5	77.0	8.2	3.0
Viennese, Bronte*	1 Biscuit/25g	106	6.2	424	4.4	45.6	24.8	0.0
Viennese, Jaffa, M & S*	1 Biscuit/17g	80	3.7	465	5.9	61.1	21.7	0.9
Viennese, Mini Pack, Paterson's*	1 Biscuit/20g	106	6.2	527	5.4	67.1	30.8	1.6
Viennese, Sandwich, Chocolate, M & S*	1 Biscuit/15g	80	4.6	535	7.2	58.0	30.6	1.7
Viennese Creams, Raspberry, M & S*	1 Biscuit/17g	90	4.9	520	4.6	60.4	28.6	1.3
Viennese Creams, Strawberry, M & S*	1 Biscuit/17g	80	3.7	485	6.4	63.0	22.2	1.7
Viennese Finger, Mr Kipling*	1 Finger/32g	167	10.2	523	4.3	54.9	31.8	0.0
Viennese Whirl, Fox's*	1 Biscuit/25g	129	6.9	518	6.7	60.1	27.8	0.0
Water, Average	1oz/28g	123	3.5	440	10.8	75.8	12.5	3.1
Yorkie, Nestle*	1 Biscuit/25g	127	6.7	510	6.7	60.4	26.8	1.3
BISON								
Raw	**1oz/28g**	**31**	**0.5**	**109**	**21.6**	**0.0**	**1.8**	**0.0**
BITTER LEMON								
Fever-Tree*	1 Glass/200ml	77	0.0	38	0.0	9.2	0.0	0.0
Low Calorie, Tesco*	1 Glass/200ml	6	0.2	3	0.1	0.3	0.1	0.1
Sainsbury's*	1 Glass/250ml	45	0.2	18	0.1	4.4	0.1	0.1
Schweppes*	1 Glass/250ml	85	0.0	34	0.0	8.2	0.0	0.0
BLACK PUDDING								
Average, Uncooked	**1 Serving/40g**	**101**	**6.0**	**252**	**10.2**	**19.0**	**14.9**	**0.6**
Slices, Grilled, Asda*	1 Slice/36g	150	10.7	417	13.3	23.2	29.7	1.9
VLH Kitchens*	1 Serving/40g	105	6.2	262	11.0	20.3	15.6	0.4

	Measure INFO/WEIGHT	per Measure KCAL	FAT	Nutrition Values per 100g / 100ml KCAL	PROT	CARB	FAT	FIBRE
BLACKBERRIES								
Fresh, Raw, Average	*1oz/28g*	*8*	*0.1*	*29*	*0.8*	*6.0*	*0.3*	*1.5*
in Fruit Juice, Average	*½ Can/145g*	*52*	*0.3*	*36*	*0.6*	*7.9*	*0.2*	*1.3*
BLACKCURRANTS								
Fresh, Raw	*1oz/28g*	*8*	*0.0*	*28*	*0.9*	*6.6*	*0.0*	*3.6*
in Fruit Juice, Average	*1 Serving/30g*	*11*	*0.0*	*37*	*0.6*	*8.6*	*0.1*	*2.4*
Stewed with Sugar	*1oz/28g*	*16*	*0.0*	*58*	*0.7*	*15.0*	*0.0*	*2.8*
Stewed without Sugar	*1oz/28g*	*7*	*0.0*	*24*	*0.8*	*5.6*	*0.0*	*3.1*
BLINIS								
Cocktail, M & S*	½ Pack/81g	154	1.9	190	6.3	35.9	2.3	2.0
Sausage, Cocktail, Waitrose*	1 Blini/16g	30	0.4	190	6.3	35.9	2.3	2.0
Smoked Salmon, M & S*	1oz/28g	67	3.6	240	11.9	18.9	13.0	1.8
BLUEBERRIES								
Dried, Whitworths*	1 Pack/75g	226	0.1	301	0.9	74.2	0.1	11.4
Dried & Sweetened, Sainsbury's*	1oz/28g	77	0.2	275	1.7	65.7	0.6	11.7
Fresh, Raw, Average	*30 Berries/50g*	*27*	*0.2*	*53*	*0.8*	*12.6*	*0.3*	*2.1*
BOAR								
Wild, Raw, Average	*1 Serving/200g*	*244*	*6.7*	*122*	*21.5*	*0.0*	*3.3*	*0.0*
BOILED SWEETS								
Average	1oz/28g	92	0.0	327	0.0	87.1	0.0	0.0
BOK CHOY								
Tesco*	1 Serving/100g	11	0.2	11	1.0	1.4	0.2	1.2
BOLOGNESE								
Al Forno, Weight Watchers*	1 Pack/354g	312	6.7	88	6.6	10.3	1.9	1.8
Beef, 2 Minute Meals, Sainsbury's*	1 Pack/200g	144	7.2	72	4.2	5.6	3.6	1.8
Beef, Asda*	1 Pack/392g	412	19.6	105	8.0	7.0	5.0	0.0
Beef, Diet Chef Ltd*	1 Serving/300g	246	6.9	82	7.7	7.6	2.3	3.4
Extra Meaty, M & S*	1oz/28g	25	0.8	90	10.4	5.5	2.7	0.0
Fusilli, Ready Meals, M & S*	1oz/28g	38	1.7	135	7.0	13.1	6.2	1.0
Meatless, Granose*	1 Pack/400g	400	16.0	100	8.0	8.0	4.0	0.0
Pasta,Solo Slim, Rosemary Conley*	1 Pack/300g	333	15.0	111	7.3	9.2	5.0	2.5
Penne, Heinz*	1 Pack/300g	213	2.7	71	3.8	11.8	0.9	0.6
Shells, Italiana, Weight Watchers*	1 Can/395g	280	5.1	71	5.2	9.6	1.3	0.7
Tagliatelle, Weight Watchers*	1 Serving/300g	300	5.4	100	5.5	15.4	1.8	0.1
Vegetarian, M & S*	1 Pack/360g	360	12.6	100	4.5	12.5	3.5	2.1
Vegetarian, Vegelicious, Tesco*	1 Pack/400g	420	10.8	105	4.6	14.9	2.7	2.0
BOMBAY MIX								
Average	1oz/28g	141	9.2	503	18.8	35.1	32.9	6.2
BON BONS								
Bassett's*	1 Sweet/7g	28	0.5	417	1.1	85.4	7.5	0.0
Fruit, Bassett's*	1 Sweet/7g	25	0.0	380	0.1	94.2	0.0	0.0
Lemon, Bassett's*	1 Sweet/7g	30	0.7	425	0.0	83.7	9.8	0.0
BOOST								
Standard Bar, Cadbury*	1 Bar/61g	305	17.0	510	5.8	57.0	28.5	0.9
Treat Size, Cadbury*	1 Bar/24g	130	7.4	535	5.3	59.6	30.5	0.0
with Glucose, Cadbury*	1 Bar/61g	315	17.8	521	5.6	58.0	29.4	4.0
with Glucose & Guarana, Cadbury*	1 Bar/61g	314	18.0	515	5.5	56.7	29.5	0.0
BOUILLON								
Beef, Benedicta*	1 fl oz/30ml	22	0.1	73	7.5	9.5	0.5	0.0
Chicken, Benedicta*	1 fl oz/30ml	22	0.9	75	4.0	8.0	3.0	5.6
Powder, Miso, Marigold*	1 Tsp/5g	12	0.5	248	7.0	34.0	9.3	1.4
Powder, Swiss Vegetable, Green Tub, Marigold*	1 Tsp/5g	12	0.4	243	10.5	29.4	8.1	0.7
Vegetable, Benedicta*	1 fl oz/30ml	30	0.1	101	7.5	17.0	0.3	0.0

INFO/WEIGHT	Measure		per Measure		Nutrition Values per 100g / 100ml				
			KCAL	FAT	KCAL	PROT	CARB	FAT	FIBRE
BOUNTY									
Calapuno, Mars*	1 Pack/175g		919	54.9	525	6.3	54.3	31.4	0.0
Dark, Mars*	1 Funsize/29g		142	8.0	488	3.7	55.7	27.6	0.0
Milk, Mars*	1 Funsize/29g		137	7.4	471	3.7	56.4	25.6	0.0
BOURNVITA									
Powder, Made Up with Semi-Skimmed Milk	1 Mug/227ml		132	3.6	58	3.5	7.8	1.6	0.0
Powder, Made Up with Whole Milk	1 Mug/227ml		173	8.6	76	3.4	7.6	3.8	0.0
BOVRIL									
Beef Extract, Drink, Made Up with Water, Bovril*	1 Serving/12g		22	0.1	184	38.9	4.6	1.2	0.0
Chicken Savoury Drink, Bovril*	1 Serving/13g		16	0.2	129	9.7	19.4	1.4	2.1
BRANDY									
37.5% Volume, Average	*1 Shot/35ml*		*72*	*0.0*	*207*	*0.0*	*0.0*	*0.0*	*0.0*
40% Volume, Average	*1 Shot/35ml*		*78*	*0.0*	*222*	*0.0*	*0.0*	*0.0*	*0.0*
Cherry, Average	*1 Shot/35ml*		*89*	*0.0*	*255*	*0.0*	*32.6*	*0.0*	*0.0*
BRAZIL NUTS									
Average	*6 Whole/20g*		*137*	*13.7*	*687*	*15.5*	*2.9*	*68.3*	*4.9*
Milk Chocolate, Tesco*	1 Nut/8g		47	3.5	585	9.9	38.0	43.7	1.9
BREAD									
50/50, Wholemeal & White, Medium Sliced, Kingsmill*	1 Slice/40g		90	0.9	225	9.9	41.2	2.3	4.9
Bagel, 4 Everything, Finest, Tesco*	1 Bagel/100g		268	1.8	268	11.1	51.9	1.8	2.5
Bagel, Baked with Marmite, Marmite*	1 Bagel/85g		240	2.6	282	12.9	49.3	3.1	2.8
Bagel, Blueberry, Sara Lee*	1 Bagel/104g		290	1.5	279	9.6	58.6	1.4	1.9
Bagel, Caramelised Onion & Poppyseed, Waitrose*	1 Bagel/86g		222	2.1	258	9.7	49.2	2.5	2.4
Bagel, Cinnamon & Raisin, New York Bagel Co*	1 Bagel/90g		231	1.0	257	10.1	49.9	1.1	3.6
Bagel, Fruit & Spice, Sainsbury's*	1 Bagel/85g		234	1.8	275	9.7	54.3	2.1	3.8
Bagel, Granary, Bagel Factory*	1 Bagel/100g		288	2.1	288	11.9	57.4	2.1	4.5
Bagel, High Bran & Seed, The Food Doctor*	1 Bagel/85g		239	6.6	281	10.7	41.3	7.8	6.3
Bagel, Multigrain, Sainsbury's*	1 Bagel/113g		293	3.5	259	10.0	49.6	3.1	2.0
Bagel, Onion, New York Bagel Co*	1 Bagel/85g		222	1.6	261	10.6	50.3	1.9	3.1
Bagel, Onion & Poppy Seed, Tesco*	1 Bagel/85g		217	2.6	255	10.0	46.7	3.1	3.6
Bagel, Original, Organic, New York Bagel Co*	1 Bagel/85g		220	1.2	259	9.3	52.2	1.4	4.1
Bagel, Plain, Average	*1 Bagel/78g*		*215*	*1.2*	*276*	*10.7*	*53.6*	*1.5*	*0.0*
Bagel, Poppy Seed, New York Bagel Co*	1 Bagel/85g		233	2.4	274	11.4	50.8	2.8	3.2
Bagel, Rye, Bagel Factory*	1 Bagel/85g		279	1.3	329	14.5	64.3	1.5	6.2
Bagel, Sesame, M & S*	1 Bagel/87g		240	2.8	275	10.2	51.2	3.2	2.1
Bagel, Sesame, New York Bagel Co*	1 Bagel/85g		226	2.6	266	10.3	49.2	3.1	4.0
Bagel, White, Asda*	1 Bagel/86g		227	2.7	264	10.0	49.0	3.1	0.0
Bagel, White, Original, Weight Watchers*	1 Bagel/67g		158	0.5	236	9.5	42.4	0.8	10.7
Bagel, Wholemeal, Multiseed, M & S*	1 Bagel/84g		215	5.6	255	13.1	35.4	6.6	8.3
Bagel, Wholemeal, New York Bagel Co*	1 Bagel/90g		223	2.1	248	11.4	41.5	2.3	7.5
Baguette, Cheese, & Onion, Asda*	¼ Loaf/42g		154	7.4	366	12.0	39.8	17.6	1.3
Baguette, Crusty Brown, M & S*	½ Loaf/71g		160	1.1	225	9.8	42.7	1.6	6.3
Baguette, Garlic, Reduced Fat, Asda*	¼ Loaf/43g		107	2.7	249	8.1	39.9	6.3	2.7
Baps, Brown, Large, Asda*	1 Bap/58g		140	0.9	242	10.0	47.0	1.6	0.0
Baps, Brown, Malted Grain, Large, Tesco*	1 Bap/93g		228	3.1	245	9.9	42.7	3.3	5.3
Baps, Cheese Top, Sainsbury's*	1 Bap/75g		218	6.4	291	12.1	41.6	8.5	2.0
Baps, Floured, M & S*	1 Bap/60g		168	3.7	280	11.5	46.8	6.2	2.0
Baps, Giant Malted, Sainsbury's*	1 Bap/109g		282	5.2	260	8.6	45.7	4.8	5.7
Baps, Malted, Large, Co-Op*	1 Bap/85g		208	2.6	245	10.2	44.3	3.1	5.0
Baps, White, Floured, Waitrose*	1 Bap/60g		147	1.2	244	8.0	48.6	2.0	1.1
Baps, White, Giant, Waitrose*	1 Bap/104g		260	3.7	250	9.5	45.0	3.6	4.8
Baps, White, Soft, Floured, M & S*	1 Bap/63g		176	3.9	280	11.5	46.8	6.2	2.0
Baps, White, Warburton's*	1 Bap/57g		144	2.5	252	9.8	43.4	4.3	2.7
Baps, White Sandwich, Kingsmill*	1 Bap/80g		209	3.2	261	10.1	46.2	4.0	2.2

B

BREAD

	Measure INFO/WEIGHT	per Measure KCAL	FAT	Nutrition Values per 100g / 100ml KCAL	PROT	CARB	FAT	FIBRE
Baps, Wholemeal, Brace's*	1 Bap/59g	137	2.6	234	10.5	42.5	4.4	4.3
Baps, Wholemeal, Giant, Rathbones*	1 Bap/110g	230	2.1	209	9.4	39.0	1.9	8.0
Baps, Wholemeal, Large, Tesco*	1 Bap/95g	223	3.9	235	10.5	39.1	4.1	7.6
Baps, Wholemeal, Tesco*	1 Bap/46g	104	2.4	227	9.6	41.4	5.3	5.6
Baps, Wholemeal, Waitrose*	1 Bap/67g	156	3.2	234	10.6	37.2	4.8	6.7
Bloomer, COU, M & S*	1 Slice/33g	78	0.5	235	9.5	45.5	1.5	3.6
Bloomer, Multiseed, Sliced, M & S*	1 Slice/54g	150	3.9	280	10.5	43.6	7.2	3.1
Bloomer, White, Sliced, Waitrose*	1 Slice/50g	129	0.9	259	8.5	52.1	1.8	2.6
Bloomer, Wholemeal, Organic, M & S*	1 Slice/50g	110	2.1	220	10.2	35.5	4.2	6.4
Brioche, Continental Classics*	1 Roll/35g	122	3.3	349	8.2	58.3	9.3	0.0
Brioche, Finest, Tesco*	1 Roll/52g	207	11.6	398	10.8	38.3	22.4	2.0
Brioche, Loaf, Butter, Sainsbury's*	1/8 Loaf/50g	173	5.2	347	8.0	55.0	10.5	2.2
Brioche, Roll	1 Roll/53g	191	7.5	361	8.8	50.1	14.1	1.5
Brown, Ciabatta, Rolls, Dietary Specials*	1 Roll/50g	137	4.0	274	5.8	36.9	8.1	8.9
Brown, Danish, Sliced, Weight Watchers*	1 Slice/20g	48	0.4	233	9.9	40.7	1.8	7.6
Brown, Deli Sub, Roll, Asda*	1 Roll/60g	142	1.9	236	0.0	35.0	3.2	0.0
Brown, Farmhouse, Linwoods*	1 Slice/25g	56	0.4	225	7.3	44.4	1.7	5.8
Brown, Gluten & Wheat Free, Sliced	1 Slice/25g	56	1.3	224	3.4	41.0	5.2	9.4
Brown, Gluten Free, Genius*	1 Slice/35g	97	4.7	277	6.7	42.2	13.3	9.5
Brown, Good Health, Warburton's*	1 Slice/35g	79	1.0	226	10.3	39.6	2.9	7.2
Brown, Granary Malted, Thick Sliced, Waitrose*	1 Slice/40g	95	0.9	238	9.4	44.8	2.3	5.1
Brown, High Fibre, Ormo*	1 Slice/24g	57	0.6	239	9.2	42.9	2.6	7.5
Brown, Irwin's Bakery*	1 Slice/64g	137	0.4	214	10.4	41.8	0.6	6.1
Brown, Kingsmill Gold, Seeds & Oats, Kingsmill*	1 Slice/45g	126	4.4	280	12.2	35.6	9.8	4.9
Brown, Malted, Farmhouse Gold, Morrisons*	1 Slice/38g	94	0.5	248	8.2	49.6	1.4	3.0
Brown, Medium Sliced	*1 Slice/34g*	*74*	*0.7*	*218*	*8.5*	*44.3*	*2.0*	*3.5*
Brown, Mixed Grain, Original, Vogel*	1 Slice/45g	102	0.6	227	9.8	47.1	1.2	6.4
Brown, Multi Grain, Wheat Free, Gluten Free	1 Slice/33g	76	1.7	229	5.1	40.8	5.1	5.6
Brown, Sainsbury's*	1 Slice/34g	81	0.7	239	8.4	46.8	2.1	4.2
Brown, Seeded Batch, Large Loaf, 800g, Warburton's*	1 Slice/46g	132	4.1	288	12.3	39.7	8.9	6.0
Brown, Sliced, By Brennans, Weight Watchers*	1 Slice/20g	51	0.4	257	9.5	45.4	2.1	6.8
Brown, Sliced, Free From, Tesco*	1 Slice/45g	121	3.7	268	5.4	43.2	8.2	3.6
Brown, Soda, M & S*	1 Slice/40g	92	1.4	229	9.2	43.6	3.6	4.9
Brown, Soy & Linseed, Vogel*	1 Slice/50g	116	2.4	232	11.2	33.3	4.9	7.0
Brown, Sunflower & Barley, Vogel*	1 Slice/42g	100	1.9	239	9.4	40.3	4.5	6.7
Brown, Thick, Warburton's*	1 Slice/38g	80	0.7	211	9.4	39.2	1.8	6.2
Brown, Toasted, Average	*1 Slice/24g*	*65*	*0.5*	*272*	*10.4*	*56.5*	*2.1*	*4.5*
Brown, Toastie, Thick Sliced, Kingsmill*	1 Slice/44g	101	1.4	230	9.5	40.5	3.3	4.7
Brown, Wholemeal, Healthy Choice, Warburton's*	1 Slice/24g	55	0.6	231	10.4	40.7	2.5	6.5
Buns, Burger, Sainsbury's*	1 Bun/56g	154	2.9	275	9.2	47.8	5.2	4.1
Buns, Burger, Sesame, Sliced, Tesco*	1 Bun/60g	168	4.0	280	7.9	47.3	6.6	2.1
Buns, White, Stay Fresh, Tesco*	1 Bun/56g	152	3.7	271	7.5	45.5	6.6	0.0
Challah, Average	*1 Slice/50g*	*143*	*3.6*	*286*	*8.9*	*53.6*	*7.1*	*3.6*
Cheese, Onion & Garlic, Tear & Share, Waitrose*	¼ Bread/112g	326	14.6	290	9.4	33.9	13.0	2.1
Cheese, Onion Mustard Seed, Cluster, Sainsbury's*	1 Cluster/100g	276	8.1	276	10.0	40.6	8.1	3.1
Cheese, Tear & Share, Tesco*	¼ Loaf/73g	225	7.8	310	8.8	44.0	10.7	0.8
Cheese & Garlic, Pizza Style, Sainsbury's*	¼ Bread/63g	199	8.1	318	10.7	39.7	13.0	2.2
Cheese & Onion, Tear & Share, Sainsbury's*	¼ Bread/71g	202	6.6	285	9.8	40.6	9.3	1.9
Cheese & Onion, Toastie, Warburton's*	1 Slice/42g	120	5.8	286	7.5	33.1	13.7	0.0
Cheese & Tomato, Tear & Share, Sainsbury's*	¼ Bread/72g	211	9.5	293	8.0	35.7	13.2	1.5
Cholla, Average	*1/10 Loaf/154g*	*421*	*14.3*	*274*	*6.9*	*40.8*	*9.3*	*1.0*
Ciabatta, Black Olive, Part Baked, Sainsbury's*	¼ Ciabatta/67g	172	2.5	257	8.8	46.8	3.8	2.4
Ciabatta, Finest, Tesco*	1 Serving/45g	124	2.7	275	10.4	44.8	5.9	2.7

BREAD

	Measure INFO/WEIGHT	per Measure		Nutrition Values per 100g / 100ml				
		KCAL	FAT	KCAL	PROT	CARB	FAT	FIBRE
Ciabatta, Garlic, Mini, Italiano, Tesco*	½ Ciabatta/47g	150	6.9	320	8.2	38.5	14.6	2.8
Ciabatta, Garlic & Herb, GFY, Asda*	¼ Ciabatta/60g	137	1.4	230	8.8	43.2	2.4	1.0
Ciabatta, Gluten & Wheat Free	1 Slice/55g	136	1.6	248	2.0	52.4	2.9	4.2
Ciabatta, Green Olive, Tesco*	¼ Ciabatta/70g	155	3.1	222	7.4	38.2	4.4	1.9
Ciabatta, Italian Style, Waitrose*	1 Ciabatta/89g	231	1.2	260	10.7	51.2	1.3	2.2
Ciabatta, Olive & Rosemary, Mini, Tesco*	1 Pack/75g	319	8.2	425	17.8	63.0	10.9	3.6
Ciabatta, Plain, Half, Waitrose*	1 Roll/80g	248	5.8	310	10.0	51.3	7.2	2.2
Ciabatta, Ready to Bake, Sainsbury's*	½ Ciabatta/66g	172	2.4	260	8.9	47.7	3.7	2.2
Ciabatta, Sun Dried Tomato & Basil, Tesco*	¼ Ciabatta/75g	193	4.3	257	8.9	42.4	5.7	2.4
Ciabatta, TTD, Sainsbury's*	¼ Pack/68g	185	4.0	274	10.4	44.8	5.9	2.7
Ciabatta Stick, Organic, M & S*	1 Stick/140g	315	2.0	225	8.9	48.5	1.4	4.2
Cinnamon & Fruit Swirl, Genesis Crafty*	1 Slice/40g	133	4.1	332	6.7	53.7	10.2	0.0
Crostini, Olive Oil, TTD, Sainsbury's*	1 Roll/4g	16	0.3	409	11.4	72.2	8.3	3.3
Danish, White, Medium Sliced, Tesco*	1 Slice/20g	47	0.3	234	9.4	45.4	1.7	3.3
Farl, Irish Soda, Irwin's Bakery*	1 Farl/150g	334	5.1	223	4.0	44.0	3.4	2.3
Farmhouse, Batch, Multiseed, Love Life, Waitrose*	1 Slice/50g	130	3.5	259	9.9	39.2	7.0	7.2
Farmhouse, Poppy Seed, Crusty, Loaf, M & S*	1 Slice/40g	104	1.3	260	9.4	47.6	3.3	2.3
Farmhouse, with Oatmeal, Batch, Finest, Tesco*	1 Slice/50g	122	2.1	245	10.5	40.8	4.3	4.9
Farmhouse Soft Grained, Sliced, Warburton's*	1 Slice/42g	109	1.7	258	10.2	44.6	4.0	5.0
Flatbread, Garlic, BGTY, Sainsbury's*	¼ Bread/56g	177	5.7	316	9.6	46.6	10.1	2.7
Flatbread, Garlic & Herb, Tear & Share, Sainsbury's*	¼ Bread/68g	201	6.3	297	10.9	42.5	9.3	3.7
Flatbread, Tomato & Garlic, Sainsbury's*	1/3 Bread/73g	191	4.9	261	8.4	41.7	6.7	3.4
Focaccia, Onion & Herb, Tesco*	½ Pack/190g	547	23.7	288	8.7	35.2	12.5	3.7
Focaccia, Roast Cherry Tomato & Olive, GFY, Asda*	½ Pack/148g	350	6.0	237	9.0	41.0	4.1	2.8
Fougasse, Garlic & Gruyere, TTD, Sainsbury's*	¼ Bread/76g	219	6.8	288	9.5	42.6	8.9	2.9
French	1.5" Slice/45g	110	0.0	244	8.9	53.3	0.0	2.2
French Stick, Average	*1 Serving/60g*	*162*	*1.6*	*270*	*9.6*	*55.4*	*2.7*	*1.5*
Fruit, Continental, Schneider Brot*	1 Slice/65g	198	3.5	305	5.4	57.0	5.4	0.0
Fruit, Raisin Swirl, Sunmaid*	1 Slice/33g	95	1.9	287	8.3	50.4	5.8	2.6
Fruit & Cinnamon Loaf, Finest, Tesco*	1 Slice/37g	134	4.9	363	6.4	54.6	13.2	1.5
Fruit Loaf, Apple, M & S*	1 Slice/39g	100	0.6	255	8.5	51.9	1.5	3.3
Fruit Loaf, Apple & Cinnamon, Soreen*	1 Slice/10g	31	0.4	307	6.9	60.5	4.2	0.0
Fruit Loaf, Banana, Soreen*	1 Slice/25g	78	1.2	313	6.8	60.9	4.7	0.0
Fruit Loaf, Cinnamon & Raisin, Soreen*	1/8 Loaf/25g	77	1.0	308	7.7	54.1	4.0	4.1
Fruit Loaf, Fruity Five, Snack Pack, Soreen*	1 Pack/61g	200	5.5	329	7.1	54.9	9.0	2.7
Fruit Loaf, Luxury, Christmas, Soreen*	1 Slice/28g	85	0.6	303	4.5	66.6	2.1	0.0
Fruit Loaf, Mixed Berry, Weight Watchers*	1 Slice/34g	79	0.9	231	7.6	44.3	2.6	7.7
Fruit Loaf, Mother's Pride*	1 Slice/36g	92	1.0	256	8.2	49.3	2.9	2.6
Fruit Loaf, Plum, Lincolnshire, Soreen*	1 Slice/25g	65	0.8	261	8.4	49.3	3.4	2.1
Fruit Loaf, Sliced, Sainsbury's*	1 Slice/40g	104	1.4	260	8.9	47.9	3.6	2.4
Fruit Loaf, Sultana & Cherry, Sainsbury's*	1 Slice/50g	178	6.1	357	2.7	59.0	12.2	1.7
Garlic, & Parsley, Tesco*	1 Loaf/230g	699	26.7	304	9.0	41.0	11.6	2.7
Garlic, & Tomato, Pizza, Italiano, Tesco*	½ Bread/140g	405	15.1	289	7.5	40.5	10.8	2.5
Garlic, Baguette, 50% Less Fat, Asda*	¼ Baguette/43g	123	3.0	287	10.0	46.0	7.0	2.5
Garlic, Baguette, Extra Strong, Sainsbury's*	½ Baguette/85g	278	12.6	327	8.4	40.0	14.8	3.4
Garlic, Baguette, Frozen, GFY, Asda*	¼ Baguette/48g	132	4.3	277	7.0	42.0	9.0	2.7
Garlic, Baguette, Organic, Tesco*	1 Serving/60g	192	8.1	320	8.5	41.1	13.5	2.5
Garlic, Baguette, Reduced Fat, Waitrose*	½ Baguette/85g	229	6.8	270	8.1	41.5	8.0	2.7
Garlic, Baguette, Waitrose*	½ Baguette/85g	290	15.2	341	7.1	37.8	17.9	0.0
Garlic, Ciabatta, Hand Stretched, Sainsbury's*	¼ Pack/75g	244	10.6	325	8.4	41.0	14.1	2.9
Garlic, Ciabatta, Italiano, Tesco*	1 Ciabatta/65g	211	9.4	324	7.7	40.9	14.4	2.2
Garlic, Ciabatta, with Herbs, Weight Watchers*	1 Pack/88g	216	3.5	245	9.2	43.0	4.0	2.9
Garlic, Finest, Tesco*	¼ Loaf/60g	187	7.9	311	7.7	40.3	13.2	1.8

B

BREAD

INFO/WEIGHT	Measure		Nutrition Values per 100g / 100ml				
	KCAL	FAT	KCAL	PROT	CARB	FAT	FIBRE
Garlic, Focaccia, & Onion, GFY, Asda*	¼ Focaccia/55g	150	2.2	272	12.0	47.0	4.0	0.0
Garlic, Focaccia, & Rosemary, Sainsbury's*	¼ Focaccia/75g	219	7.3	292	8.0	43.0	9.8	2.8
Garlic, GFY, Asda*	1 Slice/31g	108	1.4	350	12.0	65.0	4.5	4.0
Garlic, Italian Style Stone Baked, Morrisons*	½ Pack/115g	420	22.0	365	7.9	40.4	19.1	1.9
Garlic, Reduced Fat, Waitrose*	1 Pack/170g	551	18.7	324	6.9	49.4	11.0	0.9
Garlic, Slices, Chilled, Sainsbury's*	1 Pack/368g	1369	60.0	372	9.1	47.3	16.3	3.2
Garlic, Slices, Italian, Chilled, Tesco*	1 Slice/27g	110	6.0	415	6.2	46.8	22.4	2.7
Garlic, Slices, Light Choices, Tesco*	1 Slice/30g	75	1.7	250	7.3	42.3	5.7	2.9
Garlic, Slices, Morrisons*	1 Slice/30g	82	2.7	272	7.3	40.2	9.1	2.6
Garlic, Stonebaked, M & S*	1 Loaf/85g	263	10.1	310	9.3	41.4	11.9	3.1
Garlic, to Share, M & S*	¼ Loaf/82g	230	10.7	280	6.5	33.2	13.0	1.3
Garlic, with Cheese, Asda*	1 Slice/34g	130	6.1	382	11.0	44.0	18.0	0.0
Granary, Average	**1 Slice/35g**	**82**	**0.9**	**235**	**9.3**	**46.3**	**2.7**	**4.3**
Granary, Seeded, Sunflower, Hovis*	1 Slice/44g	119	2.5	271	10.1	44.9	5.7	2.9
Granary, Wholemeal, Hovis*	1 Slice/44g	104	1.1	237	10.6	39.8	2.4	6.8
Granary White, Hovis*	1 Slice/44g	102	1.5	233	9.7	40.8	3.5	5.6
Hi Bran, M & S*	1 Slice/26g	55	0.8	210	12.6	32.5	3.0	6.3
Hi Fibre, Seed, Lifefibre*	1 Slice/35g	109	3.5	313	12.5	43.6	10.1	2.7
Juvela*	1 Slice/25g	60	0.7	240	3.3	50.0	3.0	1.7
Khobez, Flatbread, White, Dina Foods Ltd*	1 Bread/56g	158	0.6	282	10.5	57.5	1.1	3.0
Malt Loaf, Fruity, Sliced, Soreen*	1 Slice/33g	101	0.7	303	7.6	62.1	2.2	3.8
Malt Loaf, Fruity, Unsliced, Soreen*	1/8 Loaf/28g	85	0.5	310	7.4	65.6	2.0	2.7
Malt Loaf, Weight Watchers*	1 Slice/23g	68	0.4	294	8.9	60.2	1.9	3.6
Malted, & Seeded, Batch, Organic, Waitrose*	1 Slice/50g	118	1.9	236	10.9	39.5	3.9	6.2
Malted, Crusty, Sainsbury's*	1 Slice/42g	109	1.4	259	8.6	48.6	3.3	4.4
Malted, Danish, Sliced, Weight Watchers*	1 Slice/20g	51	0.3	249	11.8	45.1	1.5	4.2
Malted, Floury Batch, Sainsbury's*	1 Roll/68g	190	2.9	280	8.7	51.6	4.3	4.2
Malted, Wheat Loaf, Crusty, Finest, Tesco*	1 Slice/50g	115	0.7	230	9.8	44.2	1.5	4.4
Malted Brown, Slice, BGTY, Sainsbury's*	1 Slice/22g	53	0.6	239	12.1	41.4	2.8	5.8
Malted Danish, Weight Watchers*	1 Slice/20g	49	0.3	241	12.3	44.5	1.7	4.3
Malted Grain, Good As Gold, Kingsmill*	1 Slice/47g	114	1.2	243	9.5	45.4	2.6	4.2
Malted Wheatgrain, Roberts Bakery*	1 Slice/30g	79	1.0	265	11.0	48.0	3.3	3.6
Malted Wholegrain, Nimble*	1 Slice/22g	49	0.3	222	10.4	41.9	1.4	6.7
Mixed Seed, Organic, Duchy Originals*	1 Slice/43g	114	3.4	269	10.9	39.1	8.1	5.3
Multigrain, Brown, Farmhouse Baker's, M & S*	1 Slice/51g	115	2.8	225	13.0	31.2	5.4	5.1
Multigrain, Crusty, Finest, Tesco*	1 Slice/40g	98	1.4	245	9.0	44.7	3.4	5.0
Multigrain, Gluten Free, Sainsbury's*	1 Slice/17g	39	0.8	229	5.1	40.8	5.0	5.6
Multigrain, Sunblest*	1 Slice/30g	76	0.7	254	9.0	47.0	2.5	4.5
Naan, Bombay Brassiere, Sainsbury's*	1 Naan/140g	372	4.3	266	9.8	49.6	3.1	2.9
Naan, Chilli & Mango, Finest, Tesco*	½ Naan/90g	229	5.1	255	8.4	41.9	5.7	3.2
Naan, Garlic & Coriander, Free From, Tesco*	1 Naan/90g	215	6.0	240	5.1	38.7	6.7	4.9
Naan, Garlic & Coriander, M & S*	1 Naan/150g	375	2.1	250	9.8	50.1	1.4	2.0
Naan, Garlic & Coriander, Tesco*	½ Naan/83g	235	6.4	285	7.6	45.6	7.7	2.6
Naan, Garlic & Coriander, Weight Watchers*	1 Naan/60g	155	2.6	259	8.9	46.0	4.3	3.4
Naan, Onion & Mint, M & S*	½ Naan/135g	351	11.7	260	8.9	35.8	8.7	2.5
Naan, Onion Bhaji, Sharwood's*	1 Pack/130g	378	9.9	291	7.3	48.4	7.6	2.2
Naan, Peshwari, Apple & Coconut, Mini, Sharwood's*	1 Naan/40g	112	2.7	281	6.9	46.6	6.7	3.1
Naan, Peshwari, Sharwood's*	1 Naan/130g	334	6.9	257	7.2	45.1	5.3	2.5
Naan, Plain, Average	1 Naan/160g	538	20.0	336	8.9	50.1	12.5	1.9
Naan, Take Away, Tesco*	1 Naan/39g	97	1.3	248	8.7	45.6	3.4	1.7
Naan, Tandoori, Sharwood's*	1 Naan/130g	330	6.5	254	7.3	45.0	5.0	2.0
Naan, Tandoori Baked, Waitrose*	1 Naan/140g	372	4.3	266	9.8	49.6	3.1	2.9
Oatmeal, Batch, Finest, Tesco*	1 Slice/50g	127	2.1	255	10.3	43.7	4.3	4.8

	Measure	per Measure		Nutrition Values per 100g / 100ml				
	INFO/WEIGHT	KCAL	FAT	KCAL	PROT	CARB	FAT	FIBRE

BREAD

	INFO/WEIGHT	KCAL	FAT	KCAL	PROT	CARB	FAT	FIBRE
Oatmeal, Farmhouse, Extra Special, Asda*	1 Slice/44g	102	1.1	231	11.0	41.0	2.6	6.0
Oatmeal, Farmhouse, Soft, M & S*	1 Slice/45g	110	2.0	245	11.1	39.5	4.4	5.2
Oatmeal, Farmhouse, Waitrose*	1 Slice/40g	110	2.1	276	9.4	47.9	5.2	4.6
Olive, Waitrose*	1 Slice/28g	86	3.0	306	9.0	43.6	10.6	2.0
Pea, Artisan*	1 Slice/50g	102	1.2	204	9.5	31.8	2.4	9.4
Petit Pain, Part Bake, Weight Watchers*	1 Roll/50g	111	0.4	223	6.8	43.5	0.9	6.8
Petit Pain, White, Ready to Bake, Sainsbury's*	1 Roll/50g	122	0.7	242	7.8	49.7	1.3	2.8
Pitta, Brown, Organic, Waitrose*	1 Pitta/60g	137	0.8	228	6.4	47.5	1.4	6.6
Pitta, Garlic, Sainsbury's*	1 Pitta/60g	153	0.6	255	9.5	52.0	1.0	2.5
Pitta, Garlic & Coriander, Asda*	1 Pitta/55g	116	0.5	212	7.0	44.0	0.9	1.8
Pitta, Garlic & Herb, Tesco*	1 Pitta/60g	134	1.2	223	9.6	44.6	2.0	3.0
Pitta, Mexican, Santa Maria*	1 Pitta/66g	165	0.7	250	7.5	52.0	1.0	0.0
Pitta, Multi Seed & Cereal, The Food Doctor*	1 Pitta/70g	157	1.9	224	10.1	39.9	2.7	10.2
Pitta, Organic, Tesco*	1 Pitta/60g	124	0.8	206	8.3	40.2	1.4	5.7
Pitta, Seeded, HL, Tesco*	1 Pitta/60g	153	3.6	255	10.8	39.4	6.0	12.8
Pitta, Sesame, Sainsbury's*	1 Pitta/59g	156	1.4	264	9.8	50.8	2.4	3.1
Pitta, Tex Mex Style, Mini, Morrisons*	1 Pitta/18g	43	0.2	240	9.2	48.7	0.9	3.3
Pitta, White, Average	*1 Pitta/75g*	*199*	*0.9*	*265*	*9.2*	*57.9*	*1.2*	*2.2*
Pitta, White, Free From, Tesco*	1 Pitta/55g	140	1.2	255	6.5	52.6	2.1	5.5
Pitta, White, Weight Watchers*	1 Pitta/45g	106	0.3	238	8.7	45.9	0.7	6.7
Pitta, White Picnic, Waitrose*	1 Pitta/30g	75	0.4	249	10.3	49.3	1.2	3.5
Pitta, Wholemeal, Average	*1 Pitta/64g*	*170*	*1.7*	*266*	*9.8*	*55.0*	*2.6*	*7.4*
Pitta, Wholemeal, Lemon & Pepper, Finest, Tesco*	1 Pitta/80g	215	4.8	270	10.8	42.4	6.0	6.0
Pitta, Wholemeal, Mini, M & S*	1 Pitta/18g	44	0.4	247	10.3	45.8	2.5	5.6
Pitta, Wholemeal, Weight Watchers*	1 Pitta /46g	106	0.6	229	8.7	44.5	1.2	7.6
Pitta, Wholemeal, with Extra Virgin Olive Oil, Tesco*	1 Pitta/60g	135	1.6	225	8.3	41.5	2.6	5.5
Potato Farls, M & S*	1 Farl/55g	79	0.2	144	4.2	33.8	0.4	4.7
Potato Farls, Sunblest*	1 Farl/100g	156	0.9	156	3.8	33.2	0.9	1.9
Pumpernickel, Organic, Bavarian Pumpernickel*	1 Slice/50g	90	0.5	180	6.0	38.0	1.0	10.0
Pumpernickel Rye, Kelderman*	1 Slice/50g	92	0.5	185	6.0	38.0	1.0	0.0
Pumpkin Seed, Raisin & Sunflower Seed, Sainsbury's*	1 Slice/30g	76	0.8	255	11.6	45.9	2.8	3.4
Raisin & Pumpkin Seed, Organic, Tesco*	1 Slice/30g	76	1.7	253	9.7	40.6	5.8	3.8
Roasted Onion, M & S*	1 Slice/50g	125	1.6	250	9.0	46.7	3.3	2.1
Rolls, 3 Seeded, Sandwich, Warburton's*	1 Roll/77g	242	6.7	314	13.3	41.2	8.7	6.0
Rolls, American Style Deli, Tesco*	1 Roll/65g	162	2.2	249	7.8	46.8	3.4	1.6
Rolls, Batched Sandwich, Warburton's*	1 Roll/60g	148	2.5	246	9.6	42.7	4.1	0.0
Rolls, Best of Both, Hovis*	1 Roll/62g	148	2.9	239	9.8	39.7	4.6	5.0
Rolls, Blackpool Milk, Warburton's*	1 Slice/18g	47	0.5	254	11.0	45.0	2.8	2.8
Rolls, Brioche, Plain Chocolate Chip, Sainsbury's*	1 Roll/35g	131	5.6	374	8.5	49.0	16.0	5.9
Rolls, Brioche, Sainsbury's*	1 Roll/32g	116	3.7	362	8.5	56.0	11.5	3.6
Rolls, Brown, Carb Control, Tesco*	1 Roll/45g	98	2.7	218	20.5	20.7	5.9	10.7
Rolls, Brown, Crusty	*1 Roll/50g*	*127*	*1.4*	*255*	*10.3*	*50.4*	*2.8*	*3.5*
Rolls, Brown, Soft, Average	*1 Roll/50g*	*134*	*1.9*	*268*	*10.0*	*51.8*	*3.8*	*3.5*
Rolls, Cheese Topped, Sandwich Rolls, Warburton's*	1 Roll/62g	168	4.0	270	12.1	40.7	6.5	2.6
Rolls, Ciabatta, Cheese Topped, Mini, Finest, Tesco*	1 Roll/30g	85	2.4	282	11.5	40.9	8.1	3.8
Rolls, Ciabatta, Garlic, Asda*	1 Roll/93g	333	16.7	358	9.0	40.0	18.0	2.3
Rolls, Ciabatta, M & S*	1 Roll/80g	210	3.3	262	10.3	48.1	4.1	2.1
Rolls, Ciabatta, Sun Dried Tomato, Mini, Finest, Tesco*	1 Roll/30g	79	1.9	262	8.7	42.3	6.4	2.6
Rolls, Crisp, Original, Organic, Kallo*	1 Roll/9g	34	0.5	390	11.0	74.0	5.6	3.0
Rolls, Crusty, Booths*	1 Roll/50g	123	0.6	247	8.7	50.3	1.2	2.6
Rolls, Crusty, French, M & S*	1 Roll/65g	159	0.8	245	8.1	50.5	1.2	3.3
Rolls, Finger, White, Sainsbury's*	1 Roll/40g	96	1.0	240	9.0	45.2	2.6	3.2
Rolls, Granary, Original, Hovis*	1 Roll/70g	180	2.9	257	10.7	44.3	4.1	5.3

BREAD

	Measure INFO/WEIGHT	per Measure KCAL	FAT	Nutrition Values per 100g / 100ml KCAL	PROT	CARB	FAT	FIBRE
Rolls, Granary, Waitrose*	1 Roll/59g	160	3.8	271	10.0	47.2	6.4	3.8
Rolls, Granary Malted Wheatgrain, Soft, M & S*	1 Roll/80g	208	3.1	260	9.3	47.2	3.9	2.3
Rolls, Green Olive, M & S*	1 Roll/75g	210	4.5	280	11.2	44.0	6.0	1.8
Rolls, Hot Dog, Sliced, Asda*	1 Roll/84g	197	2.8	234	7.0	44.0	3.3	0.0
Rolls, Hot Dog, Warburton's*	1 Roll/60g	137	2.8	228	8.7	37.8	4.7	1.7
Rolls, Malted, Whole Grain Rolls, Batched, Soft, M & S*	1 Roll/80g	180	3.6	225	7.8	38.5	4.5	3.1
Rolls, Malted Grain, Soft, Weight Watchers*	1 Roll/57g	142	1.0	251	11.7	47.1	1.8	4.2
Rolls, Mixed Seed, Deli, Tesco*	1 Roll/65g	165	2.1	255	9.4	46.8	3.3	5.2
Rolls, Morning, Tesco*	1 Roll/48g	117	1.2	243	10.4	44.8	2.5	4.7
Rolls, Multigrain, Torpedo, Sainsbury's*	1 Roll/112g	328	7.5	293	10.5	47.7	6.7	6.3
Rolls, Oatmeal, Ploughman's, GFY, Asda*	1 Roll/72g	181	3.2	252	10.0	43.0	4.4	3.9
Rolls, Oatmeal, Soft, M & S*	1 Roll/80g	224	5.1	280	12.3	43.4	6.4	2.7
Rolls, Pane Rustica, Waitrose*	1 Roll/114g	283	1.4	248	9.4	50.0	1.2	1.8
Rolls, Panini, Sainsbury's*	1 Roll/90g	249	5.6	276	11.0	44.1	6.2	3.0
Rolls, Poppy Seeded Knot, Waitrose*	1 Roll/60g	169	3.2	282	10.3	48.3	5.3	2.2
Rolls, Rye, Toasting, Good & Hot*	1 Roll/65g	143	0.7	220	7.3	44.6	1.1	7.1
Rolls, Seed Sensations, Deli, Hovis*	1 Roll/70g	184	5.9	263	10.3	36.5	8.5	10.6
Rolls, Seeded, Mixed Mini Loaf Pack, M & S*	1 Roll/76g	220	7.3	290	10.6	39.7	9.6	4.0
Rolls, Seeded, Sandwich, Warburton's*	1 Roll/77g	242	6.7	314	13.3	41.2	8.7	6.0
Rolls, Soft, Wholemeal, Finger, M & S*	1 Roll/66g	145	1.3	220	12.6	38.0	2.0	5.8
Rolls, Submarine, Sainsbury's*	1 Roll/117g	305	4.6	261	9.1	47.4	3.9	2.4
Rolls, Sun Dried Tomato, Homebake, Tesco*	1 Roll/50g	123	1.5	246	11.3	44.0	3.0	0.0
Rolls, Sunflower Seed, Toasting, Good & Hot*	1 Roll/65g	162	3.2	250	8.5	41.0	5.0	8.0
Rolls, Tomato & Basil, Sub, COU, M & S*	1 Roll/33g	86	0.9	265	11.0	48.7	2.7	2.4
Rolls, White, Cheese Topped, Sainsbury's*	1 Roll/75g	218	6.4	291	12.1	41.6	8.5	2.0
Rolls, White, Chunky, Hovis*	1 Roll/73g	173	2.4	237	9.4	41.7	3.3	2.5
Rolls, White, Crusty, Average	*1 Roll/50g*	*140*	*1.1*	*280*	*10.9*	*57.6*	*2.3*	*1.5*
Rolls, White, Finger, Tesco*	1 Roll/68g	170	2.4	250	8.5	45.8	3.5	2.1
Rolls, White, Floured, Warburton's*	1 Roll/50g	123	1.9	247	9.8	43.3	3.8	2.7
Rolls, White, Floury, Roberts Bakery*	1 Roll/63g	160	1.6	254	8.4	49.5	2.5	2.0
Rolls, White, Kingsmill*	1 Roll/60g	151	2.5	252	9.3	44.5	4.1	2.4
Rolls, White, Morning, Co-Op*	1 Roll/47g	134	1.4	285	12.0	53.0	3.0	2.0
Rolls, White, Organic, Sainsbury's*	1 Roll/65g	170	1.9	262	8.7	49.9	3.0	1.0
Rolls, White, Part Baked, Morrisons*	1 Roll/75g	227	1.0	303	9.6	63.0	1.4	2.6
Rolls, White, Seeded, Sainsbury's*	1 Roll/80g	217	4.7	271	10.9	43.4	5.9	4.8
Rolls, White, Soft, Average	*1 Roll/45g*	*121*	*1.9*	*268*	*9.2*	*51.6*	*4.2*	*1.5*
Rolls, White, Split, Asda*	1 Roll/45g	113	1.5	251	10.0	45.0	3.4	2.8
Rolls, White, Sub, Tesco*	1 Roll/100g	258	4.0	258	11.1	44.4	4.0	2.8
Rolls, Wholemeal	*1 Roll 45g*	*108*	*1.3*	*241*	*9.0*	*48.3*	*2.9*	*5.9*
Rolls, Wholemeal, Oat Topped, Tesco*	1 Roll/65g	166	2.9	255	11.3	42.2	4.5	5.1
Rolls, Wholemeal, Oatbran, HL, Tesco*	1 Roll/56g	115	1.4	205	11.4	33.6	2.5	7.4
Rolls, Wholemeal, Soft, Seeded, Sainsbury's*	1 Roll/75g	193	5.5	257	11.8	35.6	7.4	6.2
Rolls, Wholemeal, Submarine, Tesco*	1 Roll/100g	221	3.1	221	9.3	39.0	3.1	5.2
Rolls, Wholemeal, Sunflower & Honey, Sainsbury's*	1 Roll/85g	225	4.3	265	9.2	45.4	5.1	4.5
Rolls, Wholemeal & White, Kingsmill*	1 Roll/60g	151	2.5	251	9.5	43.7	4.2	3.5
Rolls, Wholemeal with Cracked Wheat, Allinson*	1 Roll/58g	134	2.3	231	11.0	38.0	3.9	7.0
Roti, Tesco*	1 Bread/95g	256	5.2	269	8.4	46.4	5.5	3.2
Rye, Average	*1 Slice/25g*	*55*	*0.4*	*219*	*8.3*	*45.8*	*1.7*	*4.4*
Rye, Swedish Style, Kelderman*	1 Slice/50g	92	1.6	185	7.2	31.5	3.2	4.3
Rye, Wheat Free, New York Deli, The Stamp Collection*	1 Slice/33g	61	0.5	184	6.6	43.6	1.4	7.3
Rye, with Pumpkin Seeds, Biona Organic*	1 Slice/72g	121	3.7	169	2.3	31.8	5.2	0.0
Rye, with Sunflower Seeds, Mestemacher*	1 Slice/80g	146	2.5	182	6.1	32.3	3.1	0.0
Rye, with Sunflower Seeds, Organic, Schneider Brot*	1 Slice/72g	138	2.6	191	6.2	33.4	3.6	7.9

BREAD

	Measure INFO/WEIGHT	per Measure KCAL	FAT	Nutrition Values per 100g / 100ml KCAL	PROT	CARB	FAT	FIBRE
Seeded, Batch, Finest, Tesco*	1 Slice/65g	168	4.0	259	9.3	41.8	6.1	6.1
Seeded, Farmhouse, Roberts Bakery*	1 Slice/37g	89	1.1	240	10.6	49.0	2.9	6.7
Seeded Rye, Loaf, la Brea Bakery*	1 Slice/55g	120	0.5	218	7.0	42.5	1.0	5.7
Soda	*1oz/28g*	*72*	*0.7*	*258*	*7.7*	*54.6*	*2.5*	*2.1*
Soda, Fruit, M & S*	1 Slice/40g	105	1.9	260	5.9	51.3	4.6	2.5
Soda Farls, M & S*	1 Farl/110g	267	3.0	243	9.6	50.1	2.7	2.3
Softgrain, Farmhouse, M & S*	1 Slice/25g	59	0.9	238	8.4	42.8	3.7	3.2
Softgrain, Medium Sliced, GFY, Asda*	1 Slice/35g	79	0.5	226	7.0	46.0	1.5	3.7
Softgrain, Mighty White*	1 Slice/36g	81	0.5	224	7.2	45.5	1.5	3.7
Sourdough	*1 Slice/50g*	*144*	*0.9*	*289*	*11.7*	*56.4*	*1.8*	*2.4*
Soya & Linseed, Burgen*	1 Slice/36g	99	3.6	274	15.9	29.8	10.1	6.8
Soya & Linseed, Vogel*	1 Slice/45g	107	2.7	238	12.2	34.0	5.9	5.4
Sunflower, Multi-Grain, Allinson*	1 Slice/47g	113	2.2	240	9.8	39.6	4.7	3.9
Sunflower & Honey, Organic, Cranks*	1 Slice/30g	64	0.9	215	11.6	37.2	3.0	8.3
Sunflower & Pumpkin Seed, Batched, Organic, Tesco*	1 Slice/30g	73	2.2	243	11.0	33.1	7.4	5.2
Sunflower & Pumpkin Seed, So Organic, Sainsbury's*	1 Slice/30g	76	1.6	254	11.4	40.0	5.4	12.9
Sunflower Seed, Organic, Natural, Mestemacher*	1 Slice/69g	149	2.8	216	5.6	34.7	4.0	9.4
Tiger Loaf, Tesco*	1 Slice/40g	96	0.8	239	8.7	46.6	2.0	2.6
Tomato, & Herb, Tear & Share, Tesco*	¼ Pack/73g	164	3.2	226	6.3	40.2	4.4	2.1
Tomato & Chilli, BGTY, Sainsbury's*	¼ Bread/65g	155	3.1	238	11.9	36.9	4.7	2.8
Tomato & Garlic, Italian Style, Morrisons*	½ Pack/155g	355	12.4	229	5.8	33.4	8.0	2.5
Walnut, Waitrose*	1/8 Loaf/50g	169	7.6	339	10.0	40.6	15.2	5.9
Wheat	*1 Slice/25g*	*65*	*1.0*	*260*	*9.1*	*47.2*	*4.1*	*4.3*
Wheat Rye, Wholemeal, Goldaehren, Aldi*	1 Slice/30g	68	1.2	226	8.0	36.0	4.0	7.0
Wheaten, Big Slice	1 Slice/65g	139	1.7	214	7.5	40.2	2.6	3.6
Wheaten, M & S*	1 Slice/33g	74	1.2	225	9.3	42.9	3.5	3.9
Wheaten, Sliced, Healthy, Irwin's Bakery*	1 Slice/40g	76	0.8	190	9.0	40.5	1.9	6.2
Wheatgerm, Hovis, Soft, Sliced, M & S*	1 Slice/23g	50	0.7	220	10.1	38.5	3.0	4.6
Wheatgerm, Original, Sliced, Hovis*	1 Slice/40g	85	0.9	214	10.0	38.6	2.2	5.3
Wheatgrain, Robertson*	1 Slice/30g	90	1.2	300	9.3	57.3	4.0	4.0
White, Average	*1 Slice/40g*	*94*	*0.8*	*235*	*8.4*	*49.3*	*1.9*	*1.5*
White, Commercially Prepared, Average	1oz/28g	74	0.9	266	7.6	50.6	3.3	2.4
White, Commercially Prepared, Toasted, Average	1oz/28g	82	1.1	293	9.0	54.4	4.0	2.5
White, Danish, Sliced, Weight Watchers*	1 Slice/21g	50	0.3	243	9.8	46.5	1.3	2.9
White, Danish, Soft & Light, Thick Cut, Asda*	1 Slice/26g	60	0.4	230	9.0	45.0	1.6	2.1
White, Farmhouse, Hovis*	1 Slice/44g	103	1.0	234	8.7	44.6	2.3	2.4
White, Fibre, Morrisons*	1 Slice/40g	96	0.7	240	8.0	48.4	1.7	0.3
White, Fried in Blended Oil	*1 Slice/28g*	*141*	*9.0*	*503*	*7.9*	*48.5*	*32.2*	*1.6*
White, Gluten & Wheat Free, Free From, Sainsbury's*	1 Slice/33g	75	2.8	227	1.9	35.5	8.6	1.0
White, High Fibre, Nimble*	1 Slice/22g	48	0.4	219	10.1	40.6	1.8	7.5
White, Medium Loaf, VLH Kitchens*	1 Slice/30g	72	0.6	241	8.4	49.3	1.9	1.5
White, Oatmeal, Allinson*	1 Slice/47g	111	1.4	237	9.0	43.5	3.0	2.7
White, Organic, Hovis*	1 Slice/44g	108	1.4	246	8.6	45.8	3.2	2.3
White, Sour Dough, Average	1 Slice/64g	185	1.2	289	11.7	56.4	1.8	2.4
White, Toasted, Average	*1 Slice/33g*	*87*	*0.5*	*265*	*9.3*	*57.1*	*1.6*	*1.8*
White, Wholesome, Medium Sliced, Asda*	1 Slice/35g	78	0.9	223	7.0	43.0	2.6	5.0
Whole Wheat, Nature's Own*	1 Slice/28g	66	1.0	236	14.3	39.3	3.6	10.7
Wholegrain, Average	*1 Slice/44g*	*78*	*1.1*	*178*	*8.3*	*31.6*	*2.5*	*5.2*
Wholegrain, Average, Toasted	*1 Slice/40g*	*71*	*1.0*	*178*	*8.3*	*31.6*	*2.5*	*5.2*
Wholemeal, Multigrain, Soft Batch, Sainsbury's*	1 Slice/44g	106	2.9	242	11.3	34.5	6.5	5.6
Wholemeal, Multiseed, Organic, Sainsbury's*	1 Slice/26g	75	2.5	289	13.8	36.6	9.7	6.0
Wholemeal, Nimble*	1 Slice/22g	48	0.5	219	12.2	37.0	2.5	6.8
Wholemeal, Toasted, Average	*1 Slice/26g*	*58*	*0.6*	*224*	*8.6*	*42.3*	*2.2*	*5.8*

	Measure INFO/WEIGHT	per Measure KCAL	FAT	Nutrition Values per 100g / 100ml KCAL	PROT	CARB	FAT	FIBRE
BREAD								
Wholemeal, with Seeds, Thick, Love Life, Waitrose*	1 Slice/54g	131	4.5	242	12.7	28.8	8.4	9.7
Wholemeal & Oat, Loaf, Vogel*	1 Slice/42g	86	0.6	205	8.7	34.3	1.5	9.7
Wholemeal Oatbran, Sliced, Tesco*	1 Slice/45g	90	0.7	200	10.1	35.3	1.6	7.4
BREAD & BUTTER PUDDING								
5% Fat, M & S*	1 Serving/237g	367	10.0	155	4.4	24.8	4.2	0.4
Average	1 Serving/250g	400	19.5	160	6.2	17.5	7.8	0.3
Finest, Tesco*	1 Serving/153g	379	22.0	248	4.9	24.6	14.4	0.9
Frozen, Chosen By You, Asda*	1 Serving/125g	275	10.2	220	5.5	30.4	8.2	1.4
Low Fat, Individual, BGTY, Sainsbury's*	1 Pack/125g	125	2.9	100	6.3	13.4	2.3	5.4
Reduced Fat, Waitrose*	1 Serving/205g	299	5.3	146	7.4	23.3	2.6	2.0
Tesco*	½ Pack	494	31.8	250	5.0	20.8	16.1	0.4
BREAD MIX								
Brown, Sunflower, Sainsbury's*	1 Serving/60g	151	3.7	251	10.0	38.9	6.1	4.0
Cheese & Onion, Dry Mix, Sainsbury's*	1 Serving/100g	311	2.8	311	11.9	59.5	2.8	2.6
Ciabatta, Made Up with Water & Olive Oil, Wrights*	1 Slice/45g	113	1.8	251	10.0	43.6	4.0	1.8
Crusty White, Made Up, Tesco*	1 Slice/126g	316	2.3	251	9.4	49.3	1.8	2.5
Focaccia, Garlic & Herb, Asda*	1 Serving/125g	385	10.0	308	11.0	48.0	8.0	3.3
Italian Ciabatta, Sainsbury's*	1 Slice/45g	96	0.9	213	8.7	40.0	2.0	2.4
Italian Sun Dried Tomato & Parmesan, Sainsbury's*	1 Serving/100g	247	1.7	247	8.1	50.1	1.7	2.5
Mixed Grain, Sainsbury's*	1 Serving/45g	103	0.7	228	7.7	46.0	1.5	4.4
Parmesan & Sun Dried Tomato, Made Up, Wrights*	1 Slice/45g	103	0.6	229	9.3	46.0	1.3	2.4
White Loaf, Asda*	1 Slice/60g	150	0.9	250	10.0	49.0	1.5	3.1
Wholemeal, Hovis*	1 Serving/65g	148	3.1	227	10.0	35.8	4.8	6.8
Wholemeal, Made Up, M & S*	1 Loaf/600g	1410	14.4	235	11.0	42.0	2.4	5.3
BREADCRUMBS								
Average	*1oz/28g*	**98**	**0.5**	**350**	**10.7**	**74.8**	**1.9**	**2.5**
BREADFRUIT								
Raw	*1oz/28g*	**27**	**0.1**	**95**	**1.3**	**23.1**	**0.3**	**0.0**
BREADSTICKS								
Cheese, Italian, Tesco*	4 Sticks/21g	84	1.7	399	14.2	67.5	8.0	3.4
Chive & Onion Twists, Tesco*	3 Twists/24g	115	5.3	480	11.6	57.6	22.1	2.2
Farleys*	1 Stick/12g	50	0.7	414	14.0	76.5	5.8	1.1
Grissini, Thin, with Olive Oil, Forno Bianco*	1 Stick/5g	21	0.4	420	11.0	77.0	7.5	0.0
Grissini, Waitrose*	1 Stick/6g	25	0.4	397	12.0	72.5	6.2	3.1
Mini, Sainsbury's*	4 Sticks/5g	20	0.4	404	15.6	68.7	7.4	4.8
Olive Oil & Rosemary, Finest, Tesco*	2 Sticks/10g	42	1.2	427	13.9	64.4	12.6	4.1
Original, Organic, Kallo*	1 Stick/6g	24	0.5	393	11.8	69.5	7.6	4.7
Oven Baked, Mini, Quaker Oats*	1 Pack/35g	145	3.1	415	12.9	71.0	8.8	3.7
Perfectly Balanced, Waitrose*	1 Stick/5g	20	0.1	378	13.7	77.3	1.6	3.8
Plain, Asda*	1 Stick/5g	21	0.4	412	12.0	73.0	8.0	2.9
Rosemary, Asda*	1 Stick/7g	29	1.0	439	12.0	64.0	15.0	3.5
Salted, Asda*	1 Stick/8g	36	1.4	445	13.0	60.0	17.0	4.3
BREAKFAST CEREAL								
Advantage, Weetabix*	1 Serving/30g	105	0.7	350	10.2	72.0	2.4	9.0
All Bran, Apricot Bites, Kellogg's*	1 Serving/45g	126	1.1	279	11.0	55.0	2.5	19.0
All Bran, Bran Flakes, & Fruit, Kellogg's*	1 Serving/40g	143	2.4	358	8.0	68.0	6.0	9.0
All Bran, Bran Flakes, Chocolate, Kellogg's*	1 Serving/30g	106	1.8	354	10.0	65.0	6.0	13.0
All Bran, Bran Flakes, Kellogg's*	1 Serving/30g	98	0.6	326	10.7	67.0	2.0	15.0
All Bran, Bran Flakes, Yoghurty, Kellogg's*	1 Serving/40g	141	2.0	353	10.0	67.0	5.0	12.0
All Bran, Fruit 'n' Fibre, Kellogg's*	1 Serving/30g	114	1.8	380	8.0	69.0	6.0	9.0
All Bran, Fruitful, Kellogg's*	1 Serving/40g	136	3.0	340	12.5	57.5	7.5	0.0
All Bran, Golden Crunch, Kellogg's*	1 Serving/45g	182	4.9	405	8.0	62.0	11.0	13.0
All Bran, High Fibre, Morrisons*	1 Serving/40g	109	1.4	272	14.7	45.5	3.5	27.0

BREAKFAST CEREAL	Measure INFO/WEIGHT	per Measure KCAL	FAT	Nutrition Values per 100g / 100ml KCAL	PROT	CARB	FAT	FIBRE
All Bran, Original, High Fibre, Kellogg's*	1 Serving/40g	134	1.4	334	14.0	48.0	3.5	27.0
All Bran, Splitz, Kellogg's*	1 Serving/40g	130	0.8	325	9.0	69.0	2.0	9.0
All Bran, Strawberry Medley, Kellogg's*	1 Serving/55g	170	1.5	309	9.1	80.0	2.7	1.8
Almond, Low Carb, Atkins*	1 Serving/30g	100	1.5	333	50.0	26.7	5.0	0.0
Almond, Oats & More, Nestle*	1 Serving/30g	119	2.7	398	10.7	68.7	8.9	5.5
Almond, Pecan & Cashew Muesli, Kellogg's*	1 Serving/45g	188	6.3	418	11.0	62.0	14.0	8.0
Almond, Raisin & Pecan, Nature's Pleasure, Kellogg's*	1 Serving/45g	184	5.4	408	10.0	65.0	12.0	8.0
Alpen*, Crunchy Bran*	1 Serving/40g	120	1.9	299	11.8	52.3	4.7	24.8
Amaranth, Flakes, Organic, Gillian McKeith*	1 Serving/50g	198	2.0	396	10.0	80.0	4.0	3.0
Apple, Blackberry, & Raspberry Flakes, GFY, Asda*	1 Serving/30g	103	0.5	344	9.0	73.0	1.8	11.0
Apple & Cinnamon, Crisp, Sainsbury's*	1 Serving/50g	216	7.3	433	6.2	69.1	14.7	3.4
Apple & Cinnamon, Quaker Oats*	1 Sachet/38g	136	2.1	358	8.0	68.0	5.5	2.5
Apple & Cinnamon Flakes, M & S*	1 Serving/30g	111	0.6	370	6.0	82.7	1.9	3.4
Apricot Wheats, Whole Grain, Tesco*	1 Serving/40g	130	0.6	326	7.6	70.6	1.4	8.0
Balance, Sainsbury's*	1 Serving/30g	111	0.4	370	11.4	77.7	1.5	3.2
Balance with Red Fruits, Sainsbury's*	1 Serving/40g	147	0.5	367	11.2	77.5	1.3	2.6
Banana, Papaya & Honey Oat, Crunchy, Waitrose*	1 Serving/40g	170	4.8	426	9.6	69.8	12.0	5.5
Banana & Toffee Crisp, Mornflake*	1 Serving/30g	133	4.8	443	5.7	68.8	16.1	5.4
Berry Burst, Oat So Simple, Quaker Oats*	1 Serving/39g	144	2.3	370	8.0	70.0	6.0	6.5
Berry Crunchy, Sainsbury's*	1 Serving/30g	122	3.6	408	7.7	67.3	12.0	4.8
Bitesize, Weetabix*	1 Serving/40g	135	0.8	338	11.5	68.4	2.0	10.0
Blackberry & Apple, Alpen*	1 Serving/40g	140	1.5	349	9.2	69.4	3.8	8.3
Bran, Natural, Sainsbury's*	1 Serving/30g	64	1.5	212	14.7	27.0	5.0	36.0
Bran Flakes, Crunchy Nut, Sainsbury's*	1 Serving/40g	203	3.8	507	19.7	85.7	9.5	11.0
Bran Flakes, Harvest Home, Nestle*	1 Serving/30g	99	0.7	331	10.2	67.1	2.4	14.1
Bran Flakes, HL, Tesco*	1 Serving/30g	100	0.7	335	10.2	67.0	2.4	14.1
Bran Flakes, Honey Nut, Sainsbury's*	1 Serving/40g	143	1.8	358	9.6	70.0	4.4	11.0
Bran Flakes, Kellogg's*	1 Serving/50g	163	1.0	326	10.0	67.0	2.0	15.0
Bran Flakes, Organic, Sainsbury's*	1 Serving/30g	100	0.7	332	10.2	67.4	2.4	14.1
Bran Flakes, Sultana Bran, Kellogg's*	1 Serving/30g	95	0.6	318	8.0	67.0	2.0	13.0
Bran Flakes, Whole Grain, Sainsbury's*	1 Serving/30g	99	0.7	331	10.2	67.1	2.4	14.1
Breakfast Biscuits, Aldi*	4 Biscuits/60g	213	1.5	355	13.7	69.5	2.5	7.5
Caribbean Crunch, Alpen*	1 Serving/40g	155	3.6	388	8.8	67.9	9.0	4.6
Cheerios, Honey, Nestle*	1 Serving/50g	184	1.4	369	6.6	79.2	2.8	5.8
Cheerios, Honey Nut, Nestle*	1 Serving/30g	112	1.1	374	7.0	78.3	3.7	5.2
Cheerios, Nestle*	1 Serving/30g	111	1.2	369	8.1	75.2	3.9	6.6
Choc & Nut Crisp, Tesco*	1 Serving/40g	185	8.0	462	8.3	62.5	19.9	4.8
Choco Crackles, Morrisons*	1 Serving/30g	115	0.7	383	5.5	84.8	2.4	1.9
Choco Flakes, Kellogg's*	1 Serving/30g	114	0.9	380	5.0	84.0	3.0	2.5
Choco Hoops, Asda*	1 Serving/40g	154	1.8	385	7.0	79.0	4.5	4.0
Choco Snaps, Sainsbury's*	1 Serving/30g	115	0.7	383	5.5	84.8	2.4	1.9
Choco Squares, Asda*	1 Serving/30g	130	4.2	434	10.0	67.0	14.0	4.0
Chocolate, Granola, Diet Chef Ltd*	1 Serving/40g	195	11.5	487	10.7	45.0	28.7	13.0
Chocolate Cereal, Tesco*	1 Serving/40g	169	5.6	423	8.0	66.3	14.0	6.0
Chocolate Crisp, Minis, Weetabix*	1 Serving/36g	134	1.9	371	9.0	71.7	5.3	8.5
Chocolate Wheats, Kellogg's*	1 Serving/40g	148	3.6	369	10.0	62.0	9.0	12.0
Cinnamon, Puffins, Barbara's Bakery*	1 Serving/30g	100	1.0	333	6.7	86.7	3.3	20.0
Cinnamon Grahams, Nestle*	1 Serving/40g	164	3.9	411	4.7	76.1	9.8	4.2
Clusters, Nestle*	1 Serving/30g	111	1.4	371	9.3	72.6	4.8	7.4
Coco Pops, Crunchers, Kellogg's*	1 Serving/30g	114	1.0	380	7.0	81.0	3.5	3.0
Coco Pops, Kellogg's*	1 Serving/30g	116	0.9	387	5.0	85.0	3.0	2.0
Cookie Crunch, Nestle*	1 Serving/40g	154	1.1	385	4.6	85.3	2.8	1.8
Corn Flakes, Banana Crunch, Kellogg's*	1 Serving/40g	163	3.2	408	6.0	78.0	8.0	3.0

BREAKFAST CEREAL

INFO/WEIGHT	Measure	per Measure		Nutrition Values per 100g / 100ml				
		KCAL	FAT	KCAL	PROT	CARB	FAT	FIBRE
Corn Flakes, Crispy Nut, Asda*	1 Serving/30g	117	1.3	390	7.0	81.0	4.2	2.5
Corn Flakes, Harvest Home, Nestle*	1 Serving/25g	92	0.2	367	7.3	82.7	0.8	3.6
Corn Flakes, Hint of Honey, Kellogg's*	1 Serving/30g	113	0.2	377	6.0	87.0	0.6	2.5
Corn Flakes, Honey Nut, Harvest Home, Nestle*	1 Serving/30g	118	1.3	392	7.4	81.1	4.2	2.5
Corn Flakes, Honey Nut, Sainsbury's*	1 Serving/30g	119	1.3	397	7.4	81.7	4.5	2.5
Corn Flakes, Honey Nut & Cranberries, Sainsbury's*	1 Serving/40g	166	4.0	416	7.4	74.4	9.9	3.1
Corn Flakes, Kellogg's*	1 Serving/30g	112	0.3	372	7.0	84.0	0.9	3.0
Corn Flakes, Organic, Whole Earth*	1 Serving/40g	154	0.4	386	8.6	84.2	1.0	3.0
Corn Flakes, Sainsbury's*	1 Serving/25g	93	0.2	371	7.3	83.8	0.7	3.0
Corn Flakes, with 125ml Semi Skimmed Milk, Kellogg's*	1 Serving/30g	170	2.5	567	20.0	106.7	8.3	3.0
Cornflakes, Honey Nut, Asda*	1 Serving/30g	119	1.3	397	7.4	81.7	4.5	2.5
Country Crisp, & Flakes, Red Berry, Jordans*	1 Serving/50g	203	5.8	407	7.1	68.5	11.6	7.3
Country Crisp, Four Nut Combo, Jordans*	1 Serving/50g	240	12.3	480	8.9	55.4	24.7	6.9
Country Crisp, Wild About Berries, Jordans*	1 Serving/50g	221	7.8	443	7.5	68.0	15.7	5.7
Country Crisp, with Real Raspberries, Jordans*	1 Serving/50g	214	7.9	429	7.5	64.1	15.8	7.1
Country Crisp, with Real Strawberries, Jordans*	1 Serving/50g	214	7.8	428	7.5	64.1	15.7	7.1
Country Honey, Oat So Simple, Quaker Oats*	1 Serving/36g	134	2.3	373	8.5	69.0	6.5	6.0
Cranberry Wheats, Tesco*	1 Serving/40g	130	0.6	325	7.3	70.9	1.4	7.7
Cranberry Wheats, Whole Grain, Sainsbury's*	1 Serving/50g	162	0.7	325	7.3	70.9	1.4	7.7
Crispy Rice & Wheat Flakes, Asda*	1 Serving/50g	185	0.7	370	11.0	78.0	1.5	3.2
Crunchy Bran, Weetabix*	1 Serving/40g	140	1.4	350	11.9	57.6	3.6	20.0
Crunchy Chocolate, Carrefour*	1 Serving/40g	176	6.8	440	9.0	62.0	17.0	8.0
Crunchy Nut, Clusters, Honey & Nut, Kellogg's*	1 Serving/40g	174	6.3	435	8.0	67.0	15.7	5.0
Crunchy Nut, Clusters, Milk Chocolate Curls, Kellogg's*	1 Serving/40g	183	7.2	458	8.0	66.0	18.0	4.0
Crunchy Nut, Clusters, Summer Berries, Kellogg's*	1 Serving/40g	176	6.0	439	8.0	68.0	15.0	5.0
Crunchy Nut, Corn Flakes, Kellogg's*	1 Serving/30g	118	1.2	392	6.0	83.0	4.0	2.5
Crunchy Nut, Red, Kellogg's*	1 Serving/40g	138	0.8	346	10.0	72.0	2.0	9.0
Crunchy Oat, Golden Sun*	1 Serving/50g	205	6.4	411	8.6	65.0	12.9	6.2
Crunchy Oat, with Raisins, Almonds & Fruit, Tesco*	1 Serving/50g	201	6.3	403	8.5	63.8	12.6	6.6
Crunchy Oats, with Tropical Fruits, Jordans*	1 Serving/75g	319	10.9	425	8.1	65.4	14.6	6.7
Curiously Cinnamon, Nestle*	1 Serving/30g	124	3.0	412	4.9	75.9	9.9	4.1
Fibre 1, Nestle*	1 Serving/40g	107	1.0	267	10.8	50.2	2.6	30.5
Fitnesse & Fruits, Nestle*	1 Serving/40g	148	0.4	370	6.6	83.4	1.1	3.4
Force, Nestle*	1 Serving/40g	138	0.9	344	10.6	70.3	2.3	9.2
Four Berry Crisp, Organic, Jordans*	1 Serving/50g	221	7.9	442	7.7	67.1	15.8	5.4
Frosted Flakes, Sainsbury's*	1 Serving/30g	112	0.1	374	4.9	87.8	0.4	2.4
Frosted Wheats, Kellogg's*	1 Serving/30g	104	0.6	346	10.0	72.0	2.0	9.0
Frosties, Caramel, Kellogg's*	1 Serving/30g	113	0.2	377	5.0	88.0	0.6	2.0
Frosties, Chocolate, Kellogg's*	1 Serving/40g	158	2.4	394	5.0	80.0	6.0	3.5
Frosties, Kellogg's*	1 Serving/30g	111	0.2	371	4.5	87.0	0.6	2.0
Frosties, Reduced Sugar, Kellogg's*	1 Serving/30g	111	0.2	369	6.0	85.0	0.6	2.5
Fruit & Fibre, Flakes, Waitrose*	1 Serving/40g	143	2.5	357	8.2	67.2	6.2	9.9
Fruit & Fibre, Organic, Sainsbury's*	1 Serving/40g	147	1.6	367	10.0	72.4	4.1	7.8
Fruit & Fibre, Whole Grain, Sainsbury's*	1 Serving/30g	108	1.8	361	8.1	68.7	6.0	8.9
Fruit & Nut Crisp, Minis, Weetabix*	1 Serving/40g	144	1.8	359	9.3	70.0	4.6	8.9
Fruit 'n' Fibre, Kellogg's*	1 Serving/40g	152	2.4	380	8.0	69.0	6.0	9.0
Fruit Nuts & Flakes, M & S*	1 Serving/30g	117	2.5	391	9.1	69.6	8.5	3.5
Golden Grahams, Nestle*	1 Serving/30g	112	0.9	375	6.0	81.0	3.0	3.4
Golden Honey Puffs, Tesco*	1 Serving/30g	115	0.4	382	6.6	86.3	1.2	3.0
Golden Nuggets, Nestle*	1 Serving/40g	152	0.3	381	6.2	87.4	0.7	1.5
Golden Puffs, Sainsbury's*	1 Serving/28g	107	0.3	383	6.6	86.3	1.2	3.0
Granola, Honey, Dorset Cereals*	1 Serving/40g	194	10.2	484	12.6	51.2	25.4	5.6
Granola, Low Fat, Home Farm*	1 Serving/55g	180	3.0	328	7.3	69.0	5.4	9.0

BREAKFAST CEREAL

	Measure INFO/WEIGHT	per Measure		Nutrition Values per 100g / 100ml				
		KCAL	FAT	KCAL	PROT	CARB	FAT	FIBRE
Granola, Original, Lizi's, The GoodCarb Food Company*	1 Serving/50g	248	14.6	496	10.9	46.2	29.3	10.6
Granola, Quinoa, Organic, Perfekt*	1 Serving/40g	186	6.6	466	12.4	48.5	16.4	8.9
Grape Nuts, Kraft*	1 Serving/45g	155	0.9	345	11.5	70.0	2.0	11.0
Harvest Crunch, Nut, Quaker Oats*	1 Serving/40g	184	7.8	459	8.0	62.5	19.5	6.0
Harvest Crunch, Real Red Berries, Quaker Oats*	1 Serving/50g	223	8.5	447	7.0	66.0	17.0	4.5
Harvest Crunch, Soft Juicy Raisins, Quaker Oats*	1 Serving/50g	221	8.0	442	6.0	67.0	16.0	4.0
High Fibre, Alpen*	1 Serving/45g	154	3.2	343	7.7	62.1	7.1	14.1
High Fibre Bran, Waitrose*	1 Serving/40g	112	1.5	281	14.4	47.2	3.8	26.0
High Fruit Muesli, BGTY, Sainsbury's*	1 Serving/50g	164	0.9	328	6.7	71.0	1.9	6.6
Honey, Oats & More, Nestle*	1 Serving/30g	114	1.6	379	9.7	73.1	5.3	5.9
Honey & Nut Crisp, Mini, Weetabix*	1 Serving/40g	150	0.8	375	9.4	75.1	2.0	9.3
Honey Loops, Kellogg's*	1 Serving/30g	110	0.9	367	8.0	77.0	3.0	6.0
Honey Nut & Flakes, M & S*	1 Serving/40g	164	3.5	411	9.8	73.4	8.7	2.6
Honey Raisin & Almond, Crunchy, Waitrose*	1 Serving/40g	170	4.8	425	10.5	68.8	12.0	5.7
Hooplas, Sainsbury's*	1 Serving/30g	112	1.1	375	6.5	78.6	3.8	4.6
Hoops, Multigrain, Asda*	1 Serving/30g	113	1.2	376	6.5	78.4	4.0	4.6
Hot Cereal, Flax O Meal*	1 Serving/40g	130	6.0	325	52.5	2.5	15.0	30.0
Hot Oats, Instant, Tesco*	1 Serving/30g	108	2.6	360	11.8	58.4	8.7	7.9
Just Right, Kellogg's*	1 Serving/40g	145	0.8	362	7.0	79.0	2.0	4.0
Krave, Chocolate & Hazelnut, Kellogg's*	1 Serving/30g	132	4.8	440	8.0	66.0	16.0	4.0
Lion, Nestle*	1 Serving/40g	166	3.1	415	7.2	76.9	7.7	4.3
Malt Crunchies, Co-Op*	1 Serving/50g	167	1.0	335	10.0	69.0	2.0	10.0
Malted Wheats, Waitrose*	1 Serving/32g	110	0.6	343	9.7	71.7	1.9	9.9
Malties, Sainsbury's*	1 Serving/40g	137	1.2	343	10.0	69.2	2.9	10.0
Maple & Pecan, Sainsbury's*	1 Serving/60g	318	13.2	530	13.3	69.7	22.0	5.3
Maple Frosted Flakes, Whole Earth*	1 Serving/30g	112	0.3	375	6.2	85.6	1.0	1.6
Millet Rice Oatbran Flakes, Nature's Path*	1 Serving/56g	204	3.2	365	11.3	67.0	5.8	10.0
Mini Wheats, Sainsbury's*	1 Serving/45g	157	1.0	348	11.8	69.9	2.3	11.8
Minibix, Weetabix*	1 Serving/40g	134	1.5	335	8.8	71.2	3.8	8.1
Muddles, Kellogg's*	1 Serving/30g	110	1.0	368	8.0	76.0	3.5	8.0
Muesli, Apricot, Traidcraft*	1 Serving/30g	103	1.8	344	8.0	68.0	6.0	5.0
Muesli, Berries & Cherries, Dorset Cereals*	1 Serving/70g	225	1.5	321	6.5	68.8	2.2	6.3
Muesli, Carb Control, Tesco*	1 Serving/35g	154	9.3	439	25.0	25.0	26.6	13.8
Muesli, COU, M & S*	1 Serving/60g	201	1.5	335	7.6	70.2	2.5	8.1
Muesli, Cranberry & Blueberry, Love Life, Waitrose*	1 Serving/50g	164	1.8	329	8.5	65.3	3.7	7.5
Muesli, Crunchy, Organic, Sainsbury's*	1 Serving/40g	168	5.8	420	10.6	62.0	14.4	9.2
Muesli, De Luxe, No Added Salt Or Sugar, Sainsbury's*	1 Serving/40g	161	5.6	403	11.9	57.6	13.9	8.4
Muesli, Flahavans*	1 Serving/52g	187	2.8	360	10.4	72.1	5.3	5.5
Muesli, Fruit, Luxury, Weight Watchers*	1 Serving/40g	127	0.8	318	7.2	67.7	2.0	8.1
Muesli, Fruit, Waitrose*	1 Serving/30g	101	1.4	338	7.2	66.8	4.7	6.8
Muesli, Fruit & Nut, Jordans*	1 Serving/50g	180	4.7	361	8.0	61.2	9.4	7.5
Muesli, Fruit & Nut, Luxury, Waitrose*	1 Serving/40g	145	3.8	363	9.0	60.3	9.5	6.5
Muesli, Fruit & Nut, M & S*	1 Serving/40g	128	1.1	320	7.4	74.5	2.8	7.4
Muesli, Fruit & Nut, Organic, M & S*	1 Serving/50g	166	3.0	333	8.2	61.6	6.0	7.6
Muesli, Fruit & Nut, Whole Wheat, Organic, Asda*	1 Serving/50g	171	3.5	343	10.0	60.0	7.0	7.0
Muesli, Fruit & Seeds, Organic, Pertwood Farm*	1 Serving/50g	164	3.3	328	11.4	55.5	6.7	12.6
Muesli, Fruit & Spice, Sainsbury's*	1 Serving/50g	184	3.4	368	7.4	69.4	6.8	7.7
Muesli, Fruit Sensation, M & S*	1 Serving/50g	157	1.5	315	6.0	66.0	3.0	7.4
Muesli, Fruity Fibre, Jordans*	1 Serving/50g	172	3.1	344	7.7	64.2	6.3	8.5
Muesli, Light & Crispy, Jordans*	1 Serving/50g	171	2.5	343	7.7	66.7	5.0	9.5
Muesli, Luxury, Finest, Tesco*	1 Serving/50g	197	6.5	394	8.3	60.8	13.1	5.4
Muesli, Luxury, Jordans*	1 Serving/40g	154	5.0	384	9.6	58.4	12.5	8.2
Muesli, Luxury Fruit, Perfectly Balanced, Waitrose*	1 Serving/50g	162	1.6	324	7.1	66.4	3.3	7.0

BREAKFAST CEREAL

	Measure INFO/WEIGHT	per Measure KCAL	FAT	Nutrition Values per 100g / 100ml KCAL	PROT	CARB	FAT	FIBRE
Muesli, Natural, No Added Sugar Or Salt, Jordans*	1 Serving/50g	160	2.3	321	8.9	60.7	4.7	5.2
Muesli, No Added Sugar, Waitrose*	1 Serving/40g	146	2.5	364	12.0	64.9	6.3	6.7
Muesli, No Added Sugar Or Salt, Organic, Jordans*	1 Serving/50g	175	4.4	350	9.2	58.4	8.8	9.3
Muesli, Organic, Waitrose*	1 Serving/50g	187	0.8	375	10.3	59.6	1.6	8.3
Muesli, Original, Holland & Barrett*	1 Serving/30g	105	2.5	351	11.1	61.2	8.4	7.1
Muesli, Peach & Vanilla, Sainsbury's*	1 Serving/50g	162	2.6	324	7.6	61.4	5.3	7.6
Muesli, Simply Delicious, Dorset Cereals*	1 Serving/70g	256	6.6	366	10.8	59.2	9.5	7.4
Muesli, Simply Fruity, Dorset Cereals*	1 Serving/75g	226	1.9	301	6.8	63.9	2.5	7.7
Muesli, Special, Fruit, Jordans*	1 Serving/50g	161	1.3	323	6.6	68.0	2.7	8.4
Muesli, Special, Jordans*	1 Serving/50g	183	5.3	366	7.9	59.5	10.7	8.5
Muesli, Special, Luxury Fruit & Nut, Goody*	1 Serving/50g	193	6.9	386	8.0	57.6	13.8	8.0
Muesli, Super Berry, Jordans*	1 Serving/50g	174	3.8	348	9.0	60.8	7.6	8.1
Muesli, Super High Fibre, Dorset Cereals*	1 Serving/70g	250	6.6	357	8.0	60.1	9.4	8.4
Muesli, Superfoods, Jordans*	1 Serving/50g	173	3.6	346	9.2	60.9	7.3	10.2
Muesli, Swiss Style, No Added Salt Or Sugar, Tesco*	1 Serving/50g	177	2.7	355	10.9	65.1	5.4	8.2
Muesli, Swiss Style, Organic, Whole Earth*	1 Serving/50g	172	3.5	344	9.2	60.8	7.1	11.3
Muesli, Swiss Style, Sainsbury's*	1 Serving/50g	180	2.9	361	9.2	68.1	5.8	7.1
Muesli, The Ultimate, Organic, Rude Health*	1 Serving/50g	163	4.5	326	10.8	50.5	9.0	12.3
Muesli, Tropical, Sainsbury's*	1 Serving/50g	182	3.4	365	6.5	69.4	6.8	6.4
Muesli, Tropical Fruit, Holland & Barrett*	1 Serving/60g	197	1.9	328	7.5	69.8	3.2	5.1
Muesli, Tropical Fruits, Jordans*	1 Serving/50g	164	1.4	329	6.9	68.7	2.9	7.1
Muesli, Twelve Fruit & Nut, Sainsbury's*	1 Serving/50g	166	2.3	332	8.1	64.2	4.7	7.8
Muesli, Unsweetened, M & S*	1 Serving/40g	129	1.1	322	8.1	68.0	2.7	9.4
Muesli, Whole Wheat, No Added Sugar & Salt, Tesco*	1 Serving/40g	154	5.0	386	9.5	59.1	12.4	7.4
Muesli, Whole Wheat, Organic, Asda*	1 Serving/50g	197	3.0	394	10.0	75.0	6.0	9.0
Muesli, Wild-Berry, Amaranth, Allos*	1 Serving/40g	160	4.2	401	12.5	63.3	10.6	4.3
Muesli Base, Wholesome, Waitrose*	1 Portion/50g	125	4.2	250	11.5	31.8	8.4	5.0
Muesli Mix, Perfect Start, Organic, The Food Doctor*	1 Serving/50g	196	7.1	392	12.1	55.5	14.2	7.1
Multi Fruit & Flake, COU, M & S*	1 Serving/39g	142	0.4	365	6.5	81.8	1.1	4.0
Multigrain, Fitnesse, Nestle*	1 Serving/30g	109	0.4	363	8.0	79.8	1.3	5.1
Multigrain Boulders, Tesco*	1 Serving/30g	112	0.4	375	8.2	82.3	1.3	3.6
No Added Sugar, Alpen*	1 Serving/40g	142	2.4	354	10.5	64.6	6.0	7.7
Nutty Crunch, Alpen*	1 Serving/40g	159	4.5	398	10.7	63.6	11.2	6.5
Nutty Crunch, Deliciously, M & S*	1 Serving/50g	238	11.2	476	8.8	59.6	22.5	4.4
Oat Bran, Crispies, Quaker Oats*	1 Serving/40g	153	2.6	383	11.0	69.0	6.5	9.0
Oat Crisp, Chocolate, Quaker Oats*	1 Serving/35g	135	3.9	385	10.2	57.5	11.1	12.4
Oat Crisp, Quaker Oats*	1 Serving/40g	154	2.6	385	12.0	61.0	6.5	14.0
Oat Crunchy, Blueberry & Cranberry, Waitrose*	1 Serving/60g	259	9.1	432	8.0	65.9	15.2	8.5
Oat Granola, Quaker Oats*	1 Serving/50g	205	4.4	411	8.6	73.0	8.8	5.2
Oat Krunchies, Quaker Oats*	1 Serving/30g	118	2.1	393	9.5	72.0	7.0	5.5
Oatbran & Oatgerm, Prewett's*	1 Serving/30g	103	2.9	345	14.8	49.7	9.7	15.2
Oatbran 100%, Mornflake*	1 Serving/40g	146	3.8	364	13.4	47.3	9.4	18.2
Oatbran Flakes, Nature's Path*	1 Serving/30g	124	1.4	414	8.7	83.0	4.7	6.7
Oatbran Sprinkles, Mornflake*	1 Serving/40g	146	3.8	364	13.4	47.3	9.4	18.2
Oatibix, Bitesize, Original, Weetabix*	1 Serving/36g	133	2.4	370	10.6	66.5	6.8	10.1
Oatibix, Flakes, Weetabix*	1 Serving/50g	190	2.8	381	9.5	73.2	5.6	3.5
Oatibix, Weetabix*	2 Biscuits/48g	181	3.8	377	12.5	63.7	8.0	7.3
Oatibix Bites, Cranberry, Weetabix*	1 Serving/40g	155	3.2	388	9.4	63.5	8.0	11.9
Oatiflakes, with Raisin, Cranberry & Apple, Weetabix*	1 Serving/40g	135	0.5	338	6.7	75.0	1.2	8.6
Oatmeal, Coarse, Prewett's*	1 Serving/40g	137	4.2	343	14.3	47.6	10.6	16.0
Oatmeal, Quick Oats, Dry, Quaker Oats*	1 Serving/30g	114	2.0	380	14.0	66.7	6.7	10.0
Oats, Apple Flavour, Instant, Hot, Waitrose*	1 Serving/36g	141	2.2	392	8.1	76.4	6.0	6.7
Oats, Apple Flavour, Micro, Tesco*	1 Sachet/36g	128	1.9	356	6.8	70.1	5.4	5.4

BREAKFAST CEREAL

	Measure INFO/WEIGHT	per Measure KCAL	FAT	Nutrition Values per 100g / 100ml KCAL	PROT	CARB	FAT	FIBRE
Oats, Golden Syrup Flavour, Instant, Hot, Waitrose*	1 Serving/39g	153	2.3	393	7.8	77.4	5.8	6.0
Oats, Jumbo, Organic, Waitrose*	1 Serving/50g	180	4.0	361	11.0	61.1	8.1	7.8
Oats, Original, Instant, Hot, Waitrose*	1 Sachet/27g	97	2.2	359	11.0	60.4	8.1	8.5
Oats, Superfast, Mornflake*	1 Serving/40g	144	3.2	359	11.0	60.4	8.1	8.5
Oats, Wholegrain, Organic, Quaker Oats*	1 Serving/25g	89	2.0	356	11.0	60.0	8.0	9.0
Optimum Power, Nature's Path*	1 Serving/30g	109	2.0	363	15.3	60.0	6.7	12.6
Optivita, Berry Oat Crisp, Kellogg's*	1 Serving/30g	107	1.5	357	10.0	68.0	5.0	9.0
Organic, Weetabix*	2 Biscuits/35g	116	0.8	331	10.9	66.8	2.2	11.0
Original, Crunchy, Raisins & Almonds, Jordans*	1 Serving/50g	203	6.4	407	8.7	64.0	12.9	6.6
Original, Crunchy, Tropical Fruits, Jordans*	1 Serving/50g	211	7.2	423	8.1	65.1	14.5	6.7
Original, Dry, Micro Oats, Tesco*	1 Sachet/27g	97	2.2	360	11.0	60.4	8.1	8.5
Original, Ready Brek*	1 Serving/40g	144	3.5	359	11.8	58.5	8.7	7.9
Original Granola, Diet Chef Ltd*	1 Pack/50g	248	14.6	496	10.9	46.2	29.3	10.6
Porage Oats, Old Fashioned, Dry, Scotts*	1 Serving/40g	142	3.2	355	11.0	60.0	8.0	9.0
Porage Oats, Original, Dry, Scotts*	1 Serving/40g	142	3.2	355	11.0	60.0	8.0	9.0
Porage Oats, Original, So-Easy, Dry, Scotts*	1 Serving/30g	109	2.5	364	11.0	60.0	8.5	9.0
Porage Oats, Syrup Swirl, So-Easy, Dry, Scotts*	1 Sachet/37g	135	2.2	366	8.0	70.0	6.0	6.5
Porridge, Apple, Sultana & Cinnamon, M & S*	1 Sachet/40g	144	3.0	360	10.3	62.3	7.5	8.6
Porridge, Chocolate, Oatibix, Weetabix*	1 Sachet/40g	149	3.9	372	9.9	61.3	9.7	6.2
Porridge, Free From, Sainsbury's*	1 Serving/50g	174	1.5	348	8.6	72.0	3.0	3.4
Porridge, Fruity, Apple & Raisin, Dorset Cereals*	1 Serving/70g	233	3.4	333	9.7	62.7	4.8	8.9
Porridge, Fruity, Fruit & Nut, Dorset Cereals*	1 Serving/70g	242	5.6	346	9.4	59.0	8.0	8.2
Porridge, Fruity, Mixed Berries, Dorset Cereals*	1 Serving/70g	243	4.2	347	10.8	62.6	6.0	7.9
Porridge, Golden Honey, Oatibix, Weetabix*	1 Serving/40g	145	2.6	363	9.2	66.7	6.6	7.0
Porridge, Instant, Quaker Oats*	1 Serving/34g	124	2.9	364	11.0	60.0	8.5	9.0
Porridge, Made with Semi Skimmed Milk, Waitrose*	1 Serving/50g	277	7.5	554	24.6	80.4	15.0	8.6
Porridge, Manuka Honey & Apricot, Vogel*	1 Packet/35g	122	1.0	349	10.1	66.3	2.9	7.1
Porridge, Multigrain, Jordans*	1 Serving/40g	134	2.2	335	10.4	60.9	5.5	10.0
Porridge, Oats, Golden Syrup, Sainsbury's*	1 Sachet/39g	143	2.1	367	6.3	73.6	5.3	6.7
Porridge, Original, Dry, Oat So Simple, Quaker Oats*	1 Serving/27g	98	2.3	364	11.0	60.0	8.5	9.0
Porridge, Original, Oatibix, Weetabix*	1 Sachet/30g	104	2.5	347	12.5	55.6	8.3	10.1
Porridge, Original, Simply Porridge, Asda*	1 Sachet/27g	96	2.2	356	11.0	60.0	8.0	8.0
Porridge, Perfectly, Dorset Cereals*	1 Sachet/30g	107	2.5	356	11.8	58.2	8.4	11.0
Porridge, Raspberry, Dry, Oat So Simple, Quaker Oats*	1 Sachet/35g	127	2.3	364	8.8	67.1	6.5	7.2
Porridge, Real Fruit, Raisin & Apple, Jordans*	1 Serving/40g	133	2.7	332	9.1	58.8	6.7	7.4
Porridge, Real Fruit, Sultana & Apricot, Jordans*	1 Sachet/40g	127	2.3	317	8.5	57.7	5.8	7.2
Porridge, Spiced Apple, Sultana, Oatibix, Weetabix*	1 Sachet/40g	138	2.3	345	9.7	65.4	5.7	8.5
Porridge, Superfoods, Jordans*	1 Serving/40g	145	3.6	362	10.4	59.8	9.0	8.3
Porridge, Swt Cinnamon, Oat So Simple, Quaker Oats*	1 Serving/33g	120	2.2	365	9.0	67.2	6.6	7.4
Porridge, Take Heart, Quaker Oats*	1 Serving/32g	194	5.7	606	30.9	80.3	17.8	7.8
Porridge Flakes, Organic, Barkat*	1 Serving/30g	109	0.9	362	8.5	74.1	3.0	0.0
Porridge Oats, Blueberry, Paw Ridge, Quaker Oats*	1 Sachet/28g	107	2.0	376	9.7	64.4	7.0	8.1
Porridge Oats, Honey, Paw Ridge, Quaker Oats*	1 Sachet/29g	103	2.0	361	9.6	64.7	7.0	7.9
Porridge Oats, Mornflake*	1 Serving/50g	179	4.0	359	11.0	60.4	8.1	8.5
Porridge Oats, Organic, Evernat*	1 Serving/40g	167	3.8	418	13.0	69.0	9.6	7.4
Porridge Oats, Organic, Jordans*	1 Serving/40g	146	3.7	364	11.7	58.4	9.3	9.0
Porridge Oats, Organic, Tesco*	1 Serving/28g	100	2.3	358	11.0	60.4	8.1	8.5
Porridge Oats, Original, Paw Ridge, Quaker Oats*	1 Sachet/25g	89	2.0	356	11.0	60.0	8.0	9.0
Porridge Oats, Quaker Oats*	1 Serving/45g	160	3.6	356	11.0	60.0	8.0	4.0
Porridge Oats, Rolled, Tesco*	1 Serving/50g	179	4.0	359	11.0	60.4	8.1	8.5
Porridge Oats, Scottish, Organic, Sainsbury's*	1 Serving/45g	172	2.2	383	10.0	74.4	5.0	7.9
Porridge Oats, Scottish, Tesco*	1 Serving/50g	179	4.0	359	11.0	60.4	8.1	8.5
Porridge Oats, Whole Oats, Jordans*	1 Serving/40g	146	3.7	364	11.7	58.4	9.3	9.0

B

BREAKFAST CEREAL

	Measure INFO/WEIGHT	per Measure		Nutrition Values per 100g / 100ml				
		KCAL	FAT	KCAL	PROT	CARB	FAT	FIBRE
Porridge Oats, with Bran, Scottish, Sainsbury's*	1 Serving/50g	190	2.5	380	9.6	74.1	5.0	10.3
Porridge Oats, with Oat & Wheat Bran, HL, Tesco*	1 Sachet/30g	105	1.8	350	10.8	62.3	6.1	9.2
Porridge Oats, with Wheat Bran, Tesco*	1 Serving/50g	167	3.6	334	12.3	55.0	7.2	13.0
Porridge Oats, with Wheat Bran, Waitrose*	1 Serving/50g	168	3.8	336	11.2	55.8	7.6	13.0
Precise, Sainsbury's*	1 Serving/40g	148	1.2	371	6.4	79.9	2.9	3.5
Puffed Rice, Organic, Natural, Kallo*	1 Bowl/25g	92	0.5	370	7.0	81.0	2.0	3.0
Puffed Rice, Wholegrain, Brown, Organic, Kallo*	1 Serving/25g	95	0.7	380	8.0	80.0	3.0	9.0
Puffed Rice Cereal, Honey, Organic, Kallo*	1 Serving/25g	98	0.9	392	5.0	85.0	3.5	2.1
Puffed Wheat, Quaker Oats*	1 Serving/15g	49	0.2	328	15.3	62.4	1.3	5.6
Puffed Wheat, Tesco*	1 Serving/28g	104	0.9	373	13.9	72.2	3.2	5.7
Quaker Oats Crunch, Quaker Oats*	1 Serving/40g	146	2.0	366	9.1	71.1	5.0	7.4
Quinoa, Flaked, Organic, Morning, Organic, Big OZ*	1 Serving/100g	344	7.1	344	13.6	55.7	7.1	11.5
Raisin, Bran Flakes, Asda*	1 Serving/50g	165	1.5	331	7.0	69.0	3.0	10.0
Raisin, Honey & Almond Crunch, Asda*	1 Serving/60g	238	6.8	397	8.8	64.8	11.4	7.4
Raisin, Oats and More, Nestle*	1 Serving/30g	112	1.4	373	8.9	73.7	4.7	5.8
Raisin & Almond, Crunchy, Jordans*	1 Serving/56g	230	7.0	411	8.4	66.0	12.5	5.0
Raisin & Coconut, Crunchy, Organic, Jordans*	1 Serving/50g	206	6.7	412	8.4	64.2	13.5	7.1
Raisin Wheats, Kellogg's*	1 Serving/30g	99	0.6	330	9.0	70.0	2.0	8.0
Raisin Wheats, Sainsbury's*	1 Serving/50g	166	0.7	332	8.2	71.5	1.5	8.0
Raspberry Crisp, Mornflake*	1 Serving/50g	214	7.1	428	6.5	68.2	14.3	6.8
Ready Brek, Banana, Weetabix*	1 Serving/40g	146	2.6	365	8.9	68.0	6.4	6.7
Ready Brek, Chocolate, Porridge Oats, Weetabix*	1 Serving/30g	108	2.2	361	9.9	64.2	7.2	6.6
Ready Brek, Original, Weetabix*	1 Serving/40g	158	3.5	395	11.8	58.4	8.7	7.9
Red Berry & Almond Luxury Crunch, Jordans*	1 Serving/40g	176	7.4	441	8.2	60.5	18.5	6.6
Rice & Wheat Flake, Special Choice, Waitrose*	1 Serving/30g	111	0.4	370	11.4	77.7	1.5	3.2
Rice Krispies, Honey, Kellogg's*	1 Serving/30g	114	0.2	380	4.0	89.0	0.7	1.0
Rice Krispies, Kellogg's*	1 Serving/30g	115	0.3	383	6.0	87.0	1.0	1.0
Rice Krispies, Multi-Grain Shapes, Kellogg's*	1 Serving/30g	111	0.7	370	8.0	77.0	2.5	8.0
Rice Pops, Blue Parrot Cafe, Sainsbury's*	1 Serving/30g	111	0.4	370	7.2	82.3	1.3	2.2
Rice Pops, Organic, Dove's Farm*	1 Serving/30g	107	0.2	357	6.8	86.1	0.8	2.0
Rice Pops, Sainsbury's*	1 Serving/30g	114	0.4	381	7.4	84.8	1.3	1.5
Rice Snaps, Asda*	1 Serving/28g	105	0.4	376	7.0	84.0	1.3	1.5
Rice Snaps, Harvest Home, Nestle*	1 Serving/25g	94	0.3	378	7.4	84.2	1.3	1.5
Rice Snaps, Tesco*	1 Serving/35g	135	0.5	385	7.4	84.8	1.3	1.5
Ricicles, Kellogg's*	1 Serving/30g	114	0.2	381	4.5	89.0	0.8	0.8
Right Balance, Morrisons*	1 Serving/50g	181	1.1	362	6.9	78.6	2.2	5.3
Shredded Wheat, 100% Whole Grain, Nestle*	2 Biscuits/45g	153	1.1	340	11.6	67.8	2.5	11.8
Shredded Wheat, Bitesize, Nestle*	1 Serving/45g	157	1.2	350	11.8	69.9	2.6	11.9
Shredded Wheat, Fruitful, No Added Salt, Nestle*	1 Serving/40g	142	2.0	354	8.3	68.7	5.1	8.9
Shredded Wheat, Honey Nut, Nestle*	1 Serving/40g	151	2.6	378	11.2	68.8	6.5	9.4
Shredded Wheat, Triple Berry, Nestle*	1 Serving/40g	138	0.8	344	10.6	70.6	2.1	11.1
Shreddies, Coco, Nestle*	1 Serving/45g	161	0.9	358	8.4	76.5	2.0	8.6
Shreddies, Frosted, Kellogg's*	1 Serving/50g	161	0.9	323	0.7	78.5	1.8	4.7
Shreddies, Frosted, Nestle*	1 Serving/45g	164	0.7	365	7.4	80.7	1.5	6.4
Shreddies, Frosted, Variety Pack, Nestle*	1 Pack/45g	163	0.6	363	6.7	81.1	1.3	6.8
Shreddies, Honey, Nestle*	1 Serving/45g	169	0.7	375	8.2	78.1	1.5	8.1
Shreddies, Malt Wheats, Tesco*	1 Serving/45g	151	0.9	335	8.3	70.7	2.1	9.7
Shreddies, Nestle*	1 Serving/45g	185	0.9	371	10.0	73.7	1.9	9.9
Smoothies, Strawberry, Quaker Oats*	1 Sachet/29g	117	3.5	402	6.5	67.0	12.0	5.5
Special Crunchy Luxury, Jordans*	1 Serving/50g	205	6.9	411	7.6	63.8	13.9	6.5
Special Crunchy Luxury, Maple & Pecan, Jordans*	1 Serving/50g	220	8.6	440	9.5	61.6	17.3	7.2
Special Flakes, Tesco*	1 Serving/20g	74	0.3	371	11.0	78.4	1.5	4.3
Special K, Bliss, Creamy Berry Crunch, Kellogg's*	1 Serving/30g	114	0.7	379	13.0	76.0	2.5	2.5

	Measure INFO/WEIGHT	per Measure KCAL	FAT	Nutrition Values per 100g / 100ml KCAL	PROT	CARB	FAT	FIBRE
BREAKFAST CEREAL								
Special K, Bliss, Strawberry & Chocolate, Kellogg's*	1 Serving/30g	115	0.9	383	13.0	76.0	3.0	2.5
Special K, Choco, Kellogg's*	1 Serving/40g	160	2.8	400	14.0	70.0	7.0	3.5
Special K, Kellogg's*	1 Serving/30g	112	0.3	373	16.0	75.0	1.0	2.5
Special K, Oats & Honey, Kellogg's*	1 Serving/50g	191	1.2	383	13.0	77.0	2.5	3.0
Special K, Peach & Apricot, Kellogg's*	1 Serving/30g	112	0.3	373	14.0	77.0	1.0	2.5
Special K, Protein Plus, Kellogg's*	1 Serving/29g	100	3.0	345	34.5	31.0	10.3	17.2
Special K, Purple Berries, Kellogg's*	1 Serving/30g	112	0.3	374	13.0	77.0	1.0	3.5
Special K, Red Berries, Kellogg's*	1 Serving/30g	112	0.4	374	14.0	76.0	1.5	3.0
Special K, Yoghurty, Kellogg's*	1 Serving/30g	115	0.9	383	14.0	75.0	3.0	2.5
Special K Clusters, Honey, Kellogg's*	1 Serving/45g	175	1.3	389	9.0	80.0	3.0	3.5
Start, Kellogg's*	1 Serving/30g	112	0.7	375	8.0	80.0	2.5	5.0
Start Right, Asda*	1 Serving/40g	150	2.4	376	8.0	74.0	6.0	5.0
Strawberry, Alpen*	1 Serving/40g	144	1.9	359	9.4	69.5	4.8	7.9
Strawberry & Almond Crunch, M & S*	1 Serving/40g	186	7.4	465	8.0	66.0	18.6	4.9
Sugar Puffs, Quaker Oats*	1 Serving/30g	114	0.5	379	5.3	85.8	1.6	3.7
Sultana Bran, Asda*	1 Serving/30g	98	0.9	327	9.0	66.0	3.0	11.0
Sultana Bran, Co-Op*	1 Serving/40g	130	1.2	325	9.0	66.0	3.0	11.0
Sultana Bran, HL, Tesco*	1 Serving/30g	97	0.6	325	8.2	68.0	1.9	12.0
Sultana Bran, Morrisons*	1 Serving/30g	97	0.9	325	8.8	65.8	3.0	11.4
Sultana Bran, Sainsbury's*	1 Serving/30g	97	0.6	324	8.2	68.6	1.9	11.6
Sultana Bran, Waitrose*	1 Serving/30g	97	0.6	324	8.2	68.6	1.9	11.6
Swt Cinnamon, Express, Oat So Simple, Quaker Oats*	1 Pot/57g	214	3.0	375	14.4	64.9	5.3	5.6
Toasted Multi-Grain Flakes, & Apple, Weight Watchers*	1 Serving/30g	97	0.3	323	10.4	67.8	1.1	14.4
Toffee Flavour, Oat So Simple, Quaker Oats*	1 Serving/30g	122	3.9	407	6.5	66.0	13.0	5.0
Treacle & Pecan, Granola, Diet Chef Ltd*	1 Pack/40g	196	11.3	490	9.7	47.6	28.3	11.3
Triple Chocolate Crisp, Sainsbury's*	1 Serving/40g	180	7.3	451	7.7	63.8	18.3	6.0
Ultra Bran, Soya & Linseed, Vogel*	1 Serving/45g	117	0.8	260	15.3	45.3	1.8	33.3
Vitality, Asda*	1 Serving/30g	111	0.4	370	11.0	78.0	1.5	3.2
Vitality, with Red Fruit, Asda*	1 Serving/30g	110	0.5	366	11.0	77.0	1.6	3.8
Vitality, with Tropical Fruit, Asda*	1 Serving/30g	112	1.5	373	9.0	73.0	5.0	4.9
Weet Bix, Oat Bran, Sanitarium*	2 Biscuits/40g	156	1.0	390	12.8	71.9	2.5	11.7
Weet Bix, Sanitarium*	2 Biscuits/30g	106	0.4	352	12.0	67.0	1.4	10.5
Weetabix, Chocolate, Weetabix*	2 Biscuits/45g	156	1.8	346	10.6	66.6	4.1	10.5
Weetabix*	1 Biscuit/19g	63	0.4	338	11.5	68.4	2.0	10.0
Weetaflakes, Raisin, Cranberry & Apple, Weetabix*	1 Serving/40g	135	0.5	338	6.7	75.0	1.2	8.6
Weetaflakes, Weetabix*	1 Serving/30g	102	0.4	340	8.9	72.9	1.4	11.0
Weetos, Chocolate, Weetabix*	1 Serving/30g	113	1.5	378	8.4	75.1	4.9	5.8
Wheat Biscuits, Sainsbury's*	2 Biscuits/36g	123	0.7	342	11.5	68.4	2.0	10.0
Wheat Flakes, Alpen*	1 Serving/40g	140	1.0	350	10.2	72.0	2.4	9.0
Wheat Flakes, Malted, Toasted, Suma*	1 Serving/75g	259	1.4	346	10.3	72.0	1.9	10.4
Wheats, Mini, Maple & Brown Sugar, Sainsbury's*	1 Serving/52g	99	0.5	190	4.0	44.0	1.0	5.0
Whole Wheat Biscuits, Organic, Dove's Farm*	1 Serving/30g	99	0.8	329	11.0	65.0	2.8	11.0
Whole Wheat Biscuits, Waitrose*	2 Biscuits/37g	124	0.7	336	11.8	68.0	1.9	10.1
Wholegrain, Apricot, Wheats, Sainsbury's*	1 Serving/50g	160	0.7	320	7.9	71.6	1.5	8.2
Wholegrain, Fruit & Fibre, Sainsbury's*	1 Serving/40g	109	1.8	363	8.1	69.1	6.0	8.9
Wholegrain, Sultana Bran, Sainsbury's*	1 Serving/30g	97	0.6	325	8.3	68.6	1.9	12.1
BRESAOLA								
Della Valtellina, Sainsbury's*	1 Slice/14g	23	0.4	163	34.7	0.1	2.6	0.1
Finest, Tesco*	1 Serving/35g	64	1.4	182	36.0	0.5	4.0	0.0
BROCCOLI								
Green, Boiled, Average	*1 Serving/80g*	*19*	*0.6*	*24*	*3.1*	*1.1*	*0.8*	*2.3*
Green, Raw, Average	*1 Serving/80g*	*25*	*0.6*	*31*	*3.7*	*2.1*	*0.8*	*2.4*
Purple Sprouting, Boiled, Average	*1 Serving/80g*	*15*	*0.5*	*19*	*2.1*	*1.3*	*0.6*	*2.3*

B

	Measure INFO/WEIGHT	per Measure KCAL	FAT	Nutrition Values per 100g / 100ml KCAL	PROT	CARB	FAT	FIBRE
BROCCOLI								
Purple Sprouting, Raw	*1oz/28g*	*10*	*0.3*	*35*	*3.9*	*2.6*	*1.1*	*3.5*
Purple Sprouting, Raw, Spears, TTD, Sainsbury's*	1 Serving/100g	36	1.1	36	3.9	2.6	1.1	3.5
Steamed, Average	1 Serving/100g	24	0.8	24	3.1	1.1	0.8	2.3
BROWNIES								
Average	1 Brownie/60g	243	10.1	405	4.6	0.0	16.8	0.0
Chocolate, Bites, Mini, Weight Watchers*	1 Brownie/9g	29	0.5	325	5.3	63.7	5.5	2.2
Chocolate, Cadbury*	1 Brownie/36g	145	5.7	403	6.1	59.7	15.8	0.0
Chocolate, Chewy, M & S*	1 Brownie/29g	130	6.0	455	6.5	59.8	21.1	2.0
Chocolate, Chunky, Belgian, M & S*	1 Brownie/55g	242	11.2	440	6.2	57.7	20.3	2.5
Chocolate, Fudgy, M & S*	1 Brownie/87g	400	21.9	460	4.8	56.9	25.2	3.0
Chocolate, Slices, M & S*	1 Brownie/36g	158	8.7	440	5.3	51.1	24.1	1.3
Chocolate, Tray Bake, Tesco*	1 Brownie/37g	155	6.8	420	5.5	57.1	18.4	5.7
Chocolate, Waitrose*	1 Brownie/45g	192	8.9	426	6.3	55.6	19.8	2.7
Chocolate, Weight Watchers*	1 Brownie/47g	143	1.8	304	4.8	62.5	3.8	3.2
Chocolate & Pecan, Gu*	1 Brownie/45g	200	12.0	444	6.7	44.4	26.6	5.0
BRUSCHETTA								
Cheese & Tomato, Asda*	1 Serving/38g	68	1.7	180	8.6	26.0	4.6	2.9
Pane Italia*	1 Serving/75g	367	18.8	489	12.4	53.6	25.1	1.4
Ploughman's Relish, Brunchetta, Golden Vale*	1 Pack/90g	261	15.5	290	14.2	20.2	17.2	1.6
Red Pepper & Onion, Brunchetta, Golden Vale*	1 Pack/90g	266	17.1	296	14.6	17.0	19.0	1.3
Soft Cheese & Cranberry, Brunchetta, Golden Vale*	1 Pack/95g	200	8.5	211	8.2	24.8	9.0	1.3
Toasted, Olive Oil & Sea Salt, Tesco*	1 Serving/30g	126	4.6	420	11.5	58.7	15.5	4.5
BRUSSELS SPROUTS								
& Sweet Chestnuts, Asda*	1 Serving/100g	73	1.7	73	3.1	11.0	1.7	4.2
Boiled, Average	*1 Serving/90g*	*31*	*1.2*	*35*	*3.1*	*3.2*	*1.3*	*3.5*
Button, & Chestnuts, Tesco*	1 Serving/100g	80	1.8	80	3.1	12.8	1.8	4.1
Button, Raw, Average	*1 Serving/80g*	*30*	*1.1*	*37*	*3.5*	*2.9*	*1.3*	*3.2*
Canned, Drained	*1oz/28g*	*8*	*0.3*	*28*	*2.6*	*2.4*	*1.0*	*2.6*
Frozen, Morrisons*	1 Serving/200g	70	2.6	35	3.5	2.5	1.3	4.3
Raw, Average	*1 Serving/80g*	*29*	*0.9*	*37*	*3.5*	*3.3*	*1.1*	*3.0*
Steamed, Average	1 Serving/100g	35	1.3	35	3.1	3.2	1.3	3.5
BUBBLE & SQUEAK								
Aunt Bessie's*	1 Serving/100g	145	7.1	145	2.7	17.5	7.1	1.3
Fried in Vegetable Oil	1oz/28g	35	2.5	124	1.4	9.8	9.1	1.5
Morrisons*	1 Serving/110g	168	9.6	153	2.2	16.3	8.7	0.7
Tesco*	½ Pack/325g	292	12.7	90	1.6	11.3	3.9	0.9
Waitrose*	½ Pack/225g	166	5.2	74	1.4	11.9	2.3	2.2
BUCKWHEAT								
Average	*1oz/28g*	*102*	*0.4*	*364*	*8.1*	*84.9*	*1.5*	*2.1*
BUFFALO								
Mince, Raw, Lean, Abel & Cole*	1 Serving/100g	95	0.7	95	21.7	0.4	0.7	0.0
BULGAR WHEAT								
Dry, Love Life, Waitrose*	1oz/28g	108	0.6	384	14.8	72.2	2.3	7.4
Dry Weight, Average	*1oz/28g*	*99*	*0.5*	*353*	*9.7*	*76.3*	*1.7*	*8.0*
BULGUR WHEAT								
Wholefoods, Tesco*	1 Serving/50g	180	0.8	360	9.7	76.3	1.7	9.1
BUNS								
Bath, M & S*	1 Bun/71g	217	5.7	305	8.3	49.8	8.0	1.9
Bath, Tesco*	1 Bun/80g	262	8.9	327	8.0	48.9	11.1	5.7
Belgian, Asda*	1 Bun/133g	464	19.9	350	4.8	49.0	15.0	2.2
Belgian, Co-Op*	1 Bun/118g	413	15.3	350	5.0	54.0	13.0	2.0
Belgian, Iced, Chosen By You, Asda*	1 Bun/115g	375	6.8	327	6.1	62.3	5.9	2.9
Belgian, Sainsbury's*	1 Bun/110g	398	11.3	362	6.1	61.3	10.3	1.9

	Measure	per Measure		Nutrition Values per 100g / 100ml				
	INFO/WEIGHT	KCAL	FAT	KCAL	PROT	CARB	FAT	FIBRE
BUNS								
Belgian, Tesco*	1 Bun/123g	438	15.7	356	5.2	54.9	12.8	2.2
Chelsea	1 Bun/78g	285	10.8	366	7.8	56.1	13.8	1.7
Chelsea, Sainsbury's*	1 Bun/85g	239	4.4	281	6.9	51.6	5.2	2.9
Chelsea, Tesco*	1 Bun/85g	269	6.5	316	7.9	53.9	7.6	2.3
Choux, Caramel, Asda*	1 Bun/189g	745	51.0	394	4.3	33.5	27.0	1.3
Choux, Custard, M & S*	1 Bun/85g	234	18.7	275	4.2	15.0	22.0	0.3
Choux, Fresh Cream, Tesco*	1 Bun/95g	340	23.7	358	4.9	28.5	24.9	0.9
Choux, M & S*	1 Bun/78g	247	17.3	317	5.4	25.6	22.2	0.3
Currant	1 Bun/60g	178	4.5	296	7.6	52.7	7.5	0.0
Currant, HL, Tesco*	1 Bun/63g	159	1.6	252	7.1	50.2	2.5	2.4
Currant, Sainsbury's*	1 Bun/72g	197	3.7	274	7.0	50.0	5.1	2.8
Fingers, Sticky, Iced, Chosen By You, Asda*	1 Bun/40g	132	2.4	330	7.1	62.0	5.9	2.7
Fruit, Waitrose*	1 Bun/54g	155	2.3	287	8.1	54.0	4.3	1.6
Hot Cross	1 Bun/50g	156	3.5	312	7.4	58.5	7.0	1.7
Hot Cross, Apple & Cinnamon, Large, Finest, Tesco*	1 Bun/117g	342	8.2	292	7.3	49.9	7.0	3.6
Hot Cross, Apple & Cinnamon, M & S*	1 Bun/71g	170	1.2	240	7.6	48.7	1.7	3.1
Hot Cross, Best of Both, Hovis*	1 Bun/65g	185	4.3	285	9.1	47.3	6.6	4.4
Hot Cross, BGTY, Sainsbury's*	1 Bun/70g	160	1.6	229	7.6	44.4	2.3	2.7
Hot Cross, Chocolate, Mini, Sainsbury's*	1 Bun/39g	127	4.4	325	7.7	48.1	11.3	2.5
Hot Cross, Chocolate & Raisin, Mini, Tesco*	1 Bun/40g	127	4.4	318	8.1	47.0	10.9	2.8
Hot Cross, Golden Wholemeal, 3% Fat, M & S*	1 Bun/67g	144	1.5	215	8.9	39.6	2.2	6.7
Hot Cross, Golden Wholemeal, Sainsbury's*	1 Bun/65g	180	4.0	277	9.9	45.4	6.2	4.3
Hot Cross, Less Than 3% Fat, M & S*	1 Bun/70g	175	1.3	250	8.1	49.8	1.8	2.2
Hot Cross, Luxury, M & S*	1 Bun/79g	201	3.2	255	8.6	46.2	4.0	2.1
Hot Cross, Mini, M & S*	1 Bun/41g	110	1.4	265	7.8	51.4	3.4	3.7
Hot Cross, Wholemeal, Waitrose*	1 Bun/64g	177	4.3	276	8.8	45.2	6.7	4.9
Iced, Filled with Raspberry Jam, M & S*	1 Bun/48g	155	3.2	320	6.4	58.9	6.6	1.9
Iced, Fingers, Coconut, Genesis Crafty*	1 Bun/64g	210	6.9	328	7.7	52.4	10.8	2.4
Iced, Spiced Fruit, M & S*	1 Bun/90g	270	3.3	300	7.0	60.3	3.7	1.5
Iced Finger, Tesco*	1 Bun/41g	115	1.4	280	7.1	54.7	3.4	2.9
Iced Lemon, Tesco*	1 Bun/48g	156	4.2	325	5.2	56.5	8.7	1.9
Marlborough, M & S*	1 Bun/71g	215	6.3	305	6.2	43.4	8.9	2.2
Spiced, Perfectly Balanced, Waitrose*	1 Bun/65g	177	2.2	272	8.0	52.3	3.4	2.9
Swiss, Tesco*	1 Bun/100g	334	11.9	334	4.0	52.8	11.9	1.4
Vanilla Iced, Soft, M & S*	1 Bun/39g	125	3.1	320	7.6	54.9	8.0	2.9
White Hot Cross, Sainsbury's*	1 Bun/70g	187	3.6	267	7.5	47.5	5.2	3.9
BURGERS								
American Style, Asda*	1 Burger/42g	156	10.8	374	25.0	10.0	26.0	1.1
American Style, Tesco*	1 Burger/125g	250	9.1	200	13.0	20.4	7.3	3.9
Beef, 100%, Birds Eye*	1 Burger/41g	120	10.2	292	17.3	0.0	24.8	0.0
Beef, 100%, Half Pounders, Sainsbury's*	1 Burger/148g	462	33.1	313	26.0	1.7	22.4	0.2
Beef, 100%, Mega, Birds Eye*	1 Burger/96g	280	23.8	293	17.3	0.0	24.9	0.0
Beef, 100%, Organic, Waitrose*	1 Burger/57g	140	9.6	247	23.6	0.0	16.9	0.0
Beef, 100%, Quarter Pounders, Aldi*	1 Burger/114g	320	23.3	282	24.3	0.1	20.5	1.3
Beef, 100%, Quarter Pounders, Ross*	1 Burger/74g	222	18.8	301	16.8	1.1	25.5	0.0
Beef, 100%, Sainsbury's*	1 Burger/44g	133	10.4	302	21.4	0.9	23.6	0.9
Beef, 100%, with Seasoning, No Onion, Birds Eye*	1 Burger/41g	134	11.9	326	16.1	0.2	29.0	0.0
Beef, 100%, without Onion, Sainsbury's*	1 Burger/43g	133	10.4	308	21.9	0.8	24.1	0.8
Beef, 100% Pure, Ross*	1 Burger/56g	128	9.6	229	17.1	1.4	17.1	0.0
Beef, Aberdeen Angus, ¼ Pounder, TTD, Sainsbury's*	1 Burger/91g	258	15.6	284	29.9	2.4	17.2	0.5
Beef, Aberdeen Angus, Asda*	1 Burger/112g	249	13.3	222	22.2	6.7	11.8	0.9
Beef, Aberdeen Angus, Fresh, Waitrose*	1 Burger/113g	269	21.0	238	16.4	1.2	18.6	0.0
Beef, Aberdeen Angus, Gourmet, Finest, Tesco*	1 Burger/118g	225	13.4	190	18.9	2.0	11.3	1.0

B

BURGERS

	Measure INFO/WEIGHT	per Measure KCAL	FAT	Nutrition Values per 100g / 100ml KCAL	PROT	CARB	FAT	FIBRE
Beef, Aberdeen Angus, M & S*	1 Burger/142g	298	18.9	210	18.3	4.1	13.3	0.1
Beef, Aberdeen Angus, Mega, Birds Eye*	1 Burger/101g	279	22.6	276	16.3	2.4	22.4	0.1
Beef, Aberdeen Angus, Virgin Trains*	1 Burger/240g	695	37.6	290	13.5	23.8	15.7	0.0
Beef, Asda*	1 Burger/114g	304	18.6	267	26.8	3.2	16.3	0.7
Beef, Barbecue, Tesco*	1 Burger/114g	295	22.7	260	15.6	3.5	20.0	0.5
Beef, BGTY, Sainsbury's*	1 Burger/110g	177	6.0	161	20.8	7.1	5.5	1.1
Beef, British, Finest, Tesco*	1 Burger/95g	185	11.8	195	17.2	3.3	12.4	0.9
Beef, British, Organic, Waitrose*	1 Burger/85g	226	16.6	266	19.0	3.5	19.5	1.0
Beef, British, Waitrose*	1 Burger/113g	279	21.0	247	18.6	1.2	18.6	0.0
Beef, Chargrill, Tesco*	1 Burger/114g	246	18.4	217	17.0	0.8	16.2	2.5
Beef, Chargrilled, Quarter Pounder, Morrisons*	1 Burger/227g	590	45.2	260	15.0	5.3	19.9	0.2
Beef, Filled with Gorgonzola, M & S*	1 Burger/167g	384	26.9	230	16.5	4.9	16.1	0.5
Beef, Flame Grilled, Dalepak*	1 Burger/44g	134	11.4	304	15.3	2.1	26.0	0.4
Beef, Mega, Birds Eye*	1 Burger/109g	300	25.1	275	14.3	2.7	23.0	0.3
Beef, Morrisons*	1 Burger/57g	169	14.3	298	12.3	5.5	25.2	0.6
Beef, New York Style, Grilled, Tesco*	1 Burger/35g	80	5.2	229	18.6	5.7	14.9	0.6
Beef, Organic, M & S*	1 Burger/110g	239	17.6	217	18.2	0.0	16.0	0.2
Beef, Original & Best, Birds Eye*	1 Burger/46g	115	8.9	252	14.1	5.1	19.5	0.4
Beef, Original with Onion, Birds Eye*	1 Burger/38g	110	9.5	287	13.4	2.6	24.8	0.3
Beef, Quarter Pounder, & Onion, BGTY, Sainsbury's*	1 Burger/83g	171	7.8	205	26.6	3.8	9.3	0.9
Beef, Quarter Pounder, Chilled, Morrisons*	1 Burger/115g	228	13.9	198	17.2	4.4	12.1	0.2
Beef, Quarter Pounder, with Onion, Cooked, Birds Eye*	1 Burger/100g	230	16.0	230	16.0	5.9	16.0	0.4
Beef, Quarter Pounders, Flame Grilled, Rustlers*	1 Burger/190g	557	28.7	293	14.9	24.3	15.1	0.0
Beef, Quarter Pounders, Flame Grilled, Tesco*	1 Burger/88g	246	20.4	280	13.1	4.8	23.2	0.8
Beef, Quarter Pounders, Morrisons*	1 Burger/114g	338	28.6	298	12.3	5.5	25.2	0.6
Beef, Quarter Pounders, Reduced Fat, Tesco*	1 Burger/95g	171	12.3	180	14.0	1.8	13.0	0.8
Beef, Quarter Pounders, Steak Country*	1 Burger/68g	188	15.1	276	16.3	2.4	22.2	0.1
Beef, Quarter Pounders, Tesco*	1 Burger/113g	292	23.1	258	17.8	0.7	20.4	1.3
Beef, Quarter Pounders, with Onion, Birds Eye*	1 Burger/114g	286	22.1	252	14.1	5.1	19.5	0.4
Beef, Quarter Pounders, with Onion, Sainsbury's*	1 Burger/113g	306	22.4	271	18.0	5.1	19.8	1.5
Beef, Sainsbury's*	1 Burger/57g	152	9.1	267	29.6	1.3	15.9	1.5
Beef, Scotch, Ultimate, TTD, Sainsbury's*	1 Burger/142g	284	12.2	200	26.0	4.7	8.6	1.0
Beef, Sundried Tomato, Grilled, Finest, Tesco*	1 Burger/99g	170	7.3	172	20.5	5.8	7.4	0.5
Beef, with Cheese Melt, COOK!, M & S*	1 Burger/182g	400	28.9	220	17.9	1.3	15.9	1.2
Beef, with Herbs, Finest, Tesco*	1 Burger/105g	200	11.8	190	17.3	4.5	11.2	0.7
Beef, with Jalapeno Chilli, Finest, Tesco*	1 Burger/205g	379	22.3	185	17.0	3.4	10.9	0.4
Beef, with Mediterranean Tomato & Basil, M & S*	1 Burger/169g	304	18.6	180	15.7	5.1	11.0	1.4
Beef, with Onion, Cooked, Ross*	1 Burger/41g	117	9.8	284	14.7	2.8	23.8	0.4
Beef, with Red Onion & Mustard, Finest, Tesco*	1 Burger/130g	308	24.2	237	17.2	0.2	18.6	2.6
Beef, with Shallots, Finest, Tesco*	1 Burger/84g	175	9.5	208	20.2	6.4	11.3	0.5
Beef, with West Country Cheddar, TTD, Sainsbury's*	1 Burger/112g	252	13.7	225	26.4	2.3	12.2	0.0
Beef & Mature Cheddar, Asda*	1 Burger/80g	178	10.0	223	21.5	6.2	12.5	0.5
Beef & Onion, Grilled, Asda*	1 Burger/81g	201	11.5	248	23.1	6.9	14.2	0.5
Beef Steak, British, Cooked, TTD, Sainsbury's*	1 Burger/93g	191	11.9	205	21.0	1.5	12.8	0.5
Beef with Onion, Sainsbury's*	1 Burger/42g	102	6.2	243	20.7	6.9	14.8	1.0
Cheeseburger	1 Burger/275g	706	29.0	257	13.7	25.6	10.6	1.8
Cheeseburger, American, Tesco*	1 Burger/275g	660	26.3	240	13.6	24.9	9.6	1.6
Cheeseburger, Bacon, with Bun, Chargrilled, Tesco*	1 Burger/265g	726	42.1	274	13.0	19.6	15.9	1.0
Cheeseburger, Micro Snack, Tesco*	1 Burger/115g	309	14.5	269	12.6	26.4	12.6	0.0
Cheeseburger, with Relish, American Style, Tesco*	1 Burger/61g	132	6.0	215	14.2	17.5	9.8	4.2
Cheeseburger, with Sesame Seed Bun, Tesco*	1 Burger/275g	644	32.2	234	12.2	20.1	11.7	2.0
Chicken, Crunch Crumb, Tesco*	1 Burger/57g	161	10.8	282	12.3	15.6	18.9	0.0
Chicken, Fillet, Cajun, Cooked, Birds Eye*	1 Burger/92g	128	4.3	140	20.1	4.8	4.7	0.2

BURGERS

	Measure INFO/WEIGHT	per Measure KCAL	per Measure FAT	Nutrition Values per 100g / 100ml KCAL	PROT	CARB	FAT	FIBRE
Chicken, Fresh, Non Coated, Waitrose*	1 Burger/100g	141	4.0	141	16.0	10.4	4.0	0.9
Chicken, Golden Breadcrumbs, Frozen, Birds Eye*	1 Burger/56g	130	6.9	232	13.8	16.4	12.4	0.3
Chicken, in Bun, Morrisons*	1 Burger/110g	250	4.7	228	12.7	38.1	4.3	3.8
Chicken, Quarter Pounders, Birds Eye*	1 Burger/117g	280	16.1	239	13.5	15.2	13.8	0.6
Chicken, Sainsbury's*	1 Burger/46g	115	7.0	247	15.6	12.2	15.1	1.3
Chicken, Southern Fried, Sainsbury's*	1 Burger/52g	154	10.3	297	12.6	17.2	19.8	1.3
Chicken, with Sesame Seed Bun, Breaded, Tesco*	1 Burger/205g	588	32.2	287	10.2	26.2	15.7	2.9
Chicken Fillet, Weight After Cooking, Birds Eye*	1 Burger/90g	126	4.1	140	20.0	5.1	4.6	0.2
Chilli, Quarter Pounders, Asda*	1 Burger/88g	221	14.0	252	25.0	2.0	16.0	0.0
Chilli, Quarter Pounders, Iceland*	1 Burger/84g	265	20.1	316	18.6	6.5	23.9	0.4
Classic, Eddie Rockets*	1 Burger/295g	620	35.0	210	10.8	14.9	11.9	0.0
Lamb, Minted, Asda*	1 Burger/100g	234	14.0	234	22.0	4.9	14.0	0.3
Lamb, Minted, Quarter Pounders, Asda*	1 Burger/114g	241	14.0	212	19.2	6.1	12.3	0.0
Lamb, Quarter Pounders, Asda*	1 Burger/85g	213	13.9	251	20.9	5.2	16.3	0.9
Lamb, Quarter Pounders, Birds Eye*	1 Burger/112g	232	16.9	207	13.9	3.8	15.1	0.3
Lamb, Waitrose*	1 Burger/67g	99	4.7	148	15.7	5.4	7.0	0.9
Less Than 7% Fat, Sainsbury's*	1 Burger/102g	164	5.6	161	20.8	7.1	5.5	1.1
Low Fat, Iceland*	1 Burger/85g	148	4.1	174	27.8	5.0	4.8	1.1
Meat Free, Sainsbury's*	1 Burger/57g	86	2.8	151	22.0	4.4	5.0	3.4
Mushroom & Wensleydale Cheese, Cauldron Foods*	1 Burger/87g	156	9.6	179	9.0	11.0	11.0	4.0
Ostrich, Quarter Pounder, Oslinc*	1 Burger/113g	132	1.5	117	22.9	3.5	1.3	1.1
Pork, Quarter Pounders, Birds Eye*	1 Burger/122g	292	23.2	239	13.9	3.2	19.0	0.2
Pork & Apple, Quarter Pounder, Grilled, Asda*	1 Burger/80g	147	6.4	184	23.9	4.1	8.0	0.5
Salmon, Quarter Pounders, Morrisons*	1 Burger/110g	235	13.0	214	21.4	5.5	11.8	1.7
Salmon, Quarter Pounders, Tesco*	1 Burger/114g	145	2.7	128	15.9	10.6	2.4	1.2
Salmon, Tesco*	1 Burger/100g	101	3.0	101	18.2	0.3	3.0	0.0
Spicy Bean, Ainsley Harriott*	1 Burger/200g	302	7.5	151	7.2	23.5	3.7	5.2
Spicy Bean, Cooked, Grassington's Food Co*	1 Burger/108g	201	3.8	186	6.5	32.2	3.5	2.5
Spicy Bean, Sainsbury's*	1 Burger/110g	262	13.5	240	5.0	27.1	12.4	2.0
Spicy Bean & Nacho, Morrisons*	1 Burger/113g	288	17.7	254	5.0	23.3	15.6	3.9
Steak, Rump, The Grill, M & S*	1 Burger/169g	330	20.6	195	18.7	2.6	12.2	1.1
Steak, with Cheese Melt, COOK!, M & S*	1 Burger/196g	480	35.7	245	18.4	2.3	18.2	0.2
Super Sized Beef, Big Bite, Birds Eye*	1 Burger/122g	320	25.2	262	13.1	6.0	20.6	1.0
Tuna, Quarter Pounder, Asda*	1 Burger/113g	212	11.3	188	21.0	3.4	10.0	0.0
Tuna, Quarter Pounders, Tesco*	1 Burger/114g	132	1.8	116	18.8	6.7	1.6	0.9
Turkey, Cheeseburgers, Tesco*	1 Burger/105g	252	14.8	240	15.4	12.8	14.1	1.3
Turkey, Crispy Crumb, Bernard Matthews*	1 Burger/71g	222	14.1	313	11.3	19.3	19.8	0.9
Venison, Finnebrougue Estate*	1 Burger/142g	170	7.0	120	19.9	4.2	4.9	0.5
Venison, Holme Farmed*	1 Burger/113g	119	3.4	105	21.5	2.3	3.0	0.0
Venison, TTD, Sainsbury's*	1 Burger/150g	224	6.3	149	20.4	6.5	4.2	3.2
Venison & Sweet Onion, M & S*	1 Burger/142g	163	5.0	115	19.3	1.4	3.5	0.5

BURGERS VEGETARIAN

	Measure INFO/WEIGHT	per Measure KCAL	per Measure FAT	Nutrition Values per 100g / 100ml KCAL	PROT	CARB	FAT	FIBRE
Bean, Tesco*	1 Burger/90g	192	10.9	213	4.4	21.6	12.1	5.0
Black Bean, Organic, Cauldron Foods*	1 Burger/88g	169	10.1	193	9.2	13.1	11.5	8.5
Cheese & Spring Onion, Tesco*	1 Burger/87g	178	10.3	204	4.4	20.0	11.8	3.2
Chilli, Cauldron Foods*	1 Burger/88g	148	8.1	169	11.5	8.5	9.3	3.3
Flame Grilled, Linda McCartney*	1 Burger/60g	104	3.1	174	17.9	13.8	5.2	3.3
Meat Free, Asda*	1 Burger/60g	138	6.0	230	24.0	11.0	10.0	0.3
Meat Free, Sainsbury's*	1 Burger/57g	92	4.2	161	19.6	3.9	7.4	4.8
Meat Free, Spicy, Bean & Nacho, Asda*	1 Burger/113g	288	17.7	254	5.0	23.3	15.6	3.9
Mexican Style, Bean, Meat Free, Tesco*	1 Burger/94g	206	8.7	220	4.9	28.2	9.3	3.9
Mushroom, Cauldron Foods*	1 Burger/88g	125	5.5	143	5.5	16.1	6.3	2.6
Mushroom, Meat Free, Tesco*	1 Burger/87g	151	9.5	173	3.6	15.3	10.8	3.7

	Measure INFO/WEIGHT	per Measure KCAL	FAT	Nutrition Values per 100g / 100ml KCAL	PROT	CARB	FAT	FIBRE
BURGERS VEGETARIAN								
Mushroom, Organic, Cauldron Foods*	1 Burger/88g	136	7.3	156	7.1	18.2	8.3	2.3
Quarter Pounders, Beef Style, Sainsbury's*	1 Burger/114g	216	10.8	190	20.0	6.0	9.5	2.5
Quarter Pounders, Chargrilled, Tesco*	1 Burger/114g	186	9.1	164	16.0	7.0	8.0	2.5
Quarter Pounders, HL, Tesco*	1 Burger/102g	117	1.7	114	4.0	20.7	1.7	2.0
Savoury, Cauldron Foods*	1 Burger/88g	145	8.0	166	108.0	7.9	9.2	2.4
Spicy Bean, BGTY, Sainsbury's*	1 Burger/85g	123	2.3	145	6.9	23.3	2.7	3.1
Spicy Bean, Cauldron Foods*	1 Burger/88g	203	9.8	232	5.4	27.4	11.2	6.2
Spicy Bean, Linda McCartney*	1 Burger/85g	190	9.5	223	4.3	26.2	11.2	2.9
Spicy Bean, Quarter Pounder, Dalepak*	1 Burger/115g	237	12.5	206	4.6	22.3	10.9	2.6
Tesco*	1 Burger/56g	92	4.5	164	16.0	7.0	8.0	2.5
Traditional, Fry's Special Vegetarian*	1 Burger/75g	175	9.0	233	19.2	12.9	12.0	0.2
Vegeburger, Linda McCartney*	1 Burger/59g	79	2.1	134	22.6	2.9	3.6	1.6
Vegeburger, Retail, Grilled	1oz/28g	55	3.1	196	16.6	8.0	11.1	4.2
Vegetable, Captains, Birds Eye*	1 Burger/48g	96	4.2	200	4.7	25.5	8.8	2.0
Vegetable, Organic, Goodlife*	1 Burger/67g	114	3.9	170	3.2	26.3	5.8	2.6
Vegetable, Organic, Tesco*	1 Burger/90g	108	3.9	120	2.6	17.6	4.3	2.1
Vegetable, Quarter Pounders, Crunchy, Birds Eye*	1 Burger/114g	240	11.6	211	4.8	24.9	10.2	1.8
Vegetable, Quarter Pounders, Dalepak*	1 Burger/113g	227	9.6	200	4.8	26.3	8.5	1.8
Vegetable, Quarter Pounders, Tesco*	1 Burger/108g	227	13.1	211	4.4	20.8	12.2	2.7
Vegetable, Spicy, Asda*	1 Burger/56g	108	6.2	193	3.4	20.0	11.0	0.0
BURRITO								
Beef	1 Serving/225g	430	19.0	191	9.6	18.7	8.5	2.2
BUTTER								
Brandy, Average	1 Serving/10g	56	3.8	555	0.2	46.2	38.3	0.1
Brandy, Tesco*	1oz/28g	152	10.8	543	0.3	48.3	38.7	0.5
Brandy, with Cognac, Sainsbury's*	1/8 Pot/25g	137	9.4	549	0.2	44.1	37.6	0.0
Coconut, Artisana*	2 Tbsp/32g	186	18.0	574	6.2	21.6	55.5	15.4
Creamery, Average	*1 Serving/10g*	*74*	*8.1*	*735*	*0.5*	*0.3*	*81.3*	*0.0*
Fresh, Average	*1 Thin Spread/7g*	*51*	*5.7*	*735*	*0.5*	*0.4*	*81.3*	*0.0*
Granules, Butter Buds*	1 Tsp/1.35g	5	0.1	368	1.8	77.9	6.5	2.3
Jersey, TTD, Sainsbury's*	1 Thin Spread/7g	52	5.8	744	0.5	0.6	82.2	0.0
Reduced Fat, Fresh, Average	*1 Thin Spread/7g*	*26*	*2.8*	*368*	*2.3*	*1.2*	*39.4*	*0.2*
Salted, Average	*1 Thin Spread/7g*	*51*	*5.7*	*729*	*0.4*	*0.3*	*81.1*	*0.0*
Spreadable, Butterpak, Lighter, Tesco*	1 Serving/10g	54	5.6	545	0.5	0.5	56.0	0.0
Spreadable, Fresh, Average	*1 Thin Spread/7g*	*51*	*5.7*	*730*	*0.4*	*0.3*	*80.8*	*0.0*
Spreadable, Organic, Lighter, Yeo Valley*	1 Serving/12g	66	7.3	550	0.7	0.9	60.7	0.0
Spreadable, Reduced Fat, Average	*1 Thin Spread/7g*	*38*	*4.2*	*540*	*0.5*	*0.5*	*60.0*	*0.0*
Spreadable, Slightly Salted, Lurpak*	1 Serving/10g	72	8.0	724	0.5	0.6	80.0	0.0
with Crushed Garlic, Lurpak*	1 Serving/10g	70	7.5	700	1.0	4.0	75.0	0.0
BUTTERMILK								
Average	*1 Serving/400ml*	*177*	*1.3*	*44*	*4.2*	*5.9*	*0.3*	*0.0*
BUTTONS								
Chocolate, Giant, Dairy Milk, Cadbury*	1 Button/3g	15	0.9	525	7.7	56.7	29.9	0.7
Dairy Milk, Milk Chocolate, Cadbury*	1 Pack/32ml	170	9.7	525	7.7	56.7	29.9	0.7
Milk Chocolate, Asda*	1 Bag/70g	368	21.0	526	7.0	57.0	30.0	1.5
Milk Chocolate, M & S*	1 Pack/75g	375	19.0	500	8.6	59.8	25.3	1.9
Milk Chocolate, Tesco*	1 Bag/70g	359	19.3	513	7.1	59.1	27.6	2.1
White Chocolate, Cadbury*	1 Pack/32g	180	11.0	555	4.5	58.4	33.8	0.0
White Chocolate, Co-Op*	½ Pack/35g	185	9.8	530	7.0	64.0	28.0	0.0
White Chocolate, Tesco*	1 Bag/70g	388	23.4	554	5.1	58.0	33.5	0.0

	Measure INFO/WEIGHT	per Measure KCAL	FAT	Nutrition Values per 100g / 100ml KCAL	PROT	CARB	FAT	FIBRE
CABBAGE								
Boiled, Average	*1 Serving/90g*	*14*	*0.3*	*15*	*1.0*	*2.2*	*0.3*	*1.7*
Creamed, Sainsbury's*	½ Pack/150g	88	6.3	59	1.5	3.9	4.2	2.3
Greens, Trimmed, Average	*1oz/28g*	*8*	*0.1*	*28*	*2.9*	*2.9*	*0.5*	*3.4*
Medley, Washed, Ready to Cook, Tesco*	1 Pack/200g	60	1.2	30	2.3	3.7	0.6	2.8
Raw, Average	*1 Serving/100g*	*21*	*0.4*	*21*	*1.3*	*3.1*	*0.4*	*1.8*
Red, Average	*1 Serving/90g*	*19*	*0.2*	*21*	*1.0*	*3.7*	*0.3*	*2.2*
Red, Pickled, Average	*1 Serving/100g*	*26*	*0.1*	*26*	*0.9*	*4.6*	*0.1*	*1.5*
Savoy, Boiled in Salted Water, Average	*1 Serving/90g*	*15*	*0.4*	*17*	*1.1*	*2.2*	*0.5*	*2.0*
Savoy, Raw, Average	*1 Serving/90g*	*24*	*0.4*	*27*	*2.1*	*3.9*	*0.5*	*3.1*
Steamed, Average	1 Serving/100g	15	0.3	15	1.0	2.2	0.3	1.7
White, Raw, Average	*1oz/28g*	*8*	*0.1*	*27*	*1.4*	*5.0*	*0.2*	*2.1*
CAKE								
Action Man, Birthday, Memory Lane Cakes*	1/12 Cake/83g	322	13.6	388	3.0	57.0	16.4	0.8
Alabama Chocolate Fudge, Morrisons*	1/6 Cake/58g	195	6.4	337	4.5	55.1	11.0	2.3
Almond Flavoured Rounds, Country Garden Cakes*	1 Cake/45g	183	6.7	403	4.3	62.4	14.7	2.3
Almond Slices, Lyons*	1 Slice/27g	114	6.9	426	7.1	41.3	25.8	1.6
Almond Slices, Mr Kipling*	1 Slice/33g	131	4.5	403	6.3	63.4	14.0	2.0
Almond Slices, Sainsbury's*	1 Serving/27g	120	7.1	444	5.9	45.9	26.3	1.5
Almond Slices, Weight Watchers*	1 Slice/26g	95	2.6	365	5.2	63.8	9.9	2.4
Angel, Asda*	1 Serving/46g	184	7.8	399	4.5	57.0	17.0	0.9
Angel, Sainsbury's*	1/8 Cake/41g	171	8.1	417	4.1	55.7	19.8	0.8
Angel Layer, Tesco*	1 Serving/25g	101	4.3	403	4.5	57.4	17.3	0.9
Angel Slices, Mr Kipling*	1 Slice/38g	153	7.0	403	2.9	58.8	18.3	0.6
Apple, Bramley, & Blackberry Crumble, M & S*	1/8 Cake/56g	221	10.0	395	4.4	54.1	17.9	1.5
Apple, Home Style, M & S*	1 Cake/54g	189	7.9	350	5.3	49.4	14.7	1.5
Apple & Cinnamon, Oat Break, Go Ahead, McVitie's*	1 Serving/35g	122	2.3	349	5.2	67.2	6.6	2.6
Apple Bakes, Go Ahead, McVitie's*	1 Cake/35g	126	2.7	361	2.6	70.0	7.8	2.0
Apple Crumble, Slices, Weight Watchers*	1 Slice/26g	90	2.0	346	4.5	64.8	7.7	2.3
Apple Slice, Delightful, Mr Kipling*	1 Slice/29g	92	1.1	317	4.4	66.2	3.9	1.3
Apricot & Apple, Trimlyne*	1 Cake/50g	133	1.3	267	4.3	58.4	2.7	1.9
Bakewell, The Handmade Flapjack Company*	1 Cake/75g	311	17.1	415	4.5	47.4	22.8	0.0
Bakewell Slices, Mr Kipling*	1 Slice/36g	163	7.3	454	4.2	63.4	20.4	1.2
Banana, Organic, Loaf, Respect Organics*	¼ Pack/65g	254	13.6	391	3.9	48.6	21.0	1.5
Banana, The Handmade Flapjack Company*	1 Cake/75g	290	10.8	387	5.3	59.2	14.4	0.0
Banana Loaf, Waitrose*	1 Slice/70g	236	7.5	337	5.0	55.2	10.7	1.7
Bar, Iced Rich Fruit, Finest, Tesco*	1 Serving/100g	360	10.7	360	3.8	61.3	10.7	4.2
Battenberg, Mini, Mr Kipling*	1 Cake/35g	143	3.8	410	4.6	76.2	11.0	1.3
Battenberg, Mr Kipling*	1 Serving/38g	161	4.6	421	5.0	73.3	12.0	1.6
Belgian Chocolate, Choux Bun, Sainsbury's*	1 Bun /90g	347	35.3	386	6.2	22.0	39.2	1.4
Belgian Chocolate, Slices, Weight Watchers*	1 Slice/25g	86	2.4	344	6.5	57.6	9.8	2.9
Belgian Chocolate, Waitrose*	1 Slice/47g	223	12.6	474	4.8	53.1	26.9	1.9
Birthday, M & S*	1 Serving/60g	240	7.1	400	2.3	70.9	11.9	0.8
Birthday Present, Tesco*	1 Serving/79g	347	13.9	439	3.5	66.6	17.6	0.4
Bites, Caramel, Mr Kipling*	1 Cake/14g	68	3.8	492	5.9	55.3	27.4	0.8
Bites, Chocolate Roll, Mini, Tesco*	1 Bite/18g	78	3.6	435	6.0	58.0	19.8	1.9
Butterfly, Mr Kipling*	1 Cake/29g	114	6.4	392	4.4	43.4	22.2	0.6
Buttons, Happy Birthday, Cadbury*	1 Slice/50g	235	13.5	470	4.1	52.8	27.1	0.0
Caramel, Milk Chocolate, Holly Lane*	1 Cake/25g	110	5.1	441	6.9	57.6	20.3	1.1
Caramel Shortbread, Tray Bake, Kate's Cakes Ltd*	1 Serving/100g	471	27.3	471	3.0	53.3	27.3	1.2
Caramel Shortcake Slices, McVitie's*	1 Slice /32g	146	7.7	463	4.3	56.5	24.4	1.6
Caramel Slice, M & S*	1 Slice/64g	304	16.1	475	4.9	60.4	25.2	2.6
Carrot, Arno*	1 Slice/45g	153	6.7	340	4.0	47.0	15.0	0.0
Carrot, Entenmann's*	1 Serving/40g	156	8.2	391	4.1	47.4	20.5	1.5

CAKE

	Measure INFO/WEIGHT	per Measure KCAL	FAT	Nutrition Values per 100g / 100ml KCAL	PROT	CARB	FAT	FIBRE
Carrot, Finest, Tesco*	1 Slice/72g	281	13.4	390	3.8	51.8	18.6	2.3
Carrot, Handmade, Delicious, Boots*	1 Slice/75g	292	13.5	389	4.1	53.0	18.0	1.4
Carrot, Iced, Tesco*	1 Serving/61g	246	12.0	404	3.1	53.7	19.6	1.6
Carrot, Kate's Cakes Ltd*	1 Serving/100g	405	21.4	405	4.1	47.1	21.4	2.6
Carrot, Mini, Weight Watchers*	1 Cake/31g	120	3.3	388	3.7	68.9	10.8	2.7
Carrot, Organic, Respect Organics*	1 Slice/45g	179	10.1	398	3.1	47.4	22.4	1.5
Carrot, Slices, Asda*	1 Slice/80g	302	13.2	377	3.4	53.8	16.5	1.7
Carrot, Slices, Inspirations, Mr Kipling*	1 Slice/34g	139	6.3	411	3.5	57.7	18.5	1.3
Carrot, Square, Margaret's Country Kitchen*	1 Cake/80g	307	13.5	384	3.6	54.4	16.9	2.4
Carrot, The Handmade Flapjack Company*	1 Cake/75g	295	13.0	393	6.4	53.0	17.3	0.0
Carrot, Tray Bake, Kate's Cakes Ltd*	1 Serving/100g	328	14.5	328	3.8	45.6	14.5	2.0
Carrot, Ultimate, Entenmann's*	1/8 Cake/64g	234	10.1	367	4.7	51.4	15.8	0.3
Carrot & Orange, Extra Special, Asda*	1/6 Cake/65g	240	11.7	369	4.7	47.0	18.0	0.9
Carrot & Orange, Finest, Tesco*	1/8 Cake/50g	205	10.2	410	4.6	51.2	20.5	2.1
Carrot & Orange, Waitrose*	1/6 Cake/47g	164	7.4	350	5.3	46.8	15.7	1.8
Carrot & Orange Slices, GFY, Asda*	1 Serving/23g	77	0.6	334	3.4	74.0	2.7	1.0
Carrot & Pecan, M & S*	1 Slice/90g	330	14.6	365	6.4	48.7	16.2	2.3
Carrot & Walnut, Layered, Asda*	1 Serving/42g	172	8.0	409	4.6	55.0	19.0	1.0
Carrot & Walnut, Mini Classics, Mr Kipling*	1 Cake/39g	172	9.8	440	4.5	48.6	25.2	1.0
Carrot Slices, GFY, Asda*	1 Slice/28g	83	0.6	298	2.8	66.4	2.3	2.1
Carrot Slices, Less Than 3% Fat, BGTY, Sainsbury's*	1 Slice/30g	94	0.8	313	3.4	68.7	2.7	2.4
Carrot Slices, Weight Watchers*	1 Slice/27g	84	0.2	311	2.8	73.0	0.8	0.9
Carrot Wedge, Tesco*	1 Pack/175g	532	27.6	304	3.9	36.6	15.8	1.5
Celebration, Sainsbury's*	1 Serving/100g	265	9.2	265	2.1	43.6	9.2	0.3
Cherry, Asda*	1 Slice/37g	131	4.5	351	4.7	56.0	12.0	0.6
Cherry, M & S*	1 Serving/75g	285	9.5	380	5.0	60.6	12.7	0.8
Cherry Bakewell, Delightful, Mr Kipling*	1 Cake/45g	176	5.8	390	3.9	66.4	12.9	1.2
Cherry Bakewell, Gluten Free, Bakers Delight*	1 Cake/50g	211	8.1	422	2.9	66.1	16.3	0.4
Cherry Bakewell, Layer, Asda*	1/8 Cake/50g	210	11.0	420	4.4	51.0	22.0	0.6
Cherry Bakewell, M & S*	1 Cake/44g	185	7.8	420	4.5	61.7	17.7	1.0
Cherry Bakewell, Mini, Sainsbury's*	1 Cake/27g	101	3.3	370	3.4	62.2	12.0	0.4
Cherry Bakewell, Mr Kipling*	1 Cake/45g	193	8.3	428	3.9	61.3	18.5	1.4
Cherry Bakewell, Sainsbury's*	1 Cake/46g	200	8.1	436	3.1	66.3	17.6	1.4
Cherry Bakewell, Sara Lee*	1/5 Slice/70g	228	7.9	326	4.1	51.9	11.3	1.4
Cherry Bakewell, Slices, GFY, Asda*	1 Slice/29g	98	0.7	337	3.4	75.4	2.4	0.7
Cherry Bakewell, Tesco*	1 Cake/39g	171	7.5	439	3.2	63.3	19.2	1.1
Cherry Bakewell, Waitrose*	1 Cake/44g	184	8.5	419	3.8	57.4	19.3	2.1
Chocolate	1oz/28g	128	7.4	456	7.4	50.4	26.4	0.0
Chocolate, Big, Tesco*	1 Slice/79g	311	13.1	396	7.4	54.1	16.7	1.8
Chocolate, Birthday, Tesco*	1 Serving/54g	229	13.2	425	5.9	45.5	24.4	2.1
Chocolate, Caterpillar, Tesco*	1 Serving/53g	248	13.2	468	5.7	55.3	24.9	1.1
Chocolate, Champagne, Sainsbury's*	1 Serving/75g	304	12.1	405	2.5	62.4	16.2	0.5
Chocolate, Cup, Mini, Weight Watchers*	1 Cake/17g	72	3.6	422	6.1	52.0	21.1	1.8
Chocolate, Double Dream, Nestle*	1 Serving/150g	637	37.6	425	5.0	44.7	25.1	0.9
Chocolate, Fondants, Weight Watchers*	1 Cake/19g	70	2.3	368	6.1	59.0	12.0	3.2
Chocolate, Fudge, The Cake Shop*	1 Cake/37g	178	10.8	480	3.7	50.5	29.2	1.3
Chocolate, Happy Birthday, Tesco*	1 Serving/58g	241	13.2	415	4.7	46.9	22.7	2.9
Chocolate, Iced, Tesco*	1 Serving/40g	158	6.3	395	4.7	58.5	15.8	1.8
Chocolate, Individual, with Mini Eggs, Cadbury*	1 Cake/26g	119	6.1	455	4.6	57.5	23.1	1.3
Chocolate, Large, Happy Birthday, Tesco*	1/18 Cake/63g	249	12.2	396	6.2	49.3	19.3	1.8
Chocolate, Loaf, Moist, McVitie's*	1 Slice/30g	119	6.1	398	4.8	49.0	20.3	1.9
Chocolate, Part of Tea Time Selection, Iceland*	1 Cake/31g	144	7.9	464	4.5	54.1	25.5	2.0
Chocolate, Party, Tesco*	1 Slice/62g	244	13.1	394	4.6	46.3	21.2	0.9

CAKE

INFO/WEIGHT	Measure per Measure KCAL	FAT	Nutrition Values per 100g / 100ml KCAL	PROT	CARB	FAT	FIBRE
Chocolate, Sainsbury's*	1 Serving/30g	118	5.5	395	4.1	52.6	18.5	1.3
Chocolate, Sara Lee*	¼ Cake/88g	339	14.8	385	4.1	54.3	16.8	0.0
Chocolate, Smarties, Celebration, Large, Nestle*	1/16 Cake/71g	308	17.4	432	5.4	48.9	24.4	1.2
Chocolate, The Handmade Flapjack Company*	1 Cake/75g	303	16.2	404	12.5	39.8	21.6	0.0
Chocolate, Thorntons*	1 Serving/87g	408	25.1	469	5.2	47.1	28.8	0.6
Chocolate, Triple Layer, Celebration, Tesco*	1 Slice/100g	385	18.4	385	5.4	49.0	18.4	6.4
Chocolate, White Button, Asda*	1 Cake/30g	117	6.3	390	5.0	44.0	21.0	2.0
Chocolate & Brandy Butter, Entenmann's*	1 Serving/39g	144	6.7	374	3.4	53.5	17.5	2.8
Chocolate & Caramel Tiffin Bites, Gu*	1 Tiffin/35g	168	9.9	480	3.8	51.9	28.3	2.8
Chocolate & Orange Rolls, M & S*	1 Cake/60g	228	17.0	380	3.6	27.0	28.4	1.3
Chocolate & Orange Slices, GFY, Asda*	1 Serving/30g	95	0.8	315	3.2	70.0	2.5	1.3
Chocolate & Sweetest, Beetroot, Battle Bakehouse*	1/6 Cake/49g	185	8.7	379	5.2	48.6	17.9	4.0
Chocolate Box, Asda*	1 Serving/60g	263	13.8	439	5.0	53.0	23.0	0.7
Chocolate Brownie, Fudge, Entenmann's*	1/8 Cake/55g	168	2.4	306	4.0	62.7	4.4	1.5
Chocolate Brownie, Gluten & Wheat Free, Lovemore*	1 Slice/36g	127	4.6	352	3.7	56.1	12.8	0.2
Chocolate Brownie, Tray Bake, Kate's Cakes Ltd*	1 Serving/100g	435	22.0	435	5.7	51.5	22.0	3.3
Chocolate Button, Cakes for the Connoisseur*	1 Cake/30g	145	9.8	485	5.2	42.1	32.8	2.3
Chocolate Chip, The Cake Shop*	1 Cake/35g	178	11.0	508	4.7	50.2	31.5	1.1
Chocolate Crunch, Tray Bake, Kate's Cakes Ltd*	1 Serving/80g	400	23.0	500	4.8	53.4	28.8	3.7
Chocolate Egg, Small, Tesco*	1 Cake/31g	132	6.3	425	5.4	57.2	20.2	1.7
Chocolate Flavour Slices, GFY, Asda*	1 Slice/28g	71	0.7	257	4.3	54.0	2.6	1.4
Chocolate Flower Pot, M & S*	1 Serving/69g	295	13.2	430	3.8	60.8	19.3	1.5
Chocolate Fudge	1 Serving/110g	415	19.1	377	4.4	50.4	17.4	1.4
Chocolate Fudge, & Vanilla Cream, M & S*	1/6 Cake/69g	310	17.9	450	5.2	49.8	26.0	1.3
Chocolate Fudge, Belgian, TTD, Sainsbury's*	1 Slice/66g	278	14.3	423	4.4	52.5	21.7	2.5
Chocolate Fudge, Classics, M & S*	1 Serving/71g	195	7.5	275	2.8	42.8	10.6	1.1
Chocolate Fudge, Entenmann's*	1 Serving/48g	173	7.2	361	4.4	51.8	15.1	0.9
Chocolate Fudge, Sainsbury's*	1/8 Cake/98g	402	21.9	410	5.5	47.3	22.3	1.9
Chocolate Fudge, Tea Time Treats, Asda*	1 Cake/37g	157	8.1	424	3.6	53.0	22.0	1.7
Chocolate Fudge Slice, Waitrose*	1 Slice/60g	230	9.7	383	4.7	54.6	16.2	1.5
Chocolate Heaven, Extra Special, Asda*	1/6 Cake/66g	255	13.1	388	4.0	48.0	20.0	1.0
Chocolate Indulgence, Finest, Tesco*	1 Slice/51g	207	9.1	405	4.8	55.9	17.9	1.2
Chocolate Log, Fresh Cream, Finest, Tesco*	1 Slice/85g	301	15.4	354	4.5	43.2	18.1	1.4
Chocolate Orange, Slices, Weight Watchers*	1 Slice/82g	249	2.2	304	4.9	64.9	2.7	2.6
Chocolate Orange, Sponge, Asda*	1 Serving/70g	297	18.2	425	4.9	42.9	26.0	3.0
Chocolate Party, M & S*	1 Serving/61g	240	12.6	395	4.6	46.9	20.8	1.1
Chocolate Rice Crispy, Knightsbridge*	1 Cake/24g	88	4.2	368	3.9	48.7	17.5	0.1
Chocolate Roll, Sainsbury's*	1 Slice/50g	210	10.2	420	5.0	54.0	20.4	3.3
Chocolate Sensation, Sainsbury's*	1 Serving/92g	320	17.7	348	3.7	40.0	19.2	2.3
Chocolate Slice, Go Ahead, McVitie's*	1 Slice/32g	94	2.6	293	4.5	49.4	8.2	1.9
Chocolate Slices, Mr Kipling*	1 Slice/33g	132	6.7	406	5.6	50.4	20.6	2.7
Chocolate Sponge, Less Than 5% Fat, Asda*	1 Sponge/110g	198	4.2	180	4.4	32.0	3.8	1.1
Chocolate Sponge, Tesco*	1 Serving/35g	129	5.1	373	5.3	54.4	14.9	1.5
Chocolate Truffle, Extra Special, Asda*	1 Serving/103g	402	26.8	390	5.0	34.0	26.0	1.8
Chocolate Truffle, Mini, Finest, Tesco*	1 Cake/28g	125	6.6	448	5.9	52.9	23.7	0.3
Chocolate Victoria Sponge, Co-Op*	1 Slice/61g	201	9.8	330	5.0	42.0	16.0	1.0
Chocolate with Butter Icing, Average	1oz/28g	135	8.3	481	5.7	50.9	29.7	0.0
Chorley, Asda*	1 Cake/60g	269	12.6	449	6.0	59.0	21.0	2.2
Christmas, Connoisseur, M & S*	1 Slice/60g	216	5.5	360	4.1	64.7	9.2	3.3
Christmas, Iced, Slices, Tesco*	1 Slice/45g	168	4.4	369	2.9	67.6	9.6	1.2
Christmas, Iced Rich Fruit, Finest, Tesco*	1 Serving/100g	345	7.7	345	3.1	65.3	7.7	3.7
Christmas, Knightsbridge*	1 Slice/50g	188	5.4	377	4.3	65.7	10.8	3.2
Christmas, Rich Fruit, All Iced, Sainsbury's*	1/16 Cake/85g	307	7.6	361	4.0	66.4	8.9	1.5

CAKE

	Measure INFO/WEIGHT	per Measure KCAL	FAT	Nutrition Values per 100g / 100ml KCAL	PROT	CARB	FAT	FIBRE
Christmas, Rich Fruit, Organic, Tesco*	1 Serving/76g	282	7.5	374	3.9	67.1	10.0	2.0
Christmas, Rich Fruit, Tesco*	1 Serving/75g	256	5.5	342	3.9	64.3	7.4	3.1
Christmas Pudding Slices, Mr Kipling*	1 Slice/51g	173	3.6	339	3.6	62.1	7.1	1.3
Christmas Slices, Mr Kipling*	1 Slice/52g	190	4.6	366	3.0	68.0	8.9	0.9
Christmas Slices, Weight Watchers*	1 Slice/40g	136	2.6	339	4.4	66.0	6.4	3.0
Classic Lemon Drizzle, M & S*	1/6 Cake/68g	253	10.3	375	4.7	55.0	15.3	0.6
Coconut	1 Slice/70g	304	16.7	434	6.7	51.2	23.8	2.5
Coconut & Raspberry, M & S*	1 Serving/52g	231	13.9	445	5.0	45.5	26.8	2.3
Coconut Delight, Burton's*	1 Cake/21g	89	3.5	424	4.0	63.0	16.9	2.0
Coconut Snowball, Bobby's*	1 Cake/18g	80	4.0	436	2.2	57.3	22.1	0.0
Coconut Sponge, Memory Lane Cakes*	1/6 Cake/42g	172	7.5	406	4.1	57.1	17.6	1.5
Coconut Sponge, Mini Classics, Mr Kipling*	1 Cake/38g	155	8.7	409	3.7	47.0	22.9	0.9
Coffee, Entenmann's*	1 Serving/41g	159	7.1	388	4.0	54.7	17.3	0.6
Coffee, Iced, M & S*	1 Slice/33g	135	6.5	410	4.4	54.5	19.6	1.6
Coffee, TTD, Sainsbury's*	1 Slice/68g	294	16.4	430	4.3	49.1	24.0	2.6
Coffee & Walnut, Classics, M & S*	1 Serving/71g	308	17.2	435	4.3	50.3	24.3	1.6
Coffee & Walnut, Mrs Beeton's*	1 Slice/54g	219	13.5	405	3.7	41.4	25.0	0.3
Coffee Sponge Roll, M & S*	1/6 Roll/42g	160	7.4	385	3.1	53.1	17.8	1.4
Colin the Caterpillar, M & S*	1 Slice/60g	234	12.8	390	5.3	57.2	21.3	1.3
Cornflake, Bobby's*	1/6 Cake/45g	207	9.2	461	3.9	65.5	20.4	0.0
Cornflake, Chocolate Clusters, Asda*	1 Cake/14g	64	2.6	460	8.2	65.2	18.5	2.7
Country Farmhouse, Waitrose*	1 Serving/80g	308	12.1	385	4.7	57.5	15.1	1.4
Country Slices, Asda*	1 Serving/27g	111	5.1	411	3.9	56.0	19.0	2.4
Country Slices, Mr Kipling*	1 Slice/32ml	121	4.8	380	4.4	56.7	15.0	1.2
Cream Oysters, M & S*	1 Cake/72g	227	15.3	315	3.6	27.5	21.2	3.0
Cream Slices, M & S*	1 Slice/80g	310	18.3	387	2.3	45.7	22.9	0.6
Crispy Chocolate Clusters, Mini, Tesco*	1 Cluster/8g	37	1.5	470	7.0	67.8	18.7	2.5
Date & Walnut, Slices, Light Choices, Tesco*	1 Slice/25g	72	0.3	290	5.6	63.7	1.1	1.1
Date & Walnut, Slices, Weight Watchers*	1 Slice/27g	73	0.4	271	3.5	60.6	1.6	4.2
Date & Walnut, Trimlyne*	1 Slice/50g	134	2.4	269	5.7	53.8	4.9	1.8
Date & Walnut Loaf, Sainsbury's*	1/10 Slice/40g	148	8.2	371	6.7	40.1	20.4	1.0
Date & Walnut Slices, GFY, Asda*	1 Slice/22g	62	0.3	281	5.0	61.8	1.5	1.8
D'oh Nuts, Asda*	1 Cake/50g	186	9.5	372	4.0	47.0	19.0	0.0
Double Chocolate Ganache, M & S*	1/12 Cake/61g	281	16.8	460	5.9	46.1	27.6	2.5
Dundee, Co-Op*	1/8 Cake/71g	238	7.8	335	5.0	53.0	11.0	2.0
Dundee, Tesco*	1 Serving/100g	325	8.9	325	5.3	56.0	8.9	6.0
Eccles	1 Cake/45g	214	11.9	475	3.9	59.3	26.4	1.6
Eccles, Weight Watchers*	1 Cake/48g	190	7.9	396	4.4	57.5	16.5	2.0
Fairy, Holly Lane*	1 Cake/26g	118	6.7	460	3.7	52.5	26.1	3.5
Fairy, Lemon Iced, Tesco*	1 Cake/24g	94	3.3	393	4.4	63.2	13.6	1.1
Fairy, Mini, Kids, Tesco*	1 Cake/12g	54	2.8	435	5.3	53.3	22.3	1.1
Fairy, Mini, Tesco*	1 Cake/13g	53	2.5	424	6.1	54.6	20.1	1.3
Fairy, Plain, Sainsbury's*	1 Cake/20g	84	4.3	422	4.9	46.4	21.5	1.2
Fairy, Snowman, Christmas, Tesco*	1 Cake/24g	114	6.8	471	4.6	49.8	28.1	2.9
Fairy, Strawberry Iced, Tesco*	1 Cake/24g	94	3.2	392	4.9	62.9	13.4	1.4
Fairy, Vanilla Iced, Tesco*	1 Cake/24g	93	2.9	388	4.4	65.1	12.2	1.2
Farmhouse Loaf, The Handmade Flapjack Company*	1 Cake/75g	274	12.9	365	4.5	48.4	17.2	0.0
Farmhouse Slice, Weight Watchers*	1 Slice/23g	73	0.9	317	5.5	64.9	4.0	1.3
Flake, Cadbury*	1 Cake/20g	90	4.5	445	6.3	54.5	22.3	0.0
Fondant, Dark Chocolate, Graze*	1 Pack/40g	157	5.8	393	3.5	66.2	14.5	0.0
Fondant Fancies, Lemon, Waitrose*	1 Cake/40g	176	7.1	441	2.5	67.9	17.7	0.6
Fondant Fancies, Sainsbury's*	1 Cake/27g	95	2.4	353	2.4	65.7	9.0	0.4
Fondants, with Chocolate, Mini, Delhaize*	1 Cake/20g	88	6.2	440	4.6	36.3	30.8	3.8

CAKE

	Measure INFO/WEIGHT	per Measure KCAL	FAT	Nutrition Values per 100g / 100ml KCAL	PROT	CARB	FAT	FIBRE
French Fancies, Mr Kipling*	1 Cake/28g	103	2.6	369	2.8	68.3	9.4	0.6
Fresh Cream Bramley Apple Sponge, Tesco*	1/6 Slice/43g	130	7.0	303	3.6	35.4	16.3	1.0
Fruit, Parisienne, Rich, Finest, Tesco*	1 Serving/69g	262	9.7	380	4.7	55.2	14.1	1.9
Fruit, Plain, Average	1 Slice/90g	319	11.6	354	5.1	57.9	12.9	0.0
Fruit, Rich, Average	1 Slice/70g	225	8.7	322	4.9	50.7	12.5	1.7
Fruit, Rich, Iced	1 Slice/70g	249	8.0	356	4.1	62.7	11.4	1.7
Fruit, Rich, M & S*	1 Serving/50g	157	3.2	315	3.1	60.9	6.5	4.3
Fruit, Rich, Truly Irresistible, Co-Op*	1/6 Cake/70g	235	6.0	335	3.9	59.9	8.6	2.0
Fruit, Slices, Gluten & Wheat Free, Lovemore*	1 Slice/40g	122	3.8	304	2.3	51.1	9.4	1.5
Fruit & Nut Cluster, Finest, Tesco*	1 Slice/77g	262	10.3	338	4.5	50.1	13.3	2.7
Fruit & Nut Cluster, TTD, Sainsbury's*	1 Slice/63g	239	9.2	383	5.7	56.8	14.8	4.2
Fruit Cake with Marzipan & Icing, Asda*	1/12 Cake/76g	280	6.8	369	3.9	68.0	9.0	0.0
Fruit Slices, Rich, Iced, Finest, Tesco*	1 Slice/41g	152	3.4	370	3.2	69.4	8.3	2.1
Fudge Brownie, The Handmade Flapjack Company*	1 Cake/75g	286	9.2	381	4.9	62.8	12.3	0.0
Fudgy Chocolate Slices, COU, M & S*	1 Slice/36g	95	0.8	265	4.6	66.4	2.2	2.1
Genoa, Tesco*	1 Serving/50g	162	3.7	325	3.6	60.9	7.4	4.0
Ginger Drizzle, Iced, Co-Op*	1/6 Cake/65g	226	7.7	350	3.0	58.0	12.0	1.0
Ginger Orange, The Handmade Flapjack Company*	1 Cake/75g	289	15.2	385	4.3	46.3	20.3	0.0
Glitzy Bag, Birthday, Tesco*	1 Serving/81g	314	6.9	388	2.1	75.9	8.5	0.6
Granola, Tray Bake, Kate's Cakes Ltd*	1 Serving/100g	425	16.7	425	7.3	58.2	16.7	4.7
Happy Birthday, Sainsbury's*	1 Slice/50g	207	8.0	414	2.8	64.5	16.1	0.6
Holly Hedgehog, Tesco*	1 Serving/55g	227	7.9	413	2.0	69.0	14.3	0.8
Hot Chocolate Fudge, Sainsbury's*	1/8 Cake/91g	343	15.6	376	5.1	50.3	17.1	3.5
Iced Christmas, Slice, Finest, Tesco*	1 Slice/115g	471	10.8	410	3.9	77.1	9.4	3.1
Iced Cupcake, Gluten & Wheat Free, Lovemore*	1 Cake/33g	138	6.3	418	2.1	54.5	19.0	0.4
Iced Fruit Slice, Gluten & Wheat Free, Lovemore*	1 Slice/44g	141	3.3	321	1.6	60.0	7.6	1.1
Iced Madeira, Sainsbury's*	1/8 Cake/47g	182	6.6	388	3.6	61.6	14.1	0.7
Jamaica Ginger, McVitie's*	1 Cake/291g	1056	30.6	363	3.7	63.4	10.5	1.6
Jamaica Ginger with Lemon Filling, McVitie's*	1 Cake/33g	143	8.2	434	4.0	48.3	25.0	0.8
Jammy Strawberry Rolls, Mini, Cadbury*	1 Cake/29g	119	4.8	411	4.9	59.8	16.5	0.5
Lemon, French Fancies, Mr Kipling*	1 Fancy/28g	106	2.7	378	2.5	69.9	9.8	0.5
Lemon, Half Moon, Bobby's*	1/6 Cake/60g	244	11.0	406	4.1	55.7	18.4	0.0
Lemon, Kate's Cakes Ltd*	1 Serving/100g	395	17.0	395	4.2	55.2	17.0	0.9
Lemon, Mini, Weight Watchers*	1 Cake/27g	90	3.0	333	3.7	66.7	11.1	11.1
Lemon, The Handmade Flapjack Company*	1 Cake/75g	312	16.3	416	4.5	50.5	21.8	0.0
Lemon & Orange, Finest, Tesco*	1 Serving/53g	216	10.7	410	4.5	52.4	20.3	1.1
Lemon Bakewell, Mr Kipling*	1 Cake/48g	195	7.3	407	2.6	65.0	15.2	0.7
Lemon Buttercream & Lemon Curd, The Cake Shop*	1 Cake/28g	124	7.8	444	3.5	43.4	27.8	0.6
Lemon Drizzle, M & S*	1/6 Cake/63g	230	8.8	365	4.2	55.8	13.9	1.4
Lemon Drizzle, Tray Bake, Kate's Cakes Ltd*	1 Serving/100g	324	14.4	324	4.5	44.2	14.4	1.1
Lemon Drizzle Cake, Asda*	1 Serving/50g	149	6.0	299	2.8	45.0	12.0	0.4
Lemon Drizzle Slices, Light Choices, Tesco*	1 Slice/23g	67	0.5	290	4.8	62.7	2.0	2.8
Lemon Iced Madeira, Co-Op*	1 Cake/290g	1131	52.2	390	4.0	53.0	18.0	0.6
Lemon Madeira, Half Moon, Dan Cake*	1 Slice/50g	215	10.0	430	3.5	59.0	20.0	0.0
Lemon Slice, Bakery, Tesco*	1 Slice/29g	107	3.3	370	3.7	62.7	11.3	1.6
Lemon Slices, BGTY, Sainsbury's*	1 Slice/26g	84	0.4	323	3.7	74.0	1.4	1.3
Lemon Slices, Low Fat, Weight Watchers*	1 Slice/26g	79	0.5	303	3.1	68.1	2.0	2.2
Lemon Slices, Mr Kipling*	1 Slice/29g	120	4.8	413	4.2	61.9	16.6	0.7
Lemon Smoothie Bake, Go Ahead, McVitie's*	1 Bar/35g	130	2.8	372	3.0	75.1	8.1	1.0
Lemon Tartlette, Go Ahead, McVitie's*	1 Cake/45g	161	4.3	357	3.7	67.9	9.5	1.1
Leo the Lion, Birthday, Asda*	1 Slice/81g	325	12.9	402	2.6	62.0	16.0	0.5
Loaf, Carrot, Kate's Cakes Ltd*	1 Serving/100g	322	14.9	322	4.1	42.7	14.9	2.0
Loaf, Chocolate, Kate's Cakes Ltd*	1 Serving/100g	341	16.1	341	5.4	43.7	16.1	1.1

CAKE

INFO/WEIGHT	Measure	per Measure KCAL	FAT	Nutrition Values per 100g / 100ml KCAL	PROT	CARB	FAT	FIBRE
Loaf, Golden Syrup Drizzle, Kate's Cakes Ltd*	1 Serving/100g	383	18.7	383	5.2	48.4	18.7	1.2
Loaf, Lemon, Kate's Cakes Ltd*	1 Serving/100g	376	19.0	376	5.1	46.1	19.0	1.1
Luxury Chocolate Fudge, Kate's Cakes Ltd*	1 Serving/100g	415	20.8	415	5.1	50.4	20.8	2.8
Madeira	1 Slice/40g	157	6.8	393	5.4	58.4	16.9	0.9
Madeira, All Butter, Sainsbury's*	1 Serving/30g	116	5.9	388	5.2	47.4	19.7	0.8
Madeira, Cherry, Tesco*	¼ Cake/100g	342	11.2	342	4.3	55.9	11.2	2.6
Madeira, Iced, Tesco*	1/16 Cake/56g	218	6.8	389	2.6	67.2	12.2	0.4
Madeira, Lemon Iced, Tesco*	1 Slice/30g	122	5.2	407	4.5	57.8	17.5	0.9
Madeira, Tesco*	1 Serving/50g	197	7.8	394	5.5	57.9	15.6	1.2
Magic Roundabout, Dougal, Tesco*	1 Serving/50g	214	8.0	428	2.3	68.7	16.0	0.2
Manor House, Mr Kipling*	1 Serving/69g	277	13.8	400	5.3	49.7	20.0	1.4
Marble, Tesco*	1/8 Cake/45g	184	8.4	410	4.4	55.9	18.7	1.5
Mini Battenburg, Mr Kipling*	1 Cake/32g	147	3.9	450	4.9	81.2	11.8	1.5
Mini Rolls, Blackforest, Weight Watchers*	1 Cake/24g	89	3.4	374	5.3	58.9	14.2	4.4
Mini Rolls, Cadbury*	1 Roll/27g	120	6.1	445	4.4	56.4	22.5	1.3
Mini Rolls, Chocolate, Tesco*	1 Roll/29g	135	6.7	465	5.5	58.1	23.1	1.3
Mini Rolls, Easter Selection, Cadbury*	1oz/28g	122	5.8	434	5.5	55.6	20.6	0.0
Mini Rolls, Juicy Orange, Cadbury*	1 Cake/28g	110	4.7	390	5.0	55.0	16.8	0.0
Mini Rolls, Milk Chocolate, Cadbury*	1 Roll/27g	120	6.0	445	4.4	56.5	22.2	0.0
Mini Rolls, Milk Chocolate Orange, Shapers, Boots*	1 Roll/25g	97	3.0	386	4.6	64.0	12.0	2.4
Mini Rolls, Rolo, Nestle*	1 Cake/29g	111	5.4	388	4.8	49.5	19.0	1.0
Mint Aero, Celebration, Nestle*	1 Slice/58g	232	11.8	400	4.0	49.7	20.3	1.7
Orange & Cranberry, Mini Classics, Mr Kipling*	1 Cake/36g	164	7.3	455	4.5	42.2	20.2	0.7
Orange & Ginger, Oat Break, Go Ahead, McVitie's*	1 Cake/35g	121	2.2	347	5.2	67.1	6.4	2.6
Orange Marmalade, M & S*	1 Slice/50g	195	9.1	390	3.6	53.2	18.3	1.8
Orange Marmalade Loaf, Aldi*	1 Slice/33g	88	0.7	267	4.5	57.4	2.2	1.8
Panettone, Average	1 Portion/90g	345	15.3	383	8.0	52.0	17.0	0.0
Panettone, Bauli*	1 Serving/75g	313	15.1	418	5.9	53.5	20.1	0.0
Panettone, Luxury, Christmas, Tesco*	1 Serving/83g	307	11.6	370	7.0	53.5	14.0	2.5
Panettone, M & S*	1/8 Loaf/51g	184	6.7	360	6.5	53.4	13.2	2.0
Party, Asda*	1 Serving/57g	238	9.0	421	2.3	67.0	16.0	0.4
Party Bake, M & S*	1/15 Cake/60g	230	12.1	385	4.0	46.6	20.2	0.9
Pecan Brownie, Tray Bake, Kate's Cakes Ltd*	1 Serving/100g	119	27.8	119	6.2	43.5	27.8	1.4
Piece of Cake, Birthday, M & S*	1 Serving/85g	395	24.4	465	4.3	39.7	28.7	0.9
Raisin, Dernys*	1 Cake/45g	175	7.6	388	5.0	54.0	17.0	0.0
Raisin, Sainsbury's*	1 Cake/40g	161	7.6	403	4.7	53.5	18.9	3.0
Raisin, Tesco*	1 Cake/38g	158	7.6	417	5.6	53.8	19.9	1.4
Rich Choc' Roll, Cadbury*	1/6 Portion/39g	149	6.1	381	4.8	50.2	15.6	1.0
Rich Chocolate, Christmas, Tesco*	1 Slice/82g	300	13.5	367	7.0	47.5	16.5	1.6
Rich Fruit, Iced, Finest, Tesco*	1 Slice/57g	191	4.7	335	3.6	61.2	8.3	4.4
Rich Fruit, Kate's Cakes Ltd*	1 Serving/100g	289	8.7	289	3.7	48.9	8.7	2.9
Rich Fruit, Sainsbury's*	1 Serving/100g	321	8.5	321	3.9	57.3	8.5	2.1
Rich Fruit Slices, Free From, Sainsbury's*	1 Slice/40g	144	5.0	361	4.5	57.4	12.6	3.7
Rock	1 Cake/40g	158	6.6	396	5.4	60.5	16.4	1.5
Rock, Tesco*	1 Serving/87g	311	8.4	357	7.4	60.1	9.7	1.6
Seriously Chocolatey, Large, Sainsbury's*	1/24 Cake/77g	352	19.5	457	5.4	51.0	25.3	3.0
Seriously Chocolatey Celebration, Sainsbury's*	1/8 Cake/77g	336	19.8	437	6.3	45.0	25.7	0.3
Shrek Birthday, Tesco*	1/16 Cake/72g	248	8.8	344	3.3	64.0	12.2	0.5
Simnel Slices, Mr Kipling*	1 Slice/47g	177	5.9	379	2.9	63.4	12.6	1.2
Snowballs, Sainsbury's*	1 Snowball/18g	80	4.1	445	2.5	55.6	23.0	3.6
Snowballs, Tesco*	1 Snowball/18g	79	4.0	432	2.5	55.8	22.1	5.4
Spicy Apple, Tray Bake, Kate's Cakes Ltd*	1 Serving/100g	363	20.6	363	4.4	40.0	20.6	2.4
Sponge	1 Slice/53g	243	13.9	459	6.4	52.4	26.3	0.9

	Measure INFO/WEIGHT	per Measure		Nutrition Values per 100g / 100ml				
		KCAL	FAT	KCAL	PROT	CARB	FAT	FIBRE
CAKE								
Sponge, Fatless	1 Slice/53g	156	3.2	294	10.1	53.0	6.1	0.9
Sponge, Fresh Cream & Strawberry, Asda*	1/12 Cake/60g	170	6.0	284	4.6	44.0	10.0	1.1
Sponge, Iced, M & S*	1 Serving/100g	400	17.0	400	3.4	58.4	17.0	1.3
Sponge, Jam Filled	1 Slice/65g	196	3.2	302	4.2	64.2	4.9	1.8
Sponge, Victoria, TTD, Sainsbury's*	1 Slice/57g	229	11.0	401	5.0	51.8	19.3	1.4
Sponge Roll, Chocolate, M & S*	¼ Cake/66g	251	12.1	380	3.9	50.5	18.4	1.8
Sponge with Butter Icing	1 Slice/65g	318	19.9	490	4.5	52.4	30.6	0.6
Spooky, Birthday, Memory Lane Cakes*	1 Slice/75g	295	14.6	393	3.5	50.8	19.5	0.7
St. Clements, Finest, Tesco*	1 Serving/49g	194	10.5	395	3.1	47.2	21.5	0.4
Stem Ginger, 96% Fat Free, Trimlyne*	¼ Cake/63g	170	2.2	272	4.4	58.1	3.6	1.2
Stem Ginger, Mrs Crimble's*	1 Slice/48g	158	1.1	329	2.7	73.3	2.2	2.7
Stollen, Bites, Finest, Tesco*	1 Piece/22g	81	3.2	370	6.5	52.7	14.4	4.4
Stollen, Rich Fruit, Brandy, Christmas, Finest, Tesco*	1 Slice/70g	248	8.2	355	5.6	56.4	11.7	3.1
Stollen, Slices, Finest, Tesco*	1 Slice/45g	164	5.2	365	6.9	57.3	11.6	4.2
Strawberry Sponge Roll, M & S*	1/6 Cake/49g	160	4.6	330	2.8	58.0	9.5	0.8
Sultana, Apple & Cranberry, 99% Fat Free, Trimlyne*	1/6 Cake/67g	130	0.6	195	4.6	45.5	0.9	3.3
Sultana, Fair Trade, Co-Op*	1/8 Cake/45g	155	4.0	345	5.0	60.0	9.0	1.0
Sultana & Cherry, Tesco*	1 Cake/37g	124	4.0	334	4.7	54.4	10.8	2.5
Summer Fruit Cream, GFY, Asda*	1 Serving/74g	165	3.6	223	3.6	41.0	4.9	2.5
Swiss Roll, Average	1oz/28g	77	1.2	276	7.2	55.5	4.4	0.8
Swiss Roll, Chocolate, Individual	1 Roll/26g	88	2.9	337	4.3	58.1	11.3	0.0
Swiss Roll, Chocolate, Lyons*	1 Serving/50g	189	9.6	379	4.3	47.0	19.3	0.9
Swiss Roll, Chocolate, M & S*	1 Serving/46g	168	11.1	365	4.6	32.6	24.2	1.2
Swiss Roll, Raspberry, Asda*	1/6 Roll/35g	104	0.7	298	3.0	66.9	2.0	0.4
Swiss Roll, Raspberry, Lyons*	1 Roll/175g	485	2.4	277	5.2	60.6	1.4	0.0
Swiss Roll, Raspberry, Sainsbury's*	1 Serving/35g	105	0.7	301	3.5	67.0	2.1	1.1
Swiss Roll, Raspberry, Tesco*	1 Serving/45g	132	0.9	294	3.2	65.4	2.1	1.0
Swiss Roll, Raspberry & Vanilla, Morrisons*	1 Serving/28g	98	2.7	350	4.2	61.8	9.5	0.0
Swiss Roll, Raspberry Jam, Mr Kipling*	1/6 Cake/52g	184	5.3	355	2.8	63.0	10.2	1.0
Syrup & Ginger, Tesco*	1 Serving/32g	134	7.0	420	4.5	51.4	21.8	0.7
Tangy Lemon Trickle, M & S*	1 Slice/75g	281	14.1	375	4.7	47.4	18.8	1.1
The Ultimate Carrot Passion, Entenmann's*	1 Slice/52g	210	12.6	403	4.6	42.4	24.3	1.0
Tiffin, Chocolate, Sainsbury's*	1 Cake/61g	184	11.6	301	2.7	29.8	19.0	1.3
Toffee, Iced, Tesco*	1 Serving/35g	132	5.2	376	3.3	57.2	14.9	1.6
Toffee, Slices, BGTY, Sainsbury's*	1 Slice/27g	88	0.7	327	4.3	71.7	2.5	1.8
Toffee, The Handmade Flapjack Company*	1 Cake/75g	346	18.8	462	5.1	54.0	25.1	0.0
Toffee, Thorntons*	1/6 Cake/70g	302	16.8	431	4.6	49.2	24.0	0.8
Toffee & Pecan Slices, M & S*	1 Slice/36g	160	8.5	445	4.7	54.0	23.7	1.3
Toffee Apple, McVitie's*	1 Slice/29g	104	3.2	354	3.5	60.2	11.0	1.5
Toffee Bakewell, Tesco*	1 Cake/49g	203	7.9	414	3.9	63.5	16.1	1.4
Toffee Flavour Slices, Low Fat, Weight Watchers*	1 Slice/27g	80	0.7	297	4.2	63.9	2.6	3.2
Toffee Fudge, Entenmann's*	1 Serving/65g	274	14.1	421	3.4	53.0	21.7	0.5
Toffee Snap, The Handmade Flapjack Company*	1 Cake/75g	365	19.6	487	4.6	62.2	26.1	0.0
Toffee Temptation, Finest, Tesco*	1 Serving/50g	211	11.5	423	4.7	49.0	23.1	0.6
Toffee Temptation, Tesco*	1 Slice/67g	228	12.8	340	2.9	39.1	19.1	0.3
Tray Bake, Crunchy Granola, Waitrose*	1/6 Tray/42g	187	10.1	445	5.8	51.2	24.1	4.5
Triple Chocolate Roll, Cadbury*	1 Serving/40g	165	6.7	410	4.3	60.1	16.6	1.5
Turkish Delight, Fry's*	1 Cake/26g	96	2.8	371	4.5	62.4	10.8	0.5
Vanilla Sponge, Fresh Cream, Sainsbury's*	1 Slice/50g	152	5.1	304	7.5	45.6	10.2	0.4
Very Berry, Kate's Cakes Ltd*	1 Serving/100g	346	14.6	346	3.4	50.3	14.6	1.4
Victoria Sandwich, Classic, Large, M & S*	1/10 Cake/66g	260	12.9	395	5.1	49.5	19.6	2.3
Victoria Sandwich, Co-Op*	1oz/28g	101	4.8	360	4.0	48.0	17.0	1.0
Victoria Slices, Mr Kipling*	1 Slice/28g	122	4.4	432	3.9	68.8	15.7	0.4

	Measure INFO/WEIGHT	per Measure KCAL	FAT	Nutrition Values per 100g / 100ml KCAL	PROT	CARB	FAT	FIBRE
CAKE								
Victoria Sponge, Kate's Cakes Ltd*	1 Serving/100g	410	19.7	410	4.0	52.8	19.7	0.9
Victoria Sponge, Lemon, Co-Op*	1 Slice/42g	151	8.0	360	4.0	44.0	19.0	0.7
Victoria Sponge, Mini, Bobby's*	1 Cake/35g	164	9.6	469	4.0	51.3	27.5	0.2
Victoria Sponge, Mini, Mr Kipling*	1 Cake/36g	152	6.9	420	3.9	58.5	19.0	0.8
Victoria Sponge, Mini, Weight Watchers*	1 Cake/30g	103	2.5	343	5.7	57.2	8.3	8.4
Viennese, M & S*	1 Cake/51g	250	14.1	495	4.1	58.9	28.0	2.8
Viennese Whirl, Chocolate, Mr Kipling*	1 Whirl/28g	134	7.8	484	4.6	53.1	28.0	2.1
Viennese Whirl, Lemon, Mr Kipling*	1 Cake/28g	115	4.5	409	4.2	62.2	15.9	0.7
Viennese Whirl, Mr Kipling*	1 Cake/28g	141	7.8	504	3.9	59.1	28.0	1.4
Viennese Whirl, Tesco*	1 Cake/39g	181	10.2	465	4.0	53.2	26.2	1.2
Walnut, Sandwich, Sainsbury's*	1/8 Cake/48g	182	8.3	379	5.4	53.7	17.3	1.3
Walnut & Coffee, Co-Op*	¼ Cake/65g	253	13.0	390	5.0	47.0	20.0	0.7
Welsh, Average	1oz/28g	121	5.5	431	5.6	61.8	19.6	1.5
Winnie the Pooh Birthday, Disney, Nestle*	1 Serving/100g	361	10.9	361	2.4	63.3	10.9	0.5
Xmas Pudding, Tesco*	1 Cake/17g	58	1.6	349	3.3	60.5	9.3	1.4
CAKE BAR								
Blueberry, Trimlyne*	1 Cake/50g	141	1.1	283	3.9	64.0	2.2	2.2
Bounty, McVitie's*	1 Cake/36g	166	8.8	461	5.1	55.2	24.5	0.0
Caramel, Cadbury*	1 Bar/26g	107	4.4	411	6.4	57.0	16.8	0.0
Caramel, Tesco*	1 Cake/26g	103	4.9	395	5.1	50.8	19.0	8.2
Caramel, Weight Watchers*	1 Bar/23g	89	3.0	381	5.3	56.2	12.8	9.9
Carrot, Gu*	1 Slice/38g	135	6.6	354	1.4	17.2	17.5	0.9
Carrot, Tesco*	1 Bar/68g	239	12.6	351	4.7	41.4	18.5	2.4
Carrot with Cheese Cream Icing, Kate's Cakes Ltd*	1 Serving/100g	345	15.6	345	3.3	48.3	15.6	1.5
Choc Chip, Go Ahead, McVitie's*	1 Cake/28g	100	3.5	356	6.4	56.9	12.4	1.0
Choc Chip, Mini, Go Ahead, McVitie's*	1 Bar/27g	93	3.3	343	5.7	55.3	12.1	0.9
Chocolate, Asda*	1 Bar/27g	124	5.6	461	5.0	63.0	21.0	2.5
Chocolate, High Lights, Cadbury*	1 Bar/25g	95	3.5	380	5.5	58.8	14.0	1.1
Chocolate, Snack Cakes, Penguin, McVitie's*	1 Bar/24g	122	7.2	510	4.8	54.6	30.2	1.6
Chocolate, Tesco*	1 Serving/26g	113	6.0	435	5.2	51.9	23.0	5.4
Chocolate & Orange, Go Ahead, McVitie's*	1 Cake/33g	109	2.0	330	4.3	64.9	6.0	1.0
Chocolate Chip, HL, Tesco*	1 Serving/37g	109	1.0	295	4.8	63.6	2.6	0.6
Chocolate Chip, Mr Kipling*	1 Bar/32g	151	8.4	472	5.3	53.5	26.3	1.2
Chocolate Chip, Sainsbury's*	1 Cake/25g	107	5.6	430	6.1	51.2	22.3	0.6
Chocolate Chip, Tesco*	1 Cake/30g	124	5.9	415	7.0	51.4	19.7	2.3
Chocolate Dream, Go Ahead, McVitie's*	1 Bar/36g	141	4.8	391	4.6	63.2	13.4	0.9
Chocolate with Creamy Cocoa Icing, Kate's Cakes Ltd*	1 Serving/100g	375	18.4	375	5.1	47.8	18.4	1.2
Cinder Toffee, Cadbury*	1 Cake/32g	149	8.4	465	4.2	53.4	26.2	0.9
Crunchie, Cadbury*	1 Cake/32g	147	7.2	460	5.9	58.3	22.6	0.0
Double Chocolate, Free From, Sainsbury's*	1 Cake/50g	196	7.9	391	4.2	58.2	15.7	1.0
Double Chocolate, Free From, Tesco*	1 Serving/45g	179	7.8	397	4.6	55.7	17.3	1.1
Dream, Cadbury*	1 Cake/38g	170	8.5	450	4.5	57.2	22.6	0.0
Flake, Cadbury*	1 Cake/22g	97	5.1	442	6.5	51.8	23.3	0.5
Fruit & Nut Crisp, Go Ahead, McVitie's*	1 Bar/22g	95	3.0	430	5.3	71.3	13.7	1.7
Fudge, Cadbury*	1 Pack/52g	220	9.2	420	5.7	60.3	17.6	0.0
Galaxy Caramel, McVitie's*	1 Cake/31g	137	6.5	441	5.5	57.4	21.1	0.0
Golden Syrup, McVitie's*	1 Cake/33g	127	4.8	385	3.6	60.2	14.4	1.2
Jaffa, McVitie's*	1 Bar/25g	97	3.5	390	3.2	62.4	14.2	2.4
Jaffa Cake, McVitie's*	1 Cake/31g	126	5.4	408	3.9	59.1	17.4	2.9
Jaffa Cakes, Spooky, McVitie's*	1 Bar/25g	96	3.5	390	3.2	62.1	14.2	2.7
Jamaica Ginger, McVitie's*	1 Cake/33g	128	4.9	388	3.5	60.2	14.7	1.2
Lemon Meringue, Indulgence, Weight Watchers*	1 Bar/24g	21	0.3	86	1.1	7.1	1.3	0.0
Lemon with Sugar Pearls, Kate's Cakes Ltd*	1 Serving/100g	325	15.8	325	4.2	43.4	15.8	0.9

	Measure INFO/WEIGHT	per Measure		Nutrition Values per 100g / 100ml				
		KCAL	FAT	KCAL	PROT	CARB	FAT	FIBRE
CAKE BAR								
Milk Chocolate, Cadbury*	1 Bar/35g	150	7.6	430	5.6	53.3	21.7	1.2
Milk Chocolate & Orange, Crispy, Asda*	1 Bar/22g	91	2.2	413	4.8	75.6	10.2	2.0
Milk Chocolate Orange, Sandwich Bar, Lyons*	1 Bar/28g	142	8.0	516	5.0	62.0	29.0	0.0
Milky Way, McVitie's*	1 Cake/26g	124	6.2	476	5.1	58.5	23.6	1.2
Rich Chocolate, Trimlyne*	1 Serving/40g	115	1.7	287	5.2	59.2	4.2	2.2
Toffee Cake, High Lights, Cadbury*	1 Bar/25g	95	3.5	380	7.6	56.7	14.0	0.9
CAKE MIX								
Carrot Cake, Betty Crocker*	¼ Pack/125g	504	8.4	403	5.8	78.9	6.7	1.4
Cheesecake, Original, Made Up, Asda*	1/6 Cake/85g	228	10.2	268	4.1	36.0	12.0	1.4
Cheesecake, Strawberry, Real, Green's*	1 Serving/100g	254	12.8	253	3.9	30.6	12.8	0.6
Cheesecake, Tesco*	1 Serving/76g	199	7.9	262	4.1	38.0	10.4	1.6
Chocolate Brownie, Choc Chips, Weight Watchers*	1 Pack/190g	568	13.5	299	3.2	55.6	7.1	2.1
Dennis, Green's*	1 Cake/17g	55	1.3	319	4.6	57.8	7.7	0.0
Free From, Sainsbury's*	1 Serving/50g	173	0.1	346	1.3	84.4	0.3	2.2
Yellow, Super Moist, Betty Crocker*	1 Cake/128g	517	9.5	404	3.3	81.6	7.4	1.1
CALLALOO								
Leaves, Raw, Unprepared	1 Cup/28g	6	0.1	23	2.5	4.0	0.3	0.0
CALZONE								
Bolognese, Weight Watchers*	1 Calzone/88g	178	3.0	202	11.7	31.2	3.4	4.3
Cheese & Tomato, Weight Watchers*	1 Calzone/88g	191	3.8	217	11.3	33.4	4.3	3.4
Ham & Gruyere, Asda*	1 Serving/280g	661	22.4	236	10.0	31.0	8.0	2.7
CANAPES								
Aegean Tomato, Finest, Tesco*	1 Canape/15g	45	2.2	300	7.2	34.3	14.7	2.1
Caponata, Puff Pastry, Occasions, Sainsbury's*	1 Square/12g	30	1.9	249	4.1	22.9	15.7	2.1
Salmon & Dill, Finest, Tesco*	1 Canape/15g	47	2.4	315	9.2	32.7	16.1	1.9
Smoked Salmon, Youngs*	1 Canape/10g	21	1.5	210	15.9	2.0	15.2	0.7
CANNELLONI								
Beef	1 Serving/335g	501	21.8	149	8.4	14.1	6.5	1.4
Beef, BGTY, Sainsbury's*	1 Pack/300g	249	6.9	83	5.5	10.1	2.3	1.7
Beef, Finest, Tesco*	½ Pack/300g	399	22.2	133	7.1	9.4	7.4	1.9
Beef, Great Value, Asda*	1 Pack/400g	384	10.8	96	6.0	12.0	2.7	1.6
Beef, HL, Tesco*	1 Pack/340g	323	8.2	95	6.4	11.9	2.4	1.5
Beef, Italian, Sainsbury's*	1 Pack/400g	498	26.2	124	5.9	10.5	6.5	1.6
Beef, Italian, Tesco*	1 Pack/400g	520	26.8	130	5.3	11.6	6.7	0.9
Beef, Sainsbury's*	1 Pack/400g	372	17.6	93	4.4	8.8	4.4	1.6
Beef, TTD, Sainsbury's*	1 Pack/383g	548	26.8	143	7.2	12.7	7.0	2.3
Beef & Red Wine, TTD, Sainsbury's*	½ Pack/180g	448	11.5	249	14.8	32.1	6.4	1.8
Beef & Red Wine, Waitrose*	½ Pack/170g	355	16.0	209	17.5	13.8	9.4	1.0
Chicken & Pesto, Italian, Sainsbury's*	1 Pack/450g	675	33.7	150	6.1	14.4	7.5	1.1
Mediterranean Vegetable, Waitrose*	1 Serving/170g	330	15.3	194	9.7	18.7	9.0	1.9
Mushroom, Italian, Sainsbury's*	1 Pack/450g	598	31.0	133	5.2	12.5	6.9	0.5
Parmesan & Basil, M & S*	1 Pack/360g	504	28.4	140	5.9	11.4	7.9	0.8
Ricotta & Spinach, Co-Op*	1 Pack/400g	420	20.0	105	4.0	12.0	5.0	2.0
Ricotta & Spinach, Fresh, Waitrose*	½ Pack/225g	274	16.4	122	5.1	8.8	7.3	1.2
Ricotta & Spinach, Perfectly Balanced, Waitrose*	1 Pack/400g	272	9.2	68	3.8	7.7	2.3	1.4
Roasted Vegetable, Morrisons*	1 Serving/350g	311	8.7	89	3.9	12.5	2.5	2.3
Smoked Salmon & Spinach, Sainsbury's*	1 Pack/450g	598	27.9	133	5.7	13.5	6.2	0.4
Spinach & Cheese, Finest, Tesco*	1 Pack/350g	532	31.8	152	5.4	12.1	9.1	1.5
Spinach & Ricotta, BGTY, Sainsbury's*	1 Pack/400g	372	11.6	93	4.4	12.5	2.9	1.8
Spinach & Ricotta, COU, M & S*	1 Pack/400g	360	10.0	90	4.7	10.6	2.5	2.5
Spinach & Ricotta, Finest, Tesco*	1 Serving/120g	276	13.8	230	8.4	22.1	11.5	2.1
Spinach & Ricotta, Frozen, Sainsbury's*	1 Pack/350g	513	25.8	147	6.1	13.9	7.4	1.1
Spinach & Ricotta, Healthier Choice, Co-Op*	1 Pack/400g	320	10.4	80	4.0	10.8	2.6	0.9

INFO/WEIGHT	Measure	per Measure		Nutrition Values per 100g / 100ml				
		KCAL	FAT	KCAL	PROT	CARB	FAT	FIBRE
CANNELLONI								
Spinach & Ricotta, HL, Tesco*	1 Pack/400g	320	11.2	80	4.0	10.0	2.8	1.1
Spinach & Ricotta, Italian, Sainsbury's*	1 Pack/400g	476	30.0	119	4.8	8.1	7.5	1.7
Spinach & Ricotta, Italian Style, Co-Op*	1 Pack/450g	540	27.0	120	5.0	12.0	6.0	2.0
Spinach & Ricotta, Light Choices, Tesco*	1 Pack/400g	340	11.2	85	4.0	10.0	2.8	1.1
Spinach & Ricotta, Ross*	1 Pack/299g	296	8.1	99	3.3	15.2	2.7	1.6
Spinach & Ricotta, Waitrose*	1 Pack/400g	460	26.8	115	5.1	8.7	6.7	1.3
Spinach & Wild Mushroom, Linda McCartney*	1 Pack/340g	381	13.6	112	4.9	14.1	4.0	1.7
Tubes, Dry, Average	*1oz/28g*	*101*	*1.0*	*361*	*12.5*	*69.1*	*3.6*	*1.2*
Vegetarian, Tesco*	1 Pack/400g	552	34.4	138	5.3	9.8	8.6	1.5
CAPERS								
Caperberries, Spanish, Waitrose*	1 Serving/55g	9	0.3	17	1.1	2.1	0.5	2.5
Capucines, Sainsbury's*	1 Tsp/6g	1	0.0	14	1.4	1.3	0.3	2.2
in Brine, Tesco*	1 Tsp/2g	1	0.0	29	2.4	3.5	0.6	2.7
in Vinegar, Average	1 Tsp/5g	2	0.0	34	1.7	3.0	0.6	0.0
CAPPELLETTI								
Goats Cheese & Red Pesto, Waitrose*	½ Pack/125g	374	10.9	299	11.6	43.5	8.7	2.2
Parma Ham, Fresh, Waitrose*	½ Pack/125g	367	11.5	294	14.1	38.6	9.2	2.2
CAPRI SUN								
Orange	1 Pouch/200ml	90	0.0	45	0.0	11.0	0.0	0.0
Orange, 100%, Juice	1 Pouch/200ml	75	0.0	38	0.5	9.2	0.0	0.1
CARAMAC								
Nestle*	1 Bar/30g	173	11.0	567	5.7	54.7	36.1	0.0
CARAMBOLA								
Average	*1oz/28g*	*9*	*0.1*	*32*	*0.5*	*7.3*	*0.3*	*1.3*
CARAMEL								
Egg, Cadbury*	1 Egg/39g	191	10.2	490	4.3	58.9	26.1	0.0
CARAWAY								
Seeds, Schwartz*	1 Pack/38g	170	8.1	448	23.3	40.9	21.2	0.0
CARBONARA								
Pasta, Low Fat, Solo Slim, Rosemary Conley*	1 Pack/300g	282	11.7	94	4.2	10.4	3.9	1.3
CARDAMOM								
Black, Ground, Average	*1 Tsp/2g*	*6*	*0.1*	*311*	*10.8*	*68.5*	*6.7*	*28.0*
Ground, Average	*1 Tsp/2g*	*6*	*0.1*	*314*	*10.7*	*53.6*	*7.1*	*28.6*
CAROB POWDER								
Average	*1 Tsp/2g*	*3*	*0.0*	*159*	*4.9*	*37.0*	*0.1*	*0.0*
CARP								
Fillet, Raw, Average	1 Fillet/218g	244	10.2	112	17.5	0.0	4.7	0.0
CARROT & SWEDE								
Diced, for Mashing, Average	*½ Pack/250g*	*57*	*0.7*	*23*	*0.6*	*4.7*	*0.3*	*1.9*
Mash, From Supermarket, Average	1 Serving/150g	138	7.5	92	1.3	10.4	5.0	1.3
Mash, Healthy Range, Average	1 Serving/150g	98	4.2	65	1.3	8.6	2.8	2.1
CARROTS								
Baby, Canned, Average	*1 Can/195g*	*40*	*0.5*	*21*	*0.5*	*4.2*	*0.3*	*2.1*
Baby, Fresh, Average	*1 Serving/80g*	*28*	*0.1*	*35*	*0.6*	*8.2*	*0.1*	*2.9*
Batons, Fresh, Average	*½ Pack/150g*	*41*	*0.4*	*27*	*0.6*	*5.7*	*0.3*	*2.6*
Boiled, Average	*1oz/28g*	*6*	*0.1*	*22*	*0.6*	*4.4*	*0.4*	*2.3*
Canned, Average	*1oz/28g*	*6*	*0.1*	*22*	*0.6*	*4.4*	*0.2*	*2.1*
Raw, Scrubbed, Average	1 Serving/80g	24	0.4	30	0.7	6.0	0.5	2.4
Sliced, Canned, Average	*1 Serving/180g*	*36*	*0.2*	*20*	*0.7*	*4.1*	*0.1*	*1.5*
Sliced, Fresh, Average	*1 Serving/60g*	*17*	*0.2*	*28*	*0.7*	*5.7*	*0.3*	*2.0*
Whole, Raw, Peeled, Average	*1 Carrot/75g*	*21*	*0.2*	*29*	*0.6*	*6.3*	*0.3*	*2.2*
CASHEW NUTS								
BBQ, Graze*	1 Pack/26g	142	10.8	546	13.9	37.0	41.7	0.0

	Measure INFO/WEIGHT	per Measure KCAL	FAT	Nutrition Values per 100g / 100ml KCAL	PROT	CARB	FAT	FIBRE
CASHEW NUTS								
Ca-shew! Bless You, Graze*	1 Punnet/40g	146	5.8	365	6.1	57.2	14.5	0.0
Cheese Flavour, Graze*	1 Pack/26g	140	10.8	540	15.3	35.7	41.5	0.0
Cracked Black Pepper Cashews, Graze*	1 Punnet/35g	187	14.6	535	14.0	34.5	41.6	3.0
Frosted, Graze*	1 Pack /26g	134	8.4	516	10.5	53.0	32.2	0.0
Honey, Graze*	½ Pack/13g	67	4.2	516	10.5	53.0	32.2	0.0
Hot Chilli, Graze*	1 Box/26g	139	10.9	535	14.5	33.6	41.8	0.0
Mexican Chilli, Graze*	1 Pack/26g	140	10.8	539	14.3	34.9	41.6	0.0
Plain, Average	*¼ Pack/25g*	*146*	*12.2*	*584*	*15.7*	*18.7*	*48.9*	*3.4*
Roasted & Salted, Average	*1 Serving/50g*	*306*	*25.5*	*612*	*18.8*	*19.5*	*51.1*	*3.1*
CASHEWS & PEANUTS								
Honey Roasted, Average	*1 Serving/50g*	*289*	*21.4*	*579*	*21.6*	*26.6*	*42.9*	*4.2*
Salted, Sainsbury's*	1oz/28g	169	14.2	603	24.2	12.7	50.6	6.9
CASSAVA								
Baked, Average	*1oz/28g*	*43*	*0.1*	*155*	*0.7*	*40.1*	*0.2*	*1.7*
Boiled in Unsalted Water, Average	*1oz/28g*	*36*	*0.1*	*130*	*0.5*	*33.5*	*0.2*	*1.4*
Gari, Average	*1oz/28g*	*100*	*0.1*	*358*	*1.3*	*92.9*	*0.5*	*0.0*
Raw, Average	*1oz/28g*	*40*	*0.1*	*142*	*0.6*	*36.8*	*0.2*	*1.6*
Steamed, Average	*1oz/28g*	*40*	*0.1*	*142*	*0.6*	*36.8*	*0.2*	*1.6*
CASSEROLE								
Bean, & Lentil, Morrisons*	1 Can/410g	287	1.6	70	4.1	12.5	0.4	0.0
Bean, Spicy, BGTY, Sainsbury's*	1 Pack/300g	171	2.7	57	3.0	9.1	0.9	4.2
Beef	1 Serving/336g	490	23.0	146	16.3	4.6	6.8	0.6
Beef, & Ale, Finest, Tesco*	½ Pack/300g	234	4.2	78	11.5	5.0	1.4	1.1
Beef, & Ale, with Dumplings, Sainsbury's*	1 Pack/450g	711	32.8	158	7.7	15.4	7.3	0.6
Beef, & Ale, with Mashed Potato, HL, Tesco*	1 Pack/450g	364	11.2	81	5.1	10.9	2.5	0.6
Beef, & Onion, Minced, British Classics, Tesco*	1 Pack/340g	367	19.0	108	5.0	9.3	5.6	0.8
Beef, & Red Wine, BGTY, Sainsbury's*	1 Pack/300g	192	1.8	64	8.0	6.7	0.6	0.9
Beef, Canned, Waitrose*	1 Can/400g	372	10.0	93	10.5	7.0	2.5	1.8
Beef, Diet Chef Ltd*	1 Pack/300g	177	3.0	59	7.8	4.7	1.0	2.4
Beef, Fellside, Look What We Found*	1 Pouch/300g	219	5.1	73	9.1	5.3	1.7	2.1
Beef, Meal for One, Tesco*	1 Pack/450g	425	18.9	94	3.6	10.6	4.2	1.7
Beef, Mini Favourites, M & S*	1 Pack/200g	210	8.4	105	7.1	9.3	4.2	1.4
Beef, Traditional, Control Chef, All About Weight*	1 Meal/271g	258	2.7	95	9.1	11.0	1.0	3.0
Beef, with Dumplings, GFY, Asda*	1 Pack/400g	416	8.8	104	11.0	10.0	2.2	0.9
Beef, with Herb Potatoes, Tesco*	1 Serving/475g	503	17.1	106	6.8	11.5	3.6	1.6
Beef & Red Wine, M & S*	1 Pack/420g	399	11.3	95	8.0	9.4	2.7	1.8
Beef & Red Wine, Weight Watchers*	1 Pack/330g	254	9.2	77	4.3	8.6	2.8	0.3
Chicken, & Asparagus, HL, Tesco*	1 Serving/450g	342	10.3	76	6.3	8.3	2.3	0.5
Chicken, & Asparagus, in White Wine, Finest, Tesco*	1 Pack/350g	683	42.4	195	10.0	11.6	12.1	0.3
Chicken, & Asparagus in White Wine, Tesco*	½ Pack/300g	444	23.7	148	11.5	7.7	7.9	0.8
Chicken, & Dumplings, HL, Tesco*	1 Pack/450g	441	12.1	98	7.4	11.1	2.7	0.6
Chicken, & Dumplings, Morrisons*	1 Pack/300g	291	12.6	97	3.4	11.4	4.2	1.3
Chicken, & Dumplings, Sainsbury's*	1 Serving/450g	612	32.4	136	6.8	11.0	7.2	0.6
Chicken, & Red Wine, Duchy Originals*	½ Pack/175g	187	7.5	107	14.0	5.1	4.3	1.6
Chicken, & Tomato, Asda*	¼ Pack/273g	569	41.0	208	16.0	2.2	15.0	0.5
Chicken, & Vegetable, Apetito*	1 Pack/330g	286	9.9	87	6.3	9.4	3.0	1.6
Chicken, & Vegetable, Long Life, Sainsbury's*	1 Pack/300g	186	4.5	62	4.6	7.4	1.5	0.8
Chicken, & White Wine, BGTY, Sainsbury's*	1 Serving/300g	216	6.6	72	7.2	5.9	2.2	1.3
Chicken, Carrots, Peas & Potatoes, Weight Watchers*	1 Serving/302g	193	4.2	64	4.3	8.6	1.4	0.5
Chicken, Diet Chef Ltd*	1 Pack/300g	219	2.7	73	9.0	7.2	0.9	2.5
Chicken, Green Isle*	1 Pack/400g	300	6.8	75	5.7	9.2	1.7	1.0
Chicken, Leek & Mushroom, Tesco*	1 Pack/350g	381	22.0	109	4.5	8.6	6.3	1.0
Chicken, Mediterranean, Tesco*	1 Pack/400g	260	9.2	65	6.7	4.5	2.3	0.9

C

CASEROLE

INFO/WEIGHT	Measure	per Measure KCAL	per Measure FAT	Nutrition Values per 100g / 100ml KCAL	PROT	CARB	FAT	FIBRE
Chicken, Perfectly Balanced, Waitrose*	1 Pack/400g	392	14.4	98	6.6	9.8	3.6	1.2
Chicken, Skinny Chef, All About Weight*	1 Meal/269g	277	0.8	103	11.2	11.9	0.3	3.8
Chicken, with Dumplings, M & S*	½ Pack/227g	261	10.0	115	9.7	9.0	4.4	0.9
Cowboy, Iceland*	1 Pack/400g	500	26.0	125	5.8	10.9	6.5	1.7
Ham Hock & Mash, Tesco*	1 Pack/250g	225	8.0	90	6.1	9.0	3.2	0.8
Lamb, & Rosemary, Eat Well, M & S*	1 Pack/380g	325	11.0	86	7.6	7.0	2.9	2.2
Lamb, BGTY, Sainsbury's*	1 Serving/200g	242	8.6	121	20.7	0.1	4.3	0.1
Lamb, Braised, British Classics, Tesco*	1 Pack/350g	332	18.2	95	7.5	4.6	5.2	1.2
Lamb, COU, M & S*	1 Pack/390g	253	6.6	65	5.9	6.7	1.7	1.6
Lamb, with Mint Dumplings, Minced, Sainsbury's*	1 Pack/450g	558	30.6	124	5.4	10.4	6.8	1.1
Lamb, with Rosemary Roast Potatoes, Asda*	1 Pack/450g	477	21.6	106	8.9	6.9	4.8	1.5
Mediterranean Seafood, HL, Tesco*	1 Pack/344g	292	6.9	85	5.8	10.5	2.0	3.2
Mushroom, & Onion, Iceland*	1 Pack/400g	272	12.4	68	1.3	8.8	3.1	1.9
Pork, Normandy Style, Finest, Tesco*	1 Pack/450g	405	21.6	90	7.6	4.1	4.8	2.3
Rabbit, Average	1oz/28g	29	1.4	102	11.6	2.6	5.1	0.4
Root Vegetable, with Herb Dumplings, Tesco*	1 Pack/450g	373	11.2	83	2.1	12.8	2.5	3.3
Sausage, & Potato, M & S*	1 Serving/200g	190	11.8	95	3.3	7.5	5.9	0.9
Sausage, Chosen By You, Asda*	1 Pot/400g	240	15.2	60	3.6	1.9	3.8	2.1
Sausage, Pork, Diet Chef Ltd*	1 Pack/300g	303	18.3	101	6.6	4.9	6.1	1.4
Sausage, Solo Slim, Rosemary Conley*	1 Pack/300g	312	15.0	104	5.7	9.0	5.0	3.1
Steak, & Ale, British Classics, Tesco*	1 Serving/100g	93	3.4	93	11.2	4.5	3.4	1.1
Steak, & Ale, Sainsbury's*	1 Pack/300g	288	10.5	96	10.6	5.6	3.5	0.4
Steak, & Mushroom, Asda*	½ Pack/304g	411	30.4	135	7.0	4.2	10.0	0.3
Steak, & Mushroom with Mustard Mash, Finest, Tesco*	1 Pack/550g	522	21.4	95	5.9	9.0	3.9	1.1
Steak & Kidney, Mini, Favourites, M & S*	1 Pack/200g	240	10.8	120	7.9	9.5	5.4	1.5
Three Bean, Solo Slim, Rosemary Conley*	1 Pack/300g	195	2.7	65	4.0	10.3	0.9	3.6
Vegetable, & Lentil, Canned, Granose*	1 Can/400g	272	8.0	68	3.5	9.0	2.0	3.0
Vegetable, Chunky, M & S*	1 Bag/450g	90	1.3	20	0.7	3.4	0.3	1.4
Vegetable, Country, Sainsbury's*	1 Can/400g	300	10.0	75	2.2	11.0	2.5	1.1
Vegetable, Tesco*	1 Serving/220g	66	0.7	30	0.8	6.1	0.3	1.5
Vegetable, with Herb Dumplings, COU, M & S*	1 Pack/450g	270	5.4	60	1.6	10.1	1.2	1.0
Venison, Scottish Wild, & Beaujolais, Tesco*	1 Pack/425g	365	8.9	86	11.9	4.9	2.1	0.6

CASSEROLE MIX

INFO/WEIGHT	Measure	per Measure KCAL	per Measure FAT	Nutrition Values per 100g / 100ml KCAL	PROT	CARB	FAT	FIBRE
Beef, Authentic, Schwartz*	1 Pack/43g	111	0.4	257	7.4	54.5	1.0	0.4
Beef, Colman's*	1 Pack/40g	123	0.6	308	7.5	66.0	1.5	2.5
Beef & Ale, Colman's*	1 Pack/45g	144	0.9	320	9.2	66.3	2.0	2.3
Chicken, Authentic, Schwartz*	1 Pack/36g	131	1.5	363	10.4	70.7	4.3	2.0
Chicken, Traditional, Colman's*	1 Pack/40g	124	0.5	311	5.7	69.4	1.3	1.5
Chicken Chasseur, Asda*	1 Pack/80g	273	0.8	341	9.0	74.0	1.0	1.4
Chicken Chasseur, Morrisons*	1 Pack/40g	115	0.5	288	9.2	59.8	1.2	0.0
Farmhouse Sausage, Schwartz*	1 Pack/39g	124	1.1	317	8.1	64.6	2.9	0.5
Honey Chicken, Colman's*	1 Pack/50g	128	0.5	257	3.4	58.3	1.1	1.8
Lamb, Authentic, Schwartz*	1 Pack/35g	116	1.2	332	7.7	68.0	3.3	1.3
Liver & Bacon, Colman's*	1 Pack/40g	121	0.7	303	10.3	61.6	1.7	4.7
Moroccan Lamb, Schwartz*	1 Pack/35g	124	2.0	354	6.2	74.1	5.7	4.5
Peppered Beef, Schwartz*	1 Pack/40g	129	2.0	323	7.0	62.9	4.9	7.3
Pork, Colman's*	1 Pack/40g	131	0.6	328	6.7	72.0	1.4	2.8
Pork, Morrisons*	1 Pack/36g	118	0.5	327	8.1	70.6	1.4	0.0
Sausage, Asda*	¼ Pack/25g	80	1.0	321	6.0	65.0	4.1	3.0
Sausage, Classic, Schwartz*	1 Pack/35g	96	0.9	275	12.4	50.1	2.7	14.9
Sausage, Colman's*	1 Pack/40g	144	0.6	361	8.9	77.7	1.6	1.6
Sausage & Onion, Colman's*	1 Pack/45g	143	1.2	318	9.6	64.2	2.6	2.6
Somerset Pork, Colman's*	1 Pack/45g	144	0.6	321	7.1	70.2	1.3	2.2

	Measure INFO/WEIGHT	per Measure		Nutrition Values per 100g / 100ml				
		KCAL	FAT	KCAL	PROT	CARB	FAT	FIBRE
CASSEROLE MIX								
Somerset Pork, Schwartz*	1 Pack/36g	115	1.4	320	9.4	61.9	3.8	7.7
Spicy Chicken, Colman's*	1 Pack/45g	151	0.8	336	6.5	73.4	1.8	1.5
Turkey, Colman's*	1 Pack/50g	156	0.9	313	5.9	68.0	1.9	3.5
CATFISH								
Cooked, Average	*1 Fillet/87g*	*199*	*11.6*	*229*	*18.0*	*8.0*	*13.3*	*0.7*
Raw, Average	*1oz/28g*	*27*	*0.8*	*96*	*17.6*	*0.0*	*2.8*	*0.0*
CAULIFLOWER								
Boiled, Average	*1 Serving/80g*	*22*	*0.7*	*28*	*2.9*	*2.1*	*0.9*	*1.6*
Raw, Average	*1 Serving/80g*	*25*	*0.7*	*31*	*3.2*	*2.7*	*0.8*	*1.6*
Steamed, Average	1 Serving/100g	28	0.9	28	2.9	2.1	0.9	1.6
CAULIFLOWER CHEESE								
& Bacon, Gastropub, M & S*	1 Pack/300g	318	21.0	106	6.3	4.5	7.0	1.0
& Broccoli, Morrisons*	1 Serving/500g	355	16.5	71	3.7	6.6	3.3	0.9
& Broccoli, Sainsbury's*	1 Serving/130g	83	2.1	64	4.8	7.6	1.6	2.7
Asda*	1 Pack/450g	486	36.0	108	4.6	4.3	8.0	1.5
Birds Eye*	1 Pack/329g	355	21.1	108	4.8	7.7	6.4	0.8
Extra Special, Asda*	½ Pack/200g	166	11.6	83	4.0	3.7	5.8	2.1
Finest, Tesco*	1 Serving/250g	325	22.2	130	5.7	5.9	8.9	1.2
Frozen, Tesco*	1 Pack/450g	427	30.1	95	4.2	4.3	6.7	1.3
Grills, Grassington's Food Co*	1 Grill/92g	157	4.6	171	6.1	25.3	5.0	2.6
Less Than 3% Fat, BGTY, Sainsbury's*	½ Pack/200g	98	3.4	49	3.3	5.3	1.7	1.0
M & S*	1 Serving/150g	150	9.1	100	5.5	5.9	6.1	1.1
Made with Semi-Skimmed Milk	1oz/28g	28	1.8	100	6.0	5.2	6.4	1.3
Made with Skimmed Milk	1oz/28g	27	1.7	97	6.0	5.2	6.0	1.3
Made with Whole Milk	1oz/28g	29	1.9	105	6.0	5.2	6.9	1.3
Waitrose*	1 Pack/450g	328	21.6	73	4.1	3.3	4.8	1.6
CAVATELLI								
Egg, Asda*	1 Serving/100g	203	3.4	203	9.0	34.0	3.4	3.0
King Prawn & Scallop, M & S*	1 Pack/400g	600	22.4	150	6.4	18.0	5.6	1.3
CAVIAR								
Average	*1oz/28g*	*26*	*1.3*	*92*	*11.9*	*0.5*	*4.7*	*0.0*
CELERIAC								
Boiled in Salted Water, Average	*1oz/28g*	*4*	*0.1*	*15*	*0.9*	*1.9*	*0.5*	*3.2*
Raw, Average	*1 Serving/100g*	*42*	*0.3*	*42*	*1.5*	*9.2*	*0.3*	*1.8*
CELERY								
Boiled in Salted Water	*1 Serving/50g*	*4*	*0.1*	*8*	*0.5*	*0.8*	*0.3*	*1.2*
Raw, Trimmed	*1 Stalk/40g*	*3*	*0.1*	*7*	*0.5*	*0.9*	*0.2*	*1.1*
CHAMPAGNE								
Average	*1 Glass/120ml*	*91*	*0.0*	*76*	*0.3*	*1.4*	*0.0*	*0.0*
CHANNA MASALA								
Indian, Sainsbury's*	1 Serving/149g	165	7.3	111	4.2	12.4	4.9	3.3
M & S*	1 Pack/225g	360	23.7	160	5.6	11.2	10.5	8.2
Waitrose*	1 Pack/300g	300	18.3	100	3.7	7.4	6.1	7.9
CHAPATIS								
Brown Wheat Flour, Waitrose*	1 Chapati/42g	128	3.4	305	8.6	49.4	8.0	4.6
Elephant Atta*	1 Chapati/45g	129	2.9	287	7.5	53.1	6.4	3.2
Indian Style, Asda*	1 Chapati/43g	95	0.4	221	8.0	45.0	1.0	2.9
Made with Fat	1 Chapati/60g	197	7.7	328	8.1	48.3	12.8	0.0
Made without Fat	1 Chapati/55g	111	0.5	202	7.3	43.7	1.0	0.0
Morrisons*	1 Chapati/40g	108	2.8	269	8.6	49.8	6.9	0.0
Plain, Wraps, Original, Patak's*	1 Chapati/42g	115	3.1	273	9.4	48.8	7.5	0.0
Wholemeal, Patak's*	1 Chapati/42g	130	4.0	310	11.2	44.9	9.5	9.0

C

	Measure INFO/WEIGHT	per Measure KCAL	per Measure FAT	Nutrition Values per 100g / 100ml KCAL	PROT	CARB	FAT	FIBRE
CHARD								
Average	1 Serving/80g	15	0.2	19	1.4	3.3	0.2	0.8
Swiss, Boiled in Unsalted Water	*1oz/28g*	*6*	*0.0*	*20*	*1.9*	*4.1*	*0.1*	*2.1*
Swiss, Raw	*1oz/28g*	*5*	*0.1*	*19*	*1.8*	*3.7*	*0.2*	*1.6*
CHEDDARS								
Baked, Mini, Cheese & Ham Flavour, McVitie's*	1 Bag/30g	160	8.9	534	11.0	55.5	29.8	2.0
Baked, Mini, Original, Cheddar Cheese, McVitie's*	1 Bag/30g	155	9.0	517	10.8	50.9	30.0	2.5
Baked, Mini, Peperami, McVitie's*	1 Bag/30g	160	9.1	532	9.7	55.2	30.2	2.0
Baked, Mini, Tangy Salsa, McVitie's*	1 Bag/50g	266	14.9	532	11.0	54.7	29.9	2.1
Branston Pickle, McVitie's*	1 Bag/30g	155	8.9	517	9.1	53.1	29.8	2.7
Smokey BBQ, McVitie's*	1 Pack/30g	155	8.9	516	9.3	52.8	29.8	2.6
CHEESE								
Appenzellar, Sainsbury's*	1 Serving/25g	96	7.9	386	25.4	0.0	31.6	0.0
Babybel, Emmental, Fromageries Bel*	1 Serving/20g	63	4.9	316	23.0	1.0	24.5	0.0
Babybel, Mini, Light, Fromageries Bel*	1 Cheese/20g	42	2.4	210	25.5	0.2	12.0	0.0
Babybel, Original, Mini, Fromageries Bel*	1 Cheese/20g	61	4.8	304	22.0	0.1	24.0	0.0
Babybel, with Cheddar, Mini, Fromageries Bel*	1 Cheese/20g	72	6.0	362	23.0	0.2	30.0	0.0
Blue, Castello, Soft, Castello*	¼ Pack/38g	162	15.6	432	14.0	0.5	41.5	0.0
Blue, Saint Agur*	1 Serving /30g	109	9.9	363	16.0	0.2	33.0	0.0
Brie, Average	*1 Serving/25g*	*74*	*6.0*	*296*	*19.7*	*0.3*	*24.0*	*0.0*
Brie, Reduced Fat, Average	*1 Serving/50g*	*99*	*5.7*	*198*	*23.0*	*0.8*	*11.4*	*0.0*
Caerphilly, Average	*1 Serving/50g*	*187*	*15.6*	*374*	*23.0*	*0.1*	*31.3*	*0.0*
Cambazola, Tesco*	1 Serving/30g	127	12.3	425	13.5	0.5	41.0	0.0
Camembert, Average	*1 Serving/50g*	*141*	*11.1*	*283*	*20.5*	*0.1*	*22.2*	*0.0*
Camembert, Breaded, Average	1 Serving/90g	307	20.9	341	16.6	14.2	23.2	0.4
Cantal, French, Sainsbury's*	1 Serving/30g	106	8.7	353	23.0	0.1	29.0	0.0
Cantenaar, M & S*	1 Serving/28g	84	5.4	300	32.2	0.1	19.2	0.0
Cheddar, Canadian, Average	*1 Serving/30g*	*123*	*10.3*	*409*	*25.0*	*0.1*	*34.3*	*0.0*
Cheddar, Davidstow, Mature, Average	*1 Serving/28g*	*115*	*9.6*	*410*	*25.0*	*0.1*	*34.4*	*0.0*
Cheddar, Extra Mature, Average	*1 Serving/30g*	*123*	*10.3*	*410*	*25.1*	*0.1*	*34.3*	*0.0*
Cheddar, Grated, Average	*1 Serving/50g*	*206*	*17.1*	*413*	*24.4*	*1.5*	*34.3*	*0.0*
Cheddar, Mature, Average	*1 Serving/30g*	*123*	*10.3*	*410*	*25.0*	*0.1*	*34.4*	*0.0*
Cheddar, Mature, Grated, Average	*1 Serving/28g*	*113*	*9.3*	*404*	*24.7*	*1.6*	*33.2*	*0.0*
Cheddar, Mature, Reduced Fat, Average	*1 Serving/25g*	*68*	*4.2*	*271*	*30.0*	*0.1*	*16.7*	*0.0*
Cheddar, Medium, Average	*1 Serving/30g*	*123*	*10.3*	*411*	*24.9*	*0.1*	*34.5*	*0.0*
Cheddar, Mild, Average	*1 Serving/30g*	*123*	*10.3*	*409*	*25.0*	*0.1*	*34.3*	*0.0*
Cheddar, Reduced Fat, Average	*1 Serving/30g*	*76*	*4.2*	*255*	*32.1*	*0.1*	*13.9*	*0.0*
Cheddar, Smoked, Average	*1 Serving/30g*	*123*	*10.3*	*411*	*25.2*	*0.1*	*34.4*	*0.0*
Cheddar, West Country Farmhouse, Average	*1 Serving/28g*	*115*	*9.6*	*410*	*25.0*	*0.1*	*34.4*	*0.0*
Cheddar, Wexford, Average	*1 Serving/20g*	*82*	*6.9*	*410*	*25.0*	*0.1*	*34.4*	*0.0*
Cheestrings, Cheddar, Original, Golden Vale*	1 Stick/21g	69	5.0	328	28.0	0.0	24.0	0.0
Cheestrings, Double Cheese Flavour, Golden Vale*	1 Stick/21g	69	5.0	328	28.0	0.0	24.0	0.0
Cheshire	*1oz/28g*	*106*	*8.8*	*379*	*24.0*	*0.1*	*31.4*	*0.0*
Cottage, BFY, Morrisons*	1 Pot/125g	110	1.1	88	13.0	6.9	0.9	0.0
Cottage, Crunchy Vegetable, GFY, Asda*	1 Serving/50g	37	0.6	74	11.0	4.5	1.3	0.6
Cottage, Danone*	1 Serving/100g	89	3.9	89	11.2	2.3	3.9	0.0
Cottage, Garlic & Herb, Diet, Yoplait*	1 Pot/225g	180	4.3	80	12.0	3.9	1.9	0.0
Cottage, GFY, Asda*	1oz/28g	25	0.8	88	11.5	3.4	2.7	0.0
Cottage, Healthy Choice, Nisa Heritage*	1 Pot/227g	175	4.1	77	11.8	3.4	1.8	0.3
Cottage, Jocca, Kraft*	1 Serving/50g	54	2.7	109	9.3	5.0	5.5	0.0
Cottage, Natural, COU, M & S*	½ Pot/125g	100	2.2	80	11.9	3.3	1.8	0.3
Cottage, Natural, Plain, Average	*1oz/28g*	*27*	*1.1*	*98*	*11.8*	*3.9*	*3.8*	*0.1*
Cottage, Plain, Average	*1oz/28g*	*26*	*1.0*	*93*	*12.0*	*3.3*	*3.5*	*0.1*
Cottage, Plain, Reduced Fat, Average	*1oz/28g*	*24*	*0.5*	*85*	*12.3*	*4.4*	*1.9*	*0.1*

INFO/WEIGHT	Measure		Nutrition Values per 100g / 100ml				
	KCAL	FAT	KCAL	PROT	CARB	FAT	FIBRE

CHEESE

	INFO/WEIGHT	KCAL	FAT	KCAL	PROT	CARB	FAT	FIBRE
Cottage, Red Pepper, GFY, Asda*	¼ Pot/75g	66	1.9	88	11.1	4.3	2.5	0.1
Cottage, Stilton & Celery, BGTY, Sainsbury's*	½ Pot/125g	99	2.8	79	10.8	4.0	2.2	1.5
Cottage, Tuna & Sweetcorn, GFY, Asda*	½ Pot/113g	104	2.7	92	12.4	5.3	2.4	0.3
Cottage, Virtually Fat Free, Average	1 Tbsp/20g	16	0.2	79	13.0	4.5	1.0	0.0
Cottage, West Country, Low Fat, Eat Well, M & S*	1 80g/80g	64	1.2	80	12.2	4.5	1.5	0.0
Cottage, West Country, Low Fat 1.5%, Waitrose*	1 Serving/100g	77	1.5	77	11.8	4.4	1.5	0.0
Cottage, West Country, Waitrose*	1 Serving/100g	113	6.1	113	6.1	3.3	6.1	0.0
Cottage, Whole Milk, Natural, Average	1 Serving/75g	77	3.4	103	12.5	2.7	4.5	0.0
Cottage, with Chives, Low Fat, Westacre*	1 Pot/100g	81	1.4	81	13.7	3.5	1.4	1.2
Cottage, with Chives, M & S*	1oz/28g	28	1.1	100	11.9	3.5	3.9	0.0
Cottage, with Chives, Virtually Fat Free, Longley Farm*	½ Pot/125g	87	0.1	70	14.3	2.9	0.1	0.0
Cottage, with Coronation Chicken, BGTY, Sainsbury's*	1oz/28g	25	0.3	91	11.3	8.7	1.2	0.1
Cottage, with Cucumber & Mint, COU, M & S*	1 Pot/113g	85	1.7	75	11.6	3.1	1.5	0.2
Cottage, with Cucumber & Mint, GFY, Asda*	1 Serving/75g	54	1.0	72	11.0	4.1	1.3	0.5
Cottage, with Mango & Pineapple, BGTY, Sainsbury's*	½ Pot/125g	112	0.9	90	10.7	10.4	0.7	0.2
Cottage, with Mango & Pineapple, Morrisons*	1 Pot/125g	112	0.9	90	10.7	10.4	0.7	0.0
Cottage, with Onion & Chive, GFY, Asda*	1 Serving/50g	42	0.9	85	12.0	4.4	1.9	0.1
Cottage, with Onion & Chive, HL, Tesco*	1 Serving/65g	55	1.0	85	13.9	3.6	1.5	0.3
Cottage, with Onion & Chive, Low Fat, Sainsbury's*	1oz/28g	28	1.1	99	11.6	4.4	4.0	0.1
Cottage, with Onion & Chive, M & S*	¼ Pot/65g	88	5.5	135	10.4	4.0	8.5	0.1
Cottage, with Peach & Mango, COU, M & S*	1 Pot/113g	96	1.1	85	9.1	9.7	1.0	0.4
Cottage, with Pineapple, Asda*	1oz/28g	31	1.1	109	10.0	8.0	3.9	0.0
Cottage, with Pineapple, BGTY, Sainsbury's*	1 Serving/125g	105	0.9	84	10.5	8.9	0.7	0.1
Cottage, with Pineapple, GFY, Asda*	1 Pot/227g	193	2.3	85	9.0	10.0	1.0	0.5
Cottage, with Pineapple, Less 5% Fat, Sainsbury's*	½ Pot/125g	122	4.2	98	10.0	6.8	3.4	0.1
Cottage, with Pineapple, Low Fat, Waitrose*	1 Serving/40g	34	0.7	84	10.4	6.7	1.7	0.2
Cottage, with Pineapple, Shape, Danone*	1oz/28g	20	0.1	73	9.8	8.0	0.2	0.1
Cottage, with Prawn, GFY, Asda*	1oz/28g	22	0.5	79	10.0	6.0	1.7	0.3
Cottage, with Prawn Cocktail, BGTY, Sainsbury's*	1oz/28g	25	0.3	91	12.3	8.3	0.9	0.1
Cottage, with Smoked Cheese & Onion, GFY, Asda*	1 Serving/50g	39	0.8	78	12.0	3.9	1.6	0.4
Cottage, with Sweet Chilli Chicken, M & S*	1 Serving/200g	190	4.2	95	13.8	4.7	2.1	0.5
Cottage, with Tomato & Cracked Black Pepper, Asda*	½ Pot/113g	86	2.4	76	10.0	3.1	2.1	1.3
Cottage, with Tuna & Pesto, Asda*	1 Serving/170g	184	10.2	108	10.0	3.5	6.0	0.7
Cottage, with Tuna & Sweetcorn, BGTY, Sainsbury's*	1oz/28g	25	0.3	91	12.1	8.4	0.9	0.2
Cottage, with Tuna & Sweetcorn, HL, Tesco*	1 Serving/150g	136	3.1	91	12.8	4.8	2.1	0.4
Cream, Average	*1 Portion/30g*	*132*	*14.2*	*439*	*3.1*	*0.0*	*47.4*	*0.0*
Cream, Garlic & Herbs, Light, Boursin*	1 Portion/20g	28	1.8	140	12.0	2.5	9.0	0.0
Cream, Reduced Fat, Average	*1 Serving/20g*	*23*	*1.1*	*117*	*13.0*	*4.0*	*5.3*	*0.1*
Cream, with Onion & Chives, Morrisons*	1 Serving/20g	38	3.0	190	11.0	3.0	15.0	0.0
Cream, with Pineapple, Asda*	1 Serving/40g	77	5.2	193	8.0	11.0	13.0	0.0
Cream, with Red Peppers & Onion, GFY, Asda*	1 Serving/32g	42	1.9	130	13.0	6.0	6.0	0.0
Creme de Saint Agur, Saint Agur*	1 Serving/10g	28	2.5	285	13.5	2.3	24.7	0.0
Dairylea, Light, Slices, Kraft*	1 Slice/25g	51	2.6	205	17.0	8.6	10.5	0.0
Dairylea, Rippers, Straight, Kraft*	1 Ripper/21g	60	3.9	285	28.0	1.0	18.5	0.0
Dairylea, Slices, Kraft*	1 Slice/25g	69	5.1	275	13.0	8.6	20.5	0.0
Danish Blue, Average	*1 Serving/30g*	*106*	*8.7*	*352*	*20.7*	*0.0*	*29.1*	*0.0*
Demi Pont L'eveque, Finest, Tesco*	1 Serving/46g	138	10.6	301	21.1	0.4	23.0	0.0
Dolcelatte, Average	*1 Serving/30g*	*110*	*9.7*	*366*	*17.8*	*0.4*	*32.3*	*0.4*
Double Gloucester, Average	*1 Serving/30g*	*121*	*10.2*	*404*	*24.5*	*0.1*	*34.0*	*0.0*
Doux De Montagne, Average	*1 Serving/25g*	*88*	*7.1*	*352*	*22.9*	*1.5*	*28.3*	*0.0*
Edam, Average	*1 Serving/10g*	*33*	*2.5*	*326*	*25.3*	*0.0*	*24.9*	*0.0*
Edam, Dutch, Garlic & Herb Wedge, Asda*	1 Serving/60g	197	15.0	329	26.0	0.0	25.0	0.0
Edam, Reduced Fat, Average	*1 Serving/30g*	*69*	*3.3*	*230*	*32.4*	*0.1*	*11.1*	*0.0*

CHEESE

	Measure INFO/WEIGHT	KCAL	FAT	KCAL	PROT	CARB	FAT	FIBRE
Edam, Slices, Average	*1 Slice/30g*	*96*	*7.2*	*320*	*25.0*	*0.4*	*24.1*	*0.0*
Emmental, Average	*1 Serving/10g*	*37*	*2.8*	*368*	*28.3*	*0.0*	*28.3*	*0.0*
Emmental, Light, Slices, President*	1 Slice/20g	60	3.6	298	34.0	0.0	18.0	0.0
Farmhouse, Reduced Fat, Healthy Range, Average	*1 Serving/30g*	*78*	*4.6*	*260*	*30.4*	*0.0*	*15.4*	*0.0*
Feta, Apetina, Light, 10 % Fat, Arla*	1 Serving/30g	52	3.0	173	18.4	0.6	10.1	0.0
Feta, Average	*1 Serving/30g*	*79*	*6.4*	*262*	*16.3*	*1.0*	*21.5*	*0.0*
Feta, Lemon, Asda*	1 Serving/25g	75	6.8	302	13.2	1.0	27.2	0.6
Feta, Light, Greek, Salad, 40% Reduced Fat, Attis*	1 Portion/30g	51	3.6	170	20.0	0.6	12.0	0.0
Fondue, Original, Fromalp*	1 Pack/400g	888	68.0	222	15.0	2.5	17.0	0.0
Fondue, Swiss, Easy Cook, Tesco*	¼ Pack/100g	235	17.0	235	15.5	4.0	17.0	0.0
Fontina, Average	*1 Serving/28g*	*109*	*9.0*	*389*	*25.0*	*0.0*	*32.1*	*0.0*
for Pizza, Grated	*1 Serving/50g*	*163*	*12.2*	*325*	*25.0*	*1.5*	*24.4*	*0.0*
Goats, Average	*1 Tsp/10g*	*26*	*2.1*	*262*	*13.8*	*3.8*	*21.2*	*0.0*
Goats, French, Mild, Average	*1 Serving/30g*	*49*	*3.5*	*163*	*11.2*	*3.0*	*11.8*	*0.0*
Goats, Premium, Average	*1 Serving/30g*	*98*	*7.8*	*327*	*20.5*	*0.6*	*26.1*	*0.0*
Gorgonzola, Average	*1 Serving/30g*	*100*	*8.1*	*334*	*20.0*	*0.0*	*27.0*	*0.0*
Gouda, Average	*1 Serving/30g*	*113*	*9.4*	*375*	*24.0*	*0.0*	*31.5*	*0.0*
Grana Padano, Italian Cheese, Waitrose*	1 Serving/14g	54	4.0	388	33.0	0.0	28.4	0.0
Gruyere	*1oz/28g*	*115*	*9.3*	*409*	*27.2*	*0.0*	*33.3*	*0.0*
Halloumi, Average	*1 Serving/80g*	*253*	*19.7*	*316*	*20.8*	*1.6*	*24.7*	*0.0*
Halloumi, Light, Pittas*	1 Pack/225g	589	36.0	262	27.0	2.5	16.0	0.0
Hard, Lower in Fat, Garcia Baquero*	1 Serving/20g	67	4.6	335	0.0	0.0	23.0	0.0
Italian, Grated, Average	*1 Serving/30g*	*144*	*10.0*	*481*	*44.0*	*1.1*	*33.4*	*0.0*
Jarlsberg, Slices, Average	*1 Slice/15g*	*54*	*4.0*	*360*	*27.0*	*0.0*	*27.0*	*0.0*
Lactose Free, Arla*	1 Serving/30g	103	8.1	344	25.3	1.0	27.0	0.0
Lancashire	*1oz/28g*	*104*	*8.7*	*373*	*23.3*	*0.1*	*31.0*	*0.0*
Light Salad, Discover*	1oz/28g	61	3.6	216	24.0	1.0	13.0	0.0
Manchego	*1 Serving/70g*	*339*	*30.8*	*485*	*22.2*	*0.1*	*44.0*	*0.0*
Mascarpone, 25% Less Fat, Sainsbury's*	1 Portion/30g	95	9.0	316	6.7	4.8	30.0	0.0
Mascarpone, Average	*1 Serving/30g*	*131*	*13.1*	*437*	*5.6*	*4.1*	*43.6*	*0.0*
Mature, Full Flavoured, LowLow, Kerry*	1 Serving/30g	91	6.6	302	26.0	0.2	22.0	0.0
Mature, Half Fat, Average	1 Serving/25g	66	3.9	265	29.9	0.4	15.6	0.1
Mature, Reduced Fat, Weight Watchers*	1 Serving/30g	65	3.1	217	31.0	0.1	10.3	0.0
Mild, Reduced Fat, Grated, Average	*1 Serving/30g*	*70*	*3.3*	*235*	*31.5*	*2.2*	*11.1*	*0.0*
Monterey Jack, Iga*	1 Serving/28g	110	9.0	393	25.0	0.0	32.1	0.0
Monterey Jack, Shredded, Kraft*	¼ Cup/28g	101	8.1	360	22.0	3.6	28.8	0.0
Morbier, Sainsbury's*	1 Serving/10g	33	2.4	330	28.0	0.1	24.2	0.0
Mozzarella, Average	*1 Serving/50g*	*137*	*10.3*	*275*	*21.2*	*1.2*	*20.6*	*0.0*
Mozzarella, Reduced Fat, Average	*1 Serving/50g*	*92*	*5.1*	*184*	*21.1*	*1.0*	*10.2*	*0.0*
Norvegia, Sliced Light, Tine*	1 Slice/10g	27	1.6	272	32.0	0.0	16.0	0.0
Ossau-Iraty, Average	*1 Serving/30g*	*120*	*10.2*	*400*	*22.3*	*0.2*	*34.0*	*0.0*
Parlick Fell, Hard, Sheep's, Sainsbury's*	1 Serving/30g	109	9.1	364	22.6	0.0	30.4	0.0
Parmesan, Average	*1 Tbsp/10g*	*40*	*2.9*	*401*	*35.2*	*0.0*	*29.4*	*0.0*
Parmigianino Reggiano, TTD, Sainsbury's*	1 Serving/30g	116	8.5	388	33.0	0.0	28.4	0.0
Pecorino, Italian, Tesco*	1 Serving/30g	119	9.9	397	22.0	0.0	33.0	0.0
Piccante Gorgonzola, TTD, Sainsbury's*	1 Serving/30g	108	9.0	359	22.1	0.5	29.8	0.1
Poivre, Boursin*	1oz/28g	116	11.8	414	7.0	2.0	42.0	0.0
Port Salut, M & S*	1oz/28g	90	7.3	322	21.0	1.0	26.0	0.0
Provolone Piccante, Sainsbury's*	1 Serving/30g	119	9.9	398	25.0	0.2	33.0	0.0
P'tit Louis, St Moret*	1 Serving/20g	49	4.6	247	5.0	5.0	23.0	0.0
Quark, Average	*1 Serving/20g*	*13*	*0.0*	*66*	*11.9*	*4.0*	*0.2*	*0.0*
Raclette, Richsmonts*	1 Slice/28g	100	8.0	357	25.0	0.0	28.6	0.0
Reblochon	*1 Serving/30g*	*95*	*8.0*	*318*	*19.7*	*0.0*	*26.6*	*0.0*

	Measure INFO/WEIGHT	per Measure KCAL	per Measure FAT	Nutrition Values per 100g / 100ml KCAL	PROT	CARB	FAT	FIBRE
CHEESE								
Red Leicester, Average	**1 Serving/30g**	**120**	**10.1**	**400**	**23.8**	**0.1**	**33.7**	**0.0**
Red Leicester, Reduced Fat, Average	1 Serving/30g	78	4.6	261	30.2	0.1	15.4	0.0
Ricotta, Average	**1 Serving/50g**	**67**	**4.7**	**134**	**9.3**	**2.9**	**9.5**	**0.0**
Roquefort, Average	**1oz/28g**	**105**	**9.2**	**375**	**19.7**	**0.0**	**32.9**	**0.0**
Roule, French, Sainsbury's*	1 Serving/30g	96	9.1	321	8.5	3.0	30.5	0.0
Roule, Garlic & Parsley, Light, BGTY, Sainsbury's*	1 Serving/30g	51	3.2	171	16.4	2.6	10.6	0.0
Sage Derby	**1oz/28g**	**113**	**9.5**	**402**	**24.2**	**0.1**	**33.9**	**0.0**
Shropshire, Blue, Average	**1 Serving/50g**	**195**	**17.1**	**391**	**21.0**	**0.0**	**34.2**	**0.0**
Soft, & Creamy with Onions & Garlic, GFY, Asda*	1 Serving/25g	31	1.5	126	13.0	5.0	6.0	0.0
Soft, & Creamy with Pineapple, Asda*	1 Serving/32g	62	4.2	193	8.0	11.0	13.0	0.0
Soft, Blue, Philadelphia, Kraft*	1 Serving/28g	76	7.1	270	6.8	3.4	25.5	0.2
Soft, Cracked Pepper, Less Than 5% Fat, M & S*	1 Serving/30g	30	1.3	100	11.0	4.2	4.5	0.3
Soft, Double Gloucester, & Chives, M & S*	1oz/28g	100	7.5	358	20.0	9.2	26.8	0.0
Soft, Extra Light, Average	**1 Serving/20g**	**25**	**1.2**	**125**	**14.3**	**3.5**	**5.9**	**0.1**
Soft, Fruit & Rum Halo, Discover*	1 Serving/25g	103	8.5	414	8.6	11.7	34.1	0.0
Soft, Full Fat, Average	**1 Serving/50g**	**156**	**15.2**	**312**	**8.2**	**1.7**	**30.3**	**0.0**
Soft, Garlic & Herb, Extra Light, Light Choices, Tesco*	1 Serving/38g	49	2.4	130	12.3	5.1	6.3	0.3
Soft, Garlic & Herb, Roulade, M & S*	1 Portion/100g	295	27.3	295	7.8	4.1	27.3	1.3
Soft, Garlic & Herb, Soft & Creamy, Extra Light, Asda*	¼ Pack/50g	65	3.0	130	13.0	6.0	6.0	0.0
Soft, Goats Milk	**1oz/28g**	**55**	**4.4**	**198**	**13.1**	**1.0**	**15.8**	**0.0**
Soft, Herbs & Garlic, Creamery, Light, Sainsbury's*	1 Serving/30g	54	4.6	180	7.2	3.4	15.5	0.3
Soft, Light, Average	**1 Serving/30g**	**54**	**3.9**	**179**	**12.1**	**3.2**	**13.1**	**0.0**
Soft, Light with Grilled Peppers, Philadelphia*	1 Portion/30g	44	3.1	147	7.0	5.4	10.5	0.7
Soft, Medium Fat, Average	**1 Serving/30g**	**62**	**5.4**	**207**	**8.4**	**3.0**	**17.9**	**0.0**
Soft, Onion & Chives, Less Than 5% Fat, M & S*	1 Serving/30g	30	1.4	100	10.7	4.4	4.7	1.2
Soft, Philadelphia, Extra Light, Kraft*	1 Serving/30g	33	1.4	110	11.7	5.0	4.7	0.3
Soft, Philadelphia, Garlic & Herb, Light, Kraft*	1 Serving/30g	47	3.5	157	8.3	4.0	11.7	0.3
Soft, Philadelphia, Light, Basil, Philadelphia, Kraft*	1 Serving/35g	51	3.7	146	8.0	4.0	10.5	0.5
Soft, Philadelphia, Mini Tubs, Cracked Pepper, Kraft*	1 Tub/35g	56	4.5	161	7.7	2.5	13.0	0.4
Soft, Philadelphia, Mini Tubs, Extra Light, Kraft*	1 Tub/35g	38	1.7	108	11.0	4.2	5.0	0.6
Soft, Philadelphia, Mini Tubs, Light, Kraft*	1 Tub/35g	55	4.0	158	8.7	4.0	11.5	0.4
Soft, Philadelphia, with Chives, Light, Kraft*	1 Serving/30g	48	3.6	160	8.3	4.3	12.0	0.7
Soft, Philadelphia, with Ham, Light, Kraft*	1oz/28g	52	4.2	184	7.9	4.3	15.0	0.2
Soft, Pineapple Halo, Discover*	1 Serving/25g	101	8.1	404	7.2	16.6	32.6	1.2
Soft, White, Lactofree, Arla*	1 Serving/30g	59	4.9	197	8.6	3.0	16.5	0.0
Soft, with Black Pepper, Light, Sainsbury's*	½ Pack/100g	205	16.5	205	11.0	3.0	16.5	0.0
Soft, with Garlic & Herbs, Full Fat, Deli, Boursin*	1 Serving/28g	84	8.3	299	3.5	5.0	29.5	0.0
Soft, with Garlic & Herbs, Medium Fat, Westacre*	1 Serving/30g	56	4.8	188	8.0	3.0	16.0	0.1
Soft, with Garlic & Herbs, Sainsbury's*	1 Serving/33g	89	8.6	269	6.1	2.7	26.0	0.0
Soft, with Garlic and Herbs, Lighter, Asda*	½ Pack/100g	106	4.4	106	11.8	4.3	4.4	0.1
Soft, with Onion & Chives, Lighter, Asda*	1 Serving/30g	31	1.3	105	11.6	4.5	4.3	0.2
Soya	**1oz/28g**	**89**	**7.6**	**319**	**18.3**	**0.0**	**27.3**	**0.0**
Stilton, Average	**1 Serving/30g**	**123**	**10.6**	**410**	**22.4**	**0.1**	**35.5**	**0.0**
Stilton, Blue, Average	**1 Serving/30g**	**124**	**10.7**	**412**	**22.8**	**0.1**	**35.7**	**0.0**
Stilton, White, & Apricot, M & S*	1oz/28g	94	6.5	337	13.8	18.5	23.1	0.0
Stilton, White, & Cranberry, M & S*	1oz/28g	101	7.1	362	18.2	15.5	25.3	0.0
Stilton, White, Average	**1oz/28g**	**101**	**8.8**	**362**	**19.9**	**0.1**	**31.3**	**0.0**
Stilton, White, with Cranberries, Tesco*	1 Serving/50g	184	14.8	368	15.8	9.5	29.7	0.7
Stilton, White, with Mango & Ginger, Tesco*	1/3 Pack/65g	227	14.0	350	13.1	25.8	21.6	0.6
Wedge, Leerdammer*	1 Serving/30g	112	8.6	373	28.3	0.0	28.6	0.0
Wensleydale, Average	**1 Serving/25g**	**92**	**7.8**	**369**	**22.4**	**0.1**	**31.0**	**0.0**
CHEESE ON TOAST								
Average	1oz/28g	106	7.4	380	13.8	23.8	26.3	0.7

C

CHEESE PUFFS

	Measure INFO/WEIGHT	per Measure KCAL	FAT	Nutrition Values per 100g / 100ml KCAL	PROT	CARB	FAT	FIBRE
Cheeky, Tesco*	1 Bag/20g	108	7.0	542	6.7	50.2	34.9	0.0
Morrisons*	1 Bag/25g	135	8.7	542	6.7	50.2	34.9	1.1
Sainsbury's*	1 Pack/100g	530	32.0	530	9.1	51.4	32.0	1.9
Shapers, Boots*	1 Bag/16g	80	3.8	500	7.1	64.0	24.0	0.9
CHEESE SINGLES								
50% Less Fat, Asda*	1 Slice/20g	38	2.0	190	19.0	6.0	10.0	0.0
American, 2% Milk, Kraft*	1 Slice/19g	45	3.0	237	21.0	5.3	15.8	0.0
Half Fat, Co-Op*	1 Slice/20g	47	2.4	235	25.0	7.0	12.0	0.0
Kraft*	1 Single/20g	52	3.7	260	13.5	7.6	18.5	0.0
Light Choices, Tesco*	1 Slice/20g	37	2.0	185	19.8	4.0	10.0	0.0
CHEESE SLICES								
Gouda, Tesco*	1 Slice/25g	94	7.5	375	23.0	0.1	30.0	0.0
Havarti, Tesco*	1 Slice/25g	85	6.5	340	24.0	1.4	26.0	0.0
Jarlsberg, Tesco*	1 Slice/25g	91	7.0	365	27.5	0.0	28.0	0.0
Leerdammer*	1 Slice/25g	89	7.0	358	27.0	0.1	28.0	0.0
Light, The Laughing Cow, Fromageries Bel*	1 Slice/20g	41	2.1	203	21.0	6.0	10.5	0.0
Light Choices, Tesco*	1 Slice/20g	37	2.1	185	19.8	4.0	10.6	0.0
Morrisons*	1 Slice/20g	39	2.0	196	21.0	5.4	10.0	0.0
Reduced Fat, GFY, Asda*	1 Slice/20g	38	2.0	191	21.0	4.2	10.0	0.0
CHEESE SPREAD								
60% Less Fat, Asda*	1 Serving/30g	52	2.7	174	16.0	7.3	9.0	0.0
Asda*	1 Serving/33g	92	7.9	280	9.0	7.0	24.0	0.0
BGTY, Sainsbury's*	1 Serving/25g	28	1.4	111	11.0	4.3	5.5	0.4
Cheese & Garlic, Primula*	1 Serving/20g	49	3.7	247	15.7	4.3	18.6	0.0
Cheese & Salmon with Dill, Primula*	1 Serving/30g	78	5.8	261	17.6	3.8	19.5	0.0
Dairylea, Light, Tub, Kraft*	1 Serving/30g	44	2.1	147	14.5	6.1	7.0	0.0
Dairylea, Tub, Kraft*	1 Serving/25g	60	4.9	240	11.0	5.3	19.5	0.0
Flavoured	1oz/28g	72	5.7	258	14.2	4.4	20.5	0.0
Garlic & Herbs, Light, Benecol*	1 Serving/20g	35	2.8	174	7.8	4.2	14.0	0.7
Kerrygold*	1oz/28g	60	4.2	213	11.0	8.5	15.0	0.0
Light, Primula*	1oz/28g	39	1.5	141	18.8	4.1	5.5	0.5
Low Fat, Weight Watchers*	1 Serving/50g	56	1.4	112	18.1	3.4	2.9	1.2
Mediterranean Soft & Creamy, Extra Light, Asda*	1 Serving/32g	42	1.9	130	13.0	6.0	6.0	0.0
Morrisons*	1 Serving/3g	7	0.5	225	10.0	7.0	17.5	0.0
Plain, Original, Primula*	1 Serving/30g	68	5.6	227	12.9	2.1	18.7	0.6
Soft, Low Fat, M & S*	1 Pack/100g	111	4.5	111	13.0	4.2	4.5	0.3
Squeeze, Light, The Laughing Cow, Fromageries Bel*	1 Portion/30g	42	2.1	139	12.0	7.0	7.0	5.0
Squeeze, The Laughing Cow, Fromageries Bel*	1 Portion/30g	71	6.0	236	9.0	5.0	20.0	0.0
Triangles, 50% Less Fat, Morrisons*	1 Portion/18g	29	1.4	166	15.0	8.5	8.0	0.0
with Chives, Primula*	1 Serving/30g	76	6.3	253	15.0	1.0	21.0	0.0
with Garlic & Herb, Soft, Free From, Sainsbury's*	1 Serving/30g	91	9.0	302	2.5	5.5	30.0	0.1
with Ham, Primula*	1 Serving/30g	70	5.6	232	13.5	2.1	18.8	0.3
with Shrimp, Primula*	1 Tbsp/15g	38	3.1	253	15.0	1.0	21.0	0.0
CHEESE STRAWS								
& Bacon, Party, Tesco*	1 Straw/13g	40	2.5	321	10.5	23.8	20.4	2.1
Cheddar, M & S*	1 Straw/11g	59	3.8	535	14.9	40.1	34.9	2.4
Cheese Twists, Tesco*	1 Serving/20g	99	5.6	494	14.0	46.4	28.0	4.2
Finest, Tesco*	1 Straw/7g	39	2.6	558	13.3	41.5	37.6	1.5
Fudges*	1 Serving/10g	53	3.5	534	14.9	40.1	34.9	0.0
Homemade or Bakery, Average	1 Straw/41g	173	12.6	422	11.9	24.1	30.7	0.7
Selection, Sainsbury's*	1 Straw/7g	41	2.9	558	16.6	34.5	39.3	2.8
CHEESE TRIANGLES								
Average	1 Triangle/14g	35	2.8	247	10.6	6.6	19.9	0.0

	Measure INFO/WEIGHT	per Measure KCAL	FAT	Nutrition Values per 100g / 100ml KCAL	PROT	CARB	FAT	FIBRE
CHEESE TRIANGLES								
Dairylea, Light, Kraft*	1 Triangle/20g	31	1.4	154	15.0	7.0	7.0	0.0
Extra Light, The Laughing Cow, Fromageries Bel*	1 Triangle/18g	20	0.5	116	15.0	6.5	3.0	0.0
Light, Swiss, The Laughing Cow, Fromageries Bel*	1 Triangle/18g	25	1.2	141	13.0	6.5	7.0	0.0
Light Choices, Tesco*	1 Triangle/18g	30	1.2	170	17.5	8.5	7.0	0.0
Original, The Laughing Cow, Fromageries Bel*	1 Triangle/18g	42	3.3	239	11.0	6.0	19.0	0.0
Reduced Fat, Average	1 Triangle/18g	30	1.6	170	14.8	7.4	9.0	0.0
Tri-Bites, Dairylea, Kraft*	1 Triangle/20g	60	4.6	300	20.0	3.2	23.0	0.0
CHEESE TWISTS								
All Butter, M & S*	1 Pack/125g	625	33.4	500	14.2	50.2	26.7	3.2
Asda*	1 Twist/8g	42	2.4	500	14.0	48.0	28.0	5.0
Gruyere, & Poppy Seed, Truly Irresistible, Co-Op*	1 Twist/8g	42	2.4	520	13.2	48.8	30.1	2.5
CHEESECAKE								
American Red White & Blueberry, Sainsbury's*	1/6 Cake/83g	264	15.4	318	3.8	35.1	18.5	0.4
Apple & Cinnamon, Baked, M & S*	1 Serving/116g	390	22.0	335	3.7	39.7	18.9	2.1
Apricot, Co-Op*	1 Cake/100g	230	11.0	230	4.0	29.0	11.0	0.9
Apricot, HL, Tesco*	1 Pot/100g	179	2.3	179	4.9	34.7	2.3	1.6
Autumn Berry, Waitrose*	1/6 Cake/92g	316	20.3	343	4.4	31.5	22.1	2.0
Average	1 Slice/115g	490	40.8	426	3.7	24.6	35.5	0.4
Belgian Chocolate, M & S*	1 Slice/100g	385	23.9	385	5.3	39.2	23.9	2.5
Blackcurrant, Perfectly Balanced, Waitrose*	1/6 Cake/99g	212	3.6	214	4.0	39.6	3.6	2.4
Blackcurrant, VLH Kitchens*	1 Portion/120g	341	19.7	285	3.4	32.0	16.4	0.9
Blackcurrant, Weight Watchers*	1 Cake/103g	191	2.9	185	4.6	35.4	2.8	3.5
Blackcurrant Devonshire, McVitie's*	1/6 Cake/67g	193	11.5	288	3.8	29.7	17.1	1.7
Blackcurrant Swirl, Heinz*	1/5 Cake/87g	241	13.4	277	4.1	30.3	15.4	3.6
Blueberry & Lemon Flavour Wedges, Sainsbury's*	1 Serving/80g	262	16.9	327	5.1	29.2	21.1	1.2
Blueberry & Vanilla, TTD, Sainsbury's*	1 Serving/95g	353	24.8	372	5.4	28.9	26.1	2.1
Caramel Swirl, Cadbury*	1 Slice/91g	373	23.5	410	6.0	40.1	25.8	0.0
Cherry, BGTY, Sainsbury's*	1 Serving/91g	181	3.9	199	4.6	35.5	4.3	0.5
Cherry, Low Fat, Tesco*	1 Serving/91g	185	3.7	203	3.4	38.0	4.1	0.9
Cherry, Low Saturated Fat, Waitrose*	1/6 Cake/108g	198	2.3	184	3.6	37.6	2.1	0.4
Chocolate, & Irish Cream Liqueur, Tesco*	1 Serving/93g	385	28.0	414	5.0	30.7	30.1	0.8
Chocolate, Baked, Ultimate, Entenmann's*	1 Serving/100g	331	19.0	331	5.7	34.2	19.0	2.8
Chocolate, Kate's Cakes Ltd*	1 Serving/100g	415	27.4	415	5.7	34.7	27.4	2.2
Chocolate, Pure Indulgence, Thorntons*	1 Serving/75g	307	17.5	410	5.6	44.3	23.4	0.6
Chocolate, Tesco*	1 Serving/91g	317	17.4	348	6.2	37.8	19.1	1.5
Chocolate, Weight Watchers*	1 Cake/95g	143	3.8	151	7.5	20.7	4.0	0.7
Chocolate & Hazelnut, Gold, Sara Lee*	1 Slice/65g	205	12.8	316	5.9	28.7	19.7	1.1
Chocolate & Hazelnut, Sara Lee*	1 Serving/65g	224	13.9	345	6.5	31.2	21.4	1.2
Chocolate & Vanilla, Gu*	1 Cake/90g	323	22.4	359	4.1	29.6	24.9	1.4
Chocolate & Vanilla, Reduced Fat, M & S*	1 Serving/114g	319	13.7	280	7.0	37.9	12.0	1.5
Chocolate Swirl, Deeply Delicious, Heinz*	1/5 Cake/82g	221	9.4	271	4.6	37.4	11.5	4.7
Chocolate Truffle, HL, Tesco*	1 Slice/96g	250	13.2	260	10.3	23.7	13.8	6.5
Citrus, Good Choice, Mini, Iceland*	1 Cake/111g	198	4.7	178	3.5	31.6	4.2	0.4
Commercially Prepared	1/6 Cake/80g	257	18.0	321	5.5	25.5	22.5	0.4
Creamy Vanilla, New York, Slices, Tesco*	1 Slice/106g	371	26.7	350	4.6	25.9	25.2	2.2
Devonshire Strawberry, McVitie's*	1/6 Cake/66g	192	10.7	291	4.4	31.8	16.2	3.6
Double Chocolate Wedge, Sainsbury's*	1 Serving/75g	327	24.7	436	5.7	29.0	33.0	1.7
Fudge, Tesco*	1 Serving/102g	384	23.6	376	4.6	37.5	23.1	0.5
Irish Cream, McVitie's*	1/4 Slice/190g	616	36.9	324	4.4	33.0	19.4	0.4
Lemon, Asda*	1 Slice/90g	319	21.2	354	4.3	31.2	23.5	1.1
Lemon, BGTY, Sainsbury's*	1/6 Cake/71g	142	2.7	200	4.4	37.0	3.8	0.5
Lemon, Carb Control, Tesco*	1 Serving/85g	269	23.0	316	8.6	9.6	27.1	11.1
Lemon, Sainsbury's*	1 Serving/180g	650	37.1	361	4.0	39.9	20.6	1.3

CHEESECAKE

	Measure INFO/WEIGHT	per Measure KCAL	FAT	Nutrition Values per 100g / 100ml KCAL	PROT	CARB	FAT	FIBRE
Lemon, Swirl, Asda*	1 Pack/125g	445	29.9	356	3.1	32.1	23.9	1.8
Lemon, Tesco*	1 Slice/93g	315	21.0	339	5.2	28.6	22.6	0.3
Lemon, Weight Watchers*	1 Serving/100g	211	5.0	211	6.3	30.1	5.0	1.8
Lemon Creamy & Light, M & S*	1/6 Cake/68g	236	13.8	350	3.5	32.3	20.4	0.4
Lemon Meringue, Tesco*	1 Slice/94g	352	25.0	375	3.8	30.1	26.6	0.3
Mandarin, Co-Op*	1 Slice/99g	297	16.8	300	4.0	32.0	17.0	0.3
Mandarin, GFY, Asda*	1/6 Cake/92g	178	4.0	194	3.6	35.0	4.4	1.2
Mandarin, Light Choices, Tesco*	1/6 Cake/92g	170	3.5	185	4.1	33.1	3.8	1.5
Mandarin, Low Fat, Tesco*	1 Serving/70g	145	3.3	207	3.3	37.0	4.7	1.4
Mandarin, Morrisons*	1 Serving/135g	335	16.9	248	3.8	32.2	12.5	0.8
Mandarin, Weight Watchers*	1 Cake/103g	180	2.9	175	4.6	32.9	2.8	1.5
Praline, Asda*	1/8 Cake/62g	226	14.9	364	7.0	30.0	24.0	3.2
Raspberry, BGTY, Sainsbury's*	1 Pot/95g	154	2.5	163	6.6	28.2	2.6	2.8
Raspberry, Creamy, Tesco*	1 Serving/100g	365	23.4	365	5.9	32.1	23.4	0.9
Raspberry, Light Choices, Tesco*	1 Cake/95g	185	4.1	195	4.3	34.7	4.3	1.3
Raspberry, Low Saturated Fat, Waitrose*	1/6 Cake/108g	187	2.1	174	3.6	35.4	2.0	0.4
Raspberry, M & S*	1 Slice/105g	331	21.5	315	5.0	32.2	20.5	1.0
Raspberry, Perfectly Balanced, Waitrose*	1 Serving/106g	212	3.7	200	4.0	36.2	3.5	1.7
Raspberry, Weight Watchers*	1 Cake/100g	213	4.3	213	5.9	29.7	4.3	1.9
Raspberry & Mascarpone, Best, Morrisons*	1 Cake/84g	257	14.0	306	3.9	34.8	16.7	1.0
Raspberry & Strawberry, M & S*	1 Slice/105g	340	21.1	325	3.9	33.4	20.2	1.2
Raspberry Brulee, M & S*	1 Serving/100g	255	12.9	255	5.7	29.7	12.9	2.1
Raspberry Rapture, Slices, Tesco*	1 Slice/110g	341	20.3	310	4.2	30.8	18.5	1.8
Raspberry Swirl, Heinz*	1 Serving/100g	266	14.5	266	3.9	30.1	14.5	2.8
Rhubarb Crumble, Sainsbury's*	1 Serving/114g	268	10.6	235	3.1	34.8	9.3	2.4
Rocky Road, Chosen By You, Asda*	1 Serving/75g	301	17.3	402	4.5	43.4	23.1	1.4
Sticky Toffee, Tesco*	1 Slice/66g	247	16.0	375	4.0	35.3	24.2	0.5
Strawberries & Cream, Finest, Tesco*	1 Serving/104g	325	22.4	312	4.3	25.3	21.5	0.5
Strawberries & Devonshire Cream, Heinz*	1/6 Cake/66g	184	10.1	279	3.9	31.4	15.3	3.7
Strawberry, Baked New York, Sara Lee*	1 Serving/100g	248	9.9	248	4.7	34.9	9.9	0.7
Strawberry, Creamy, Weight Watchers*	1 Cake/105g	187	2.6	178	4.7	34.2	2.5	2.2
Strawberry, Finest, Tesco*	1 Slice/113g	383	25.1	339	4.8	30.1	22.2	0.9
Strawberry, Fresh, M & S*	¼ Cake/125g	300	19.2	240	2.8	23.1	15.4	1.1
Strawberry, Frozen, Sainsbury's*	1/6 Cake/84ml	277	14.2	332	4.3	40.4	17.0	2.3
Strawberry, Heinz*	1 Pack/245g	588	31.1	240	3.4	28.1	12.7	2.4
Strawberry, Tesco*	1 Serving/100g	254	12.0	254	3.9	32.5	12.0	0.0
Strawberry Shortcake, Sara Lee*	1/6 Slice/68g	230	15.7	337	4.9	27.6	23.0	0.5
Strawberry Swirl, Chosen By You, Asda*	1 Serving/100g	329	15.9	329	4.5	41.5	15.9	1.0
Summerfruit, GFY, Asda*	1/6 Cake/92g	175	3.8	191	3.7	34.5	4.2	1.4
The Ultimate New York Baked, Entenmann's*	1 Cake/100g	347	21.3	347	4.2	35.7	21.3	0.9
Toffee, American Style, Asda*	1 Serving/75g	269	15.7	359	4.5	38.0	21.0	3.8
Toffee, Asda*	1 Cake/87g	295	19.1	339	4.3	31.0	22.0	3.5
Toffee, M & S*	1 Serving/105g	357	22.6	340	5.2	37.2	21.5	0.9
Toffee, Mini, Asda*	1 Cake/20g	57	2.4	286	4.6	40.0	12.0	2.1
Toffee, Morrisons*	1 Serving/100g	341	17.4	341	5.5	40.4	17.4	0.0
Toffee, Tesco*	1 Serving/100g	265	12.9	265	4.3	33.1	12.9	0.8
Toffee & Pecan, Wedge, Sainsbury's*	1 Serving/75g	296	21.7	395	5.4	28.1	29.0	3.1
Toffee Swirl, Chosen By You, Asda*	1 Serving/100g	334	16.1	334	5.5	41.4	16.1	0.9
Vanilla	1 Serving/100g	395	26.2	395	5.3	42.8	26.2	1.1
Vanilla, Tesco*	1 Serving/115g	417	28.4	363	5.7	29.4	24.7	0.6
Vanilla Chocolate, Baked, Slice, Sainsbury's*	1 Slice/90g	349	23.0	388	5.7	33.8	25.6	2.7
Zesty Lemon, M & S*	1/6 Cake/97g	325	18.9	335	4.0	38.7	19.5	2.6

	Measure INFO/WEIGHT	per Measure		Nutrition Values per 100g / 100ml				
		KCAL	FAT	KCAL	PROT	CARB	FAT	FIBRE
CHERRIES								
Black, Fresh, Average	*1 Serving/80g*	*41*	*0.1*	*51*	*0.9*	*11.5*	*0.1*	*1.6*
Black, in Syrup, Average	*1 Serving/242g*	*160*	*0.0*	*66*	*0.6*	*16.0*	*0.0*	*0.7*
Black, in Syrup, Pitted, Canned, Drained, Waitrose*	1 Can/213g	128	0.0	60	0.6	14.4	0.0	0.6
Dried, Love Life, Waitrose*	1 Portion/10g	35	0.1	348	0.2	84.3	1.1	2.1
Dried, Sainsbury's*	1 Tbsp/14g	45	0.2	319	3.8	72.4	1.5	6.2
Dried, Wholefoods, Tesco*	1 Serving/25g	86	0.2	345	1.9	81.6	0.8	4.6
Glace, Average	*1oz/28g*	*79*	*0.0*	*280*	*0.3*	*71.2*	*0.1*	*1.1*
Morello, Dried, Graze*	1 Pack/30g	100	0.4	335	4.5	82.0	1.5	0.0
Raw, Average	*1oz/28g*	*14*	*0.0*	*49*	*0.9*	*11.2*	*0.1*	*1.4*
Stewed, with Sugar, Average	*1oz/28g*	*23*	*0.0*	*82*	*0.7*	*21.0*	*0.1*	*0.7*
Stewed, without Sugar, Average	*1oz/28g*	*12*	*0.0*	*42*	*0.8*	*10.1*	*0.1*	*0.8*
CHESTNUTS								
Roasted, Peeled, Average	*1 Nut/10g*	*17*	*0.3*	*170*	*2.0*	*36.6*	*2.7*	*4.1*
CHEWING GUM								
Airwaves, Sugar Free, Wrigley's*	1 Pack/15g	23	0.0	155	0.0	62.0	0.0	0.0
Extra, Cool Breeze, Wrigley's*	1 Piece/2g	3	0.0	153	0.0	64.0	0.0	0.0
Extra, Peppermint, Sugar Free, Wrigley's*	1 Piece/2g	3	0.0	155	0.0	39.0	0.0	0.0
Peppermint, Soft, Sugar Free, Trident*	1 Stick/3g	4	0.0	155	0.4	62.3	0.4	0.0
Spearmint, Extra, Wrigley's*	1 Piece/1g	1	0.0	143	0.0	64.3	0.0	0.0
Spearmint, Wrigley's*	1 Piece/3g	9	0.0	295	0.0	73.0	0.0	0.0
Splash, Raspberry & Peach, Trident*	1 Piece/2g	4	0.0	180	1.6	68.5	0.5	0.0
Sugar Free Peppermint, Active, Aldi*	2 Pieces/3g	4	0.0	146	0.0	61.0	0.0	0.0
CHICK PEAS								
Dried, Average	*1 Serving/100g*	*319*	*5.4*	*319*	*21.7*	*47.4*	*5.4*	*8.0*
Dried, Boiled, Average	*1 Serving/75g*	*85*	*1.7*	*114*	*7.3*	*16.4*	*2.2*	*2.5*
Dried, Cooked, Waitrose*	1 Serving /80g	101	1.7	126	8.5	18.2	2.1	4.2
Dried, Dry Weight, Wholefoods, Tesco*	1 Serving/50g	167	2.7	335	21.3	49.6	5.4	10.7
in Salted Water, Canned, Average	*1 Can/179g*	*204*	*5.2*	*114*	*7.2*	*14.9*	*2.9*	*4.1*
in Water, Canned, Average	*1 Can/250g*	*282*	*6.5*	*113*	*7.2*	*15.3*	*2.6*	*4.8*
CHICKEN								
Barbeque, Meal For One, Chosen By You, Asda*	1 Pot/350g	423	6.6	121	7.1	18.1	1.9	1.5
BBQ Slices, Morrisons*	½ Pack/75g	101	0.8	135	23.9	7.5	1.1	0.0
Bites, Battered, Tesco*	1 Pack/200g	440	28.6	220	15.2	7.6	14.3	2.0
Bites, Hot & Spicy, Tesco*	1 Pack/110g	143	1.8	130	18.9	9.6	1.6	2.5
Bites, in Light Batter, Captain Birds Eye, Birds Eye*	1 Piece/15g	31	1.9	210	18.6	5.8	12.5	0.2
Bites, Southern Fried, Tesco*	1 Pack/300g	720	33.3	240	18.1	16.9	11.1	2.1
Bites, Tikka, Average	1 Serving/50g	96	5.3	193	20.7	3.8	10.5	1.9
Breast, Chargrilled, Lemon & Herb, Bernard Matthews*	1 Serving/100g	154	4.5	154	23.7	4.7	4.5	0.0
Breast, Chargrilled, Lime & Coriander, Asda*	1 Breast/159g	260	11.2	163	25.0	0.1	7.0	1.5
Breast, Chargrilled, Premium, Average	1 Piece/10g	20	1.1	197	21.6	1.5	11.2	0.3
Breast, Chargrilled, Sliced, Average	1 Slice/19g	24	0.5	124	24.4	0.5	2.7	0.4
Breast, Chilli & Ginger, COU, M & S*	1 Breast/120g	156	2.4	130	19.5	8.6	2.0	1.7
Breast, Chinese Style, Cooked, Sliced, Sainsbury's*	½ Pack/65g	96	1.2	148	28.3	4.7	1.8	0.1
Breast, Diced, Average	*1 Serving/188g*	*215*	*3.8*	*114*	*25.0*	*0.1*	*2.0*	*0.1*
Breast, Eastern Spices, Birds Eye*	1 Portion/175g	308	20.8	176	13.5	3.8	11.9	1.5
Breast, Escalope, Pesto Chargrilled, M & S*	1 Serving/100g	135	6.2	135	19.6	0.7	6.2	0.6
Breast, Escalope, Plain, Average	*1 Serving/100g*	*110*	*2.2*	*110*	*22.3*	*0.7*	*2.2*	*0.5*
Breast, Fillet, Mesquite, KP Snacks*	1 Serving/85g	130	7.0	153	20.0	1.2	8.2	0.0
Breast, Fillets, Breaded, Average	1 Fillet/112g	246	11.6	220	17.5	14.0	10.4	1.3
Breast, Fillets, Breaded, Lemon & Pepper, Average	1 Fillet/89g	133	2.0	150	22.0	10.1	2.3	1.3
Breast, Fillets, Cajun, Average	1 Fillet/93g	124	2.6	134	23.6	3.5	2.8	0.3
Breast, Fillets, Chargrilled, Average	1 Serving/100g	120	1.1	120	27.3	0.3	1.1	0.3
Breast, Fillets, Garlic & Herb, Tesco*	1 Fillet/135g	290	12.1	215	18.9	14.4	9.0	1.3

CHICKEN

	Measure INFO/WEIGHT	per Measure KCAL	per Measure FAT	Nutrition Values per 100g / 100ml KCAL	PROT	CARB	FAT	FIBRE
Breast, Fillets, Korma Style, Average	1 Serving/100g	131	2.7	131	27.4	0.8	2.7	0.5
Breast, Fillets, Lemon Parsley, M & S*	½ Pack/145g	232	3.5	160	14.3	20.7	2.4	4.3
Breast, Fillets, Lime & Coriander, Just Add, M & S*	1 Pack/140g	182	2.4	130	26.1	2.7	1.7	0.1
Breast, Fillets, Mexican Style, Cooked, Asda*	½ Pack/100g	147	1.5	147	27.8	5.5	1.5	0.1
Breast, Fillets, Mini, Raw, Average	*1oz/28g*	*34*	*0.4*	*121*	*26.9*	*0.2*	*1.5*	*0.1*
Breast, Fillets, Organic, Average	*1 Serving/150g*	*153*	*1.1*	*102*	*23.9*	*0.0*	*0.7*	*0.0*
Breast, Fillets, Skin On, Free Range, TTD, Sainsbury's*	1 Fillet/162g	235	7.6	145	25.7	0.0	4.7	0.0
Breast, Fillets, Skinless & Boneless, Raw, Average	*1 Serving/100g*	*126*	*2.3*	*126*	*25.1*	*1.2*	*2.3*	*0.2*
Breast, Fillets, Slices, Red Thai, Mini, Tesco*	2 Slices/65g	81	0.6	125	25.8	2.4	0.9	0.5
Breast, Fillets, Smokey Maple, Roast, Waitrose*	1 Fillet/96g	140	1.9	146	27.9	4.2	2.0	0.1
Breast, Fillets, Smoky Chilli, Tesco*	1 Fillet/92g	111	1.2	121	21.2	6.0	1.3	0.1
Breast, Fillets, Sundried Tomato & Basil, M & S*	½ Pack/110g	165	4.5	150	22.5	4.7	4.1	1.1
Breast, Fillets, Tikka, Mini, Ready to Eat, Tesco*	½ Pack/95g	120	1.8	125	22.4	4.2	1.9	0.2
Breast, Garlic & Herb, Premium, Bernard Matthews*	1 Serving/50g	50	1.2	101	17.9	1.6	2.5	1.8
Breast, Garlic & Herb Flavour, Co-Op*	1 Serving/170g	280	15.3	165	19.0	2.0	9.0	0.3
Breast, Grilled, Average	*1 Breast/130g*	*192*	*2.9*	*148*	*32.0*	*0.0*	*2.2*	*0.0*
Breast, Joint, Lemon & Tarragon, Finest, Tesco*	1 Serving/175g	247	11.0	141	18.8	2.3	6.3	0.2
Breast, Latino Style, Asda*	1 Breast/65g	99	2.0	152	27.0	4.1	3.1	0.5
Breast, Meat & Skin, Raw, Average	*1 Serving/145g*	*249*	*13.4*	*172*	*20.8*	*0.0*	*9.2*	*0.0*
Breast, Meat & Skin, Weight with Bone, Raw, Average	*1oz/28g*	*48*	*2.6*	*172*	*20.8*	*0.0*	*9.2*	*0.0*
Breast, Meat Only, Fried	*1 Serving/50g*	*93*	*2.4*	*187*	*33.4*	*0.5*	*4.7*	*0.0*
Breast, Nacho, Fresh Tastes, Asda*	½ Pack/159g	243	9.9	153	18.2	6.0	6.2	1.9
Breast, Pieces, Tikka, Average	1 Serving/100g	154	3.3	154	28.2	2.7	3.3	0.4
Breast, Roast, Sliced, From Supermarket, Average	*1 Slice/13g*	*17*	*0.4*	*139*	*25.0*	*1.8*	*3.5*	*0.2*
Breast, Roast, without Skin, Average	*1oz/28g*	*42*	*1.3*	*149*	*25.4*	*1.0*	*4.7*	*0.2*
Breast, Roll, Average	*1 Slice/10g*	*17*	*1.0*	*167*	*16.1*	*3.2*	*10.0*	*0.2*
Breast, Short Sliced, Mexican, Sainsbury's*	1 Pack/130g	177	2.9	136	26.4	2.5	2.2	0.1
Breast, Sliced, Mexican Style, Cooked, Asda*	1 Pack/234g	307	5.1	131	25.5	4.3	2.2	0.1
Breast, Slices, Roast, Hot 'n' Spicy, Sainsbury's*	½ Pack/65g	91	1.0	139	27.1	3.9	1.6	0.1
Breast, Smoked, Sliced, Average	*1 Slice/20g*	*22*	*0.5*	*110*	*20.7*	*0.9*	*2.6*	*0.1*
Breast, Southern Fried, in Breadcrumbs, Birds Eye*	1 Breast/100g	240	14.0	240	15.0	14.0	14.0	0.7
Breast, Southern Fried, Premium, Bernard Matthews*	1 Serving/60g	70	1.7	117	19.6	3.1	2.9	0.6
Breast, Strips, Raw, Average	*1 Serving/280g*	*358*	*5.7*	*128*	*27.1*	*0.3*	*2.0*	*0.3*
Breast, Tandoori Style, Average	1 Serving/180g	237	6.7	131	22.3	2.3	3.7	1.0
Breast, Tikka, Sliced, Average	1oz/28g	34	0.5	120	24.9	2.0	1.7	0.6
Chargrills, Garlic, Weight After Cooking, Birds Eye*	1 Chargrill/95g	182	10.4	192	19.0	4.0	11.0	0.1
Chargrills, Garlic, Weight Before Cooking, Birds Eye*	1 Chargrill/95g	190	10.7	200	20.3	4.2	11.3	0.1
Chargrills, Original, Weight Before Cooking, Birds Eye*	1 Chargrill/95g	156	8.5	164	17.5	3.2	9.0	0.1
Chargrills, Weight After Cooking, Baked, Birds Eye*	1 Chargrill/90g	160	8.7	178	18.9	3.4	9.7	0.1
Cooked, Sliced, Average	*1 Slice/15g*	*18*	*0.4*	*118*	*22.4*	*1.6*	*2.4*	*0.1*
Dippers, Crispy, Average	5 Dippers/93g	231	14.3	249	13.2	14.4	15.4	0.6
Drumsticks, BBQ Flavour, Average	1 Serving/200g	348	16.0	174	22.6	3.1	8.0	0.4
Drumsticks, Breaded, Fried, Average	1oz/28g	70	4.1	248	19.6	9.9	14.6	0.6
Drumsticks, Chinese Style, Average	1 Serving/100g	177	8.1	177	22.5	3.5	8.1	0.7
Drumsticks, Free Range, TTD, Sainsbury's*	1 Piece/67g	126	6.7	188	24.4	0.0	10.0	0.0
Drumsticks, Hoi Sin, Co-Op*	1 Pack/750g	1012	42.0	135	19.8	1.3	5.6	1.3
Drumsticks, Roast, without Skin, Average	*1 Serving/100g*	*163*	*7.8*	*163*	*22.6*	*0.5*	*7.8*	*0.2*
Drumsticks, Southern Fried, Sainsbury's*	1 Serving/87g	190	8.6	218	20.8	11.2	9.9	0.7
Drumsticks, with Skin, Average	*1 Piece/125g*	*268*	*16.6*	*215*	*22.1*	*1.8*	*13.3*	*0.3*
Escalope, Breaded, Average	1 Piece/128g	361	21.6	282	13.4	19.1	16.9	0.7
Escalope, Cheese Topped, Asda*	1 Piece/173g	411	22.5	237	12.0	18.0	13.0	1.9
Escalope, Lemon & Pepper, Sainsbury's*	1 Piece/143g	428	27.6	299	12.8	18.7	19.3	1.9
Fillet, Thigh, TTD, Sainsbury's*	1 Piece/60g	96	3.5	160	26.8	0.0	5.9	0.0

CHICKEN

	Measure INFO/WEIGHT	per Measure KCAL	FAT	Nutrition Values per 100g / 100ml KCAL	PROT	CARB	FAT	FIBRE
Fillet Strips, Barbeque, Birds Eye*	4 Strips/100g	180	8.7	179	18.9	6.5	8.6	0.2
Fillet Strips, Dijon Mustard, Birds Eye*	4 Strips/113g	155	5.9	137	18.9	3.7	5.2	0.1
Fillet Strips, Red Pesto, Birds Eye*	4 Strips/100g	135	5.1	135	19.1	3.2	5.1	0.2
Fillet Strips, Tomato & Basil, Birds Eye*	4 Strips/101g	150	5.4	149	19.4	5.6	5.4	0.3
Fillets, Battered, Average	1 Fillet/90g	199	10.4	221	16.1	13.3	11.5	0.5
Fillets, Breaded, Average	1 Piece/98g	214	10.5	219	14.2	15.9	10.7	1.9
Fillets, Chilli & Mango, Tesco*	1 Serving/100g	130	0.7	130	27.1	3.7	0.7	1.0
Fillets, Chinese Style, Average	1oz/28g	37	0.5	131	24.4	4.6	1.7	0.5
Fillets, Coronation, BGTY, Sainsbury's*	1 Fillet/100g	136	2.6	136	27.1	2.4	2.6	1.0
Fillets, Hickory Barbecue & Chilli, BGTY, Sainsbury's*	1 Fillet/100g	133	1.2	133	26.9	3.6	1.2	0.9
Fillets, Hickory Style BBQ, Tesco*	1 Fillet/80g	112	1.8	140	28.4	1.5	2.2	0.5
Fillets, Honey & Maple, Roast, Mini, Waitrose*	½ Pack/100g	131	0.5	131	23.0	8.6	0.5	1.5
Fillets, Honey & Mustard, Average	1 Serving/100g	138	3.7	138	18.4	7.5	3.7	0.8
Fillets, Hot & Spicy, Average	1oz/28g	58	3.1	206	16.4	10.5	11.0	1.1
Fillets, Lime & Coriander, Mini, Average	1 Fillet/42g	49	0.5	118	24.3	2.6	1.3	0.6
Fillets, Mango Salsa, Mini, Sainsbury's*	½ Pack/100g	132	1.2	132	24.7	5.6	1.2	0.0
Fillets, Mini, Green Thai Marinated, Love Life, Waitrose*	½ Pack/138g	153	3.3	111	21.2	1.2	2.4	0.6
Fillets, Piri Piri Style, Mini, Ready to Eat, Tesco*	1 Pack/190g	256	2.1	135	22.7	7.6	1.1	0.8
Fillets, Red Pepper, Mini, BGTY, Sainsbury's*	1 Serving/100g	126	0.6	126	26.5	3.7	0.6	0.7
Fillets, Red Thai, Mini, Average	1oz/28g	36	0.6	127	21.7	5.4	2.0	0.6
Fillets, Roast, Sweet Chilli, Mini, Waitrose*	1 Pack/200g	314	1.0	157	29.4	8.8	0.5	1.0
Fillets, Southern Fried, Meat Only, Average	1 Piece/100g	222	12.0	222	16.4	12.2	12.0	1.1
Fillets, Sweet Chilli, Mini, Sainsbury's*	½ Pack/100g	119	1.1	119	21.8	5.4	1.1	0.9
Fillets, Sweet Chilli & Lime, Mini, M & S*	1 Serving/50g	77	1.1	155	28.3	5.1	2.2	0.0
Fillets, Tandoori Style, Mini, Average	1 Serving/100g	127	2.0	127	24.7	2.5	2.0	0.3
Fillets, Thai, COU, M & S*	1 Fillet/120g	160	1.9	133	19.5	10.4	1.6	1.3
Fillets, Tikka, Average	1 Serving/100g	141	5.0	141	22.4	1.7	5.0	1.1
Fillets, Tikka, Mini, Average	1oz/28g	35	0.6	124	25.1	1.3	2.1	1.1
Fillets, Tomato & Basil, Mini, Average	1oz/28g	34	0.6	123	23.4	2.5	2.1	0.3
Fingers, Average	1 Serving/75g	187	9.9	250	13.7	18.7	13.2	1.1
Free Range, Large, TTD, Sainsbury's*	1 Serving/187g	354	17.2	189	26.6	0.0	9.2	0.0
Garlic, Frozen, Tesco*	1 Serving/95g	182	8.3	192	15.6	12.9	8.7	1.0
Garlic Basted, Morrisons*	1 Serving/100g	231	13.1	231	23.3	0.7	13.1	0.4
Goujons, Breaded, Average	1 Serving/114g	293	17.1	258	15.8	15.2	15.0	1.0
Goujons, Breast, Fresh, Average	1oz/28g	36	0.5	127	28.0	0.0	1.6	0.0
Goujons, Cracked Black Pepper, American, Asda*	1 Serving/150g	333	21.0	222	16.0	8.0	14.0	2.5
Goujons, Garlic & Herb, Breaded, American, Asda*	½ Pack/150g	376	22.5	251	17.0	12.0	15.0	2.1
Goujons, Hot & Spicy, Sainsbury's*	½ Pack/125g	252	9.6	202	20.0	13.1	7.7	1.2
Griddlers, BBQ, Captain Birds Eye, Birds Eye*	1 Serving/77g	161	9.6	209	18.3	5.7	12.5	0.5
Honey Roast, Sliced, Average	1 Slice/13g	15	0.3	117	21.5	2.1	2.4	0.1
Leg, Meat Only, Raw, Average	*1oz/28g*	*34*	*1.1*	*120*	*20.1*	*0.0*	*3.8*	*0.0*
Leg, Meat Only, Raw, with Skin & Bone, Average	*1oz/28g*	*38*	*1.2*	*134*	*22.5*	*0.0*	*4.3*	*0.0*
Leg, Meat Only, Stewed, with Bone & Skin, Average	*1oz/28g*	*52*	*2.3*	*185*	*26.3*	*0.0*	*8.1*	*0.0*
Leg, with Skin, Raw, Average	*1oz/28g*	*48*	*2.9*	*172*	*19.1*	*0.0*	*10.4*	*0.0*
Leg, with Skin, Roasted, Average	*1oz/28g*	*66*	*4.6*	*234*	*21.5*	*0.1*	*16.4*	*0.0*
Leg or Thigh, Hot & Spicy, Average	1oz/28g	50	3.0	179	19.4	1.0	10.8	0.4
Leg Portion, Roast, with Bone, without Skin	1 Portion/114g	246	15.5	216	43.5	0.0	13.6	0.0
Leg Portion, Roasted Dry, with Skin, No Bone, Average	1 Quarter/120g	*244*	*15.3*	*203*	*21.6*	*0.3*	*12.7*	*0.2*
Legs, Free Range, TTD, Sainsbury's*	1 Serving/188g	384	23.3	204	23.1	0.0	12.4	0.0
Light Meat, Raw	*1oz/28g*	*30*	*0.3*	*106*	*24.0*	*0.0*	*1.1*	*0.0*
Light Meat, Roasted	*1oz/28g*	*43*	*1.0*	*153*	*30.2*	*0.0*	*3.6*	*0.0*
Meat, Roasted, Average	*1oz/28g*	*50*	*2.1*	*177*	*27.3*	*0.0*	*7.5*	*0.0*
Meat & Skin, Raw, Average	*1oz/28g*	*64*	*5.0*	*230*	*17.6*	*0.0*	*17.7*	*0.0*

C

CHICKEN

	Measure INFO/WEIGHT	per Measure KCAL	FAT	Nutrition Values per 100g / 100ml KCAL	PROT	CARB	FAT	FIBRE
Meat & Skin, Roasted, Average	*1oz/28g*	*60*	*3.9*	*216*	*22.6*	*0.0*	*14.0*	*0.0*
Meat & Skin Portions, Deep Fried, Average	1oz/28g	73	4.7	259	26.9	0.0	16.8	0.0
Mexican Chilli, Sliced, Eat Well, M & S*	1 Pack/130g	169	3.4	130	25.9	0.8	2.6	0.5
Mince, Average	*1oz/28g*	*39*	*1.7*	*140*	*20.9*	*0.1*	*6.0*	*0.2*
Nuggets, Battered, Average	1 Nugget/20g	50	2.9	251	13.5	16.9	14.4	0.9
Nuggets, Breaded, Average	1 Nugget/14g	37	2.0	263	14.8	19.8	13.8	1.9
Nuggets, Free From Gluten & Wheat, Sainsbury's*	1 Nugget/19g	47	2.5	251	13.4	19.7	13.2	0.8
Pieces, Boneless, Breaded, Fried, From Restaurant	1 Piece/17g	51	3.3	301	17.0	14.4	19.4	0.0
Pieces, Garlic, Crunchy, Birds Eye*	1 Piece/99g	259	15.0	262	14.4	16.9	15.2	0.9
Pieces, Spicy, Mexican, Birds Eye*	1 Piece/103g	254	14.0	247	14.6	16.5	13.6	0.6
Pops, Southern Fried, Frozen, Tesco*	1 Pack/225g	517	25.9	230	13.1	18.1	11.5	1.9
Roast, Lemon, City Kitchen, Tesco*	1 Pack/385g	470	15.0	122	8.2	13.4	3.9	1.2
Seasoned & Basted, M & S*	1oz/28g	38	1.3	137	17.3	6.7	4.5	0.5
Shashlik, Patak's*	1 Serving/250g	203	3.6	81	12.4	4.4	1.4	0.0
Soy Braised, M & S*	1 Serving/100g	130	7.0	130	13.1	3.4	7.0	0.7
Spatchcock, Poussin, Sainsbury's*	1 Serving/122g	168	6.6	138	21.1	0.1	5.4	0.2
Spatchcock, Salt & Cracked Pepper, Sainsbury's*	1 Serving/122g	168	6.6	138	21.1	0.1	5.4	0.2
Spicy, Fried, Sainsbury's*	1 Serving/150g	414	24.9	276	28.8	2.9	16.6	2.1
Steaks, Average	*1 Serving/100g*	*205*	*9.4*	*205*	*21.1*	*9.0*	*9.4*	*0.7*
Steaks, Garlic & Herb, Tesco*	1 Serving/138g	354	23.2	257	14.1	12.2	16.9	1.7
Sticks, Chilli, Southern Fried, Tesco*	5 Sticks/52g	167	11.4	322	13.4	17.8	21.9	1.1
Strips, Breast, Grilled, KP Snacks*	1 Serving/84g	90	1.5	107	25.0	0.0	1.8	0.0
Strips, Mexican, Sliced, M & S*	½ Pack/70g	77	0.4	110	24.3	2.3	0.6	0.5
Strips Or Tenders, Chinese Style, Average	1oz/28g	41	1.1	145	19.6	7.9	4.1	1.0
Tenders, Tex Mex, Jumbo, M & S*	1 Serving/200g	250	6.8	125	22.8	0.7	3.4	0.6
Tex Mex, Skinny Chef, All About Weight*	1 Meal/270g	192	2.2	71	12.9	1.1	0.8	3.8
Thigh, Fillets, Tesco*	1 Serving/100g	165	9.8	165	18.3	0.0	9.8	0.0
Thigh, Meat & Skin, Average	*1 Serving/100g*	*218*	*14.7*	*218*	*21.4*	*0.0*	*14.7*	*0.0*
Thigh, Meat & Skin, Casseroled, Average	*1oz/28g*	*65*	*4.6*	*233*	*21.5*	*0.0*	*16.3*	*0.0*
Thigh, Meat Only, Diced, Casseroled	*1oz/28g*	*50*	*2.4*	*180*	*25.6*	*0.0*	*8.6*	*0.0*
Thigh, Meat Only, Raw, Average	*1 Thigh/90g*	*113*	*4.9*	*126*	*19.4*	*0.0*	*5.4*	*0.0*
Thigh, Roast, Average	*1 Serving/100g*	*238*	*15.6*	*238*	*23.8*	*0.4*	*15.6*	*0.0*
Wafer Thin, Average	1 Slice/10g	12	0.4	120	19.0	2.8	3.6	0.1
Wafer Thin, Coronation, Sainsbury's*	½ Pack/50g	67	2.2	135	19.1	4.5	4.5	0.1
Whole, Roast, Average	*1oz/28g*	*59*	*3.7*	*211*	*21.2*	*1.5*	*13.4*	*0.2*
Whole, Roasted, Brown Sugar Marinade, Tesco*	1 Serving/100g	195	11.3	195	22.1	0.1	11.3	0.1
Wing, Breaded, Fried, Average	1oz/28g	82	5.2	294	18.4	14.0	18.5	0.4
Wing, Meat & Skin, Cooked, Average	*1oz/28g*	*67*	*4.4*	*241*	*23.3*	*1.9*	*15.6*	*0.3*
Wing Quarter, Meat Only, Casseroled	*1oz/28g*	*46*	*1.8*	*164*	*26.9*	*0.0*	*6.3*	*0.0*
Wings, BBQ Flavour, Average	1oz/28g	61	3.5	219	20.3	6.5	12.4	0.6
Wings, Chinese Style, Average	1oz/28g	72	4.3	256	24.2	5.1	15.5	0.6
Wings, Hickory Smoke Flavour, Nibbles, Sainsbury's*	1 Wing/100g	245	15.3	245	23.5	3.5	15.3	0.5
Wings, Hot & Spicy, Average	1oz/28g	65	3.8	231	21.8	5.1	13.6	0.8
Wings, Meat & Skin, Raw, Average	*1oz/28g*	*52*	*3.3*	*184*	*19.0*	*0.5*	*11.8*	*0.2*

CHICKEN &

	Measure INFO/WEIGHT	per Measure KCAL	FAT	Nutrition Values per 100g / 100ml KCAL	PROT	CARB	FAT	FIBRE
Apricot Rice, COU, M & S*	1 Pack/400g	360	3.6	90	9.4	10.6	0.9	0.7
Asparagus, in a Champagne Sauce, Finest, Tesco*	1 Pack/500g	615	33.5	123	8.8	7.0	6.7	0.9
Asparagus with Rice, Frozen, Low Fat, Waitrose*	1 Pack/380g	403	7.6	106	8.5	13.6	2.0	0.6
Bacon, Easy Steam, Tesco*	1 Pack/400g	728	36.4	182	11.7	13.6	9.1	0.8
Bacon Parcels, Finest, Tesco*	1 Pack/233g	379	21.6	163	16.1	3.7	9.3	0.5
Bacon Parcels, Sainsbury's*	½ Pack/170g	406	28.6	239	21.9	0.1	16.8	0.0
Balsamic Roasted Pepper Pasta, M & S*	1 Pack/310g	418	11.5	135	7.8	17.2	3.7	1.7
Black Bean, Chinese, Tesco*	1 Pack/350g	381	17.2	109	8.9	7.4	4.9	0.7

	Measure INFO/WEIGHT	per Measure KCAL	per Measure FAT	Nutrition Values per 100g / 100ml KCAL	PROT	CARB	FAT	FIBRE
CHICKEN &								
Black Bean, Chinese Takeaway, Tesco*	1 Serving/200g	190	6.6	95	8.3	8.0	3.3	0.5
Black Bean, Special Fried Rice, HL, Tesco*	1 Pack/450g	360	6.3	80	6.8	9.5	1.4	0.9
Black Bean, with Chinese Rice, COU, M & S*	1 Pack/400g	320	9.6	80	7.4	7.6	2.4	1.1
Black Bean, with Noodles, Tesco*	1 Pack/475g	470	7.6	99	7.6	13.6	1.6	0.2
Black Bean, with Rice, Chinese, Tesco*	1 Serving/450g	459	9.5	102	5.3	15.4	2.1	0.5
Black Bean, with Rice, HL, Tesco*	1 Pack/450g	463	7.2	103	6.9	19.6	1.6	0.6
Black Bean, with Vegetable Egg Rice, COU, M & S*	1 Packet/400g	360	6.4	90	7.2	12.0	1.6	1.4
Black Bean Noodles, Sainsbury's*	1 Serving/130g	155	0.9	119	4.3	23.9	0.7	0.8
Broccoli, with Herb Potatoes, Tesco*	1 Pack/475g	499	10.9	105	7.8	12.5	2.3	1.5
Butternut Squash, Curry Pot, Weight Watchers*	1 Pot/250g	232	3.5	93	6.6	12.5	1.4	1.6
Cashew Nuts, Asda*	1 Pack/400g	528	36.4	132	8.2	4.2	9.1	0.8
Cashew Nuts, Chinese, Cantonese, Sainsbury's*	½ Pack/175g	171	8.7	98	8.4	4.9	5.0	1.3
Cashew Nuts, Chinese, Tesco*	1 Pack/350g	378	19.6	108	9.5	4.9	5.6	0.6
Cashew Nuts, Easy Steam, Tesco*	1 Serving/400g	460	19.2	115	8.7	9.2	4.8	1.0
Cashew Nuts, Oriental, HL, Tesco*	1 Pack/450g	436	4.5	97	7.0	15.1	1.0	0.7
Cashew Nuts, with Egg Fried Rice, HL, Tesco*	1 Pack/450g	441	5.8	98	8.9	12.7	1.3	1.3
Cashew Nuts, with Egg Rice, GFY, Asda*	1 Pack/396g	396	8.7	100	7.0	13.0	2.2	1.3
Chargrilled Vegetable Roll, HL, Tesco*	1 Pack/221g	336	6.0	152	10.1	21.8	2.7	2.3
Chips, BBQ, BGTY, Sainsbury's*	1 Pack/381g	423	6.9	111	7.9	15.9	1.8	2.5
Chorizo Paella, Go Cook, Asda*	½ Pack/475g	591	10.5	124	10.2	15.9	2.2	2.6
Cranberry, Perfectly Balanced, Waitrose*	1 Pack/240g	161	1.0	67	11.8	4.1	0.4	1.1
Fries, Southern Fried, Sainsbury's*	½ Pack/250g	562	21.7	225	10.5	26.2	8.7	0.8
Fries, Southern Fried Style, Tesco*	1 Pack/500g	930	40.0	186	11.5	16.0	8.0	1.4
Gravy, COU, M & S*	1 Pack/300g	216	3.9	72	7.2	7.8	1.3	1.6
Herb Pasta with Lemon, HL, Tesco*	1 Pack/400g	520	8.0	130	8.2	18.8	2.0	1.6
King Prawn Special Fried Rice, Finest, Tesco*	1 Pack/450g	733	31.9	163	7.7	17.0	7.1	0.7
Mushroom, Chinese, Iceland*	1 Pack/400g	276	9.2	69	8.2	3.8	2.3	0.4
Mushroom, Chinese, Sainsbury's*	½ Pack/175g	115	3.5	66	7.6	4.4	2.0	0.9
Mushroom, Chinese, Tesco*	1 Pack/460g	474	12.9	103	5.7	13.8	2.8	1.0
Mushroom, in White Wine Sauce, GFY, Asda*	1 Pack/400g	272	7.2	68	6.0	7.0	1.8	1.2
Mushroom, with Egg Fried Rice, Iceland*	1 Pack/500g	410	6.0	82	4.9	13.0	1.2	0.7
Mushroom, with Vegetable Rice, BGTY, Sainsbury's*	1 Pack/400g	376	7.2	94	6.4	13.0	1.8	0.9
Mushrooms, Skinny Chef, All About Weight*	1 Meal/268g	204	2.7	76	12.1	3.0	1.0	3.1
Peppers, in a Black Bean Sauce, M & S*	1 Pack/320g	256	4.8	80	9.4	7.3	1.5	1.2
Peppers, M & S*	1 Serving/240g	264	10.8	110	14.7	2.3	4.5	0.6
Pineapple, Chilled, Tesco*	1 Pack/350g	364	8.4	104	9.6	11.1	2.4	5.5
Pineapple, with Egg Fried Rice, HL, Tesco*	1 Pack/450g	414	3.1	92	6.0	15.4	0.7	0.6
Pineapple, with Egg Fried Rice, Tesco*	1 Pack/450g	450	10.8	100	7.6	12.1	2.4	1.2
Pineapple, with Rice, HL, Tesco*	1 Pack/450g	400	7.2	89	6.6	12.0	1.6	1.0
Pineapple, with Vegetable Rice, M & S*	1 Pack/400g	400	7.6	100	7.2	13.0	1.9	1.6
Stuffing, Roast, HL, Tesco*	1 Serving/17g	19	0.2	111	23.3	1.3	1.4	0.2
Tomato & Basil, COU, M & S*	½ Pack/200g	180	4.6	90	14.3	3.4	2.3	0.8
Tomato Saag, with Pilau Rice, BGTY, Sainsbury's*	1 Pack/400g	404	4.0	101	7.3	15.6	1.0	1.0
Vegetable Pasta, Steam Meal, Light Choices, Tesco*	1 Meal/400g	340	2.8	85	6.8	12.6	0.7	1.9
Vegetables in Gravy, Chosen By You, Asda*	1 Pack/420g	441	10.9	105	13.9	6.0	2.6	0.8
CHICKEN ALFREDO								
BGTY, Sainsbury's*	1 Serving/200g	208	5.4	104	18.0	1.9	2.7	0.5
CHICKEN ARRABBIATA								
Al Forno, Sainsbury's*	1 Pack/900g	1026	22.5	114	6.5	16.4	2.5	1.4
Bistro, Waitrose*	½ Pack/175g	156	5.2	89	12.9	2.5	3.0	0.5
Easy Steam, HL, Tesco*	1 Pack/400g	284	3.2	71	8.4	7.6	0.8	1.2
GFY, Asda*	1 Pack/448g	394	3.1	88	5.2	15.1	0.7	1.1
Perfectly Balanced, Waitrose*	1 Serving/240g	211	5.8	88	12.4	4.0	2.4	0.6

	Measure INFO/WEIGHT	per Measure		Nutrition Values per 100g / 100ml				
		KCAL	FAT	KCAL	PROT	CARB	FAT	FIBRE
CHICKEN ARRABBIATA								
Weight Watchers, Heinz*	1 Serving/300g	222	1.8	74	5.4	11.5	0.6	0.8
CHICKEN BANG BANG								
Oriental Express*	½ Pack/200g	170	3.4	85	6.4	11.0	1.7	3.2
Waitrose*	1 Pack/350g	367	17.2	105	9.4	5.9	4.9	1.2
CHICKEN BUTTER								
& Rice, Indian, Finest, Tesco*	1 Serving/475g	660	28.3	139	7.1	14.0	6.0	1.6
Curry, Fresh, Tesco*	1 Pack/350g	486	24.5	139	11.8	7.1	7.0	1.8
Indian, with Pilau Rice, Asda*	1 Pack/500g	770	23.5	154	7.0	21.0	4.7	1.3
Rich & Aromatic, Sainsbury's*	1 Pack/400g	592	36.4	148	12.1	4.4	9.1	1.2
Tesco*	1 Pack/350g	515	33.0	147	11.7	3.7	9.4	0.7
CHICKEN CAJUN								
& Potato Hash, HL, Tesco*	1 Pack/450g	427	6.3	95	6.5	14.1	1.4	1.5
Breast, Chargrilled, Iceland*	1 Serving/80g	114	1.5	142	27.4	3.9	1.9	0.0
Breast, Morrisons*	½ Pack/180g	328	16.9	182	16.6	7.7	9.4	2.0
CHICKEN CANTONESE								
& Rice, Sizzler, Tesco*	1 Serving/450g	639	25.6	142	7.7	14.9	5.7	0.9
Breast, Fillets, Sainsbury's*	1 Serving/154g	168	2.3	109	20.3	3.6	1.5	0.6
Chinese, Tesco*	½ Pack/175g	196	6.5	112	10.3	9.4	3.7	0.4
Honey, Sesame, Sainsbury's*	1/3 Pack/135g	116	3.6	86	9.8	5.5	2.7	0.8
Honey Pepper, Sainsbury's*	½ Pack/175g	124	3.9	71	6.6	6.1	2.2	0.9
CHICKEN CARIBBEAN								
Fruity, with Rice & Peas, New, BGTY, Sainsbury's*	1 Pack/400g	352	3.6	88	6.9	13.1	0.9	2.2
Style, Breasts, COU, M & S*	1 Serving/205g	205	3.1	100	14.6	7.3	1.5	1.3
CHICKEN CHASSEUR								
BGTY, Sainsbury's*	1 Pack/320g	243	3.5	76	6.8	9.5	1.1	1.0
Breast Fillets, Morrisons*	1 Pack/380g	384	11.4	101	15.7	2.9	3.0	0.8
Finest, Tesco*	½ Pack/200g	200	6.4	100	14.3	2.4	3.2	1.1
Mix, Colman's*	1 Pack/38g	120	0.4	316	8.6	68.2	1.0	3.7
CHICKEN CHILLI								
& Lemongrass, with Egg Noodles, BGTY, Sainsbury's*	1 Pack/450g	499	15.3	111	10.0	10.2	3.4	1.2
Sweet, & Egg Fried Rice, HL, Tesco*	1 Serving/450g	446	8.1	99	5.7	15.0	1.8	0.4
Sweet, Findus*	1 Pack/350g	420	12.2	120	6.0	15.0	3.5	1.5
Sweet, Just Cook, Sainsbury's*	½ Pack/191g	200	1.3	105	15.2	9.4	0.7	0.5
Sweet, with Noodles, Frozen, HL, Tesco*	1 Pack/369g	340	5.1	92	6.7	13.1	1.4	1.0
with Lime, Breast, Simple Solutions, Tesco*	1 Pack/400g	564	21.2	141	22.5	0.8	5.3	1.4
CHICKEN CHINESE								
& Prawns, Sizzler, House Special, Tesco*	1 Serving/450g	684	23.4	152	7.5	18.8	5.2	1.2
Balls, M & S*	1 Ball/16g	45	2.2	280	10.8	29.2	13.6	2.1
Battered, with Plum Sauce, Tesco*	1 Pack/350g	647	20.3	185	6.7	26.5	5.8	0.8
Crispy Aromatic, Half, Tesco*	1 Serving/233g	524	24.2	225	16.3	16.7	10.4	1.7
Fillets, with Sweet Chilli Sauce, Tesco*	1 Serving/350g	591	22.0	169	8.8	19.2	6.3	0.7
Stir Fry, Morrisons*	1 Serving/319g	341	5.4	107	5.7	17.0	1.7	1.5
Style Sauce, Breast Fillets, Morrisons*	½ Pack/200g	162	2.0	81	13.5	4.6	1.0	1.2
with Ginger & Spring Onion, Tesco*	1 Serving/350g	299	10.1	85	7.6	7.3	2.9	0.6
CHICKEN CIDER								
COU, M & S*	1 Pack/400g	300	9.2	75	7.2	6.7	2.3	0.8
with Colcannon, Perfectly Balanced, Waitrose*	1 Pack/401g	353	12.4	88	6.2	8.9	3.1	1.1
CHICKEN CORDON BLEU								
Breast, Fillets, Sainsbury's*	1 Serving/150g	304	14.3	203	17.5	11.5	9.5	1.6
Waitrose*	1 Serving/160g	325	15.4	203	20.1	9.1	9.6	2.4
CHICKEN CORONATION								
COU, M & S*	1oz/28g	34	0.6	120	16.3	8.6	2.2	0.7
M & S*	1 Serving/200g	420	26.4	210	12.6	10.6	13.2	1.3

	Measure INFO/WEIGHT	per Measure KCAL	FAT	Nutrition Values per 100g / 100ml KCAL	PROT	CARB	FAT	FIBRE
CHICKEN CURRIED								
with Vegetables, Plumrose*	1 Serving/196g	253	16.1	129	5.8	8.0	8.2	0.0
CHICKEN DINNER								
Breast, with Pork, Sage & Onion Stuffing, Tesco*	1 Serving/180g	277	14.8	154	19.4	0.7	8.2	0.5
Kershaws*	1 Pack/350g	210	3.5	60	4.3	8.4	1.0	1.2
Tesco*	1 Serving/400g	388	7.2	97	9.2	10.9	1.8	1.2
with Gravy, The Crafty Cook*	1 Serving/320g	330	6.7	103	5.6	15.3	2.1	1.9
CHICKEN EN CROUTE								
Asda*	½ Pack/174g	393	17.4	226	14.0	20.0	10.0	1.5
Breast, Tesco*	1 Serving/215g	555	33.1	258	9.4	20.4	15.4	0.6
Just Cook, Sainsbury's*	1 Serving/180g	481	27.2	267	16.8	15.9	15.1	0.4
CHICKEN ESCALOPE								
Cheese & Chive, Asda*	1 Piece/159g	377	21.1	237	11.5	15.9	13.3	0.7
Creamy Peppercorn, Sainsbury's*	1 Serving/150g	367	24.5	245	13.3	11.2	16.3	1.1
Lemon, & Herb, Waitrose*	1 Serving/200g	242	6.4	121	22.0	1.0	3.2	0.6
Sour Cream & Chive, Tesco*	1 Piece/143g	390	24.8	274	13.3	16.1	17.4	2.0
Spinach & Ricotta, Sainsbury's*	1 Piece/150g	354	22.9	236	13.1	11.5	15.3	0.9
Topped with Cheese, Ham & Mushrooms, Asda*	½ Pack/149g	217	9.0	145	22.0	0.8	6.0	0.4
CHICKEN FLORENTINE								
Asda*	1 Serving/200g	322	18.0	161	18.0	2.1	9.0	0.9
Finest, Tesco*	½ Pack/225g	358	19.1	159	11.0	9.7	8.5	1.3
HL, Tesco*	1 Pack/400g	340	10.8	85	12.1	3.0	2.7	0.9
CHICKEN FU YUNG								
Chinese Takeaway, Tesco*	1 Pack/350g	315	3.5	90	5.6	14.5	1.0	0.8
CHICKEN GINGER								
& Plum, with Rice, Perfectly Balanced, Waitrose*	1 Pack/400g	492	2.0	123	6.3	23.5	0.5	1.0
& Spring Onion, with Rice, Sharwood's*	1 Pack/375g	347	6.4	93	5.1	14.2	1.7	1.7
CHICKEN HARISSA								
BGTY, Sainsbury's*	1 Serving/250g	211	3.0	84	10.4	8.0	1.2	1.5
with Cous Cous, Perfectly Balanced, Waitrose*	1 Pack/400g	348	8.0	87	7.6	9.5	2.0	1.7
CHICKEN HONEY & MUSTARD								
HL, Tesco*	1 Serving/375g	424	8.6	113	5.8	17.3	2.3	1.4
with Baby Potatoes, BGTY, Sainsbury's*	1 Pack/450g	391	3.1	87	8.5	11.7	0.7	0.8
with Spring Vegetable Rice, Slim Fast*	1 Pack/375g	375	5.2	100	5.8	15.5	1.4	0.8
CHICKEN IN								
Bacon, Mushroom & Red Wine Sauce, Asda*	1 Serving/151g	145	3.9	96	16.0	2.2	2.6	0.5
Barbecue Sauce, COU, M & S*	1 Pack/352g	370	5.6	105	8.6	13.8	1.6	1.2
Barbeque Sauce, Breasts, COU, M & S*	1 Pack/350g	420	6.7	120	8.5	20.6	1.9	0.6
BBQ Sauce, Breast, Sainsbury's*	1 Serving/170g	199	1.2	117	14.5	13.1	0.7	1.3
BBQ Sauce, Chargrilled, Breast, GFY, Asda*	1 Serving/166g	214	6.1	129	19.0	5.0	3.7	1.0
BBQ Sauce, GFY, Asda*	1 Pack/380g	494	2.7	130	18.0	13.0	0.7	0.2
BBQ Sauce, Weight Watchers*	1 Pack/339g	332	11.9	98	5.8	10.8	3.5	0.9
Black Bean, with Egg Fried Rice, Tesco*	1 Pack/450g	652	26.1	145	7.0	16.1	5.8	1.2
Black Bean Sauce, & Rice, Morrisons*	1 Pack/400g	408	9.2	102	3.9	16.4	2.3	1.2
Black Bean Sauce, Canned, BGTY, Sainsbury's*	1 Can/400g	308	3.6	77	9.3	7.9	0.9	0.7
Black Bean Sauce, Chinese Takeaway, Iceland*	1 Pack/400g	348	12.8	87	9.3	5.3	3.2	0.7
Black Bean Sauce, Frozen, BGTY, Sainsbury's*	1 Pack/400g	380	4.4	95	4.5	16.6	1.1	0.5
Black Bean Sauce, M & S*	1 Pack/350g	297	7.0	85	8.7	8.0	2.0	1.1
Black Bean Sauce, Sainsbury's*	1 Pack/465g	484	7.9	104	5.0	17.3	1.7	0.3
Black Bean Sauce, Tinned, Tesco*	1 Serving/200g	164	2.6	82	10.0	7.7	1.3	1.1
Black Bean Sauce, Waitrose*	1 Pack/300g	243	3.6	81	10.9	6.6	1.2	0.8
Black Bean Sauce, with Egg Fried Rice, GFY, Asda*	1 Serving/416g	320	4.2	77	5.0	12.0	1.0	0.9
Black Bean Sauce, with Noodles, Pro Cuisine*	1 Pack/600g	366	3.6	61	5.6	8.5	0.6	0.0
Black Bean Sauce, with Rice, Asda*	1 Pack/400g	500	7.6	125	7.0	20.0	1.9	0.6

	Measure INFO/WEIGHT	per Measure		Nutrition Values per 100g / 100ml				
		KCAL	FAT	KCAL	PROT	CARB	FAT	FIBRE

CHICKEN IN

	Measure INFO/WEIGHT	KCAL	FAT	KCAL	PROT	CARB	FAT	FIBRE
Black Bean Sauce, with Rice, Iceland*	1 Pack/400g	388	6.0	97	5.1	15.8	1.5	0.8
Broccoli & Mushroom, Good Choice, Iceland*	1 Pack/500g	590	11.0	118	6.4	18.1	2.2	0.6
Cheese & Bacon, Wrapped, Breast, Tesco*	1 Serving/300g	474	23.4	158	20.7	1.2	7.8	0.5
Chilli & Lemon Grass with Rice, Sainsbury's*	1 Pack/450g	526	11.2	117	6.2	17.4	2.5	0.7
Coconut, Sizzler, HL, Tesco*	1 Pack/350g	280	7.7	80	9.8	4.5	2.2	2.1
Creamy Madeira Sauce, HL, Tesco*	1 Pack/400g	320	6.8	80	12.8	2.3	1.7	1.0
Creamy Mushroom Sauce, HL, Tesco*	1 Pack/400g	296	6.0	74	13.2	1.8	1.5	0.5
Creamy Mushroom Sauce, Weight Watchers*	1 Pack/330g	343	9.6	104	7.0	12.5	2.9	0.6
Creamy Mustard Sauce, GFY, Asda*	1 Pack/400g	468	9.2	117	6.0	18.0	2.3	0.4
Creamy Tikka Style Sauce, Tesco*	1 Breast/190g	215	10.4	113	15.1	0.7	5.5	0.8
Creamy Tomato & Mascarpone Sauce, Waitrose*	1 Serving/400g	492	23.2	123	7.9	9.9	5.8	0.8
Creamy White Wine Sauce, Sainsbury's*	1 Pack/324g	285	12.0	88	8.9	4.7	3.7	1.0
Garlic & Cream Sauce, Breast Fillet, Morrisons*	1 Serving/180g	262	15.8	146	14.9	1.8	8.8	0.6
Garlic & Herbs, Breast, Sainsbury's*	1 Serving/200g	316	5.2	158	28.3	5.4	2.6	0.1
Ginger & Chilli with Veg Noodles, COU, M & S*	1 Pack/400g	300	2.4	75	6.4	10.7	0.6	1.1
Gravy, Breast, Sainsbury's*	1 Box/200g	124	1.0	62	11.8	2.9	0.5	0.2
Gravy, Chunky, M & S*	1 Can/489g	465	19.1	95	13.6	1.4	3.9	0.8
Honey Mustard & Parsnip Mash, Light Choices, Tesco*	1 Pack/400g	340	6.8	85	8.0	9.0	1.7	2.0
Hot Ginger Sauce, with Thai Sticky Rice, Sainsbury's*	1 Pack/450g	603	20.7	134	6.8	16.3	4.6	0.5
Hunter's BBQ Sauce, Asda*	½ Pack /190g	348	14.1	183	19.1	10.3	7.4	0.0
Leek & Bacon Sauce, Chilled, Co-Op*	1 Pack/400g	460	20.0	115	15.0	2.0	5.0	0.2
Leek & Bacon Sauce, with Mash, HL, Tesco*	1 Pack/450g	337	8.1	75	6.7	8.0	1.8	1.6
Lemon & Garlic Marinade, Thighs, Go Cook, Asda*	½ Pack/265g	493	30.2	186	19.7	1.2	11.4	0.8
Lemon Sauce with Rice, Sainsbury's*	1 Pack/450g	513	6.7	114	8.1	17.0	1.5	0.7
Lime & Coriander Marinade, Chargrilled, Asda*	½ Pack/163g	286	14.7	175	23.0	0.5	9.0	0.0
Madeira Sauce, with Mushrooms, Finest, Tesco*	½ Pack/200g	210	8.3	105	13.8	2.9	4.1	0.9
Masala with Spiced Indian Lentils, M & S*	1 Pack/330g	297	8.2	90	10.3	6.1	2.5	5.9
Mediterranean Sauce, Breasts, BGTY, Sainsbury's*	½ Pack/170g	148	3.4	87	14.5	2.7	2.0	0.9
Mediterranean Sauce, Iceland*	1 Pack/500g	640	6.0	128	7.4	21.8	1.2	0.5
Mexican Salsa, Tesco*	1 Pack/320g	368	8.6	115	19.5	3.1	2.7	0.6
Mexican Style Sauce, Tesco*	1 Serving/180g	128	1.4	71	13.3	2.6	0.8	0.7
Mushroom & White Wine Sauce, Breasts, Asda*	1 Breast/168g	232	9.4	138	20.5	1.4	5.6	0.5
Mushroom & White Wine Sauce, Fillets, Morrisons*	1 Serving/190g	243	10.4	128	18.8	0.9	5.5	0.5
Mushroom Sauce, Diet Chef Ltd*	1 1pack/300g	225	6.9	75	7.9	5.7	2.3	0.1
Oyster Sauce, & Mushrooms, Tesco*	1 Pack/350g	252	5.6	72	8.0	6.3	1.6	0.7
Oyster Sauce, with Mushrooms, Tesco*	1 Pack/350g	189	3.1	54	8.0	3.5	0.9	0.8
Peanut Sauce, Cafe Classics, Lean Cuisine	1 Pack/255g	300	9.0	118	7.8	13.7	3.5	1.2
Peppercorn Sauce, GFY, Asda*	1 Serving/399g	431	7.2	108	6.0	17.0	1.8	0.5
Peppers, Fillets, Sainsbury's*	1 Pack/360g	378	13.3	105	13.7	4.2	3.7	1.1
Pesto Style Dressing, Asda*	1 Serving/150g	210	10.0	140	18.7	1.3	6.7	0.0
Red Pepper Dressing, Tesco*	1 Serving/140g	228	13.3	163	19.2	0.1	9.5	0.5
Red Wine Sauce, Breasts, Fresh Tastes, Asda*	½ Pack/190g	245	8.0	129	20.5	2.4	4.2	0.5
Reggae Reggae Sauce, Drumsticks, Levi Roots*	1 Serving/100g	165	7.3	165	21.5	3.4	7.3	0.0
Smoky Barbecue Sauce, Breast, Fresh Tastes, Asda*	1 Breast/160g	258	6.2	161	21.9	9.6	3.9	0.9
Smoky Barbeque Sauce, Tesco*	1 Serving/185g	229	3.9	124	16.3	9.9	2.1	1.0
Spicy Chilli Sauce, Topped with Cheese, Breast, Asda*	½ Pack/190g	241	7.0	127	20.0	3.4	3.7	0.0
Sun Dried Tomato & Basil Sauce, Breast, Iceland*	1 Serving/156g	134	2.5	86	14.6	3.3	1.6	1.0
Sweet Chilli Sauce, Breast, Fresh Tastes, Asda*	½ Pack/180g	288	9.0	160	18.4	10.3	5.0	0.5
Tarragon Sauce, Lean Cuisine*	1 Pack/338g	270	6.7	80	4.0	11.0	2.0	1.5
Tomato & Basil Sauce, Breast, Fresh Tastes, Asda*	½ Pack/130g	136	2.7	105	19.3	2.3	2.1	0.7
Tomato & Basil Sauce, Breast, GFY, Asda*	1 Pack/392g	447	13.3	114	12.0	9.0	3.4	1.5
Tomato & Basil Sauce, Breast Fillets, Morrisons*	½ Pack/171g	231	7.5	135	21.3	2.5	4.4	1.4
Tomato & Basil Sauce, GFY, Asda*	½ Pack/189g	231	6.1	122	22.0	1.2	3.2	2.0

	Measure INFO/WEIGHT	per Measure KCAL	FAT	Nutrition Values per 100g / 100ml KCAL	PROT	CARB	FAT	FIBRE
CHICKEN IN								
Tomato & Basil Sauce, Good Choice, Iceland*	½ Pack/170g	153	4.4	90	13.3	3.3	2.6	0.6
Tomato & Basil Sauce, HL, Tesco*	1 Breast/200g	154	2.4	77	12.4	4.2	1.2	0.6
Tomato & Herb Sauce, Breasts, Tesco*	½ Pack/173g	155	2.4	90	15.0	3.6	1.4	0.5
Tomato & Wine Sauce, Steamfresh, Birds Eye*	1 Pack/400g	280	5.6	70	7.7	6.7	1.4	1.6
White Sauce, BGTY, Sainsbury's*	1 Can/200g	162	4.2	81	1.2	2.4	2.1	1.1
White Sauce, Canned, Asda*	½ Can/400g	644	44.0	161	12.0	3.5	11.0	0.0
White Sauce, Canned, HL, Tesco*	½ Can/200g	180	5.8	90	14.3	1.3	2.9	5.4
White Wine, with Pasta, Perfectly Balanced, Waitrose*	1 Pack/400g	400	10.0	100	8.2	12.1	2.5	2.5
White Wine & Asparagus Panzerotti, Asda*	½ Pack/150g	238	2.5	159	8.0	28.0	1.7	0.0
White Wine & Mushroom Sauce, M & S*	1 Serving/200g	260	13.6	130	15.6	1.6	6.8	1.0
White Wine & Tarragon Sauce, Breasts, Finest, Tesco*	½ Pack/200g	326	20.2	163	16.8	1.3	10.1	0.0
White Wine & Tarragon Sauce, Waitrose*	½ Pack/225g	281	17.3	125	10.7	3.1	7.7	0.3
White Wine Sauce, Breasts, Tesco*	1 Serving/370g	388	14.1	105	16.9	0.8	3.8	0.6
White Wine Sauce, Wild Rice, Pub Specials, Birds Eye*	1 Pack/450g	335	5.9	74	7.1	8.4	1.3	2.1
Wild Mushroom Sauce, Breasts, HL, Tesco*	1 Serving/212g	191	5.1	90	15.1	2.1	2.4	1.5
Wild Mushroom Sauce, Extra Special, Asda*	1 Serving/225g	319	19.0	142	14.2	2.2	8.4	0.3
Zesty Orange Sauce, Asda*	1 Serving/200g	340	12.0	170	16.0	13.0	6.0	0.4
Zesty Orange Sauce, Breast, Asda*	1 Serving/200g	326	14.0	163	16.0	9.0	7.0	0.0
CHICKEN ITALIAN								
Style, BGTY, Sainsbury's*	1 Pack/400g	364	4.4	91	6.0	14.5	1.1	0.9
Style, Dinner, Asda*	1 Pack/400g	244	4.0	61	6.0	7.0	1.0	1.1
Style, Meal, Asda*	1 Pack/408g	241	3.3	59	6.0	7.0	0.8	0.8
Style, Sainsbury's*	½ Pack/190g	222	7.6	117	16.3	3.9	4.0	0.1
with a Spicy Tomato, Chilli & Herb Sauce, Slim Fast*	1 Pack/371g	390	4.1	105	7.1	16.6	1.1	0.4
CHICKEN JEERA								
Sainsbury's*	½ Pack/201g	247	14.1	123	10.5	4.6	7.0	1.8
CHICKEN KUNG PO								
Sainsbury's*	½ Pack/175g	131	4.4	75	9.2	4.0	2.5	1.0
Waitrose*	1 Pack/350g	318	3.9	91	8.2	12.1	1.1	1.2
with Egg Fried Rice, Asda*	1 Pack/450g	688	22.5	153	6.0	21.0	5.0	1.0
CHICKEN LEMON								
Balls, Asda*	1 Ball/15g	42	2.5	279	14.0	19.0	17.0	1.6
Battered, Cantonese, Sainsbury's*	1 Pack/350g	560	19.6	160	10.7	16.6	5.6	0.9
Battered, Chinese Meal for Two, Tesco*	½ Serving/175g	294	12.9	168	6.6	18.8	7.4	2.0
Breast, Fillets, BGTY, Sainsbury's*	1 Fillet/113g	195	2.4	173	18.4	19.9	2.1	1.9
Cantonese, Sainsbury's*	½ Pack/140g	218	8.8	156	11.0	13.9	6.3	0.6
Chinese, Tesco*	1 Serving/350g	563	11.2	161	7.0	26.0	3.2	0.3
COU, M & S*	1 Pack/150g	150	1.3	100	17.9	5.6	0.9	0.8
Tesco*	½ Pack/175g	213	7.3	122	11.0	10.1	4.2	0.6
Waitrose*	1 Serving/400g	596	23.2	149	12.7	11.7	5.8	0.9
with Vegetable Rice, BGTY, Sainsbury's*	1 Pack/400g	428	6.4	107	6.5	16.8	1.6	0.8
CHICKEN LUNCH								
French Style, Light, John West*	1 Pack/240g	194	6.5	81	7.2	6.9	2.7	2.1
Italian Style, Light, John West*	1 Pack/240g	209	6.2	87	6.9	9.0	2.6	0.7
CHICKEN MEXICAN								
Style, BGTY, Sainsbury's*	1 Serving/260g	255	6.5	98	6.9	12.1	2.5	2.2
Style, Combo, Asda*	1 Pack/380g	562	16.7	148	21.0	6.0	4.4	2.0
Style, GFY, Asda*	½ Pack/200g	256	10.0	128	17.0	3.7	5.0	0.3
Style, with Rice, BFY, Morrisons*	1 Pack/400g	360	5.2	90	5.1	14.1	1.3	0.8
Style Sauce, Breast, Tesco*	1 Serving/180g	128	1.4	71	13.3	2.6	0.8	0.7
CHICKEN MOROCCAN								
Style, Sainsbury's*	½ Pack/269g	334	7.0	124	14.7	10.4	2.6	3.1
Style, with Spicy Cous Cous, BGTY, Sainsbury's*	1 Serving/225g	304	3.8	135	9.2	20.6	1.7	0.0

C

	Measure INFO/WEIGHT	per Measure KCAL	FAT	Nutrition Values per 100g / 100ml KCAL	PROT	CARB	FAT	FIBRE
CHICKEN MOROCCAN								
with Cous Cous, GFY, Asda*	1 Serving/450g	414	5.8	92	8.0	12.0	1.3	0.8
with Cous Cous & Fruity Sauce, BGTY, Sainsbury's*	1 Pack/400g	440	8.0	110	10.0	13.1	2.0	2.6
CHICKEN MUSTARD								
with Gratin Potatoes, HL, Tesco*	1 Pack/450g	463	12.1	103	9.0	10.7	2.7	2.5
CHICKEN ORIENTAL								
& Pineapple, HL, Tesco*	1 Serving/450g	414	3.1	92	6.0	15.4	0.7	0.6
with Noodles, Steamfresh, Birds Eye*	1 Pack/400g	336	8.8	84	7.1	9.0	2.2	0.3
CHICKEN PAPRIKA								
COU, M & S*	1 Pack/400g	380	6.4	95	9.0	11.7	1.6	2.0
with Savoury Rice & Vegetables, BGTY, Sainsbury's*	1 Pack/400g	383	2.4	96	7.1	15.5	0.6	1.1
CHICKEN PARMESAN								
& Sun Dried Tomato, Fillets, Mini, Sainsbury's*	1 Pack/200g	278	5.8	139	22.1	6.0	2.9	0.5
Sun Dried Tomato, Fillets, BGTY, Sainsbury's*	½ Pack/100g	138	2.9	138	22.1	6.0	2.9	0.5
CHICKEN PENANG								
Waitrose*	1 Pack/400g	364	10.8	91	10.1	6.6	2.7	0.8
CHICKEN PIRI PIRI								
Breast, Fillets, Mini, Tesco*	½ Pack/100g	135	1.1	135	22.7	7.6	1.1	0.0
GFY, Asda*	1 Pack/400g	406	2.8	102	5.8	18.0	0.7	1.4
M & S*	1 Pack/300g	420	23.1	140	10.0	7.3	7.7	1.3
Sainsbury's*	½ Pack/200g	248	10.8	124	14.0	4.8	5.4	0.5
with Rice, BGTY, Sainsbury's*	1 Serving/399g	395	4.4	99	10.3	11.9	1.1	1.6
CHICKEN RENDANG								
Sainsbury's*	1 Pack/350g	689	53.5	197	9.6	5.1	15.3	1.7
CHICKEN ROAST								
in a Pot, Sainsbury's*	1 Pack/450g	477	13.0	106	9.6	10.3	2.9	0.7
CHICKEN SAFFRON								
& Rice, M & S*	1 Pack/400g	360	4.8	90	7.6	11.6	1.2	1.1
CHICKEN SIZZLER								
GFY, Asda*	1 Pack/350g	289	5.0	83	12.9	4.6	1.4	1.4
HL, Tesco*	1 Serving/350g	273	7.0	78	11.1	3.8	2.0	4.3
CHICKEN SPANISH								
Style, Asda*	½ Pack/275g	322	13.5	117	14.0	4.1	4.9	0.7
CHICKEN STUFFED								
with Moroccan Style Cous Cous, GFY, Asda*	½ Pack/180g	259	4.9	144	20.0	10.0	2.7	0.0
with Mushrooms, Finest, Tesco*	1 Serving/150g	177	7.6	118	15.9	2.0	5.1	0.6
CHICKEN SUPREME								
BGTY, Sainsbury's*	1 Pack/350g	416	4.9	119	9.4	17.2	1.4	0.5
Breast, Sainsbury's*	1 Serving/187g	421	29.5	225	20.6	0.3	15.8	0.6
with Rice, Asda*	1 Pack/450g	616	31.5	137	15.0	3.4	7.0	1.1
with Rice, Birds Eye*	1 Pack/376g	470	9.8	125	6.6	18.8	2.6	0.5
with Rice, Weight Watchers*	1 Pack/300g	255	4.8	85	5.6	11.9	1.6	0.5
CHICKEN SZECHUAN								
Chilli & Peppercorn, Sainsbury's*	1 Pack/400g	352	16.0	88	9.9	3.2	4.0	0.5
Tesco*	1 Pack/350g	385	10.5	110	7.2	13.6	3.0	0.3
with Noodles, Sainsbury's*	1 Pack/450g	423	13.9	94	6.0	10.4	3.1	0.9
CHICKEN TANDOORI								
Finest, Tesco*	1 Pack/450g	495	18.4	110	7.4	10.2	4.1	1.3
Fresh Tastes, Asda*	1 Pack/400g	356	5.6	89	6.4	12.7	1.4	2.1
GFY, Asda*	1 Pack/400g	324	9.6	81	7.5	7.3	2.4	1.7
Masala, & Rice, HL, Tesco*	1 Serving/450g	409	7.6	91	6.6	12.9	1.7	0.6
Masala, Asda*	1 Pack/400g	580	20.0	145	7.0	18.0	5.0	1.3
Masala, Indian, Tesco*	1 Serving/350g	430	25.9	123	10.2	4.0	7.4	1.8
Masala, Sainsbury's*	1 Pack/400g	536	27.2	134	13.2	5.0	6.8	0.5

	Measure INFO/WEIGHT	per Measure KCAL	FAT	Nutrition Values per 100g / 100ml KCAL	PROT	CARB	FAT	FIBRE
CHICKEN TANDOORI								
Sizzler, HL, Tesco*	1 Pack/350g	275	7.0	79	11.1	3.8	2.0	4.3
Sizzler, Sainsbury's*	1 Pack/400g	536	29.2	134	12.8	4.3	7.3	1.7
Sizzler, Tesco*	1 Serving/175g	243	11.5	139	10.0	10.0	6.6	1.0
Tesco*	1 Serving/175g	198	8.6	113	10.6	6.7	4.9	1.0
with Rice, Easy Steam, Tesco*	1 Pack/400g	484	12.0	121	8.7	14.7	3.0	0.7
with Vegetable Pilau Rice, HL, Tesco*	1 Pack/348g	400	9.0	115	8.4	14.1	2.6	1.9
CHICKEN TERIYAKI								
& Noodles, Asda*	½ Pack/340g	445	8.8	131	9.0	18.0	2.6	0.9
Asda*	1 Pack/360g	299	5.0	83	9.1	8.6	1.4	0.8
Japanese, with Ramen Noodles, Sainsbury's*	1 Pack/450g	481	9.4	107	6.5	15.5	2.1	0.8
CHICKEN THAI								
& Vegetables, Eat Positive, Birds Eye*	1 Packet/400g	412	12.0	103	5.9	13.0	3.0	1.0
Chiang Mai, & Noodles, BGTY, Sainsbury's*	1 Pack/448g	484	17.9	108	6.9	11.0	4.0	1.7
Green, Fillets, Mini, Sainsbury's*	½ Pack/100g	130	1.6	130	27.9	0.9	1.6	0.8
Style, with Noodles, Tesco*	1 Pack/400g	332	6.8	83	7.5	9.5	1.7	1.0
Style Marinade, Breast, Chargrilled, GFY, Asda*	½ Pack/178g	178	5.3	100	17.0	1.3	3.0	0.5
with Rice, Steamfresh, Birds Eye*	1 Serving/400g	380	7.6	95	6.7	12.7	1.9	0.9
CHICKEN TIKKA								
& Coriander Rice, Weight Watchers*	1 Pack/400g	348	2.4	87	6.2	14.3	0.6	1.6
& Cous Cous, Boots*	1 Pack/160g	307	17.6	192	6.2	17.0	11.0	1.3
& Lemon Rice, Deli Meal, M & S*	1 Pack/360g	342	7.2	95	9.8	10.2	2.0	0.7
BGTY, Sainsbury's*	1 Serving/188g	265	3.0	141	10.5	21.2	1.6	0.0
Creamy, Breast, Tesco*	1 Breast/190g	215	10.4	113	15.1	0.7	5.5	0.8
Masala, COU, M & S*	½ Pack/175g	245	12.9	140	12.5	5.6	7.4	1.6
Masala, with Pilau Rice, Hot, Tesco*	1 Pack/550g	797	31.9	145	7.4	15.0	5.8	1.4
Masala, with Rice & Naan, Big Dish, Tesco*	1 Pack/600g	960	40.4	160	6.7	18.1	6.7	1.2
Masala, with Yellow Rice, Light Choices, Tesco*	1 Pack/441g	485	8.8	110	4.9	17.4	2.0	1.0
Masala & Pilau Rice, Asda*	1 Serving/500g	720	20.0	144	6.2	20.7	4.0	0.9
with Basmati Rice, GFY, Asda*	1 Pack/400g	592	7.2	148	9.0	24.0	1.8	1.6
with Pilau Rice, GFY, Asda*	1 Pack/450g	382	2.7	85	7.0	13.0	0.6	1.8
CHICKEN VINDALOO								
Average	1 Serving/410g	787	51.2	192	18.5	2.6	12.5	0.3
CHICKEN WITH								
a Sea Salt & Black Pepper Crust, Breasts, Asda*	1 Serving/154g	186	4.3	121	19.0	5.0	2.8	0.0
a Sticky Honey & Chilli Sauce, Breast, Asda*	1 Serving/175g	247	5.6	141	20.0	8.0	3.2	0.0
Asparagus & Rice, BGTY, Sainsbury's*	1 Pack/400g	428	5.6	107	9.1	14.5	1.4	0.9
Bacon & Leeks, GFY, Asda*	1 Pack/400g	328	8.0	82	13.0	3.0	2.0	0.6
Basil, Puy Lentils & Spelt, Roasted, The Food Doctor*	1 Pack/350g	210	7.3	60	9.6	0.7	2.1	10.2
Broccoli & Pesto Pasta, BGTY, Sainsbury's*	1 Pack/301g	328	5.1	109	10.3	13.2	1.7	2.5
Caesar Melt & Prosciutto, Breast, M & S*	1 Pack/375g	487	18.7	130	19.6	1.3	5.0	1.0
Caramelised Peppers, Chargrilled, M & S*	½ Pack/237g	225	9.0	95	12.9	2.1	3.8	1.3
Cheese, Leek & Ham, Breast, Fresh Tastes, Asda*	1 Pack/430g	658	30.5	153	18.9	3.4	7.1	0.7
Cheese & Bacon, Tesco*	½ Pack/175g	262	11.9	150	18.9	2.6	6.8	0.4
Cheese & Chive Sauce, Carb Control, Tesco*	1 Serving/400g	400	25.6	100	8.4	2.0	6.4	1.6
Cheese Croutons & Onion, Asda*	1 Serving/200g	200	6.4	100	16.0	2.0	3.2	0.9
Cherrywood Barbecue Sauce, Simply Cook, Tesco*	1 Serving/147g	165	2.5	112	16.6	7.6	1.7	0.4
Chorizo, & Patatas Bravas, COU, M & S*	1 Pack/400g	380	9.2	95	7.8	10.8	2.3	1.7
Chorizo & Tomato Sauce, Catalan, Bighams*	1 Pack/479g	407	15.8	85	10.9	2.8	3.3	0.7
Coriander & Lime, Asda*	1 Serving/105g	122	0.9	116	24.0	2.9	0.9	0.2
Cous Cous, Lemon & Herb, Finest, Tesco*	1 Pack/370g	492	18.5	133	10.5	11.5	5.0	0.9
Cranberry & Orange Stuffing, Sainsbury's*	1 Serving/100g	201	10.3	201	23.0	4.1	10.3	0.8
Cranberry Stuffing, Breast, Finest, Tesco*	½ Pack/200g	252	4.8	126	16.2	9.9	2.4	0.9
Creamy Spinach & Parmesan, M & S*	1 Pack/390g	468	17.2	120	10.8	12.3	4.4	2.5

CHICKEN WITH

	Measure INFO/WEIGHT	per Measure KCAL	FAT	Nutrition Values per 100g / 100ml KCAL	PROT	CARB	FAT	FIBRE
Fresh Mango, Chilli & Coriander, British, COU, M & S*	1 Pack/169g	270	3.9	160	12.1	22.8	2.3	1.9
Fusilli & Courgette, Sainsbury's*	1 Pack/450g	675	28.8	150	8.6	14.6	6.4	0.5
Garlic & Chilli Balti, Tesco*	1 Pack/400g	320	7.6	80	11.0	4.4	1.9	0.8
Garlic & Herbs, Asda*	1 Slice/25g	28	0.4	114	23.9	1.1	1.5	0.0
Garlic Mushrooms, Asda*	1 Serving/320g	342	16.0	107	13.7	1.7	5.0	2.2
Garlic Mushrooms, Breast, Simply Cook, Tesco*	½ Pack/125g	170	6.6	136	22.0	0.1	5.3	0.1
Garlic Mushrooms, Breast, Tesco*	1 Breast/125g	149	5.9	119	19.0	0.2	4.7	0.1
Grapes & Asparagus, Sainsbury's*	½ Pack/200g	240	13.2	120	13.3	1.8	6.6	1.0
Gravy & Stuffing, Breasts, Tesco*	½ Pack/173g	257	11.1	149	14.4	8.3	6.4	2.2
Gruyere Cheese & Parma Ham, Breast, COOK!, M & S*	1 Breast/194g	349	21.3	180	18.0	2.5	11.0	0.9
Hoi Sin Sauce, Ooodles of Noodles, Oriental Express*	1 Pack/425g	399	9.4	94	5.3	13.2	2.2	1.7
Honey & Mustard Sauce, Breasts, Simply Cook, Tesco*	½ Pack/219g	230	1.3	105	16.3	8.0	0.6	0.3
Honey & Sesame, with Rice, Light Choices, Tesco*	1 Pack/400g	432	12.0	108	5.3	14.9	3.0	2.2
Lemon Grass, Thai Greens & Baby Corn, Sainsbury's*	1 Serving/200g	196	6.8	98	10.0	6.9	3.4	1.4
Lime & Coriander, Chargrilled, Asda*	1 Serving/190g	351	17.1	185	24.0	2.0	9.0	1.1
Lime & Coriander, Easy, Waitrose*	½ Pack/168g	203	7.9	121	18.9	0.7	4.7	0.5
Lime & Tequila, Asda*	1 Serving/150g	193	2.7	129	24.0	4.3	1.8	0.5
Lyonnaise Potatoes, M & S*	½ Pack/260g	286	8.1	110	12.6	8.0	3.1	0.9
Madeira Wine & Porcini Mushrooms, Waitrose*	1 Pack/415g	378	11.2	91	8.8	7.9	2.7	2.8
Mango, Lime & Coriander, Asda*	1 Pack/400g	416	6.0	104	6.6	15.9	1.5	1.4
Mango Salsa & Potato Wedges, BGTY, Sainsbury's*	1 Pack/400g	336	6.4	84	7.0	10.4	1.6	1.5
Mascarpone, Bacon & Roasted Onions, Finest, Tesco*	1 Serving/200g	312	17.6	156	14.5	4.7	8.8	0.5
Mozzarella & Pancetta, Breast, Finest, Tesco*	½ Pack/225g	326	13.9	145	14.4	7.9	6.2	1.1
Mozzarella & Pesto Melt, Breasts, COOK!, M & S*	½ Pack/165g	206	10.2	125	16.4	1.3	6.2	0.7
Mushroom & Bacon, Fillets, M & S*	½ Pack/188g	225	11.2	120	15.5	0.5	6.0	1.7
Mushroom & Garlic Butter, Breasts, Sainsbury's*	½ Pack/195g	388	20.1	199	20.0	4.6	10.3	0.1
Mushroom & Tomato Sauce, GFY, Asda*	1 Serving/175g	180	3.7	103	19.0	2.0	2.1	2.7
Mushroom Pilaff, BGTY, Sainsbury's*	1 Serving/400g	320	2.0	80	8.0	10.5	0.5	1.4
Mushroom Risotto, M & S*	1 Pack/400g	480	11.6	120	6.9	16.7	2.9	0.8
Mushroom Sauce & Herby Rice, Fillets, M & S*	1 Pack/380g	475	19.4	125	7.7	12.0	5.1	1.3
Mushrooms & Bacon in a Wine Sauce, Breasts, M & S*	½ Pack/189g	255	13.8	135	15.7	1.1	7.3	0.6
Pancakes & Plum Sauce, COU, M & S*	1 Pack/245g	257	5.6	105	7.9	12.7	2.3	0.3
Pasta, Chianti & Balsamic, BGTY, Sainsbury's*	1 Pack/400g	372	7.6	93	9.4	9.5	1.9	1.9
Pesto & Linguine Pasta, Steamfresh Meal, Birds Eye*	1 Pack/400g	440	16.0	110	8.5	10.0	4.0	1.3
Plum Sauce, Battered, Tesco*	1 Serving/175g	324	10.2	185	6.7	26.5	5.8	0.8
Plum Tomatoes & Basil, Breast, Birds Eye*	1 Serving/172g	200	8.1	116	13.3	5.0	4.7	0.6
Pork, Parsnip Herb Stuffing, Sainsbury's*	1 Serving/100g	181	9.0	181	22.9	2.1	9.0	0.7
Pork, Sage & Onion Stuffing, Mini Roasts, Tesco*	1 Serving/240g	353	20.6	147	14.7	2.6	8.6	0.2
Pork Stuffing, Breast, Roast, M & S*	1 Serving/100g	165	6.5	165	24.1	3.0	6.5	0.0
Pork Stuffing & Chipolatas, Breast Joint, Tesco*	½ Pack/340g	524	27.9	154	16.7	3.4	8.2	0.5
Potato & Smoked Bacon Topping, M & S*	1 Serving/175g	227	8.4	130	17.8	3.2	4.8	1.2
Potato Wedges, Tomato & Basil, Weight Watchers*	1 Pack/330g	247	6.9	75	4.7	9.3	2.1	1.3
Prosciutto, Dolcelatte & 3 Cheese Sauce, Asda*	½ Pack/195g	355	11.7	182	30.0	1.9	6.0	1.2
Rice, Breast, Chargrilled, Spicy, Asda*	1 Pack/400g	372	2.4	93	6.0	16.0	0.6	1.0
Rice, Fiesta, Weight Watchers*	1 Pack/330g	307	6.6	93	6.1	12.8	2.0	0.4
Rice 'n' Peas, Sainsbury's*	1 Pack/300g	489	18.3	163	12.5	14.4	6.1	2.1
Sage & Onion Stuffing, Breast, Roast, Sliced, M & S*	1 Slice/17g	27	1.1	165	24.1	3.0	6.5	0.0
Soy & Ginger Noodles, Love Life, Waitrose*	1 Pot/360g	212	4.7	59	5.0	6.7	1.3	2.3
Spinach, Honey Mustard, American Style, Asda*	1 Serving/240g	394	24.0	164	14.0	4.4	10.0	0.3
Spirelli, Steam Meal, Tesco*	1 Serving/400g	400	10.8	100	6.6	12.0	2.7	1.2
Spring Vegetables, Chargrilled, COU, M & S*	1 Pack/414g	290	3.7	70	8.8	7.3	0.9	1.8
Stilton & Port Sauce, Breasts, Finest, Tesco*	1 Serving/400g	668	34.4	167	18.5	3.9	8.6	0.7
Stuffing, TTD, Sainsbury's*	1 Slice/34g	50	2.0	148	22.7	1.3	5.8	0.9

	Measure INFO/WEIGHT	per Measure		Nutrition Values per 100g / 100ml				
		KCAL	FAT	KCAL	PROT	CARB	FAT	FIBRE
CHICKEN WITH								
Sun Dried Tomato & Basil Butter, Sainsbury's*	1 Breast/185g	363	17.6	196	25.0	2.5	9.5	0.2
Sun Dried Tomato & Basil Sauce, Bistro, Waitrose*	½ Pack/175g	254	14.2	145	14.2	3.7	8.1	0.3
Sweet Chilli & Garlic, Chinese, Asda*	1 Serving/400g	436	2.4	109	8.0	18.0	0.6	2.1
Sweet Chilli & Noodles, Healthier Choice, Co-Op*	1 Pack/400g	320	4.4	80	7.6	9.5	1.1	1.9
Sweet Chilli Noodles, Morrisons*	1 Pack/400g	325	4.4	81	4.8	13.1	1.1	1.3
Sweet Chilli Sauce & Egg Fried Rice, Tesco*	1 Pack/380g	494	10.3	130	7.5	18.2	2.7	1.3
Sweet Potato Mash, Jerk, Super Naturals, Sainsbury's*	1 Pack/400g	284	4.4	71	6.1	9.2	1.1	2.2
Tagine, Cous Cous, Perfectly Balanced, Waitrose*	1 Pack/400g	516	14.0	129	8.2	16.2	3.5	1.0
Tangy Lemon Sauce, Breasts, Just Cook, Sainsbury's*	1 Serving/164g	244	3.0	149	16.2	16.9	1.8	0.1
Tomato & Basil, GFY, Sainsbury's*	1 Pack/400g	300	3.2	75	13.6	3.4	0.8	1.4
Tomato & Basil, Steam Cuisine, M & S*	1 Pack/400g	460	13.6	115	9.6	11.6	3.4	2.0
CHICORY								
Fresh, Raw, Average	*1 Head/150g*	*30*	*0.9*	*20*	*0.6*	*2.8*	*0.6*	*0.9*
CHILLI								
& Potato Wedges, Good Choice, Iceland*	1 Pack/400g	368	13.6	92	5.5	9.8	3.4	1.2
& Potato Wedges, Sainsbury's*	1 Pack/371g	393	15.2	106	7.2	10.1	4.1	2.2
& Rice, Birds Eye*	1 Serving/285g	305	7.7	107	3.4	17.2	2.7	1.0
& Rice, Frozen, Sainsbury's*	1 Pack/400g	436	7.6	109	4.8	18.4	1.9	0.6
& Rice, GFY, Asda*	1 Pack/400g	352	1.6	88	5.0	16.0	0.4	1.8
& Rice, Low Fat, Solo Slim, Rosemary Conley*	1 Serving/100g	89	2.8	89	8.3	7.8	2.8	3.5
& Rice, Morrisons*	1 Serving/500g	630	15.5	126	5.7	18.9	3.1	1.1
& Wedges, BBQ, HL, Tesco*	1 Pack/420g	391	10.9	93	5.4	12.2	2.6	1.9
& Wedges, GFY, Asda*	1 Pack/400g	364	10.0	91	7.0	10.1	2.5	2.5
Beef, & Potato Crush, Weight Watchers*	1 Pack/400g	232	6.0	58	5.0	5.9	1.5	3.4
Beef, Asda*	½ Pack/200g	190	7.8	95	7.0	8.0	3.9	1.2
Beef, with Rice, GFY, Asda*	1 Serving/402g	354	6.0	88	4.7	14.0	1.5	0.9
Beef, with Rice, Sainsbury's*	1 Serving/300g	360	5.1	120	5.6	20.6	1.7	1.1
Beef & Mushrooms, GFY, Asda*	1 Pack/400g	364	6.0	91	9.1	10.2	1.5	1.2
Beef & Rice Pot, Shapers, Boots*	1 Pot/301g	250	4.5	83	4.0	12.0	1.5	2.1
Bowl, American Style, Sainsbury's*	½ Pack/300g	255	10.5	85	8.8	4.6	3.5	2.0
Chicken Grande, Stagg*	1 Serving/205g	168	1.2	82	9.7	9.4	0.6	1.6
Con Carne, & Rice, Light Choices, Tesco*	1 Pack/500g	485	7.5	97	6.1	14.8	1.5	2.3
Con Carne, 2 Minute Meals, Sainsbury's*	1 Pouch/200g	146	3.2	73	6.0	8.6	1.6	2.7
Con Carne, Asda*	1 Can/392g	376	13.7	96	7.0	9.0	3.5	0.0
Con Carne, Baked Bean, Heinz*	1 Can/390g	324	5.8	83	7.0	10.3	1.5	2.8
Con Carne, BGTY, Sainsbury's*	1 Serving/400g	384	8.8	96	5.3	13.8	2.2	2.8
Con Carne, Canned, la Caldera*	¼ Can/200g	240	12.8	120	6.9	8.6	6.4	0.0
Con Carne, Canned, Morrisons*	1 Can/392g	368	11.8	94	8.8	8.0	3.0	2.4
Con Carne, Canned, Sainsbury's*	½ Can/200g	162	4.2	81	6.6	8.9	2.1	2.5
Con Carne, Canned, Tesco*	½ Can/200g	220	11.4	110	7.8	6.4	5.7	4.7
Con Carne, Diet Chef Ltd*	1 Pack/300g	306	14.4	102	8.6	6.2	4.8	4.4
Con Carne, Dynamite Hot, Stagg*	1 Serving/250g	310	15.5	124	7.6	9.6	6.2	2.5
Con Carne, Fluffy White Rice, COU, M & S*	1 Pack/400g	360	7.6	90	5.7	12.3	1.9	1.5
Con Carne, From Restaurant, Average	1 Serving/253g	256	8.3	101	9.7	8.7	3.3	0.0
Con Carne, Frozen, Co-Op*	1 Pack/340g	306	3.4	90	6.0	15.0	1.0	1.0
Con Carne, Good Choice, Iceland*	1 Pack/400g	476	4.0	119	5.5	21.9	1.0	1.0
Con Carne, Homepride*	1 Can/390g	234	2.3	60	2.5	11.2	0.6	0.0
Con Carne, M & S*	1 Pack/285g	285	10.5	100	8.7	7.4	3.7	2.0
Con Carne, Recipe Mix, Colman's*	1 Pack/50g	158	1.2	316	10.4	62.9	2.5	6.8
Con Carne, Restaurant, Sainsbury's*	1 Serving/100g	80	2.7	80	6.9	7.0	2.7	1.5
Con Carne, Slim Fast*	1 Pack/375g	394	7.1	105	5.5	16.2	1.9	1.5
Con Carne, with Rice, Birds Eye*	1 Pack/285g	291	7.1	102	3.3	16.6	2.5	0.8
Con Carne, with Rice, Weight Watchers*	1 Serving/301g	262	3.3	87	4.6	14.7	1.1	0.4

	Measure INFO/WEIGHT	per Measure KCAL	FAT	Nutrition Values per 100g / 100ml KCAL	PROT	CARB	FAT	FIBRE
CHILLI								
Con Carne & Rice, Healthy Living, Co-Op*	1 Pack/400g	400	6.8	100	7.8	13.9	1.7	2.1
Con Carne with Long Grain Rice, COU, M & S*	1 Pack/400g	380	7.6	95	5.0	13.9	1.9	1.9
Con Carne with Rice, GFY, Asda*	1 Serving/400g	456	6.4	114	6.0	19.0	1.6	0.9
Con Carne with Rice, Healthy Choice, Asda*	1 Pack/400g	412	8.4	103	6.0	15.0	2.1	0.9
Con Carne with Rice, Organic, Sainsbury's*	1 Pack/400g	472	10.8	118	5.0	18.5	2.7	1.8
Con Carne with Rice, Perfectly Balanced, Waitrose*	1 Pack/400g	404	7.2	101	5.8	15.3	1.8	1.7
Mealpack, Flavoured, All About Weight*	1 Pack/35g	120	2.8	343	31.4	34.9	8.0	9.1
Medium, Uncle Ben's*	1 Jar/500g	305	4.0	61	1.8	11.1	0.8	0.0
Mexican, Rice Time, Uncle Ben's*	1 Pot/300g	339	3.0	113	2.5	22.8	1.0	1.3
Mexican Chilli with Potato Wedges, Weight Watchers*	1 Pack/400g	388	11.2	97	5.4	11.2	2.8	2.5
Minced, Master Foods*	1 Tsp/7g	7	0.1	103	1.6	20.8	1.4	0.0
Mixed Vegetable, Tesco*	1 Pack/400g	352	11.6	88	3.9	11.0	2.9	3.2
Non Carne, Linda McCartney*	1 Pack/340g	275	7.8	81	5.8	9.2	2.3	1.7
Peruvian, Hot, in Sunflower Oil, Barts*	1 Serving/100g	62	1.5	62	1.5	10.7	1.5	0.0
Spicy, & Wedges, Healthy Options, Birds Eye*	1 Pack/350g	259	6.3	74	4.7	9.7	1.8	1.4
Three Bean, Diet Chef Ltd*	1 Pack/300g	195	2.7	65	4.0	10.3	0.9	3.6
Uncle Ben's*	1oz/28g	17	0.2	59	1.8	11.1	0.8	0.0
Vegetable	1oz/28g	16	0.2	57	3.0	10.8	0.6	2.6
Vegetable, Canned, Sainsbury's*	1 Can/400g	368	2.0	92	5.1	16.7	0.5	4.9
Vegetable, Diet Chef Ltd*	1 Pack/300g	258	4.8	86	3.4	14.5	1.6	4.4
Vegetable, Retail	1oz/28g	20	0.6	70	4.0	9.4	2.1	0.0
Vegetable, Tinned, GFY, Asda*	½ Can/200g	140	1.8	70	3.5	12.0	0.9	3.5
Vegetable & Rice, BGTY, Sainsbury's*	1 Pack/450g	409	4.9	91	3.5	16.7	1.1	3.5
Vegetable Garden, Stagg*	1 Can/410g	254	2.0	62	3.6	10.8	0.5	2.3
Vegetarian, with Rice, Tesco*	1 Pack/500g	575	13.0	115	4.0	19.0	2.6	1.8
CHINESE LEAF								
Fresh, Raw, Average	**1oz/28g**	**4**	**0.1**	**14**	**1.5**	**1.5**	**0.2**	**1.7**
CHINESE MEAL								
Duck, Crispy, & Pancakes, Kit, Asda*	½ Pack/59g	173	12.9	294	12.0	12.0	22.0	0.5
for One, GFY, Asda*	1 Pack/570g	946	16.5	166	7.0	28.0	2.9	0.0
for Two, Tesco*	1 Pack/500g	480	8.0	96	4.4	16.0	1.6	1.1
House Special, HL, Tesco*	1 Pack/450g	369	7.2	82	6.5	10.5	1.6	1.1
House Special, with Egg Fried Rice, Tesco*	1 Pack/450g	562	8.5	125	7.2	19.7	1.9	0.8
My Very Own, Asda*	1 Pack/297g	416	5.3	140	7.0	24.0	1.8	0.6
CHIPS								
& Curry Sauce, Tesco*	1 Serving/400g	440	20.0	110	2.1	14.1	5.0	1.0
11mm Fresh, Deep Fried, McCain*	1oz/28g	66	3.0	235	3.2	31.8	10.6	0.0
14mm Fresh, Deep Fried, McCain*	1oz/28g	59	1.9	209	2.7	34.2	6.8	0.0
14mm Friers Choice, Deep Fried, McCain*	1oz/28g	56	2.2	199	3.5	29.3	8.0	0.0
9/16" Straight Cut Caterpack, Deep Fried, McCain*	1oz/28g	63	2.6	225	3.1	32.1	9.4	0.0
American Style, Oven, Co-Op*	1 Serving/150g	255	9.0	170	2.0	26.0	6.0	3.0
American Style, Oven, Sainsbury's*	1 Serving/165g	313	13.7	190	5.4	23.6	8.3	1.3
American Style, Thin, Oven, Tesco*	1 Serving/125g	210	8.1	168	2.7	24.6	6.5	2.1
Beefeater, Deep Fried, McCain*	1oz/28g	71	2.8	253	3.3	37.7	9.9	0.0
Beefeater, Oven Baked, McCain*	1oz/28g	55	1.6	195	4.0	32.2	5.6	0.0
British Classics, HL, Tesco*	½ Pack/200g	250	1.6	125	2.6	26.9	0.8	1.3
Chippy, Microwave, McCain*	1oz/28g	49	2.0	176	2.6	25.2	7.2	1.7
Chunky, Baked, Organic, M & S*	1 Serving/100g	150	3.7	150	1.7	27.1	3.7	2.2
Chunky, COU, M & S*	1 Serving/150g	157	2.4	105	2.1	20.5	1.6	2.3
Chunky, Fresh, Chilled, Finest, Tesco*	1 Pack/450g	607	18.0	135	2.1	22.3	4.0	2.7
Chunky, Gastropub, M & S*	1 Pack/400g	520	12.4	130	2.6	22.4	3.1	2.3
Chunky, Ready to Bake, M & S*	1 Serving/200g	310	8.4	155	2.2	26.8	4.2	2.0
Chunky, Waitrose*	1 Portion/155g	200	8.8	129	1.9	17.6	5.7	2.8

CHIPS

INFO/WEIGHT	Measure	per Measure		Nutrition Values per 100g / 100ml				
		KCAL	FAT	KCAL	PROT	CARB	FAT	FIBRE
Chunky Oven, Harry Ramsden's*	1 Serving/150g	184	5.4	123	2.8	19.9	3.6	1.6
Crinkle Cut, Frozen, Fried in Corn Oil	1oz/28g	81	4.7	290	3.6	33.4	16.7	2.2
Crinkle Cut, M & S*	1 Serving/150g	270	8.1	180	3.3	29.5	5.4	2.4
Crinkle Cut, Oven, Asda*	1 Serving/100g	134	3.8	134	2.0	23.0	3.8	8.0
Crinkle Cut, Oven Baked, Aunt Bessie's*	1 Serving/100g	206	9.2	206	2.9	28.0	9.2	3.2
Crisscuts, Conagra Foods*	1 Serving/100g	192	9.6	192	2.6	24.0	9.6	2.2
Family Fries, Oven, Tesco*	1 Serving/125g	164	4.6	131	2.0	22.4	3.7	1.8
Fat, with Fluffy Centres, M & S*	1 Serving/200g	210	9.0	105	1.6	14.2	4.5	1.8
Fine Cut, Frozen, Fried in Blended Oil	1oz/28g	102	6.0	364	4.5	41.2	21.3	2.4
Fine Cut, Frozen, Fried in Corn Oil	1oz/28g	102	6.0	364	4.5	41.2	21.3	2.7
Fried, Average	1 Serving/130g	296	12.3	228	4.4	33.3	9.5	1.7
Fried, Chip Shop, Average	1 Serving/100g	239	12.4	239	3.2	30.5	12.4	2.2
Frozen, Crinkle Cut, Aunt Bessie's*	1 Serving/100g	163	7.3	163	3.1	21.3	7.3	2.2
Frying, Crinkle Cut, Tesco*	1 Serving/125g	161	4.1	129	2.6	22.2	3.3	1.9
Homefries, Chunky, Weighed Baked, McCain*	1 Serving/100g	153	3.1	153	3.2	28.0	3.1	2.3
Homefries, Chunky, Weighed Frozen, McCain*	1 Serving/100g	123	2.5	123	2.5	22.6	2.5	1.6
Homefries, Crinkle Cut, Weighed Baked, McCain*	1 Serving/100g	176	5.0	176	2.6	30.1	5.0	2.3
Homefries, Crinkle Cut, Weighed Frozen, McCain*	1 Serving/100g	142	5.1	142	1.9	22.2	5.1	1.3
Homefries, Jacket Oven, McCain*	1 Serving/100g	220	7.4	220	3.9	37.9	7.4	0.0
Homefries, Straight Cut, Weighed Baked, McCain*	1 Serving/100g	181	6.2	181	3.1	28.1	6.2	2.4
Homefries, Straight Cut, Weighed Frozen, McCain*	1 Serving/100g	134	4.6	134	2.2	21.0	4.6	1.7
Homefries, Thin & Crispy, Weighed Frozen, McCain*	1 Serving/100g	143	4.1	143	2.6	24.0	4.1	1.5
Homemade, Fried in Blended Oil, Average	1oz/28g	53	1.9	189	3.9	30.1	6.7	2.2
Homemade, Fried in Corn Oil, Average	1oz/28g	53	1.9	189	3.9	30.1	6.7	2.2
Homemade, Fried in Dripping, Average	1oz/28g	53	1.9	189	3.9	30.1	6.7	2.2
Homestyle, Frozen, Aunt Bessie's*	1 Serving/200g	260	11.2	130	2.2	17.6	5.6	2.7
Homestyle, Oven Cooked, Aunt Bessie's*	1 Serving/100g	191	7.8	191	3.1	27.0	7.8	2.9
Homestyle Oven, Sainsbury's*	1 Serving/125g	206	5.4	165	2.4	29.2	4.3	2.1
Micro, Asda*	1 Serving/112g	221	7.8	197	3.5	30.0	7.0	4.0
Micro, Crinkle Cut, Tesco*	1 Serving/100g	203	8.0	203	3.3	29.5	8.0	1.8
Micro Chips, Crinkle Cut, Cooked, McCain*	1 Pack/100g	166	4.2	166	2.9	28.9	4.2	2.4
Micro Chips, Straight Cut, Cooked, McCain*	1 Pack/100g	163	4.8	163	2.3	27.7	4.8	2.0
Microwave, Cooked	1oz/28g	62	2.7	221	3.6	32.1	9.6	2.9
Oven, 5% Fat, Frozen, McCain*	1 Serving/200g	238	6.0	119	1.9	21.0	3.0	1.6
Oven, American Style, Champion*	1 Serving/200g	372	14.4	186	2.2	28.2	7.2	2.0
Oven, Best in the World, Iceland*	1 Serving/175g	332	11.7	190	3.4	28.9	6.7	3.5
Oven, Champion*	1 Pack/133g	210	6.0	158	2.5	27.0	4.5	0.0
Oven, Chunky, Extra Special, Asda*	1 Serving/125g	237	7.0	190	3.4	31.5	5.6	3.2
Oven, Chunky, Ross*	1 Serving/100g	177	6.5	177	3.1	26.6	6.5	3.9
Oven, Chunky, TTD, Sainsbury's*	1 Serving/166g	250	5.3	151	2.0	28.6	3.2	2.3
Oven, Cooked, Weight Watchers*	1 Serving/100g	150	3.0	150	2.8	33.7	3.0	5.9
Oven, Crinkle Cut, 5% Fat, Weighed Baked, McCain*	1 Serving/100g	163	4.3	163	3.1	27.9	4.3	3.0
Oven, Crinkle Cut, 5% Fat, Weighed Frozen, McCain*	1 Serving/100g	134	3.6	134	2.4	23.2	3.6	2.4
Oven, Crinkle Cut, Sainsbury's*	1 Serving/165g	297	9.1	180	3.3	29.5	5.5	2.4
Oven, Frozen, Baked	1 Portion/80g	130	3.4	162	3.2	29.8	4.2	2.0
Oven, Frozen, BGTY, Sainsbury's*	1 Serving/165g	226	4.6	137	2.9	25.0	2.8	2.7
Oven, Homefries, McCain*	1 Serving/100g	134	4.6	134	2.2	21.0	4.6	1.7
Oven, Morrisons*	1 Serving/100g	134	3.9	134	2.4	22.2	3.9	0.0
Oven, Organic, Waitrose*	1 Serving/165g	233	6.3	141	1.5	25.1	3.8	1.6
Oven, Original, McCain*	1 Serving/100g	158	3.8	158	2.5	28.5	3.8	2.3
Oven, Original, Straight Cut, 5% Fat, Cooked, McCain*	1 Serving/100g	172	4.9	172	3.4	32.4	4.9	2.3
Oven, Original, Straight Cut, 5% Fat, Frozen, McCain*	1 Serving/100g	138	4.0	138	2.5	26.2	4.0	1.9
Oven, Steak Cut, Asda*	1 Serving/100g	153	4.1	153	2.0	27.0	4.1	2.5

	INFO/WEIGHT	KCAL	FAT	KCAL	PROT	CARB	FAT	FIBRE
CHIPS								
Oven, Steak Cut, Frozen, Champion*	1 Serving/100g	130	3.5	130	1.9	22.6	3.5	3.3
Oven, Steak Cut, Sainsbury's*	1 Serving/165g	266	7.8	161	2.6	27.1	4.7	2.8
Oven, Steak Cut, Waitrose*	1 Serving/165g	218	5.6	132	2.7	22.7	3.4	1.7
Oven, Steakhouse, Frozen, Tesco*	1 Serving/125g	165	4.2	132	2.7	22.7	3.4	1.7
Oven, Straight Cut, 5% Fat, Sainsbury's*	1 Serving/165g	280	8.1	170	3.4	28.0	4.9	2.5
Oven, Straight Cut, Asda*	1 Serving/100g	199	5.0	199	3.5	35.0	5.0	3.0
Oven, Straight Cut, BFY, Morrisons*	1 Serving/165g	249	5.8	151	2.8	27.1	3.5	2.1
Oven, Straight Cut, Frozen Weight, HL, Tesco*	1 Serving/125g	132	2.4	106	2.1	20.0	1.9	2.3
Oven, Straight Cut, Iceland*	1 Serving/100g	197	6.2	197	3.6	31.6	6.2	2.3
Oven, Straight Cut, Low Fat, HL, Tesco*	1 Serving/100g	132	2.8	132	2.7	23.9	2.8	2.8
Oven, Straight Cut, Nisa Heritage*	1 Serving/150g	186	5.2	124	1.8	21.3	3.5	0.0
Oven, Straight Cut, Reduced Fat, Tesco*	1 Serving/100g	127	3.0	127	2.3	22.7	3.0	2.1
Oven, Straight Cut, Waitrose*	1 Serving/165g	219	6.1	133	2.0	23.0	3.7	1.7
Oven, Thick Cut, Frozen, Baked	1oz/28g	44	1.2	157	3.2	27.9	4.4	1.8
Oven, Thin & Crispy, Tesco*	1 Portion/100g	205	4.9	205	2.7	37.6	4.9	5.8
Oven, Thin Cut, American Style, Asda*	1 Serving/100g	240	10.0	240	3.4	34.0	10.0	3.0
Oven, Thin Fries, Morrisons*	1 Serving/100g	161	6.1	161	2.9	23.6	6.1	1.2
Real Homemade, 1 Spoonful, Actifry*	1 Portion/250g	217	3.6	87	2.0	16.9	1.4	1.0
Rustic, TTD, Sainsbury's*	½ Pack/122g	176	2.9	144	2.8	27.9	2.4	2.8
Steak Cut, Frying, Asda*	1 Serving/97g	181	6.8	187	2.9	28.0	7.0	2.8
Steak Cut, Oven, Tesco*	1 Serving/165g	233	6.4	141	2.0	24.4	3.9	2.0
Steakhouse, Fry, Tesco*	1 Serving/125g	278	15.1	222	3.1	25.2	12.1	2.0
Straight Cut, Frozen, Fried in Blended Oil	1oz/28g	76	3.8	273	4.1	36.0	13.5	2.4
Straight Cut, Frozen, Fried in Corn Oil	1oz/28g	76	3.8	273	4.1	36.0	13.5	2.4
Straight Cut, Low Fat, Tesco*	1 Serving/125g	159	3.7	127	2.3	22.7	3.0	2.1
Straight Cut, Oven, BGTY, Sainsbury's*	1 Portion/165g	226	3.5	137	2.7	26.8	2.1	4.1
The Big Chip, Frozen, Tesco*	1 Serving/200g	220	4.8	110	1.8	20.3	2.4	2.1
Thick Cut, Frozen, Fried in Corn Oil, Average	1oz/28g	66	2.9	234	3.6	34.0	10.2	2.4
Three Way Cook, Skinny, Co-Op*	1 Serving/100g	175	7.0	175	2.0	26.0	7.0	3.0
Waffle, Birds Eye*	1 Serving/75g	156	8.4	208	2.5	24.3	11.2	2.6
CHIVES								
Fresh, Average	**1 Tsp/2g**	**0**	**0.0**	**23**	**2.8**	**1.7**	**0.6**	**1.9**
CHOC ICES								
Chocolate, Dark, Seriously Creamy, Waitrose*	1 Ice/82g	195	12.9	238	2.6	21.6	15.7	1.7
Chocolate, Real Milk, Sainsbury's*	1 Ice/48g	151	9.5	312	3.5	30.3	19.7	0.8
Chunky, Wall's Ice Cream*	1 Ice/81g	162	10.6	200	2.6	18.9	13.1	0.0
Dark, Sainsbury's*	1 Ice/43g	136	9.5	315	3.8	25.5	22.0	0.4
Dark, Tesco*	1 Ice/43g	141	9.1	325	2.8	30.2	21.0	0.1
Morrisons*	1 Ice/31g	86	6.0	279	3.0	24.7	19.3	0.4
Neapolitan Chocolate, Co-Op*	1 Ice/62g	120	8.2	194	2.0	16.9	13.2	0.4
White Chocolate, Sainsbury's*	1 Ice/48g	140	8.9	292	3.8	27.3	18.6	0.1
CHOCOLATE								
Advent Calendar, Dairy Milk, Cadbury*	1 Chocolate/4g	22	1.3	525	7.5	56.6	30.1	0.7
Advent Calendar, Magic of Christmas, Cadbury*	1 Chocolate/9g	48	2.7	510	7.0	57.7	28.0	0.7
Advent Calendar, Maltesers, Mars*	1 Chocolate/4g	21	1.2	537	6.8	57.9	30.9	0.0
Advent Calendar, Milky Bar, Nestle*	1 Chocolate/4g	22	1.3	547	7.3	58.4	31.7	0.0
Advent Calendar, Pirates of the Caribbean, Kinnerton*	1 Chocolate/4g	19	1.0	525	5.4	61.2	28.6	1.6
Advent Calendar, The Simpsons, Kinnerton*	1 Chocolate/4g	20	1.1	526	5.3	63.2	28.9	1.6
Advent Calendar, The Snowman, M & S*	1 Chocolate/4g	21	1.2	550	6.6	60.4	31.0	0.0
Almond & Honey, Dairy Milk, Cadbury*	1 Bar/54g	281	15.6	520	8.0	57.1	28.9	1.0
Animal Bar, Nestle*	1 Bar/19g	97	5.0	513	5.8	63.6	26.1	0.0
Baking, Belgian, Milk, for Cakes, Luxury, Sainsbury's*	1 Chunk/8g	44	2.7	556	7.6	56.5	33.3	1.5
Baking, Continental, for Home Baking, Luxury, Tesco*	1 Pack/150g	822	67.6	548	2.7	27.7	45.1	0.9

CHOCOLATE

	Measure INFO/WEIGHT	per Measure KCAL	FAT	Nutrition Values per 100g / 100ml KCAL	PROT	CARB	FAT	FIBRE
Baking, Milk, for Home Baking, Luxury, Tesco*	1 Pack/150g	838	54.3	559	7.0	51.4	36.2	1.7
Bar, Apricot & Raisin, Thorntons*	1 Bar/40g	185	10.9	462	8.0	46.0	27.3	3.5
Bar, Bliss, Hazelnut Truffle, Cadbury*	1 Serving/100g	565	37.9	565	7.2	47.7	37.9	2.6
Bar, Bliss, Toffee Flavour Truffle, Cadbury*	2 Chunks/23g	128	8.1	555	6.9	51.6	35.3	1.6
Bar, Bliss, Truffle, Cadbury*	1 Bar/40g	226	14.9	565	6.6	48.8	37.3	2.8
Bar, Cappuccino, Thorntons*	1 Bar/38g	201	13.2	529	5.2	49.7	34.7	0.5
Bar, Dark, 60% Cocoa, with Macadamia, Thorntons*	1 Bar/70g	183	12.8	523	6.5	42.3	36.5	12.6
Bar, Dark, Thorntons*	1 Bar/48g	250	17.7	521	7.3	39.9	36.9	10.9
Bar, Dark, with Ginger, Thorntons*	1 Bar/100g	509	35.1	509	5.8	44.3	35.1	8.8
Bar, Dark Chocolate, Diabetic, Thorntons*	1 Bar/75g	345	26.8	460	5.4	28.5	35.8	8.1
Bar, Extra Dark, 60% Cocoa, Lindor, Lindt*	1 Bar/150g	900	73.5	600	5.0	35.0	49.0	2.0
Bar, Flake Allure, Cadbury*	1 Bar/30g	170	10.9	567	6.7	51.0	36.3	0.7
Bar, Hazel Nut & Cashew, Dairy Milk, Cadbury*	3 Chunks/18g	96	6.0	540	8.8	50.6	33.5	1.8
Bar, Jazz Orange, Thorntons*	1 Bar/56g	304	18.1	543	6.8	55.7	32.3	1.2
Bar, Milk, Thorntons*	1 Bar/50g	269	16.0	538	7.5	54.8	32.0	1.0
Bar, Milk Chocolate, Diabetic, Thorntons*	½ Bar/37g	174	12.2	470	7.3	43.0	33.1	2.2
Bar, Twisted, Creme Egg, Cadbury*	1 Bar/45g	210	9.4	465	5.2	64.6	20.8	0.5
Bar, Very Peculiar, Milk with Marmite Flavour, Marmite*	4 Squares/13g	70	4.2	540	6.9	54.9	32.1	2.0
Bar, Viennese, Continental, Thorntons*	1 Bar/38g	206	13.0	542	4.2	53.9	34.2	0.8
Bar, White, Thorntons*	1 Bar/50g	273	15.6	547	6.5	59.5	31.3	0.0
Beans, Coffee, Dark, Solid, M & S*	1 Serving/10g	53	3.8	532	4.7	42.4	37.6	11.6
Beans, Non Dairy, Graze*	1 Pack/40g	196	8.8	491	3.3	70.0	22.0	0.0
Beans, Plain, Carl Brandt*	4 Beans/5g	25	1.4	501	5.7	54.6	28.9	0.0
Bear, Lindt*	1 Bear/11g	60	3.6	572	7.5	57.7	34.6	0.0
Belgian, Kschocolat*	4 Pieces/40g	212	12.2	530	6.0	57.5	30.5	2.3
Belgian, Milk, Mini Eggs, M & S*	1 Egg/8g	43	2.5	535	7.0	55.8	31.7	2.7
Belgian Milk, TTD, Sainsbury's*	1 Piece/10g	55	3.5	549	9.6	48.3	35.3	2.0
Black Magic, Nestle*	1oz/28g	128	5.8	456	4.4	62.6	20.8	1.6
Breakaway, Nestle*	1 Bar/20g	100	5.0	499	6.5	61.1	25.2	0.0
Bubbly, Dairy Milk, Cadbury*	1 Bar/35g	185	10.5	525	7.7	56.9	29.7	0.7
Bubbly Santa, M & S*	1 Santa/23g	124	7.3	540	7.0	55.8	31.7	2.7
Bunny, Easter, Mars*	1 Bunny/29g	155	9.2	535	6.2	56.2	31.7	0.0
Bunny, Lindt*	1 Bunny/11g	60	3.6	572	7.5	57.5	34.6	0.0
Cappuccino, Nestle*	1 Serving/20g	109	6.6	545	6.1	56.0	32.9	0.0
Caramel, Chunk, Dairy Milk, Cadbury*	1 Chunk/33g	158	7.6	480	5.0	63.0	23.0	0.0
Caramel, Dairy Milk, Cadbury*	1 Bar/47g	225	10.9	479	4.9	62.8	23.2	0.4
Choco Swing, Kraft*	1 Square/16g	89	5.5	555	5.7	54.0	34.5	0.0
Chocolat Noir, Lindt*	1/6 Bar/17g	87	5.4	510	6.0	50.0	32.0	0.0
Chocolate Favourites, Tesco*	½ Box/227g	1015	43.6	447	4.2	64.3	19.2	0.3
Chomp, Cadbury*	1 Bar/24g	112	4.8	465	3.3	67.9	20.0	0.2
Christmas Tree Decoration, Cadbury*	1 Piece/12g	60	3.4	525	7.6	56.2	29.9	0.0
Chunk Bar, Dairy Milk, Cadbury*	1 Chunk/7g	35	2.0	525	7.5	57.0	29.8	0.1
Chunky Hazelnut Bar, M & S*	1 Bar/52g	293	19.4	563	8.8	48.1	37.3	1.7
Coconut, White, Excellence, Lindt*	1 Square/10g	61	4.4	610	6.0	48.0	44.0	0.0
Coins, Milk, Sainsbury's*	1 Coin/5g	26	1.4	502	5.5	58.8	27.1	2.5
Cool & Delicious, Dairy Milk, Cadbury*	1 Bar/21g	110	6.3	525	7.6	56.1	30.1	0.0
Counters, Galaxy, Mars*	4 Counters/10g	53	2.9	529	6.8	59.4	29.1	1.4
Crispies, Chunk, Dairy Milk, Cadbury*	1 Chunk/31g	158	8.5	510	7.6	58.6	27.4	0.0
Crispies, Dairy Milk, Cadbury*	1 Bar/49g	250	13.4	510	7.6	58.6	27.4	0.0
Crispy, Sainsbury's*	4 Squares/19g	99	5.4	521	9.1	56.9	28.5	2.1
Dairy Milk, Cadbury*	1 Bar/49g	255	14.6	520	7.5	56.9	29.8	0.6
Dark, & Hazelnuts & Currant, Organic, Green & Black's*	1 Bar/100g	513	33.5	513	7.6	45.4	33.5	9.2
Dark, & Orange & Spices, Maya Gold, Green & Black's*	1 Bar/35g	184	11.8	526	7.3	48.2	33.8	8.2

CHOCOLATE

INFO/WEIGHT	Measure	per Measure KCAL	FAT	KCAL	PROT	CARB	FAT	FIBRE
Dark, 70% Cocoa Solida, Extra Fine, Lindt*	1 Square/10g	54	4.1	537	8.0	33.0	41.0	0.0
Dark, 70% Cocoa Solids, Organic, Green & Black's*	1 Bar/35g	193	14.4	551	9.3	36.0	41.1	11.5
Dark, 70% Cocoa Solids, Organic, Morrisons*	½ Bar/50g	265	20.5	531	7.9	31.6	41.1	11.0
Dark, 75% Cacao, Rausch*	1 Row/31g	163	12.9	522	8.8	28.5	41.1	15.0
Dark, 85% Cocoa, Excellence, Lindt*	1 Serving/40g	212	18.4	530	11.0	19.0	46.0	0.0
Dark, 85% Cocoa, TTD, Sainsbury's*	1 Serving/25g	142	12.8	569	9.7	17.0	51.4	14.1
Dark, 99% Cocoa, Excellence, Lindt*	1 Serving/25g	132	12.5	530	13.0	8.0	50.0	8.0
Dark, Belgian, Extra Special, Asda*	2 Squares/20g	102	8.0	508	11.0	26.0	40.0	16.0
Dark, Belgian, Luxury Continental, Sainsbury's*	1 Bar/100g	490	38.7	490	11.1	24.2	38.7	7.4
Dark, Bittersweet, with Cherries, Green & Black's*	1 Bar/100g	477	28.2	477	7.9	48.0	28.2	8.7
Dark, Chilli, Excellence, Lindt*	1 Serving/40g	202	12.8	506	5.4	49.0	32.0	0.0
Dark, Classic, Bourneville, Cadbury*	1 Bar/18g	87	4.6	495	4.0	61.1	26.3	6.0
Dark, Continental, Luxury, Tesco*	1 Bar/100g	571	37.8	571	11.3	46.5	37.8	0.1
Dark, Co-Op*	1 Bar/50g	252	14.5	505	4.0	57.0	29.0	6.0
Dark, Espresso, Coffee, Organic, Green & Black's*	1 Bar/150g	823	62.4	549	9.8	33.8	41.6	11.7
Dark, Fair Trade, Co-Op*	1 Bar/45g	214	13.0	475	4.0	49.0	29.0	6.0
Dark, Feuilles, with Orange, Nestle*	1 Piece/8g	42	2.6	524	4.6	54.4	32.0	0.0
Dark, Luxury Continental, Sainsbury's*	½ Bar/50g	252	20.0	504	10.7	25.5	40.0	16.1
Dark, Orange with Slivered Almonds, Excellence, Lindt*	1 Square/10g	50	3.0	500	6.0	46.0	30.0	0.0
Dark, Plain, Average	**1oz/28g**	**143**	**7.8**	**510**	**5.0**	**63.5**	**28.0**	**2.5**
Dark, Rich, Tesco*	1 Serving/20g	98	6.1	491	5.8	60.0	30.4	11.5
Dark, Smooth, Bar, Galaxy, Mars*	1 Bar/125g	651	42.0	521	6.2	48.0	33.6	9.3
Dark, Special, Hershey*	1 Pack/41g	180	12.0	439	4.9	61.0	29.3	7.3
Dark, Whole Nut, Tesco*	1 Serving/13g	67	4.5	539	6.1	48.3	35.7	6.5
Dark, with Chilli, Thorntons*	4 Squares/20g	107	7.9	533	7.2	36.3	39.5	10.4
Diet, Ritter Sport*	1 Square/6g	25	1.8	412	6.0	44.0	30.0	0.0
Divine, Milk, Co-Op*	1 Bar/45g	243	14.4	540	7.0	57.0	32.0	2.0
Double Blend, Nestle*	1 Piece/11g	61	3.6	553	7.3	55.9	33.0	0.0
Double Chocolate, Nestle*	1 Serving/25g	133	8.3	532	9.1	49.4	33.1	0.0
Dream, with Real Strawberries, Cadbury*	1 Bar/45g	250	14.9	555	4.5	59.6	33.1	0.0
Egg, Double Cream, Nestle*	1 Egg/28g	163	11.1	582	6.9	49.2	39.7	0.4
Egg, Mars*	1 Egg/33g	166	9.3	503	4.5	57.3	28.2	0.0
Egg, Truffle Filled, Dark Chocolate, Black Magic, Nestle*	1 Egg/28g	144	8.9	522	5.8	52.0	32.3	3.4
Freddo, Caramel, Dairy Milk, Cadbury*	1 Bar/20g	95	4.8	485	5.5	60.2	24.6	0.0
Freddo, Dairy Milk, Cadbury*	1 Freddo/18g	95	5.4	525	7.5	57.0	29.8	0.7
Fruit & Nut, Belgian, Waitrose*	1 Serving/50g	254	14.6	508	8.6	54.6	29.2	3.4
Fruit & Nut, Dark, Tesco*	4 Squares/25g	123	7.0	494	5.8	54.8	27.9	6.5
Fudge, Keto Bar*	1 Serving/65g	250	7.0	385	36.9	36.9	10.8	32.3
Ginger, Traidcraft*	1 Bar/50g	212	7.4	424	3.9	68.2	14.8	0.0
Hazelnut & Walnut, Dark, Organic, Seeds of Change*	1 Bar/100g	559	41.7	559	8.4	37.5	41.7	9.2
Kinder, Bueno Bar, Ferrero*	1 Bar/22g	121	8.1	563	9.8	46.6	37.5	0.0
Kinder, Riegel, Ferrero*	1 Bar/21g	117	7.1	558	10.0	53.0	34.0	0.0
Kinder Maxi, Ferrero*	1 Bar/21g	115	7.1	550	10.0	51.0	34.0	0.0
Kinder Surprise, Ferrero*	1 Egg/20g	110	6.8	550	10.0	51.0	34.0	0.4
King Size, Dairy Milk, Cadbury*	1 Serving/85g	446	25.2	525	7.6	56.4	29.7	0.0
Kitten, Milk Chocolate, Lindt*	1 Kitten/11g	60	3.6	572	7.5	57.7	34.6	0.0
Lait Intense, Experiences, Cote D'or*	3 Squares/100g	575	40.0	575	7.2	44.5	40.0	5.0
Light & Whippy, Bite Sized, Sainsbury's*	1 Bar/15g	66	2.4	439	3.3	69.7	16.3	0.1
Little Bars, Dairy Milk, Cadbury*	1 Bar/21g	110	6.3	530	7.7	56.6	30.1	0.7
Macadamia Nut, Excellence, Lindt*	1 Bar/100g	560	37.0	560	7.0	51.0	37.0	0.0
Maciek Adwokat, Wawel*	1 Bar/40g	197	9.9	492	6.0	57.3	24.7	0.0
Matchmakers, Mint, Nestle*	1 Stick/4g	20	0.8	477	4.3	69.7	20.1	0.9
Milk, a Darker Shade, Green & Black's*	1 Bar/35g	183	10.4	523	9.9	54.0	29.7	3.7

CHOCOLATE

	Measure INFO/WEIGHT	per Measure KCAL	FAT	Nutrition Values per 100g / 100ml KCAL	PROT	CARB	FAT	FIBRE
Milk, Average	1oz/28g	146	8.6	520	7.7	56.9	30.7	0.8
Milk, Bars, M & S*	1 Bar/40g	214	12.8	535	7.8	54.0	32.0	1.9
Milk, Bubbly, Swiss, M & S*	1 Serving/40g	218	13.7	545	8.0	52.0	34.3	2.5
Milk, Extra Au Lait, Milch Extra, Lindt*	½ Bar/50g	267	15.5	535	6.5	57.0	31.0	0.0
Milk, Extra Creamy, Excellence, Lindt*	1 Bar/100g	560	37.1	560	6.0	51.1	37.1	0.0
Milk, Extra Fine, Swiss, M & S*	1 Serving/25g	141	9.2	565	7.2	50.9	36.7	2.3
Milk, Figures, Hollow, Dairyfine, Aldi*	1 Serving/11g	58	3.2	523	5.5	59.9	29.0	3.1
Milk, Fimbles Bar, Kinnerton*	1 Bar/12g	65	3.8	539	5.8	57.0	31.8	1.9
Milk, Honey, Traidcraft*	1 Bar/50g	272	16.5	545	6.0	54.0	33.0	0.0
Milk, Italian, Low Sugar, Groder*	1 Serving/40g	199	14.6	498	6.9	51.2	36.5	1.9
Milk, Less Than 99 Calories, M & S*	1 Bar/16g	85	4.6	531	7.5	61.2	28.7	0.6
Milk, Lindor, Lindt*	1 Square/11g	68	5.2	615	4.7	43.0	47.0	0.0
Milk, Santas, Tesco*	1 Bag/90g	433	21.8	481	4.5	61.4	24.2	1.4
Milk, Soft Caramel Centre, Organic, Green & Black's*	1 Bar/100g	495	26.4	495	8.3	56.2	26.4	2.8
Milk, Super Naturals, Sainsbury's*	4 Pieces/40g	85	4.9	212	2.4	23.0	12.2	0.9
Milk, Swiss, Diabetic with Fruit and Nuts, Boots*	½ Bar/21g	97	6.7	462	7.0	55.0	32.0	2.7
Milk, Swiss Made, Organic, Traidcraft*	4 Squares/17g	91	5.6	550	7.0	50.0	34.0	0.0
Milk, Whole Nut, Tesco*	1 Serving/25g	129	8.4	517	8.7	53.4	33.8	9.0
Milk, with Biscuit Pieces, Asda*	2 Squares/14g	73	4.1	521	8.0	57.0	29.0	1.9
Milk, with Crisped Rice, Dubble*	1 Bar/40g	211	11.8	528	6.4	59.6	29.4	0.0
Milk, with Honey & Almond Nougat, Swiss, Toblerone*	1 Piece/8g	42	2.4	525	5.4	59.0	29.5	2.2
Milk, with Peanut Butter Filling, Ghirardelli*	1 Serving/45g	250	17.0	556	8.9	48.9	37.8	2.2
Milk, with Raisins & Hazelnuts, Green & Black's*	1 Bar/100g	556	36.9	556	9.2	46.8	36.9	3.2
Milk, with Whole Almonds, Organic, Green & Black's*	1 Bar/100g	578	42.2	578	11.8	37.7	42.2	5.2
Mini, Toblerone*	1 Serving/6g	31	1.8	525	5.6	57.5	30.0	3.5
Mint Chips, Chunk, Dairy Milk, Cadbury*	1 Chunk/32g	162	8.4	505	6.5	61.2	26.1	0.0
Mint Chips, Dairy Milk, Cadbury*	1 Bar/49g	247	12.8	505	6.6	61.6	26.1	0.6
Mint Creme, Sainsbury's*	1 Serving/20g	93	4.9	467	2.8	62.7	24.5	2.1
Mint Crisp, Sainsbury's*	4 Squares/19g	95	4.7	501	5.0	63.7	25.0	3.6
Mountain Bar, Swiss, M & S*	1 Bar/100g	555	35.3	555	6.5	55.2	35.3	0.2
Mountain Bar, with Orange, Swiss, M & S*	½ Bar/50g	267	16.4	535	8.0	52.2	32.8	3.2
Natural Orange, Excellence, Lindt*	1 Bar/100g	560	37.0	560	7.0	50.0	37.0	0.0
Natural Vanilla, Excellence, Lindt*	1 Bar/100g	590	40.0	590	6.0	51.0	40.0	0.0
Nibs, Raw, Cacao, Organic, Navitas Naturals*	1 Serving/28g	130	12.0	464	14.3	35.7	42.9	32.1
Noir, Special, Frey*	1 Bar/35g	197	15.7	562	8.0	30.0	45.0	0.0
NutRageous, Reese's, Hershey*	1 Bar/51g	260	16.0	510	11.8	54.9	31.4	3.9
Nuts About Caramel, Cadbury*	1 Bar/55g	272	15.1	495	5.8	56.6	27.4	0.0
Nutty Nougat, Bite Sized, Sainsbury's*	1 Bar/23g	111	5.5	481	7.6	59.0	23.8	0.6
Old Jamaica, Cadbury*	4 Squares/23g	107	5.4	465	4.2	59.6	23.4	0.0
Orange, Fair Trade, Divine Foods*	4 Squares/17g	92	5.4	541	6.5	57.7	31.5	0.0
Orange, Sainsbury's*	4 Squares/19g	100	5.8	531	9.2	54.3	30.7	2.2
Orange Cream, Cadbury*	1 Bar/51g	217	7.9	425	2.6	68.6	15.4	0.0
Orange Cream, Fry's*	1 Bar/50g	210	6.8	420	2.8	72.3	13.7	0.0
Panna Cotta & Raspberry, M & S*	1 Bar/36g	190	12.1	528	4.7	51.4	33.6	0.3
Peppermint, Ritter Sport*	1 Bar/100g	483	26.0	483	3.0	60.0	26.0	0.0
Peppermint Cream, Fry's*	1 Bar/51g	217	7.9	425	2.6	68.8	15.4	0.0
Plain, 50% Cocoa Solids Minimum, Tesco*	4 Squares/22g	115	6.2	523	7.4	60.0	28.1	1.8
Plain, 72% Cocoa Solids, Finest, Tesco*	1 Square/10g	60	4.4	603	7.7	44.0	44.0	3.7
Plain, Belgian, Organic, Waitrose*	1 Bar/100g	505	37.6	505	9.6	32.0	37.6	5.6
Plain, Belgian, TTD, Sainsbury's*	1 Piece/10g	57	4.7	570	7.0	29.3	47.2	10.2
Plain, Continental, Waitrose*	1 Square/4g	23	1.8	558	7.7	32.9	44.0	5.9
Plain, Dark, Fruit & Nut, Rich, Sainsbury's*	4 Squares/25g	122	7.0	489	5.2	53.9	27.9	5.7
Plain, Fair Trade, Tesco*	1 Bar/40g	200	11.8	501	4.8	53.8	29.6	6.6

CHOCOLATE

	Measure INFO/WEIGHT	per Measure KCAL	FAT	Nutrition Values per 100g / 100ml KCAL	PROT	CARB	FAT	FIBRE
Plain, Whole Nut, Belgian, Waitrose*	4 Squares/25g	135	9.5	540	6.3	45.4	38.0	7.8
Plain, Wholenut, Sainsbury's*	1 Serving/25g	142	9.0	567	5.7	54.6	36.2	2.5
Plain, with Ginger, Swiss, Waitrose*	4 Squares/17g	88	5.0	519	5.3	58.3	29.4	2.0
Plain, with Hazelnuts, Tesco*	4 Squares/25g	135	8.9	539	6.1	48.3	35.7	6.5
Praline, M & S*	1 Bar/34g	185	12.0	545	7.3	49.6	35.2	3.1
Snack Bar, Kinder*	1 Bar/21g	116	7.1	554	10.0	52.0	34.0	0.0
Snack Size, Dairy Milk, Cadbury*	1 Bar/30g	159	9.0	530	7.8	57.1	29.9	0.0
Snickers, More Nuts, Snickers*	1 Bar/58g	299	17.3	515	10.1	52.8	29.8	0.0
Tasters, Dairy Milk, Cadbury*	1 Bag/45g	238	13.7	530	7.6	56.4	30.5	0.0
Taz Chocolate Bar, Cadbury*	1 Bar/25g	121	6.0	485	4.8	62.0	24.0	0.0
Treatsize, Dairy Milk, Cadbury*	1 Bar/14g	73	4.2	525	7.5	57.0	29.8	0.7
Turkish Delight, Large Bar, Dairy Milk, Cadbury*	1 Square/8g	35	1.6	470	5.6	63.2	21.4	0.5
Wafer, Dairy Milk, Cadbury*	1 Bar/46g	235	12.9	510	7.7	57.0	28.0	0.0
White, Average	*1oz/28g*	*148*	*8.7*	*529*	*8.0*	*58.3*	*30.9*	*0.0*
White, Creamy Vanilla, Green & Black's*	1 Bar/35g	201	12.8	573	7.4	53.5	36.6	0.1
White, Crispy, Fair Trade, Co-Op*	½ Bar/50g	277	17.5	555	9.0	51.0	35.0	0.1
White, Double Berry, Nestle*	¼ Bar/30g	167	10.3	556	6.6	54.9	34.5	0.0
White, No Added Sugar, Belgian, Boots*	1 Serving/30g	146	10.8	488	6.0	47.8	36.0	7.0
White, with Honey & Almond Nougat, Toblerone*	1 Serving/25g	132	7.2	530	6.2	60.5	29.0	0.2
White, with Strawberries, Divine*	1 Piece/3g	16	0.9	534	7.6	59.9	29.3	0.1
White, with Strawberry Pieces, Under 99 Cals, M & S*	1 Bar/16g	86	4.9	540	6.6	60.4	30.4	0.3
Whole Nut, Dairy Milk, Cadbury*	1 Bar/49g	270	17.4	550	8.9	49.5	35.4	1.7
Whole Nut, Sainsbury's*	4 Chunks/25g	141	9.4	566	8.5	48.5	37.6	2.6
Wildlife Bar, Cadbury*	1 Bar/21g	109	6.2	520	7.8	56.8	29.3	0.0
with Almonds, Nestle*	1 Square/20g	109	7.0	547	9.2	48.7	35.1	0.1
with Creme Egg, Dairy Milk, Cadbury*	1 Bar/45g	210	9.3	470	5.2	64.8	20.9	0.5
with Crunchie Bits, Dairy Milk, Cadbury*	1 Bar/200g	1000	48.8	500	6.2	63.3	24.4	0.0
with Shortcake Biscuit, Dairy Milk, Cadbury*	1 Square/6g	31	1.7	520	7.5	59.0	28.0	0.0

CHOCOLATE NUTS

Almonds, Dark Chocolate Covered, Bolero*	2 Almonds/3g	15	1.0	510	2.6	48.8	33.5	0.0
Peanuts, Assorted, Thorntons*	1 Bag/140g	785	57.1	561	13.8	34.8	40.8	3.6
Peanuts, Belgian Coated, M & S*	1 Serving/20g	109	7.6	545	14.7	35.6	38.0	5.8
Peanuts, Milk, Tesco*	1 Bag/227g	1221	86.0	538	17.5	31.8	37.9	4.4

CHOCOLATE ORANGE

Bar, Montana*	1 Serving/25g	131	6.8	523	7.0	62.2	27.4	0.0
Crunchball, Terry's*	1 Segment/9g	45	2.4	520	6.9	59.8	28.1	2.0
Dark, Terry's*	1 Segment/9g	45	2.6	511	4.3	57.0	29.3	6.2
Egg & Spoon, Terry's*	1 Egg/34g	195	12.9	575	5.5	51.6	38.0	1.7
Goes Minty, Terry's*	3 Slices/26g	133	7.7	510	4.3	57.0	29.5	6.2
Milk, Mini Segments, Terry's*	1 Segment/8g	42	2.4	527	7.7	57.9	29.4	2.1
Milk, Terry's*	1 Orange/175g	931	51.6	532	7.4	57.8	29.5	2.1
Plain, Terry's*	1 Orange/175g	889	51.4	508	3.8	56.8	29.4	6.2
Segsations, Terry's*	1 Segsation/8g	43	2.3	520	6.9	58.5	28.5	2.8
White, Terry's*	1 Segment/11g	61	3.4	535	6.3	60.9	29.4	0.0

CHOCOLATE RAISINS

Assorted, Thorntons*	1 Bag/140g	601	27.6	429	4.2	58.8	19.7	2.9
Bonds Sweetstars*	1 Serving/28g	109	4.5	391	4.7	57.0	16.0	0.0
Californian, Belgian White Chocolate, M & S*	1 Pack/100g	450	20.9	450	4.3	60.6	20.9	0.8
Californian, Tesco*	¼ Bag/57g	268	11.7	472	5.2	66.2	20.7	1.3
Coated, Californian, M & S*	1 Bag/130g	520	19.1	400	4.3	63.2	14.7	1.9
Co-Op*	¼ Pack/50g	205	7.5	410	4.0	64.0	15.0	1.0
Jameson's*	1 Serving/23g	96	3.8	418	4.7	62.7	16.5	1.4
Milk, Asda*	1 Serving/28g	127	5.6	452	6.0	62.0	20.0	1.2

	Measure INFO/WEIGHT	per Measure		Nutrition Values per 100g / 100ml				
		KCAL	FAT	KCAL	PROT	CARB	FAT	FIBRE
CHOCOLATE RAISINS								
Milk, Co-Op*	½ Bag/100g	420	17.0	420	5.0	63.0	17.0	6.0
Milk, Tesco*	1 Lge Bag/227g	933	35.0	411	4.8	63.3	15.4	0.9
CHOCOLATE SPREAD								
& Caramel, Chosen By You, Asda*	1 Serving/100g	564	34.7	564	2.5	60.1	34.7	0.8
Average	*1 Tsp/12g*	*68*	*4.5*	*569*	*4.1*	*57.1*	*37.6*	*0.0*
Hazelnut, Nutella, Ferrero*	1oz/28g	148	8.7	530	6.4	56.4	31.0	3.5
Snickers, Mars*	1 Serving/7g	38	2.6	548	8.7	43.3	37.8	0.0
with Nuts	*1 Tsp/12g*	*66*	*4.0*	*549*	*6.2*	*60.5*	*33.0*	*0.8*
CHOCOLATES								
All Gold, Dark, Terry's*	1 Serving/30g	151	8.7	505	4.0	57.5	29.0	4.3
All Gold, Milk, Terry's*	1 Serving/30g	157	9.1	525	4.8	58.0	30.5	1.5
Almond Marzipan, Milk, Thorntons*	1 Chocolate/13g	60	2.9	464	6.6	59.4	22.6	5.6
Almond Mocca Mousse, Thorntons*	1 Chocolate/14g	76	5.3	543	8.5	40.7	37.9	2.9
Alpini, Thorntons*	1 Chocolate/13g	70	4.2	538	7.0	54.6	32.3	2.3
Assortment, Occasions, Tesco*	1 Chocolate/15g	70	3.1	470	4.6	65.8	20.9	0.5
Bites, Galaxy*	1 Pack/40g	197	9.7	492	5.0	63.0	24.2	0.8
Bittermint, Bendicks*	1 Mint/18g	80	3.0	440	4.3	68.9	16.3	2.4
Brandy Liqueurs, Asda*	1 Chocolate/8g	34	1.4	409	4.0	60.0	17.0	0.8
Brazil Nut Assortment, M & S*	1oz/28g	163	12.7	581	9.6	37.5	45.3	1.5
Cafe Au Lait, Continental Selection, Thorntons*	1 Chocolate/16g	77	4.0	481	5.3	58.1	25.0	0.6
Cappuccino, Continental Selection, Thorntons*	1 Chocolate/13g	70	4.7	538	5.9	48.5	36.2	0.8
Caramels, Sainsbury's*	1 Sweet/12g	57	2.6	490	3.5	69.0	22.2	0.2
Celebrations, Mars*	1 Sweet/8g	41	2.2	512	5.7	61.5	27.0	1.7
Cherry Liqueur, M & S*	1 Chocolate/10g	39	1.8	395	2.9	52.8	17.8	4.3
Chocolate Mousse, Thorntons*	1 Chocolate/13g	67	4.7	515	7.5	40.0	36.2	3.1
Classic Collection, Thorntons*	1 Chocolate/12g	58	2.8	472	4.3	62.7	22.8	2.4
Coffee Creme, Dark, Thorntons*	1 Chocolate/13g	52	1.4	400	3.0	71.5	10.8	0.8
Coffee Creme, Milk, Thorntons*	1 Chocolate/13g	52	1.3	400	2.8	74.6	10.0	0.8
Continental, Belgian, Thorntons*	1 Chocolate/13g	67	3.9	514	5.8	53.5	30.3	2.9
Continental, Thorntons*	1 Chocolate/15g	76	4.4	506	5.6	54.5	29.3	2.7
Country Caramel, Milk, Thorntons*	1 Chocolate/9g	45	2.4	500	4.6	62.2	26.7	0.0
Dairy Box, Milk, Nestle*	1 Piece/11g	50	2.1	456	4.4	65.9	19.4	0.7
Dark, Elegant, Elizabeth Shaw*	1 Chocolate/8g	38	1.8	469	2.9	62.5	23.1	0.0
Dark, Swiss Thins, Lindt*	1 Pack/125g	681	46.2	545	4.7	49.2	37.0	0.0
Drops, Plain, Sainsbury's*	1 Serving/125g	637	34.5	510	5.3	60.1	27.6	4.0
Eclipse, Truffle, Plain, Dark, Montezuma*	1 Truffle/16g	93	8.5	581	0.6	21.9	53.1	0.0
Ferrero Rocher, Ferrero*	1 Chocolate/13g	74	5.1	593	7.0	49.0	41.0	0.0
Fondant, Chocolate Coated, Average	1 Chocolate/11g	40	1.0	366	2.2	80.4	9.3	2.1
Golf Balls, Milk Chocolate, Lindt*	1 Packet/110g	619	39.5	563	6.5	53.6	35.9	0.0
Gorgeous, Bendicks*	3 Sweets/15g	82	5.0	550	6.6	55.3	33.3	1.1
Italian Collection, Amaretto, M & S*	1 Chocolate/13g	60	3.1	480	4.4	59.7	25.1	2.3
Italian Collection, Cappuccino, M & S*	1 Bag/100g	545	37.0	545	6.3	46.7	37.0	1.8
Italian Collection, Favourites, M & S*	1 Chocolate/14g	74	4.7	530	5.7	50.4	33.7	1.6
Italian Collection, Panna Cotta, M & S*	1 Chocolate/13g	70	4.7	545	5.3	49.4	36.4	0.1
Liqueur, Barrels, Cointreau	1 Chocolate/10g	43	1.8	435	3.5	57.0	18.0	0.0
Liqueurs, Cognac Truffle, Thorntons*	1 Chocolate/14g	65	3.8	464	7.3	40.0	27.1	2.9
Milk, Shapes, Easter Friends, Tesco*	1 Chocolate/13g	67	4.3	540	8.0	52.3	34.2	2.3
Milk, Swiss Thins, Lindt*	1 Pack/125g	687	43.3	550	5.8	53.6	34.6	0.0
Milk, Winnie the Pooh, Solid Shapes, M & S*	1 Chocolate/6g	32	1.9	540	8.1	54.1	32.4	1.3
Milk Tray, Cadbury*	1 Chocolate/9g	47	2.4	495	4.7	61.5	25.8	0.7
Milky Bar, Giant Buttons, Mars*	1 Sweet/2g	11	0.6	546	7.5	57.7	31.6	0.0
Mingles, Bendicks*	1 Chocolate/5g	27	1.6	540	6.5	58.6	31.3	0.1
Mini Bites, Chunky, Moments, Fox's*	1 Roll/20g	90	4.9	450	5.7	52.4	24.6	2.2

C

CHOCOLATES

	Measure INFO/WEIGHT	per Measure KCAL	FAT	Nutrition Values per 100g / 100ml KCAL	PROT	CARB	FAT	FIBRE
Mini Eggs, Cadbury*	1 Egg/3g	16	0.7	485	4.6	67.8	21.9	1.3
Mini Eggs, Caramel, Cadbury*	1 Egg/11g	55	2.9	485	5.7	59.0	25.7	0.4
Mini Eggs, Lindor, Lindt*	3 Eggs/15g	90	7.0	600	6.7	46.7	46.7	0.0
Mini Eggs, with Soft White Truffle Centre, M & S*	1 Egg/6g	33	2.0	550	6.5	56.3	33.9	1.4
Mint Crisp, Bendicks*	1 Mint/8g	38	2.3	494	5.2	55.0	29.9	0.0
Mint Crisp, Dark, Elizabeth Shaw*	1 Chocolate/6g	27	1.2	458	1.9	68.0	20.7	0.0
Mint Crisp, Milk, Elizabeth Shaw*	1 Chocolate/6g	30	1.3	493	4.0	70.9	21.4	0.0
Mint Crisp, Thorntons*	1 Chocolate/7g	34	2.2	486	7.7	40.0	31.4	4.3
Mints, After Eight, Dark, Nestle*	1 Sweet/7g	32	0.9	461	5.0	63.0	12.9	2.0
Mints, After Eight, Orange, Nestle*	1 Sweet/7g	29	0.9	417	2.5	72.6	12.9	1.1
Mints, After Eight, Straws, Nestle*	1 Sweet/5g	24	1.4	526	5.1	56.6	31.0	4.0
Misshapes, Assorted, Cadbury*	1 Chocolate/8g	41	2.3	515	5.2	57.5	29.1	0.0
Mistletoe Kisses, Mars*	1 Packet /42g	209	11.5	498	5.3	57.0	27.3	0.0
Moments, Thorntons*	1 Chocolate/7g	37	2.0	511	5.4	59.9	27.8	1.9
Neapolitans, Terry's*	1oz/28g	146	8.3	522	6.0	57.3	29.7	4.1
Orange Crisp, Elizabeth Shaw*	1 Chocolate/6g	29	1.3	478	2.9	68.2	21.5	0.0
Peanut Butter Cup, Big Cup, Reese's, Hershey*	1 Cup/39g	210	12.0	538	10.3	53.8	30.8	2.6
Peanut Butter Cup, Miniature, Reese's, Hershey*	1 Cup/9g	44	2.6	500	9.1	59.1	29.5	2.3
Peanut Butter Cup, Reese's, Hershey*	1 Cup/21g	105	6.5	500	11.9	57.1	30.9	5.9
Peanut Butter Cup, White, Mini, Reese's, Hershey*	5 Cups/39g	210	12.0	538	12.8	53.8	30.8	2.6
Peppermint Patty, Hershey*	3 Patties/41g	160	3.0	390	2.4	80.5	7.3	0.0
Planets, Mars*	1 Pack/37g	178	8.3	481	4.9	65.4	22.4	0.0
Praline, Coffee, Thorntons*	1 Chocolate/7g	37	2.4	529	7.0	47.1	34.3	2.9
Praline, Hazelnut, Thorntons*	1 Chocolate/5g	27	1.8	540	7.0	48.0	36.0	4.0
Praline, Marzipan, Thorntons*	1 Chocolate/14g	63	3.0	450	5.9	58.6	21.4	2.1
Praline, Roast Hazelnut, Thorntons*	1 Chocolate/13g	70	4.4	538	6.0	51.5	33.8	3.1
Quality Street, Nestle*	1 Sweet/9g	44	1.9	470	3.5	67.3	20.5	1.5
Rafaello, Roche, Ferrero*	1 Sweet/10g	60	4.7	600	9.7	35.4	46.6	0.0
Reese's, Fast Break, Candy Bar, Hershey*	1 Bar/56g	260	12.0	464	8.9	62.5	21.4	3.6
Reese's Pieces, Bite Size, Minis, Hershey*	11 Pieces/39g	200	12.0	513	7.7	59.0	30.8	2.6
Rocher, Continental, Thorntons*	1 Chocolate/15g	76	5.0	507	6.8	45.3	33.3	2.0
Rocky Road, Clusters, Tesco*	1 Serving/32g	160	9.5	500	7.1	51.0	29.7	6.7
Roses, Cadbury*	1 Chocolate/9g	42	2.2	495	4.8	62.6	25.3	0.7
Sea Shells, Belgian, Guylian*	1 Shell/11g	65	4.4	574	8.0	49.0	39.0	0.0
Seashells, Milk & White, Belgian, Waitrose*	1 Serving/15g	77	4.6	511	5.0	53.1	31.0	2.8
Shots, Cadbury*	1 Pack/160g	752	37.1	470	5.9	59.7	23.2	0.0
Snaps, Hazelnut, Cadbury*	1 Curl/4g	20	1.1	520	6.8	57.8	28.8	0.0
Snaps, Milk, Cadbury*	1 Snap/3g	15	0.8	505	6.3	60.5	27.0	1.0
Snaps, Orange, Cadbury*	1 Snap/3g	15	0.8	505	6.3	60.4	27.0	1.0
Speckled Eggs, M & S*	1 Egg/6g	25	1.0	440	6.6	63.1	18.2	1.5
Strawberries & Cream, Thorntons*	1 Chocolate/12g	64	3.9	533	5.1	54.2	32.5	0.8
Swiss Tradition, De Luxe, Lindt*	1 Packet/250g	1387	90.7	555	6.3	51.9	36.3	0.0
Swiss Tradition, Mixed, Lindt*	1 Packet/392g	2215	149.4	565	6.1	49.8	38.1	0.0
Tartufo, Thorntons*	1 Chocolate/15g	77	5.4	513	7.4	40.0	36.0	3.3
Teddy Bear, Milk Chocolate, Thorntons*	1 Teddy/250g	1357	83.7	543	7.6	52.6	33.5	1.0
Toffifee, Storck*	1 Sweet/6g	32	1.9	535	6.0	58.0	31.0	0.0
Truffle, Amaretto, Thorntons*	1 Chocolate/14g	66	3.6	471	5.5	55.0	25.7	2.9
Truffle, Belgian, Flaked, Tesco*	1 Truffle/14g	80	5.4	575	4.4	52.7	38.5	2.3
Truffle, Belgian Milk, Waitrose*	1 Truffle/14g	73	4.8	525	5.8	52.9	34.1	1.2
Truffle, Brandy, Thorntons*	1 Chocolate/14g	68	3.8	486	6.1	52.1	27.1	0.7
Truffle, Caramel, Thorntons*	1 Chocolate/14g	67	3.6	479	4.2	57.9	25.7	2.1
Truffle, Champagne, Petit, Thorntons*	1 Chocolate/6g	31	1.9	517	7.5	48.3	31.7	3.3
Truffle, Champagne, Premier, Thorntons*	1 Chocolate/17g	88	5.6	518	6.9	45.3	32.9	2.4

	Measure INFO/WEIGHT	per Measure KCAL	per Measure FAT	Nutrition Values per 100g / 100ml KCAL	PROT	CARB	FAT	FIBRE
CHOCOLATES								
Truffle, Cherry, Thorntons*	1 Chocolate/14g	58	3.0	414	4.2	50.7	21.4	1.4
Truffle, Continental Champagne, Thorntons*	1 Chocolate/16g	78	4.5	488	6.1	51.3	28.0	0.6
Truffle, Dark Chocolate, Balls, Lindor, Lindt*	1 Ball/12g	76	6.2	630	3.4	38.5	51.4	0.0
Truffle, French Cocoa Dusted, Sainsbury's*	1 Truffle/10g	57	4.5	570	4.0	37.0	45.0	0.0
Truffle, Grand Marnier, Thorntons*	1 Chocolate/15g	77	5.1	513	7.2	40.7	34.0	4.0
Truffle, Hazelnut, Balls, Lindor, Lindt*	1 Ball/12g	76	6.1	632	5.0	39.1	50.6	0.0
Truffle, Irish Milk Chocolate Cream, Elizabeth Shaw*	1 Chocolate/12g	57	2.7	477	3.9	63.4	22.8	0.0
Truffle, Lemon, White, Thorntons*	1 Chocolate/14g	63	3.5	450	4.6	64.3	25.0	0.7
Truffle, Milk Chocolate, Balls, Lindor, Lindt*	1 Ball/12g	73	6.0	611	5.6	41.7	50.0	2.7
Truffle, Rum, Average	1 Truffle/11g	57	3.7	521	6.1	49.7	33.7	1.9
Truffle, Rum, Thorntons*	1 Chocolate/13g	63	3.2	485	4.8	58.5	24.6	4.8
Truffle, Selection, Tesco*	1 Chocolate/14g	75	4.2	539	5.1	62.0	29.8	0.5
Truffle, Seville, Thorntons*	1 Chocolate/14g	76	4.7	543	7.1	53.6	33.6	1.4
Truffle, Thorntons*	1 Chocolate/7g	33	1.9	471	6.0	48.6	27.1	1.4
Truffle, Vanilla, Thorntons*	1 Chocolate/13g	64	3.5	492	4.8	57.7	26.9	1.5
Truffle, Viennese, Dark, Thorntons*	1 Chocolate/10g	53	3.6	530	5.9	47.0	36.0	3.0
Truffle, Viennese, Milk, Thorntons*	1 Chocolate/10g	56	3.6	560	4.9	54.0	36.0	0.0
Truffle, White Chocolate, Balls, Lindor, Lindt*	1 Ball/12g	78	6.2	649	5.2	40.2	51.9	0.0
Truffle Filled, Swiss, Balls, Finest, Tesco*	3 Balls/37g	240	19.0	640	5.0	40.7	50.8	1.5
Truffle Hearts, Baileys*	1 Chocolate/15g	76	4.3	506	5.2	52.6	28.9	1.3
Truffles, Mini Milk Chocolate Balls, Lindor, Lindt*	3 Balls/15g	90	7.0	600	6.7	40.0	46.7	0.0
Twilight, Dark, with Mint, Terry's*	1 Chocolate/6g	33	1.9	530	3.1	59.5	30.5	4.2
Valentine, Thorntons*	1 Chocolate/11g	60	3.8	542	5.7	52.0	34.5	2.1
Winter Selection, Thorntons*	1 Chocolate/10g	51	3.1	506	6.2	51.3	30.6	3.8
CHOP SUEY								
Chicken, with Noodles, Sainsbury's*	1 Pack/300g	300	7.5	100	5.7	13.6	2.5	1.2
Chinese, Vegetable, Stir Fry, Sharwood's*	1 Pack/310g	223	3.4	72	1.5	13.9	1.1	0.6
Vegetable, M & S*	½ Pack/150g	90	6.1	60	2.0	3.1	4.1	2.9
CHOW MEIN								
Beef, Sainsbury's*	1 Pack/450g	499	11.2	111	6.6	15.5	2.5	0.8
Cantonese Vegetable Stir Fry, Sainsbury's*	¼ Pack/100g	85	3.8	85	2.2	10.6	3.8	1.2
Char Sui, Cantonese, Sainsbury's*	½ Pack/225g	205	7.0	91	5.7	10.0	3.1	1.1
Chicken, Ainsley Harriott*	1 Serving/250g	447	11.8	179	14.0	21.2	4.7	2.0
Chicken, Chinese Takeaway, Sainsbury's*	1 Pack/316g	338	8.5	107	9.1	11.6	2.7	0.7
Chicken, Chinese Takeaway, Tesco*	1 Serving/350g	294	8.4	84	8.1	7.5	2.4	1.1
Chicken, Chosen By You, Asda*	1 Pack/400g	312	2.8	78	8.3	9.2	0.7	0.9
Chicken, COOK!, M & S*	1 Pack/375g	356	7.9	95	7.9	10.5	2.1	1.7
Chicken, Co-Op*	1 Pack/300g	270	9.0	90	8.0	9.0	3.0	0.9
Chicken, COU, M & S*	1 Pack/200g	180	4.6	90	9.3	8.1	2.3	1.1
Chicken, Frozen, Sainsbury's*	1 Pack/404g	424	12.1	105	6.1	13.4	3.0	0.9
Chicken, Great Value, Asda*	1 Pack/400g	408	11.6	102	5.0	14.0	2.9	0.8
Chicken, Less Than 3% Fat, BGTY, Sainsbury's*	1 Pack/450g	355	10.3	79	5.8	8.7	2.3	1.4
Chicken, Morrisons*	1 Pack/400g	368	9.2	92	5.8	13.0	2.3	1.1
Chicken, New, BGTY, Sainsbury's*	1 Pack/450g	373	6.3	83	6.0	11.4	1.4	1.1
Chicken, New Improved Recipe, Sainsbury's*	1 Pack/449g	395	9.0	88	5.7	11.7	2.0	1.2
Chicken, Sainsbury's*	1 Serving/400g	364	8.4	91	5.2	12.9	2.1	1.0
Chicken, Waitrose*	1 Serving/400g	384	11.6	96	6.0	11.4	2.9	1.3
Chicken with Vegetable Spring Roll, Oriental Express*	1 Pack/300g	213	1.8	71	5.5	12.4	0.6	1.9
Pork, Perfectly Balanced, Waitrose*	½ Pack/310g	332	2.8	107	7.6	17.2	0.9	1.6
Special, COU, M & S*	1 Pack/400g	320	4.0	80	7.4	9.9	1.0	1.0
Special, HL, Tesco*	1 Pack/450g	351	5.4	78	6.3	10.6	1.2	0.6
Special, Perfectly Balanced, Waitrose*	1 Pack/400g	316	4.4	79	7.4	10.0	1.1	0.9
Stir Fry, Asda*	1 Pack/350g	269	17.5	77	2.1	6.0	5.0	0.0

C

	Measure INFO/WEIGHT	per Measure KCAL	per Measure FAT	Nutrition Values per 100g / 100ml KCAL	PROT	CARB	FAT	FIBRE
CHOW MEIN								
Stir Fry, Tesco*	½ Pack/240g	180	3.4	75	2.8	12.0	1.4	1.6
Vegetable, Asda*	1 Pack/400g	520	15.2	130	2.4	21.5	3.8	3.0
Vegetable, Take Away, Meal for One, Tesco*	1 Serving/345g	262	7.6	76	6.7	7.3	2.2	1.3
Vegetable, Waitrose*	1 Pack/300g	216	2.7	72	2.9	13.1	0.9	1.9
Vesta*	1 Pack/433g	585	10.0	135	5.4	23.1	2.3	2.9
CHRISTMAS PUDDING								
Average	1oz/28g	81	2.7	291	4.6	49.5	9.7	1.3
BGTY, Sainsbury's*	1 Serving/114g	302	2.8	266	2.8	58.2	2.5	4.6
Retail	1oz/28g	92	3.3	329	3.0	56.3	11.8	1.7
Rich Fruit, Laced with Brandy, Tesco*	1 Serving/100g	305	9.7	305	3.7	50.8	9.7	1.3
Rich Fruit, Tesco*	1 Serving/114g	331	6.7	290	2.4	55.0	5.9	0.0
Sticky Toffee, Tesco*	¼ Pud/114g	372	7.3	326	2.5	64.5	6.4	0.8
Toffee Sauce Coated, Morrisons*	1 Pudding/100g	324	6.4	324	2.5	64.5	6.4	0.0
Traditional Style, Asda*	1 Pudding/100g	296	6.0	296	2.6	58.0	6.0	1.6
VLH Kitchens*	1 Slice/114g	310	2.9	272	3.1	59.3	2.5	4.6
with Cider & Sherry, Waitrose*	¼ Pud/113g	344	7.2	303	2.5	59.0	6.3	3.2
CHUTNEY								
Albert's Victorian, Baxters*	1 Serving/25g	37	0.0	150	35.0	6.0	0.1	0.0
Apple, Tomato & Sultana, Tesco*	1 Serving/50g	88	0.1	176	1.1	42.4	0.2	1.3
Apple & Pear, TTD, Sainsbury's*	1 Serving/20g	38	0.2	190	0.6	45.2	0.8	1.7
Apple & Walnut, Waitrose*	1 Serving/20g	49	0.5	243	12.0	53.8	2.6	3.8
Apricot, Sharwood's*	1 Tsp/16g	21	0.0	131	0.6	32.0	0.1	2.3
Bengal Spice Mango, Sharwood's*	1 Tsp/5g	12	0.0	236	0.5	58.0	0.2	1.2
Caramelised Onion, Sainsbury's*	1 Serving/25g	28	0.3	111	1.1	23.5	1.4	1.1
Caramelised Onion, TTD, Sainsbury's*	1 Serving/20g	31	0.1	157	0.8	37.3	0.5	2.1
Caramelised Red Onion, Loyd Grossman*	1 Serving/10g	11	0.0	111	0.5	27.2	0.0	0.5
Cranberry & Caramelised Red Onion, Baxters*	1 Serving/20g	31	0.0	154	0.3	38.0	0.1	0.3
Fruit, Spiced, Baxters*	1 Tsp/16g	23	0.0	143	6.0	34.8	0.1	0.0
Indian Appetisers, Pot, Waitrose*	1 Pot/158g	330	2.2	209	1.8	47.3	1.4	1.8
Lime & Chilli, Geeta's*	1 Serving/25g	69	0.3	277	2.0	64.0	1.4	1.9
Mango, Cottage*	1 Tsp/10g	27	0.0	268	0.3	59.7	0.2	0.0
Mango, Green Label, Sharwood's*	1 Tsp/10g	23	0.0	234	0.3	57.8	0.2	0.9
Mango, Hot, Patak's*	1 Jar/340g	877	0.7	258	0.4	67.1	0.2	0.7
Mango, Indian Takeaway, Asda*	1 Pack/70g	145	0.1	207	0.3	50.9	0.2	1.0
Mango, Major Grey, Patak's*	1 Tbsp/15g	38	0.0	255	0.4	66.0	0.2	0.7
Mango, Sensations, Walkers*	¼ Jar/57g	122	0.1	214	0.3	53.0	0.1	0.6
Mango, Spiced, M & S*	1 Serving/15g	26	0.1	175	1.2	42.3	0.4	3.2
Mango, Spicy, Sainsbury's*	1 Tbsp/15g	24	0.1	160	0.7	37.0	0.7	1.3
Mango, Sweet	**1 Tsp/16g**	**30**	**0.0**	**189**	**0.7**	**48.3**	**0.1**	**0.0**
Mango, Tesco*	1 Serving/20g	45	0.0	224	0.4	55.5	0.1	1.3
Mango, Waitrose*	1 Serving/20g	43	0.3	215	1.0	49.0	1.5	2.0
Mango & Ginger, Baxters*	1 Jar/320g	598	0.6	187	5.0	45.7	0.2	2.0
Mango & Mint, Cofresh*	1 Tbsp/20g	31	0.1	155	1.7	36.4	0.3	2.0
Mixed Fruit	**1 Tsp/16g**	**25**	**0.0**	**155**	**0.6**	**39.7**	**0.0**	**0.0**
Peach, Spicy, Waitrose*	1 Serving/20g	43	0.3	215	1.0	49.0	1.5	1.5
Ploughman's Plum, The English Provender Co.*	1 Tsp/10g	16	0.0	160	1.3	38.1	0.2	1.6
Red Onion & Sherry Vinegar, Sainsbury's*	1 Serving/10g	24	0.1	236	0.5	57.1	0.6	1.4
Spicy Fruit, Baxters*	1 Serving/15g	22	0.0	146	0.6	35.4	0.2	0.0
Spicy Onion, Organic, The English Provender Co*	1 Serving/10g	24	0.0	245	1.2	59.0	0.5	3.5
Sweet Mango, Patak's*	1 Tbsp/15g	39	0.0	259	0.3	67.4	0.1	0.7
Sweet Tomato & Chilli, The English Provender Co.*	1 Tsp/10g	19	0.0	189	0.9	46.0	0.2	1.7
Tomato	**1 Tsp/16g**	**20**	**0.0**	**128**	**1.2**	**31.0**	**0.2**	**1.3**
Tomato, Waitrose*	1 Pot/100g	195	0.3	195	1.3	46.8	0.3	0.0

	Measure INFO/WEIGHT	per Measure KCAL	per Measure FAT	Nutrition Values per 100g / 100ml KCAL	PROT	CARB	FAT	FIBRE
CHUTNEY								
Tomato & Red Pepper, Baxters*	1 Jar/312g	512	1.2	164	2.0	38.0	0.4	1.5
CIDER								
Cyder, Organic, Aspall*	1 Glass/200ml	120	0.2	60	0.1	3.1	0.1	0.0
Cyder, Perronelle's Blush, Aspall*	1 Glass/200ml	122	0.2	61	0.1	5.4	0.1	0.5
Cyder, Premier Cru, Aspall*	1 Glass/200ml	120	0.0	60	0.0	3.1	0.0	0.0
Cyder, Suffolk, Medium, Aspall*	1 Glass/200ml	134	0.0	67	0.1	4.4	0.0	0.0
Dry, Average	*1 Pint/568ml*	*205*	*0.0*	*36*	*0.0*	*2.6*	*0.0*	*0.0*
Light, Bulmers*	1 Can/500ml	140	0.0	28	0.0	0.8	0.0	0.0
Low Alcohol	*1 Pint/568ml*	*97*	*0.0*	*17*	*0.0*	*3.6*	*0.0*	*0.0*
Low Carb, Stowford*	1 Bottle/500ml	140	0.0	28	0.0	0.2	0.0	0.0
Magner's*	½ Pint/284ml	105	0.0	37	0.0	2.0	0.0	0.0
Pear, Average	*1 Glass/200ml*	*86*	*0.0*	*43*	*0.0*	*3.6*	*0.0*	*0.0*
Pear, Non Alcoholic, Kopparberg*	1 Bottle/500ml	170	0.5	34	0.0	8.4	0.1	0.0
Scrumpy, Average	*1 Glass/200ml*	*93*	*0.0*	*46*	*0.0*	*2.3*	*0.0*	*0.0*
Sweet, Average	*1 Pint/568ml*	*239*	*0.0*	*42*	*0.0*	*4.3*	*0.0*	*0.0*
Vintage	*1 Pint/568ml*	*574*	*0.0*	*101*	*0.0*	*7.3*	*0.0*	*0.0*
CINNAMON								
Ground, Average	*1 Tsp/3g*	*8*	*0.1*	*261*	*3.9*	*55.5*	*3.2*	*0.0*
Stick, Schwartz*	1 Stick/2g	7	0.0	339	4.7	79.3	0.3	0.0
CLAMS								
in Brine, Average	*1oz/28g*	*22*	*0.2*	*79*	*16.0*	*2.4*	*0.6*	*0.0*
Raw, Average	*20 Sm/180g*	*133*	*1.7*	*74*	*12.8*	*2.6*	*1.0*	*0.0*
CLEMENTINES								
Raw, Weighed with Peel, Average	*1 Med/60g*	*22*	*0.1*	*36*	*0.8*	*11.3*	*0.1*	*1.6*
Raw, Weighed without Peel, Average	*1 Med/46g*	*22*	*0.0*	*47*	*0.8*	*12.0*	*0.1*	*1.7*
COCKLES								
Boiled	*1 Cockle/4g*	*2*	*0.0*	*53*	*12.0*	*0.0*	*0.6*	*0.0*
Bottled in Vinegar, Drained	*1oz/28g*	*17*	*0.2*	*60*	*13.3*	*0.0*	*0.7*	*0.0*
COCOA BUTTER								
Average	*1oz/28g*	*251*	*27.9*	*896*	*0.0*	*0.0*	*99.5*	*0.0*
COCOA POWDER								
Cadbury*	1 Tbsp/16g	52	3.3	322	23.1	10.5	20.8	0.0
Dry, Unsweetened, Average	1 Tbsp/5g	12	0.7	229	19.6	54.3	13.7	33.2
Organic, Green & Black's*	1 Tbsp/15g	52	3.3	350	23.6	13.6	22.3	0.0
Valrhona*	1 Tsp/5g	22	1.0	450	25.0	45.0	20.0	30.0
COCONUT								
Chips, Organic, Infinity Foods*	1 Serving/100g	604	62.0	604	5.6	6.4	62.0	13.7
Creamed, Average	*1oz/28g*	*186*	*19.2*	*665*	*6.0*	*6.7*	*68.4*	*7.0*
Desiccated, Average	*1oz/28g*	*169*	*17.4*	*604*	*5.6*	*6.4*	*62.0*	*13.7*
Desiccated, Whitworths*	1oz/28g	170	17.4	606	5.6	6.4	62.0	13.7
Fresh, Flesh Only, Average	*1oz/28g*	*98*	*10.1*	*351*	*3.2*	*3.7*	*36.0*	*7.3*
Ice, Average	*1oz/28g*	*104*	*3.6*	*371*	*1.7*	*66.7*	*12.7*	*2.6*
Milk, Average	*1 Can/400ml*	*698*	*69.7*	*174*	*1.4*	*2.9*	*17.4*	*2.9*
Milk, Reduced Fat, Average	*1 Serving/100g*	*103*	*10.0*	*103*	*0.9*	*2.4*	*10.0*	*0.4*
COD								
Baked, Average	*1oz/28g*	*27*	*0.3*	*96*	*21.4*	*0.0*	*1.2*	*0.0*
Beer Battered, Crispy, Finest, Tesco*	1 Portion/250g	575	35.0	230	12.0	13.4	14.0	1.3
Dried, Salted, Average	*1oz/28g*	*82*	*0.7*	*290*	*62.8*	*0.0*	*2.4*	*0.0*
Dried, Salted, Boiled, Average	*1oz/28g*	*39*	*0.3*	*138*	*32.5*	*0.0*	*0.9*	*0.0*
Fillets, Battered, Average	1 Serving/90g	158	7.3	175	12.5	12.9	8.1	1.0
Fillets, Breaded, Average	1 Serving/97g	200	9.4	206	13.0	16.7	9.7	1.0
Fillets, Breaded, Chunky, Average	1 Piece/135g	204	8.0	151	13.7	10.9	5.9	1.4
Fillets, Breaded, Chunky, Prime, HL, Tesco*	1 Fillet/125g	162	3.1	130	12.9	12.8	2.5	0.7

	Measure INFO/WEIGHT	per Measure KCAL	per Measure FAT	Nutrition Values per 100g / 100ml KCAL	PROT	CARB	FAT	FIBRE
COD								
Fillets, Breaded, Light, Healthy Range, Average	1 Fillet/135g	209	6.9	154	13.6	13.3	5.1	1.2
Fillets, Chunky, Average	*1 Fillet/198g*	*267*	*7.3*	*135*	*17.1*	*8.2*	*3.7*	*0.8*
Fillets, Skinless & Boneless, Raw, Average	*1 Portion/92g*	*90*	*1.6*	*98*	*17.8*	*2.7*	*1.7*	*0.4*
Fillets, Smoked, Average	*1 Serving/150g*	*151*	*2.4*	*101*	*21.6*	*0.0*	*1.6*	*0.0*
Loin, Skinless, TTD, Sainsbury's*	1 Serving/100g	83	0.9	83	18.6	0.0	0.9	0.0
Loins, Average	*1 Serving/145g*	*116*	*1.2*	*80*	*17.9*	*0.1*	*0.8*	*0.2*
Loins, Beer Battered, TTD, Sainsbury's*	1 Fillet/93g	182	10.8	196	14.4	8.5	11.6	2.7
Loins, Steaks, Skinless & Boneless, TTD, Sainsbury's*	1 Steak/100g	105	0.4	105	25.2	0.1	0.4	0.1
Poached, Average	*1oz/28g*	*26*	*0.3*	*94*	*20.9*	*0.0*	*1.1*	*0.0*
Smoked, Raw, Average	*1oz/28g*	*22*	*0.2*	*79*	*18.3*	*0.0*	*0.6*	*0.0*
Steaks, Battered, Chip Shop Style, Average	1 Serving/150g	321	18.0	214	12.5	14.3	12.0	1.1
Steamed, Average	*1oz/28g*	*23*	*0.3*	*83*	*18.6*	*0.0*	*0.9*	*0.0*
COD &								
Cauliflower Bake, Asda*	1 Pack/400g	492	28.0	123	9.5	5.5	7.0	1.0
Cauliflower Cheese, Fillets, Iceland*	½ Pack/176g	234	13.5	133	12.7	3.3	7.7	1.7
Parsley Sauce, Frozen, M & S*	1 Pack/184g	156	7.2	85	11.1	1.9	3.9	1.0
Salmon, Steam Cuisine, COU, M & S*	1 Pack/400g	340	7.2	85	6.8	8.9	1.8	1.2
COD IN								
a Sweet Red Pepper Sauce, Fillets, GFY, Asda*	½ Pack/170g	143	2.7	84	15.0	2.3	1.6	0.1
Butter Sauce, Ross*	1 Serving/150g	126	5.8	84	9.1	3.2	3.9	0.1
Butter Sauce, Steaks, Birds Eye*	1 Pack/170g	185	9.3	109	9.8	5.0	5.5	0.1
Butter Sauce, Steaks, Frozen, Asda*	1 Pouch/152g	163	4.0	107	16.0	5.0	2.6	0.8
Butter Sauce, Steaks, Morrisons*	1 Steak/170g	153	5.6	90	10.9	4.1	3.3	0.4
Butter Sauce, Steaks, Sainsbury's*	1 Serving/170g	184	10.0	108	10.5	3.1	5.9	0.1
Butter Sauce, Tesco*	1 Pack/150g	123	5.4	82	9.4	2.9	3.6	0.5
Cheese Sauce, BGTY, Sainsbury's*	1 Serving/170g	144	4.1	85	12.8	3.1	2.4	0.0
Cheese Sauce, Steaks, Birds Eye*	1 Pack/182g	175	6.4	96	10.9	5.2	3.5	0.1
Mushroom Sauce, BGTY, Sainsbury's*	1 Serving/170g	112	2.9	66	9.9	2.8	1.7	0.1
Parsley Sauce, COU, M & S*	1 Pack/185g	129	4.6	70	10.6	1.4	2.5	0.6
Parsley Sauce, Fillets, BGTY, Sainsbury's*	1 Pack/351g	316	15.1	90	11.6	1.3	4.3	0.7
Parsley Sauce, Frozen, Morrisons*	1 Serving/170g	131	4.6	77	9.6	3.2	2.7	0.5
Parsley Sauce, GFY, Asda*	½ Pack/149g	124	5.2	83	12.0	1.5	3.5	0.6
Parsley Sauce, Portions, Asda*	1 Serving/150g	115	3.0	77	11.0	3.8	2.0	0.1
Parsley Sauce, Portions, Ocean Trader*	1 Serving/120g	112	4.7	93	9.4	4.0	3.9	0.1
Parsley Sauce, Steaks, Birds Eye*	1 Steak/172g	155	4.8	90	10.5	5.6	2.8	0.1
Parsley Sauce, Steaks, Iceland*	1 Serving/151g	130	7.0	86	9.1	2.1	4.6	0.7
Parsley Sauce, Steaks, Sainsbury's*	1 Portion/150g	121	4.6	81	10.2	3.0	3.1	0.2
Parsley Sauce, Tesco*	1 Serving/150g	121	4.6	81	10.0	3.3	3.1	0.3
Red Pepper Sauce, Steamfresh, Birds Eye*	1 Serving/125g	115	2.4	92	14.4	4.7	1.9	0.3
Rich Butter Sauce, Steaks, Ocean Trader*	1 Pouch/150g	136	6.1	91	10.3	3.3	4.1	0.1
COD MEDITERRANEAN								
Perfectly Balanced, Waitrose*	1 Serving/370g	255	3.7	69	13.1	1.9	1.0	1.2
Style, Fillets, GFY, Asda*	1 Pack/397g	274	9.9	69	9.0	2.5	2.5	0.9
Style, Fillets, Herb, Tesco*	1 Serving/115g	163	11.0	142	13.8	0.1	9.6	0.1
COD WITH								
a Mediterranean Pepper Sauce, Fillets, Waitrose*	1 Pack/370g	240	4.8	65	12.2	1.1	1.3	0.9
a Thai Crust, Perfectly Balanced, Waitrose*	1 Pack/280g	249	7.0	89	15.1	1.6	2.5	0.6
Chunky Chips, M & S*	1 Serving/340g	510	20.4	150	6.5	17.5	6.0	1.5
Fish Pesto, Fillets, COOK!, M & S*	½ Pack/165g	210	5.1	127	16.4	8.4	3.1	4.2
Mediterranean Butter, Sainsbury's*	1 Pack/170g	196	8.9	115	17.0	0.1	5.2	0.1
Parma Ham & Sardinian Chick Peas, M & S*	½ Pack/255g	268	12.5	105	9.8	5.3	4.9	0.5
Roasted Vegetables, M & S*	1 Serving/280g	238	10.6	85	8.0	4.9	3.8	1.7
Salsa & Rosemary Potatoes, BGTY, Sainsbury's*	1 Pack/450g	355	4.0	79	4.7	13.1	0.9	1.6

	Measure INFO/WEIGHT	per Measure KCAL	per Measure FAT	Nutrition Values per 100g / 100ml KCAL	PROT	CARB	FAT	FIBRE
COD WITH								
Sunblush Tomato Sauce, GFY, Asda*	½ Pack/177g	117	2.7	66	13.0	0.1	1.5	1.0
Sweet Chilli, COU, M & S*	1 Pack/400g	360	2.0	90	7.7	13.1	0.5	1.6
Tomato Sauce, Fillets, Asda*	1 Serving/181g	210	10.9	116	13.0	2.6	6.0	2.3
COFFEE								
Alternative, Wake Up, Whole Earth*	1 Cup/5g	19	0.0	377	5.5	88.4	0.2	0.0
Black, Average	1 Mug/270ml	5	0.0	2	0.2	0.3	0.0	0.0
Cafe Caramel, Cafe Range, Nescafe*	1 Sachet/17g	72	2.4	423	9.2	64.6	14.1	1.3
Cafe Hazelnut, Nescafe*	1 Sachet/17g	73	2.4	428	9.3	66.0	14.1	0.0
Cafe Irish Cream, Cafe Range, Nescafe*	1 Sachet/23g	98	3.2	425	8.2	65.2	14.1	1.2
Cafe Latte, Dry, Douwe Egberts*	1 Serving/12g	58	2.6	480	10.0	60.0	22.0	0.0
Cafe Latte, Instant, Maxwell House*	1 Serving/16g	67	3.0	420	17.0	45.5	18.9	0.1
Cafe Mocha, Cafe Range, Nescafe*	1 Sachet/22g	92	2.9	418	8.5	66.6	13.1	0.0
Cafe Vanilla, Cafe Range, Nescafe*	1 Sachet/19g	79	2.8	429	9.3	64.6	14.9	1.2
Cappuccino, Cafe Mocha, Dry, Maxwell House*	1 Serving/23g	100	2.5	434	4.3	78.2	10.8	0.0
Cappuccino, Cafe Specials, Dry, M & S*	1 Serving/14g	55	1.6	395	14.0	59.0	11.5	0.7
Cappuccino, Cappio, Iced, Kenco*	1 Can/200ml	138	6.0	69	3.0	7.0	3.0	0.0
Cappuccino, Cappio, Kenco*	1 Sachet/18g	79	1.9	439	11.7	73.9	10.6	0.6
Cappuccino, Co-Op*	1 Serving/13g	55	2.0	440	16.0	64.0	16.0	8.0
Cappuccino, Decaff, Instant, Made Up, Nescafe*	1 Mug/200ml	68	2.3	34	0.9	5.0	1.1	0.0
Cappuccino, Decaff, Nescafe*	1 Sachet/16g	68	2.3	428	11.6	62.6	14.6	0.0
Cappuccino, Decaff, Unsweetened, Nescafe*	1 Sachet/16g	70	3.1	437	14.5	51.2	19.4	4.3
Cappuccino, Dreamy, Cafe, Options*	1 Serving/30g	77	5.1	256	12.9	58.1	16.9	0.0
Cappuccino, Dry, Maxwell House*	1 Mug/15g	52	1.4	350	12.0	64.0	9.6	0.4
Cappuccino, Dry, Waitrose*	1 Sachet/13g	58	2.3	439	15.1	56.0	17.2	4.4
Cappuccino, for Filter Systems, Kenco*	1 Sachet/6g	22	0.8	375	19.0	44.0	13.5	0.0
Cappuccino, Instant, Aldi*	1 Sachet/13g	49	1.7	393	12.5	55.1	13.6	0.0
Cappuccino, Instant, Asda*	1 Sachet/15g	60	2.3	399	13.0	53.0	15.2	0.9
Cappuccino, Instant, Kenco*	1 Sachet/20g	80	2.8	401	13.5	55.7	13.8	0.0
Cappuccino, Instant, Made Up, Maxwell House*	1 Serving/280g	123	5.3	44	0.6	5.8	1.9	0.0
Cappuccino, Instant, Unsweetened, Douwe Egberts*	1 Serving/12g	48	1.9	400	11.0	53.0	16.0	0.0
Cappuccino, Low Sugar, Tesco*	1 Serving/13g	55	2.6	425	18.4	43.3	19.8	0.4
Cappuccino, M & S*	1 Serving/164g	66	2.6	40	1.5	4.4	1.6	0.0
Cappuccino, Made up, Dolce Gusto, Nescafe*	1 Serving/240g	84	3.7	35	1.1	4.0	1.5	0.3
Cappuccino, Organic Chocolate, Traidcraft*	1 Serving/25g	139	9.5	555	7.0	43.0	38.0	0.0
Cappuccino, Original, Sachets, Nescafe*	1 Sachet/18g	80	3.1	444	11.7	60.3	17.4	0.0
Cappuccino, Original Mugsticks, Maxwell House*	1 Serving/18g	73	2.8	406	14.4	52.8	15.6	0.0
Cappuccino, Premium Quality, Ernesto*	1 Sachet/13g	46	0.4	372	12.0	71.0	3.0	1.0
Cappuccino, Reduced Sugar, Sainsbury's*	1 Serving/12g	48	2.3	418	18.0	41.0	20.0	0.0
Cappuccino, Sainsbury's*	1 Serving/12g	49	1.9	411	14.9	52.9	15.5	0.4
Cappuccino, Semi Skim Milk, Average	1 Serving/200ml	48	2.1	24	1.6	2.6	1.1	0.0
Cappuccino, Skinny, Nescafe*	1 Sachet/16g	51	0.7	318	23.6	43.9	4.4	10.6
Cappuccino, Swiss Chocolate, Nescafe*	1 Sachet/20g	81	2.3	404	10.5	65.3	11.5	2.9
Cappuccino, to Go, Original, Nescafe*	1 Serving/19g	84	3.3	444	11.7	60.3	17.4	0.0
Cappuccino, to Go, Unsweetened, Nescafe*	1 Serving/17g	79	4.0	464	15.0	47.3	23.8	0.0
Cappuccino, Unsweetened, Cappio, Kenco*	1 Serving/18g	73	1.8	406	12.2	66.7	10.0	0.6
Cappuccino, Unsweetened, Nescafe*	1 Sachet/16g	74	3.8	464	15.0	47.3	23.8	0.0
Cappuccino, Unsweetened Taste, Maxwell House*	1 Serving/15g	65	2.9	434	17.4	47.6	19.3	0.3
Columbian, Nescafe*	1 Serving/2g	2	0.0	111	16.7	11.1	0.0	5.6
Compliment*	1 Serving/14ml	20	1.8	143	1.4	6.4	12.9	0.0
Dandelion, Symingtons*	1 Tsp/6g	19	0.0	320	2.8	79.3	0.0	0.0
Double Choca Mocha, Cafe Range, Nescafe*	1 Sachet/23g	94	2.5	408	9.2	68.0	11.0	2.8
Espresso, Made up, Dolce Gusto, Nescafe*	1 Serving/60ml	1	0.1	2	0.1	0.0	0.1	0.3
Fermented Milk Flavoured Unsweetened LC1, Nestle*	1 Bottle/100g	80	0.9	80	2.8	13.4	0.9	0.0

	Measure INFO/WEIGHT	per Measure KCAL	FAT	Nutrition Values per 100g / 100ml KCAL	PROT	CARB	FAT	FIBRE
COFFEE								
Frappe Iced, Nestle*	1 Sachet/24g	92	1.0	384	15.0	72.0	4.0	0.5
Gold Blend, Decaffeinated, Nescafe*	1 Tsp/5g	3	0.0	63	7.0	9.0	0.2	27.0
Gold Blend, Nescafe*	1 Tsp/5g	3	0.0	63	7.0	9.0	0.2	27.0
Ice Mocha Drink, Nescafe, Nestle*	1 Bottle/280ml	160	3.4	57	1.1	10.5	1.2	0.0
Infusion, Average with Semi-Skimmed Milk	1 Cup/220ml	15	0.4	7	0.6	0.7	0.2	0.0
Infusion, Average with Single Cream	1 Cup/220ml	31	2.6	14	0.4	0.3	1.2	0.0
Infusion, Average with Whole Milk	1 Cup/220ml	15	0.9	7	0.5	0.5	0.4	0.0
Instant, Alta Rica, Nescafe*	1 Tsp/2g	2	0.0	98	13.8	10.0	0.3	21.0
Instant, Decaffeinated, Nescafe*	1 Tsp/2g	2	0.0	101	14.9	10.0	0.2	8.4
Instant, Made with Skimmed Milk	1 Serving/270ml	15	0.0	6	0.6	0.8	0.0	0.0
Instant, Made with Water & Semi-Skimmed Milk	1 Serving/350ml	24	1.4	7	0.4	0.5	0.4	0.0
Instant, Original, Nescafe*	1 Tsp/2g	1	0.0	63	7.0	9.0	0.2	27.0
Instant, with Skimmed Milk, Costa Rican, Kenco*	1 Mug/300ml	17	0.1	6	0.6	0.8	0.0	0.0
Latte, Cafe, M & S*	1 Serving/190g	142	5.3	75	4.3	8.3	2.8	0.0
Latte, Instant, Skinny, Douwe Egberts*	1 Serving/12g	35	1.3	290	11.0	38.0	11.0	29.0
Latte, Luscious, Options*	1 Serving/14g	62	2.4	443	14.3	57.9	17.1	3.6
Latte, Macchiato, Tassimo*	1 Cup/275ml	135	7.7	49	2.3	3.6	2.8	0.0
Latte, Nescafe*	1 Sachet/22g	110	6.3	498	14.5	45.7	28.5	0.0
Latte, No Sugar, in Cup, From Machine, Kenco*	1 Cup/4g	17	0.9	400	7.6	44.0	22.0	0.0
Latte, Skinny, Nescafe*	1 Sachet/20g	72	1.1	359	24.1	54.3	5.3	1.1
Latte Macchiato, Made up, Dolce Gusto, Nescafe*	1 Serving/220g	89	4.2	40	1.9	4.1	1.9	0.3
Mocha, Instant, Skinny, Douwe Egberts*	1 Serving/12g	37	1.3	308	10.8	40.8	10.8	5.0
Mocha, Made up, Dolce Gusto, Nescafe*	1 Serving/210g	117	5.1	56	2.4	6.1	2.4	0.6
Mocha, Sainsbury's*	1 Serving/22g	84	3.0	383	14.0	51.0	13.7	1.3
Mocha, Skinny, Made Up, Nescafe*	1 Sachet/21g	77	0.7	367	13.6	70.3	3.5	4.3
Regular, Ground or Instant	1 Cup/177g	6	0.0	4	0.2	0.7	0.0	0.0
Skinny Cappuccino, Made Up, Dolce Gusto, Nescafe*	1 Mug/15g	49	0.1	337	33.3	48.8	0.9	2.3
COFFEE MATE								
Original, Nestle*	1 Tsp/4g	19	1.2	547	2.4	56.7	34.4	0.0
Virtually Fat Free, Nestle*	1 Tsp/5g	10	0.1	200	1.0	42.0	3.0	0.0
COFFEE SUBSTITUTE								
Bambu, Vogel*	1 Tsp/3g	10	0.0	320	3.5	75.3	0.5	0.0
COFFEE WHITENER								
Half Fat, Co-Op*	1 Tsp/5g	21	0.6	430	0.9	78.0	13.0	0.0
Light, Asda*	1 Serving/3g	13	0.4	433	0.9	78.0	13.0	0.0
Light, Tesco*	1 Tsp/3g	13	0.4	429	0.9	77.7	12.7	0.0
Morrisons*	1 Serving/10g	53	3.3	535	2.6	57.5	32.8	0.0
Tesco*	1 Tsp/3g	16	0.9	533	1.2	61.3	31.4	0.0
COGNAC								
40% Volume	**1 Shot/35ml**	**78**	**0.0**	**222**	**0.0**	**0.0**	**0.0**	**0.0**
French, All Flavours, Alize*	1 fl oz/30ml	69	0.0	230	0.0	6.7	0.0	0.0
COLA								
Average	1 Can/330ml	135	0.0	41	0.0	10.9	0.0	0.0
Coke, Cherry, Coca-Cola*	1 Bottle/500ml	225	0.0	45	0.0	11.2	0.0	0.0
Coke, Coca-Cola*	1 Can/330ml	142	0.0	43	0.0	10.7	0.0	0.0
Coke, Diet, Caffeine Free, Coca-Cola*	1 Can/330ml	1	0.0	0	0.0	0.1	0.0	0.0
Coke, Diet, Coca-Cola*	1 Can/330ml	1	0.0	0	0.0	0.0	0.0	0.0
Coke, Diet, with Cherry, Coca-Cola*	1 Bottle/500ml	5	0.0	1	0.0	0.0	0.0	0.0
Coke, Vanilla, Coca-Cola*	1 Bottle/500ml	215	0.0	43	0.0	10.7	0.0	0.0
Coke, with Lemon, Diet, Coca-Cola*	1 Can/330ml	5	0.0	1	0.0	0.0	0.0	0.0
Coke, with Vanilla, Diet, Coca-Cola*	1 Glass/200ml	1	0.0	0	0.0	0.1	0.0	0.0
Curiosity, Fentiman's*	1 Bottle/275ml	129	0.0	47	0.1	11.6	0.0	0.0
Diet, Asda*	1 Glass/200ml	0	0.0	0	0.0	0.0	0.0	0.0

	Measure INFO/WEIGHT	per Measure		Nutrition Values per 100g / 100ml				
		KCAL	FAT	KCAL	PROT	CARB	FAT	FIBRE
COLA								
Diet, Classic, Sainsbury's*	1 Can/330ml	1	0.0	0	0.0	0.0	0.0	0.0
Diet, Just, Asda*	1 Bottle/250ml	0	0.0	0	0.0	0.0	0.0	0.0
Diet, M & S*	1 Can/330ml	3	0.0	1	0.0	0.3	0.0	0.0
Diet, Morrisons*	1 Glass/250ml	2	0.0	1	0.0	0.0	0.0	0.0
Diet, Pepsi*	1 Can/330ml	1	0.0	0	0.0	0.0	0.0	0.0
Diet, Tesco*	1 Glass/200ml	2	0.2	1	0.1	0.1	0.1	0.0
Diet, Virgin Trains*	1 Glass/250ml	1	0.2	0	0.1	0.1	0.1	0.0
M & S*	1 Bottle/500ml	225	0.0	45	0.0	11.0	0.0	0.0
Max, Pepsi*	1 Can/330ml	2	0.0	1	0.1	0.1	0.0	0.0
Pepsi*	1 Can/330ml	145	0.0	44	0.0	11.1	0.0	0.0
Royal Crown*	1 Glass/200ml	1	0.0	0	0.1	0.1	0.0	0.0
Tesco*	1 Can/330ml	145	0.0	44	0.0	10.8	0.0	0.0
Twist, Light, Pepsi*	1 Bottle/500ml	4	0.0	1	0.0	0.1	0.0	0.0
Twist, Pepsi*	1 Bottle/500ml	235	0.0	47	0.0	11.7	0.0	0.0
Zero, Coca-Cola*	1 Can/330	2	0.0	0	0.0	0.0	0.0	0.0
COLCANNON								
Chosen By You, Asda*	1 Serving/100g	90	4.2	90	1.5	11.5	4.2	0.0
COLESLAW								
20% Less Fat, Asda*	1 Serving/100g	88	6.0	88	1.5	7.0	6.0	1.7
99% Fat Free, Kraft*	1 Serving/40ml	50	0.4	126	1.0	28.9	1.0	0.0
Cheese, M & S*	1 Serving/57g	185	19.1	325	4.2	2.0	33.5	1.7
Cheese, Sainsbury's*	1 Serving/75g	174	16.3	232	3.4	5.6	21.8	0.6
Cheese, Supreme, Waitrose*	¼ Pack/88g	197	18.2	225	4.5	5.0	20.8	1.2
Coronation, Sainsbury's*	¼ Pot/75g	135	10.6	180	1.2	11.9	14.2	2.4
COU, M & S*	½ Pack/125g	75	3.4	60	1.3	7.4	2.7	1.7
Creamy, 30% Less Fat, Sainsbury's*	1 Tub/300g	378	33.0	126	1.0	5.5	11.0	1.4
Creamy, Light Choices, Tesco*	1/3 Pot/100g	105	8.8	105	1.2	4.9	8.8	1.6
Creamy, Tesco*	1 Serving/75g	142	13.3	190	1.0	5.5	17.8	1.5
Deli Style, BGTY, Sainsbury's*	1 Serving/75g	64	4.6	85	1.5	6.0	6.1	1.7
Deli Style, M & S*	1 Serving/50g	110	10.6	220	1.0	4.8	21.2	1.9
Deli Style, Sainsbury's*	½ Pot/150g	291	28.2	194	0.9	5.2	18.8	1.5
Fruity, M & S*	1 Serving/63g	151	14.3	240	1.1	8.3	22.7	3.1
Garlic & Herb, Asda*	1 Tbsp/15g	22	2.0	147	0.9	5.8	13.3	1.7
GFY, Asda*	1 Serving/50g	27	1.4	55	1.3	6.0	2.9	2.3
Half Fat, Waitrose*	1 Serving/100g	64	4.5	64	1.0	4.8	4.5	2.0
Less Than 5% Fat, Side Salad, M & S*	1 Serving/80g	44	3.4	55	1.0	3.4	4.2	3.9
Light, Reduced Fat, Morrisons*	1 Serving/30g	37	3.1	125	0.8	7.4	10.2	0.0
Luxury, Asda*	1 Serving/50g	108	10.5	217	0.9	6.0	21.0	0.0
Luxury, Morrisons*	1 Serving/50g	136	13.5	273	1.2	6.4	27.0	0.0
Premium, Co-Op*	1 Serving/50g	160	17.0	320	1.0	3.0	34.0	2.0
Reduced Calorie, Iceland*	1 Serving/50g	51	3.7	102	0.7	7.8	7.5	1.6
Reduced Calorie Dressing, Retail	1 Serving/40g	27	1.8	67	0.9	6.1	4.5	1.4
Reduced Fat, Asda*	1 Pot/250g	217	15.7	87	1.5	6.0	6.3	1.6
Reduced Fat, Co-Op*	1 Serving/50g	45	3.5	90	0.9	6.0	7.0	2.0
Reduced Fat, Creamy, Morrisons*	1 Portion/100g	163	14.5	163	1.3	7.2	14.5	1.7
Reduced Fat, Healthy Living, Co-Op*	1 Serving/50g	47	3.5	95	0.8	8.0	7.0	2.0
Reduced Fat, M & S*	½ Tub/112g	230	22.4	205	1.1	5.4	20.0	2.8
Sainsbury's*	1 Serving/75g	103	9.0	138	1.4	6.1	12.0	1.7
Tesco*	1 Serving/50g	79	7.1	158	2.2	5.2	14.3	1.6
Three Cheese, Asda*	1 Serving/78g	203	18.7	260	5.0	6.0	24.0	1.7
Three Cheese, Finest, Tesco*	1/3 Pack/100g	255	22.7	255	6.4	5.8	22.7	1.1
TTD, Sainsbury's*	¼ Pot/75g	218	22.5	291	1.5	3.5	30.1	2.8
with 60% Less Fat, GFY, Asda*	1 Serving/41g	36	2.5	88	1.5	7.0	6.0	1.7

	Measure INFO/WEIGHT	per Measure KCAL	FAT	Nutrition Values per 100g / 100ml KCAL	PROT	CARB	FAT	FIBRE
COLESLAW MIX								
Average	*1oz/28g*	*8*	*0.2*	*30*	*0.8*	*4.9*	*0.8*	*2.0*
COLEY								
Portions, Raw, Average	*1 Serving/92g*	*75*	*0.7*	*81*	*18.4*	*0.0*	*0.7*	*0.0*
Steamed, Average	*1oz/28g*	*29*	*0.4*	*105*	*23.3*	*0.0*	*1.3*	*0.0*
CONCHIGLIE								
Cooked, Average	*1 Serving/185g*	*247*	*1.6*	*133*	*4.8*	*26.6*	*0.8*	*0.5*
Dry Weight, Average	*1 Serving/100g*	*352*	*1.7*	*352*	*12.5*	*71.6*	*1.7*	*2.6*
Shells, Dry, Average	*1 Serving/100g*	*345*	*1.5*	*345*	*12.3*	*70.4*	*1.5*	*3.0*
Whole Wheat, Dry Weight, Average	*1 Serving/75g*	*237*	*1.5*	*316*	*12.6*	*62.0*	*2.0*	*10.7*
CONCHIGLIONI								
Dry, Waitrose*	1 Serving/75g	256	1.0	341	12.5	69.8	1.3	3.7
CONSERVE								
Apricot, Average	*1 Tbsp/15g*	*37*	*0.0*	*244*	*0.5*	*59.3*	*0.2*	*1.5*
Apricot, Reduced Sugar, Streamline*	1 Tbsp/20g	37	0.0	184	0.5	45.0	0.2	0.0
Apricot, TTD, Sainsbury's*	1 Tbsp/15g	43	0.0	285	0.4	70.5	0.1	0.5
Black Cherry, with Amaretto, Finest, Tesco*	1 Tsp/10g	26	0.0	261	0.5	64.4	0.1	0.8
Blackcurrant, Average	*1 Tbsp/15g*	*37*	*0.0*	*245*	*0.6*	*60.0*	*0.1*	*1.9*
Blackcurrant, TTD, Sainsbury's*	1 Tbsp/15g	42	0.0	281	0.6	69.4	0.1	0.5
Blueberry, M & S*	1 Tsp/8g	15	0.0	206	0.3	51.1	0.1	1.3
Hedgerow, TTD, Sainsbury's*	1 Tbsp/15g	41	0.0	276	0.5	68.2	0.1	0.5
Morello Cherry, Waitrose*	1 Tbsp/15g	39	0.0	258	0.4	64.2	0.0	1.4
Plum, TTD, Sainsbury's*	1 Tbsp/15g	44	0.0	295	0.3	73.1	0.1	0.5
Raspberry, Average	*1 Tbsp/15g*	*37*	*0.1*	*249*	*0.6*	*61.0*	*0.3*	*1.3*
Raspberry, TTD, Sainsbury's*	1 Tbsp/15g	43	0.0	290	0.7	71.5	0.1	0.5
Red Cherry, Finest, Tesco*	1 Tbsp/15g	42	0.0	277	0.6	67.6	0.1	0.8
Red Cherry, TTD, Sainsbury's*	1 Tbsp/15g	43	0.0	283	0.4	70.2	0.1	0.5
Rhubarb & Ginger, M & S*	1 Tbsp/15g	29	0.0	194	0.3	47.9	0.1	1.0
Strawberry, 60% Fruit, Reduced Sugar, M & S*	1 Tsp/7g	9	0.0	135	0.4	30.1	0.2	1.9
Strawberry, Average	*1 Tbsp/15g*	*37*	*0.0*	*250*	*0.4*	*61.6*	*0.1*	*0.5*
Strawberry, TTD, Sainsbury's*	1 Tbsp/15g	43	0.0	287	0.4	71.1	0.1	0.5
CONSOMMÉ								
Average	*1oz/28g*	*3*	*0.0*	*12*	*2.9*	*0.1*	*0.0*	*0.0*
COOKIES								
All Butter, Almond, Italian Style, M & S*	1 Cookie/23g	120	6.4	515	6.7	59.4	27.6	3.6
All Butter, Ginger Bread, M & S*	1 Cookie/23g	102	5.0	445	4.3	57.5	21.8	2.4
All Butter, Italian Style Sorrento Lemon, M & S*	1 Cookie/24g	120	6.4	500	4.9	60.4	26.7	2.1
All Butter, Melting Moment, M & S*	1 Cookie/23g	110	6.4	470	4.5	51.5	27.5	3.4
All Butter, Sultana, TTD, Sainsbury's*	1 Cookie/17g	79	3.8	476	5.4	62.7	22.6	2.0
Almond, Ose*	1 Cookie/10g	46	1.4	456	8.4	74.0	14.0	0.0
Apple & Raisin, Go Ahead, McVitie's*	1 Cookie/15g	66	1.9	443	5.3	76.8	12.7	3.4
Apple Crumble, M & S*	1 Cookie/26g	90	0.5	345	4.6	76.8	2.0	2.9
Apple Pie, The Biscuit Collection*	1 Cookie/19g	90	4.2	474	3.9	65.0	22.1	0.0
Big Milk Chocolate Chunk, Cookie Coach*	1 Cookie/35g	174	8.8	497	6.2	61.4	25.1	0.0
Brazil Nut, Organic, Traidcraft*	1 Cookie/17g	91	5.4	547	5.8	57.7	32.6	2.1
Brazil Nut, Prewett's*	1 Cookie/50g	122	7.4	244	2.6	25.2	14.8	1.0
Butter & Sultana, Sainsbury's*	1 Cookie/13g	61	2.6	473	4.5	68.4	20.1	1.6
Cherry Bakewell, COU, M & S*	1 Cookie/25g	90	0.6	355	6.0	77.2	2.5	3.4
Choc Chunk, Fabulous Bakin' Boys*	1 Cookie/60g	270	12.6	450	5.0	59.0	21.0	3.0
Choc Chunk, Finest, Tesco*	1 Cookie/80g	355	14.1	445	5.7	65.3	17.7	1.8
Choc Chunk & Hazelnut, Co-Op*	1 Cookie/17g	89	5.3	525	6.0	56.0	31.0	3.0
Chocolate, Belgian, Extra Special, Asda*	1 Cookie/26g	138	8.0	535	6.0	58.0	31.0	2.0
Chocolate, Milk, Free From, Tesco*	1 Cookie/20g	100	6.1	500	5.6	50.4	30.7	4.1
Chocolate, Quadruple, Sainsbury's*	1 Cookie/20g	117	6.6	585	6.0	66.5	33.0	1.5

COOKIES

	Measure INFO/WEIGHT	KCAL	FAT	KCAL	PROT	CARB	FAT	FIBRE
Chocolate, Triple, Half Coated, Finest, Tesco*	1 Cookie/25g	131	7.3	525	5.7	58.7	29.3	2.3
Chocolate & Nut, Organic, Evernat*	1 Cookie/69g	337	15.6	489	7.2	64.1	22.6	0.0
Chocolate & Orange, COU, M & S*	1 Cookie/26g	90	0.7	350	5.7	77.2	2.6	3.2
Chocolate Chip, Average	1 Cookie/10g	49	2.5	489	5.5	64.1	24.7	2.9
Chocolate Chip, BGTY, Sainsbury's*	1 Cookie/17g	72	2.0	428	4.5	75.6	11.9	2.5
Chocolate Chip, Carb Check, Heinz*	1 Cookie/20g	91	5.0	457	7.2	43.1	24.9	7.2
Chocolate Chip, Gluten & Wheat Free, Lovemore*	1 Cookie/17g	81	4.5	483	3.8	57.8	26.8	3.5
Chocolate Chip, Gluten Free, Organic, Dove's Farm*	1 Cookie/17g	77	3.1	451	4.3	66.9	18.5	0.0
Chocolate Chip, Handbaked, Border*	1 Cookie/15g	72	3.4	480	5.9	67.4	22.6	0.0
Chocolate Chip, M & S*	1 Cookie/12g	59	3.0	495	5.7	62.1	24.8	2.7
Chocolate Chip, McVitie's*	1 Cookie/11g	54	2.8	496	5.8	60.2	25.8	3.0
Chocolate Chip, Organic, Sainsbury's*	1 Cookie/17g	89	4.9	530	5.0	61.8	29.2	0.3
Chocolate Chip, Organic, Tesco*	1 Cookie/17g	88	4.7	520	4.0	63.3	27.4	2.8
Chocolate Chip, Weight Watchers*	1 Cookie/11g	49	1.9	443	7.6	65.4	17.2	4.6
Chocolate Chip & Hazelnut, Extra Special, Asda*	1 Cookie/25g	130	8.1	516	6.0	51.0	32.0	2.5
Chocolate Chunk, All Butter, COU, M & S*	1 Cookie/24g	110	4.3	460	5.7	69.1	17.9	2.3
Chocolate Chunk, All Butter, M & S*	1 Cookie/24g	120	6.0	500	5.2	62.4	25.2	2.9
Chocolate Chunk, Cadbury*	1 Cookie/22g	119	6.9	540	6.5	58.0	31.2	0.0
Chocolate Chunk & Hazelnut, Tesco*	1 Cookie/22g	118	6.7	538	6.2	60.2	30.3	1.9
Chocolate Chunk & Hazelnut, TTD, Sainsbury's*	1 Cookie/17g	88	5.2	528	6.5	54.8	31.4	2.8
Chocolate Fruit & Nut, Extra Special, Asda*	1 Cookie/25g	125	7.1	509	6.0	56.0	29.0	2.0
Chocolate Orange, Half Coated, Finest, Tesco*	1 Cookie/22g	107	5.6	488	4.9	59.6	25.5	1.2
Chocolate Thin Crisp, Simply Food, M & S*	1 Pack/23g	100	2.0	435	4.3	78.3	8.7	4.3
Chunkie Extremely Chocolatey, Fox's*	1 Cookie/26g	130	6.8	506	6.2	61.0	26.3	2.6
Cocoa, Organic, Bites, No Junk, Organix*	1 Bag/25g	105	3.2	421	7.0	69.0	13.0	5.5
Coconut, Gluten-Free, Sainsbury's*	1 Cookie/20g	103	6.1	516	5.6	54.4	30.7	4.1
Coconut & Raspberry, Gluten Free, Sainsbury's*	1 Cookie/20g	102	5.9	511	5.9	56.0	29.3	6.7
Cranberry & Orange, Finest, Tesco*	1 Cookie/26g	125	5.8	490	4.1	67.4	22.6	3.2
Cranberry & Orange, Go Ahead, McVitie's*	1 Cookie/17g	77	2.2	452	5.3	78.0	13.2	2.4
Crunchy Muesli, Mini, Shapers, Boots*	1 Pack/30g	134	4.5	448	6.7	71.0	15.0	1.8
Danish Butter, Tesco*	1 Cookie/26g	133	6.6	516	4.7	66.7	25.6	1.3
Dark Chocolate Chunk & Ginger, The Best, Morrisons*	1 Cookie/25g	126	6.4	503	4.6	63.7	25.5	2.8
Dark Treacle, Weight Watchers*	1 Cookie/11g	49	1.7	423	5.2	66.7	15.1	1.7
Double Choc, Cadbury*	1 Cookie/11g	55	2.5	485	7.3	64.3	22.2	0.0
Double Choc, Maryland*	1 Cookie/10g	51	2.6	510	5.2	64.4	25.7	0.0
Double Choc Chip, Giant, Paterson's*	1 Cookie/60g	293	15.2	489	0.3	61.3	25.3	3.7
Double Choc Chip, Mini, M & S*	1 Cookie/22g	108	5.2	490	5.3	63.6	23.7	1.8
Double Choc Chip, Tesco*	1 Cookie/11g	55	2.7	500	4.2	65.3	24.7	3.0
Double Choc Chip, Weight Watchers*	1 Cookie/11g	49	1.9	443	7.6	65.4	17.2	4.6
Double Chocolate, Organic, Dove's Farm*	1 Cookie/17g	80	3.4	468	4.5	67.5	20.1	0.3
Double Chocolate, Premium, Co-Op*	1 Cookie/17g	86	4.6	505	5.0	62.0	27.0	2.0
Double Chocolate & Walnut, Soft, Tesco*	1 Cookie/25g	116	6.4	463	5.8	52.1	25.7	4.7
Double Chocolate Chip, Co-Op*	1 Cookie/17g	87	4.6	510	5.0	63.0	27.0	2.0
Double Chocolate Chip, Organic, Waitrose*	1 Cookie/18g	96	5.6	535	5.1	58.6	31.0	1.9
Double Chocolate Chip, Traidcraft*	1 Cookie/22g	114	5.9	520	5.8	64.1	26.7	2.4
Double Fudge & Chocolate, Sugar Free, Murray*	1 Cookie/12g	47	2.3	400	5.7	65.7	20.0	5.7
Fortune, Average	1 Cookie/8g	30	0.2	378	4.2	84.0	2.7	1.6
Fruit, Giant, Cookie Coach*	1 Cookie/60g	280	13.2	466	4.9	62.0	22.0	0.0
Fruity Shrewsbury, Giant, Paterson's*	1 Cookie/60g	298	15.2	496	4.8	62.6	25.4	1.7
Fudge Brownie, Maryland*	1 Cookie/11g	56	2.7	510	5.8	63.0	25.0	0.0
Fudge Brownie American Cream, Sainsbury's*	1 Cookie/12g	60	2.8	499	4.8	67.9	23.2	2.2
Ginger, Gluten Free, Barkat*	1 Cookie/17g	85	4.4	501	3.2	63.8	25.9	0.0
Ginger, Half Coated, Finest, Tesco*	1 Cookie/25g	124	6.1	495	4.7	64.2	24.4	3.8

COOKIES	Measure INFO/WEIGHT	per Measure KCAL	FAT	Nutrition Values per 100g / 100ml KCAL	PROT	CARB	FAT	FIBRE
Ginger, Low Fat, M & S*	1 Cookie/23g	82	1.0	358	5.1	74.9	4.3	2.4
Ginger & Brazil Nut, Organic, Dove's Farm*	1 Cookie/17g	79	3.5	464	5.0	65.0	20.5	4.8
Ginger & Choc Chip, BGTY, Sainsbury's*	1 Cookie/17g	69	3.2	415	5.8	55.3	19.0	12.1
Glace Cherry, Border*	1 Cookie/15g	74	3.8	493	5.4	64.3	25.6	0.0
Hazelnut, Gluten Free, Organic, Dove's Farm*	1 Cookie/17g	79	3.7	463	4.8	61.5	21.9	1.8
Hazelnut & Choc Chip 'n' Chunk, McVitie's*	1 Cookie/11g	55	3.0	505	6.1	57.8	27.7	3.5
Lemon & Ginger, Weight Watchers*	1 Cookie/11g	49	2.0	450	6.4	65.0	18.2	5.0
Lemon Meringue, COU, M & S*	1 Cookie/25g	89	0.6	355	5.6	77.6	2.6	3.0
Lemon Zest, Gluten Free, Organic, Dove's Farm*	1 Cookie/17g	80	3.1	473	3.3	73.7	18.3	0.0
Milk Chocolate, Classic, Millie's Cookies*	1 Cookie/45g	190	10.2	422	5.1	49.3	22.7	1.3
Oat, Giant Jumbo, Paterson's*	1 Cookie/60g	299	16.2	499	0.4	58.4	27.0	3.2
Oat & Cranberry, BGTY, Sainsbury's*	1 Cookie/28g	126	5.0	449	6.8	65.0	18.0	5.1
Oatflake & Honey, Organic, Sainsbury's*	1 Cookie/17g	82	3.6	480	6.3	66.0	21.2	2.6
Oatflake & Raisin, Waitrose*	1 Cookie/17g	80	3.8	469	5.8	61.7	22.1	4.7
Oatmeal, Chocolate Chip, Chewy, Dad's*	1 Cookie/15g	70	3.0	467	6.7	66.7	20.0	3.3
Oreo, Nabisco*	1 Cookie/11g	52	2.3	471	5.9	70.6	20.6	2.9
Praline Nougatine, Belle France*	1 Cookie/17g	84	4.1	506	8.0	63.0	25.0	0.0
Quadruple Chocolate, TTD, Sainsbury's*	1 Cookie/20g	104	5.7	518	6.2	59.8	28.2	1.6
Raisin & Cinnamon, Low Fat, M & S*	1 Cookie/22g	78	0.9	355	6.2	73.0	4.1	3.2
Raspberry Spritz, Heaven Scent*	1 Cookie/19g	90	6.0	474	5.3	52.6	31.6	0.0
Rolo, Nestle*	1 Cookie/73g	242	11.1	331	3.4	46.0	15.2	0.6
Spiced Apple, COU, M & S*	1 Cookie/25g	82	0.6	330	5.0	72.8	2.5	2.1
Spiced Apple, M & S*	1 Cookie/25g	90	0.7	360	5.2	75.6	2.8	2.0
Stem Ginger, Aldi*	1 Cookie/13g	58	2.4	463	3.6	68.5	19.4	0.0
Stem Ginger, BGTY, Sainsbury's*	1 Cookie/17g	73	2.0	431	4.5	76.5	11.9	1.7
Stem Ginger, Free From, Sainsbury's*	1 Cookie/17g	84	4.8	489	6.5	58.0	28.0	6.8
Stem Ginger, Half Coated, Finest, Tesco*	1 Cookie/25g	127	6.7	508	4.4	62.4	26.8	3.6
Stem Ginger, Less Than 5% Fat, M & S*	1 Cookie/22g	79	0.9	360	6.2	73.9	4.3	3.0
Stem Ginger, Reduced Fat, Waitrose*	1 Cookie/17g	75	2.7	448	4.5	71.0	16.2	1.6
Stem Ginger, Tesco*	1 Cookie/20g	98	4.8	489	4.2	64.0	24.0	2.0
Stem Ginger, TTD, Sainsbury's*	1 Cookie/17g	79	3.7	476	5.2	64.3	22.0	2.3
Sultana, All Butter, Reduced Fat, M & S*	1 Cookie/17g	70	2.4	420	4.9	68.6	14.2	2.6
Sultana, Soft & Chewy, Sainsbury's*	1 Cookie/25g	103	3.5	414	4.4	67.8	13.9	2.5
Sultana & Cinnamon, Weight Watchers*	1 Cookie/12g	46	1.4	398	5.0	67.1	12.1	1.8
Tennessee American Style, Stiftung & Co*	1 Cookie/19g	96	4.6	504	6.0	66.0	24.0	0.0
Toffee, Weight Watchers*	1 Cookie/12g	52	1.9	456	5.2	71.1	16.8	2.9
Triple Chocolate Chunk, Bakery, Finest, Tesco*	1 Cookie/80g	360	15.9	450	7.4	59.2	19.9	2.1
White Chocolate, Asda*	1 Cookie/54g	256	11.9	474	5.0	64.0	22.0	2.1
White Chocolate, Maryland*	1 Cookie/10g	51	2.5	512	5.7	64.0	25.0	0.0
White Chocolate, TTD, Sainsbury's*	1 Cookie/25g	126	6.4	504	5.5	62.5	25.8	1.2
White Chocolate & Raspberry, Finest, Tesco*	1 Cookie/76g	304	9.6	400	5.2	66.3	12.6	2.4
White Chocolate & Raspberry, McVitie's*	1 Cookie/17g	87	4.4	512	4.7	64.1	25.9	1.8
COQ AU VIN								
Diet Chef Ltd*	1 Pack/300g	285	13.2	95	7.7	6.1	4.4	2.2
Finest, Tesco*	1 Serving/273g	251	9.8	92	14.3	0.7	3.6	1.8
HL, Tesco*	½ Pack/200g	172	3.8	86	15.2	2.1	1.9	0.4
M & S*	1 Serving/295g	398	22.7	135	14.2	1.5	7.7	1.0
Perfectly Balanced, Waitrose*	1 Pack/500g	445	15.5	89	12.6	2.7	3.1	0.6
Sainsbury's*	1 Pack/400g	484	17.6	121	16.8	3.5	4.4	0.2
with Potatoes, Diet Chef Ltd*	1 Pack/300g	285	13.2	95	7.7	6.1	4.4	2.2
CORDIAL								
Blackcurrant, New Zealand Honey Co*	1 Serving/30ml	109	0.3	363	1.0	88.0	1.0	0.0
Elderflower, Made Up, Bottle Green*	1 Glass/200ml	46	0.0	23	0.0	5.6	0.0	0.0

	Measure INFO/WEIGHT	per Measure KCAL	FAT	Nutrition Values per 100g / 100ml KCAL	PROT	CARB	FAT	FIBRE
CORDIAL								
Elderflower, Undiluted, Waitrose*	1 Serving/20ml	22	0.0	110	0.0	27.5	0.0	0.0
Lemon & Lime: High Juice, M & S*	1 Glass/250ml	75	0.0	30	0.0	7.0	0.0	0.0
Lime, Juice, Diluted, Rose's*	1 Serving/30ml	6	0.0	21	0.0	4.9	0.0	0.0
Lime, Sainsbury's*	1 Serving/50ml	13	0.0	27	0.0	6.2	0.0	0.0
Lime, with Aromatic Bitters & Ginger, Sainsbury's*	1 Serving/40ml	12	0.1	29	0.0	6.9	0.3	0.3
Lime Juice, Concentrated	1 Serving/20ml	22	0.0	112	0.1	29.8	0.0	0.0
Lime Juice, Diluted	1 Glass/250ml	55	0.0	22	0.0	6.0	0.0	0.0
Lime Juice, Waitrose*	1 Serving/20ml	21	0.0	104	10.0	23.7	0.0	0.0
Pomegreat, Original, Pomegreat*	1 Serving/50ml	16	0.0	32	0.0	7.6	0.0	0.0
CORIANDER								
Leaves, Dried, Average	*1oz/28g*	*78*	*1.3*	*279*	*21.8*	*41.7*	*4.8*	*0.0*
Leaves, Fresh, Average	*1 Bunch/20g*	*5*	*0.1*	*23*	*2.1*	*3.7*	*0.5*	*2.8*
Seeds, Ground, Schwartz*	1 Tsp/5g	22	0.9	446	14.2	54.9	18.8	0.0
CORN								
Baby, & Asparagus Tips, Tesco*	1 Pack/150g	37	0.7	25	2.6	2.5	0.5	1.9
Baby, & Mange Tout, Tesco*	1 Serving/100g	27	0.2	27	2.9	3.3	0.2	2.1
Baby, Average	*1 Serving/80g*	*21*	*0.3*	*26*	*2.5*	*3.1*	*0.4*	*1.7*
Cobs, Boiled, Weighed with Cob, Average	*1 Ear/200g*	*132*	*2.8*	*66*	*2.5*	*11.6*	*1.4*	*1.3*
Creamed Style, Green Giant*	1 Can/418g	238	2.1	57	1.2	11.9	0.5	3.0
CORN CAKES								
M & S*	½ Pack/85g	238	17.0	280	6.4	19.8	20.0	3.4
Organic, Kallo*	1 Cake/5g	16	0.2	340	12.7	74.3	4.1	11.2
Slightly Salted, Mrs Crimble's*	1 Pack/28g	104	0.9	380	7.9	80.0	3.4	5.4
Thick Slices, Orgran*	1 Cake/11g	42	0.4	385	13.2	79.0	3.7	14.2
CORN SNACKS								
Crispy, Bugles*	1 Bag/20g	102	5.6	508	4.8	60.7	28.0	1.4
Light Bites, Cheese Flavour, Special K, Kellogg's*	1 Packet/28g	116	2.2	416	9.0	77.0	8.0	1.0
Light Bites, Tikka Flavour, Special K, Kellogg's*	1 Pack/28g	116	2.2	416	7.0	79.0	8.0	1.5
Paprika Flavour, Shapers, Boots*	1 Pack/13g	64	3.5	494	8.7	54.0	27.0	2.2
Scampi, Smiths, Walkers*	1 Bag/27g	134	7.0	496	13.0	52.5	26.0	0.0
Toasted, Holland & Barrett*	1 Serving/100g	412	12.1	412	8.1	69.7	12.1	4.0
CORNED BEEF								
Average	*1 Slice/35g*	*75*	*4.3*	*214*	*25.9*	*0.7*	*12.1*	*0.0*
Lean, Healthy Range, Average	*1 Slice/30g*	*57*	*2.6*	*191*	*27.0*	*1.0*	*8.7*	*0.0*
Sliced, Premium, Average	*1 Slice/31g*	*69*	*3.9*	*222*	*26.6*	*0.5*	*12.6*	*0.0*
CORNFLOUR								
Average	*1 Tsp/5g*	*18*	*0.1*	*355*	*0.6*	*86.9*	*1.2*	*0.1*
COURGETTE								
Boiled in Unsalted Water, Average	*1oz/28g*	*5*	*0.1*	*19*	*2.0*	*2.0*	*0.4*	*1.2*
Fried, Average	*1oz/28g*	*18*	*1.3*	*63*	*2.6*	*2.6*	*4.8*	*1.2*
Raw, Average	*1 Med/224g*	*40*	*0.9*	*18*	*1.8*	*1.8*	*0.4*	*0.9*
COUS COUS								
& Chargrilled Vegetables, M & S*	1 Serving/200g	200	3.0	100	3.9	17.3	1.5	1.6
& Chickpeas, TTD, Sainsbury's*	¼ Pot/72g	121	6.8	167	4.7	15.8	9.4	1.4
& Wok Oriental, Findus*	½ Pack/300g	510	25.5	170	4.5	19.0	8.5	0.0
Alle Spices Mediterraneo, Antony Worrall Thompson's*	½ Pack/100g	352	2.8	352	10.7	71.0	2.8	3.8
Chargrilled Red & Yellow Pepper, Tesco*	1 Pack/200g	212	3.6	106	4.6	17.8	1.8	0.5
Chargrilled Vegetable, Morrisons*	1 Serving/225g	227	5.4	101	3.3	16.5	2.4	1.3
Chargrilled Vegetables & Olive Oil, Delphi*	½ Pot/75g	105	2.9	140	3.8	22.5	3.9	1.9
Citrus Kick, Cooked, Ainsley Harriott*	1 Serving/130g	182	1.6	140	4.3	27.9	1.2	2.4
Citrus Kick, Dry, Ainsley Harriott*	½ Sachet/50g	184	1.2	368	11.6	77.0	2.4	9.2
Cooked, Average	*1 Cup/157g*	*249*	*2.9*	*158*	*4.3*	*31.4*	*1.9*	*1.3*
Coriander & Lemon, Morrisons*	1 Serving/100g	159	3.4	159	4.4	27.7	3.4	1.4

C

	Measure INFO/WEIGHT	per Measure KCAL	FAT	Nutrition Values per 100g / 100ml KCAL	PROT	CARB	FAT	FIBRE
COUS COUS								
Coriander & Lemon, Sainsbury's*	½ Pack/137g	205	5.9	150	4.3	23.4	4.3	2.7
Dry, Average	*1 Serving/50g*	*178*	*0.7*	*356*	*13.7*	*72.8*	*1.5*	*2.6*
Garlic & Coriander, Dry, Waitrose*	1 Serving/70g	235	2.5	336	11.7	64.2	3.6	6.2
Giant, Tesco*	1 Pack/220g	350	14.4	160	4.1	20.7	6.6	1.2
Harissa Style Savoury, Sainsbury's*	1 Serving/260g	434	12.0	167	4.7	26.8	4.6	1.3
Hot & Spicy Flavour, Dry, Amazing Grains, Haldane's*	1 Serving/50g	182	2.1	365	12.5	67.0	4.2	3.1
in Soy Sauce, with Sesame Ginger, Amazing Grains*	½ Sachet/50g	180	1.3	360	11.2	73.0	2.6	3.1
Indian Style, Sainsbury's*	½ Pack/143g	204	3.9	143	4.5	25.1	2.7	1.0
Israeli & Sardinian, TTD, Sainsbury's*	¼ Pot/55g	69	2.6	126	3.2	17.7	4.7	1.6
Lemon & Coriander, Cooked, Tesco*	1 Serving/137g	207	3.3	151	4.0	28.3	2.4	2.0
Lemon & Coriander, Dry, Tesco*	1 Pack/110g	375	3.0	341	11.0	68.2	2.7	6.1
Mediterranean Style, Cooked, Tesco*	1 Serving/146g	215	3.8	147	4.4	26.5	2.6	1.3
Mediterranean Style, Dry, Tesco*	1 Pack/110g	368	3.3	335	11.9	65.1	3.0	5.6
Mediterranean Tomato, GFY, Asda*	½ Pack/141g	192	1.3	136	5.0	27.0	0.9	1.7
Mint & Coriander Flavour, Dry, Amazing Grains*	1 Sachet/99g	349	2.7	353	12.2	70.0	2.7	3.2
Moroccan, Roast Chicken, Delicious, Shapers, Boots*	1 Pack/250g	247	3.7	99	9.2	12.0	1.5	2.6
Moroccan Medley, Ainsley Harriott*	½ Sachet/130g	178	1.9	137	5.4	25.4	1.5	2.2
Moroccan Style, Break, GFY, Asda*	1 Pack/150g	215	2.7	143	5.6	26.1	1.8	1.8
Moroccan Style, Finest, Tesco*	1 Tub/225g	292	5.6	130	4.3	22.6	2.5	3.7
Moroccan Style, Fruity, M & S*	1 Serving/200g	370	5.4	185	3.4	36.7	2.7	3.4
Moroccan Style, Sainsbury's*	½ Pack/150g	195	4.0	130	5.0	21.5	2.7	1.0
Moroccan Style, Savoury, Sainsbury's*	½ Pack/151g	196	4.1	130	5.0	21.5	2.7	1.0
Moroccan Style, TTD, Sainsbury's*	1 Pot/200g	364	7.2	182	4.4	30.3	3.6	5.5
Moroccan Sultana & Pine Nuts, Dry, Sammy's*	1 Serving/50g	171	1.5	343	12.0	72.0	3.0	6.0
Morrisons*	1 Serving/100g	126	1.2	126	5.5	23.2	1.2	3.5
Mushroom & Garlic, Cooked, Morrisons*	1 Serving/100g	164	3.0	164	5.7	28.7	3.0	1.7
Mushrooms, Onion, Garlic & Herbs, Dry, Tesco*	½ Pack/50g	166	1.3	333	11.3	66.2	2.6	4.9
Plain, Dry Weight, Tesco*	1 Serving/50g	182	0.5	365	15.1	73.1	1.1	0.8
Red Pepper & Chilli, Waitrose*	1 Pack/200g	344	13.8	172	4.5	23.0	6.9	1.3
Roasted Vegetable, Cooked, Ainsley Harriott*	1 Serving/130g	180	2.0	138	5.6	25.5	1.5	2.6
Roasted Vegetable, Dry, Ainsley Harriott*	½ Sachet/50g	180	2.0	360	14.6	66.4	4.0	6.8
Roasted Vegetable, Snack Salad Pot, HL, Tesco*	1 Pack/60g	213	2.4	355	15.1	64.6	4.0	4.2
Roasted Vegetables, Waitrose*	1 Serving/200g	328	13.2	164	3.9	22.0	6.6	0.9
Spice Fusion, Lyttos*	1 Serving/100g	134	1.5	134	4.3	23.9	1.5	3.4
Spice Sensation, Dry, Ainsley Harriott*	½ Sachet/50g	166	1.2	332	11.6	66.2	2.4	9.2
Spicy Moroccan Chicken & Veg, COU, M & S*	1 Pack/400g	380	6.8	95	9.1	10.3	1.7	1.9
Spicy Vegetable, GFY, Asda*	½ Pack/55g	71	0.6	129	4.7	25.0	1.1	2.0
Spicy Vegetable, Morrisons*	1 Pack/110g	187	5.5	170	5.1	26.2	5.0	2.9
Sun Dried Tomato, & Mediterranean Herbs, Sammy's*	1 Serving/63g	210	1.8	333	13.2	70.5	2.9	6.7
Sweet Vegetable, Chosen By You, Asda*	1 Serving/100g	120	0.0	120	2.9	14.8	0.0	0.0
Tangy Tomato, Dry, Ainsley Harriott*	½ Sachet/50g	166	0.8	332	12.2	67.2	1.6	8.8
Tomato & Basil, Made Up, Tesco*	1 Serving/200g	348	16.6	174	3.9	21.0	8.3	3.4
Tomato & Onion, Dry Weight, Waitrose*	1 Pack/110g	376	4.0	342	12.6	64.9	3.6	5.1
Tomato & Vegetable, Snack Pack, Dry, Sammy's*	1 Serving/70g	228	2.4	326	12.0	67.9	3.5	6.3
Vegetable, Roast, Veg Pot, Summer Special, Innocent*	1 Pot/400g	460	9.2	115	3.6	17.5	2.3	4.3
Wholewheat, Tesco*	1 Serving/50g	177	1.0	355	12.0	72.0	2.0	5.0
with Balsamic Roasted Vegetables, TTD, Sainsbury's*	1/3 Pack/80g	94	4.3	117	2.8	14.3	5.4	1.1
with Sun Dried Tomato, Chosen By You, Asda*	1 Pack/310g	515	12.1	166	4.6	26.2	3.9	4.0
Zesty Lemon & Coriander, Dry, Sammy's*	1 Serving/50g	171	1.4	342	13.0	74.0	2.8	6.0
CRAB								
Boiled, Meat Only, Average	*1 Tbsp/40g*	*51*	*2.2*	*128*	*19.5*	*0.0*	*5.5*	*0.0*
Brown, Cornish, Seafood & Eat It*	1 Pack/100g	171	10.7	171	17.9	1.9	10.7	0.0
Claws, Asda*	1oz/28g	25	0.3	89	11.0	9.0	1.0	0.2

	Measure INFO/WEIGHT	per Measure KCAL	per Measure FAT	Nutrition Values per 100g / 100ml KCAL	PROT	CARB	FAT	FIBRE
CRAB								
Cocktail, Waitrose*	1 Serving/100g	217	17.6	217	10.8	3.8	17.6	0.4
Cornish 50/50, Seafood & Eat It*	1 Pot/100g	144	5.8	144	21.6	1.2	5.8	0.5
Cornish Potted, Seafood & Eat It*	1 Pack/100g	235	17.5	235	15.0	5.1	17.5	0.8
Dressed, Average	*1 Serving/43g*	*66*	*3.4*	*154*	*16.8*	*4.1*	*7.9*	*0.2*
Meat, in Brine, Average	*½ Can/60g*	*46*	*0.3*	*76*	*17.2*	*0.9*	*0.4*	*0.1*
Meat, Raw, Average	*1oz/28g*	*28*	*0.2*	*100*	*20.8*	*2.8*	*0.6*	*0.0*
White Cornish, Seafood & Eat It*	1 Pack/100g	81	0.5	81	19.0	0.1	0.5	0.0
CRAB CAKES								
Goan, M & S*	1 Pack/190g	228	7.6	120	8.0	12.9	4.0	1.8
Iceland*	1 Serving/18g	52	3.2	288	7.2	25.6	18.0	1.3
Tesco*	1 Serving/130g	281	16.0	216	11.0	15.4	12.3	1.1
Thai, TTD, Sainsbury's*	½ Pack/106g	201	9.5	189	9.5	17.8	8.9	1.4
CRAB STICKS								
Average	1 Stick/15g	14	0.0	94	9.1	13.9	0.3	0.0
CRACKERBREAD								
Original, Ryvita*	1 Slice/5g	21	0.2	380	10.3	76.9	3.5	3.5
Rice, Asda*	1 Slice/5g	19	0.1	374	9.1	79.4	2.2	1.9
Sainsbury's*	1 Slice/5g	19	0.2	380	10.0	80.0	4.0	2.0
Wholegrain, Ryvita*	1 Slice/6g	20	0.2	360	12.4	68.7	3.9	9.8
CRACKERS								
Bath Oliver, Jacob's*	1 Cracker/12g	52	1.6	432	9.6	67.6	13.7	2.6
Black Olive, M & S*	1 Cracker/4g	20	1.0	485	8.3	59.4	23.5	4.3
Black Pepper, for Cheese, Ryvita*	1 Cracker/7g	27	0.2	384	13.2	72.9	2.9	6.8
Bran, Jacob's*	1 Cracker/7g	32	1.3	454	9.7	62.8	18.2	3.2
Butter Puff, Sainsbury's*	1 Cracker/10g	54	2.7	523	10.4	60.7	26.5	2.5
Chapati Chips, Tikka, Medium Spicy, Patak's*	1 Serving/25g	127	7.0	508	8.0	56.0	28.0	4.0
Cheddars, McVitie's*	1 Cracker/4g	22	1.3	543	10.0	55.1	31.3	2.6
Cheese, Cheese Heads, Walkers*	1 Pack/27g	128	6.0	475	10.8	58.0	22.3	2.8
Cheese, Mini, Heinz*	1 Pack/25g	108	3.6	433	9.4	68.6	14.6	0.6
Cheese, Ritz*	1 Cracker/4g	17	0.9	486	10.1	55.9	24.7	2.2
Cheese, Trufree*	1 Cracker/8g	42	2.6	524	9.0	50.0	32.0	0.5
Cheese Thins, Asda*	1 Cracker/4g	21	1.3	532	12.0	49.0	32.0	0.0
Cheese Thins, Co-Op*	1 Cracker/4g	21	1.3	530	12.0	49.0	32.0	3.0
Cheese Thins, Mini, Snack Rite*	1 Bag/30g	144	6.8	480	12.9	55.9	22.7	2.5
Cheese Thins, Waitrose*	1 Cracker/4g	21	1.2	545	11.9	52.6	31.9	2.5
Chinese, Pop Pan*	1 Cracker/8g	40	2.5	533	13.3	53.3	33.3	0.0
Chives, Jacob's*	1 Cracker/6g	28	1.0	457	9.5	67.5	16.5	2.7
Choice Grain, Jacob's*	1 Cracker/8g	32	1.1	427	9.0	65.5	14.3	5.4
Corn Thins, 97% Fat Free, Real Foods*	1 Cracker/6g	23	0.2	378	10.2	81.7	3.0	8.6
Cream, 45% Less Fat, Morrisons*	1 Cracker/8g	32	0.6	403	10.5	74.2	7.1	3.3
Cream, Average	1 Cracker/7g	31	1.1	440	9.5	68.3	16.3	2.2
Cream, Choice Grain, Jacob's*	1 Cracker/7g	30	0.9	400	9.0	64.5	11.8	7.0
Cream, Jacob's*	1 Cracker/8g	34	1.1	431	10.0	67.5	13.5	3.8
Cream, Light, Jacob's*	1 Cracker/8g	31	0.5	388	10.6	72.2	6.3	4.1
Cream, Roasted Onion, Jacob's*	1 Cracker/8g	35	1.2	441	10.2	66.8	14.8	2.9
Cream, Sun Dried Tomato Flavour, Jacob's*	1 Cracker/8g	35	1.1	434	10.2	66.7	14.0	3.0
Crispy Cheese, M & S*	1 Cracker/4g	20	1.0	470	9.4	58.1	22.1	3.0
Extra Wheatgerm, Hovis*	1 Serving/6g	27	1.1	447	10.2	60.0	18.5	4.4
Garden Herbs, Jacob's*	1 Cracker/6g	28	1.0	457	9.5	67.5	16.5	2.7
Goan Curry, Graze*	1 Pack/15g	80	4.2	532	4.5	65.5	28.0	0.9
Golden Rye, for Cheese, Ryvita*	1 Cracker/7g	27	0.2	384	13.2	72.9	2.9	6.5
Harvest Grain, Sainsbury's*	1 Cracker/6g	27	1.1	458	8.5	64.5	18.4	4.1
Herb & Onion, 99% Fat Free, Rakusen's*	1 Cracker/5g	18	0.0	360	9.1	82.6	1.0	3.9

	Measure INFO/WEIGHT	per Measure KCAL	FAT	Nutrition Values per 100g / 100ml KCAL	PROT	CARB	FAT	FIBRE
CRACKERS								
Herb & Onion, Trufree*	1 Cracker/6g	25	0.7	418	2.5	75.0	12.0	10.0
Herb & Spice, Jacob's*	1 Cracker/6g	27	1.0	457	9.5	67.5	16.5	2.7
Herbs & Spice Selection, Jacob's*	1 Cracker/6g	27	0.9	451	9.5	68.0	15.7	2.7
Krackawheat, McVitie's*	1 Cracker/7g	33	1.4	446	9.7	60.0	18.6	5.8
Light & Crispy, Sainsbury's*	1 Cracker/11g	42	1.2	384	11.3	61.0	10.5	13.0
Lightly Salted, Crispy, Sainsbury's*	1 Cracker/5g	25	1.3	533	7.8	62.6	27.9	2.1
Lightly Salted, Italian, Jacob's*	1 Cracker/6g	26	0.8	429	10.3	67.6	13.0	2.9
Mediterranean, Jacob's*	1 Cracker/6g	27	1.0	450	9.7	66.5	16.1	2.7
Mixed Seed, Multi Grain, Asda*	1 Cracker/6g	28	1.1	445	11.0	62.0	17.0	4.4
Multi-grain, Aldi, Savour Bakes, Aldi*	1 Cracker/5g	20	0.8	404	8.3	55.0	16.8	5.1
Multigrain, Corn Thins, Real Foods*	1 Cracker/6g	23	0.2	388	10.9	71.0	3.7	10.3
Multigrain, Snack Crackers, Special K, Kellogg's*	1 Pack/30g	120	3.0	400	10.0	73.3	10.0	6.7
Multigrain, Tesco*	1 Cracker/6g	27	1.1	458	8.5	64.5	18.4	4.1
Oat & Wheat, Weight Watchers*	4 Crackers/20g	74	0.4	368	8.3	78.9	2.1	3.5
Olive Oil & Oregano, Mediterreaneo, Jacob's*	1 Cracker/6g	25	0.7	412	12.4	65.5	11.2	6.0
Passionately Pizza, Jacobites, Jacob's*	1 Pack/150g	708	38.1	472	5.7	55.3	25.4	1.7
Peanut, Wasabi, Graze*	1 Pack/26g	125	5.6	479	15.2	53.8	21.4	5.4
Pesto, Jacob's*	1 Cracker/6g	27	1.0	450	9.7	66.5	16.1	2.7
Poppy & Sesame Seed, Sainsbury's*	1 Cracker/4g	21	1.1	530	9.6	58.9	28.4	3.4
Ritz, Mini, Kraft*	1 Bag/25g	126	6.0	504	7.9	63.0	24.0	2.0
Ritz, Original, Jacob's*	1 Cracker/3g	17	1.0	509	6.9	55.6	28.8	2.0
Rye, Organic, Dove's Farm*	1 Cracker/7g	28	1.0	393	7.0	58.4	14.6	8.7
Salt & Black Pepper, Eat Well, M & S*	1 Pack/25g	105	3.7	422	9.6	62.9	14.7	5.1
Salt & Black Pepper, Jacob's*	1 Cracker/6g	27	1.0	457	9.5	67.5	16.5	2.7
Salted, Ritz, Nabisco*	1 Cracker/3g	17	0.9	493	7.0	57.5	26.1	2.9
Sesame & Poppy Thins, Tesco*	1 Cracker/4g	20	1.0	485	9.9	57.6	23.5	4.4
Spicy, Trufree*	1 Cracker/6g	25	0.8	412	3.8	70.0	13.0	12.5
Spicy Indonesian Vegetable, Waitrose*	1 Pack/60g	295	16.3	492	1.2	60.6	27.2	2.2
Sweet Chilli, Thins, Savours, Jacob's*	1 Cracker/4g	21	0.9	472	8.0	62.3	21.2	3.6
Thai Spicy Vegetable, Sainsbury's*	1 Pack/50g	231	10.4	462	7.2	61.5	20.8	2.6
Tom Yum Yum, Graze*	1 Pack/23g	90	0.6	390	7.2	84.8	2.4	1.4
Tuc, Cheese Sandwich, Jacob's*	1 Cracker/14g	72	4.3	531	8.4	53.8	31.4	0.0
Tuc, Jacob's*	1 Cracker/5g	24	1.3	522	7.0	60.5	28.0	2.9
Tuc, Mini, with Sesame Seeds, Jacob's*	1 Cracker/2g	10	0.5	523	9.7	63.1	25.8	3.9
Unsalted, Tops, Premium Plus, Impress*	1 Cracker/3g	13	0.3	448	10.3	75.9	10.3	0.0
Vegetable, Oriental Snack Selection, Sainsbury's*	1 Cracker/20g	42	1.9	209	4.5	26.2	9.6	3.4
Veggie, Heinz*	1 Pack/25g	110	3.0	440	7.0	76.0	12.0	3.6
Wasapeas, Graze*	1 Pack/25g	101	1.9	406	14.8	65.2	7.8	0.0
Waterthins, Wafers, Philemon*	1 Crackers/2g	7	0.1	392	10.6	77.9	3.6	5.0
Wheaten, M & S*	1 Cracker/4g	20	0.9	450	10.2	57.0	20.2	5.0
Whole Wheat, 100%, Oven Baked, Master Choice*	1 Cracker/4g	17	0.4	429	10.0	75.0	9.6	12.1
Wholemeal, Tesco*	1 Cracker/7g	29	1.0	414	9.4	60.6	14.9	10.4
Wholewheat, Saiwa*	1 Pack/31g	128	3.9	414	12.5	62.9	12.5	7.9
Wholmeal, Organic, Nairn's*	1 Cracker/14g	58	2.0	413	9.0	61.4	14.6	8.7
with Onion, Cumin Seed, & Garlic, GFY, Asda*	1 Cracker/6g	22	0.2	380	11.0	78.0	2.7	1.7
CRANBERRIES								
Dried, Sweetened, Average	**1 Serving/10g**	**34**	**0.1**	**335**	**0.3**	**81.1**	**0.8**	**4.4**
Dried, Wholesome, Love Life, Waitrose*	¼ Pack/25g	92	0.2	370	0.3	86.8	0.8	4.6
Fresh, Raw	**1oz/28g**	**4**	**0.0**	**15**	**0.4**	**3.4**	**0.1**	**3.0**
Organic, Infinity Foods*	1 Serving/100g	334	0.6	334	0.9	80.3	0.6	7.2
CRAYFISH								
Raw	**1oz/28g**	**19**	**0.2**	**67**	**14.9**	**0.0**	**0.8**	**0.0**
Tails, Chilli & Garlic, Asda*	1 Serving/140g	133	4.3	95	16.0	1.1	3.1	0.8

	Measure INFO/WEIGHT	per Measure		Nutrition Values per 100g / 100ml				
		KCAL	FAT	KCAL	PROT	CARB	FAT	FIBRE
CRAYFISH								
Tails, in Brine, Luxury, The Big Prawn Co*	½ Tub/90g	46	0.6	51	10.1	1.0	0.7	0.0
CREAM								
Aerosol, Average	**1oz/28g**	**87**	**8.7**	**309**	**1.7**	**6.2**	**30.9**	**0.0**
Aerosol, Reduced Fat, Average	**1 Serving/55ml**	**33**	**3.0**	**59**	**0.6**	**1.9**	**5.4**	**0.0**
Brandy, Pourable, with Remy Martin*, Finest, Tesco*	½ Pot/125ml	460	35.5	368	2.7	19.8	28.4	0.0
Brandy, Really Thick, Finest, Tesco*	½ Pot/125ml	579	49.5	463	1.3	19.7	39.6	0.0
Brandy, Really Thick, Tesco*	1 Pot/250ml	1162	98.2	465	1.4	21.3	39.3	0.0
Chantilly, TTD, Sainsbury's*	2 Tbsp/30g	136	14.0	455	1.4	6.9	46.8	0.0
Clotted, Fresh, Average	**1 Serving/28g**	**162**	**17.5**	**579**	**1.6**	**2.3**	**62.7**	**0.0**
Clotted, TTD, Sainsbury's*	1 Serving/30g	176	19.0	587	1.6	2.2	63.5	0.0
Double, Average	**1 Serving/25ml**	**110**	**11.7**	**438**	**1.8**	**2.7**	**46.7**	**0.0**
Double, Reduced Fat, Average	**1 Serving/30g**	**73**	**7.0**	**243**	**2.7**	**5.6**	**23.3**	**0.1**
Extra Thick, 99% Real Dairy Cream, Anchor*	1 Serving/13g	51	5.4	409	1.7	3.9	43.0	0.0
Extra Thick, Reduced Fat, Weight Watchers*	1 Serving/30g	42	3.4	140	2.5	6.7	11.5	0.8
Oat Alternative, Dairy Free, Oatly*	1 Carton/250ml	375	32.5	150	1.0	6.0	13.0	0.8
Single, Average	**1 Tbsp/15ml**	**18**	**1.6**	**123**	**2.6**	**4.4**	**10.5**	**0.1**
Single, Extra Thick, Average	**1 Serving/38ml**	**72**	**6.9**	**192**	**2.7**	**4.1**	**18.4**	**0.0**
Soured, Fresh, Average	**1 Tbsp/15ml**	**29**	**2.8**	**191**	**2.7**	**3.9**	**18.4**	**0.0**
Soured, Reduced Fat, Average	**1 fl oz/30ml**	**36**	**2.6**	**119**	**5.2**	**6.7**	**8.6**	**0.4**
Strawberry, Light, Real Dairy, Uht, Anchor*	1 Serving/13g	25	2.1	198	2.6	8.7	17.0	0.0
Thick, Sterilised, Average	**1 Tbsp/15ml**	**35**	**3.5**	**233**	**2.6**	**3.6**	**23.1**	**0.0**
Uht, Double, Average	**1 Tbsp/15g**	**41**	**3.9**	**274**	**2.2**	**7.3**	**26.3**	**0.0**
Uht, Reduced Fat, Average	**1 Serving/25ml**	**15**	**1.4**	**62**	**0.5**	**2.2**	**5.6**	**0.0**
Uht, Single, Average	**1 Tbsp/15ml**	**29**	**2.8**	**194**	**2.6**	**4.0**	**18.8**	**0.0**
Whipping, Average	**1 Tbsp/15ml**	**52**	**5.5**	**348**	**2.1**	**3.2**	**36.4**	**0.0**
CREAM SODA								
American, with Vanilla, Tesco*	1 Glass/313ml	75	0.0	24	0.0	5.9	0.0	0.0
No Added Sugar, Sainsbury's*	1 Can/330ml	2	0.3	0	0.1	0.1	0.1	0.1
Traditional Style, Tesco*	1 Can/330ml	139	0.0	42	0.0	10.4	0.0	0.0
CREME BRULEE								
Average	1 Serving/100g	313	26.0	313	3.8	15.7	26.0	0.2
CREME CARAMEL								
Average	1 Serving/128g	140	2.8	109	3.0	20.6	2.2	0.0
Carmelle, Green's*	1 Pack/70g	82	2.8	117	3.0	17.0	4.0	0.0
CREME EGG								
Cadbury*	1 Egg/39g	174	6.2	445	3.0	71.0	16.0	0.0
Minis, Cadbury*	1 Egg/11g	50	1.8	445	4.1	67.5	16.4	0.4
CREME FRAICHE								
Average	**1 Pot/295g**	**1067**	**112.2**	**362**	**2.2**	**2.6**	**38.0**	**0.0**
Cucumber & Mint, Triangles, Sainsbury's*	1 Serving/25g	105	2.4	421	11.0	72.3	9.7	2.5
Extra Light, President*	1 Tub/200g	182	10.0	91	2.7	8.7	5.0	0.0
Half Fat, Average	**1 Serving30g**	**54**	**4.9**	**181**	**3.1**	**5.5**	**16.2**	**0.0**
CREPES								
Chocolate Filled, Tesco*	1 Crepe/32g	140	5.8	437	5.9	62.5	18.1	1.6
Lobster, Finest, Tesco*	1 Serving/160g	250	10.2	156	10.7	14.0	6.4	1.2
Mushroom, M & S*	1 Pack/186g	195	4.5	105	5.7	17.1	2.4	2.5
CRISPBAKES								
Broccoli & Leek, Asda*	1 Bake/132g	263	13.2	199	6.3	21.0	10.0	2.0
Bubble & Squeak, M & S*	1 Bake/47g	79	4.1	170	2.7	19.6	8.8	1.5
Cheese, Spring Onion & Chive, Sainsbury's*	1 Bake/114g	287	16.8	253	7.1	24.5	14.8	1.7
Cheese & Onion, Dalepak*	1 Bake/98g	239	12.6	243	7.2	24.1	12.8	1.7
Cheese & Onion, M & S*	1 Bake/114g	285	18.5	250	6.4	19.4	16.2	1.7
Cheese & Onion, Tesco*	1 Bake/109g	275	17.2	252	7.9	19.6	15.8	2.1

C

	Measure INFO/WEIGHT	per Measure KCAL	FAT	Nutrition Values per 100g / 100ml KCAL	PROT	CARB	FAT	FIBRE
CRISPBAKES								
Dutch, Asda*	1 Bake/8g	31	0.3	388	14.7	74.9	3.3	4.2
Dutch, HL, Tesco*	1 Bake/8g	30	0.2	385	14.7	74.9	2.7	4.2
Dutch, Sainsbury's*	1 Bake/10g	38	0.5	392	14.5	72.3	5.0	5.8
Minced Beef, M & S*	1 Bake/113g	226	12.3	200	10.0	15.6	10.9	1.5
Mushroom, Uncooked, Dalepak*	1 Bake/84g	141	7.4	168	3.8	18.5	8.8	2.1
Roast Vegetable & Basil, Cauldron Foods*	1 Bake/115g	241	11.0	210	3.5	26.0	9.6	2.9
Spinach, Cheese & Sweetcorn, Cauldron Foods*	1 Bake/115g	233	12.2	203	5.6	21.3	10.6	2.1
Vegetable, Sainsbury's*	1 Bake/114g	246	13.0	216	2.0	26.2	11.4	2.0
CRISPBREAD								
3 Seed, Classic, Gourmet, Dr Karg*	1 Bread/25g	107	4.9	430	16.5	46.6	19.7	10.9
3 Seed, Organic, Gourmet	1 Bread/25g	101	4.7	405	15.8	48.8	18.8	14.6
Corn, Orgran*	1 Bread/5g	18	0.1	360	7.5	83.0	1.8	3.0
Cracked Black Pepper, Ryvita*	1 Bread/11g	35	0.2	315	9.0	66.2	1.6	13.7
Crisp 'n' Light, Wasa*	1 Bread/7g	24	0.1	360	12.0	73.0	2.2	5.3
Dark Rye, Ryvita*	1 Bread/10g	34	0.1	342	8.5	66.5	1.2	15.2
Emmental Cheese & Pumpkin Seed, Gourmet, Dr Karg*	1 Bread/25g	100	4.1	402	17.7	45.5	16.6	12.3
Emmental Cheese & Pumpkin Seed, Organic, Dr Karg*	1 Bread/25g	107	3.7	428	17.7	50.7	14.9	9.6
Gluten Free	1 Bread/8g	25	0.1	331	6.4	72.9	1.5	0.0
Mildly Seasoned, Gourmet, Dr Karg*	1 Bread/25g	101	4.0	405	16.2	48.8	16.1	11.6
Multigrain, Ryvita*	1 Bread/11g	41	0.8	370	11.2	56.0	7.2	18.3
Multigrain, Wasa*	1 Bread/13g	43	0.3	320	12.0	62.0	2.6	14.0
Original, Ryvita*	1 Bread/10g	35	0.2	350	8.5	66.9	1.7	16.5
Original Rye, Thin, Finn Crisp*	1 Slice/13g	47	0.3	360	11.0	60.0	2.4	19.0
Original Rye, Wasa*	1 Bread/11g	35	0.2	315	9.0	67.0	1.4	14.0
Poppyseed, Wasa*	1 Bread/13g	45	1.0	350	13.0	56.0	8.0	14.0
Provita*	1 Bread/6g	26	0.6	416	12.5	68.4	9.9	0.0
Pumpkin Seeds & Oats, Ryvita*	1 Slice/13g	45	1.2	362	12.5	55.6	9.9	14.5
Rice, & Cracked Pepper, Orgran*	1 Bread/5g	18	0.1	388	8.4	81.9	1.8	2.0
Rice, Original, Sakata*	1 Bread/25g	102	0.6	410	6.9	88.0	2.6	1.3
Rice, Sakata*	1 Bread/25g	25	0.2	102	1.7	22.0	0.7	0.3
Roasted Onion, Gourmet, Dr Karg*	1 Bread/25g	100	4.1	399	15.9	46.6	16.5	11.1
Roasted Onion, Organic, Dr Karg*	1 Bread/25g	97	3.7	390	15.8	48.5	14.8	12.9
Rounds, Multigrain, Finn Crisp*	1 Bread/13g	41	0.7	330	13.0	56.0	6.0	18.0
Rounds, Original, Rye, Finn Crisp*	1 Bread/14g	45	0.4	320	11.0	60.0	2.7	16.0
Rounds, Wholegrain Wheat, Finn Crisp*	1 Bread/13g	45	0.7	360	11.0	66.0	5.9	10.0
Scan Bran, Slimming World*	1 Bread/10g	31	0.5	310	14.9	29.0	5.3	42.1
Seeded, Spelt, Organic, Dr Karg*	1 Bread/25g	102	4.5	408	17.2	44.4	18.0	10.4
Sesame, Ryvita*	1 Bread/10g	37	0.7	373	10.5	58.3	7.0	17.5
Sesame, Savour Bakes, Aldi*	1 Bread/9g	33	0.5	366	12.3	57.2	5.2	20.6
Snacks, Caribbean Chicken, Seasons, Quaker Oats*	1 Pack/28g	118	2.5	421	7.9	77.1	8.9	2.1
Snacks, Cheese, Onion & Chive Flavour, Quaker Oats*	1 Pack/28g	118	2.5	420	8.3	76.0	9.1	2.4
Snacks, Lime & Coriander, Seasons, Quaker Oats*	1 Pack/28g	115	2.5	410	7.5	75.0	9.0	2.3
Spelt, Cheese, Sunflower Seeds, Organic, Dr Karg*	1 Bread/25g	103	4.5	411	19.2	42.8	18.1	10.4
Spelt, Muesli, Organic, Dr Karg*	1 Bread/25g	94	2.8	375	14.2	54.4	11.2	10.6
Spelt, Sesame, Sunflower, Amisa*	1 Bread/29g	85	4.3	297	11.7	28.5	15.1	5.0
Sport, Wasa*	1 Bread/15g	46	0.2	310	9.0	64.0	1.5	16.0
Sunflower Seeds & Oats, Ryvita*	1 Bread/12g	46	1.1	384	9.7	58.4	9.0	15.3
Sweet Onion, Ryvita*	1 Bread/12g	43	0.2	356	9.0	70.6	1.4	12.6
Thin Crisps, Original Taste, Finn Crisp*	1 Bread/6g	20	0.2	320	11.0	63.0	2.4	19.0
Trufree*	1 Bread/6g	22	0.1	370	6.0	82.0	2.0	1.0
Whole Grain, Classic, Organic, Dr Karg*	1 Bread/25g	89	4.1	355	13.4	38.2	16.5	10.2
Whole Grain, Crispy, Thin, Kavli*	3 Breads/15g	50	0.3	333	10.0	70.0	1.7	12.7
Wholegrain, Classic Three Seed, Organic, Dr Karg*	1 Bread/25g	101	4.5	405	15.8	44.8	18.0	14.6

	Measure INFO/WEIGHT	per Measure KCAL	per Measure FAT	Nutrition Values per 100g / 100ml KCAL	PROT	CARB	FAT	FIBRE
CRISPBREAD								
Wholemeal, Light, Allinson*	1 Bread/5g	17	0.1	349	11.7	69.7	2.6	11.0
Wholemeal, Organic, Allinson*	1 Bread/5g	17	0.1	336	14.2	66.0	1.7	12.2
Wholemeal, Rye with Milk, Grafschafter*	1 Bread/9g	29	0.1	316	11.4	64.0	1.6	15.0
Wholemeal Rye, Organic, Kallo*	1 Bread/10g	31	0.2	314	9.7	65.0	1.7	15.4
CRISPS								
Apple, Dried, Snapz*	1 Packet/15g	52	0.0	344	2.0	77.0	0.0	14.7
Apple, The Fruit Factory*	1 Packet/10g	33	0.0	334	1.3	81.1	0.5	12.4
Apple, Thyme & Sage, M & S*	1 Bag/55g	253	13.4	460	5.5	55.3	24.3	6.1
Argentinean Flame Grilled Steak, Walkers*	1 Bag/35g	182	11.3	520	6.5	50.7	32.4	4.2
Bacon, Shapers, Boots*	1 Bag/23g	99	3.4	431	8.0	66.0	15.0	3.0
Bacon & Cheddar, Baked, Walkers*	1 Pack/38g	149	3.2	397	6.5	73.7	8.5	4.7
Bacon Crispies, Sainsbury's*	1 Bag/25g	117	5.7	468	19.9	45.8	22.8	4.8
Bacon Flavour Rashers, BGTY, Sainsbury's*	1 Pack/10g	34	0.2	340	10.8	70.3	1.6	3.5
Bacon Pillows, Light, Shapers, Boots*	1 Pack/12g	44	0.3	367	3.7	83.0	2.3	4.0
Bacon Rashers, Blazin, Tesco*	1 Bag/25g	121	6.6	485	16.5	45.7	26.3	3.8
Bacon Rashers, COU, M & S*	1 Pack/20g	72	0.6	360	9.4	77.5	2.9	3.5
Bacon Rashers, Iceland*	1 Bag/75g	330	13.2	440	8.3	61.9	17.6	2.9
Bacon Rashers, Tesco*	1 Serving/25g	125	6.4	500	7.1	59.8	25.5	4.0
Bacon Rice Bites, Asda*	1 Bag/30g	136	4.8	452	7.0	70.0	16.0	0.4
Bacon Sizzler, Ridge Cut, McCoys*	1 Bag/32g	165	9.7	516	7.1	53.6	30.3	3.9
Baked, Ready Salted, Walkers*	1 Packet/38g	146	3.0	390	6.0	74.0	8.0	5.5
Baked, Sour Cream & Chive, Walkers*	1 Packet/38g	148	3.2	395	7.0	73.0	8.5	5.0
Baked Bean Flavour, Walkers*	1 Bag/35g	184	11.5	525	6.5	50.0	33.0	4.0
Banging BBQ, Shots, Walkers*	1 Pack/18g	87	4.5	485	5.5	60.0	25.0	1.3
Barbecue, Handcooked, Tesco*	1 Bag/40g	187	10.0	468	6.6	53.8	25.1	5.2
Barbecue, Savoury Snacks, Weight Watchers*	1 Pack/22g	81	1.9	366	18.6	61.0	8.7	6.1
Barbecue, Snack Rite*	1 Bag/25g	131	8.3	524	5.1	51.3	33.2	0.0
Barbecue, Sunseed Oil, Walkers*	1 Pack/25g	131	8.2	525	6.5	50.0	33.0	4.0
Barbecue Beef, Select, Tesco*	1 Pack/25g	134	8.7	536	6.4	49.2	34.8	4.4
Barbecue Flavour Waffles, American, Shapers, Boots*	1 Pack/20g	95	4.4	476	4.5	65.0	22.0	3.7
BBQ Rib, Sunseed, Walkers*	1 Bag/25g	131	8.2	525	6.5	50.0	33.0	4.0
Beef, Squares, Walkers*	1 Bag/25g	105	4.5	420	6.0	59.0	18.0	4.6
Beef & Onion, Asda*	1 Bag/25g	129	7.8	516	5.7	53.3	31.1	3.9
Beef & Onion, Morrisons*	1 Pack/25g	131	8.2	524	5.9	51.2	32.9	4.2
Beef & Onion, Potato, M & S*	1 Bag/25g	130	8.5	530	6.6	48.2	34.5	5.0
Beef & Onion, Tayto*	1 Bag/35g	184	11.9	526	7.6	47.3	34.0	4.5
Beef & Onion, Walkers*	1 Bag/35g	184	11.5	525	6.5	50.0	33.0	4.0
Beefy, Smiths, Walkers*	1 Bag/25g	133	9.2	531	4.3	45.2	37.0	0.0
Beetroot Chips, Crunchy, Apple Snapz*	1 Bag/20g	52	0.2	260	14.7	76.0	1.0	28.0
Builders Breakfast, Walkers*	1 Sm Bag/25g	131	8.3	524	5.6	50.8	33.2	4.0
Butter & Chive, COU, M & S*	1 Bag/26g	95	0.5	365	7.7	77.3	1.9	4.6
Cajun Squirrel, Walkers*	1 Sm Bag/25g	130	8.2	522	5.8	51.2	32.7	4.2
Chargrilled Chicken, Ridge Cut, McCoys*	1 Pack/32g	167	10.0	521	7.0	52.9	31.3	4.0
Chargrilled Chicken Crinkles, Shapers, Boots*	1 Bag/20g	96	4.8	482	6.6	60.0	24.0	4.0
Chargrilled Steak, Max, Walkers*	1 Bag/55g	289	18.1	525	6.5	50.0	33.0	4.0
Cheddar & Onion, Ridge Cut, McCoys*	1 Bag/32g	165	9.8	516	7.0	53.2	30.6	3.9
Cheddar & Red Onion Chutney, Sensations, Walkers*	1 Bag/40g	198	11.2	495	6.5	54.0	28.0	4.5
Cheddar & Spring Onion, 35% Less Fat, Sainsbury's*	1 Pack/20g	93	4.2	463	6.3	62.4	20.9	0.9
Cheddar Cheese & Bacon, Walkers*	1 Bag/25g	131	8.2	523	5.9	50.6	33.0	4.1
Cheese, Space Raiders, KP Snacks*	1 Bag/16g	76	3.5	473	7.1	61.6	22.0	3.1
Cheese & Branston Pickle, Walkers*	1 Bag/35g	181	11.4	525	6.5	50.0	33.0	4.0
Cheese & Chive Flavour, GFY, Asda*	1 Bag/25g	119	6.0	476	6.0	59.0	24.0	6.0
Cheese & Chives, Walkers*	1 Bag/35g	185	11.5	530	6.5	50.0	33.0	4.1

CRISPS

INFO/WEIGHT	Measure	per Measure KCAL	FAT	Nutrition Values per 100g / 100ml KCAL	PROT	CARB	FAT	FIBRE
Cheese & Onion, 30% Less Fat, Sainsbury's*	1 Pack/25g	115	5.4	459	7.5	58.1	21.8	5.4
Cheese & Onion, Baked, Walkers*	1 Bag/25g	99	2.1	396	6.5	73.8	8.3	4.7
Cheese & Onion, BGTY, Sainsbury's*	1 Bag/25g	120	6.2	479	7.0	57.0	24.8	5.7
Cheese & Onion, Crinkle Cut, Low Fat, Waitrose*	1 Bag/25g	122	5.8	490	7.7	62.6	23.2	4.7
Cheese & Onion, Flavour Crinkles, Shapers, Boots*	1 Bag/20g	96	4.8	482	6.6	60.0	24.0	4.0
Cheese & Onion, GFY, Asda*	1 Pack/26g	122	5.7	470	7.0	61.0	22.0	4.2
Cheese & Onion, Golden Wonder*	1 Bag/25g	131	8.4	524	6.1	49.2	33.6	2.0
Cheese & Onion, KP Snacks*	1 Bag/25g	133	8.7	534	6.6	48.7	34.8	4.8
Cheese & Onion, Lights, Walkers*	1 Bag/24g	113	5.0	470	7.5	62.0	21.0	5.0
Cheese & Onion, M & S*	1 Bag/25g	134	8.9	535	5.5	48.8	35.5	5.0
Cheese & Onion, Max, Walkers*	1 Pack/50g	262	16.0	525	6.8	52.0	32.0	5.2
Cheese & Onion, Organic, Tesco*	1 Bag/25g	128	8.1	514	5.2	49.9	32.6	7.0
Cheese & Onion, Oven Baked, Asda*	1 Bag/25g	95	2.0	380	5.1	72.0	8.0	3.3
Cheese & Onion, Oven Baked, Tesco*	1 Bag/25g	102	1.6	410	5.3	74.7	6.6	7.7
Cheese & Onion, Potato Heads, Walkers*	1 Pack/23g	108	5.3	470	6.0	60.0	23.0	5.5
Cheese & Onion, Sainsbury's*	1 Bag/25g	132	8.7	527	4.6	48.8	34.8	3.9
Cheese & Onion, Snack Rite*	1 Pack/25g	132	8.3	527	5.3	51.3	33.4	0.0
Cheese & Onion, Sprinters*	1 Bag/25g	137	9.1	549	5.4	49.4	36.6	0.0
Cheese & Onion, Squares, Walkers*	1 Bag/25g	107	4.5	430	6.5	61.0	18.0	5.5
Cheese & Onion, Sunseed Oil, Walkers*	1 Bag/35g	181	11.4	525	7.0	50.0	33.0	4.0
Cheese & Onion, Tayto*	1 Bag/25g	131	8.5	526	7.6	47.3	34.0	4.5
Cheese & Onion, Tesco*	1 Pack/25g	132	8.3	530	5.8	51.6	33.2	4.4
Cheese & Onion Flavour, Asda*	1 Bag/25g	130	7.8	519	5.6	53.6	31.4	3.7
Cheese & Onion Rings, Crunchy, Shapers, Boots*	1 Bag/15g	56	0.4	374	5.9	81.0	2.9	2.0
Cheese Bites, Weight Watchers*	1 Pack/18g	73	1.0	406	13.9	71.1	5.6	2.2
Cheese Curls, Morrisons*	1 Bag/14g	71	4.5	510	4.5	51.0	32.0	2.6
Cheese Curls, Red Mill*	½ Bag/50g	276	18.0	553	6.6	50.6	36.0	2.0
Cheese Curls, Shapers, Boots*	1 Pack/14g	68	3.8	489	4.5	57.0	27.0	2.7
Cheese Curls, Sprinters*	1 Bag/14g	68	3.8	483	4.1	56.4	26.8	0.0
Cheese Curls, Tesco*	1 Bag/14g	75	4.5	520	4.5	54.4	31.1	1.9
Cheese Curls, Weight Watchers*	1 Pack/20g	78	1.7	392	5.0	73.8	8.6	3.4
Cheese Moments, Smiths*	1 Pack/28g	148	9.2	530	8.0	50.0	33.0	2.0
Cheese Puffs, Weight Watchers*	1 Pack/18g	80	1.9	444	7.8	77.2	10.6	3.3
Cheese Tasters, M & S*	1 Bag/30g	154	8.8	515	8.1	55.0	29.3	1.7
Cheese Twirls, Boulevard, Simply Delicious*	1 Pack/25g	137	8.7	550	12.1	46.7	35.0	0.0
Cheeses with Onion, Soulmates, Kettle Chips*	1 Pack/40g	195	11.6	488	7.7	50.2	29.0	5.4
Cheesy & Oniony, Potato, Tasty Little Numbers*	1 Pack/19g	100	6.1	527	7.9	51.6	32.1	2.6
Cheesy Curls, Bobby's*	1 Bag/40g	225	14.8	563	7.6	50.1	36.9	0.0
Cheesy Curls, Tesco*	1 Pack/17g	90	5.4	530	3.5	56.0	32.0	1.9
Cheesy Puffs, Co-Op*	1 Bag/60g	321	20.4	535	3.0	54.0	34.0	2.0
Chicken, Firecracker, McCoys*	1 Bag/35g	177	10.3	506	6.2	54.0	29.5	4.0
Chicken, Oven Roasted with Lemon & Thyme, Walkers*	1 Bag/40g	200	11.2	500	6.5	55.0	28.0	4.5
Chicken, Potato Heads, Walkers*	1 Pack/23g	106	4.8	460	8.5	58.0	21.0	6.0
Chicken & Thyme, Oven Roasted, Tesco*	1 Pack/150g	727	40.5	485	6.5	54.0	27.0	4.5
Chilli & Chocolate, Walkers*	1 Pack/25g	131	8.3	523	6.1	50.1	33.1	4.2
Chilli & Lemon, Walkers*	1 Pack/25g	131	8.2	525	6.3	51.0	33.0	3.8
Chinese Sizzling Beef, McCoys*	1 Bag/35g	178	10.6	506	6.9	51.8	30.2	4.0
Chinese Spare Rib, Walkers*	1 Bag/25g	131	8.2	525	6.5	50.0	33.0	4.0
Cider Vinegar & Sea Salt, Tyrrells*	1 Pack/40g	192	9.8	481	7.2	60.1	24.6	2.4
Cool Cheese Curly, Tesco*	1 Bag/14g	71	4.5	510	4.5	51.0	32.0	2.6
Corn Chips, Fritos*	1 Pack/43g	240	15.0	565	4.7	56.5	35.3	0.0
Coronation Chicken, Walkers*	1 Bag/25g	131	8.2	525	6.5	50.0	33.0	4.0
Crinkle Cut, Lower Fat, No Added Salt, Waitrose*	1 Bag/40g	193	10.0	483	6.5	58.0	25.0	3.9

CRISPS

INFO/WEIGHT	Measure	per Measure		Nutrition Values per 100g / 100ml				
		KCAL	FAT	KCAL	PROT	CARB	FAT	FIBRE
Crinkles, Cheddar & Onion, Walkers*	1 Pack/28g	150	9.3	537	6.0	51.5	33.3	3.5
Crispy Duck & Hoi Sin, Walkers*	1 Bag/25g	131	8.1	523	5.8	51.5	32.6	4.0
Crushed Natural Sea Salt, Darling Spuds*	1 Bag/40g	195	12.0	488	5.6	53.4	30.0	4.5
Curls, Cheesy, Asda*	1 Pack/17g	87	4.9	511	3.8	59.7	28.6	1.7
D'lites, Cheddar & Red Onion Bites, The Real Crisp Co.*	1 Pack/20g	83	2.0	414	2.1	78.8	10.0	2.7
Dutch Edam Cheese, Walkers*	1 Bag/25g	131	8.3	523	6.1	50.2	33.1	4.0
English Cheddar & Red Onion, Red Sky*	1 Pack/40g	183	8.4	457	6.9	60.2	21.0	5.1
English Roast Beef, & Yorkshire Pudding, Walkers*	1 Bag/35g	180	11.3	522	6.6	50.4	32.7	4.0
Extra Crunchy, Salt & Malt Vinegar, Walkers*	1 Pack/30g	139	6.2	463	6.6	59.9	20.8	4.8
Feta Cheese Flavour, Mediterranean, Walkers*	1 Pack/25g	127	8.2	510	6.5	49.0	33.0	4.5
Flame Grilled Steak, Extra Crunchy, Walkers*	1 Bag /150g	702	31.6	468	6.9	60.0	21.1	5.0
Flame Grilled Steak, Ridge Cut, McCoys*	1 Bag/32g	165	9.8	516	7.0	53.0	30.7	4.0
Four Cheese & Red Onion, Sensations, Walkers*	1 Bag/40g	194	10.8	485	6.5	54.0	27.0	4.5
French Garlic Baguette, Walkers*	1 Packet/25g	131	8.2	523	5.9	50.8	32.9	4.1
Garlic & Herbs Creme Fraiche, Kettle Chips*	1 Bag/50g	248	14.1	497	6.0	54.7	28.3	4.2
Greek Kebab, Mediterranean, Walkers*	1 Pack/25g	127	8.2	510	6.0	49.0	33.0	4.5
Grilled Chicken, Golden Lights, Golden Wonder*	1 Bag/21g	93	3.8	444	4.4	66.2	18.0	4.3
Heinz Tomato Ketchup, Sunseed, Walkers*	1 Bag/35g	179	11.0	520	6.5	51.0	32.0	4.0
Honey Roasted Ham, Sensations, Walkers*	1 Bag/40g	196	10.8	490	6.5	55.0	27.0	4.0
Hoops, Ready Salted, Weight Watchers*	1 Bag/20g	73	0.3	365	3.4	82.7	1.4	4.1
Hot & Spicy Salami, Tesco*	1 Bag/50g	215	17.9	431	26.2	0.7	35.9	0.0
Irish Cheddar with Onion Chutney, Phileas Fogg*	1 Pack/38g	195	11.2	512	7.1	54.3	29.6	4.3
Jalapeno Peppers, Fire Roasted, Darling Spuds*	1 Pack/40g	191	11.4	478	6.3	53.4	28.5	4.5
Lamb & Mint, Slow Roasted, Sensations, Walkers*	1 Bag/35g	170	9.4	485	6.5	54.0	27.0	4.5
Lamb & Mint, Sunseed Oil, Walkers*	1 Pack/35g	181	11.4	525	6.5	50.0	33.0	4.0
Lightly Salted, Baked, COU, M & S*	1 Bag/25g	87	0.6	350	8.5	76.4	2.3	5.7
Lightly Salted, Crinkle Cut, Low Fat, Waitrose*	1 Pack/35g	163	8.0	466	5.2	60.1	22.8	5.1
Lightly Salted, Crinkles, Shapers, Boots*	1 Pack/20g	96	4.8	482	6.6	60.0	24.0	4.0
Lightly Salted, Handcooked, Finest, Tesco*	½ Pack/150g	708	39.1	472	6.4	52.9	26.1	5.1
Lightly Salted, Hoops, Mini, Weight Watchers*	1 Pack/20g	71	0.2	355	4.0	82.0	1.0	3.5
Lightly Salted, Low Fat, Waitrose*	1 Bag/25g	125	6.2	500	7.5	61.3	25.0	4.8
Lightly Salted, Potato Bakes, Weight Watchers*	1 Pack/20g	78	1.8	392	5.0	72.0	9.0	5.0
Lightly Salted, Reduced Fat, Crinkles, Eat Well, M & S*	1 Pack/30g	140	6.6	460	6.7	59.4	21.8	4.5
Lightly Sea Salted, Jonathan Crisp*	1 Bag/35g	176	10.1	503	6.5	52.0	29.0	5.4
Lightly Sea Salted, Potato Chips, Hand Fried, Burts*	¼ Bag/50g	252	13.8	504	6.4	57.4	27.7	0.0
Lightly Sea Salted, Tyrrells*	1 Pack/40g	204	10.2	510	5.9	49.0	25.4	5.3
Lime & Thai Spices, Infused, Sensations, Walkers*	1 Pack/40g	200	11.6	500	6.5	54.0	29.0	4.0
Lincolnshire Sausage, Tyrrells*	1 Pack/100g	530	28.2	530	8.6	60.8	28.2	3.0
Mango & Chilli, Baked, Walkers*	1 Packet/38g	147	3.0	392	6.4	74.0	8.0	4.8
Marmite, Sunseed, Walkers*	1 Bag/35g	179	11.4	520	6.5	49.0	33.0	4.0
Mature Cheddar & Chive, Kettle Chips*	1 Serving/50g	239	12.7	478	8.1	54.4	25.4	5.0
Mature Cheddar & Chive, Tyrrells*	1 Bag/40g	194	10.0	485	8.4	58.7	25.1	2.4
Mature Cheddar & Red Onion, Kettle Chips*	1 Bag/40g	187	10.2	467	7.5	52.2	25.4	6.2
Mature Cheddar & Shallot, Temptations, Tesco*	1/6 Bag/25g	131	8.5	524	6.6	47.4	34.2	4.4
Mediterranean Baked Potato, COU, M & S*	1 Pack/25g	90	0.6	360	7.6	74.0	2.4	6.8
Mexican Chilli, Ridge Cut, McCoys*	1 Bag/32g	164	9.8	514	6.9	53.0	30.5	4.5
Mexican Chilli & Cheese, Golden Wonder*	1 Pack/45g	230	14.1	511	6.6	50.7	31.3	0.0
Mixed Pepper Flavour Burst, M & S*	1 Bag/55g	286	18.4	520	6.0	50.1	33.5	4.0
Naked, Tyrrells*	1 Pack/150g	748	41.2	499	7.7	56.5	27.5	0.0
New York Cheddar, Kettle Chips*	1 Bag/50g	241	13.3	483	6.7	53.9	26.7	4.5
Olive Oil, Mozzarella & Oregano, Walkers*	1 Serving/30g	151	8.7	505	6.5	54.0	29.0	4.0
Onion Bhaji, Walkers*	1 Pack/25g	130	8.2	522	6.1	50.7	32.7	4.3
Onion Rings, Crunchy, Shapers, Boots*	1 Bag/12g	61	3.4	507	2.5	62.0	28.0	2.6

CRISPS

INFO/WEIGHT		per Measure KCAL	FAT	Nutrition Values per 100g / 100ml KCAL	PROT	CARB	FAT	FIBRE
Onion Rings, M & S*	1 Pack/40g	186	8.6	465	5.2	62.1	21.5	4.3
Onion Rings, Maize Snacks, Sainsbury's*	¼ Bag/25g	122	6.6	488	5.6	56.9	26.4	1.7
Onion Rings, Tayto*	1 Pack/17g	82	4.1	484	3.0	63.4	24.0	2.4
Onion Rings, Tesco*	1 Serving/30g	148	7.6	495	8.4	57.8	25.5	2.5
Oriental Ribs, Ridge Cut, McCoys*	1 Pack/50g	255	15.0	511	7.3	52.7	30.1	4.2
Paprika, Handcooked, Shapers, Boots*	1 Bag/20g	99	4.8	493	7.2	62.0	24.0	5.0
Paprika, Max, Walkers*	1 Bag/50g	260	15.9	520	6.5	52.0	31.9	5.1
Paprika, Mini Hoops, Shapers, Boots*	1 Bag/13g	64	3.5	494	8.7	54.0	27.0	2.2
Parsnip, Passions, Snack Rite*	1 Serving/25g	123	9.4	494	4.5	34.5	37.6	18.8
Parsnip & Black Pepper, Sainsbury's*	1 Serving/35g	166	11.1	473	3.2	43.6	31.8	15.2
Pastrami & Cheese, Crinkle, M & S*	1 Bag/25g	120	5.9	485	6.5	61.0	24.0	3.5
Peri Peri Chicken, Nando's*	½ Bag/75g	410	20.2	547	5.1	57.4	27.0	3.4
Pickled Onion, Beastie Bites, Asda*	1 Bag/20g	100	5.2	498	6.0	60.0	26.0	0.0
Pickled Onion, Golden Wonder*	1 Bag/25g	131	8.5	524	5.6	49.0	34.0	2.0
Pickled Onion, M & S*	1 Bag/20g	70	0.3	345	5.0	81.7	1.5	3.7
Pickled Onion, Monster Bites, Sainsbury's*	1 Bag/20g	107	6.7	535	5.2	53.5	33.3	1.0
Pickled Onion, Stompers, Morrisons*	1 Pack/25g	129	7.9	518	6.1	52.2	31.6	1.3
Pickled Onion, Sunseed, Walkers*	1 Bag/35g	181	11.4	525	6.5	50.0	33.0	4.0
Pickled Onion, Tesco*	1 Bag/20g	104	7.0	520	6.5	50.0	35.0	1.0
Pickled Onion Flavour Rings, BGTY, Sainsbury's*	1 Serving/10g	34	0.1	345	5.0	81.7	1.5	3.7
Pickled Onion Rings, COU, M & S*	1 Bag/20g	69	0.3	345	5.0	81.7	1.5	3.7
Potato	1oz/28g	148	9.6	530	5.7	53.3	34.2	5.3
Potato, Baked, COU, M & S*	1 Bag/25g	87	0.6	350	8.5	76.4	2.3	5.7
Potato, Cheddar & Onion, Hand Cooked, Aldi*	1 Pack/150g	753	41.8	502	7.7	54.9	27.9	4.0
Potato, Low Fat	1oz/28g	128	6.0	458	6.6	63.5	21.5	5.9
Potato, Tyrrells*	1 Pack/261g	1362	72.8	522	6.1	56.5	27.9	0.0
Potato Chips, Anglesey Sea Salt, Red Sky*	1 Pack/40g	185	8.7	463	6.8	59.8	21.8	5.0
Potato Chips, Roasted Red Pepper & Lime, Red Sky*	1 Pack/40g	187	9.0	467	6.8	59.5	22.4	4.8
Potato Chips, Sour Cream & Green Herbs, Red Sky*	1 Pack/40g	188	9.4	471	6.8	58.4	23.4	4.8
Potato Squares, Ready Salted, Sainsbury's*	1 Bag/50g	192	7.9	384	6.5	53.8	15.9	7.8
Potato Thins, Lightly Salted, Light Choices, Tesco*	1 Pack/20g	72	0.4	360	5.1	79.5	2.0	4.2
Potato Triangles, Ready Salted, Sainsbury's*	½ Pack/50g	243	11.7	486	9.4	59.7	23.4	3.4
Potato Zoo, Crispy Potato Animals, Kids, Tesco*	1 Bag/30g	57	1.9	190	2.5	24.5	6.3	2.1
Prawn Cocktail, 30% Less Fat, Sainsbury's*	1 Pack/25g	117	5.9	470	6.3	58.9	23.6	5.7
Prawn Cocktail, Asda*	1 Bag/25g	134	8.7	535	6.0	49.0	35.0	4.3
Prawn Cocktail, BGTY, Sainsbury's*	1 Bag/25g	118	5.9	473	6.3	58.6	23.7	5.7
Prawn Cocktail, Boots*	1 Pack/21g	99	4.6	470	6.8	60.0	22.0	4.3
Prawn Cocktail, Golden Wonder*	1 Bag/25g	130	8.4	521	5.8	49.0	33.5	2.0
Prawn Cocktail, KP Snacks*	1 Bag/25g	133	8.7	531	5.9	48.4	34.9	4.7
Prawn Cocktail, Lites, Advantage, Tayto*	1 Pack/21g	96	4.1	455	5.3	65.1	19.3	3.8
Prawn Cocktail, Lites, Shapers, Boots*	1 Bag/21g	92	3.8	438	5.1	64.0	18.0	4.1
Prawn Cocktail, M & S*	1 Bag/30g	155	8.6	515	6.2	58.0	28.6	2.2
Prawn Cocktail, Sainsbury's*	1 Bag/25g	130	8.7	521	4.3	47.5	34.9	3.9
Prawn Cocktail, Seabrook*	1 Bag/32g	150	7.1	472	5.3	66.7	22.3	3.8
Prawn Cocktail, Snack Rite*	1 Bag/25g	129	8.3	516	5.0	49.2	33.2	0.0
Prawn Cocktail, Sunseed Oil, Walkers*	1 Bag/35g	181	11.4	525	6.5	50.0	33.0	4.0
Prawn Cocktail, Tayto*	1 Bag/35g	185	12.3	526	7.5	46.6	35.0	4.5
Prawn Cocktail, Tesco*	1 Pack/25g	135	8.2	540	5.2	52.0	32.8	4.0
Prawn Cocktail Flavour, Morrisons*	1 Bag/25g	131	8.2	525	5.1	51.9	33.0	4.1
Prawn Crackers, Tesco*	1 Bag/60g	316	17.5	527	3.2	62.8	29.2	0.8
Ready Salted, BGTY, Sainsbury's*	1 Bag/25g	121	6.5	486	6.8	55.7	26.2	6.6
Ready Salted, Co-Op*	1 Bag/25g	131	8.5	525	6.0	51.0	34.0	3.0
Ready Salted, GFY, Asda*	1 Bag/23g	109	5.3	475	7.0	60.0	23.0	4.3

	Measure INFO/WEIGHT	per Measure		Nutrition Values per 100g / 100ml				
		KCAL	FAT	KCAL	PROT	CARB	FAT	FIBRE

CRISPS

	Measure INFO/WEIGHT	KCAL	FAT	KCAL	PROT	CARB	FAT	FIBRE
Ready Salted, Golden Wonder*	1 Bag/25g	135	8.8	539	5.5	49.9	35.3	2.0
Ready Salted, KP Snacks*	1 Bag/24g	131	8.8	545	5.6	47.9	36.8	4.9
Ready Salted, Lower Fat, Asda*	1 Bag/25g	120	6.2	481	6.0	58.0	25.0	4.8
Ready Salted, Lower Fat, Sainsbury's*	1 Bag/25g	111	5.4	444	7.0	55.0	21.8	5.1
Ready Salted, M & S*	1 Bag/25g	136	9.1	545	5.6	47.8	36.6	4.9
Ready Salted, Morrisons*	1 Bag/25g	134	8.7	536	4.9	50.9	34.8	4.3
Ready Salted, Organic, Tesco*	1 Bag/25g	130	8.5	520	4.3	49.0	34.1	7.3
Ready Salted, Oven Baked, Asda*	1 Bag/25g	95	1.9	379	4.4	73.1	7.7	2.6
Ready Salted, Oven Baked, Tesco*	1 Bag/25g	95	1.9	380	4.4	73.1	7.7	8.4
Ready Salted, Potato Chips, Tesco*	1 Bag/25g	131	8.2	526	5.6	51.7	33.0	3.8
Ready Salted, Reduced Fat, Tesco*	1 Pack/25g	114	6.2	456	6.3	52.0	24.7	5.9
Ready Salted, Ridge Cut, McCoys*	1 Bag/49g	257	15.6	524	6.6	52.6	31.9	4.1
Ready Salted, Sainsbury's*	1 Bag/25g	134	9.2	538	4.3	47.4	36.8	4.1
Ready Salted, Select, Tesco*	1 Bag/25g	136	9.1	544	6.2	47.9	36.6	4.5
Ready Salted, Snack Rite*	1 Bag/25g	136	9.0	545	4.9	50.3	36.0	0.0
Ready Salted, Squares, M & S*	1 Bag/35g	150	6.3	430	6.8	63.5	18.1	3.9
Ready Salted, Squares, Walkers*	1 Pack/25g	109	4.7	435	6.5	60.0	19.0	6.0
Ready Salted, Sunseed Oil, Walkers*	1 Bag/35g	183	11.7	530	6.5	49.0	34.0	4.0
Red Leicester & Spring Onion, Handcooked, M & S*	1 Pack/40g	194	10.6	485	6.8	55.0	26.4	5.1
Ridge, Thick & Chunky, Ready Salted, Eastmans*	1 Pack/30g	155	9.2	515	5.9	53.5	30.6	4.1
Roast Beef, KP Snacks*	1 Bag/25g	133	8.8	534	6.6	47.5	35.3	4.7
Roast Beef & Mustard, Thick Cut, Brannigans*	1 Bag/40g	203	12.0	507	7.6	51.7	30.0	3.7
Roast Chicken, 30% Less Fat, Sainsbury's*	1 Pack/25g	115	5.5	460	7.4	58.3	21.9	5.2
Roast Chicken, Golden Wonder*	1 Bag/25g	130	8.4	522	6.2	48.6	33.6	2.0
Roast Chicken, Highlander*	1 Bag/25g	138	9.7	554	5.3	46.0	38.9	5.1
Roast Chicken, Morrisons*	1 Pack/25g	131	8.2	525	5.5	51.7	32.9	4.2
Roast Chicken, Select, Tesco*	1 Bag/25g	134	8.7	536	6.6	48.6	35.0	4.4
Roast Chicken, Snack Rite*	1 Bag/25g	131	8.3	526	5.3	51.3	33.3	0.0
Roast Chicken, Sunseed Oil, Walkers*	1 Bag/35g	181	11.4	525	6.5	50.0	33.0	4.0
Roast Chicken, Tayto*	1 Bag/35g	184	11.9	526	7.6	47.3	34.0	4.5
Roast Chicken & Sage Flavour, M & S*	1 Bag/25g	135	8.6	540	5.9	50.6	34.6	4.6
Roast Chicken Flavour, BGTY, Sainsbury's*	1 Bag/25g	118	5.9	473	6.2	58.9	23.6	5.7
Roast Chicken Flavour, Crinkle, Weight Watchers*	1 Pack/16g	76	3.3	475	5.6	63.1	20.6	6.2
Roast Ham & Mustard, Ridge Cut, McCoys*	1 Pack/35g	181	10.7	518	7.1	53.5	30.6	3.9
Roast Pork & Apple Sauce, Select, Tesco*	1 Bag/25g	136	8.8	544	6.5	50.0	35.3	3.7
Salt & Balsamic Vinegar, Perfectly Balanced, Waitrose*	1 Bag/20g	69	0.5	347	4.2	76.4	2.7	5.2
Salt & Black Pepper, Handcooked, M & S*	1 Bag/40g	180	9.2	450	5.7	55.0	22.9	5.2
Salt & Cracked Black Pepper, Shapers, Boots*	1 Bag/20g	91	4.4	453	7.2	57.0	22.0	5.0
Salt & Malt Vinegar, Ridge Cut, McCoys*	1 Bag/32g	164	9.7	514	6.7	53.2	30.4	3.9
Salt & Malt Vinegar Flavour, Sainsbury's*	1 Bag/25g	134	8.8	538	4.9	50.3	35.2	2.3
Salt & Shake, Walkers*	1 Bag/30g	162	10.5	540	6.5	50.0	35.0	4.0
Salt & Vinegar, 30% Less Fat, Sainsbury's*	1 Bag/25g	114	5.4	458	7.2	58.3	21.8	5.1
Salt & Vinegar, Baked, Walkers*	1 Packet/38g	146	3.0	390	6.0	73.0	8.0	5.0
Salt & Vinegar, BGTY, Sainsbury's*	1 Bag/25g	120	6.3	482	6.5	57.3	25.2	5.2
Salt & Vinegar, Crinkle, M & S*	1 Pack/25g	120	5.9	485	6.5	61.0	24.0	3.5
Salt & Vinegar, Crinkle Cut, Low Fat, Waitrose*	1 Bag/25g	121	5.8	484	7.1	61.3	23.4	4.5
Salt & Vinegar, Crinkle Cut, Seabrook*	1 Bag/32g	181	11.7	569	5.4	54.4	36.7	3.9
Salt & Vinegar, Crinkles, Shapers, Boots*	1 Pack/20g	96	4.8	482	6.6	60.0	24.0	4.0
Salt & Vinegar, Crispy Discs, Shapers, Boots*	1 Bag/92g	404	17.5	439	4.8	63.0	19.0	4.9
Salt & Vinegar, Everyday, Co-Op*	1 Bag/17g	77	3.4	455	6.0	62.0	20.0	2.0
Salt & Vinegar, GFY, Asda*	1 Bag/26g	120	5.7	466	6.0	61.0	22.0	4.1
Salt & Vinegar, Golden Lights, Golden Wonder*	1 Bag/21g	94	3.9	446	4.2	65.7	18.5	3.7
Salt & Vinegar, Golden Wonder*	1 Bag/25g	130	8.5	522	5.4	48.5	34.0	2.0

CRISPS

	Measure INFO/WEIGHT	per Measure KCAL	FAT	Nutrition Values per 100g / 100ml KCAL	PROT	CARB	FAT	FIBRE
Salt & Vinegar, KP Snacks*	1 Bag/25g	133	8.7	532	5.5	48.7	35.0	4.7
Salt & Vinegar, Lights, Walkers*	1 Bag/28g	133	6.2	475	7.0	62.0	22.0	4.5
Salt & Vinegar, Lower Fat, Asda*	1 Bag/25g	120	6.2	481	5.0	58.0	25.0	4.8
Salt & Vinegar, M & S*	1 Bag/25g	131	8.6	525	5.4	48.8	34.5	4.6
Salt & Vinegar, Morrisons*	1 Bag/25g	129	7.8	515	4.9	53.9	31.1	3.6
Salt & Vinegar, Oven Baked, Asda*	1 Bag/25g	95	2.0	380	5.1	72.0	8.0	2.9
Salt & Vinegar, Potato Bakes, Weight Watchers*	1 Bag/20g	81	1.8	404	5.3	76.0	8.8	2.3
Salt & Vinegar, Red Mill*	1 Bag/40g	174	7.0	436	3.9	65.8	17.5	2.4
Salt & Vinegar, Rough Cuts, Tayto*	1 Bag/30g	152	9.2	506	4.6	56.8	30.8	0.0
Salt & Vinegar, Sainsbury's*	1 Bag/25g	130	8.8	522	4.1	46.9	35.3	3.9
Salt & Vinegar, Select, Tesco*	1 Bag/25g	132	8.7	529	5.9	47.8	34.9	4.3
Salt & Vinegar, Snack Rite*	1 Bag/25g	127	8.2	508	4.7	48.1	33.0	0.0
Salt & Vinegar, Space Raiders, KP Snacks*	1 Bag/17g	81	3.8	478	6.9	61.7	22.6	2.2
Salt & Vinegar, Squares, Walkers*	1 Bag/25g	107	4.5	430	6.5	61.0	18.0	5.5
Salt & Vinegar, Sunseed Oil, Walkers*	1 Bag/35g	181	11.4	525	6.5	50.0	33.0	4.0
Salt & Vinegar, Tayto*	1 Bag/35g	184	11.9	526	7.6	47.3	34.0	4.5
Salt & Vinegar, Tubes, HL, Tesco*	1 Bag/17g	61	0.3	357	3.2	82.4	1.6	3.0
Salt & Vinegar, Waitrose*	1 Pack/25g	132	8.4	529	6.3	50.5	33.8	4.4
Salt & Vinegar, Walkers*	1 Pack/25g	131	8.3	524	6.4	50.0	33.2	4.0
Salt & Vinegar Flavour, Asda*	1 Bag/25g	130	8.5	522	6.0	48.0	34.0	4.2
Salt & Vinegar Flavour, Half Fat, M & S*	1 Bag/40g	168	6.8	420	5.8	61.0	17.0	7.7
Salt & Vinegar Flavour, Sprinters*	1 Bag/25g	133	8.8	532	4.8	49.1	35.2	0.0
Salt & Vinegar Fries, COU, M & S*	1 Bag/25g	85	0.4	340	5.0	80.0	1.6	4.0
Salt & Vinegar Spirals, Shapers, Boots*	1 Pack/15g	71	3.4	475	3.1	64.0	23.0	1.7
Salt Your Own, Excluding Salt, Aldi*	1 Pack/24g	130	8.1	536	6.0	52.6	33.5	4.5
Salt Your Own, Jacket, 35% Less Fat, Sainsbury's*	1 Bag/20g	98	4.5	490	7.5	64.5	22.5	9.5
Salt Your Own, Sainsbury's*	1 Pack/24g	127	7.9	520	5.0	52.2	32.3	3.7
Salt Your Own, Snackrite, Aldi*	1 Pack/24g	130	8.1	536	6.0	52.6	33.5	4.5
Salted Tubes, Shapers, Boots*	1 Bag/15g	67	3.0	448	5.1	62.0	20.0	3.6
Sausage & Tomato, Sainsbury's*	1 Pack/25g	131	8.4	525	6.0	49.3	33.8	3.8
Sausage & Tomato Flavour, Golden Wonder*	1 Bag/35g	174	10.6	505	6.1	51.3	30.6	4.5
Scotch Bonnet Flavour, Mackies of Scotland*	1 Pack/150g	732	369.0	488	78.0	574.0	246.0	42.0
Sea Salt, Golden Lights, Golden Wonder*	1 Bag/21g	94	3.9	448	3.9	66.4	18.5	4.4
Sea Salt, Gourmet, TTD, Sainsbury's*	1/3 Pack/50g	249	15.0	498	5.7	51.4	30.0	6.4
Sea Salt, Handcooked, Extra Special, Asda*	1 Pack/31g	149	7.8	477	7.0	56.0	25.0	4.1
Sea Salt, Original, Crinkle Cut, Seabrook*	1 Bag/32g	181	11.7	569	5.4	54.4	36.7	3.9
Sea Salt & Balsamic Vinegar, Kettle Chips*	1 Bag/40g	190	10.0	476	5.9	56.8	25.0	4.5
Sea Salt & Black Pepper, GFY, Asda*	1 Bag/100g	476	24.0	476	6.0	59.0	24.0	6.0
Sea Salt & Black Pepper, Shapers, Boots*	1 Bag/20g	96	4.8	482	6.6	60.0	24.0	4.0
Sea Salt & Black Pepper, Tyrrells*	1/4 Pack/38g	182	9.3	480	7.3	59.9	24.5	2.4
Sea Salt & Cider Vinegar, TTD, Sainsbury's*	1/3 Pack/50g	245	14.3	489	5.5	52.7	28.5	6.1
Sea Salt & Cracked Black Pepper, Lights, Walkers*	1 Bag/24g	115	5.3	480	7.0	63.0	22.0	5.0
Sea Salt & Indian Black Pepper, Pipers Crisps*	1 Pack/40g	195	11.6	487	6.6	49.9	29.0	0.0
Sea Salt & Malt Vinegar, Sensations, Walkers*	1 Bag/40g	194	10.8	485	6.5	54.0	27.0	4.5
Sea Salt & Modena Balsamic Vinegar, Darling Spuds*	1 Bag/40g	190	11.4	475	5.4	54.3	28.5	4.2
Shells, Prawn Cocktail, Asda*	1 Bag/18g	90	5.3	501	4.6	54.9	29.2	6.2
Simply Salted, Extra Crunchy, Walkers*	1 Bag/30g	142	6.5	473	6.8	59.8	21.8	5.0
Simply Salted, Lights, Walkers*	1 Bag/24g	113	5.3	470	7.0	61.0	22.0	5.0
Sizzling Beef, Spice, McCoys*	1 Bag/35g	175	10.4	501	6.4	51.7	29.8	4.0
Sizzling King Prawn, Ridge Cut, McCoys*	1 Pack/50g	259	15.1	518	6.6	54.7	30.3	4.0
Smoked Ham & Pickle, Thick Cut, Brannigans*	1 Bag/40g	203	11.9	507	7.0	52.8	29.8	3.8
Smokey Bacon, Crinkle, Shapers, Boots*	1 Pack/20g	96	4.8	482	6.6	60.0	24.0	4.0
Smokey Bacon, Seabrook*	1 Bag/32g	181	11.7	569	5.4	54.4	36.7	3.9

CRISPS

INFO/WEIGHT	per Measure KCAL	per Measure FAT	KCAL	PROT	CARB	FAT	FIBRE

	Measure INFO/WEIGHT	per Measure KCAL	per Measure FAT	Nutrition Values per 100g / 100ml KCAL	PROT	CARB	FAT	FIBRE
Smokey Bacon, Select, Tesco*	1 Bag/25g	134	8.7	536	6.4	49.0	34.9	4.3
Smokey Bacon Potato Hoops, COU, M & S*	1 Pack/16g	58	0.4	360	5.6	78.7	2.7	4.5
Smoky Bacon, 30% Lower Fat, Sainsbury's*	1 Bag/25g	118	5.9	471	6.5	58.4	23.6	5.7
Smoky Bacon, Asda*	1 Bag/25g	132	8.5	530	6.0	50.0	34.0	4.5
Smoky Bacon, BGTY, Sainsbury's*	1 Bag/25g	118	5.9	472	6.5	58.5	23.6	5.7
Smoky Bacon, Golden Wonder*	1 Bag/25g	131	8.4	523	5.9	49.1	33.7	2.0
Smoky Bacon, Sainsbury's*	1 Bag/25g	132	8.5	529	5.7	49.5	34.2	4.4
Smoky Bacon, Snack Rite*	1 Bag/25g	131	8.3	525	5.5	51.2	33.1	0.0
Smoky Bacon, Sunseed Oil, Walkers*	1 Bag/35g	183	11.4	530	6.5	51.0	33.0	4.0
Smoky Bacon, Tayto*	1 Bag/35g	184	11.9	526	7.6	47.3	34.0	4.5
Snaps, Spicy Tomato Flavour, Walkers*	1 Bag/18g	91	4.8	508	1.5	65.5	26.8	0.0
Snax, Tayto*	1 Pack/17g	82	3.7	483	2.4	70.0	21.5	1.6
Sour Cream & Chive, Crinkle, Reduced Fat, M & S*	1 Bag/40g	178	8.2	445	5.6	58.8	20.6	5.6
Sour Cream & Chive, Lights, Walkers*	1 Bag/24g	114	5.3	475	7.5	62.0	22.0	5.0
Sour Cream & Chive, Perfectly Balanced, Waitrose*	1 Pack/20g	69	0.5	347	4.4	76.3	2.7	5.2
Sour Cream & Chive, Potato Bakes, Weight Watchers*	1 Bag/20g	83	1.8	417	3.8	80.7	8.8	3.6
Sour Cream & Chive, Potato Bites, BGTY, Sainsbury's*	1 Pack/20g	73	0.6	365	7.2	77.8	2.8	3.9
Sour Cream & Chive Baked Potato, COU, M & S*	1 Pack/24g	84	0.7	350	7.5	73.2	2.8	7.9
Sour Cream & Chive Crispy Discs, Shapers, Boots*	1 Bag/21g	94	4.0	448	5.7	61.9	19.0	4.3
Sour Cream & Chives, Jordans*	1 Bag/30g	125	3.6	417	7.3	69.9	12.0	2.7
Sour Cream & Onion, Golden Lights, Golden Wonder*	1 Bag/21g	93	3.8	442	4.1	66.0	17.9	4.4
Space Raiders, Pickled Onion, KP Snacks*	1 Bag/16g	77	3.7	480	6.7	61.3	23.3	4.0
Spare Rib Flavour, Chinese, Walkers*	1 Bag/35g	181	11.4	525	6.5	50.0	33.0	4.0
Spiced Chilli, McCoys*	1 Bag/35g	175	10.1	500	6.1	54.2	28.8	4.2
Spicy Chilli, Sunseed, Walkers*	1 Pack/35g	183	11.4	530	6.5	51.0	33.0	4.0
Spring Onion, Seabrook*	1 Bag/32g	182	11.7	569	5.4	54.4	36.7	3.9
Spring Onion Flavour, M & S*	1 Bag/40g	210	13.7	525	5.9	48.7	34.3	5.1
Spring Onion Flavour, Tayto*	1 Bag/35g	184	11.9	526	7.6	47.3	34.0	4.5
Steak & Onion, Walkers*	1 Pack/35g	179	11.4	520	6.5	49.0	33.0	4.0
Sun Bites, Wholegrain, Lightly Sea Salted, Walkers*	1 Bag/25g	120	5.4	481	7.5	60.7	21.7	6.6
Sun Dried Tomato & Basil, Jonathan Crisp*	1 Pack/35g	176	10.1	503	5.6	52.0	29.0	5.4
Sun Dried Tomato & Chilli, Asda*	1 Pack/150g	700	34.5	467	7.0	58.0	23.0	4.1
Sunbites, Cheddar & Caramelised Onion, Walkers*	1 Bag/25g	120	5.4	480	7.6	60.8	21.6	6.4
Sunbites, Sweet Chilli, Sun Ripened, Walkers*	1 Bag/25g	120	5.4	480	7.6	60.8	21.6	6.4
Superbly Spiced, Cassava, Gluten Free, Hale & Hearty*	1 Bag/30g	136	7.0	453	3.3	56.7	23.3	6.7
Sweet Chill, Mexican, Phileas Fogg*	1 Bag/38g	193	11.0	507	6.7	54.8	29.0	4.2
Sweet Chilli, Baked Potato, COU, M & S*	1 Bag/26g	91	0.7	350	7.6	73.9	2.8	8.5
Sweet Chilli, Crinkle Cut, Weight Watchers*	1 Bag/20g	80	1.9	400	4.5	74.5	9.5	4.0
Sweet Chilli, Hand Cooked, Asda*	1 Pack/25g	120	7.1	479	5.7	54.5	28.3	4.5
Sweet Chilli & Red Peppers, Fusion, Tayto*	1 Bag/28g	140	8.3	500	4.9	52.2	29.8	4.6
Sweet Chilli Chicken, Extra Crunchy, Walkers*	1 Bag/30g	143	6.7	477	6.5	59.9	22.5	4.8
T Bone Steak, Roysters*	1 Pack/28g	148	9.0	530	5.2	55.3	32.0	3.0
Tangy Malaysian Chutney, Sensations, Walkers*	1 Bag/24g	116	6.2	485	0.9	62.0	26.0	0.0
Tangy Tom & Red Pepper Salsa, Sensations, Walkers*	1 Bag/35g	168	9.4	480	6.5	53.0	27.0	4.5
Tangy Toms, Red Mill*	1 Bag/15g	76	4.1	507	6.0	60.0	27.3	0.7
Thai Curry & Coriander, Tyrrells*	1 Pack/50g	261	13.9	522	6.1	56.5	27.9	5.4
Thai Sweet Chicken, Ridge Cut, McCoys*	1 Bag/50g	257	15.0	514	7.0	54.0	30.0	4.1
Thai Sweet Chilli, Sensations, Walkers*	1 Bag/40g	194	10.4	485	6.0	57.0	26.0	4.2
Thai Sweet Chilli Flavour, Velvet Crunch, King*	1 Pack/20g	81	1.9	404	1.6	77.5	9.7	2.0
Tomato & Basil, Mediterranean, Walkers*	1 Pack/25g	127	8.2	510	6.5	49.0	33.0	4.5
Tomato & Herb, Shapers, Boots*	1 Bag/20g	94	4.2	468	3.7	66.0	21.0	3.9
Tomato Sauce, Golden Wonder*	1 Bag/25g	130	8.4	521	5.7	49.2	33.5	2.0
Tortillas, Nacho Cheese Flavour, Weight Watchers*	1 Pack/18g	78	2.9	433	6.1	66.7	16.1	3.9

C

	Measure INFO/WEIGHT	per Measure KCAL	per Measure FAT	Nutrition Values per 100g / 100ml KCAL	PROT	CARB	FAT	FIBRE
CRISPS								
Traditional, Hand Cooked, Finest, Tesco*	1 Bag/150g	708	39.1	472	6.4	52.9	26.1	5.1
Turkey & Paxo, Walkers*	1 Bag/35g	181	11.4	525	6.4	50.1	33.0	4.1
Vegetable, Crunchy, Asda*	½ Bag/50g	251	12.0	502	1.4	70.0	24.0	6.0
Vegetable, TTD, Sainsbury's*	½ Pack/52g	254	17.9	490	4.8	39.9	34.5	12.8
Vegetable, Waitrose*	1 Pack/100g	490	35.2	490	4.7	38.5	35.2	13.0
Wild Chilli, McCoys*	1 Bag/50g	255	15.1	510	6.0	53.2	30.3	4.8
Wild Paprika Flavour, Croky*	1 Pack/45g	234	13.0	521	6.0	58.0	29.0	0.0
Worcester Sauce, Sunseed Oil, Walkers*	1 Bag/35g	183	11.4	530	6.5	52.0	33.0	4.0
Worcester Sauce Flavour, Hunky Dorys*	1 Bag/45g	211	12.9	469	6.3	49.3	28.7	0.0
Wotsits, Really Cheesy, Walkers*	1 Pack/17g	93	5.6	547	5.5	56.0	33.0	1.1
CRISPY PANCAKE								
Beef Bolognese, Findus*	1 Pancake/65g	104	2.6	160	6.5	25.0	4.0	1.0
Chicken, Bacon & Sweetcorn, Findus*	1 Pancake/63g	101	2.5	160	5.5	26.0	4.0	1.1
Minced Beef, Findus*	1 Pancake/63g	100	2.5	160	6.5	25.0	4.0	1.0
Three Cheeses, Findus*	1 Pancake/62g	118	4.0	190	7.0	25.0	6.5	0.9
CROISSANT								
All Butter, BGTY, Sainsbury's*	1 Croissant/44g	151	6.5	343	9.3	42.7	14.8	1.8
All Butter, Finest, Tesco*	1 Croissant/77g	328	18.2	426	8.6	44.9	23.6	1.9
All Butter, M & S*	1 Croissant/54g	222	12.8	415	7.4	45.2	23.8	1.6
All Butter, Mini, Sainsbury's*	1 Croissant/35g	150	8.6	428	9.2	42.6	24.5	1.2
All Butter, Mini, Tesco*	1 Croissant/35g	150	8.2	430	9.3	45.2	23.5	2.0
All Butter, Reduced Fat, Tesco*	1 Croissant/52g	164	5.5	315	7.5	47.4	10.6	1.8
All Butter, Sainsbury's*	1 Croissant/44g	188	10.8	428	9.2	42.6	24.5	1.2
All Butter, Tesco*	1 Croissant/48g	192	10.4	400	8.5	41.7	21.6	2.6
Average	1 Croissant/50g	180	10.1	360	8.3	38.3	20.3	1.6
Butter, Asda*	1 Croissant/46g	191	11.0	416	8.0	42.0	24.0	1.9
Butter, GFY, Asda*	1 Croissant/44g	153	7.0	352	6.0	46.0	16.0	2.0
Butter, Morrisons*	1 Croissant/44g	196	12.5	446	9.3	38.2	28.4	2.0
Butter, Part Bake, Morrisons*	1 Croissant/45g	179	8.5	397	7.3	49.6	18.8	1.9
Butter, Part Baked, De Graaf*	1 Croissant/45g	170	8.4	378	7.3	45.2	18.7	0.0
Cheese & Ham, Mini, Waitrose*	1 Croissant/17g	64	4.1	383	13.2	28.1	24.5	3.0
Continental, Mini, Chosen By You, Asda*	1 Croissant/35g	150	8.9	427	9.2	40.6	25.3	1.6
Flaky Pastry with a Plain Chocolate Filling, Tesco*	1 Croissant/78g	318	19.0	408	6.5	41.0	24.3	2.0
Heart Shaped, Breakfast in Bed, M & S*	1 Croissant/54g	230	13.6	430	8.2	43.7	25.5	1.2
Homebake, Long Life, Stay Fresh Range, Harvestime*	1 Croissant/44g	159	6.0	362	7.6	51.9	13.7	1.9
Low Fat, M & S*	1 Croissant/45g	180	9.1	400	8.2	46.0	20.2	1.8
Organic, Tesco*	1 Croissant/45g	195	11.6	433	8.2	42.0	25.8	2.2
Reduced Fat, Sainsbury's*	1 Croissant/44g	173	7.7	393	9.8	49.2	17.5	2.2
TTD, Sainsbury's*	1 Croissant/70g	289	16.1	413	8.1	43.4	23.0	2.5
Wholesome, Sainsbury's*	1 Croissant/44g	192	12.1	436	8.8	38.3	27.5	4.0
CROQUETTES								
Morrisons*	1 Serving/150g	231	8.1	154	3.3	23.1	5.4	1.1
Potato, Birds Eye*	1 Croquette/29g	44	1.7	152	2.6	22.6	5.7	1.2
Potato, Chunky, Aunt Bessie's*	1 Serving/41g	62	2.5	152	2.3	23.9	6.1	1.8
Potato, Fried in Blended Oil, Average	1 Croquette/80g	171	10.5	214	3.7	21.6	13.1	1.3
Potato, M & S*	1 Croquette/41g	68	3.6	165	2.4	19.3	8.8	2.2
Potato, Sainsbury's*	1 Croquette/28g	50	2.4	180	2.8	22.6	8.6	2.5
Potato, Waitrose*	1 Croquette/30g	47	2.4	157	3.0	17.9	8.1	1.5
Vegetable, Sainsbury's*	1 Serving/175g	392	20.8	224	5.8	23.3	11.9	2.2
CROUTONS								
Fresh, M & S*	1 Serving/10g	53	3.3	530	11.4	50.0	32.8	3.2
Garlic, Waitrose*	1 Serving/40g	209	12.0	522	10.8	52.1	30.0	2.7
Herb, Sainsbury's*	1 Serving/15g	64	1.7	429	13.4	68.2	11.4	2.8

	Measure INFO/WEIGHT	per Measure KCAL	FAT	Nutrition Values per 100g / 100ml KCAL	PROT	CARB	FAT	FIBRE
CROUTONS								
Herb & Garlic, La Rochelle*	¼ Pack/18g	106	7.2	587	6.9	49.8	40.0	2.1
Italian Salad, Sainsbury's*	1 Pack/40g	204	10.0	510	8.5	62.7	25.0	2.5
La Rochelle*	1 Bag/70g	400	28.0	572	7.0	49.0	40.0	0.0
Lightly Sea Salted, Asda*	1 Serving/20g	83	1.9	414	12.9	69.7	9.3	4.3
Migros*	1 Serving/15g	56	0.4	375	14.0	72.0	3.0	3.5
Sun Dried Tomato, Sainsbury's*	¼ Pack/15g	75	3.8	497	11.7	55.2	25.5	2.5
CRUDITE								
Platter, Sainsbury's*	1 Pack/275g	96	0.8	35	1.4	6.6	0.3	1.6
Selection, Prepared, M & S*	1 Serving/250g	75	1.0	30	1.4	5.8	0.4	2.0
Vegetable Sticks, Average	1 Serving/100g	24	0.2	24	0.7	4.5	0.2	1.9
CRUMBLE								
Apple, Co-Op*	¼ Crumble/110g	269	7.7	245	2.0	43.0	7.0	2.0
Apple, Fresh, Chilled, Tesco*	¼ Pack/150g	367	13.3	245	2.8	38.0	8.9	1.4
Apple, Frozen, Iceland*	1 Serving/97g	240	9.8	247	2.1	36.9	10.1	1.8
Apple, Frozen, Tesco*	¼ Pack/150g	345	16.3	230	2.1	30.7	10.9	3.9
Apple, Iceland*	1 Pie/45g	175	7.0	389	4.0	58.4	15.6	2.0
Apple, Sainsbury's*	1 Crumble/565g	1034	32.8	183	2.3	30.5	5.8	2.9
Apple, Sara Lee*	1 Serving/200g	606	18.0	303	2.3	53.3	9.0	1.2
Apple, Waitrose*	1 Serving/125g	310	2.9	248	2.2	54.5	2.3	1.2
Apple, with Sultanas, Weight Watchers*	1 Dessert/110g	196	4.3	178	1.4	34.2	3.9	1.3
Apple & Blackberry, Asda*	1 Serving/175g	427	15.7	244	2.7	38.0	9.0	1.2
Apple & Blackberry, M & S*	1 Serving/135g	398	15.1	295	3.5	44.9	11.2	1.6
Apple & Blackberry, Sainsbury's*	1 Serving/110g	232	6.2	211	3.0	37.1	5.6	2.1
Apple & Blackberry, Tesco*	1 Crumble/335g	737	32.2	220	2.8	30.7	9.6	2.0
Apple & Custard, Asda*	1 Serving/125g	250	8.7	200	2.3	32.0	7.0	0.0
Apple & Toffee, Weight Watchers*	1 Pot/98g	190	4.5	194	1.6	36.6	4.6	0.0
Apple with Custard, Green's*	1 Serving/79g	171	5.3	216	1.9	37.0	6.7	1.2
Apple with Custard, Individual, Sainsbury's*	1 Pudding/120g	286	13.9	238	2.0	31.4	11.6	2.4
Bramley Apple, Chosen By You, Asda*	1 Serving/100g	257	8.4	257	2.5	41.8	8.4	2.3
Bramley Apple, Favourites, M & S*	1 Serving/140g	390	13.8	279	4.6	43.2	9.9	1.2
Bramley Apple, M & S*	1 Serving/149g	387	13.7	260	4.3	40.3	9.2	1.1
Bramley Apple, Tesco*	1/3 Pack/155g	378	14.9	244	2.8	36.7	9.6	1.8
Cauliflower & Camembert, Sainsbury's*	1 Pack/400g	588	43.2	147	5.5	6.9	10.8	0.7
Fish & Prawn, Youngs*	1 Pie/375g	476	27.0	127	5.8	9.7	7.2	1.3
Fruit	1 Portion/170g	337	11.7	198	2.0	34.0	6.9	1.7
Fruit, Wholemeal	1oz/28g	54	2.0	193	2.6	31.7	7.1	2.7
Fruit with Custard	1 Serving/270g	463	17.6	171	2.4	27.0	6.5	1.3
Gooseberry, M & S*	1 Serving/133g	379	14.2	285	3.5	43.3	10.7	1.7
Ocean, Low Fat, Light & Easy, Youngs*	½ Pie/150g	130	2.8	87	4.6	12.9	1.9	1.7
Ocean, Low Fat, Ross*	1 Crumble/300g	219	2.4	73	5.1	11.4	0.8	0.4
Rhubarb, Asda*	½ Crumble/200g	460	24.0	230	2.4	28.0	12.0	5.0
Rhubarb, Co-Op*	¼ Crumble/110g	269	7.7	245	2.0	42.0	7.0	1.0
Rhubarb, M & S*	1 Serving/133g	366	13.2	275	3.4	42.6	9.9	1.4
Rhubarb, Sainsbury's*	1 Serving/50g	112	2.8	224	3.1	40.4	5.6	1.8
Rhubarb, with Custard, Sainsbury's*	1 Serving/120g	288	13.9	240	2.4	31.4	11.6	2.3
Salmon, Youngs*	1 Pie/360g	367	14.4	102	5.4	11.1	4.0	1.0
CRUMPETS								
Asda*	1 Crumpet/45g	85	0.4	188	6.0	39.0	0.9	2.1
Co-Op*	1 Crumpet/40g	70	0.3	175	7.0	35.0	0.7	2.0
Essential, Waitrose*	1 Crumpet/41g	77	0.4	187	5.9	38.8	0.9	2.3
Fruit, From Bakery, Tesco*	1 Crumpet/73g	161	1.7	220	6.2	43.2	2.3	1.1
Gluten, Wheat & Milk Free, Free From, Livwell*	1 Crumpet/55g	83	1.7	151	3.6	26.9	3.1	2.0
Kingsmill*	1 Crumpet/55g	99	0.4	180	5.8	37.5	0.8	1.7

CRUMPETS								
Less Than 2% Fat, M & S*	1 Crumpet/61g	116	0.8	190	8.0	36.9	1.3	2.1
Morning Fresh*	1 Crumpet/20g	36	0.3	180	7.3	34.8	1.3	5.2
Morrisons*	1 Crumpet/40g	70	0.3	174	6.6	35.3	0.7	1.8
Mother's Pride*	1 Crumpet/43g	80	0.4	185	5.6	38.3	1.0	2.3
Perfectly Balanced, Waitrose*	1 Crumpet/55g	94	0.2	171	6.1	36.1	0.3	4.4
Premium, Sainsbury's*	1 Crumpet/50g	95	0.7	191	6.1	38.6	1.4	1.7
Sainsbury's*	1 Crumpet/46g	86	0.3	186	5.8	39.1	0.7	2.5
Soldier, Mother's Pride*	1 Crumpet/30g	58	0.5	193	7.8	37.1	1.6	1.6
Square, SpongeBob Square Pants*	1 Crumpet/50g	93	0.5	186	7.0	37.2	1.0	1.0
Square, Tesco*	1 Crumpet/60g	101	0.5	168	6.3	33.8	0.8	2.7
Toasted, Average	1 Crumpet/40g	80	0.4	199	6.7	43.4	1.0	2.0
Toasted, Tesco*	1 Crumpet/65g	120	0.6	185	5.2	37.9	0.9	3.7
Toaster, Organic, Waitrose*	1 Crumpet/55g	95	0.3	172	7.3	34.4	0.6	4.6
TTD, Sainsbury's*	1 Crumpet/65g	124	1.0	191	5.9	38.5	1.5	2.3
Waitrose*	1 Crumpet/62g	116	0.7	188	6.3	37.9	1.2	2.1
Warburton's*	1 Crumpet/55g	95	0.4	173	5.6	36.1	0.7	2.3
CRUNCHIE								
Blast, Cadbury*	1 Serving/42g	199	8.3	480	4.7	69.6	20.1	0.7
Cadbury*	1 Bar/40g	186	7.6	465	4.0	69.5	18.9	0.5
Nuggets, Cadbury*	1 Bag/125g	569	20.5	455	3.8	73.1	16.4	0.0
Treat Size, Cadbury*	1 Treat Bar/17g	80	3.1	470	4.0	71.5	18.4	0.0
CRUNCHY STICKS								
Ready Salted, M & S*	1 Pack/75g	397	24.7	530	5.6	52.2	33.0	3.8
Ready Salted, Tesco*	1 Serving/25g	119	5.9	475	5.6	60.3	23.5	3.0
Salt & Vinegar, Sainsbury's*	1 Bag/25g	118	6.1	474	5.9	58.0	24.3	2.4
Salt & Vinegar, Shapers, Boots*	1 Pack/21g	96	3.8	457	5.7	66.7	18.1	2.4
Salt & Vinegar, Tesco*	1 Serving/25g	117	6.1	470	6.9	55.7	24.4	2.7
CUCUMBER								
Average	*1 Serving/80g*	*8*	*0.1*	*10*	*0.7*	*1.5*	*0.1*	*0.6*
CUMIN								
Seeds, Ground, Schwartz*	1 Tsp/5g	22	1.2	446	19.0	40.3	23.2	0.0
Seeds, Whole, Average	*1 Tsp/2g*	*7*	*0.5*	*375*	*17.8*	*44.2*	*22.7*	*10.5*
CUPCAKES								
Assorted, Sainsbury's*	1 Cake/38g	130	2.3	341	2.2	69.3	6.1	0.4
Chocolate, 5% Fat, Sainsbury's*	1 Cake/38g	133	1.7	349	2.5	74.8	4.4	1.7
Chocolate, BGTY, Sainsbury's*	1 Cake/38g	121	1.7	318	2.5	66.5	4.6	0.8
Chocolate, COU, M & S*	1 Cake/45g	130	1.3	290	4.6	62.2	2.8	4.3
Chocolate, Fabulous Bakin' Boys*	1 Cupcake/34g	152	8.1	448	4.0	54.0	24.0	1.0
Chocolate, Lyons*	1 Cake/39g	125	1.8	321	2.4	67.5	4.6	0.8
Chocolate, Mini, Weight Watchers*	1 Cupcake/20g	87	4.3	426	6.1	52.0	21.1	1.8
Lemon, COU, M & S*	1 Cupcake/43g	130	0.9	305	3.3	68.1	2.1	2.0
Lemon, Mini, Weight Watchers*	1 Cupcake/17g	56	0.8	333	2.4	63.3	4.9	12.1
Mini, Jack O' Lantern, Vanilla Iced, The Cookieman Ltd*	1 Cupcake/25g	105	3.8	419	2.4	66.8	15.3	2.0
Pink, M & S*	1 Cupcake/39g	160	3.3	410	2.5	81.3	8.5	0.6
CURACAO								
Average	*1 Shot/35ml*	*109*	*0.0*	*311*	*0.0*	*28.3*	*0.0*	*0.0*
CURLY WURLY								
Cadbury*	1 Bar/26g	115	4.5	442	3.5	69.2	17.3	0.8
Squirlies, Cadbury*	1 Squirl/3g	13	0.5	442	3.5	69.2	17.3	0.8
CURRANTS								
Average	*1oz/28g*	*75*	*0.1*	*267*	*2.3*	*67.8*	*0.4*	*1.9*
CURRY								
Aubergine	1oz/28g	33	2.8	118	1.4	6.2	10.1	1.5

CURRY

INFO/WEIGHT	Measure	per Measure KCAL	per Measure FAT	Nutrition Values per 100g / 100ml KCAL	PROT	CARB	FAT	FIBRE
Beef, Hot, Canned, M & S*	1 Can/425g	446	21.7	105	12.2	2.8	5.1	1.0
Beef, Sainsbury's*	1 Serving/400g	552	32.8	138	10.7	5.4	8.2	0.9
Beef, Thai, Finest, Tesco*	1 Serving/500g	770	29.0	154	9.0	16.5	5.8	1.2
Beef, with Rice, Asda*	1 Pack/406g	548	15.8	135	6.0	19.0	3.9	1.2
Beef, with Rice, Birds Eye*	1 Pack/388g	524	10.9	135	6.9	20.8	2.8	0.8
Beef, with Rice, Healthy Choice, Asda*	1 Pack/400g	476	10.4	119	6.0	18.0	2.6	0.9
Beef, with Rice, Iceland*	1 Pack/400g	404	6.8	101	6.7	14.7	1.7	1.0
Beef, with Rice, Morrisons*	1 Serving/400g	480	20.0	120	6.0	12.6	5.0	0.6
Beef, with Rice, Tesco*	1 Pack/400g	456	13.2	114	4.5	16.7	3.3	0.6
Beef, with Rice, Weight Watchers*	1 Pack/328g	249	3.3	76	4.2	12.5	1.0	0.3
Beef & Rice, Chosen By You, Asda*	1 Pack/400g	452	7.6	113	4.6	18.6	1.9	1.6
Biryani, Lamb	1 Serving/100g	195	9.7	195	7.3	20.9	9.7	0.0
Blackeye Bean, Gujerati	1oz/28g	36	1.2	127	7.2	16.1	4.4	2.8
Bombay Butternut Squash, Veg Pot, Innocent*	1 Pot/380g	403	9.9	106	3.1	15.4	2.6	4.1
Bombay Squash, Innocent*	1 Pot/380g	296	4.2	78	2.6	12.5	1.1	4.1
Cabbage	1oz/28g	23	1.4	82	1.9	8.1	5.0	2.1
Cauliflower & Chickpea, Lovely Vegetables, M & S*	1 Serving/390g	351	13.6	90	2.9	11.2	3.5	3.7
Cauliflower & Potato	1oz/28g	17	0.7	59	3.4	6.6	2.4	1.8
Chana Dahl, Curry Special*	1 Pack/350g	434	22.7	124	6.0	10.5	6.5	5.9
Chick Pea, Red Pepper & Spinach, Cranks*	1 Pack/300g	249	13.5	83	3.0	7.6	4.5	2.8
Chick Pea, Whole, Average	1oz/28g	50	2.1	179	9.6	21.3	7.5	4.5
Chick Pea, Whole, Basic, Average	1oz/28g	30	1.0	108	6.0	14.2	3.6	3.3
Chicken, & Rice, International Cuisine*	1 Serving/400g	420	11.6	105	3.3	16.4	2.9	0.8
Chicken, Asda*	1 Can/200g	210	10.0	105	10.0	5.0	5.0	0.0
Chicken, Canned, Sainsbury's*	1 Serving/100g	136	6.1	136	11.1	9.1	6.1	1.0
Chicken, Chinese with Egg Fried Rice, Morrisons*	1 Pack/500g	600	15.5	120	5.7	17.4	3.1	0.9
Chicken, Diet Chef Ltd*	1 Portion/300g	342	13.2	114	9.1	9.5	4.4	1.0
Chicken, Green Thai, BGTY, Sainsbury's*	1 Pack/400g	316	10.4	79	10.6	3.4	2.6	1.9
Chicken, Green Thai, Birds Eye*	1 Pack/450g	535	19.8	119	4.7	15.2	4.4	0.3
Chicken, Green Thai, Breasts, Finest, Tesco*	1 Serving/200g	292	16.0	146	16.5	2.0	8.0	0.7
Chicken, Green Thai, Jasmine Rice, Weight Watchers*	1 Pack/320g	291	3.2	91	6.1	14.3	1.0	0.5
Chicken, Green Thai, Sainsbury's*	½ Pack/200g	264	13.6	132	13.0	4.8	6.8	0.9
Chicken, Green Thai Style, & Sticky Rice, Asda*	1 Pack/450g	585	10.8	130	7.0	20.0	2.4	0.1
Chicken, Healthy Options, Birds Eye*	1 Pack/350g	336	3.1	96	5.1	16.8	0.9	0.5
Chicken, Hot, Can, Tesco*	1 Can/418g	514	26.3	123	9.7	6.9	6.3	0.9
Chicken, Hot, Canned, Asda*	1 Can/398g	501	23.9	126	11.0	7.0	6.0	0.5
Chicken, Hot, Iceland*	1 Can/392g	492	20.4	126	9.9	9.8	5.2	0.7
Chicken, Kashmiri, Waitrose*	1 Serving/400g	640	36.4	160	14.5	5.0	9.1	0.6
Chicken, Medium Hot, M & S*	1 Serving/200g	310	14.2	155	7.8	14.3	7.1	0.8
Chicken, Mild, Asda*	½ Can/190g	239	11.4	126	11.0	7.0	6.0	0.5
Chicken, Mild, BGTY, Sainsbury's*	1 Serving/200g	184	5.2	92	10.0	7.2	2.6	0.5
Chicken, Mild, Canned, Bilash*	½ Can/200g	180	7.6	90	9.5	4.5	3.8	0.7
Chicken, Mild, Iceland*	½ Can/200g	234	9.0	117	10.6	8.5	4.5	0.7
Chicken, Mild, Sainsbury's*	1 Can/400g	472	27.6	118	10.5	3.5	6.9	1.3
Chicken, Mild, Tinned, Sainsbury's*	1 Serving/200g	214	7.0	107	12.7	6.1	3.5	1.1
Chicken, Red Thai, 97% Fat Free, Birds Eye*	1 Pack/366g	425	7.0	116	5.7	19.0	1.9	0.5
Chicken, Red Thai, Asda*	1 Pack/360g	461	27.7	128	9.1	5.5	7.7	1.0
Chicken, Red Thai, COU, M & S*	1 Pack/400g	420	9.2	105	7.1	13.4	2.3	1.4
Chicken, Red Thai, Tesco*	1 Serving/175g	215	11.5	123	10.5	5.5	6.6	1.4
Chicken, Red Thai, with Rice, Tesco*	1 Serving/475g	746	32.3	157	7.2	16.8	6.8	1.1
Chicken, Reduced Fat, Asda*	1 Pack/400g	476	10.4	119	6.0	18.0	2.6	0.9
Chicken, Thai, Red, GFY, Asda*	1 Serving/400g	364	8.4	91	6.0	12.0	2.1	1.6
Chicken, Thai, Tom Yum, Sainsbury's*	1 Pot/400g	416	20.4	104	11.1	3.5	5.1	1.9

CURRENT

INFO/WEIGHT	Measure	per Measure KCAL	FAT	Nutrition Values per 100g / 100ml KCAL	PROT	CARB	FAT	FIBRE

CURRY

	Measure INFO/WEIGHT	per Measure KCAL	FAT	KCAL	PROT	CARB	FAT	FIBRE
Chicken, Thai, with Rice, Oriental Express*	1 Pack/340g	303	4.4	89	4.1	15.3	1.3	1.2
Chicken, Thai Green, Nutritionally Balanced, M & S*	1 Pack/400g	400	5.2	100	9.2	12.4	1.3	1.4
Chicken, Thai Mango, Sainsbury's*	½ Pack/200g	288	17.8	144	11.2	4.8	8.9	1.9
Chicken, Thai Peanut, Sainsbury's*	½ Pack/200g	314	19.2	157	12.8	4.9	9.6	1.2
Chicken, Weight Watchers*	1 Pack/320g	307	4.8	96	5.3	15.4	1.5	0.1
Chicken, with Naan Bread, Iceland*	1 Portion/260g	484	16.4	186	10.1	22.3	6.3	1.4
Chicken, with Potatoes, Diet Chef Ltd*	1 Pack/300g	291	13.2	97	7.5	6.9	4.4	2.8
Chicken, with Rice, Asda*	1 Pack/400g	492	12.0	123	6.0	18.0	3.0	1.0
Chicken, with Rice, Birds Eye*	1 Pack/400g	468	11.2	117	4.5	18.4	2.8	0.6
Chicken, with Rice, Dunnes Stores*	1 Pack/375g	400	6.3	107	4.2	20.2	1.7	0.8
Chicken, with Rice, Fresh, Co-Op*	1 Pack/300g	270	9.0	90	3.0	13.0	3.0	1.0
Chicken, with Rice, Frozen, Sainsbury's*	1 Pack/400g	528	10.0	132	6.5	20.8	2.5	1.7
Chicken, with Rice, Frozen, Tesco*	1 Pack/400g	488	15.6	122	4.6	17.2	3.9	0.7
Chicken, with Rice, Fruity, HL, Tesco*	1 Pack/450g	495	5.4	110	6.5	18.2	1.2	1.2
Chicken, with Rice, Hot, Asda*	1 Pack/400g	476	12.0	119	5.0	18.0	3.0	1.0
Chicken, with Rice, Iceland*	1 Pack/500g	566	14.8	113	5.2	16.4	3.0	1.2
Chicken, with Rice, Malaysian, Bernard Matthews*	1 Pack/400g	512	15.6	128	6.1	17.0	3.9	0.0
Chicken, with Rice, Morrisons*	1 Pack/300g	345	6.0	115	5.5	18.7	2.0	0.4
Chicken, with Rice, Ross*	1 Serving/320g	275	3.8	86	3.7	14.8	1.2	0.5
Chicken, with Rice, Tesco*	1 Pack/300g	390	12.6	130	4.4	17.5	4.2	1.2
Chicken, with Vegetables, Morrisons*	1 Can/392g	392	15.7	100	9.0	7.0	4.0	1.0
Chicken, Yellow Thai Style, HL, Tesco*	1 Pack/450g	504	12.1	112	9.3	12.6	2.7	0.5
Chicken & Vegetable, Big Eat, Heinz*	1 Pot/350g	392	18.2	112	5.4	10.9	5.2	4.3
Chicken Biryani, Recipe Mix, Schwartz*	1 Pack/30g	75	2.4	249	14.6	58.1	8.1	28.6
Chicken Katsu, City Kitchen, Tesco*	1 Pack/385g	465	13.2	121	6.0	16.3	3.4	1.3
Chicken Korma, Diet Chef Ltd*	1 Pack/300g	324	15.0	108	11.1	4.6	5.0	0.6
Chinese Chicken, Morrisons*	1 Pack/340g	347	15.6	102	10.3	5.0	4.6	0.8
Chinese Chicken, Oriental Express*	1 Pack/340g	286	2.0	84	4.8	16.2	0.6	0.8
Chinese Chicken, with Rice, GFY, Asda*	1 Pack/400g	444	11.6	111	10.7	10.6	2.9	0.5
Chinese Chicken, with Vegetable Rice, M & S*	1 Pack/400g	320	8.0	80	7.1	8.4	2.0	1.3
Courgette & Potato	1oz/28g	24	1.5	86	1.9	8.7	5.2	1.2
Creamy Chicken, Control Chef, All About Weight*	1 Meal/270g	232	2.7	86	9.8	7.7	1.0	3.5
Dudhi, Kofta	1oz/28g	32	2.1	113	2.6	9.4	7.4	2.8
Fish, & Vegetable, Bangladeshi, Average	1oz/28g	33	2.4	117	9.1	1.4	8.4	0.5
Fish, Bangladeshi, Average	1oz/28g	35	2.2	124	12.2	1.5	7.9	0.3
Fish, Red Thai, Waitrose*	1 Pack/500g	275	11.0	55	5.2	3.7	2.2	1.0
Gobi Aloo Sag, Retail	1oz/28g	27	1.9	95	2.2	7.1	6.9	1.4
Indian Daal, Tasty Veg Pot, Innocent*	1 Pot/380g	319	9.9	84	2.8	9.7	2.6	5.3
Indian Vegetable, Sainsbury's*	½ Pack/200g	206	14.6	103	2.5	6.8	7.3	4.6
King Prawn, Coconut & Lime, Sainsbury's*	½ Pack/351g	207	8.8	59	3.7	5.4	2.5	1.0
King Prawn, Malay with Rice, Sainsbury's*	1 Pack/400g	608	20.4	152	5.0	21.5	5.1	1.4
King Prawn, Red Thai, City Kitchen, Tesco*	1 Pack/385g	460	14.4	119	4.5	16.7	3.7	1.0
King Prawn Malay, Waitrose*	1 Pack/350g	364	19.2	104	6.6	7.1	5.5	0.9
Lamb, Hot, M & S*	½ Can/213g	320	19.6	150	14.9	6.0	9.2	2.3
Lamb, Kefthedes, Waitrose*	½ Pack/200g	294	17.6	147	9.0	8.0	8.8	2.1
Lamb, with Rice, Birds Eye*	1 Pack/382g	520	13.0	136	5.6	20.8	3.4	0.9
Masala, Aubergine, TTD, Sainsbury's*	½ Pack/115g	135	11.4	117	2.9	4.1	9.9	5.8
Masala, Indian, Veg Pot, Innocent*	1 Pot/380g	331	10.3	87	2.9	11.6	2.7	3.6
Masala with Babycorn & Asparagus, Waitrose*	½ Pack/125g	92	5.6	74	3.1	5.3	4.5	5.0
Matar Paneer, Peas & Cheese, Ashoka*	½ Pack/150g	183	10.0	122	5.3	10.0	6.7	2.0
Medium, with Rice, Rice Time, Uncle Ben's*	1 Pot/300g	396	9.0	132	2.3	23.2	3.0	1.2
Mild Chicken Tikka Masala, Diet Chef Ltd*	1 Meal/300g	291	6.6	97	10.4	9.0	2.2	0.6
Mushroom & Pea, Masala, Indian, Sainsbury's*	1 Pack/300g	264	14.7	88	3.3	5.2	4.9	5.1

CURRENT

INFO/WEIGHT	per Measure KCAL	per Measure FAT	KCAL	PROT	CARB	FAT	FIBRE

CURRY

	Measure INFO/WEIGHT	per Measure KCAL	per Measure FAT	KCAL	PROT	CARB	FAT	FIBRE
Paste, Green, Maesri*	1 Tbsp/15g	10	0.0	65	4.3	13.0	0.0	4.3
Paste, Red, Maesri*	1 Tbsp/20g	17	0.4	84	3.8	8.6	1.9	0.0
Potato & Pea	1oz/28g	26	1.1	92	2.9	13.0	3.8	2.4
Prawn, & Mushroom	1oz/28g	47	4.0	168	7.3	2.5	14.4	1.0
Prawn, King, Goan, M & S*	1 Pack/400g	680	44.4	170	5.1	11.6	11.1	1.5
Prawn, Red Thai, Sainsbury's*	1 Pack/300g	546	39.6	182	6.3	9.4	13.2	1.7
Prawn, Red Thai Sauce, Youngs*	1 Pack/255g	197	8.7	77	4.8	6.5	3.4	0.8
Prawn, Thai, with Jasmine Rice, BGTY, Sainsbury's*	1 Serving/401g	353	6.0	88	4.2	14.5	1.5	2.0
Prawn, with Rice, Asda*	1 Pack/400g	420	10.4	105	3.5	17.0	2.6	1.1
Prawn, with Rice, Birds Eye*	1 Pack/375g	442	0.0	118	3.5	20.6	0.0	0.0
Prawn, with Rice, Frozen, Sainsbury's*	1 Pack/400g	552	7.6	138	3.9	26.4	1.9	2.1
Prawn, with Rice, Iceland*	1 Pack/450g	468	14.4	104	3.2	16.4	3.2	1.5
Prawn, with Rice, Light & Easy, Youngs*	1 Pack/310g	248	3.4	80	3.3	14.2	1.1	0.9
Red Kidney Bean, Punjabi	1oz/28g	30	1.6	106	4.7	10.1	5.6	3.8
Red Thai, with Rice, Finest, Tesco*	1 Pack/500g	660	15.5	132	8.0	17.8	3.1	0.6
Salmon, Green, Waitrose*	1 Pack/401g	581	40.5	145	9.1	4.5	10.1	2.7
Spicy Paneer, Lovely Vegetables, M & S*	1 Pot/300g	330	12.0	110	4.3	11.9	4.0	4.0
Thai Chicken, Diet Chef Ltd*	1 Pack/300g	291	12.6	97	5.8	9.0	4.2	2.4
Thai Chicken, Low Fat, Solo Slim, Rosemary Conley*	1 Serving/100g	79	2.5	79	21.6	7.0	2.5	2.3
Thai Green Chicken, Charlie Bigham's*	½ Pack/300g	402	26.7	134	9.9	3.6	8.9	0.8
Vegetable, & Pilau Rice, BGTY, Sainsbury's*	1 Pack/400g	272	1.6	68	2.0	14.0	0.4	2.3
Vegetable, & Rice, Microwaveable, M & S*	1 Pot/325g	390	7.2	120	2.3	22.3	2.2	2.2
Vegetable, Asda*	1 Pack/350g	329	21.0	94	1.9	8.0	6.0	1.9
Vegetable, Canned, Sainsbury's*	½ Can/200g	200	12.2	100	1.4	9.8	6.1	1.8
Vegetable, Diet Chef Ltd*	1 Pack/300g	153	3.6	51	2.0	8.0	1.2	2.1
Vegetable, Frozen, Mixed Vegetables, Average	1oz/28g	25	1.7	88	2.5	6.9	6.1	0.0
Vegetable, in a Mild & Creamy Curry Sauce, Waitrose*	1 Pack/400g	388	26.4	97	2.6	6.9	6.6	1.5
Vegetable, in Sweet Sauce, Average	1 Serving/330g	162	6.9	49	1.4	6.7	2.1	1.3
Vegetable, Indian, Canned, Tesco*	1 Can/400g	320	18.0	80	2.0	6.7	4.5	1.1
Vegetable, Indian, Tesco*	1 Serving/225g	257	17.8	114	2.1	8.6	7.9	1.6
Vegetable, Indian Meal for One, Tesco*	1 Serving/200g	218	14.4	109	2.0	9.0	7.2	1.2
Vegetable, Light Choices, Tesco*	1 Pack/350g	350	4.2	100	2.3	19.4	1.2	1.5
Vegetable, Medium, Tesco*	1 Pack/350g	325	21.7	93	2.3	7.1	6.2	1.9
Vegetable, Mild, COU, M & S*	1 Pack/400g	340	2.0	85	2.6	17.0	0.5	2.8
Vegetable, Mild, Tesco*	1 Can/425g	314	10.6	74	2.1	10.7	2.5	1.7
Vegetable, Mixed, Organic, Pure & Pronto*	1 Pack/400g	368	11.6	92	4.2	12.4	2.9	4.8
Vegetable, Pakistani, Average	1oz/28g	17	0.7	60	2.2	8.7	2.6	2.2
Vegetable, Sabzi Tarkari, Patak's*	1 Pack/400g	500	31.2	125	2.5	11.1	7.8	2.2
Vegetable, Solo Slim, Rosemary Conley*	1 Pack/300g	153	3.6	51	2.0	8.0	1.2	2.1
Vegetable, Takeaway, Average	1 Serving/330g	346	24.4	105	2.5	7.6	7.4	0.0
Vegetable, Tinned, Asda*	½ Can/200g	206	12.0	103	2.2	10.0	6.0	2.5
Vegetable, Way to Five, Sainsbury's*	½ Pack/344g	227	3.8	66	2.5	11.6	1.1	1.4
Vegetable, with Pilau Rice, Linda McCartney*	1 Pack/339g	224	2.0	66	1.6	13.5	0.6	0.5
Vegetable, with Rice, Asda*	1 Pack/393g	432	12.2	110	2.6	18.0	3.1	1.4
Vegetable, with Rice, Birds Eye*	1 Pack/414g	455	9.5	110	2.3	19.6	2.3	1.1
Vegetable, with Rice, Co-Op*	1 Pack/340g	289	3.4	85	2.0	17.0	1.0	0.7
Vegetable, with Rice, HL, Tesco*	1 Pack/450g	486	12.1	108	2.7	18.2	2.7	1.1
Vegetable, with Rice, Light Choices, Tesco*	1 Pack/350g	340	4.0	97	2.3	19.3	1.1	1.5
Vegetable, with Rice, Retail, Average	1oz/28g	29	0.8	102	3.3	16.4	3.0	0.0
Vegetable, with Rice, Tesco*	1 Pack/400g	440	12.0	110	2.1	18.7	3.0	1.0
Vegetable, with Yoghurt, Average	1oz/28g	17	1.1	62	2.6	4.6	4.1	1.4
Vegetable, Yellow, Tesco*	1 Pack/356g	324	17.4	91	1.9	9.9	4.9	1.4
Vegetable, Yellow Thai, Sainsbury's*	1 Pack/400g	624	48.8	156	2.2	9.4	12.2	1.1

	Measure INFO/WEIGHT	per Measure KCAL	FAT	Nutrition Values per 100g / 100ml KCAL	PROT	CARB	FAT	FIBRE
CURRY								
Vegetable Masala, Light Choices, Tesco*	1 Pack/350g	297	5.9	85	3.8	13.6	1.7	3.4
CURRY LEAVES								
Fresh	*1oz/28g*	*27*	*0.4*	*97*	*7.9*	*13.3*	*1.3*	*0.0*
CURRY PASTE								
Balti, Asda*	1 Tube/100g	220	14.7	220	4.7	17.2	14.7	1.9
Balti, Sharwood's*	¼ Pack/73g	328	28.7	453	5.0	19.2	39.6	3.1
Balti, Tomato & Coriander, Original, Patak's*	1 Tbsp/15g	58	5.1	388	4.0	14.6	34.0	3.7
Bhuna, Tomato & Tamarind, Patak's*	1 Serving/10g	40	5.6	397	4.3	17.5	56.2	6.3
Garam Masala, Cinnamon & Ginger, Hot, Patak's*	1 Serving/30g	121	10.6	403	3.2	17.9	35.4	0.6
Green, Thai, Asda*	1 Tbsp/25g	28	2.0	114	1.6	10.0	8.0	5.0
Green Thai, Mild, Sainsbury's*	1 Tbsp/15g	23	1.5	156	2.2	14.5	9.9	2.7
Green Thai, Tesco*	1 Tbsp/15g	17	1.2	115	2.1	8.7	7.9	3.1
Jalfrezi, Patak's*	1 Serving/30g	96	8.1	320	3.7	14.2	26.9	5.6
Korma, Asda*	1 Tube/100g	338	23.5	338	5.1	26.6	23.5	1.2
Korma, Coconut & Coriander, Original, Patak's*	1 Serving/30g	124	11.7	415	3.5	11.6	39.0	5.2
Madras, Cumin & Chilli, Hot, Patak's*	¼ Jar/70g	202	18.1	289	4.7	7.6	25.9	10.8
Medium, Asda*	1 Tsp/5ml/5g	18	1.6	364	5.0	14.0	32.0	5.0
Medium, Barts Spices*	1 Serving/30g	88	6.4	295	4.5	19.2	21.5	5.5
Mild, Asda*	¼ Jar/46g	206	18.9	448	3.8	16.0	41.0	7.0
Mild, Coriander & Cumin, Original, Patak's*	1 Serving/30g	169	15.7	562	4.8	16.8	52.5	2.8
Red, Thai, Asda*	1 Tbsp/25g	31	2.5	124	1.6	7.0	10.0	5.0
Red Thai, M & S*	½ Jar/100g	150	10.8	150	1.3	11.9	10.8	2.8
Red Thai, Sainsbury's*	1 Jar/250g	385	31.0	154	2.2	8.5	12.4	3.5
Red Thai, Tesco*	1 Tsp/5g	5	0.4	110	1.5	8.9	7.3	3.7
Rogan Josh, Tomato & Paprika, Patak's*	1 Serving/30g	119	11.0	397	4.1	12.7	36.7	5.9
Tamarind & Ginger, Original, Patak's*	1 Tbsp/15g	20	0.3	133	3.4	23.1	2.0	2.9
Tandoori, Sharwood's*	1oz/28g	64	4.4	228	5.9	15.5	15.8	1.9
Tandoori, Tamarind & Ginger, Patak's*	1 Serving/30g	33	0.5	110	3.1	20.4	1.8	2.6
Tikka, Asda*	½ Tube/50g	117	8.5	235	4.5	16.1	17.0	1.6
Tikka Masala, Coriander & Lemon, Medium, Patak's*	1 Serving/30g	111	9.5	369	3.8	16.9	31.8	2.9
Tom Yum, Thai Taste*	1 Tsp/13g	35	2.0	269	5.4	30.8	15.4	7.7
CURRY POWDER								
Average	*1 Tsp/2g*	*6*	*0.3*	*325*	*12.7*	*41.8*	*13.8*	*0.0*
CURRY SAUCE								
Asda*	1 Tbsp/15g	62	2.1	414	13.0	59.0	14.0	1.3
Balti, Asda*	¼ Jar/125g	155	12.5	124	1.6	7.0	10.0	1.7
Balti, Loyd Grossman*	½ Jar/175g	173	11.7	99	1.3	8.4	6.7	1.7
Chinese Style, Cooking, Asda*	1 Jar/560g	465	24.1	83	1.5	9.6	4.3	1.7
Dopiaza, Finest, Tesco*	1 Jar/350g	234	10.5	67	1.3	8.5	3.0	3.7
Green Curry, Thai, Stir Fry, Blue Dragon*	1 Sachet/120g	74	4.8	62	0.9	5.7	4.0	0.5
Green Thai, Asda*	1 Jar/340g	309	27.2	91	0.5	4.3	8.0	0.2
Green Thai, Express, Uncle Ben's*	1 Pack/170g	131	9.9	77	1.1	5.4	5.8	0.0
Jalfrezi, Loyd Grossman*	½ Jar/213g	270	20.2	127	2.1	8.2	9.5	1.2
Jalfrezi, Piri Piri, Finest, Tesco*	1 Serving/175g	145	10.8	83	1.2	5.7	6.2	1.5
Jalfrezi, Tesco*	1 Jar/500g	450	32.5	90	1.3	6.6	6.5	2.4
Korma, Loyd Grossman*	½ Jar/222g	542	37.7	244	3.6	19.1	17.0	0.6
Korma, Uncle Ben's*	1 Jar/500g	630	42.0	126	1.4	11.1	8.4	0.0
Madras, Aldi*	1 Serving/113g	68	2.3	60	1.5	9.0	2.0	0.0
Madras, Cooking, Asda*	¼ Jar/142g	109	6.2	77	1.3	8.0	4.4	1.0
Madras, Cooking, Sharwood's*	1 Tsp/2g	2	0.1	86	1.5	6.9	5.8	1.3
Madras, Cooking, Tesco*	1/3 Jar/161g	145	9.2	90	1.9	6.9	5.7	2.5
Madras, Cumin & Chilli, Original, in Glass Jar, Patak's*	1 Jar/540g	648	38.3	120	2.1	11.9	7.1	1.8
Madras, Indian, Sharwood's*	1 Jar/420g	433	26.5	103	1.8	9.7	6.3	1.9

	Measure INFO/WEIGHT	per Measure		Nutrition Values per 100g / 100ml				
		KCAL	FAT	KCAL	PROT	CARB	FAT	FIBRE
CURRY SAUCE								
Madras, Sharwood's*	1 Jar/420g	521	38.2	124	1.7	8.9	9.1	1.4
Madras, Tesco*	½ Jar/200g	168	13.0	84	1.1	5.2	6.5	1.3
Makhani, Sharwood's*	1 Jar/420g	399	29.0	95	0.9	7.2	6.9	0.4
Malaysian Rendang, Loyd Grossman*	1 Serving/100g	143	10.1	143	2.6	10.4	10.1	1.4
Masala, Red Pepper & Mango, Sainsbury's*	½ Jar/175g	142	8.6	81	1.4	7.8	4.9	1.1
Medium, Uncle Ben's*	1 Jar/500g	330	10.0	66	0.9	10.9	2.0	0.0
Moglai Pasanda, Asda*	½ Jar/170g	277	21.0	163	2.9	10.0	12.3	1.1
Oven Bake Biryani, Medium & Aromatic, Patak's*	½ Jar/175g	135	9.3	77	1.1	6.1	5.3	1.7
Red Curry, Thai, Stir Fry, Blue Dragon*	1 Sachet/120g	112	9.6	93	0.9	4.4	8.0	0.5
Rogan Josh, Loyd Grossman*	1 Serving/106g	206	16.7	194	2.4	10.5	15.8	1.5
Rogan Josh, Worldwide Sauces*	1 Jar/500g	255	1.5	51	1.1	11.0	0.3	0.0
Sri Lankan Devil Curry, Sharwood's*	1 Jar/380g	220	11.4	58	0.5	7.2	3.0	2.1
Tikka, Cooking, Tesco*	1 Jar/500g	617	42.1	123	1.7	10.1	8.4	2.0
Tikka Masala, Cooking, HL, Tesco*	¼ Jar/125g	94	3.7	75	2.6	8.2	3.0	1.2
Tikka Masala, COU, M & S*	½ Pack/100g	80	2.6	80	4.5	9.9	2.6	1.7
Tikka Masala, Loyd Grossman*	½ Jar/213g	438	34.4	206	2.6	12.5	16.2	1.0
Vindaloo, Cooking, Chosen By You, Asda*	½ Jar/160g	128	5.4	80	1.5	10.4	3.4	1.0
Vindaloo, Hot, Patak's*	1 Jar/540g	643	46.4	119	1.7	8.5	8.6	2.1
CUSTARD								
Banana Flavour, Ambrosia*	1 Pot/135g	139	3.9	103	2.9	16.1	2.9	0.0
Chocolate, COU, M & S*	1 Pot/140g	147	3.1	105	3.1	18.6	2.2	1.0
Chocolate Flavour, Ambrosia*	1 Pot/150g	177	4.3	118	3.0	20.0	2.9	0.7
Dairy Free, Sainsbury's*	1 Serving/250g	210	4.2	84	3.0	14.2	1.7	0.2
Instant, Just Add Water, Weight Watchers*	1 Serving/145g	93	0.6	64	1.2	13.9	0.4	0.9
Low Fat, Average	*1/3 Pot/141g*	*116*	*1.6*	*82*	*2.9*	*15.0*	*1.2*	*0.0*
Pot, Forest Fruits Flavour, Hot 'n' Fruity, Bird's*	1 Pot/174g	171	4.2	98	0.9	18.5	2.4	0.1
Powder	*1 Tsp/5g*	*18*	*0.0*	*354*	*0.6*	*92.0*	*0.7*	*0.1*
Ready To Eat, Chocolate, Tesco*	1 Pot/150g	150	3.4	100	3.2	16.2	2.3	0.3
Ready to Serve, Average	*1 Serving/50g*	*59*	*2.3*	*118*	*3.3*	*16.1*	*4.6*	*0.2*
Strawberry Flavoured, Ambrosia*	1 Serving/135g	139	3.8	103	2.8	16.7	2.8	0.0
Strawberry Style, Shapers, Boots*	1 Pot/148g	83	1.2	56	4.0	8.2	0.8	0.1
Summer, Ambrosia*	1 Pack/500g	490	15.0	98	2.7	15.0	3.0	0.0
Toffee Flavour, Ambrosia*	1 Pot/150g	156	4.2	104	2.8	17.0	2.8	0.0
Vanilla, COU, M & S*	1 Pot/140g	147	3.5	105	4.3	16.6	2.5	0.6
Vanilla, Fresh, Waitrose*	1 Serving/100g	214	15.3	214	3.2	15.8	15.3	1.1
Vanilla, TTD, Sainsbury's*	1 Pot/150g	312	23.2	208	2.5	14.7	15.5	0.1
Vanilla with Apple Crunch, Ambrosia*	1 Pack/193g	276	8.7	143	3.4	22.4	4.5	0.8
with Strawberry Sauce, Ambrosia*	1 Pot/160g	171	3.8	107	2.4	19.0	2.4	0.1
CUSTARD APPLE								
Weighed without Skin & Seeds, Average	1 Fruit/312g	234	2.1	75	1.6	17.7	0.7	3.0
CUTLETS								
Nut, Goodlife*	1 Cutlet/88g	283	19.4	322	9.1	21.8	22.0	3.4
Nut, Meat Free, Tesco*	1 Cutlet/83g	224	14.0	270	8.1	20.5	16.9	4.3
Nut, Retail, Fried in Vegetable Oil, Average	1 Cutlet/90g	260	20.1	289	4.8	18.7	22.3	1.7
Nut, Retail, Grilled, Average	1 Cutlet/90g	191	11.7	212	5.1	19.9	13.0	1.8
Vegetable & Nut, Asda*	1 Cutlet/88g	296	20.3	335	10.0	22.0	23.0	4.6
CUTTLEFISH								
Raw	*1oz/28g*	*20*	*0.2*	*71*	*16.1*	*0.0*	*0.7*	*0.0*

C

	Measure INFO/WEIGHT	per Measure KCAL	FAT	Nutrition Values per 100g / 100ml KCAL	PROT	CARB	FAT	FIBRE
DAB								
Fillets, Lightly Dusted, M & S*	1 Fillet/112g	190	9.7	170	12.8	9.7	8.7	0.5
Raw	*1oz/28g*	*21*	*0.3*	*74*	*15.7*	*0.0*	*1.2*	*0.0*
DAIRYLEA DUNKERS								
Baked Crisps, Dairylea, Kraft*	1 Pack/45g	101	4.0	225	9.2	26.0	9.0	1.1
Jumbo Munch, Dairylea, Kraft*	1 Serving/50g	150	9.2	300	7.2	26.5	18.5	1.2
Salt & Vinegar, Dairylea, Kraft*	1 Tub/42g	115	8.2	275	6.7	17.5	19.5	0.3
with Jumbo Tubes, Kraft*	1 Pack/43g	108	5.1	255	9.1	27.0	12.0	0.9
with Ritz Crackers, Dairylea, Kraft*	1 Tub/46g	122	6.4	265	9.6	25.0	13.9	0.6
DAIRYLEA LUNCHABLES								
Ham & Cheese Pizza, Dairylea, Kraft*	1 Pack/97g	247	10.7	255	11.5	26.0	11.0	1.6
Harvest Ham, Dairylea, Kraft*	1 Pack/110g	313	18.7	285	16.5	16.5	17.0	0.3
Tasty Chicken, Dairylea, Kraft*	1 Pack/110g	313	18.1	285	17.0	17.5	16.5	0.3
DAMSONS								
Raw, Weighed with Stones, Average	*1oz/28g*	*10*	*0.0*	*34*	*0.5*	*8.6*	*0.0*	*1.6*
Raw, Weighed without Stones, Average	*1oz/28g*	*11*	*0.0*	*38*	*0.5*	*9.6*	*0.0*	*1.8*
DANDELION & BURDOCK								
Fermented, Botanical, Fentiman's*	1 Bottle/275ml	130	0.0	47	0.0	11.6	0.0	0.0
Original, Ben Shaws*	1 Can/440ml	128	0.0	29	0.0	7.0	0.0	0.0
Sparkling, Diet, Morrisons*	1 Glass/200ml	2	0.0	1	0.0	0.3	0.0	0.0
DANISH PASTRY								
Apple, Bar, Sara Lee*	1/6 Bar/70g	160	4.0	229	4.3	42.1	5.7	1.7
Apple, Fresh Cream, Sainsbury's*	1 Pastry/67g	248	14.6	368	3.1	40.2	21.6	0.4
Apple, Iceland*	¼ Pastry/95g	223	5.0	235	5.3	41.5	5.3	2.3
Apple & Cinnamon, Danish Twist, Entenmann's*	1 Serving/52g	150	1.0	288	5.6	62.0	1.9	1.5
Apple & Sultana, Tesco*	1 Pastry/72g	293	16.4	407	5.4	45.0	22.8	1.4
Average	1 Pastry/110g	411	19.4	374	5.8	51.3	17.6	1.6
Cherry, Bar, Sainsbury's*	¼ Bar/88g	220	10.0	252	4.2	33.2	11.4	1.7
Cherry & Custard, Bar, Tesco*	1 Bar/350g	910	49.0	260	3.5	29.9	14.0	7.7
Custard, Bar, Sara Lee*	¼ Bar/100g	228	6.4	228	6.6	36.1	6.4	0.8
Fruit Filled, Average	1 Pastry/94g	335	15.9	356	5.1	47.9	16.9	0.0
Pecan, M & S*	1 Serving/67g	287	17.4	428	6.2	45.0	26.0	1.3
Toasted Pecan, Danish Twist, Entenmann's*	1 Slice/48g	171	7.6	351	7.0	47.2	15.6	1.4
DATES								
Bite Size, Snack Pack, Whitworths*	1 Pack/35g	119	0.6	340	2.0	74.7	1.8	8.2
Deglet Nour, Graze*	1 Pack/60g	181	0.3	301	2.1	72.0	0.5	0.0
Deglet Nour, Love Life, Waitrose*	1 Portion/50g	143	0.1	287	3.3	68.0	0.2	8.0
Dried, Average	*1 Date/5g*	*14*	*0.0*	*272*	*2.8*	*65.4*	*0.4*	*4.2*
Dried, Medjool, Average	*1 Date/20g*	*56*	*0.1*	*279*	*2.2*	*69.3*	*0.3*	*4.3*
Fresh, Raw, Yellow, Average	*1 Date/20g*	*23*	*0.0*	*115*	*1.4*	*29.1*	*0.1*	*1.6*
Medjool, Stuffed with Walnuts, Tesco*	2 Dates/40g	98	2.3	245	4.4	44.0	5.7	3.4
Milk Chocolate Coated, Julian Graves*	1 Pack/200g	768	22.6	384	4.5	66.0	11.3	2.6
Organic, Medjool, Pitted, Love Life, Waitrose*	1 Date/18g	52	0.0	291	3.3	68.0	0.2	6.7
Stoned, Wholefoods, Tesco*	1 Pack/500g	1600	13.0	320	4.4	69.2	2.6	8.4
DELI FILLER								
Chicken, Caesar Style, Sainsbury's*	1 Pack/80g	212	18.2	265	14.0	1.0	22.7	2.6
Chicken & Bacon, Co-Op*	1 Pack/200g	420	29.6	210	17.6	1.0	14.8	2.6
King Prawn & Avocado, M & S*	1 Pack/170g	425	38.8	250	9.5	1.4	22.8	0.5
Prawn & Mayonnaise, M & S*	1 Serving/60g	150	13.8	250	11.3	1.0	23.0	0.5
Smoked Salmon & Soft Cheese, M & S*	1 Serving/85g	208	17.3	245	11.7	3.3	20.4	0.5
DELIGHT								
Butterscotch Flavour, No Added Sugar, Tesco*	1 Pack/49g	225	10.0	460	4.8	63.3	20.5	0.0
Chocolate Flavour, Dry, Tesco*	1 Pack/49g	220	9.0	450	6.2	64.2	18.4	2.3
Ravishing Raspberry, Made Up, Asda*	1/3 Pack/100g	112	3.9	112	3.2	16.0	3.9	0.0

	Measure INFO/WEIGHT	per Measure KCAL	FAT	Nutrition Values per 100g / 100ml KCAL	PROT	CARB	FAT	FIBRE
DELIGHT								
Strawberry, No Added Sugar, Dry, Tesco*	1 Pack/49g	51	1.8	105	3.4	13.7	3.7	0.1
Strawberry, Shapers, Boots*	1 Pot/122g	96	1.2	79	4.5	13.0	1.0	0.1
Vanilla, No Added Sugar, Dry, Tesco*	1 Pack/49g	51	1.8	105	3.4	13.7	3.7	0.1
DESSERT								
Almond, Naturgreen*	1 Serving/130g	143	6.2	110	2.3	14.5	4.8	0.2
Apple Crumble, Sainsbury's*	1 Pot/136g	291	10.5	214	3.2	33.0	7.7	2.7
Baked Lemon, COU, M & S*	1 Serving/100g	140	2.5	140	6.8	22.0	2.5	0.8
Banana Split	1 Serving/175g	368	25.5	210	2.2	18.0	14.6	0.1
Banoffee, Sainsbury's*	1 Pot/140g	360	19.1	257	2.7	30.9	13.6	1.3
Banoffee, Shape, Danone*	1 Pot/120g	175	2.8	146	3.3	28.0	2.3	0.5
Banoffee, Weight Watchers*	1 Dessert/81g	170	3.6	210	4.9	37.7	4.4	1.4
Banoffee Layered, Sainsbury's*	1 Pot/115g	270	14.7	235	2.2	27.8	12.8	1.0
Black Cherry, Dragana, Waitrose*	1 Pot/125g	236	11.4	189	2.1	24.7	9.1	0.5
Black Cherry & Chocolate, COU, M & S*	1 Pack/115g	132	1.6	115	3.6	22.6	1.4	1.2
Black Forest, Light Choices, Tesco*	1 Pot/145g	188	2.3	130	3.2	25.8	1.6	0.9
Black Forest, Tesco*	1 Pot/100g	287	14.4	287	3.5	35.8	14.4	2.4
Blissful Banana, Asda*	1/3 Pack/100g	122	4.3	122	3.7	17.0	4.3	0.0
Blueberry Muffin, Tesco*	1 Pot/91g	265	18.7	291	2.0	24.5	20.6	3.0
Bounty, Mars*	1 Pot/110g	253	15.0	230	5.3	23.2	13.6	0.0
Butterscotch Flavour Whip, Co-Op*	1 Pack/64g	241	0.1	377	0.6	93.4	0.1	0.0
Buttons, Milk Chocolate, Cadbury*	1 Pot/100g	280	14.9	280	6.2	30.8	14.9	0.0
Cafe Latte, COU, M & S*	1 Pot/120g	162	2.6	135	5.0	24.0	2.2	0.9
Cafe Mocha, COU, M & S*	1 Dessert/115g	155	3.1	135	5.5	21.8	2.7	1.0
Cappuccino, Italian, Co-Op*	1 Pack/90g	256	10.8	285	5.0	39.0	12.0	0.1
Caramel, Delights, Shape, Danone*	1 Pot/110g	109	2.5	99	3.3	16.3	2.3	0.1
Caramel Crunch, Weight Watchers*	1 Serving/89g	174	2.6	196	4.6	37.9	2.9	1.7
Caramel Flavour, Soya, Dairy Free, Organic, Provamel*	1 Pot/125g	122	2.1	98	3.0	17.5	1.7	0.6
Caramel Shortcake, Luxury, Weight Watchers*	1 Pot/100ml	103	3.5	103	1.9	17.9	3.5	0.8
Catalan Cream, Sainsbury's*	1 Pot/95g	375	35.1	395	4.2	11.2	37.0	0.1
Cheeky & Saucy Little Pots Au Chocolat, Gu*	1 Pot/45g	199	16.6	443	3.3	24.1	36.9	2.3
Cherry & Vanilla, BGTY, Sainsbury's*	1 Pot/115g	225	7.6	196	1.6	32.6	6.6	1.0
Chocolate, Campina*	1 Pot/125g	186	8.6	149	3.2	18.5	6.9	0.0
Chocolate, Custardz, Chosen By You, Asda*	1 Pot/90g	97	2.0	108	3.2	18.8	2.2	0.0
Chocolate, Delights, Shape, Danone*	1 Pot/110g	109	2.4	99	3.3	16.3	2.2	0.6
Chocolate, Frappe, Skinny, COU, M & S*	1 Pot/100g	115	2.0	115	5.7	18.3	2.0	0.5
Chocolate, HL, Tesco*	1 Pot/95g	87	2.2	92	3.7	14.1	2.3	1.1
Chocolate, M & S*	1 Serving/120g	168	2.5	140	5.6	26.4	2.1	1.1
Chocolate, Triple Delight, Weight Watchers*	1 Dessert/110g	183	2.9	166	4.9	30.8	2.6	2.6
Chocolate, Weight Watchers*	1 Serving/82g	145	2.5	177	5.2	32.3	3.0	2.9
Chocolate & Coconut, COU, M & S*	1 Pot/125g	169	2.7	135	3.6	25.6	2.2	0.7
Chocolate & Mallow, Weight Watchers*	1 Pot/150ml	140	1.8	93	2.0	18.7	1.2	2.3
Chocolate Banoffee, Gu*	1 Pot/85g	325	21.5	382	3.9	35.0	25.3	1.0
Chocolate Brownie, M & S*	1/4 Pack/144g	610	39.5	425	4.7	39.6	27.5	1.0
Chocolate Buttons, Cadbury*	1 Pack/100g	275	14.5	275	5.0	30.5	14.5	0.0
Chocolate Desire, Magnum, Wall's Ice Cream*	1 Dessert/85g	374	24.0	440	5.3	40.0	28.2	0.0
Chocolate Dream, Co-Op*	1 Pot/110g	184	7.7	167	4.1	22.0	7.0	0.0
Chocolate Duetto, Weight Watchers*	1 Pot/85g	99	2.4	117	4.4	18.4	2.8	0.0
Chocolate Fudge Brownie, Tesco*	1 Pot/125g	374	16.6	299	4.6	40.2	13.3	1.3
Chocolate Hazelnut, Charolait, Aldi*	1 Serving/200g	270	11.0	135	3.3	18.1	5.5	0.0
Chocolate Honeycomb Crisp, COU, M & S*	1 Serving/71g	110	2.1	155	4.6	27.6	2.9	1.0
Chocolate Marshmallow, Weight Watchers*	1 Serving/50g	97	2.3	194	3.2	34.5	4.7	1.3
Chocolate Mint Torte, Weight Watchers*	1 Dessert/88g	174	4.1	198	4.7	34.3	4.7	5.2
Chocolate Mocha, BGTY, Sainsbury's*	1 Pot/100g	115	2.6	115	3.8	19.2	2.6	2.8

DESERT

INFO/WEIGHT	Measure		Nutrition Values per 100g / 100ml				
	per Measure						
	KCAL	FAT	KCAL	PROT	CARB	FAT	FIBRE
Chocolate Mousse Cake, Weight Watchers*	1 Dessert/75g	148	2.2	198	5.9	37.1	2.9	1.0
Chocolate Muffin, COU, M & S*	1 Pot/110g	154	2.7	140	6.1	26.1	2.5	1.5
Chocolate Muffin, Light Choices, Tesco*	1 Pot/108g	140	2.4	130	4.3	22.6	2.2	1.3
Chocolate Muffin, Tesco*	1 Serving/104g	354	21.2	340	3.5	35.5	20.4	2.1
Chocolate Toffee, Weight Watchers*	1 Dessert/89g	177	4.0	197	4.3	34.9	4.5	2.2
Chocolate Top, Weight Watchers*	1 Pot/75g	162	7.4	216	4.2	29.3	9.9	2.8
Crazy Chocolate Overload, M & S*	1 Pot/120g	402	27.0	335	3.1	30.0	22.5	0.5
Creme Caramel, Sainsbury's*	1 Pot/100g	116	1.6	116	2.6	22.9	1.6	0.0
Crunchie, Dairy Milk, Cadbury*	1 Pot/100g	260	12.2	260	4.4	33.4	12.2	0.0
Custard, with Caramel, Layers, Ambrosia*	1 Pot/161g	183	4.7	114	2.5	19.6	2.9	0.0
Double Chocolate Brownie, Weight Watchers*	1 Pot/86g	163	3.3	189	5.1	33.7	3.8	2.4
Double Chocolate Fudge, M & S*	1 Pot/119g	387	25.5	325	3.0	30.6	21.4	1.6
Dreamy Vanilla, BGTY, Sainsbury's*	1 Serving/58g	146	8.2	252	3.5	27.6	14.2	5.3
Flake, Milk Chocolate, Cadbury*	1 Pot/100g	275	14.6	275	6.2	29.8	14.6	0.0
Fruit & Nut, Cadbury*	1 Pot/100g	285	12.5	285	6.4	36.3	12.5	0.0
Fudge, Cadbury*	1 Pot/90g	216	11.2	240	4.1	28.5	12.4	0.0
Galaxy, Mars*	1 Pot/75g	166	9.2	221	4.9	22.7	12.3	0.0
Gulabjam Indian, Waitrose*	1 Pot/180g	479	15.5	266	4.8	42.9	8.6	0.6
Hot Chocolate & Raspberry Truffle Bakes, M & S*	1 Truffle/92g	363	15.5	395	3.2	30.9	16.9	2.0
Irish Cream Cafe Latte, COU, M & S*	1 Pot/120g	160	2.6	133	5.0	24.0	2.2	0.9
Jaffa Cake, COU, M & S*	1 Serving/120g	138	3.1	115	2.4	20.1	2.6	1.0
Key Lime Pie	1 Serving/125g	431	25.0	344	4.1	37.9	20.0	1.4
Lemon, Sainsbury's*	1 Pot/115g	136	1.7	118	2.8	23.2	1.5	0.9
Lemon & Sultana Sponge, COU, M & S*	1 Pot/130g	169	1.6	130	2.8	26.5	1.2	0.5
Lemon Meringue, Weight Watchers*	1 Pot/85g	161	0.4	189	2.4	43.1	0.5	0.6
Lemon Mousse Cake, Weight Watchers*	1 Serving/90g	130	2.4	144	3.2	26.7	2.7	0.5
Lemoncello, Italian, Co-Op*	1 Pot/90g	265	14.4	295	3.0	34.0	16.0	0.1
Mandarin, COU, M & S*	1 Serving/150g	195	5.7	130	1.0	22.0	3.8	0.1
Maple & Pecan, American Style, Sainsbury's*	1 Pot/110g	287	15.6	261	2.6	30.6	14.2	1.2
Mars, Mars*	1 Pot/110g	214	7.4	195	6.0	28.2	6.7	0.7
Millionaire's Shortbread, M & S*	1 Dessert/120g	425	25.7	355	2.6	38.3	21.5	1.4
Mini Frozen Raspberry, Easycuisine*	1 Glass/49g	137	9.7	280	2.3	23.2	19.8	1.2
Mint Chocolate Top, Weight Watchers*	1 Pot/75g	160	6.9	214	4.0	31.4	9.2	3.5
Mississippi Mud Pie	1 Serving/125g	480	32.0	384	5.3	33.1	25.6	1.8
Peach & Raspberry, COU, M & S*	1 Pot/90g	135	1.4	150	2.6	30.5	1.6	1.0
Pineapple & Passionfruit, M & S*	1 Pot/100g	130	3.8	130	0.8	21.7	3.8	0.3
Raspberry, Frappe, Skinny, COU, M & S*	1 Pot/95g	109	1.3	115	3.1	22.0	1.4	0.5
Raspberry & Chardonnay, COU, M & S*	1 Serving/135g	155	0.7	115	1.6	25.5	0.5	2.7
Raspberry Flavour Whip, Co-Op*	1 Whip/64g	241	0.1	377	1.2	92.5	0.2	0.0
Raspberry Royale, Essential, Waitrose*	1 Pot/150g	216	10.6	144	1.1	18.9	7.1	0.5
Raspberry Royale, Finest, Tesco*	½ Pack/170g	314	15.8	185	1.7	22.8	9.3	1.4
Raspberry with Lemon Sponge, Weight Watchers*	1 Dessert/85g	152	3.7	178	4.1	30.4	4.4	2.8
Rich Chocolate, Weight Watchers*	1 Pot/70g	62	1.7	89	3.5	13.4	2.4	1.4
Rocky Road, Sainsbury's*	1 Pot/110g	328	21.6	298	3.6	26.8	19.6	2.1
Rolo, Nestle*	1 Pot/77g	187	9.5	243	3.1	30.0	12.3	0.5
Simply Strawberry, Sainsbury's*	1 Pot/150g	126	0.1	84	0.6	19.3	0.1	0.9
Skinny Dippers, Minis, Skinny Cow*	1 Lolly/40ml	65	2.0	162	3.4	24.3	5.0	3.3
Skinny Raspberry, Frappe, COU, M & S*	1 Pot/95g	109	1.3	115	3.1	22.0	1.4	0.5
Skinny Raspberry Latte, COU, M & S*	1 Serving/100g	125	1.9	125	4.1	22.8	1.9	0.5
Soya, Mocha Flavour, Provamel*	1 Serving/125g	117	2.2	94	3.0	16.3	1.8	0.6
Splijies, Vanilla, Tip Top, Nestle*	1 Tube/85g	97	3.1	114	4.0	16.1	3.7	0.0
Strawberries & Cream, BFY, Morrisons*	1 Serving/200g	244	2.2	122	2.2	26.0	1.1	0.1
Strawberry, BGTY, Sainsbury's*	1 Pot/115g	133	1.6	116	2.7	23.1	1.4	1.3

	Measure INFO/WEIGHT	per Measure KCAL	per Measure FAT	Nutrition Values per 100g / 100ml KCAL	PROT	CARB	FAT	FIBRE
DESSERT								
Strawberry, HL, Tesco*	1 Pot/122g	94	2.3	77	2.7	12.3	1.9	1.1
Strawberry & Rhubarb, COU, M & S*	1 Pot/110g	104	0.8	95	1.5	20.1	0.7	0.9
Strawberry Meringue, Iced, Luxury, Weight Watchers*	1 Pot/100ml	86	0.7	162	2.4	34.2	1.4	1.0
Strawberry Mousse Cake, Weight Watchers*	1 Serving/90g	124	2.4	138	3.0	25.5	2.7	0.5
Summer Berry, HL, Tesco*	1 Pot/93g	120	2.1	130	2.8	24.5	2.3	1.5
Summer Fruits, COU, M & S*	1 Serving/105g	110	1.2	105	2.1	21.6	1.1	1.2
Summer Fruits, Marbled Cream, Waitrose*	1 Serving/125g	214	11.4	171	2.1	20.2	9.1	1.1
Tantalising Toffee, COU, M & S*	¼ Pot/85g	144	2.5	170	3.1	32.8	2.9	0.5
Tantalising Toffee Flavour, Weight Watchers*	1 Serving/57g	93	2.7	163	2.7	26.2	4.8	0.2
Tiramisu	1 Serving/150g	420	20.8	280	4.4	34.0	13.9	0.8
Toffee, with Biscuit Pieces, Iced, Weight Watchers*	1 Pot/57g	93	2.7	163	2.7	26.2	4.8	0.2
Toffee, with Biscuit Pieces, Weight Watchers*	1 Pot/57g	93	2.7	163	2.7	26.2	4.8	0.2
Toffee & Vanilla, Weight Watchers*	1 Pot/67g	107	0.5	159	3.1	34.8	0.8	3.9
Toffee Chocolate, Weight Watchers*	1 Pot/100g	197	4.5	197	4.3	34.9	4.5	2.2
Toffee Flavour Custard, Ambrosia*	1 Pack/135g	139	3.9	103	2.7	16.4	2.9	0.1
Toffee Muffin, COU, M & S*	1 Serving/100g	180	2.2	180	3.7	35.8	2.2	0.3
Trifle, Chocolate, Light, Cadbury*	1 Pot/93g	130	4.0	140	4.6	20.4	4.3	0.0
Triple Chocolate, Delice, Sainsbury's*	1 Serving/105g	399	27.4	380	3.8	32.4	26.1	0.7
Triple Chocolate Layered, BGTY, Sainsbury's*	1 Pot/105g	147	2.9	140	4.2	24.4	2.8	0.5
Triple Chocolate Truffle, Entenmann's*	1 Serving/100g	304	19.1	304	4.5	28.4	19.1	2.2
Vanilla, Exquisa*	1 Serving/100g	103	0.2	103	5.2	20.0	0.2	0.0
Vanilla, Luxury, Charolait*	1 Serving/200g	248	10.2	124	3.0	16.6	5.1	0.0
Vanilla & Caramel, Little Desserts, Petits Filous, Yoplait*	1 Pot/50g	75	2.6	150	4.7	21.0	5.3	0.2
Vanilla & Chocolate Twist, Desira, Aldi*	1 Pack/150g	182	7.2	121	0.0	15.0	4.8	0.0
Vanilla & Strawberry Compote, Weight Watchers*	1 Pot/57g	81	2.2	142	2.5	23.4	3.9	0.2
Vanilla & Toffee, Heavenly Swirls, Tesco*	1 Pot/73g	106	1.8	145	2.5	28.1	2.5	0.5
Vanilla Creamed Rice, Weight Watchers*	1 Pot/130g	112	0.6	86	3.2	16.9	0.5	0.4
Vanilla Flavour, Soya, Dairy Free, Organic, Provamel*	1 Pot/125g	105	2.2	84	3.2	13.4	1.8	0.5
Vanilla Supreme, Sainsbury's*	1 Pot/95g	116	3.8	122	3.0	18.0	4.0	0.0
Vanilla with Strawberries Swirl, Weight Watchers*	1 Pot/57g	46	1.3	81	1.5	13.3	2.2	0.2
Whip, Banoffee, Prep with Skim Milk, Weight Watchers*	½ Packet/69g	49	1.2	71	3.1	10.5	1.8	0.5
White Chocolate, Delights, Shape, Danone*	1 Pot/110g	109	2.6	99	3.5	15.9	2.4	0.1
White Chocolate & Raspberry, Tesco*	1 Dessert/88g	180	8.9	204	3.4	25.0	10.1	3.1
Zabaglione	1 Serving/100g	278	18.3	278	3.6	24.3	18.3	2.3
DESSERT SAUCE								
Chocolate, M & S*	1 Dtsp/11g	35	1.0	330	2.1	59.3	9.4	1.9
Raspberry, M & S*	1 Serving/20g	24	0.1	120	0.5	28.7	0.3	2.6
Toffee, Old English, Asda*	1 Serving/28g	99	1.7	355	2.3	73.0	6.0	0.0
DHAL								
Black Gram, Average	1oz/28g	21	1.0	74	4.2	7.0	3.4	1.7
Blackeye Bean, Patak's*	1oz/28g	29	1.3	102	3.6	12.4	4.6	1.8
Chick Pea	1oz/28g	42	1.7	149	7.4	17.7	6.1	3.8
Chick Pea, Asda*	1 Serving/400g	404	12.0	101	4.5	14.0	3.0	3.0
Chick Pea, Canned, Asda*	½ Can/194g	198	6.2	102	4.3	14.0	3.2	2.9
Chick Pea, Sainsbury's*	½ Can/200g	432	18.2	216	10.8	22.7	9.1	7.1
Chickpea, Canned, Sainsbury's*	½ Can/432g	933	39.3	216	10.8	22.7	9.1	7.1
Lentil, Patak's*	1 Can/283g	156	2.8	55	2.8	9.3	1.0	1.0
Lentil, Red, Way to Five, Sainsbury's*	½ Pack/273g	254	4.1	93	5.5	14.4	1.5	1.4
Lentil, Red Masoor, Punjabi, Average	1oz/28g	39	1.3	139	7.2	19.2	4.6	2.0
Lentil, Red Masoor & Tomato with Butter, Average	1oz/28g	26	1.4	94	4.0	9.7	4.9	0.9
Lentil, Red Masoor & Vegetable, Average	1oz/28g	31	1.1	110	5.8	14.7	3.8	1.8
Lentil, Red Masoor with Vegetable Oil, Average	1oz/28g	48	2.2	172	7.6	19.2	7.9	1.8
Lentil, Red Masoorl & Mung Bean, Average	1oz/28g	32	1.9	114	4.8	9.9	6.7	1.6

D

	Measure INFO/WEIGHT	per Measure		Nutrition Values per 100g / 100ml				
		KCAL	FAT	KCAL	PROT	CARB	FAT	FIBRE
DHAL								
Lentil, Tesco*	1 Serving/200g	248	13.2	124	5.1	10.6	6.6	2.5
Mung Bean, Bengali	1oz/28g	20	0.9	73	4.2	7.4	3.3	1.7
Mung Beans, Dried, Boiled in Unsalted Water	1oz/28g	26	0.1	92	7.8	15.3	0.4	0.0
Mung Beans, Dried, Raw	1oz/28g	81	0.3	291	26.8	46.3	1.1	0.0
Regular, Eastern Essence*	1 Serving/113g	105	4.0	93	7.1	19.5	3.5	2.6
Split Peas, Yellow, Chana, Asda*	1 Serving/275g	300	19.2	109	2.6	9.0	7.0	1.8
Tarka, Asda*	½ Pack/150g	216	12.0	144	6.0	12.0	8.0	6.0
Vegetable Spicy, & Lentil, Solo Slim, Rosemary Conley*	1 Serving/100g	79	2.0	79	4.2	11.3	2.0	3.5
DHANSAK								
Chicken, Ready Meals, M & S*	1oz/28g	50	3.2	180	12.4	6.6	11.5	1.6
Chicken with Bagara Rice, Waitrose*	1 Pack/450g	549	8.1	122	8.2	18.2	1.8	1.2
Vegetable, Sainsbury's*	1 Serving/200g	148	5.6	74	3.1	8.9	2.8	2.8
DILL								
Dried	*1 Tsp/1g*	*3*	*0.0*	*253*	*19.9*	*42.2*	*4.4*	*13.6*
Fresh, Average	*1 Tbsp/3g*	*1*	*0.0*	*25*	*3.7*	*0.9*	*0.8*	*2.5*
DIM SUM								
From Restaurant, Average	1 Piece/12g	50	2.4	433	28.9	31.3	20.4	0.0
Steamed, Prawn, M & S*	6 Pieces/120g	222	3.2	185	1.1	39.0	2.7	1.5
DIME								
Terry's*	1oz/28g	154	9.5	550	4.6	68.5	33.8	0.6
DIP								
Aubergine, Fresh, Waitrose*	1 Serving/85g	159	12.7	187	2.5	10.5	15.0	1.7
Bean & Cheese, Asda*	1 Serving/50g	78	4.5	157	7.0	12.0	9.0	1.7
Blue Cheese, Fresh, Sainsbury's*	1/5 Pot/34g	115	11.7	337	3.6	3.1	34.5	0.1
Cajun Red Pepper, Sainsbury's*	1 Serving/50g	25	0.9	50	1.4	7.0	1.8	1.4
Cheddar & Onion, M & S*	1oz/28g	88	8.3	315	5.1	7.5	29.5	0.5
Cheddar & Spring Onion, M & S*	1 Pack/125g	581	60.4	465	3.6	4.7	48.3	0.5
Cheese & Chive, 50% Less Fat, Asda*	1 Pot/125g	261	21.5	209	4.5	9.0	17.2	0.0
Cheese & Chive, 50% Less Fat, Morrisons*	1 Serving/50g	86	6.3	172	8.8	5.2	12.7	0.2
Cheese & Chive, Asda*	1 Serving/43g	190	19.5	447	4.9	3.4	46.0	0.0
Cheese & Chive, Fresh, Sainsbury's*	1oz/28g	109	11.3	390	3.9	2.7	40.4	0.0
Cheese & Chive, M & S*	1oz/28g	120	12.3	430	4.5	3.9	44.1	0.5
Cheese & Chive, Tesco*	¼ Pack/50g	267	27.5	535	4.3	4.3	55.1	0.1
Chilli, M & S*	1 Pot/35g	103	0.1	295	0.4	73.2	0.2	0.4
Chilli Cheese, Asda*	1 Serving/50g	131	11.0	262	8.0	8.0	22.0	1.1
Chilli Cheese, Max, Walkers*	1 Jar/300g	390	27.3	130	3.3	9.4	9.1	0.3
Cucumber & Mint, Fresh, Sainsbury's*	1oz/28g	34	2.8	123	4.5	3.7	10.0	0.0
Feta Cheese, Fresh, Tesco*	1oz/28g	81	7.1	288	6.8	7.9	25.5	0.7
Frijolemole, Tesco*	¼ Pot/50g	105	8.1	210	3.6	12.3	16.2	2.0
Garlic & Herb	1 Serving/100g	583	62.3	583	1.3	4.1	62.3	0.2
Garlic & Herb, Big Dipper, Morrisons*	¼ Pot/75g	277	28.1	370	1.3	6.9	37.5	0.4
Garlic & Herb, Reduced Fat, M & S*	1 Serving/10g	9	0.4	95	6.0	8.1	4.0	0.5
Garlic & Herb, Tesco*	¼ Pack/43g	257	27.8	604	0.9	3.2	65.4	0.3
Garlic Herb & Rocket, M & S*	1 Serving/25g	104	10.7	415	2.4	4.5	43.0	0.5
Guacamole, Reduced Fat, BGTY, Sainsbury's*	½ Pot/65g	75	7.2	116	1.3	2.7	11.1	4.0
Guacamole, Supreme, Waitrose*	½ Pot/85g	105	10.3	124	1.6	2.1	12.1	4.3
Guacamole Style, Topping, Discovery*	1 Serving/37g	29	2.1	79	1.2	6.0	5.6	1.2
Hot Salsa, Doritos, Walkers*	1 Jar/300g	87	0.6	29	0.9	5.8	0.2	1.6
Mature Cheddar Cheese & Chive, Fresh, Waitrose*	½ Pot/85g	393	40.5	462	5.8	2.4	47.7	1.7
Mexican Bean, Doritos, Walkers*	1 Tbsp/20g	18	0.7	89	2.7	12.1	3.3	2.4
Mild Salsa, Doritos, Walkers*	1 Tbsp/30g	9	0.1	30	0.8	6.0	0.3	1.5
Mustard & Honey, Fresh, Sainsbury's*	1oz/28g	100	10.2	356	2.2	5.1	36.3	0.0
Mustard Mash, M & S*	1oz/28g	25	0.9	90	2.6	12.7	3.1	1.0

DIP

	Measure INFO/WEIGHT	per Measure KCAL	FAT	Nutrition Values per 100g / 100ml KCAL	PROT	CARB	FAT	FIBRE
Nacho Cheese, From Multipack Selection, Tesco*	1 Tub/125g	619	62.0	495	5.9	5.8	49.6	0.0
Nacho Cheese, M & S*	1oz/28g	76	6.6	270	9.8	3.8	23.7	0.4
Nacho Cheese, Primula*	1 Serving/57g	144	14.2	253	2.7	3.6	24.9	2.1
Nacho Cheese, Sainsbury's*	1 Serving/50g	243	25.1	487	4.8	3.9	50.2	0.0
Onion & Garlic, 50% Less Fat, Asda*	1oz/28g	59	4.8	209	4.5	9.0	17.2	0.0
Onion & Garlic, Classic, Tesco*	1 Serving/30g	133	13.9	442	1.7	4.6	46.3	0.2
Onion & Garlic, Fresh, BGTY, Sainsbury's*	1oz/28g	56	5.1	201	4.4	4.8	18.2	0.8
Onion & Garlic, GFY, Asda*	1/5 Pot/34g	56	4.8	166	2.1	8.0	14.0	0.2
Onion & Garlic, HL, Tesco*	1 Serving/43g	80	7.2	188	2.5	6.3	17.0	0.1
Onion & Garlic, Tesco*	1oz/28g	177	18.8	632	2.5	4.4	67.2	0.1
Pea, Yogurt & Mint, Sainsbury's*	1/4 Pack/50g	119	10.8	238	3.4	7.5	21.6	2.1
Peanut, Satay Selection, Occasions, Sainsbury's*	1 Serving/2g	4	0.2	186	7.1	13.8	11.4	1.1
Pecorino, Basil & Pine Nut, Fresh, Waitrose*	1/2 Pot/85g	338	33.7	398	5.1	5.1	39.7	0.0
Raita, Indian, Asda*	1 Pot/70g	120	11.5	172	2.6	3.6	16.4	0.5
Red Pepper, Nando's*	1 Serving/260g	550	13.2	211	5.2	36.3	5.1	1.8
Red Pepper, Sainsbury's*	1 Pot/100g	103	4.0	103	2.3	14.6	4.0	0.0
Roast Onion, Garlic & Rocket, Reduced Fat, Waitrose*	1 Serving/25g	50	4.7	202	2.7	5.4	18.8	1.5
Salsa, Chunky, Fresh, Sainsbury's*	1 Serving/100g	51	1.7	51	1.1	7.8	1.7	1.2
Salsa, Chunky Tomato, Tesco*	1 Pot/170g	68	2.2	40	1.1	5.9	1.3	1.1
Salsa, GFY, Asda*	1 Pot/170g	68	0.7	40	1.2	8.0	0.4	1.5
Salsa Mild, Asda*	1 Portion/100g	47	0.3	47	1.4	8.7	0.3	1.8
Smoked Salmon & Dill, Fresh, Waitrose*	1/2 Pot/85g	373	38.0	439	5.1	4.1	44.7	0.1
Smoked Salmon & Dill, Reduced Fat, Waitrose*	1/2 Pot/85g	184	16.7	217	3.9	6.1	19.7	1.1
Sour Cream, Co-Op*	1oz/28g	137	14.6	490	2.0	3.0	52.0	0.0
Sour Cream, Tesco*	1 Serving/38g	111	11.2	297	3.4	3.9	29.8	0.2
Sour Cream & Chive, BGTY, Sainsbury's*	1oz/28g	46	4.1	165	4.9	3.4	14.6	0.7
Sour Cream & Chive, Doritos, Walkers*	1 Tbsp/20g	52	4.9	258	1.9	6.9	24.7	1.9
Sour Cream & Chive, Fresh, Tesco*	1/2 Pot/75g	305	31.8	407	2.1	4.1	42.4	0.0
Sour Cream & Chive, Half Fat, Waitrose*	1/2 Pot/85g	133	9.9	157	5.5	7.6	11.6	0.1
Sour Cream & Chive, Primula*	1 Serving/57g	169	17.4	297	4.3	1.3	30.5	1.0
Sour Cream & Chive, Sainsbury's*	1 Serving/50g	141	13.7	282	3.1	5.4	27.5	0.1
Sour Cream & Chives, Mexican Style, Morrisons*	1/4 Pack/25g	68	7.0	274	2.2	3.4	27.9	0.4
Soured Cream & Chive, 95% Fat Free, M & S*	1oz/28g	25	0.8	90	6.5	9.6	2.8	0.5
Soured Cream & Chive, BGTY, Sainsbury's*	1 Serving/170g	253	17.5	149	4.2	9.9	10.3	0.1
Soured Cream & Chive, Classic, Tesco*	1 Serving/25g	81	8.4	323	1.7	3.2	33.7	0.2
Soured Cream & Chive, for Skins, Tesco*	1 Serving/12g	36	3.6	297	3.4	3.9	29.8	0.2
Soured Cream & Chive, HL, Tesco*	1 Serving/31g	45	3.3	145	3.8	7.5	10.6	0.2
Soured Cream & Chive, Light Choices, Tesco*	1/4 Pot/50g	65	4.5	130	4.3	7.4	9.0	0.1
Soured Cream & Chive, Morrisons*	1 Serving/100g	317	32.6	317	2.6	3.3	32.6	0.0
Spiced Mango, Ginger & Chilli Salsa, Weight Watchers*	1 Serving/56g	48	0.1	85	1.0	19.9	0.2	2.6
Spicy Moroccan, BGTY, Sainsbury's*	1/2 Pot/85g	56	1.7	66	2.1	10.0	2.0	1.7
Sweet & Sour, M & S*	1oz/28g	36	0.0	130	0.7	31.4	0.1	0.5
Sweet & Sour, Primula*	1 Serving/57g	76	0.1	133	0.4	32.8	0.2	0.0
Sweet Chilli, Chinese Snack Selection, Morrisons*	1/2 Pot/20g	64	0.0	320	0.1	79.4	0.2	0.6
Sweet Chilli, Oriental Selection, Waitrose*	1/2 Pot/35g	88	0.3	250	1.3	59.4	0.8	0.4
Sweet Chilli Mango, Encona*	1 Tbsp/15ml	22	0.1	148	0.4	35.4	0.6	0.0
Thai Sweet Chilli, Primula*	1 Serving/57g	126	0.1	221	0.6	54.4	0.1	0.2
Thousand Island, HL, Tesco*	1 Serving/31g	57	4.6	183	2.5	9.6	14.9	0.3
Thousand Island, M & S*	1oz/28g	69	6.2	245	2.1	9.4	22.2	0.7
Tomato Ketchup, Asda*	1 Pack/25g	18	0.0	71	1.6	16.0	0.1	1.0
Tortilla Chips, Cool Flavour, Big, Morrisons*	1/2 Pack/100g	453	22.0	453	6.4	57.4	22.0	8.1
Yoghurt & Cucumber Mint, Tesco*	1oz/28g	34	2.0	121	7.0	7.2	7.1	0.6

D

	Measure INFO/WEIGHT	per Measure KCAL	FAT	Nutrition Values per 100g / 100ml KCAL	PROT	CARB	FAT	FIBRE
DISCOS								
Beef, KP Snacks*	1 Pack/28g	145	8.2	518	5.1	58.7	29.3	2.4
Cheese & Onion, KP Snacks*	1 Pack/28g	146	8.2	520	5.1	59.1	29.3	2.5
Salt & Vinegar, KP Snacks*	1 Bag/28g	145	8.3	517	4.7	58.3	29.5	2.3
DOLLY MIXTURES								
M & S*	1 Pack/115g	431	1.6	375	1.8	89.2	1.4	0.0
Sainsbury's*	1 Serving/10g	40	0.2	401	1.4	94.4	1.9	0.1
Tesco*	1 Pack/100g	376	1.5	376	1.6	88.9	1.5	0.0
DOPIAZA								
Chicken, M & S*	1 Pack/350g	402	21.3	115	11.5	3.7	6.1	2.5
Chicken, Sainsbury's*	½ Pack/200g	272	15.8	136	13.2	3.1	7.9	0.8
Chicken, Tesco*	1 Pack/350g	448	24.8	128	10.8	5.3	7.1	0.6
Chicken, with Pilau Rice, Sharwood's*	1 Pack/375g	472	17.2	126	5.3	15.8	4.6	0.8
Chicken, with Pilau Rice, Tesco*	1 Pack/400g	424	15.2	106	5.7	12.3	3.8	1.5
Mushroom, Retail	1oz/28g	19	1.6	69	1.3	3.7	5.7	1.1
Mushroom, Waitrose*	½ Pack/150g	81	4.6	54	2.2	4.3	3.1	2.3
DORITOS								
Chargrilled BBQ, Walkers*	1 Bag/35g	170	8.7	485	5.5	59.0	25.0	3.5
Cheesy 3d's, Doritos, Walkers*	1 Pack/20g	89	3.2	445	7.0	68.0	16.0	3.0
Chilli Heatwave, Walkers*	1 Bag/35g	175	9.1	500	7.0	60.0	26.0	3.0
Cool, Ranch Chips, Walkers*	1 Pack/50g	250	13.0	504	8.1	64.5	26.2	4.0
Cool Original, Walkers*	1 Bag/40g	200	10.8	500	7.5	58.0	27.0	3.0
Cool Spice 3ds, Walkers*	1 Bag/24g	108	4.3	450	8.0	64.0	18.0	4.4
Dippas, Hint of Chilli, Dipping Chips, Walkers*	1 Bag/35g	173	8.7	495	7.0	61.0	25.0	3.5
Dippas, Hint of Garlic, Dipping Chips, Walkers*	1 Serving/35g	175	8.7	500	7.0	61.0	25.0	3.5
Dippas, Hint of Lime, Walkers*	1 Bag/35g	173	8.7	495	7.0	60.0	25.0	3.5
Dippas, Lightly Salted, Dipping Chips, Walkers*	1 Serving/35g	178	9.4	510	6.5	60.0	27.0	3.0
Latinos, Chargrilled BBQ, Walkers*	1 Serving/35g	170	8.7	485	5.5	59.0	25.0	3.5
Latinos, Mexican Grill, Walkers*	1 Serving/35g	170	8.7	485	6.5	59.0	25.0	3.5
Latinos, Sour Cream & Sweet Pepper, Walkers*	1 Pack/40g	194	10.0	485	5.5	60.0	25.0	3.5
Lightly Salted Dippas, Doritos, Walkers*	1 Serving/40g	204	10.8	510	6.5	60.0	27.0	3.0
Mexican Hot, Walkers*	1 Bag/40g	202	10.8	505	8.0	57.0	27.0	3.5
Tangy Cheese, Walkers*	1 Bag/40g	200	10.8	500	7.0	57.0	27.0	3.0
DOUBLE DECKER								
Cadbury*	1 Bar/60g	276	11.3	460	4.4	68.4	18.9	0.6
Snack Size, Cadbury*	1 Bar/36g	165	7.4	465	4.8	64.5	20.9	0.0
with Nuts, Cadbury*	1 Bar/60g	291	14.7	485	7.9	58.6	24.5	0.0
DOUGH BALLS								
Cheese & Garlic, Occasions, Sainsbury's*	1 Ball/12g	41	2.2	341	10.3	33.4	18.5	2.1
Garlic, GFY, Asda*	1 Ball/8g	21	0.2	250	9.0	49.0	2.0	2.0
Garlic, HL, Tesco*	1 Serving/40g	110	3.2	274	8.8	42.0	7.9	2.3
Garlic, Tesco*	1 Serving/10g	40	2.3	400	7.0	40.0	23.0	1.0
Garlic, Waitrose*	1 Ball/11g	38	1.8	347	8.5	41.4	16.4	3.3
Garlic & Herb, Asda*	4 Balls/48g	173	8.5	361	9.2	40.9	17.8	3.6
Garlic & Herb, Occasions, Sainsbury's*	1 Ball/12g	41	2.1	343	8.4	38.7	17.2	2.2
Sainsbury's*	1 Ball/12g	41	2.1	343	8.4	38.7	17.2	2.2
Supermarket, Pizza Express*	8 Balls/100g	363	1.7	363	14.3	72.9	1.7	3.3
with Garlic & Herb Butter, Aldi*	1 Ball/12g	45	2.2	365	7.7	46.7	18.2	1.8
DOUGHNUTS								
Apple & Fresh Cream, Sainsbury's*	1 Doughnut/79g	216	11.4	273	5.4	30.5	14.4	1.9
Baked, HL, Tesco*	1 Doughnut/67g	166	3.9	248	6.4	42.2	5.9	1.4
Cream & Jam, Assorted Box, Sainsbury's*	1 Doughnut/71g	229	12.7	322	6.2	34.2	17.9	2.2
Cream & Jam, Tesco*	1 Doughnut/90g	288	14.1	320	5.4	39.4	15.7	2.0
Custard, Sainsbury's*	1 Doughnut/70g	172	7.5	246	5.1	32.3	10.7	2.3

	Measure INFO/WEIGHT	per Measure KCAL	FAT	Nutrition Values per 100g / 100ml KCAL	PROT	CARB	FAT	FIBRE
DOUGHNUTS								
Custard, Tesco*	1 Doughnut/91g	266	14.4	292	4.1	33.4	15.8	1.1
Custard & Bramley Apple, Sainsbury's*	1 Doughnut/91g	256	12.6	282	4.5	34.6	13.9	1.0
Custard Filled, Average	1 Doughnut/75g	268	14.2	358	6.2	43.3	19.0	0.0
Finger, Co-Op*	1 Doughnut/82g	299	14.8	365	4.0	45.0	18.0	2.0
Jam, American Style, Sainsbury's*	1 Doughnut/65g	220	20.6	339	4.9	49.6	31.8	3.5
Jam, Fresh Cream, Sweet Fresh, Tesco*	1 Doughnut/74g	248	12.1	335	5.5	40.7	16.4	1.9
Jam, M & S*	1 Doughnut/49g	141	2.0	287	5.0	57.6	4.0	1.3
Jam, Mini, Frozen, Party, Tesco*	2 Doughnut/25g	101	5.5	405	5.3	45.0	22.1	2.0
Jam Filled, Average	1 Doughnut/75g	252	10.9	336	5.7	48.8	14.5	0.0
Mini, Chocolate Topped, Chosen By You, Asda*	1 Serving/100g	393	19.5	393	5.2	49.1	19.5	2.0
Mini, Sainsbury's*	1 Doughnut/14g	53	2.7	379	5.2	47.9	18.9	2.1
Original, Glazed, Krispy Kreme*	1 Doughnut/52g	217	13.0	417	6.0	43.0	25.0	4.0
Plain, Ring, Average	1 Doughnut/60g	238	13.0	397	6.1	47.2	21.7	0.0
Raspberry Jam, Sainsbury's*	1 Doughnut/77g	266	15.7	345	4.7	35.7	20.4	1.3
Ring, Iced, Average	1 Doughnut/70g	268	12.2	383	4.8	55.1	17.5	0.0
Strawberry Jam & Cream, Sainsbury's*	1 Doughnut/80g	299	18.5	374	5.3	36.2	23.2	1.3
Toffee, Tesco*	1 Doughnut/75g	235	8.7	313	8.0	44.2	11.6	1.6
Yum Yums, Glazed, Sweet, Waitrose*	1 Doughnut/45g	172	10.0	382	4.0	41.6	22.2	2.0
Yum Yums, M & S*	1 Doughnut/37g	155	8.9	420	4.9	45.7	23.9	1.6
Yum Yums, Tesco*	1 Doughnut/61g	232	10.1	380	6.1	51.6	16.6	1.7
DOVER SOLE								
Raw, Average	*1oz/28g*	*25*	*0.5*	*89*	*18.1*	*0.0*	*1.8*	*0.0*
DR PEPPER*								
Coca-Cola*	1 Bottle/500ml	210	0.0	42	0.0	10.9	0.0	0.0
Z, Coca-Cola*	1 Glass/250ml	10	0.0	4	0.0	0.0	0.0	0.0
Zero, Coca-Cola*	1 Can/330ml	2	0.0	0	0.0	0.0	0.0	0.0
DRAGON FRUIT								
Raw, Edible Portion, Average	1 Serving/100g	41	0.5	41	0.7	9.6	0.5	3.6
DRAMBUIE								
39% Volume	*1 Shot/35ml*	*95*	*0.0*	*272*	*0.0*	*23.0*	*0.0*	*0.0*
DREAM								
Double Fudge, Cadbury*	1oz/28g	139	7.1	495	6.3	61.4	25.2	0.0
Snowbites, Cadbury*	1 Serving/31g	170	10.2	545	3.1	59.7	32.7	0.0
White Chocolate, Cadbury*	1 Piece/8g	44	2.7	555	4.5	59.7	33.3	0.0
DREAM TOPPING								
Dry, Bird's*	1oz/28g	193	16.4	690	6.7	32.5	58.5	0.5
Made Up, Skimmed Milk, Bird's*	1oz/28g	21	1.5	75	2.0	4.8	5.3	0.0
Sugar Free, Dry, Bird's*	1oz/28g	195	16.9	695	7.3	30.5	60.5	0.5
DRESSING								
Balsamic, Fresh Olive Co*	1 Tbsp/15g	42	0.1	282	1.5	67.8	0.5	0.6
Balsamic, Light Choices, Tesco*	1 Tbsp/14g	12	0.2	85	0.3	16.7	1.5	0.2
Balsamic, M & S*	1 Tbsp/15g	73	7.2	490	0.3	9.7	48.0	0.5
Balsamic, Sainsbury's*	1 Tbsp/15ml	47	4.3	316	0.4	13.8	28.8	0.4
Balsamic, Schwartz*	1 Tbsp/15ml	12	0.3	77	0.5	14.2	2.0	0.0
Balsamic, Sweet, Finest, Tesco*	1 Serving/10ml	15	0.0	155	0.4	36.9	0.1	0.4
Balsamic, Weight Watchers*	1 Serving/15ml	12	0.3	81	0.1	16.0	1.8	0.5
Balsamic Bliss, Ainsley Harriott*	1 Tbsp/15g	41	3.2	272	0.8	19.3	21.1	0.0
Balsamic Vinegar, Asda*	1 Pack/44ml	121	11.9	275	0.9	7.0	27.0	0.0
Balsamic Vinegar, Light, Kraft*	1 Serving/15ml	15	0.9	100	0.3	9.6	6.3	0.5
Balsamic Vinegar, Olives & Herb, COU, M & S*	1 Serving/30g	22	0.6	75	0.5	14.3	2.0	0.5
Basil & Pesto, COU, M & S*	1 Serving/50ml	30	1.1	60	0.6	8.3	2.2	0.8
Blue Cheese, 60% Less Fat, BGTY, Sainsbury's*	1 Tbsp/15ml	26	2.3	172	1.9	7.3	15.1	0.2
Blue Cheese, Fresh, Sainsbury's*	1 Dtsp/10ml	42	4.6	423	2.3	0.5	45.7	0.1

DRESSING

INFO/WEIGHT	Measure	per Measure KCAL	FAT	Nutrition Values per 100g / 100ml KCAL	PROT	CARB	FAT	FIBRE
Blue Cheese, Hellmann's*	1 Tbsp/15g	69	7.1	459	0.7	6.3	47.2	1.1
Blue Cheese, Sainsbury's*	1 Serving/20g	64	6.0	321	2.3	10.6	29.9	0.4
Blue Cheese, Salad, Waitrose*	1 Serving/50g	265	25.1	530	2.1	17.3	50.3	4.1
Caesar, 95% Fat Free, Tesco*	1 Tsp/6g	5	0.2	88	4.1	8.9	3.7	0.3
Caesar, Asiago, Briannas*	1 Tbsp/15ml	70	7.5	467	3.3	3.3	50.0	
Caesar, Chilled, Reduced Fat, Tesco*	1 Tsp/5ml	13	1.2	252	6.5	3.1	23.7	0.1
Caesar, Classic, Sainsbury's*	1 Tsp/5ml	22	2.3	442	2.7	4.6	45.9	0.5
Caesar, Finest, Tesco*	1 Tbsp/15ml	72	7.6	477	1.9	2.8	50.9	0.2
Caesar, Fresh, Asda*	1 Dtsp/10ml	45	4.8	454	2.4	3.2	48.0	0.0
Caesar, Fresh, M & S*	1 Tsp/6g	31	3.4	525	2.0	1.8	56.4	0.2
Caesar, Hellmann's*	1 Tsp/6g	30	3.1	499	2.5	4.5	51.7	0.3
Caesar, Less Than 3% Fat, BGTY, Sainsbury's*	1 Serving/20g	10	0.4	48	0.8	7.0	1.9	0.3
Caesar, Light, Kraft*	1 Tbsp/15g	14	0.5	95	1.7	13.0	3.6	0.2
Caesar, Light Choices, Tesco*	1 Tbsp/15g	9	0.2	60	1.5	9.5	1.5	0.5
Caesar, Loyd Grossman*	1 Dtsp/10g	34	3.4	342	2.1	7.0	33.9	0.0
Caesar, Luxury, Hellmann's*	1 Tsp/4g	20	2.1	498	2.5	4.4	51.7	0.3
Caesar, Original, Cardini's*	1 Serving/10g	55	6.0	555	2.3	1.5	60.0	0.2
Caesar, Waitrose*	1 Serving/15ml	72	7.6	479	4.5	0.9	50.8	0.2
Caesar Style, GFY, Asda*	1 Sachet/44ml	34	1.0	77	5.0	9.0	2.3	0.0
Champagne, For Smoked Haddock Tian, Waitrose*	½ Pack/38g	195	21.1	513	1.1	2.3	55.5	0.8
Citrus Salad, BGTY, Sainsbury's*	1 Tbsp/15ml	13	0.5	90	0.3	14.4	3.1	0.3
Classic French, Fresh, M & S*	1 Serving/10ml	51	5.3	515	0.6	8.2	53.1	0.2
Classic Italian, Get Dressed, Kraft*	1 Serving/25ml	30	2.6	120	0.1	5.6	10.3	0.5
Cream Cheese & Chive, Creamy Ranch, Kraft*	1 Serving/15ml	31	2.5	205	1.2	11.0	17.0	0.0
Creamy, Waistline, 93% Fat Free, Crosse & Blackwell*	1 Tsp/6g	7	0.4	120	1.0	14.4	6.4	0.2
Creamy Caesar, Waistline, Crosse & Blackwell*	1 Dtsp/11g	15	1.0	135	1.5	11.1	9.2	0.3
Creamy Ranch, 95% Fat Free, Kraft*	1 Tsp/6ml	7	0.3	111	1.4	14.5	5.0	0.3
Creamy Roasted Garlic, GFY, Asda*	1 Tbsp/15g	10	0.6	70	0.8	8.0	3.9	0.6
Creme Fraiche, Salad, Kraft*	1 Tbsp/15ml	12	0.4	78	0.8	12.5	2.5	0.0
Dijon Honey Mustard, Briannas*	1 Tbsp/15ml	65	6.0	433	0.0	20.0	40.0	0.0
Fire Roasted Garlic & Thyme, Tesco*	1 Serving/10ml	45	4.7	447	0.9	4.7	47.2	0.0
Fire Roasted Red Pepper, M & S*	1 Serving/30g	13	0.0	45	0.5	10.7	0.1	0.9
Fire Roasted Tomato Basil, COU, M & S*	1 Serving/30g	13	0.3	45	0.6	8.1	0.9	1.1
French, BGTY, Organic, Sainsbury's*	1 Tbsp/15ml	11	0.6	71	0.2	8.3	4.1	0.5
French, BGTY, Sainsbury's*	1 Tbsp/15ml	12	0.7	79	1.1	8.8	4.4	0.5
French, Chilled, Tesco*	1 Tbsp/15ml	63	5.9	421	1.1	15.1	39.6	0.0
French, Cider Vinegar & Mustard, Tesco*	1 Tbsp/15ml	45	4.2	300	0.7	9.9	28.1	0.3
French, Classic, Fat Free, Kraft*	1 Tsp/5ml	2	0.0	39	0.1	8.7	0.0	0.5
French, Classic, Sainsbury's*	1 Tbsp/15ml	71	7.4	473	1.0	5.7	49.6	0.5
French, Classic, The English Provender Company*	1 Sachet/25g	21	0.6	84	0.8	14.7	2.4	0.0
French, Classics, M & S*	1 Tbsp/15ml	77	8.0	516	0.6	8.2	53.1	0.2
French, COU, M & S*	1/3 Bottle/105g	73	2.7	70	0.7	11.5	2.6	0.7
French, Finest, Tesco*	1 Tbsp/15g	55	5.8	370	0.4	5.1	38.7	1.0
French, Fresh, Organic, Sainsbury's*	1 Tbsp/15ml	45	4.6	301	0.4	5.5	31.0	0.3
French, Fresh, Sainsbury's*	1 Tbsp/15ml	64	6.7	429	0.6	6.6	44.6	0.6
French, GFY, Asda*	1 Tbsp/15g	7	0.3	50	0.7	7.0	2.1	0.1
French, Less Than 3% Fat, M & S*	1 Tbsp/15ml	10	0.4	68	0.7	11.5	2.6	0.7
French, Light, Heinz*	1 Sachet/12g	13	0.6	111	0.7	15.4	5.4	0.0
French, Light Choices, Tesco*	1 Serving/20g	10	0.3	48	0.8	7.6	1.6	1.1
French, Luxury, Hellmann's*	1 Tbsp/15g	45	3.9	297	0.4	14.9	25.9	0.3
French, Oil Free, French, Waitrose*	1 Tsp/5ml	4	0.1	76	1.5	13.1	2.0	0.6
French, Oil Free, Perfectly Balanced, Waitrose*	1 Serving/15ml	11	0.2	72	2.2	12.2	1.6	1.1
French, Organic, M & S*	1 Tbsp/15g	98	10.4	655	0.2	7.5	69.4	0.3

DRESSING

INFO/WEIGHT	Measure	per Measure KCAL	per Measure FAT	Nutrition per 100g/100ml KCAL	PROT	CARB	FAT	FIBRE
French, Reduced Fat, M & S*	1 Tbsp/15g	10	0.4	70	0.7	11.5	2.8	0.7
French, Sainsbury's*	1 Tbsp/15ml	33	2.9	219	0.6	9.8	19.1	0.5
French, Tesco*	1 Serving/25ml	110	11.2	441	0.7	7.2	44.9	0.2
French, Virtually Fat Free, Aldi*	1 Serving/10g	3	0.0	33	0.9	6.7	0.3	1.1
French Salad, M & S*	1 Serving/25ml	156	16.8	625	0.5	3.8	67.3	0.1
French Style Calorie-Wise Salad, Kraft*	1 Tbsp/15ml	24	1.6	160	0.0	18.7	10.7	0.0
Garlic & Herb, Perfectly Balanced, Waitrose*	1 Serving/50ml	67	0.7	135	0.6	29.9	1.4	0.8
Garlic & Herb, Reduced Calorie, Hellmann's*	1 Tbsp/15ml	35	2.9	232	0.6	12.8	19.3	0.4
Garlic & Herb, Tesco*	1 Tbsp/15g	31	3.0	210	0.9	5.8	20.2	0.8
Green Olive, M & S*	1oz/28g	40	4.0	144	1.5	2.2	14.4	1.3
Green Thai, Coconut & Lemon Grass, Loyd Grossman*	1oz/28g	49	3.0	174	0.2	19.3	10.6	0.5
Green Thai, Finest, Tesco*	1 Bottle/250ml	940	81.8	376	0.3	19.1	32.7	0.3
Herb & Garlic, Light, 5% Fat, Get Dressed, Kraft*	1 Serving/25ml	29	1.3	116	1.3	15.5	5.1	0.2
Honey, Orange & Mustard, BGTY, Sainsbury's*	1 Tbsp/15ml	16	0.4	105	1.8	18.6	2.5	1.8
Honey & Mustard, BGTY, Sainsbury's*	1 Tbsp /20g	14	0.1	71	0.4	16.1	0.5	0.2
Honey & Mustard, Fresh, M & S*	1 Serving/10ml	43	4.2	430	1.7	9.7	42.4	0.5
Honey & Mustard, GFY, Asda*	1 Tbsp/15g	13	0.5	89	1.5	13.0	3.4	0.8
Honey & Mustard, Light Choices, Tesco*	1 Tbsp/14g	9	0.2	65	1.3	11.6	1.1	0.6
Honey & Mustard, M & S*	1 Tbsp/15ml	64	6.4	427	1.7	9.7	42.4	0.6
Honey & Mustard, Sainsbury's*	1 Serving/10ml	37	3.3	366	1.0	15.4	33.0	0.1
Honey & Mustard, Tesco*	1 Serving/10ml	38	3.6	378	0.8	13.1	35.8	0.6
Honey & Mustard, The English Provender Co.*	1 Tbsp/15ml	17	0.2	111	2.5	21.8	1.5	1.0
Hot Lime & Coconut, BGTY, Sainsbury's*	1 Tbsp/15ml	8	0.4	51	0.7	5.7	2.9	1.2
Italian, Light, Low Fat, Newman's Own*	1 Serving/15g	9	0.4	57	0.1	6.7	2.8	0.5
Italian, Low Fat, Heinz*	1 Pot/30ml	26	1.9	86	0.9	6.3	6.3	2.7
Italian, M & S*	1 Tbsp/15ml	62	6.2	415	0.9	8.9	41.5	1.0
Italian, Reduced Calorie, Hellmann's*	1 Serving/25ml	67	5.2	269	0.5	19.5	20.8	0.3
Italian, Waistline, 99% Fat Free, Crosse & Blackwell*	1 Tsp/6g	2	0.1	39	0.7	7.0	0.9	0.3
Italian Balsamic, Loyd Grossman*	1 Serving/10g	36	3.3	357	0.9	13.1	33.5	0.1
Italian Balsamic, The English Provender Co.*	1 Serving/30ml	20	0.8	67	0.8	9.9	2.7	0.2
Italian Salad, Hellmann's*	1 Serving/50g	103	8.3	206	0.7	12.8	16.7	0.0
Lemon, Feta & Oregano, M & S*	1 Tbsp/15ml	24	2.0	160	1.3	8.2	13.4	0.6
Lemon & Cracked Black Pepper, GFY, Asda*	1 Tbsp/15g	9	0.0	57	0.2	14.0	0.0	0.3
Lemon & Watercress, COU, M & S*	1 Serving/28g	14	0.5	50	0.4	8.5	1.8	0.5
Lime & Coriander, Oil Free, Waitrose*	1 Tsp/5ml	3	0.1	65	1.5	11.9	1.3	0.4
Lime & Coriander, Sainsbury's*	1 Tbsp/15ml	61	6.1	409	0.4	10.0	40.8	0.5
Lime & Coriander, The English Provender Co.*	1 Serving/50g	28	0.1	57	0.3	13.3	0.3	0.0
Mayonnaise Style, 90% Fat Free, Weight Watchers*	1 Tsp/11g	14	1.0	125	1.7	8.9	9.2	0.0
Mild Mustard, Low Fat, Weight Watchers*	1 Tbsp/10g	6	0.4	63	2.0	5.7	3.6	0.0
Mint & Tomato, Mary Berry*	1 Serving/100g	399	37.1	399	0.8	14.8	37.1	0.3
Mustard & Dill, Perfectly Balanced, Waitrose*	1 Tbsp/15ml	24	0.5	159	1.1	31.5	3.2	1.1
Oil & Lemon	1 Tbsp/15g	97	10.6	647	0.3	2.8	70.6	0.0
Olive Oil & Balsamic Vinegar, Sainsbury's*	1 Serving/25ml	104	10.4	415	0.9	9.4	41.8	0.2
Orange & Cracked Pepper, Tesco*	1 Tbsp/15ml	17	0.0	114	0.5	27.8	0.1	0.3
Orange & Honey, Luxury, Hellmann's*	1 Serving/15ml	16	0.5	110	0.8	17.5	3.5	0.8
Parmesan & Peppercorn, Loyd Grossman*	1oz/28g	98	9.9	349	2.1	5.9	35.2	0.5
Ranch Style, Asda*	1 Serving/44ml	37	1.7	85	3.5	9.0	3.9	0.0
Red Pepper, BGTY, Sainsbury's*	1 Bottle/250g	107	0.7	43	0.2	9.8	0.3	0.2
Red Pepper, M & S*	1 Tbsp/15ml	58	5.9	385	0.6	7.6	39.2	0.5
Rich Poppy Seed, Briannas*	1 Tbsp/15ml	65	6.5	433	0.0	20.0	43.3	0.0
Salad, Caesar, Light, Fry Light*	1 Spray/0.2ml	1	0.1	321	0.4	9.2	30.7	0.1
Salad, Catalina, Kraft*	1 Serving/34g	100	6.0	294	0.0	29.4	17.6	0.0
Salad, Honey & Mustard, Light, Kraft*	1 Tbsp/15ml	19	0.7	126	1.2	19.0	4.6	1.1

DRESSING

	Measure INFO/WEIGHT	per Measure		Nutrition Values per 100g / 100ml				
		KCAL	FAT	KCAL	PROT	CARB	FAT	FIBRE
Salad, Italian, Light, Kraft*	1 Tbsp/15ml	5	0.0	31	0.1	6.8	0.0	0.6
Salad, Italian, Newman's Own*	1 Tbsp/10g	54	6.0	545	0.2	1.0	59.8	0.0
Salad, Kickin' Mango, Oil Free, Ainsley Harriott*	1 Tbsp/15ml	14	0.0	92	0.1	21.1	0.1	0.0
Salad, Light, Heinz*	1 Serving/10g	24	2.0	244	1.8	13.5	19.9	0.0
Salad, Low Fat, Weight Watchers*	1 Tbsp/10g	10	0.4	106	1.5	15.4	4.3	0.0
Salad, Mary Berry*	1 Serving/15g	77	6.6	513	0.8	28.5	44.0	0.1
Salad, Raspberry Balsamic, GFY, Asda*	1 Tbsp/15ml	6	0.1	40	0.7	9.3	0.7	1.3
Salad, Sun Dried Tomato & Chilli, Loyd Grossman*	1 Tsp/5g	18	1.9	361	0.9	5.3	37.3	0.9
Salad, Thousand Island, 95% Fat Free, Asda*	1 Tsp/6g	6	0.3	99	1.6	12.6	4.7	0.5
Salad, Thousand Island, Hellmann's*	1oz/28g	97	8.7	347	0.9	15.2	31.0	1.0
Salad, Thousand Island, Reduced Calorie, Hellmann's*	1oz/28g	73	5.4	259	1.0	19.0	19.4	0.9
Salad, Vinaigrette Style, 95% Fat Free, Asda*	1 Tbsp/15ml	6	0.0	42	0.1	10.6	0.0	0.3
Seafood, M & S*	1 Tsp/7g	39	4.2	555	0.9	4.9	59.3	0.9
Sicilian Lemon, M & S*	1 Tbsp/15ml	73	7.4	485	0.1	10.5	49.1	0.0
Smoked Garlic & Parmesan, Sainsbury's*	1 Serving/20ml	83	8.2	415	3.0	4.0	41.1	0.3
Special Mustard, & Daughter, Mary Berry*	1 Tbsp/15g	75	7.0	499	1.5	23.2	46.4	0.4
Sun Dried Tomato, Sainsbury's*	1 Serving/15ml	27	2.2	179	1.5	10.9	14.4	0.6
Sweet Balsamic & Smoked Garlic, BGTY, Sainsbury's*	1 Serving/20g	10	0.1	51	0.2	11.9	0.3	0.2
Sweet Chilli, COU, M & S*	1 Tbsp/15ml	9	0.1	60	0.5	14.5	0.5	0.4
Texas Ranch, Frank Cooper*	1 Pot/28g	128	12.8	457	1.9	9.4	45.8	0.2
Thai Lime & Coriander, The English Provender Co.*	1 Serving/25g	26	0.2	104	1.6	22.3	0.9	1.1
Thousand Island	1 Tsp/6g	19	1.8	323	1.1	12.5	30.2	0.4
Thousand Island, BGTY, Sainsbury's*	1 Serving/20g	19	1.4	95	0.4	7.3	7.2	0.5
Thousand Island, COU, M & S*	1 Serving/30g	25	0.8	85	1.4	14.2	2.6	1.1
Thousand Island, Light, Kraft*	1 Tbsp/15ml	14	0.0	94	0.6	21.5	0.2	3.0
Thousand Island, Original, Kraft*	1oz/28g	102	8.8	365	0.9	19.0	31.5	0.4
Thousand Island, Reduced Calorie	1 Tsp/6g	12	0.9	195	0.7	14.7	15.2	0.0
Thousand Island, Tesco*	1 Tbsp/15g	55	4.7	360	1.1	19.5	30.5	0.3
Tomato & Basil, HL, Tesco*	½ Pot/75ml	41	1.1	55	0.8	9.0	1.5	0.5
Tomato & Herb, Less Than 1% Fat, Asda*	1 Tbsp/15g	6	0.1	43	0.7	8.0	0.9	0.4
Tomato & Red Pepper, BGTY, Sainsbury's*	1 Serving/50ml	41	2.1	83	1.1	10.0	4.3	0.6
Tomato Basil, Light, Kraft*	1 Serving/15ml	10	0.1	68	1.0	14.5	0.4	2.5
True Blue Cheese, Briannas*	2 Tbsp/30ml	120	11.0	400	3.3	16.7	36.7	0.0
Vinaigrette, BGTY, Sainsbury's*	1 Dtsp/20g	13	0.5	64	1.1	9.3	2.4	2.5
Waistline, Reduced Fat, Crosse & Blackwell*	1oz/28g	29	1.7	105	0.8	11.6	6.0	0.3
Whole Grain Dijon Mustard & Honey, Loyd Grossman*	1oz/28g	93	8.9	331	1.2	9.9	31.8	1.3
Yoghurt & Mint, HL, Tesco*	1 Serving/50g	31	1.2	62	4.1	6.9	2.5	0.2
Yoghurt & Mint Dressing Less Than 3% Fat, Asda*	1 Tbsp/16g	12	0.3	76	2.8	11.7	2.0	0.4
Yoghurt Mint Cucumber, M & S*	1 Tsp/5ml	6	0.4	115	1.0	8.7	8.0	0.0

DRIED FRUIT

	Measure INFO/WEIGHT	per Measure		Nutrition Values per 100g / 100ml				
		KCAL	FAT	KCAL	PROT	CARB	FAT	FIBRE
Banana, Bites, Kiddylicious, Babylicious*	1 Serving/15g	43	2.9	285	10.8	43.6	19.3	6.1
Beach Bum, Graze*	1 Pack/35g	127	4.3	363	3.3	61.5	12.4	9.7
Exotic, Ready to Eat, Sainsbury's*	1/3 Pack/85g	241	0.1	284	0.2	70.6	0.1	2.4
Figgy Pop, Graze*	1 Pack/40g	100	0.4	251	2.5	61.6	1.1	0.0
Honey Coated Banana Chips, Whitworths*	1 Serving/25g	131	7.8	526	1.0	59.9	31.4	1.7
Jewel of The Nile, Graze*	1 Pack/45g	112	0.4	248	2.5	61.3	0.8	0.0
Juicy Sprinkle, Nature's Harvest*	1 Serving/20g	79	2.0	397	4.9	71.9	10.0	4.2
Jus Fruit, Mango Pieces, Yu!*	1 Pack/24g	87	0.1	364	1.0	84.7	0.4	0.0
Jus Fruit Blueberry Pieces, Yu!*	1 Pack/24g	84	0.1	350	0.8	80.8	0.4	0.0
Prunes, Juicy, Whitworths*	1 Pack/500g	740	2.0	148	2.5	34.0	0.4	5.7
Strawberry, Banana & Cherry, Sunshine Mix, Graze*	1 Pack/50g	78	0.2	157	9.7	37.2	0.4	0.0
Top Banana, Graze*	1 Serving/40g	115	0.4	287	2.6	70.1	0.9	0.0
Trail Mix, Kick Start, Wholefoods, Asda*	1 Serving/50g	193	10.2	387	10.9	40.0	20.4	10.7

	Measure INFO/WEIGHT	per Measure KCAL	FAT	KCAL	PROT	CARB	FAT	FIBRE
DRIED FRUIT MIX								
5 Fruits, Ready to Eat, Sundora*	½ Pack/100g	233	0.4	233	1.6	58.4	0.4	6.8
Agadoo, Pineapple, Jumbo & Green Raisins, Graze*	1 Pack/40g	110	0.4	275	2.1	69.0	0.9	0.0
Albert Heijn*	1 Serving/50g	110	0.2	220	2.1	51.0	0.5	0.0
Apple Strudel, Graze*	1 Pack/40g	99	0.3	247	2.2	58.7	0.7	5.9
Average	1 Tbsp/25g	67	0.1	268	2.3	68.1	0.4	2.2
Berry, Love Life, Waitrose*	1 Serving/30g	89	0.3	296	1.9	70.0	0.9	3.0
Berry, Whole Foods, Tesco*	1 Serving/25g	66	0.2	265	3.3	60.0	0.7	7.5
Dates, Raisins & Apricots, Wholefoods, Tesco*	1 Serving/20g	52	0.1	260	3.1	59.0	0.4	4.0
Eden, Graze*	1 Punnet /25g	69	0.2	275	2.0	63.7	1.0	8.1
Exotic Mix, Sundora*	1 Sm Pack/50g	138	1.3	276	2.3	60.6	2.7	3.8
Fruit & Oat Bites, Mixed Berry, Planet Lunch*	1 Bar/20g	53	0.6	265	3.9	56.0	2.8	8.0
Fruit & Oat Bites, Strawberry, Planet Lunch*	1 Bar/20g	54	0.5	270	4.0	57.0	2.5	7.2
Fruit Salad, Whitworths*	1 Serving/62g	113	0.3	183	2.9	41.8	0.5	6.6
Fruit Sangria, Graze*	1 Punnet/36g	110	0.6	306	3.8	70.3	1.8	2.6
Hanging Gardens of Babylon, Graze*	1 Punnet/49g	114	0.2	232	3.2	57.1	0.5	7.6
Little Figgy Went to Market, Graze*	1 Punnet/37g	101	0.3	273	1.8	63.9	0.7	7.9
Luxury, Co-Op*	1 Serving/40g	114	0.2	285	2.0	68.0	0.6	4.0
Medley, Shapers, Boots*	1 Serving/50g	131	0.3	262	3.2	61.0	0.6	5.5
Raisins Mix, Wholesome, Love Life, Waitrose*	1 Serving/30g	88	0.3	293	2.1	69.0	0.9	3.7
Scrumptious Blueberry Swirl, Graze*	1 Punnet/39g	149	2.7	381	1.2	78.8	6.9	3.5
Sultanas, Currants, Raisins & Citrus Peel, Asda*	1 Serving/100g	283	0.5	283	2.6	67.0	0.5	1.7
Taste of Hawaii, Extra Special, Asda*	1 Serving/100g	314	0.8	314	1.7	75.0	0.8	4.4
Tropical, Morrisons*	1 Pack/200g	368	1.0	184	1.7	50.6	0.5	6.3
Vine Fruit, Wholesome, Waitrose*	1 Serving/30g	87	0.1	289	2.1	69.3	0.4	5.3
DRIFTER								
Nestle*	1 Finger/20g	98	4.8	488	4.8	62.7	24.2	0.7
DRINK MIX								
Chocolate, Flavia*	1 Serving/18g	64	0.7	368	15.6	67.2	4.0	0.0
Chocolate Orange, Clipper*	1 Pack/28g	98	0.4	350	14.6	69.7	1.5	0.0
Milk Chocolate, Instant Break, Cadbury*	4 Tsp/28g	119	3.9	425	10.9	64.2	14.0	0.0
DRINKING CHOCOLATE								
Cadbury*	1 Tbsp/16g	64	0.4	402	4.4	89.3	2.4	0.0
Dry, Asda*	1 Serving/30g	111	1.8	370	6.0	73.0	6.0	0.0
Dry, M & S*	3 Tsp/20g	73	0.9	365	8.4	66.0	4.4	13.0
Dry, Tesco*	3 Tsp/25g	92	1.4	368	6.4	72.6	5.8	4.2
Dry, Waitrose*	3 Tsp/12g	48	0.7	403	7.2	79.9	6.1	2.9
Dry Powder, Cocodirect*	1 Serving/18g	67	1.5	372	8.9	65.1	8.4	0.0
Fairtrade, Truly Irresistible, Co-Op*	1 Serving/20g	73	1.9	365	10.0	60.3	9.4	13.8
Granules, Dry, Impress*	1oz/28g	102	1.0	365	5.6	77.0	3.7	6.0
Hot Chocolate, Light Choices, Tesco*	1 Cup/11g	38	0.8	345	13.8	54.9	7.7	13.1
Made Up, BGTY, Sainsbury's*	1 Serving/178g	114	0.4	64	3.9	11.4	0.2	0.7
Made Up with Semi-Skimmed Milk, Average	1 Mug/227ml	129	4.3	57	3.5	7.0	1.9	0.2
Made Up with Skimmed Milk, Average	1 Mug/227ml	100	1.1	44	3.5	7.0	0.5	0.0
Made Up with Whole Milk, Average	1 Mug/227ml	173	9.5	76	3.4	6.8	4.2	0.2
Maxpax, Light, Suchard*	1 Serving/11g	37	0.6	355	20.0	56.0	5.5	9.3
Powder, Made Up with Skimmed Milk	1 Mug/227ml	134	1.4	59	3.5	10.8	0.6	0.0
Powder, Made Up with Whole Milk	1 Mug/227ml	204	9.3	90	3.4	10.6	4.1	0.0
DRIPPING								
Beef	**1oz/28g**	**249**	**27.7**	**891**	**0.0**	**0.0**	**99.0**	**0.0**
DUCK								
Breast, Meat Only, Cooked, Average	**1oz/28g**	**48**	**2.0**	**172**	**25.3**	**1.8**	**7.0**	**0.0**
Breast, Meat Only, Raw, Average	**1 Serving/160g**	**206**	**6.8**	**128**	**22.5**	**0.0**	**4.2**	**0.2**
Fillets, Gressingham, Mini, TTD, Sainsbury's*	½ Pack/90g	127	2.4	141	29.0	0.0	2.7	0.6

D

	Measure INFO/WEIGHT	per Measure KCAL	per Measure FAT	Nutrition Values per 100g / 100ml KCAL	PROT	CARB	FAT	FIBRE
DUCK								
Leg, Meat & Skin, Average	*1oz/28g*	*80*	*5.6*	*286*	*17.2*	*9.5*	*20.0*	*0.4*
Raw, Meat, Fat & Skin	*1oz/28g*	*109*	*10.4*	*388*	*13.1*	*0.0*	*37.3*	*0.0*
Roasted, Meat, Fat & Skin	*1oz/28g*	*118*	*10.7*	*423*	*20.0*	*0.0*	*38.1*	*0.0*
DUCK &								
Plum Sauce, Roasted, Sainsbury's*	½ Pack/150g	174	3.7	116	6.9	16.0	2.5	1.8
DUCK A L' ORANGE								
Roast, M & S*	½ Pack/270g	553	42.1	205	12.5	4.1	15.6	0.6
DUCK AROMATIC								
Crispy, Asda*	1/3 Pack/166g	469	24.9	283	19.0	18.0	15.0	0.8
Crispy, Half, with Hoisin Sauce & 12 Pancakes, Tesco*	1/6 Pack/70g	162	7.4	232	18.3	15.9	10.6	1.1
Crispy, Half Duck & Pancakes, M & S*	½ Pack/311g	590	26.7	190	13.9	14.0	8.6	2.1
with a Plum Sauce, Finest, Tesco*	1 Serving/250g	400	14.0	160	16.1	11.3	5.6	4.6
with Plum Sauce, Tesco*	½ Pack/250g	350	11.5	140	9.3	15.2	4.6	0.3
DUCK CANTONESE								
Style, Roast, Tesco*	1 Pack/300g	375	6.9	125	8.2	17.9	2.3	0.5
DUCK IN								
Chinese Barbecue, Wings, Sainsbury's*	1 Serving/175g	430	25.0	246	19.4	9.7	14.3	0.0
Orange Sauce, Iceland*	1 Serving/200g	336	20.8	168	11.3	7.4	10.4	1.2
Orange Sauce, Legs, Extra Special, Asda*	1oz/28g	39	1.6	141	18.0	4.3	5.7	1.3
Oriental Sauce, Iceland*	1 Pack/201g	352	22.7	175	12.0	6.3	11.3	1.5
Plum & Chilli Sauce, Legs, Aldi*	½ Pack/200g	342	11.6	171	5.7	24.0	5.8	0.6
Plum Sauce, Crispy, M & S*	1 Pack/325g	569	31.2	175	10.7	11.2	9.6	0.9
Plum Sauce, Legs, Asda*	1 Leg/200g	452	23.0	226	24.1	6.4	11.5	0.5
Red Wine Sauce, Free Range Fillets, Waitrose*	½ Pack/250g	377	19.2	151	16.4	4.1	7.7	2.2
DUCK PEKING								
Crispy, Aromatic, Sainsbury's*	½ Pack/300g	1236	110.7	412	19.5	0.6	36.9	0.1
Crispy, Cherry Valley*	1 Serving/270g	702	35.9	260	17.5	17.8	13.3	0.7
DUCK WITH								
Hoisin & Noodles, Fuller for Longer, M & S*	1 Pack/370g	335	7.4	91	8.2	10.0	2.0	2.0
Noodles, Shanghai Roast, Sainsbury's*	1 Pack/450g	580	17.1	129	5.6	18.0	3.8	1.2
Pancakes, Shredded, Iceland*	1 Pack/220g	471	5.9	214	20.4	27.0	2.7	1.5
Pancakes, with Hoisin Sauce, M & S*	1 Pack/80g	136	3.2	170	13.0	19.9	4.0	0.9
DUMPLING MIX								
Farmhouse, Goldenfry Foods Ltd*	1 Serving/35g	152	5.3	434	6.5	61.5	18.0	0.0
DUMPLINGS								
Average	1oz/28g	58	3.3	208	2.8	24.5	11.7	0.9
Dried Mix, Tesco*	1 Pack/137g	404	16.7	295	5.4	39.9	12.2	2.8
Homestyle, Baked Weight, Frozen, Aunt Bessie's*	1 Dumpling/49g	188	8.6	384	9.7	44.4	17.6	2.8
Pork & Garlic Chive, Waitrose*	1 Pack/115g	215	8.1	187	9.4	20.4	7.0	1.1
Prawn, Cantonese, Crispy, Sainsbury's*	1 Dumpling/11g	27	1.5	241	9.3	20.9	13.4	1.1
Prawn, Siu Mai, Chinese, M & S*	8 Pieces/170g	170	2.9	100	7.8	13.1	1.7	1.3

D

	Measure INFO/WEIGHT	per Measure KCAL	FAT	Nutrition Values per 100g / 100ml KCAL	PROT	CARB	FAT	FIBRE
EASTER EGG								
Aero Bubbles, Nestle*	1 Egg/235g	1264	72.4	538	6.6	57.6	30.8	2.2
Buttons, Chocolate Egg Shell Only, Cadbury*	1 Egg/153g	803	45.9	525	7.5	56.8	30.0	0.7
Caramel, Chocolate Egg Shell Only, Cadbury*	1 Egg/336g	1764	100.8	525	7.5	56.8	30.0	0.7
Chick, Dairy Milk, Chocolate Egg Shell Only, Cadbury*	1 Egg/167g	885	50.3	530	7.5	56.7	30.1	0.7
Chocolate Egg Shell Only, Dairy Milk, Cadbury*	1 Egg/178g	934	53.4	525	7.5	56.8	30.0	0.7
Chocolate Orange, Terry's*	1 Egg/120g	636	36.6	530	7.4	57.0	30.5	2.4
Creme Egg, Chocolate Egg Shell Only, Cadbury*	½ Shell/60g	315	18.0	525	7.5	56.8	30.0	0.7
Crunchie, Cadbury*	1 Egg/120g	630	36.0	525	7.5	56.8	30.0	0.7
Dark Chocolate, 70%, Green & Black's*	1 Egg/110g	606	45.2	551	9.3	36.0	41.1	0.0
Dark Chocolate, Thorncroft's*	1 Egg/360g	1890	134.6	525	6.8	39.4	37.4	9.8
Disney, Nestle*	1 Egg/65g	342	18.9	526	6.3	59.7	29.1	0.6
Flake, Chocolate Egg Shell Only, Cadbury*	1 Egg/153g	803	45.9	525	7.5	56.8	30.0	0.7
Kit Kat, Chunky, Nestle*	1 Egg/220g	1170	63.4	532	5.5	61.7	28.8	1.7
Mars*	1 Serving/63g	281	10.9	449	4.2	69.0	17.4	0.0
Milk Chocolate, Nestle*	½ Egg/42g	205	9.7	489	5.0	65.2	23.1	0.5
Milk Chocolate, Swiss, Hollow, M & S*	1 Egg/18g	100	6.3	555	6.7	53.2	34.8	2.5
Milky Bar, Nestle*	1 Egg/40g	182	6.9	454	4.2	70.8	17.2	0.0
Roses, Chocolate Egg Shell Only, Cadbury*	1 Egg/200g	1050	60.0	525	7.5	56.8	30.0	0.7
Smarties, Nestle*	1 Sm Egg/90g	480	26.1	533	5.6	61.0	29.0	1.7
Twirl, Chocolate Egg Shell Only, Cadbury*	1 Lge Egg/325g	1706	97.5	525	7.5	56.8	30.0	0.7
White Chocolate, Thorntons*	1 Egg/360g	1958	109.1	544	5.5	62.2	30.3	2.1
Wispa, Chocolate Egg Shell Only, Cadbury*	1 Lge Egg/313g	1643	93.9	525	7.5	56.8	30.0	0.7
ECLAIR								
Belgian Chocolate, Weight Watchers*	1 Eclair/30g	81	3.5	271	3.9	37.6	11.7	6.6
Chocolate, 25% Less Fat, Sainsbury's*	1 Eclair/58g	171	9.3	295	6.8	31.1	16.0	1.2
Chocolate, Asda*	1 Eclair/33g	144	11.0	436	6.7	27.3	33.3	4.8
Chocolate, Cream, Fresh, Tesco*	1 Eclair/66g	285	20.5	430	6.0	31.1	30.9	1.8
Chocolate, Cream Filled, VLH Kitchens*	1 Eclair/66g	286	19.3	434	7.0	36.4	29.2	1.8
Chocolate, Dairy Cream, Co-Op*	1 Eclair/59g	227	17.1	385	5.0	26.0	29.0	0.3
Chocolate, Fresh Cream, M & S*	1 Eclair/44g	170	12.2	390	6.3	28.4	27.9	2.0
Chocolate, Fresh Cream, Sainsbury's*	1 Eclair/59g	212	13.9	360	4.2	32.7	23.6	0.5
Chocolate, Frozen, Morrisons*	1 Eclair/31g	116	9.6	374	5.0	18.8	31.0	1.3
Chocolate, Mini, Iceland*	1 Eclair/13g	55	4.6	426	4.9	21.5	35.6	0.4
Chocolate & Fresh Cream, Tempting, Tesco*	1 Eclair/39g	158	11.2	405	6.5	29.1	28.8	1.1
Double Chocolate, with Fresh Cream, Tesco*	1 Eclair/69g	275	18.6	400	5.9	33.4	27.0	1.6
EEL								
Cooked Or Smoked, Dry Heat, Average	*1 Serving/100g*	*236*	*14.9*	*236*	*23.6*	*0.0*	*14.9*	*0.0*
Jellied, Average	*1oz/28g*	*27*	*2.0*	*98*	*8.4*	*0.0*	*7.1*	*0.0*
Raw, Average	*1oz/28g*	*47*	*3.2*	*168*	*16.6*	*0.0*	*11.3*	*0.0*
EGG SUBSTITUTE								
99% Real Eggs, The Crafty Cook*	¼ Cup/61g	30	0.0	49	10.0	2.0	0.0	0.0
Original, The Crafty Cook*	¼ Cup 1oz/28g	30	0.0	107	21.4	3.6	0.0	0.0
EGGS								
Dried, White, Average	*1 Tbsp/14g*	*41*	*0.0*	*295*	*73.8*	*0.0*	*0.0*	*0.0*
Dried, Whole, Average	*1oz/28g*	*159*	*11.6*	*568*	*48.4*	*0.0*	*41.6*	*0.0*
Duck, Boiled & Salted, Average, Weight with Shell	1 Egg/75g	169	13.2	225	16.6	0.0	17.6	0.0
Duck, Whole, Raw, Average, Weight with Shell	*1 Egg/75g*	*139*	*10.0*	*185*	*16.2*	*0.0*	*13.4*	*0.0*
Free Range, Large, Average, Weight with Shell	*1 Egg/68g*	*109*	*7.6*	*161*	*14.1*	*0.9*	*11.2*	*0.0*
Free Range, Medium, Average, Weight with Shell	1 Egg/58g	93	6.5	161	14.1	0.9	11.2	0.0
Fried in Veg Oil, Average	1 Med/60g	107	8.3	179	13.6	0.0	13.9	0.0
Fried without Fat, Average	1 Med/60g	104	7.6	174	15.0	0.0	12.7	0.0
Goose, Whole, Fresh, Raw, Average, with Shell	*1 Egg/144g*	*267*	*19.1*	*185*	*13.9*	*1.3*	*13.3*	*0.0*
Large, Average, Weight with Shell	*1 Egg/68g*	*112*	*8.2*	*165*	*14.0*	*0.6*	*12.1*	*0.1*

E

	Measure INFO/WEIGHT	per Measure KCAL	FAT	Nutrition Values per 100g / 100ml KCAL	PROT	CARB	FAT	FIBRE
EGGS								
Medium, Average, Weight with Shell	*1 Egg/58g*	*93*	*6.5*	*161*	*14.1*	*0.9*	*11.2*	*0.0*
Medium, Boiled, Average, Weight with Shell	1 Egg/50g	83	6.1	165	14.0	0.6	12.1	0.1
Poached, Weight with Shell	1 Med/50g	83	6.1	165	14.0	0.6	12.1	0.6
Quail, Whole, Raw, Weight with Shell	*1 Egg/13g*	*21*	*1.6*	*164*	*14.0*	*0.4*	*12.1*	*0.0*
Scrambled, Average	1 Egg/68g	109	7.9	160	13.8	0.0	11.6	0.0
Scrambled with Milk, Average	1 Egg/60g	154	14.0	257	10.9	0.7	23.4	0.0
Turkey, Whole, Raw, Weight with Shell	*1 Egg/79g*	*154*	*10.9*	*194*	*15.5*	*1.3*	*13.9*	*0.0*
Very Large, Average, Weight with Shell	1 Egg/78g	125	8.7	161	14.1	0.9	11.2	0.0
Whites, Free Range, Liquid, Two Chicks*	3 Tbsp/45g	23	0.0	50	10.5	1.0	0.0	0.0
Whites Only, Raw, Average	*1 Lge Egg/33g*	*12*	*0.2*	*36*	*10.9*	*0.3*	*0.6*	*0.0*
Whole, Raw, Weight with Shell	*1 Small/48g*	*79*	*5.8*	*165*	*14.0*	*0.0*	*12.1*	*0.0*
Yolks, Raw	*1 Yolk/14g*	*47*	*4.3*	*339*	*16.1*	*0.0*	*30.5*	*0.0*
ELDERBERRIES								
Average	*1oz/28g*	*10*	*0.1*	*35*	*0.7*	*7.4*	*0.5*	*0.0*
ELICHE								
Dry Weight, Buitoni*	1 Serving/80g	282	1.5	352	11.2	72.6	1.9	0.0
ENCHILADAS								
Beef, Light Choices, Tesco*	1 Pack/400g	412	9.2	103	7.0	13.5	2.3	2.2
Chicken	1 Serving/295g	483	18.8	164	11.6	16.0	6.4	1.7
Chicken, American, HL, Tesco*	1 Serving/240g	353	4.3	147	10.4	22.5	1.8	1.2
Chicken, Asda*	1 Serving/500g	690	30.0	138	10.0	17.0	6.0	1.0
Chicken, Diner Specials, M & S*	½ Pack/227g	340	12.0	150	9.9	15.4	5.3	2.0
Chicken, in a Spicy Salsa & Bean Sauce, Asda*	½ Pack/212g	373	17.0	176	10.0	16.0	8.0	0.0
Chicken, Perfectly Balanced, Waitrose*	1 Pack/450g	481	14.4	107	6.9	12.7	3.2	1.1
Three Bean, Vegetarian, Tesco*	1 Pack/440g	572	24.6	130	4.9	14.1	5.6	3.3
Vegetable, GFY, Asda*	1 Pack/350g	399	15.7	114	4.4	14.0	4.5	1.3
ENDIVE								
Raw	*1oz/28g*	*4*	*0.1*	*13*	*1.8*	*1.0*	*0.2*	*2.0*
ENERGY DRINK								
Blue Bolt, Sainsbury's*	1 Can/250ml	105	0.0	42	0.0	10.0	0.0	0.0
Burn, Coca-Cola*	1 fl oz/30ml	13	0.0	44	0.0	10.5	0.0	0.0
Cherry, Lucozade*	1 Bottle/500ml	345	0.0	69	0.0	17.1	0.0	0.0
Citrus, Isotonic, Umbro*	1 Bottle/500ml	139	0.0	28	0.0	6.5	0.0	0.0
Coffee & Guarana, Self Heat Can, Rocket Fuel*	1 Can/200ml	70	1.0	35	1.4	4.1	0.5	0.1
Juiced Berry, Relentless*	1 Can/500g	230	0.0	46	0.0	10.7	0.0	0.0
Juiced Orange & Tropical Fruit, Relentless*	1 Can/500ml	230	0.0	46	0.0	10.4	0.0	0.0
Lemon, Active Sport, Tesco*	1 Bottle/500ml	135	0.0	27	0.0	6.5	0.0	0.0
Libertus, Blue, Sugar Free, Relentless*	1 Can/500ml	20	0.0	4	0.0	0.0	0.0	0.0
Monster*	1 Can/500ml	240	0.0	48	0.0	12.0	0.0	0.0
Orange, Active Sport, Tesco*	1 Bottle/500ml	135	0.0	27	0.0	6.5	0.0	0.0
Original, Rockstar*	1 Can/500ml	290	0.0	60	0.4	13.6	0.0	0.0
Powerade, Aqua+*	1 Bottle/500ml	80	0.0	16	0.0	3.7	0.0	0.0
Red Devil, Britvic*	1 Can/250ml	160	0.0	64	0.4	15.1	0.0	0.0
Red Rooster, Hi Energy Mixer, Cott Beverages Ltd*	1 Can/250ml	112	0.0	45	0.6	10.3	0.0	0.0
Red Thunder, Diet, Low Calorie, Aldi*	1 Can/250ml	5	0.0	2	0.1	0.0	0.0	0.0
Redcard, Britvic*	1 Can/330ml	96	0.0	29	0.1	7.0	0.0	0.0
Relentless, Sugar Free, Coca-Cola*	1 Can/500ml	20	0.0	4	0.0	0.0	0.0	0.0
SoBe, Appleberry Burst, Britvic*	1 Can/250ml	135	0.0	54	0.4	12.0	0.0	0.0
Sparkling Orange, Dual Energy, Powerade*	1 Bottle/500ml	225	0.0	45	0.0	10.5	0.0	0.0
Sugar Free, Boost Drinks Ltd*	1 Can/250ml	5	0.0	2	0.0	0.0	0.0	0.0
Sugar Free, Diet, Mountain Dew, Britvic*	1 Can/440ml	3	0.0	1	0.0	0.0	0.0	0.0
V, Frucor Beverages*	1 Can/250ml	112	0.0	45	0.0	11.2	0.0	0.0

	Measure INFO/WEIGHT	per Measure KCAL	FAT	Nutrition Values per 100g / 100ml KCAL	PROT	CARB	FAT	FIBRE
FAGGOTS								
in Rich Gravy, Iceland*	1 Faggot/81g	116	5.2	143	6.5	15.9	6.4	1.1
Mushy Peas & Mash, Sainsbury's*	1 Pack/450g	576	19.3	128	6.0	16.3	4.3	1.6
FAJITA								
Beef, GFY, Asda*	½ Pack/208g	354	9.8	170	11.0	21.0	4.7	1.6
Chicken	1 Serving/275g	501	17.0	182	10.2	21.5	6.2	1.7
Chicken, American Style, Tesco*	1 Pack/275g	388	14.0	141	9.5	14.2	5.1	1.0
Chicken, Asda*	½ Pack/225g	371	10.1	165	11.0	20.0	4.5	3.5
Chicken, BGTY, Sainsbury's*	1 Pack/172g	256	4.3	149	10.8	20.9	2.5	1.7
Chicken, Boots*	1 Pack/223g	448	16.1	201	9.1	25.0	7.2	3.9
Chicken, Co-Op*	1 Serving/230g	391	16.1	170	11.0	15.0	7.0	3.0
Chicken, COU, M & S*	1 Pack/230g	287	5.3	125	10.0	16.5	2.3	1.5
Chicken, Finest, Tesco*	½ Pack/288g	457	19.5	159	9.9	14.4	6.8	2.1
Chicken, GFY, Asda*	½ Pack/225g	233	4.1	104	9.3	12.9	1.8	2.0
Chicken, Just Cook, Sainsbury's*	½ Pack/200g	200	3.0	100	18.5	3.1	1.5	2.0
Chicken, M & S*	1 Pack/230g	345	12.2	150	8.6	17.7	5.3	1.0
Chicken, Mexican, No Mayo, Foo-Go*	1 Pack/198g	360	11.1	182	9.6	23.3	5.6	2.4
Chicken, Morrisons*	1 Serving/300g	370	15.2	123	7.4	12.2	5.1	1.9
Chicken, Sainsbury's*	½ Pack/275g	396	14.6	144	9.5	14.5	5.3	1.9
Chicken, Salt Balanced, COU, M & S*	1 Pack/230g	253	5.3	110	9.5	13.2	2.3	1.7
Chicken, Tesco*	½ Pack /275g	382	14.3	139	9.2	13.9	5.2	1.9
Gammon Steaks, Tesco*	1 Serving/250g	367	15.5	147	17.5	5.3	6.2	0.0
Meal Kit, Tesco*	1 Serving/100g	210	3.4	210	6.1	38.2	3.4	2.1
Mini Chicken, Tesco*	1 Fajita/18g	37	1.1	205	8.7	27.8	6.3	3.4
Vegetable	1 Serving/275g	472	14.9	171	4.9	25.5	5.4	1.9
Vegetable, Tesco*	1 Fajita/112g	133	5.6	119	4.2	14.3	5.0	1.1
FALAFEL								
12 Pack, Sainsbury's*	1 Falafel/17g	44	2.5	259	7.3	20.6	14.8	7.2
Asda*	½ Pack/50g	140	9.5	281	8.3	18.9	19.1	8.2
Fried in Vegetable Oil, Average	1 Falafel/25g	45	2.8	179	6.4	15.6	11.2	3.4
Gourmet, Meat Free, Vegideli, The Redwood Co*	1 Patty/17g	26	1.4	159	6.1	20.5	8.5	8.1
Mini, M & S*	1 Falafel/14g	43	2.5	310	7.9	28.1	18.4	2.6
Mini, Sainsbury's*	1 Serving/168g	499	29.6	297	8.0	26.8	17.6	3.2
Mix, Asda*	1 Packet/120g	313	15.0	261	6.4	30.8	12.5	2.6
Mix, Authentic, Al'fez*	1 Serving/100g	235	13.8	235	7.1	26.3	13.8	8.8
Mix, Lebanese Style, Al'fez*	½ Pack/200g	470	27.6	235	7.1	26.3	13.8	0.0
Mix, Organic, Quick & Easy, Hale & Hearty*	1 Pack/200g	646	11.0	323	19.2	43.8	5.5	10.7
Mix, Organic, Wheat & Gluten Free, Hale & Hearty*	1 Falafel/11g	75	1.4	301	19.2	43.8	5.5	10.7
Organic, Cauldron Foods*	1 Falafel/25g	51	2.4	203	8.4	20.3	9.8	7.2
Vegab Mat Ab, Vegab*	1 Falafel/20g	62	3.4	309	11.0	28.0	17.0	0.0
Vegetarian, Organic, Waitrose*	1 Falafel/25g	55	2.6	220	8.0	23.3	10.5	7.6
FANTA								
Apple, Z, Coca-Cola*	1 Can/330ml	13	0.0	4	0.0	0.6	0.0	0.0
Fruit Twist, Coca-Cola*	1 Glass/250ml	132	0.0	53	0.0	13.0	0.0	0.0
Icy Lemon, Coca-Cola*	1 Can/330ml	165	0.0	50	0.0	12.2	0.0	0.0
Icy Lemon, Zero, Coca-Cola*	1 Can/330ml	7	0.0	2	0.0	0.2	0.0	0.0
Lemon, Coca-Cola*	1 Can/330ml	165	0.0	50	0.0	12.0	0.0	0.0
Light, Coca-Cola*	1 Glass/250ml	5	0.0	2	0.0	0.5	0.0	0.0
Orange, Coca-Cola*	1 Glass/251ml	75	0.0	30	0.0	7.1	0.0	0.0
Orange, Z, Coca-Cola*	1 Can/330ml	10	0.0	3	0.0	0.5	0.0	0.0
Peach, Singapore, Coca-Cola*	1 Bottle/500ml	230	0.0	46	0.0	11.0	0.0	0.0
Summer Fruits, Z, Coca-Cola*	1 fl oz/30ml	1	0.0	3	0.0	0.6	0.0	0.0
FARFALLE								
Bows, Dry, Average	*1 Serving/75g*	*265*	*1.4*	*353*	*11.4*	*72.6*	*1.9*	*1.9*

F

	INFO/WEIGHT	KCAL	FAT	KCAL	PROT	CARB	FAT	FIBRE
FENNEL								
Florence, Boiled in Salted Water	*1oz/28g*	*3*	*0.1*	*11*	*0.9*	*1.5*	*0.2*	*2.3*
Florence, Raw, Unprepared	*1 Bulb/250g*	*30*	*0.5*	*12*	*0.9*	*1.8*	*0.2*	*2.4*
Florence, Steamed	*1 Serving/80g*	*9*	*0.2*	*11*	*9.0*	*1.5*	*0.2*	*2.3*
FENUGREEK								
Leaves, Raw, Fresh, Average	*1 Serving/80g*	*28*	*0.2*	*35*	*4.6*	*4.8*	*0.2*	*1.1*
FETTUCINI								
Cajun Chicken, COU, M & S*	1 Pack/400g	380	8.0	95	8.0	10.8	2.0	2.9
Chicken, Cajun, GFY, Asda*	1 Pack/400g	384	7.6	96	8.9	9.7	1.9	2.4
Chicken Mushroom, GFY, Asda*	1 Pack/400g	359	7.0	90	7.2	11.2	1.7	0.7
Dry Weight, Buitoni*	1 Serving/90g	326	1.5	362	12.2	74.4	1.7	0.0
with Tomato & Mushroom, Easy Cook, Napolina*	1 Pack/120g	461	8.6	384	11.8	67.9	7.2	0.0
FIG ROLLS								
Asda*	1 Biscuit/19g	71	1.7	372	4.8	68.0	9.0	0.0
Bolands*	1 Biscuit/18g	69	1.6	382	2.9	73.5	8.8	2.9
Go Ahead, McVitie's*	1 Biscuit/15g	55	0.7	365	4.2	76.8	4.6	2.9
Jacob's*	1 Biscuit/18g	68	1.5	380	4.0	71.4	8.5	3.3
Sainsbury's*	1 Biscuit/19g	70	1.7	377	4.8	68.3	9.4	2.6
Vitalinea, Jacob's*	1 Biscuit/18g	61	1.0	339	3.7	68.2	5.8	3.8
FIGS								
Dried, Average	*1 Fig/14g*	*32*	*0.1*	*232*	*3.6*	*53.2*	*1.1*	*8.6*
In Light Syrup, Asda*	1 Serving/100g	75	0.1	75	0.4	18.0	0.1	0.7
Raw, Fresh, Average	*1 Fresh Fig/35g*	*16*	*0.1*	*45*	*1.3*	*9.8*	*0.2*	*1.5*
Smyrna, Soft, Dried, Waitrose*	1 Fig/25g	49	0.3	197	2.4	44.0	1.3	10.6
FISH								
Balls, Gefilte, M & S*	1 Pack/200g	280	7.8	140	14.1	11.9	3.9	1.0
Battered, Portion, Ross*	1 Serving/110g	223	11.9	203	10.4	16.1	10.8	0.8
Breaded, Asda*	1 Serving/150g	351	21.0	234	15.0	12.0	14.0	0.5
Dried, Small, Ogura*	1 Serving/10g	32	0.3	320	69.0	0.3	3.0	0.0
Fillet, Dinner, Light & Easy, Youngs*	1 Pack/385g	362	15.8	94	6.2	8.2	4.1	1.4
Fillets, Garlic & Herb, Youngs*	1 Fillet/118g	261	14.8	222	11.0	16.2	12.6	1.4
Fillets, Lemon & Pepper, Youngs*	1 Fillet/130g	283	16.7	218	10.3	15.3	12.9	4.3
Fillets, White, Breaded, Tesco*	1 Piece/95g	198	10.4	208	10.6	16.9	10.9	1.0
Fillets, White, Natural, Tesco*	1 Fillet/100g	72	0.6	72	16.6	0.0	0.6	0.0
Goujons, Asda*	1 Serving/125g	240	8.0	192	12.8	20.8	6.4	0.2
in Batter, Morrisons*	1 Fish/140g	235	8.1	168	14.0	15.0	5.8	0.2
in Batter, Youngs*	1 Serving/100g	315	19.7	315	14.9	20.4	19.7	0.8
Medley, Steamfresh, Birds Eye*	1 Bag/170g	170	6.3	100	13.0	2.3	3.7	0.1
Melts with Tomato & Mozzarella Filling, Birds Eye*	1 Fillet/100g	255	15.0	255	13.0	17.0	15.0	0.6
Portion, Chip Shop, Youngs*	1 Portion/135g	315	19.7	233	11.0	15.1	14.6	0.6
Salted, Chinese, Steamed	1oz/28g	43	0.6	155	33.9	0.0	2.2	0.0
Seaside Shapes, Birds Eye*	2 Pieces/80g	197	11.2	246	11.0	19.0	14.0	1.1
Steaks, Chip Shop, Youngs*	1 Serving/100g	198	10.4	198	11.0	14.9	10.4	0.9
White, Breaded, Fillets, Ocean Pure*	1 Fillet/113g	276	11.5	245	20.8	16.9	10.2	1.2
White, Smoked, Average	1 Serving/100g	108	0.9	108	23.4	0.0	0.9	0.0
FISH & CHIPS								
Cod, Asda*	1 Serving/280g	450	14.0	161	8.0	21.0	5.0	1.1
Cod, HL, Tesco*	1 Pack/400g	492	7.2	123	5.3	21.4	1.8	1.7
Ross*	1 Serving/250g	415	19.0	166	6.2	18.1	7.6	1.6
Tesco*	1 Serving/300g	489	18.6	163	5.5	21.2	6.2	1.6
with Mushy Peas, Kershaws*	1 Pack/315g	450	18.3	143	6.4	16.4	5.8	1.6
FISH BAKE								
Cheese & Leek, HL, Tesco*	1 Pack/400g	340	8.0	85	11.0	5.8	2.0	0.8
Cheese Pastry, Birds Eye*	1 Serving/171g	390	23.3	228	9.3	17.2	13.6	1.9

F

	Measure INFO/WEIGHT	per Measure KCAL	FAT	Nutrition Values per 100g / 100ml KCAL	PROT	CARB	FAT	FIBRE
FISH BAKE								
Haddock & Prawn, COU, M & S*	1 Pack/340g	289	9.5	85	7.3	7.3	2.8	0.4
Italiano, Birds Eye*	1 Pack/400g	404	16.4	101	12.0	3.9	4.1	0.4
FISH CAKES								
Breaded, Sainsbury's*	1 Cake/42g	75	3.4	179	10.0	16.2	8.1	0.7
Bubbly Batter, Youngs*	1 Cake/44g	109	6.7	247	7.1	20.5	15.1	1.4
Captain's Coins, Mini, Captain Birds Eye, Birds Eye*	1 Cake/20g	38	1.7	188	9.5	18.7	8.3	1.1
Cod, & Pancetta, Cafe Culture, M & S*	1 Cake/85g	166	13.2	195	9.2	7.2	15.5	2.0
Cod, Big Time, Birds Eye*	1 Cake/114g	223	11.6	196	8.3	17.8	10.2	1.0
Cod, Birds Eye*	1 Cake/51g	93	4.4	182	10.0	16.0	8.7	1.1
Cod, Cheese & Chive, Finest, Tesco*	1 Cake/100g	212	11.5	212	9.7	18.3	11.5	1.7
Cod, Chunky, Breaded, Chilled, Youngs*	1 Cake/90g	192	11.5	213	9.5	14.9	12.8	1.2
Cod, Fresh, Asda*	1 Cake/75g	164	8.2	219	7.0	23.0	11.0	1.6
Cod, Homemade, Average	1 Cake/50g	120	8.3	241	9.3	14.4	16.6	0.7
Cod, in Crunch Crumb, Birds Eye*	1 Cake/50g	93	4.3	187	11.4	16.0	8.6	1.0
Cod, King Prawn & Pancetta, Extra Special, Asda*	1 Cake/115g	202	7.7	176	11.0	17.8	6.7	15.0
Cod, M & S*	1 Cake85g	153	7.8	180	8.9	15.4	9.2	1.3
Cod, Tesco*	1 Cake/90g	202	9.4	224	8.9	23.8	10.4	0.2
Cod & Parsley, Waitrose*	1 Cake/85g	147	6.5	173	9.2	16.9	7.6	1.1
Crab, & Prawn, Thai, Tesco*	1 Cake/115g	269	16.6	234	8.8	17.4	14.4	1.2
Fried in Blended Oil	1 Cake/50g	109	6.7	218	8.6	16.8	13.4	0.0
Frozen, Average	1 Cake/85g	112	3.3	132	8.6	16.7	3.9	0.0
Grilled, Average	1 Cake/50g	77	2.2	154	9.9	19.7	4.5	0.0
Haddock, Asda*	1 Cake/88g	181	8.8	206	8.0	21.0	10.0	1.5
Haddock, Fresh Tastes, Asda*	1 Cake/75g	141	5.0	188	9.6	22.2	6.7	1.8
Haddock, Sainsbury's*	1 Cake/83g	166	6.8	199	11.4	20.1	8.1	1.8
Haddock, Smoked, Breaded, Asda*	1 Cake/90g	202	11.7	225	9.0	18.0	13.0	1.6
Haddock, Smoked, Frozen, Waitrose*	1 Cake/85g	186	10.3	219	9.6	17.8	12.1	0.8
Haddock, Smoked, M & S*	1 Cake/85g	153	8.0	180	10.6	13.4	9.4	2.6
Haddock in Breadcrumbs, Sainsbury's*	1 Cake/88g	158	6.2	179	10.8	18.2	7.0	1.4
Halibut Cod Loin, Finest, Tesco*	1 Cake/115g	213	8.3	185	8.8	21.3	7.2	1.4
M & S*	1 Cake/80g	180	10.6	225	8.0	18.0	13.2	0.0
Pollock with Chives & Cream, Jamie Oliver, Youngs*	1 Cake/84g	160	7.0	190	9.1	18.7	8.3	1.8
Prawn, Battered, Asda*	1 Cake/90g	182	10.0	202	10.0	15.6	11.1	1.0
Prawn, Sainsbury's*	1 Cake/90g	184	7.8	204	9.6	21.7	8.7	1.2
Prawn, Thai Style, Finest, Tesco*	1 Cake/145g	305	13.5	210	6.7	24.2	9.3	1.0
Ross*	1 Cake/52g	83	3.8	160	7.4	15.9	7.4	1.2
Salmon, & Broccoli, Morrisons*	1 Cake/60g	126	7.1	210	9.8	17.2	11.9	1.3
Salmon, & Dill, Waitrose*	1 Cake/85g	206	11.9	242	11.5	17.5	14.0	1.8
Salmon, & Leek, Northern Catch, Aldi*	1 Cake/114g	212	9.0	186	9.5	19.3	7.9	0.9
Salmon, & Tarragon, Waitrose*	1 Cake/85g	179	10.0	211	11.9	14.3	11.8	2.2
Salmon, Birds Eye*	1 Cake/50g	84	4.5	168	9.5	12.2	9.0	1.4
Salmon, Breaded, Crispy, Frozen, Sainsbury's*	1 Cake/60g	140	8.7	234	12.2	13.7	14.5	1.9
Salmon, Chunky, Sainsbury's*	1 Cake/84g	192	10.5	228	13.2	15.8	12.5	2.9
Salmon, Homemade, Average	1 Cake/50g	136	9.8	273	10.4	14.4	19.7	0.7
Salmon, in Crunch Crumb, Birds Eye*	1 Cake/50g	107	6.4	216	9.7	15.0	13.0	1.4
Salmon, M & S*	1 Cake/86g	180	10.9	210	9.1	15.1	12.7	1.7
Salmon, Sainsbury's*	1 Cake/88g	171	7.6	194	12.6	16.5	8.6	1.6
Salmon, Spinach & Sicilian Lemon, Finest, Tesco*	1 Cake/114g	251	13.5	220	10.0	18.3	11.8	4.2
Salmon, VLH Kitchens*	1 Cake/56g	155.6	11.2	278	10.5	14.4	20.0	0.6
Salmon, with Lemon Butter Sauce, Finest, Tesco*	1 Cake/220g	524	40.3	238	7.3	10.9	18.3	1.0
Salmon, with Lemon Butter Sauce, Gastropub, M & S*	1 Cake/108g	188	13.3	175	7.8	8.5	12.4	1.2
Thai, Finest, Tesco*	1 Cake/65g	149	8.6	230	7.5	20.3	13.2	1.6
Thai, Frozen, Sainsbury's*	1 Cake/15g	28	1.1	187	21.3	9.3	7.3	0.7

F

	Measure INFO/WEIGHT	per Measure KCAL	per Measure FAT	Nutrition Values per 100g / 100ml KCAL	PROT	CARB	FAT	FIBRE
FISH CAKES								
Thai, Oriental Selection, Waitrose*	1 Cake/11g	18	0.3	161	17.8	15.8	3.0	1.5
Thai Prawn, Morrisons*	1 Cake/90g	211	9.6	234	7.9	26.4	10.7	0.3
Thai Style, Sainsbury's*	1 Cake/49g	69	2.1	141	12.0	13.8	4.2	1.7
Tuna, & Red Pepper, Waitrose*	1 Cake/85g	175	10.0	206	9.5	15.4	11.8	1.6
Tuna, Asda*	1 Cake/75g	185	10.1	247	14.9	16.5	13.5	1.4
Tuna, Lime & Coriander, BGTY, Sainsbury's*	1 Cake/91g	200	10.7	220	10.7	17.7	11.8	2.6
Tuna, Sainsbury's*	1 Cake/90g	183	7.5	203	13.7	18.4	8.3	2.1
FISH FINGERS								
Atlantis*	1 Finger/30g	52	2.2	172	12.0	14.0	7.5	0.4
Brilliant, 10 Pack, Jamie Oliver, Youngs*	3 Fingers/86g	177	7.9	205	11.7	18.4	9.1	1.2
Chip Shop, Youngs*	1 Finger/30g	75	4.9	251	9.3	16.6	16.4	1.2
Cod, 100% Cod Fillet, Tesco*	1 Finger/30g	53	2.2	177	12.4	14.9	7.5	1.4
Cod, Chunky, Tesco*	1 Finger/40g	70	3.0	175	12.3	14.3	7.6	1.6
Cod, Fillet, Chunky, M & S*	1 Finger/40g	70	2.4	175	12.0	17.2	6.0	1.0
Cod, Fillet, Chunky, TTD, Sainsbury's*	2 Fingers/114g	209	9.3	183	10.4	17.2	8.1	2.9
Cod, Fillet, Waitrose*	1 Finger/30g	55	2.2	183	11.9	16.9	7.5	0.7
Cod, Fried in Blended Oil, Average	1 Finger/28g	67	3.9	238	13.2	15.5	14.1	0.6
Cod, Frozen, Average	1 Finger/28g	48	2.2	170	11.6	14.2	7.8	0.6
Cod, Grilled, Average	1 Finger/28g	56	2.5	200	14.3	16.6	8.9	0.7
Cod, Sainsbury's*	1 Finger/28g	53	2.1	190	12.5	17.7	7.7	1.0
Free From, Sainsbury's*	1 Finger/30g	56	2.3	188	11.4	18.0	7.8	0.7
Haddock, Fillet, Asda*	1 Finger/30g	61	2.7	205	14.0	17.0	9.0	0.0
Haddock, in Crispy Batter, Birds Eye*	1 Finger/30g	56	2.3	188	14.3	15.1	7.8	0.7
Haddock, in Crunchy Crumb, Morrisons*	1 Finger/30g	57	2.4	190	13.1	16.3	8.0	1.1
Hoki, Fillet, Birds Eye*	1 Finger/30g	58	2.7	193	12.6	15.6	8.9	0.7
Iceland*	1 Finger/23g	44	2.0	192	11.5	17.3	8.5	1.3
in Batter, Crispy, Jumbo, Morrisons*	1 Finger/71g	146	8.9	205	11.3	12.2	12.5	0.6
Omega 3, Tesco*	1 Finger/30g	58	2.5	195	12.7	16.3	8.3	1.6
Ross*	1 Finger/26g	50	2.3	193	10.7	17.7	8.8	0.8
Salmon, Birds Eye*	1 Finger/28g	63	2.7	225	13.2	21.7	9.5	0.9
FISH IN								
Butter Sauce, Steaks, Ross*	1 Serving/150g	126	5.8	84	9.1	3.2	3.9	0.1
Butter Sauce, Steaks, Youngs*	1 Steak/150g	115	4.2	77	10.2	2.8	2.8	0.8
Parsley Sauce, Steaks, Ross*	1 Serving/150g	123	5.5	82	9.1	3.1	3.7	0.1
FIVE SPICE								
Powder, Sharwood's*	1 Tsp/2g	3	0.2	172	12.2	11.6	8.6	23.4
FLAKE								
Cadbury*	1 Bar/32g	170	9.9	530	8.1	55.6	30.8	0.7
Dipped, Cadbury*	1 Bar/41g	215	12.5	530	7.6	56.1	30.8	0.8
Luxury, Cadbury*	1 Bar/45g	240	13.6	533	7.3	57.8	30.2	0.0
Praline, Cadbury*	1 Bar/38g	201	12.9	535	7.7	49.5	34.3	0.0
Snow, Cadbury*	1 Bar/36g	198	11.1	550	7.2	60.1	30.9	0.0
FLAN								
Cauliflower, Cheese & Broccoli, Hot, Sainsbury's*	¼ Flan/100g	303	19.8	303	6.4	24.7	19.8	1.2
Cheese & Potato, Hot, Tesco*	¼ Flan/100g	282	19.7	282	6.0	20.0	19.7	2.3
Chicken & Smoked Bacon, Hot, Sainsbury's*	¼ Flan/100g	293	18.5	293	10.2	21.5	18.5	1.2
Mediterranean Vegetable, Co-Op*	¼ Flan/88g	188	10.5	215	4.0	22.0	12.0	3.0
Pastry, with Fruit	1oz/28g	33	1.2	118	1.4	19.3	4.4	0.7
Sponge with Fruit	1oz/28g	31	0.4	112	2.8	23.3	1.5	0.6
FLAN CASE								
Sponge, Average	**1oz/28g**	**90**	**1.5**	**320**	**7.0**	**62.5**	**5.4**	**0.7**
FLAPJACK								
7 Fruits, Graze*	1 Punnet/55g	223	10.5	406	5.1	54.9	19.1	4.3

F

	Measure INFO/WEIGHT	per Measure		Nutrition Values per 100g / 100ml				
		KCAL	FAT	KCAL	PROT	CARB	FAT	FIBRE
FLAPJACK								
90% Fat Free, Cookie Coach*	1 Flapjack/75g	287	7.4	383	7.0	66.2	9.9	0.0
All Butter, Blackcurrant Jam, M & S*	1 Serving/65g	279	12.1	430	4.8	60.5	18.6	2.2
All Butter, Organic, Sainsbury's*	1 Serving/35g	156	8.0	446	5.3	54.5	23.0	2.7
All Butter, Squares, M & S*	1 Flapjack/34g	150	7.2	441	6.2	56.2	21.2	4.4
All Butter, Waitrose*	1 Flapjack/34g	126	9.0	376	3.8	52.4	26.8	1.2
Apple & Cinnamon, Graze*	1 Punnet/55g	235	11.4	428	0.0	56.6	20.8	3.2
Apple & Raisin, Lite, Crazy Jack*	1 Flapjack70g	227	1.5	324	9.8	72.0	2.1	0.0
Apple & Raspberry, Fox's*	1 Flapjack/26g	105	5.0	403	4.8	52.5	19.4	3.7
Apple & Sultana, Mr Kipling*	1 Flapjack/27g	123	6.0	456	4.6	59.0	22.4	3.6
Apricot, The Handmade Flapjack Company*	1 Flapjack/90g	321	4.8	357	5.5	71.6	5.3	0.0
Apricot & Raisin, Waitrose*	1 Flapjack/38g	143	4.2	376	4.7	64.3	11.1	5.8
Average	1 Flapjack/50g	242	13.3	484	4.5	60.4	26.6	2.7
Banana, The Handmade Flapjack Company*	1 Flapjack/90g	379	13.1	421	5.3	67.2	14.6	0.0
Brazil Nut Cluster, The Handmade Flapjack Company*	1 Flapjack/90g	353	9.1	392	6.6	68.7	10.1	0.0
Butter, Mr Kipling*	1 Flapjack/75g	337	15.9	450	5.4	59.6	21.2	3.2
Caramel Bake, The Handmade Flapjack Company*	1 Flapjack/90g	375	13.0	417	6.0	65.6	14.5	0.0
Chocolate, McVitie's*	1 Flapjack/85g	422	23.0	496	6.6	56.6	27.1	3.2
Chocolate, The Handmade Flapjack Company*	1 Flapjack/90g	391	17.6	435	6.0	58.6	19.5	0.0
Chocolate & Hazelnut, M & S*	1 Flapjack/71g	330	18.1	465	7.3	55.6	25.5	3.8
Chocolate Chip, Boots*	1 Flapjack/75g	313	11.2	417	5.6	65.0	15.0	3.5
Chocolate Dipped, M & S*	1 Flapjack/96g	442	21.5	460	6.1	61.3	22.4	3.0
Chocolate Special, The Handmade Flapjack Company*	1 Flapjack/90g	392	17.8	436	5.7	58.7	19.8	0.0
Chunky Chocolate, M & S*	1 Flapjack/80g	348	15.1	435	5.8	59.9	18.9	2.2
Cranberry, Apple & Raisin, Light Choices, Tesco*	1 Flapjack/30g	97	1.7	325	5.7	63.1	5.6	5.7
Date & Walnut, The Handmade Flapjack Company*	1 Flapjack/90g	360	13.5	400	6.1	60.2	14.9	0.0
Fruit, GFY, Asda*	1 Flapjack/45g	173	3.6	384	6.0	72.0	8.0	3.4
Fruit, Mr Kipling*	1 Flapjack/75g	306	13.6	408	4.8	56.7	18.1	3.0
Fruit, Tesco*	1 Flapjack/33g	136	5.2	412	5.7	62.0	15.7	4.0
Hob Nobs, Milk Chocolate, McVitie's*	1 Flapjack/35g	159	7.5	454	5.7	59.4	21.4	4.0
Milk Chocolate Digestive, McVitie's*	1 Flapjack/65g	293	13.8	451	5.4	59.7	21.2	3.4
Plain, The Handmade Flapjack Company*	1 Flapjack/90g	398	19.2	442	5.4	57.1	21.3	0.0
Really Raspberry, Fabulous Bakin' Boys*	1 Flapjack/90g	378	16.2	420	6.0	60.0	18.0	0.0
Snickers, McVitie's*	1 Flapjack/65g	315	18.5	484	7.9	49.0	28.5	6.0
Sultana, Tesco*	1 Flapjack/50g	173	10.0	346	5.0	36.2	20.1	3.7
Toffee, Finest, Tesco*	1 Flapjack/35g	156	6.7	446	4.9	63.6	19.1	1.3
Toffeemac, The Handmade Flapjack Company*	1 Flapjack/90g	411	19.7	457	6.1	59.0	21.9	0.0
Tropical Mix, Reduced Fat, Fabulous Bakin' Boys*	1 Flapjack/90g	346	10.8	385	6.0	63.0	12.0	3.0
Weight Watchers*	1 Flapjack/30g	109	1.8	363	6.7	71.0	6.0	4.0
FLATBREAD								
BBQ Chicken, Improved, Shapers, Boots*	1 Pack/165g	268	3.8	162	10.0	25.0	2.3	1.2
Cheese & Onion Swedish Style, Shapers, Boots*	1 Bread/127g	265	10.3	209	10.0	24.0	8.1	1.3
Cheese & Tomato, Tesco*	¼ Pack/56g	134	3.7	240	8.7	36.1	6.6	2.7
Chicken & Mango Salad, Sainsbury's*	1 Pack/100g	251	2.5	251	16.9	40.4	2.5	2.5
Chicken Tikka, BGTY, Sainsbury's*	1 Bread/188g	241	2.6	128	10.3	18.5	1.4	2.0
Chicken Tikka, Shapers, Boots*	1 Bread/164g	269	4.1	164	11.0	24.0	2.5	1.5
Chinese Chicken, COU, M & S*	1 Bread/156g	281	4.4	180	13.9	24.3	2.8	2.2
Chinese Chicken, Shapers, Boots*	1 Pack/159g	274	2.1	172	11.0	29.0	1.3	1.8
Feta Cheese, Shapers, Boots*	1 Pack/166g	255	6.5	154	6.7	23.0	3.9	1.4
Gluten, Wheat & Milk Free, 4 Pack, Free From, Livwell*	1 Bread/55g	148	2.9	269	6.4	53.6	5.3	4.5
Greek Feta Salad, Boots*	1 Pack/158g	241	5.7	153	6.4	24.0	3.6	1.2
Greek Style Salad, Waitrose*	1 Pack/172g	280	8.4	163	7.4	22.3	4.9	3.3
Italian Chicken, Improved, Shapers, Boots*	1 Pack/151g	263	6.8	174	11.0	22.0	4.5	1.8
King Prawn Tikka, Waitrose*	1 Pack/165g	257	3.3	156	9.4	25.1	2.0	1.5

F

	Measure INFO/WEIGHT	per Measure KCAL	FAT	Nutrition Values per 100g / 100ml KCAL	PROT	CARB	FAT	FIBRE
FLATBREAD								
Mature Cheddar & Garlic, Finest, Tesco*	¼ Bread/66g	188	6.3	285	7.2	41.8	9.6	2.6
Mediterranean Chicken, Ginsters*	1 Pack/168g	302	6.7	180	10.6	25.5	4.0	0.0
Mediterranean Tuna, Ginsters*	1 Pack/167g	297	6.3	178	10.3	25.6	3.8	0.0
Mexican, Chicken, Stonebaked, Finest, Tesco*	1 Pack/155g	280	5.1	180	11.7	25.1	3.3	1.6
Mexican Style Chicken, GFY, Asda*	1 Pack/161g	241	3.2	150	13.0	20.0	2.0	2.5
Peking Duck, Less Than 3% Fat, Shapers, Boots*	1 Pack/156g	246	3.7	158	7.2	27.0	2.4	1.9
Rancher's Chicken, COU, M & S*	1 Pack/174g	270	3.5	155	10.9	23.0	2.0	1.5
Ranchers Chicken, Shapers, Boots*	1 Pack/194g	303	4.3	156	12.0	22.0	2.2	1.5
Salsa Chicken, Shapers, Boots*	1 Pack/191g	328	8.4	172	11.0	22.0	4.4	1.6
Spicy Chicken, Shapers, Boots*	1 Pack/181g	292	4.5	161	11.0	23.0	2.5	0.0
Spicy Mexican, New, Shapers, Boots*	1 Pack/184g	281	5.0	153	8.0	24.0	2.7	1.9
Spicy Mexican, Shapers, Boots*	1 Pack/190g	296	7.6	156	7.0	23.0	4.0	3.7
Sticky BBQ Style Chicken, Shapers, Boots*	1 Pack/158g	274	7.3	173	10.0	23.0	4.6	2.8
Tomato & Chilli, Sainsbury's*	¼ Bread/65g	155	3.1	238	11.9	36.9	4.7	2.8
FLAXSEED								
Milled, Organic, Linwoods*	2 Dtsp/30g	153	13.9	510	21.9	1.7	46.2	28.9
Organic, Premium Ground, Prewett's*	1 Tbsp/15g	73	6.0	489	24.0	2.0	40.0	23.0
FLOUR								
00 Grade, Pasta, TTD, Sainsbury's*	1 Bag/1000g	3390	13.0	339	11.5	70.3	1.3	3.0
Arrowroot, Average	*1oz/28g*	*100*	*0.0*	*357*	*0.3*	*88.1*	*0.1*	*3.4*
Bread, Brown, Strong, Average	*1 Serving/100g*	*311*	*1.8*	*311*	*14.0*	*61.0*	*1.8*	*6.4*
Bread, White, Strong, Average	*1oz/28g*	*94*	*0.4*	*336*	*11.8*	*68.4*	*1.5*	*3.4*
Brown, Chapati, Average	*1 Tbsp/20g*	*67*	*0.2*	*333*	*11.5*	*73.7*	*1.2*	*0.0*
Brown, Wheat	*1oz/28g*	*90*	*0.5*	*323*	*12.6*	*68.5*	*1.8*	*6.4*
Chick Pea	*1oz/28g*	*88*	*1.5*	*313*	*19.7*	*49.6*	*5.4*	*10.7*
Millet	*1oz/28g*	*99*	*0.5*	*354*	*5.8*	*75.4*	*1.7*	*0.0*
Plain, Average	*1oz/28g*	*98*	*0.4*	*349*	*10.3*	*73.8*	*1.5*	*2.2*
Potato	*1oz/28g*	*92*	*0.3*	*328*	*9.1*	*75.6*	*0.9*	*5.7*
Quinoa	1 Serving/100g	349	5.2	349	14.1	61.4	5.2	3.4
Rice	*1 Tsp/5g*	*18*	*0.0*	*366*	*6.4*	*80.1*	*0.8*	*2.0*
Rye, Whole	*1oz/28g*	*94*	*0.6*	*335*	*8.2*	*75.9*	*2.0*	*11.7*
Soya, Full Fat, Average	*1oz/28g*	*118*	*6.1*	*421*	*37.9*	*19.7*	*21.7*	*11.6*
Soya, Low Fat, Average	*1oz/28g*	*99*	*2.0*	*352*	*45.3*	*28.2*	*7.2*	*13.5*
Spelt, Average	*1 Serving/57g*	*216*	*1.7*	*381*	*14.3*	*74.5*	*2.9*	*6.3*
Strong, Wholemeal, Average	*1 Serving/100g*	*315*	*2.2*	*315*	*13.2*	*60.5*	*2.2*	*9.0*
White, Average	*1oz/28g*	*89*	*0.3*	*319*	*9.8*	*66.8*	*1.0*	*2.9*
White, Chapati, Average	*1 Tbsp/20g*	*67*	*0.1*	*335*	*9.8*	*77.6*	*0.5*	*0.0*
White, Self Raising, Average	*1oz/28g*	*94*	*0.4*	*336*	*9.9*	*71.8*	*1.3*	*2.9*
White, Wheat, Average	*1oz/28g*	*95*	*0.4*	*341*	*10.4*	*76.5*	*1.3*	*3.1*
Wholemeal, Average	*1oz/28g*	*87*	*0.6*	*312*	*12.6*	*61.9*	*2.2*	*9.0*
FLYING SAUCERS								
Asda*	1 Bag/23g	82	0.6	355	0.1	83.0	2.5	0.8
Co-Op*	1 Sweet/1g	4	0.0	370	0.5	90.0	1.0	0.6
FLYTE								
Mars*	1 Bar/23g	99	3.2	441	3.4	74.8	14.2	0.0
Snacksize, Mars*	1 Bar/23g	98	3.3	436	3.8	72.5	14.5	0.0
FOOL								
Apricot, Fruit, Tesco*	1 Pot/113g	200	12.7	177	2.6	16.4	11.2	0.3
Blackcurrant, Asda*	1 Pot/114g	89	3.0	78	3.6	10.0	2.6	0.6
Blackcurrant, BGTY, Sainsbury's*	1 Pot/113g	89	2.9	79	3.5	10.4	2.6	0.6
Fruit	1oz/28g	46	2.6	163	1.0	20.2	9.3	1.2
Gooseberry, BFY, Morrisons*	1 Pot/114g	99	3.9	87	3.4	10.7	3.4	0.4
Gooseberry, Fruit, BGTY, Sainsbury's*	1 Pot/121g	93	3.4	77	2.9	10.0	2.8	0.8

	Measure INFO/WEIGHT	per Measure KCAL	FAT	Nutrition Values per 100g / 100ml KCAL	PROT	CARB	FAT	FIBRE
FOOL								
Gooseberry, Fruit, Co-Op*	1 Pot/114g	211	11.4	185	3.0	22.0	10.0	1.0
Gooseberry, Perfectly Balanced, Waitrose*	1 Pot/113g	125	2.9	111	3.6	18.3	2.6	0.7
Gooseberry, Sainsbury's*	1 Pot/113g	214	12.9	189	2.6	19.1	11.4	1.1
Gooseberry, Tesco*	1 Pot/113g	225	14.1	200	3.0	17.8	12.5	0.7
Lemon, BFY, Morrisons*	1 Pot/114g	96	3.9	84	3.4	10.1	3.4	0.3
Lemon, Fruit, BGTY, Sainsbury's*	1 Pot/113g	94	3.8	83	3.4	9.7	3.4	0.3
Lemon, Fruit, Morrisons*	1 Pot/114g	226	12.9	198	0.0	20.5	11.3	0.0
Raspberry, Fruit, Tesco*	1 Pot/113g	234	12.8	207	2.6	23.6	11.3	0.3
Rhubarb, Fruit, BGTY, Sainsbury's*	1 Pot/120g	91	3.1	76	3.5	9.5	2.6	0.3
Rhubarb, Fruit, Waitrose*	1 Pot/114g	182	12.9	160	2.7	11.9	11.3	0.3
Rhubarb, Perfectly Balanced, Waitrose*	1 Pot/113g	101	2.9	89	3.5	13.0	2.6	0.3
Rhubarb, Sainsbury's*	1 Pot/113g	180	12.9	159	2.6	11.5	11.4	0.4
Strawberry, Fruit, BGTY, Sainsbury's*	1 Pot/120g	100	3.1	83	3.7	11.1	2.6	0.8
Strawberry, Fruit, Co-Op*	1 Pot/114g	188	10.3	165	2.0	18.0	9.0	0.8
Strawberry, GFY, Asda*	1 Pot/114g	95	3.0	83	3.8	11.0	2.6	0.8
FRANKFURTERS								
Average	*1 Sausage/42g*	*123*	*11.2*	*292*	*12.0*	*1.3*	*26.6*	*0.0*
FRANKFURTERS VEGETARIAN								
Asda*	1 Sausage/27g	54	3.4	199	18.0	3.5	12.5	2.5
Tivall*	1 Sausage/30g	73	4.8	244	18.0	7.0	16.0	3.0
FRAZZLES								
Bacon, Smith's, Walkers*	1 Bag/23g	112	5.3	485	6.5	62.0	23.0	1.3
FRENCH FRIES								
Cheese & Onion, Walkers*	1 Pack/22g	95	3.5	430	5.0	66.0	16.0	5.0
Ready Salted, Walkers*	1 Bag/22g	93	3.5	425	5.0	65.0	16.0	5.0
Salt & Vinegar, BGTY, Sainsbury's*	1 Bag/15g	51	0.2	340	6.0	80.1	1.5	4.1
Salt & Vinegar, Walkers*	1 Bag/22g	95	3.5	430	5.0	66.0	16.0	5.0
Worcester Sauce, Walkers*	1 Bag/22g	93	3.7	425	4.5	64.0	17.0	4.1
FRENCH TOAST								
Asda*	1 Toast/8g	30	0.4	381	10.0	74.0	5.0	4.0
Co-Op*	1 Toast/8g	31	0.5	385	10.0	72.0	6.0	5.0
Morrisons*	1 Toast/8g	31	0.5	393	11.0	72.5	6.6	3.0
Sainsbury's*	1 Toast/8g	31	0.5	382	10.0	72.0	6.6	5.0
Tesco*	1 Toast/100g	393	6.6	393	11.0	72.5	6.6	3.0
FRIES								
9/16" Straight Cut Home, Deep Fried, McCain*	1oz/28g	65	2.8	233	3.2	32.7	9.9	0.0
9/16" Straight Cut Home, Oven Baked, McCain*	1oz/28g	53	1.5	188	3.2	31.5	5.5	0.0
American Style, Frozen, Thin, Tesco*	1 Serving/125g	207	10.1	166	2.2	21.1	8.1	1.9
American Style, Slim, Iceland*	1 Serving/100g	187	6.1	187	2.4	30.6	6.1	2.4
Crispy French, Weighed Deep Fried, McCain*	1 Serving/100g	193	8.5	193	1.9	27.4	8.5	0.9
Curly, Cajun, Weighed Frozen, McCain*	1 Portion/100g	156	8.7	156	1.6	17.7	8.7	1.8
Curly, Southern Style, Tesco*	1 Serving/50g	124	3.6	248	3.8	41.7	7.3	3.8
Curly, Twisters, Frozen, Conagra Foods*	1 Serving/150g	273	13.9	182	2.5	22.0	9.3	2.2
Extra Chunky, Oven Baked, Homefries, McCain*	1 Serving/200g	306	6.2	153	3.2	28.0	3.1	2.3
Oven, American Style, Frozen, Asda*	1 Serving/180g	407	14.4	226	3.9	34.6	8.0	4.0
Oven, Straight Cut, Morrisons*	1 Serving/100g	149	4.3	149	2.8	24.6	4.3	2.6
Seasoned, Conagra Foods*	1 Serving/150g	247	12.0	165	2.4	20.8	8.0	1.9
Southern, Oven Cook, Baked, Potato Winners, McCain*	1 Serving/100g	232	8.3	232	3.6	35.7	8.3	2.4
Southern Spicy Spiral, Deep Fried, McCain*	1oz/28g	58	2.9	208	2.7	26.4	10.2	0.0
Southern Spicy Spiral, Oven Baked, McCain*	1oz/28g	46	1.8	165	1.7	24.6	6.6	0.0
FRISPS								
Tangy Salt & Vinegar, KP Snacks*	1 Bag/30g	160	10.0	532	5.0	52.6	33.5	2.9
Tasty Cheese & Onion, KP Snacks*	1 Bag/28g	150	9.4	537	5.5	53.2	33.6	3.2

	Measure INFO/WEIGHT	per Measure		Nutrition Values per 100g / 100ml				
		KCAL	FAT	KCAL	PROT	CARB	FAT	FIBRE
FROG								
Legs, Raw, Meat Only	*1oz/28g*	*20*	*0.1*	*73*	*16.4*	*0.0*	*0.3*	*0.0*
FROMAGE FRAIS								
0% Fat, Vitalinea, Danone*	1 Tbsp/28g	14	0.0	50	7.4	4.7	0.1	0.0
Apple Pie, Low Fat, Sainsbury's*	1 Pot/90g	108	2.3	120	6.7	17.3	2.6	0.3
Apricot, Layered, Weight Watchers*	1 Pot/100g	46	0.1	46	5.4	5.8	0.1	0.2
Apricot, Tesco*	1 Pot/100g	77	3.0	77	6.5	6.0	3.0	1.3
Bakewell Tart Flavour, BGTY, Sainsbury's*	1 Pot/100g	54	0.2	54	7.6	5.5	0.2	1.1
Banana, Organic, Yeo Valley*	1 Pot/90g	118	5.4	131	6.6	12.6	6.0	0.2
Black Cherry, Asda*	1 Pot/100g	113	5.0	113	4.1	13.0	5.0	0.0
Blackberry, Layered, Weight Watchers*	1 Pot/100g	47	0.2	47	5.5	5.7	0.2	0.4
Blackcurrant, GFY, Asda*	1 Pot/100g	43	0.2	43	6.0	4.2	0.2	0.0
Blue Parrot Cafe, Sainsbury's*	1 Serving/50g	49	1.5	98	6.6	11.0	3.1	0.2
Cherries & Chocolate, Finest, Tesco*	1 Serving/165g	299	14.5	181	5.4	20.1	8.8	0.7
Cherry, 0% Fat, Vitalinea, Danone*	1 Serving/150g	88	0.2	59	6.1	8.0	0.1	1.6
Danone*	1 Serving/100g	73	3.1	73	7.2	3.9	3.1	0.0
Fat Free, Average	*1 Pot/60g*	*35*	*0.1*	*58*	*7.7*	*6.8*	*0.2*	*0.0*
Forest Fruits, Layered, Weight Watchers*	1 Pot/100g	47	0.2	47	5.5	5.7	0.2	0.4
Fruit, Balanced Lifestyle, Aldi*	1 Pot/100g	52	0.2	52	5.4	7.1	0.2	0.7
Fruit on the Bottom, BFY, Morrisons*	1 Pot/100g	66	0.1	66	5.6	10.6	0.1	0.0
Kids, Yeo Valley*	1 Serving/90g	111	4.8	123	6.6	12.6	5.3	0.0
Lemon, Balanced Lifestyle, Aldi*	1 Serving/100g	52	0.3	52	5.6	6.6	0.3	0.6
Lemon Pie, Low Fat, Sainsbury's*	1 Pot/90g	108	2.4	120	6.7	17.3	2.7	0.2
Mandarin & Orange, HL, Tesco*	1 Pot/100g	55	0.2	55	6.2	7.0	0.2	0.3
Mandarin & Orange, Tesco*	1 Pot/100g	75	3.0	75	6.5	5.6	3.0	2.3
Morello Cherries, Perfectly Balanced, Waitrose*	½ Pot/250ml	260	4.7	104	2.5	19.1	1.9	1.8
Morrisons*	1 Serving/28g	17	0.0	59	9.8	4.8	0.0	0.0
Munch Bunch, Nestle*	1 Pot/42g	44	1.3	105	6.7	12.6	3.0	0.0
Natural, Creamy, Co-Op*	1 Pot/200g	204	14.6	102	6.1	2.9	7.3	0.0
Natural, Fat Free, M & S*	1 Serving/100g	60	0.1	60	9.8	4.8	0.1	0.0
Natural, GFY, Asda*	½ Pot/100g	52	0.3	52	7.3	5.0	0.3	0.0
Natural, HL, Tesco*	1 Serving/65g	30	0.1	46	7.8	3.3	0.2	0.0
Natural, Plain, Fat Free, Normandy, BGTY, Sainsbury's*	1 Serving/30g	15	0.0	49	8.0	4.2	0.1	0.0
Natural, Virtually Fat Free, French, Waitrose*	1 Tub/500g	260	1.5	52	7.3	5.0	0.3	0.0
Normandy, Light Choices, Tesco*	1 Serving/100g	46	0.2	46	7.8	3.3	0.2	0.0
Normandy, Sainsbury's*	1 Serving/25g	29	2.0	116	7.7	3.4	8.1	0.0
Organic, Vrai*	1 Serving/100g	83	3.6	83	8.1	4.5	3.6	0.0
Peach, BGTY, Sainsbury's*	1 Pot/100g	53	0.2	53	7.2	5.5	0.2	0.5
Peach, Layered, Weight Watchers*	1 Pot/100g	46	0.1	46	5.0	8.0	0.1	0.0
Petit Dessert, Co-Op*	1 Pot/60g	74	2.6	123	6.3	14.5	4.4	0.0
Pineapple & Passion Fruit, HL, Tesco*	1 Pot/100g	55	0.2	55	6.2	7.1	0.2	0.1
Plain, Average	*1oz/28g*	*32*	*2.0*	*113*	*6.8*	*5.7*	*7.1*	*0.0*
Raspberry, COU, M & S*	1 Pot/100g	60	0.2	60	7.0	8.1	0.2	0.5
Raspberry, GFY, Asda*	1 Pot/100g	43	0.2	43	6.0	4.2	0.2	0.0
Raspberry, Healthy Choice, Asda*	1 Pot/100g	41	0.2	41	6.0	3.8	0.2	0.0
Raspberry, Layered, Weight Watchers*	1 Pot/100g	47	0.2	47	5.5	5.7	0.2	0.4
Raspberry, Little Stars, Muller*	1 Pot/60g	66	2.4	110	5.0	12.7	4.0	0.4
Raspberry, Organic, Yeo Valley*	1 Pot/100g	127	6.5	127	6.1	11.1	6.5	0.4
Raspberry & Redcurrant, BGTY, Sainsbury's*	1 Pot/100g	51	0.1	51	7.4	5.4	0.1	1.6
Real Fruit, Tesco*	1 Pot/100g	54	0.1	54	5.6	7.6	0.1	0.1
Rhubarb & Crumble, Low Fat, Sainsbury's*	1 Pot/90g	96	2.3	107	6.7	14.1	2.6	0.4
Strawberry, 0% Fat, Vitalinea, Danone*	1 Serving/150g	82	0.2	55	6.0	7.4	0.1	1.6
Strawberry, 99.9% Fat Free, Onken*	1 Serving/50g	45	0.0	91	6.9	15.3	0.1	0.0
Strawberry, Balanced Lifestyle, Aldi*	1 Serving/100g	52	0.2	52	5.4	7.1	0.2	0.7

F

	Measure INFO/WEIGHT	per Measure KCAL	FAT	Nutrition Values per 100g / 100ml KCAL	PROT	CARB	FAT	FIBRE
FROMAGE FRAIS								
Strawberry, COU, M & S*	1 Pot/100g	60	0.2	60	6.5	8.0	0.2	0.5
Strawberry, GFY, Asda*	1 Pot/100g	58	0.2	58	6.0	8.0	0.2	0.0
Strawberry, Layered, Weight Watchers*	1 Pot/100g	50	0.1	50	5.4	6.2	0.1	0.8
Strawberry, Low Fat, St Ivel*	1 Pot/100g	69	1.2	69	6.9	6.8	1.2	0.0
Strawberry, Organic, Yeo Valley*	1 Pot/90g	116	5.4	129	6.3	12.5	6.0	0.2
Strawberry, Tesco*	1 Pot/100g	75	3.0	75	6.5	5.5	3.0	2.5
Strawberry, Thomas the Tank Engine, Yoplait*	1 Pot/50g	50	0.6	101	6.8	15.4	1.3	0.0
Strawberry & Raspberry, Organic, Yeo Valley*	1 Pot/90g	118	5.4	131	6.3	12.9	6.0	0.2
Strawberry Tart, Sainsbury's*	1 Pot/100g	54	0.2	54	7.6	5.5	0.2	1.1
Toffee & Pecan Pie, Smooth & Creamy, Tesco*	1 Pot/100g	148	6.8	148	6.9	14.8	6.8	0.2
Tropical Fruit, COU, M & S*	1 Pot/100g	60	0.2	60	6.5	8.4	0.2	0.5
Vanilla, Danone*	1 Serving/200g	274	8.2	137	5.3	19.6	4.1	0.0
Virtually Fat Free, Tesco*	1 Pot/100g	56	0.1	56	5.6	8.2	0.1	0.0
Wildlife, Strawberry, Raspberry Or Peach, Yoplait*	1 Pot/50g	46	0.6	93	7.1	13.2	1.3	0.2
FROZEN DESSERT								
Banoffee, HL, Tesco*	1 Serving/60g	92	1.6	153	2.5	29.9	2.6	0.6
Vanilla, BGTY, Sainsbury's*	1 Serving/75g	89	2.2	119	3.0	19.9	3.0	3.7
Vanilla, GFY, Asda*	1 Serving/52g	72	2.3	139	2.7	22.0	4.5	0.0
Vanilla, Too Good to Be True, Wall's Ice Cream*	1 Serving/50ml	35	0.2	70	2.0	14.9	0.4	0.1
Vanilla Choc Fudge, Non Dairy Soya, Tofutti*	1 Tub/500ml	825	45.0	165	1.6	20.0	9.0	0.4
FROZEN YOGHURT								
Black Cherry, M & S*	1 Pot/125g	164	1.4	131	3.1	27.1	1.1	0.5
Raspberry, Handmade Farmhouse, Sainsbury's*	1 Serving/100g	132	3.8	132	2.7	21.8	3.8	2.2
Raspberry, Orchard Maid*	1 Serving/80ml	89	1.7	111	2.8	19.9	2.1	0.0
Strawberry, Organic, Yeo Valley*	1 Serving/100g	140	3.0	140	4.8	23.5	3.0	0.1
Strawberry, Tesco*	1 Pot/60g	82	1.3	136	2.6	26.5	2.2	0.8
Vanilla, Less Than 5% Fat, Tesco*	1 Pot/120g	179	2.9	149	8.1	23.8	2.4	0.7
FRUIT								
Apple, Pineapple & Grape, Ready to Eat, Sainsbury's*	1 Pack/180g	94	0.2	52	0.5	8.3	0.1	1.3
Apple & Pear, Snack Pack, Great Stuff, Asda*	1 Pack/80g	42	0.1	52	0.4	11.0	0.1	2.6
Baked, Nibbles, Cherry Berry, We Are Bear*	1 Packet/30g	87	0.0	290	1.2	76.0	0.1	10.3
Baked, Nibbles, Mango Pineapple, We Are Bear*	1 Bag/30g	85	0.0	285	1.4	73.0	0.1	11.0
Berry Medley, Freshly Prepared, M & S*	1 Pack/180g	90	0.4	50	0.7	10.9	0.2	2.9
Bites, Apple & Grape, Food Explorers, Waitrose*	1 Pack/80g	44	0.1	55	0.4	13.2	0.1	1.4
Bites, Raspberry, Mini, HL, Tesco*	1 Bag/25g	87	0.7	350	4.5	76.8	2.7	4.4
Black Forest, Frozen, Tesco*	1 Serving/80g	37	0.0	46	0.7	10.5	0.0	1.7
Black Forest, Shearway*	1oz/28g	12	0.0	44	0.7	9.9	0.1	0.0
Cempedak	1 Serving/100g	116	0.4	116	3.0	28.6	0.4	0.0
Citrus Selection, Fresh, Sainsbury's*	1 Pack/240g	79	0.2	33	0.9	7.1	0.1	1.6
Deluxe, Fresh, Rindless, Shapers, Boots*	1 Pack/168g	64	0.3	38	0.7	8.3	0.2	0.7
Exotic, M & S*	1 Pack/425g	212	1.3	50	0.7	11.8	0.3	0.0
Exotic Fruit Frenzy, Freshly Prepared, Tesco*	1 Pack/300g	132	0.6	44	0.6	9.8	0.2	1.6
Fabulous Fruity Fingers, Melon & Mango, M & S*	1 Pack/240g	96	0.5	40	0.6	8.2	0.2	1.0
Fingers, Melon & Pineapple, Sainsbury's*	1 Pack/240g	74	0.2	31	0.5	6.5	0.1	0.8
Fingers, Sunmaid*	1 Pack/50g	162	2.1	325	3.5	68.3	4.3	4.3
Frozen, Garden, M & S*	1 Serving/30g	7	0.1	25	0.7	4.6	0.2	1.8
Grapefruit & Orange Segments, Breakfast, Del Monte*	1 Can/411g	193	0.4	47	1.0	10.2	0.1	1.0
Mango, Slices, in Juice, SPC Nature's Finest*	1 Pot/400g	224	0.8	56	5.0	12.3	0.2	1.5
Melon, Kiwi Fruit & Strawberries, Fresh Tastes, Asda*	1 Pack/240g	96	0.5	40	0.8	7.7	0.2	2.1
Melon & Grape Munchies, Eat Well, M & S*	½ Pack/200g	70	0.2	35	0.5	8.3	0.1	0.7
Melon & Grape Pot, Co-Op*	1 Pot/125g	44	0.1	35	0.6	7.0	0.1	0.9
Melon Medley, Average	1 Pack/240g	66	0.3	27	0.6	6.0	0.1	0.5
Mix for Pie or Crumble, Frozen, Sainsbury's*	1 Pack/400g	128	0.8	32	0.8	5.7	0.2	2.1

F

	Measure INFO/WEIGHT	per Measure KCAL	per Measure FAT	Nutrition Values per 100g / 100ml KCAL	PROT	CARB	FAT	FIBRE
FRUIT								
Mixed, Fresh, 5 a Day, Tesco*	1 Pack/400g	136	0.8	34	0.8	7.4	0.2	1.4
Mixed, Fresh, Tesco*	1 Pack/200g	70	0.4	35	0.8	7.4	0.2	1.4
Mixed, Fruitime, Pieces, Tesco*	1 Can/140g	84	0.0	60	0.4	14.0	0.0	1.0
Mixed, Pieces, in Orange Jelly, Fruitini, Del Monte*	1 Can/140g	94	0.1	67	0.3	15.8	0.1	0.0
Mixed, Tropical, Fruit Express, Del Monte*	1 Pot/185g	89	0.2	48	0.2	11.2	0.1	1.2
Mixed, Vine, Crazy Jack*	1 Serving/10g	31	0.0	309	2.8	74.0	0.3	4.7
Mount Pleasant, Graze*	1 Pack/21g	87	5.1	415	2.5	46.9	24.2	9.2
Nectarine, White Flesh, Waitrose*	1 Peach/130g	56	0.1	43	1.4	9.0	0.1	1.6
Outrageously Orange Melon, M & S*	1 Pack/180g	36	0.2	20	0.6	4.2	0.1	0.8
Peach, Slices, Frozen, Sainsbury's*	1 Serving/80g	30	0.0	37	1.0	7.6	0.0	1.5
Peach Pieces in Fruit Juice, Tesco*	1 Pot/125g	60	0.0	48	0.4	11.7	0.0	1.0
Pieces, Mixed in Fruit Juice, Fruitini, Del Monte*	1 Serving/120g	61	0.1	51	0.4	12.0	0.1	0.5
Pineapple, Grape & Kiwi, Asda*	1 Serving/200g	98	0.6	49	0.6	11.0	0.3	1.7
Pineapple & Mango Tango, Eat Well, M & S*	1 Pack/200g	100	0.8	50	1.0	22.2	0.4	2.6
Pineapple Pot, Chosen By You, Asda*	1 Pot/200g	106	0.0	53	0.4	12.5	0.0	0.7
Prunes, Stoned, Ready To Eat, Asda*	6 Prunes/30g	46	0.1	154	2.5	35.2	0.4	8.5
Rolls, Peach, Yo Yo, Bear*	1 Roll/10g	27	0.0	275	1.4	72.0	0.2	10.0
Snack, Apple & Grape, Blue Parrot Cafe, Sainsbury's*	1 Pack/80g	42	0.1	53	0.4	12.5	0.1	2.1
Snack, Sweet Grape, Shapers, Boots*	1 Pack/80g	53	0.1	66	0.4	15.0	0.1	1.0
Snack Pack, Fresh, Sainsbury's*	1 Serving/120g	54	0.1	45	0.1	11.0	0.1	1.3
Strawberries, Apple & Grapes, Fresh Tastes, Asda*	1 Pot/190g	91	0.2	48	0.5	10.6	0.1	0.0
Summer Berries, M & S*	1 Pack/160g	80	0.3	50	0.7	10.0	0.2	3.0
Tayberry	1 Serving/100g	25	0.0	25	1.2	12.0	0.0	7.0
to Go, Del Monte*	1 Can/113g	80	0.0	71	0.0	17.7	0.0	0.0
Tropical, in Juice, Dole*	1 Pot/113g	59	0.0	52	0.3	14.2	0.0	1.8
Tropical, Tesco*	1 Pack/180g	85	0.4	47	0.6	10.8	0.2	1.9
Tutti Frutti Collection, Freshly Prepared, Tesco*	1 Pack/200g	82	0.4	41	0.6	9.1	0.2	1.4
FRUIT & NUT MIX								
Almond, Raisin & Berry, Sainsbury's*	1 Bag/50g	188	7.1	377	6.1	57.6	14.3	4.2
Almonds & Raisins, Love Life, Waitrose*	1 Pack/150g	681	42.6	454	11.6	38.1	28.4	4.7
Bakewell Tart, Graze*	1 Pack/37g	154	8.1	416	8.9	48.3	21.8	4.7
Banana Split, Graze*	1 Punnet/35g	160	8.6	458	12.3	50.3	24.7	2.8
Banoffee Pie, Graze*	1 Punnet/33g	154	9.1	468	6.9	48.0	27.6	6.6
Billionaire's Shortbread, Graze*	1 Punnet/38g	177	9.5	465	7.8	53.0	24.9	4.3
Born in The USA, Graze*	1 Pack/50g	285	21.9	570	10.6	33.8	43.8	0.0
Bounty Hunter, Graze*	1 Punnet/43g	206	13.2	479	4.6	46.0	30.6	0.0
Cacao Vine, Graze*	1 Punnet/45g	187	9.4	416	8.5	51.4	20.8	0.0
Cheeky Monkey, Graze*	1 Punnet/30g	130	6.4	435	6.4	54.7	21.2	0.0
Cherish, Graze*	1 Punnet/40g	148	9.3	369	4.4	35.8	23.2	6.6
Cherries, Raisins & Nuts, Love Life, Waitrose*	1 Serving/30g	132	7.5	439	7.7	45.8	25.0	3.4
Cinnamon & Praline, Christmas, Finest, Tesco*	¼ Pot/106g	470	26.7	442	8.2	45.9	25.1	11.5
Dried, Bear Necessities, Graze*	1 Pack/35g	126	8.1	361	4.6	34.9	23.2	6.5
Dried, Selection, Wholesome, Love Life, Waitrose*	1 Serving/30g	144	9.6	479	9.8	38.0	32.0	4.4
Eleanor's Apple Crumble, Graze*	1 Pack/31g	108	3.9	349	6.3	56.2	12.6	6.7
Exotic, Waitrose*	1 Serving/50g	207	8.8	414	9.0	54.6	17.7	4.6
Fajita, Graze*	1 Box/55g	255	17.0	463	15.1	38.0	30.9	0.0
Flapjack, Fruit & Seed, Graze*	1 Punnet/55g	229	11.2	417	5.2	54.7	20.4	4.3
Fruit & Nut Case, Graze*	1 Punnet/40g	168	8.8	420	5.8	52.1	22.1	2.9
Fruit Squash, Graze*	1 Pack/40g	180	9.5	451	13.4	47.5	23.8	6.4
Fruitabulous, You Are What You Eat*	1 Bag/40g	155	7.8	388	7.2	46.0	19.5	5.5
Grandma's Apple Crumble, Graze*	1 Punnet/40g	154	7.8	385	0.0	48.9	19.6	4.0
Hazelnut Espresso, Natural Treats, Graze*	1 Punnet/39g	191	12.3	490	8.4	42.9	31.6	4.2
Himalayas & Beyond, Graze*	1 Pack/30g	139	9.2	465	5.0	44.1	30.7	6.7

	Measure INFO/WEIGHT	per Measure KCAL	per Measure FAT	Nutrition Values per 100g / 100ml KCAL	PROT	CARB	FAT	FIBRE
FRUIT & NUT MIX								
Honeycomb Crunch, Graze*	1 Punnet/40g	181	10.2	452	9.8	48.0	25.4	3.2
Jaffa Cake, Graze*	1 Punnet/44g	210	13.7	476	6.8	43.1	31.0	5.1
Johnny Come Lately, Graze*	1 Pack/65g	262	14.8	403	10.0	41.4	22.8	0.0
Jungle Fever, Graze*	1 Pack/30g	135	8.3	449	7.4	42.3	27.8	6.8
Lemon Meringue Pie, Graze*	1 Punnet/45g	177	6.0	393	5.0	66.3	13.4	2.0
Limoncello, Graze*	1 Punnet/41g	162	8.4	396	6.3	50.6	20.6	4.3
Lost, Coconut, Banana & Raisins, Graze*	1 Punnet/30g	115	5.8	382	3.5	51.0	19.2	5.8
Luxury, Asda*	1 Serving/50g	225	15.2	451	9.0	33.5	30.5	7.4
M & S*	1 Serving/30g	135	7.6	450	12.4	44.3	25.3	6.0
Macadamias & Dried Cranberries, Love Life, Waitrose*	1 Serving/30g	143	9.2	477	3.3	47.1	30.8	6.2
Mayan Mocha, Graze*	1 Punnet/40g	185	11.1	462	10.4	46.4	27.8	6.0
New World, Graze*	1 Serving/50g	206	11.7	413	16.8	45.2	23.4	0.0
Nuts & Raisins, Mixed, Natural, Love Life, Waitrose*	1 Serving/50g	256	16.4	513	16.5	38.4	32.8	7.2
Ooh La La, Graze*	1 Punnet/45g	181	7.2	402	5.0	63.6	15.9	1.0
Organic, Love Life, Waitrose*	1 Serving/30g	115	6.1	383	9.8	40.4	20.2	5.8
Organic, Waitrose*	1 Pack/100g	489	32.6	489	15.0	33.8	32.6	5.4
Papaya & Cranberry, Sainsbury's*	1 Serving/75g	300	10.9	400	4.1	63.1	14.6	7.3
Peanuts, Cashews & Mango, Fair Trade, Tesco*	1/6 Pack	130	8.7	520	16.4	33.2	34.8	4.8
Port & Winter Spice, Christmas, Finest, Tesco*	¼ Pot/90g	379	23.8	421	7.8	37.9	26.5	13.9
Seed, Nut & Sultana Sprinkle, Love Life, Waitrose*	1 Serving/30g	177	15.4	591	17.2	15.4	51.2	4.3
Strawberry Milkshake, Graze*	1 Pack/35g	135	4.0	385	3.6	66.6	11.3	5.2
Sun Dance, Graze*	1 Punnet/38g	136	3.8	358	4.3	67.2	9.9	4.5
Swallows & Amazons, Graze*	1 Pack/60g	252	11.8	420	6.3	56.3	19.7	0.0
The Mix, Whitworths*	1 Pot/90g	341	13.1	379	4.1	63.1	14.6	7.3
The Waldorf, Graze*	1 Punnet/28g	109	6.2	389	6.0	43.5	22.1	5.7
Trail Mix, Average	1oz/28g	121	8.0	432	9.1	37.2	28.5	4.3
Trail Mix, Love Life, Waitrose*	1 Portion/30g	126	9.3	506	14.2	28.5	37.2	6.3
Tropical Praline, Graze*	1 Punnet/35g	121	4.2	347	4.2	59.2	12.1	2.0
Unsalted, Tesco*	1 Serving/25g	112	4.6	449	12.6	58.1	18.5	12.2
Walnut Whip, Graze*	1 Pack/37g	181	12.0	489	9.9	41.4	32.3	4.6
Ying & Yang, Graze*	1 Pack/60g	296	19.5	493	6.8	41.2	32.5	0.0
FRUIT COCKTAIL								
Fresh, Morrisons*	1oz/28g	12	0.1	44	0.6	11.3	0.2	1.0
Fresh & Ready, Sainsbury's*	1 Pack/300g	117	0.3	39	0.6	9.0	0.1	1.2
in Apple Juice, Asda*	1/3 Can/80g	40	0.1	50	0.3	12.0	0.1	1.6
in Fruit Juice, Heinz*	1 Pot/125g	77	0.0	62	0.5	15.0	0.0	1.0
in Fruit Juice, Morrisons*	1 Can/140g	64	0.0	46	0.4	11.0	0.0	0.0
in Fruit Juice, Sainsbury's*	1 Serving/198g	97	0.2	49	0.3	11.9	0.1	1.3
in Fruit Juice, Waitrose*	1 Can/142g	71	0.0	50	0.4	12.0	0.0	1.0
in Grape Juice, Tesco*	1oz/28g	12	0.0	43	0.4	10.0	0.0	1.0
in Juice, Del Monte*	1 Can/415g	203	0.4	49	0.4	11.2	0.1	0.0
in Light Syrup, Princes*	1 Serving/206g	64	0.0	31	0.4	7.3	0.0	1.0
in Light Syrup, Sainsbury's*	½ Can/125g	72	0.1	58	0.4	14.0	0.1	1.3
in Light Syrup, Valfrutta*	1 Serving/206g	95	0.0	46	0.2	11.4	0.0	1.5
in Syrup, Del Monte*	1 Can/420g	315	0.4	75	0.4	18.0	0.1	0.0
in Syrup, Morrisons*	½ Can/205g	129	0.2	63	0.3	14.9	0.1	0.0
in Syrup, Tesco*	1 Serving/135g	85	0.0	63	0.4	15.0	0.0	1.0
No Added Sugar, Asda*	1 Serving/134g	67	0.1	50	0.3	12.0	0.1	1.6
Tropical, Asda*	½ Can/135g	81	0.0	60	0.0	15.0	0.0	1.6
Tropical, Canned, Asda*	½ Can/200g	120	0.0	60	0.0	15.0	0.0	1.6
Tropical, Heinz*	1 Pot/113g	61	0.0	54	0.5	13.0	0.0	1.0
Tropical, in Juice, Morrisons*	1 Serving/100g	56	0.0	56	0.0	14.0	0.0	0.0
Tropical, in Syrup, Sainsbury's*	½ Can/130g	95	0.1	73	0.5	17.6	0.1	1.4

F

	Measure INFO/WEIGHT	per Measure KCAL	per Measure FAT	Nutrition Values per 100g / 100ml KCAL	PROT	CARB	FAT	FIBRE
FRUIT COMPOTE								
& Vanilla Sponge, Weight Watchers*	1 Pack/140g	202	2.9	144	2.2	29.0	2.1	1.8
Apple, Strawberry & Blackberry, Organic, Yeo Valley*	½ Pot/112g	73	0.1	65	0.5	15.5	0.1	1.9
Apricot & Prune, Yeo Valley*	1 Pot/225g	207	0.2	92	0.6	22.3	0.1	1.6
Black Cherry & Creme Fraiche, Extra Special, Asda*	1 Pot/118g	188	9.4	159	1.7	20.0	8.0	0.8
Hartley's*	1 Serving/95g	63	0.1	66	0.8	15.5	0.1	2.4
Orchard Fruits, GFY, Asda*	1 Pot/180g	113	0.2	63	0.5	15.0	0.1	0.0
Spiced, Tesco*	1 Serving/112g	122	0.6	109	1.7	24.4	0.5	3.1
Strawberry & Raspberry, M & S*	1 Serving/80g	72	0.1	90	0.7	23.5	0.1	2.3
Summerfruit, M & S*	¼ Pot/125g	119	0.7	95	0.9	22.7	0.6	0.8
FRUIT DRINK								
Alive Tropical Torrent, Coca-Cola*	1 Glass/200ml	88	0.0	44	0.0	11.0	0.0	0.0
Cherryade, No Added Sugar, Morrisons*	1 Glass/250ml	2	0.0	1	0.0	0.1	0.0	0.0
Lemon & Lime, Diet, Carbonated, M & S*	1 Glass/250ml	5	0.0	2	0.0	0.2	0.0	0.0
Multivitamin, Rejuvenation, Active Life, Purdy's*	1 Bottle/330ml	125	0.0	38	0.0	9.5	0.0	0.0
Pineapple, Sparkling, KA, Barr's*	1 Can/330ml	168	0.0	51	0.0	12.5	0.0	0.0
FRUIT FILLING								
Cherry & Amaretto, Asda*	¼ Pack/100g	105	0.2	105	0.9	23.0	0.2	0.0
Red Cherry, Morton*	1 Serving/70g	69	0.0	98	0.4	23.9	0.0	0.0
FRUIT FLAKES								
Blackcurrant, with Yoghurt Coating, Fruit Bowl*	1 Bag/25g	112	5.1	449	1.7	64.2	20.6	0.0
Raisins, with Yoghurt Coating, Fruit Bowl*	1 Pack/30g	133	5.5	444	2.9	66.6	18.4	0.0
Raspberry, with Yoghurt Coating, Fruit Bowl*	1 Serving/25g	112	5.1	449	1.7	64.2	20.6	0.0
Strawberry, Fruit Bowl*	1 Pack/20g	66	0.4	330	1.0	78.0	2.0	2.0
Strawberry, with Yoghurt Coating, Fruit Bowl*	1 Serving/25g	112	5.1	449	1.7	64.2	20.6	0.0
FRUIT GUMS								
Fruit Salad, Tesco*	6 Sweets/30g	100	0.1	335	8.3	73.4	0.5	0.3
No Added Sugar, Boots*	1 Sweet/2g	1	0.0	88	0.0	22.0	0.0	0.0
Rowntree's*	1 Tube/49g	170	0.1	344	4.8	81.3	0.2	0.0
Sugar Free, Sainsbury's*	1 Serving/30g	63	0.1	209	7.7	71.3	0.2	0.1
FRUIT MEDLEY								
Dried, Tropical, Soft, Love Life, Waitrose*	1 Serving/30g	86	0.0	288	0.2	70.6	0.0	2.5
Exotic, Co-Op*	1 Serving/120g	54	0.2	45	0.6	10.0	0.2	0.0
Fresh, Tesco*	1 Pack/200g	86	0.2	43	0.4	10.0	0.1	1.1
in Fresh Orange Juice, Co-Op*	1 Serving/140g	49	0.0	35	0.5	9.0	0.0	0.0
Mango, Melon, Kiwi & Blueberry, Fresh, M & S*	1 Pack/260g	104	0.8	40	0.7	9.1	0.3	1.6
Mixed, Fruit Harvest, Whitworths*	1 Pack/50g	165	0.3	331	1.8	79.4	0.7	4.8
Nectarine, Mango & Blueberry, Fresh, M & S*	1 Pack/245g	122	0.5	50	1.0	11.1	0.2	2.1
Pineapple, Papaya & Mango, Waitrose*	1 Pack/550g	297	0.5	54	0.6	12.8	0.1	1.1
Raisin, Fruit Harvest, Whitworths*	1 Pack/50g	157	0.6	315	1.8	74.4	1.3	4.3
Shapers, Boots*	1 Pack/140g	55	0.3	39	0.7	8.6	0.2	1.0
FRUIT MIX								
Apple Strudel, Graze*	1 Pack/55g	172	0.4	312	2.6	63.5	0.7	0.0
Banana, Coconut & Mango, Dried, Graze*	1 Punnet/45g	144	3.7	320	18.7	57.1	8.2	0.0
Banana Coins, Graze*	1 Serving/20g	49	0.1	245	2.4	54.0	0.6	0.0
Beach Bum, Graze*	1 Pack/40g	168	3.4	419	2.2	59.8	8.4	0.0
Berry, Sainsbury's*	1 Serving/20g	64	0.4	319	1.0	78.1	1.9	5.5
Caribbean, Dried, Graze*	1 Box/50g	187	6.4	374	1.2	67.6	12.8	0.0
Cherish, Graze*	1 Pack/50g	221	10.0	443	5.2	52.5	20.0	0.0
Date To Remember, Graze*	1 Punnet/40g	131	1.8	327	3.3	68.3	4.4	6.3
Fig & Cherry Fruit Bake, Graze*	1 Punnet/44g	116	0.4	263	2.9	64.6	0.9	7.6
Fig Roll, Graze*	1 Punnet/35g	110	0.6	313	1.6	23.1	1.7	2.0
Forest Fruit, Dried, Graze*	1 Pack/50g	159	0.4	319	1.8	76.0	0.8	0.0
Frozen, Blueberries & Strawberries, Sainsbury's*	1 Portion/75g	25	0.1	34	0.7	6.5	0.2	1.5

F

	Measure INFO/WEIGHT	per Measure KCAL	per Measure FAT	Nutrition Values per 100g / 100ml KCAL	PROT	CARB	FAT	FIBRE
FRUIT MIX								
Go Goji Go Go Go, Graze*	1 Punnet/40g	112	0.3	279	2.2	69.0	0.8	0.0
Golden Pineapple Rings, Graze*	1 Punnet/20g	53	0.1	263	0.6	72.0	0.6	8.1
Italian Stallion, Graze*	1 Punnet/40g	118	0.4	296	1.7	71.0	0.9	2.6
Juicy Orange Raisins, Graze*	1 Pack/40g	110	0.4	275	2.1	69.0	0.9	0.0
Loco in Acapulco, Graze*	1 Pack /30g	123	6.4	410	4.0	53.2	21.4	0.0
Love Mix, Graze*	1 Pack/40g	98	0.4	245	4.0	58.0	0.9	5.9
Luxury, Sainsbury's*	1 Serving/30g	78	0.1	261	1.8	62.3	0.5	2.7
Mango & Cranberry, Way to Five, Sainsbury's*	1 Serving/50g	165	0.3	331	1.8	79.4	0.7	4.8
Melon, Strawberry & Grape, Sainsbury's*	1 Pack/180g	58	0.4	32	0.5	7.0	0.2	0.4
Muffin, Dried, Graze*	1 Box/60g	221	6.8	368	1.7	65.8	11.3	1.7
Nectarine, Raspberry & Blueberry, Seasonal, M & S*	1 Pack/160g	72	0.3	45	1.3	8.3	0.2	2.7
Pina Colada, Graze*	1 Punnet/20g	74	2.7	369	2.8	64.2	13.4	8.8
Pineapple, Kiwi, Mango & Blueberry, Waitrose*	1 Pack/330g	208	1.0	63	0.7	14.5	0.3	1.9
Pineapple, Melon, Mango, Tesco*	1 Pack/440g	242	0.9	55	1.1	11.4	0.2	1.3
Pumpkin Pie, Graze*	1 Pack/65g	274	11.2	422	11.4	48.2	17.2	0.0
Raisins & Apricots, Great Stuff, Asda*	1 Pack/40g	112	0.1	281	2.6	66.9	0.3	6.0
Rocky Mountain, Graze*	1 Pack/50g	264	19.3	529	3.2	38.2	38.6	0.0
Sour Mango Tangtastic, Graze*	1 Pack/34g	110	0.2	323	1.3	79.8	0.6	2.0
Strawberries & Cream, Graze*	1 Pack/70g	303	11.4	433	3.7	66.9	16.3	0.0
Strawberry Fields Forever, Graze*	1 Punnet /40g	117	0.4	292	1.9	70.9	0.9	2.5
Summer Fruits, British, Frozen, Waitrose*	1 Pack/380g	99	0.8	26	1.0	5.2	0.2	5.5
Summer Pudding, Graze*	1 Punnet/31g	106	0.4	342	1.6	81.2	1.2	4.2
Super Berry Detox, Graze*	1 Punnet/43g	129	0.3	299	1.7	73.9	0.7	3.4
Super Dried, Graze*	1 Pack/55g	176	0.9	320	5.6	76.4	1.6	0.0
Tropical, Fresh, Waitrose*	1 Pack/240g	122	0.5	51	0.6	11.6	0.2	1.9
FRUIT PUREE								
Apple, & Blueberry, Organix*	1 Pot/100g	54	0.6	54	0.4	11.6	0.6	2.5
Apple, & Peach, Organix*	1 Pot/100g	49	0.3	49	0.6	11.0	0.3	2.1
Apple & Blueberry, Organic, Clearspring*	1 Tub/100g	76	0.3	76	0.4	17.8	0.3	0.0
Banana, Apple, & Apricot, Organix*	1 Pot/100g	68	0.4	68	0.8	15.4	0.4	2.0
FRUIT SALAD								
Autumn, Fresh, M & S*	½ Pack/160g	64	0.2	40	0.7	9.4	0.1	2.9
Berry, Asda*	1 Pack/250g	122	0.2	49	0.6	10.9	0.1	0.0
Berry, Seasonal, Asda*	1 Pack/300g	93	0.3	31	0.6	7.0	0.1	2.1
Chunky, in Fruit Juice, Canned, John West*	1 Can/411g	193	0.8	47	0.4	11.0	0.2	0.8
Citrus, Asda*	1 Serving/265g	88	0.3	33	0.9	7.2	0.1	1.5
Citrus, Fresh, M & S*	½ Pack/225g	79	0.2	35	0.9	7.7	0.1	1.5
Classic, Co-Op*	1 Box/285g	142	0.3	50	0.6	11.0	0.1	2.3
Classic, Fresh, Sainsbury's*	1 Pack/400g	148	0.8	37	0.6	8.6	0.2	1.8
Classic, Shapers, Boots*	1 Pack/200g	75	0.2	37	0.7	8.5	0.1	1.3
Dried, M & S*	½ Pack/125g	269	0.5	215	1.8	51.4	0.4	5.9
Exotic, Fresh, Tesco*	1 Serving/225g	85	0.4	38	0.7	8.4	0.2	1.5
Exotic, Fully Prepared, Sainsbury's*	1 Serving/200g	74	0.4	37	0.6	8.3	0.2	1.3
Exotic, Morrisons*	1 Serving/150g	78	0.3	52	0.6	12.2	0.2	0.0
Exotic, Waitrose*	1 Pack/300g	126	0.6	42	0.6	9.5	0.2	1.1
Exotic, with Melon, Mango, Kiwi Fruit & Grapes, Asda*	1 Pot/300g	141	0.9	47	0.6	10.5	0.3	1.4
Fresh, Morrisons*	1 Tub/350g	150	0.3	43	0.7	9.9	0.1	0.0
Fresh, Sweet, Ripe & Moist, Tesco*	1 Serving/750g	345	0.7	46	0.7	10.6	0.1	1.6
Fresh, Tesco*	1 Pack/200g	84	0.4	42	0.7	9.3	0.2	1.5
Fresh, Washed, Ready to Eat, Tesco*	1 Pack/200g	92	0.2	46	0.7	10.6	0.1	1.6
Fresh for You, Tesco*	1 Pack/160g	59	0.3	37	0.6	8.2	0.2	1.1
Freshly Prepared, M & S*	1 Pack/350g	140	0.7	40	0.5	9.3	0.2	1.0
Fruit, Mediterranean Style, Shapers, Boots*	1 Pack/142g	61	0.1	43	0.6	10.0	0.1	1.5

F

FRUIT SALAD

	Measure INFO/WEIGHT	per Measure KCAL	FAT	Nutrition Values per 100g / 100ml KCAL	PROT	CARB	FAT	FIBRE
Fruit Crunch, Salad Bowl, M & S*	½ Pack/120g	174	4.1	145	3.1	25.5	3.4	0.6
Golden, Fresh, Asda*	1 Pot/147g	69	0.1	47	0.6	11.0	0.1	1.6
Grapefruit & Orange, Fresh, M & S*	1 Serving/250g	87	0.2	35	0.9	7.4	0.1	1.6
Green, M & S*	1 Pack/400g	200	0.8	50	0.6	10.9	0.2	1.2
Homemade, Unsweetened, Average	1 Serving/140g	77	0.1	55	0.7	13.8	0.1	1.5
Juicy Melon, Pineapple & Grapes, Asda*	1 Pot/300g	111	0.3	37	0.5	8.4	0.1	0.9
Kiwi, Pineapple & Grape, Fresh Tastes, Asda*	1 Pack/200g	106	0.6	53	0.6	11.0	0.3	1.8
Layered, Tropical Rainbow, Freshly Prepared, M & S*	1 Pack/375g	206	1.1	55	0.7	12.6	0.3	1.7
Luxury, Fresh, Tesco*	1 Serving/400g	164	0.8	41	0.7	9.2	0.2	1.6
Luxury, Frozen, Boylans*	1 Serving/100g	54	0.2	54	0.7	12.7	0.2	0.0
Luxury, Frozen, Tesco*	½ Pack/250g	115	0.2	46	0.7	10.7	0.1	1.3
Luxury, M & S*	1oz/28g	11	0.0	40	0.6	9.2	0.1	1.1
Mango, Kiwi, Blueberry & Pomegranate, Fresh, M & S*	1 Pack/350g	210	1.0	60	0.9	13.4	0.3	2.4
Melon, Kiwi, Grapes & Pomegranate Seeds, Morrisons*	1 Pack/400g	152	1.2	38	0.7	8.2	0.3	1.2
Melon, Kiwi, Strawberry, Way to Five, Sainsbury's*	1 Pack/245g	73	0.5	30	0.8	6.3	0.2	1.3
Melon, Pineapple & Grapes, Fresh, Tesco*	1 Pack/300g	120	0.3	40	0.5	9.2	0.1	1.0
Melon & Grapes, Shapers, Boots*	1 Pack/220g	75	0.2	34	0.6	7.7	0.1	0.8
Melon & Red Grape, Freshly Prepared, M & S*	1 Pack/450g	157	0.4	35	0.5	8.4	0.1	0.7
Mixed, Food to Go, M & S*	1 Pack/400g	400	1.2	100	0.9	23.3	0.3	2.8
Mixed, Fresh, Sainsbury's*	1 Pack/200g	84	0.4	42	0.7	9.4	0.2	1.9
Mixed, Tesco*	1 Pack/225g	85	0.4	38	0.7	8.3	0.2	1.3
Oranges, Apple, Pineapple & Grapes, Fresh, Asda*	1 Pack/260g	120	0.3	46	0.6	10.5	0.1	2.1
Peaches & Pears, Fruit Express, Del Monte*	1 Serving/185g	87	0.2	47	0.4	10.8	0.1	0.9
Pineapple, Apple, Melon & Grape, Shapers, Boots*	1 Serving/100g	49	0.1	49	0.4	10.5	0.1	1.2
Pineapple, Apple & Strawberries, Tesco*	1 Pack/190g	80	0.2	42	0.4	9.8	0.1	1.4
Pineapple, Mandarin & Grapefruit, Asda*	1 Serving/200g	86	0.2	43	0.6	10.0	0.1	0.0
Pineapple, Mango, Apple & Grape, Waitrose*	1 Pack/300g	186	0.6	62	0.5	14.7	0.2	1.7
Pineapple, Mango & Passion Fruit, Prepared, M & S*	1 Pack/400g	200	0.8	50	0.7	10.8	0.2	1.8
Radiant Rainbow, Layered, Eat Well, M & S*	1 Pack/350g	140	0.7	40	0.5	9.1	0.2	0.9
Rainbow, Asda*	1 Pack/350g	140	1.0	40	0.6	8.8	0.3	1.4
Rainbow, Fresh, Tesco*	1 Tub/270g	105	0.5	39	0.5	8.8	0.2	0.9
Rainbow Layers, Tesco*	1 Pack/270g	121	0.5	45	0.5	9.8	0.2	1.1
Seasonal, Fresh, Asda*	1 Pack/125g	55	0.1	44	0.5	10.4	0.1	1.2
Seasonal, M & S*	1 Serving/200g	100	0.4	50	0.5	11.8	0.2	2.1
Seasonal Melon & Grapes, Asda*	½ Pack/200g	66	1.0	33	0.5	7.5	0.5	0.4
Shapers, Boots*	1 Pack/140g	55	0.3	39	0.7	8.6	0.2	1.0
Sharing, Fresh Tastes, Asda*	1 Pack/450g	220	0.9	49	0.4	10.4	0.2	0.0
Strawberry & Blueberry, Asda*	1 Pack/240g	86	0.2	36	0.9	7.0	0.1	1.5
Summer, Red, Fresh, M & S*	1 Pack/400g	160	0.8	40	0.0	10.0	0.2	1.2
Summer, Sainsbury's*	1 Pack/240g	84	0.5	35	0.7	7.8	0.2	1.3
Sunshine, Fresh, M & S*	1 Serving/200g	70	0.2	35	0.0	8.3	0.1	1.3
Tropical, Australian Gold*	1 Pot/130g	92	0.1	71	0.6	17.2	0.1	0.0
Tropical, Co-Op*	1 Serving/150g	67	0.3	45	0.6	9.0	0.2	1.0
Tropical, Fresh, Asda*	1 Pack/400g	164	0.8	41	0.7	9.0	0.2	1.8
Tropical, Fruit Snacks, Frozen, Sainsbury's*	1 Serving/175g	79	0.2	45	0.7	10.4	0.1	1.6
Tropical, in Light Syrup, Passion Fruit Juice, Tesco*	½ Can/216g	130	0.2	60	0.3	14.1	0.1	1.1
Tropical, Tropical Harvest*	1 Serving/100g	52	0.0	52	0.3	12.8	0.0	1.4
Tutti Frutti, Freshly Prepared, Tesco*	1 Pack/300g	132	0.6	44	0.7	9.8	0.2	1.7
Virgin Trains*	1 Serving/140g	56	0.1	40	0.4	10.0	0.1	0.8
Weight Watchers*	1 Serving/135g	50	0.1	37	0.2	9.0	0.1	0.7

FRUIT SHOOT

	Measure INFO/WEIGHT	per Measure KCAL	FAT	Nutrition Values per 100g / 100ml KCAL	PROT	CARB	FAT	FIBRE
Apple, Low Sugar, Robinson's*	1 Bottle/200ml	14	0.0	7	0.0	1.2	0.0	0.0
Apple & Blackcurrant, Robinson's*	1 Bottle/200ml	10	0.0	5	0.1	0.8	0.0	0.0

	Measure	per Measure		Nutrition Values per 100g / 100ml				
	INFO/WEIGHT	KCAL	FAT	KCAL	PROT	CARB	FAT	FIBRE
FRUIT SHOOT								
Hydro Orange & Pineapple, Spring Water, Robinson's*	1 Bottle/350ml	3	0.0	1	0.0	0.0	0.0	0.0
Orange, Pure, Robinson's*	1 Bottle/250ml	115	0.2	46	0.5	9.9	0.1	0.2
FRUIT SPREAD								
Apricot, Pure, Organic, Whole Earth*	1 Serving/20g	33	0.1	167	0.8	40.0	0.4	0.9
Blackcurrant, Carb Check, Heinz*	1 Tbsp/15g	8	0.0	54	0.5	12.8	0.1	2.7
Blackcurrant, Weight Watchers*	1 Tsp/6g	6	0.0	106	0.2	26.3	0.0	0.9
Cherries & Berries, Organic, Meridian Foods*	1 Tbsp/15g	16	0.0	109	0.5	26.0	0.3	1.1
Cherry & Berry, Meridian Foods*	1 Serving/10g	14	0.1	138	0.7	33.7	0.6	3.2
High, Blueberry, St Dalfour*	1 Tsp/15g	34	0.0	228	0.5	56.0	0.2	2.2
Raspberry, Weight Watchers*	1 Tsp/6g	7	0.0	111	0.4	27.1	0.1	0.9
Raspberry & Cranberry, No Added Sugar, Superjam*	1 Spread/10g	22	0.0	216	2.1	47.0	0.3	0.0
Seville Orange, Weight Watchers*	1 Tsp/15g	17	0.0	111	0.2	27.5	0.0	0.3
Strawberry, Weight Watchers*	1 Tbsp/15g	23	0.0	156	0.7	39.8	0.1	1.8
FU YUNG								
Egg, Average	1oz/28g	67	5.8	239	9.9	2.2	20.6	1.3
FUDGE								
All Butter, Finest, Tesco*	1 Sweet/10g	43	1.4	429	1.3	73.4	14.5	0.0
Butter, Milk, Thorntons*	1 Sweet/13g	60	2.5	462	3.7	68.5	19.2	0.0
Butter Tablet, Thorntons*	1oz/28g	116	3.1	414	0.9	77.6	11.1	0.0
Cadbury*	1 Bar/25g	115	4.0	440	2.3	73.7	15.3	0.4
Cherry & Almond, Thorntons*	1 Bag/100g	464	19.1	464	3.2	70.5	19.1	0.4
Chocolate, Average	1 Sweet/30g	132	4.1	441	3.3	81.1	13.7	0.0
Chocolate, Thorntons*	1 Bag/100g	459	19.1	459	3.1	69.0	19.1	0.6
Chunks, Home Cooking, Asda*	1 Portion/10g	45	1.3	446	1.5	79.7	13.2	1.1
Chunks for Baking	1 Serving/100g	427	12.2	427	1.7	77.2	12.2	0.5
Clotted Cream, M & S*	1oz/28g	133	6.2	474	1.7	67.6	22.1	0.0
Clotted Cream, Sainsbury's*	1 Sweet/8g	35	0.9	430	1.9	81.5	10.7	0.7
Dairy, Co-Op*	1 Sweet/9g	39	1.2	430	2.0	76.0	13.0	0.0
Double Chocolate Bar, M & S*	1 Bar/43g	202	9.0	470	4.2	66.9	21.0	0.7
Mini Chunks, Sainsbury's*	1 Pack/100g	409	11.3	409	1.9	74.8	11.3	0.0
Pure Indulgence, Thorntons*	1 Bar/45g	210	9.9	466	1.8	65.9	21.9	0.0
Vanilla, Bar, Diabetic, Thorntons*	1 Bar/34g	121	6.7	356	3.2	69.7	19.7	0.6
Vanilla, Bar, M & S*	1 Bar/43g	205	10.0	476	3.7	63.0	23.3	0.4
Vanilla, Thorntons*	1 Bag/100g	465	21.9	465	1.8	65.9	21.9	0.0
Vanilla, Whipped, M & S*	1 Serving/43g	210	10.3	490	3.8	65.4	23.9	0.3
FUSE								
Cadbury*	1 Bar/49g	238	12.2	485	7.6	58.2	24.8	0.0
FUSILLI								
Carb Check, Heinz*	1 Serving/75g	219	1.7	292	52.7	15.2	2.3	20.8
Carb Options, Knorr*	1oz/28g	98	0.4	350	28.5	34.0	1.5	21.0
Cooked, Average	*1 Serving/210g*	*248*	*1.4*	*118*	*4.1*	*23.8*	*0.6*	*1.1*
Dry, Average	*1 Serving/90g*	*316*	*1.4*	*351*	*12.3*	*72.0*	*1.6*	*2.2*
Fresh, Cooked, Average	*1 Serving/200g*	*329*	*3.6*	*164*	*6.4*	*30.6*	*1.8*	*1.7*
Fresh, Dry, Average	*1 Serving/75g*	*208*	*2.0*	*277*	*10.9*	*53.4*	*2.7*	*2.1*
Tricolore, Dry, Average	*1 Serving/75g*	*264*	*1.3*	*351*	*12.2*	*71.8*	*1.7*	*2.7*
Whole Wheat, Dry Weight, Average	*1 Serving/90g*	*290*	*2.1*	*322*	*13.1*	*62.3*	*2.3*	*9.0*
FYBOGEL								
Lemon, Reckitt Benckiser*	1 Serving/4g	4	0.0	95	2.4	11.3	1.1	64.8
Orange, Reckitt Benckiser*	1 Serving/4g	5	0.0	106	2.3	12.7	1.1	64.3

F

	Measure INFO/WEIGHT	per Measure KCAL	per Measure FAT	Nutrition Values per 100g / 100ml KCAL	PROT	CARB	FAT	FIBRE
GALAXY								
Amicelli, Mars*	1 Serving/13g	66	3.5	507	6.2	59.7	27.1	0.0
Caramel, Mars*	1 Bar/49g	254	13.0	518	5.8	64.2	26.4	0.0
Caramel Crunch, Promises, Mars*	1 Bar/100g	540	31.8	540	6.1	57.5	31.8	0.0
Cookie Crumble, Mars*	1 Bar/119g	651	39.6	547	6.2	55.6	33.3	1.8
Fruit & Hazelnut, Milk, Mars*	1 Bar/47g	235	13.2	501	7.1	55.2	28.0	0.0
Hazelnut, Mars*	1 Piece/6g	37	2.5	582	7.8	49.4	39.2	0.0
Hazelnut, Roast, Promises, Mars*	1 Bar/100g	544	32.9	544	6.4	55.6	32.9	0.0
Liaison, Mars*	1 Bar/48g	233	11.9	485	5.4	60.3	24.7	0.0
Swirls, Mars*	1 Bag/150g	747	39.7	498	4.9	60.2	26.5	0.0
GAMMON								
Breaded, Average	1oz/28g	34	0.9	120	22.5	1.0	3.0	0.0
Dry Cured, Ready to Roast, M & S*	½ Joint/255g	255	3.8	100	20.5	0.5	1.5	0.5
Honey & Mustard, Average	½ Pack/190g	294	13.5	155	19.1	3.6	7.1	0.1
Joint, Boiled, Average	*1 Serving/60g*	*122*	*7.4*	*204*	*23.3*	*0.0*	*12.3*	*0.0*
Joint, Raw, Average	*1 Serving/100g*	*138*	*7.5*	*138*	*17.5*	*0.0*	*7.5*	*0.0*
Joint, Unsmoked, Tesco*	2 Slices/150g	247	15.6	165	16.8	0.2	10.4	0.0
Steaks, Average	*1 Steak/97g*	*157*	*7.1*	*161*	*23.3*	*0.4*	*7.4*	*0.0*
Steaks, Healthy Range, Average	*1 Serving/110g*	*107*	*3.5*	*97*	*18.0*	*0.4*	*3.2*	*0.2*
Steaks, Honey Roast, Average	*1 Steak/100g*	*142*	*5.3*	*142*	*21.5*	*2.3*	*5.3*	*0.0*
Steaks, Smoked, Average	*1 Steak/110g*	*150*	*5.5*	*137*	*22.7*	*0.1*	*5.0*	*0.1*
GAMMON &								
Parsley Sauce, Steak, Tesco*	½ Pack/140g	217	7.3	155	23.7	2.9	5.2	0.5
Pineapple, Roast, Dinner, Iceland*	1 Pack/400g	360	6.4	90	6.2	12.7	1.6	1.7
GAMMON IN								
Creamy Cheddar Sauce, Steaks, Fresh Tastes, Asda*	½ Pack/143g	270	14.4	189	19.1	5.4	10.1	1.5
GAMMON WITH								
Cheese Sauce & Crumb, Steaks, Simply Cook, Tesco*	½ Pack/156g	218	12.0	140	14.2	3.1	7.7	1.0
Egg & Fries, Steak	1 Serving/540g	684	26.9	127	10.3	10.1	5.0	0.0
Pineapple, Steaks, Asda*	½ Pack/195g	253	2.7	130	17.8	11.5	1.4	0.7
Three Cheese & Mustard Crust, Joint, Asda*	1 Serving/270g	351	11.6	130	21.7	1.2	4.3	0.0
GARAM MASALA								
Dry, Ground, Average	*1 Tbsp/15g*	*57*	*2.3*	*379*	*15.6*	*45.2*	*15.1*	*0.0*
GARGANELLI								
Egg, Dry, Waitrose*	1 Serving/125g	450	5.2	360	13.5	66.9	4.2	3.5
GARLIC								
Crushed, Frozen, Taj*	1 Block/18g	18	0.1	102	7.5	14.0	0.6	4.0
Minced, Nishaan*	1 Tsp/5g	5	0.0	97	6.0	16.2	0.9	0.0
Pickled, Bevellini*	1 Serving/12g	5	0.0	42	2.5	0.8	0.1	0.0
Powder, Average	*1 Tsp/3g*	*7*	*0.0*	*246*	*18.7*	*42.7*	*1.2*	*9.9*
Raw, Average	*1 Clove/3g*	*4*	*0.0*	*149*	*6.4*	*33.1*	*0.5*	*2.1*
Spice Blend, Gourmet Garden*	1 Serving/10ml	31	2.4	210	4.5	10.8	16.2	10.3
Very Lazy, The English Provender Co.*	1 Tsp/3g	3	0.0	111	6.0	20.9	0.4	3.0
Wild	1 Clove/3g	1	0.0	23	2.8	1.7	0.6	1.9
GARLIC & GINGER								
Minced, Paste, Nishaan*	1 Tsp/5g	4	0.1	71	2.4	8.5	1.6	0.0
GARLIC PUREE								
Average	*1 Tbsp/18g*	*68*	*6.0*	*380*	*3.5*	*16.9*	*33.6*	*0.0*
in Vegetable Oil, GIA*	1 Tsp/5g	20	2.1	391	3.3	1.6	41.3	0.0
with Tomato, GIA*	1 Tsp/10g	7	0.1	70	5.1	0.5	1.2	0.0
GATEAU								
Au Fromage Blanc, Ligne Et Plaisir*	1 Serving/80g	128	2.1	160	8.0	26.0	2.6	0.0
Black Forest, Sara Lee*	1 Serving/80g	221	9.8	276	3.6	37.9	12.3	1.2
Blackforest, Sainsbury's*	1/8 Cake/63g	163	10.8	259	3.9	27.7	17.1	3.5

G

	Measure INFO/WEIGHT	per Measure KCAL	FAT	Nutrition Values per 100g / 100ml KCAL	PROT	CARB	FAT	FIBRE
GATEAU								
Chocolate, Asda*	1 Serving/100g	176	10.0	176	2.4	19.0	10.0	0.4
Chocolate, Swirl, Tesco*	1 Serving/83g	230	13.3	277	3.8	29.3	16.0	0.2
Chocolate Layer, M & S*	1 Serving/86g	278	15.7	323	4.2	35.9	18.3	0.9
Chocolate Orange, Co-Op*	1 Serving/97g	320	17.5	330	5.0	37.0	18.0	1.0
Coffee, Tesco*	1 Serving/100g	300	17.0	300	4.2	32.5	17.0	0.6
Double Chocolate, Light, Sara Lee*	1/5 Cake/59g	139	2.7	237	5.7	43.3	4.6	2.0
Double Chocolate, Sara Lee*	1oz/28g	93	4.6	331	5.6	41.3	16.5	0.9
Double Strawberry, Sara Lee*	1/8 Cake/199g	533	24.3	268	3.2	36.2	12.2	0.6
Lemon & Lime, M & S*	1 Serving/100g	295	15.6	295	3.2	35.0	15.6	0.3
Orange & Lemon, Iceland*	1 Serving/90g	220	9.9	245	2.6	33.8	11.0	0.3
Strawberry, Co-Op*	1 Serving/77g	222	12.9	288	5.1	29.2	16.7	1.0
Strawberry, Family Size, Tesco*	1 Serving/84g	197	11.4	235	2.9	25.2	13.6	0.6
Swiss, Cadbury*	1/6 Cake/60g	228	10.1	380	5.2	52.0	16.8	0.9
Triple Chocolate, Heinz*	¼ Cake/85g	209	9.5	245	5.1	31.2	11.1	2.4
GELATINE								
Average	*1oz/28g*	*95*	*0.0*	*338*	*84.4*	*0.0*	*0.0*	*0.0*
GEMELLI								
Durum Wheat, Tesco*	1 Serving/100g	354	2.0	354	13.2	68.5	2.0	2.9
GHEE								
Butter	*1oz/28g*	*251*	*27.9*	*898*	*0.0*	*0.0*	*99.8*	*0.0*
Palm	*1oz/28g*	*251*	*27.9*	*897*	*0.0*	*0.0*	*99.7*	*0.0*
Vegetable	*1oz/28g*	*251*	*27.8*	*895*	*0.0*	*0.0*	*99.4*	*0.0*
GHERKINS								
Pickled, Average	*1 Gherkin/36g*	*5*	*0.0*	*14*	*0.9*	*2.5*	*0.1*	*1.2*
GIN								
& Diet Tonic, Can, Greenalls*	1 Can/250ml	95	0.0	38	0.0	0.0	0.0	0.0
37.5% Volume	*1 Shot/35ml*	*72*	*0.0*	*207*	*0.0*	*0.0*	*0.0*	*0.0*
40% Volume	*1 Shot/35ml*	*78*	*0.0*	*222*	*0.0*	*0.0*	*0.0*	*0.0*
Gordons & Bitter Lemon, Premixed, Canned, Gordons*	1 Can/250ml	170	0.0	68	0.0	71.0	0.0	0.0
London Dry, Bombay Sapphire*	1 Serving/25ml	59	0.0	236	0.0	0.0	0.0	0.0
GINGER								
Chunks, Crystallised, Julian Graves*	1 Serving/10g	28	0.0	283	0.2	70.1	0.2	1.5
Crystallised, Suma*	1 Serving/30g	104	0.0	348	0.2	82.0	0.1	0.3
Ground, Average	*1 Tsp/2g*	*5*	*0.1*	*258*	*7.4*	*60.0*	*3.3*	*0.0*
Lazy, Minced, The English Provender Co.*	1 Tsp/5g	1	0.0	15	0.2	3.2	0.2	1.5
Root, Raw, Pared, Average	*1 Tsp/2g*	*2*	*0.0*	*86*	*2.0*	*19.1*	*0.8*	*2.1*
Root, Raw, Unprepared, Average	*1oz/28g*	*22*	*0.2*	*80*	*1.8*	*17.8*	*0.7*	*2.0*
Stem in Syrup, Waitrose*	1 Jar/350g	1071	7.7	306	0.1	70.4	2.2	0.7
GINGER ALE								
1870, Silver Spring*	1 Glass/100ml	18	0.0	18	0.0	4.2	0.0	0.0
American, Low Calorie, Tesco*	1 fl oz/30ml	0	0.0	1	0.0	0.0	0.0	0.0
American, Tesco*	1 Glass/250ml	57	0.0	23	0.0	5.5	0.0	0.0
Dry	1 Glass/250ml	37	0.0	15	0.0	3.9	0.0	0.0
Low Calorie, Asda*	1 Serving/100ml	2	0.0	2	0.0	0.0	0.0	0.0
GINGER BEER								
Alcoholic, Crabbies*	1 Bottle/500ml	254	0.0	51	0.0	7.1	0.0	0.0
Asda*	1 Can/330ml	144	0.0	44	0.0	10.9	0.0	0.0
Classic, Schweppes*	1 Can/330ml	115	0.0	35	0.0	8.4	0.0	0.0
D & G Old Jamaican*	1 Can/330ml	211	0.0	64	0.0	16.0	0.0	0.0
Gastropub, M & S*	1 Bottle/1038ml	675	0.0	65	0.0	15.4	0.0	0.0
Jamaican, Boots*	1 Bottle/500ml	5	0.0	1	0.0	0.0	0.0	0.0
Light, Waitrose*	1 Glass/250ml	2	0.2	1	0.0	0.0	0.1	0.1
No Added Sugar, Aldi*	1 Glass/250ml	5	0.0	2	0.0	0.0	0.0	0.0

G

	Measure INFO/WEIGHT	per Measure KCAL	per Measure FAT	Nutrition Values per 100g / 100ml KCAL	PROT	CARB	FAT	FIBRE
GINGER BEER								
Sainsbury's*	1 Can/330ml	69	0.0	21	0.0	5.1	0.0	0.0
Sparkling, Organic, Whole Earth*	1 Can/330ml	115	0.0	35	0.0	8.2	0.0	0.0
Traditional, Fentiman's*	1 Bottle/275ml	130	0.0	47	0.0	11.3	0.0	0.0
GINGERBREAD								
Average	1oz/28g	106	3.5	379	5.7	64.7	12.6	1.2
Decorate Your Own, Chosen By You, Asda*	1 Serving/100g	414	12.6	414	4.8	70.4	12.6	2.3
Men, Mini, M & S*	1 Biscuit/17g	78	3.1	470	6.2	63.9	18.6	1.7
Men, Mini, Sainsbury's*	1 Biscuit/12g	56	1.4	463	5.7	83.4	11.8	1.5
GNOCCHI								
Di Patate, Italfresco*	½ Pack/200g	296	0.4	148	3.3	33.2	0.2	0.0
Fresh, Italian, Chilled, Sainsbury's*	¼ Pack/125g	190	0.4	152	3.8	33.6	0.3	1.4
Potato, Average	*1 Serving/150g*	*199*	*0.0*	*133*	*0.0*	*33.2*	*0.0*	*0.0*
GOAT								
Meat, Uncooked	1 Portion/100g	109	2.3	109	20.0	0.0	2.3	0.0
Raw	*1oz/28g*	*31*	*0.6*	*109*	*20.6*	*0.0*	*2.3*	*0.0*
GOJI BERRIES								
Average	*1 Serving/100g*	*287*	*0.7*	*287*	*6.6*	*65.1*	*0.7*	*6.8*
GOOSE								
Leg, with Skin, Fire Roasted	*1 Leg/174g*	*482*	*29.8*	*277*	*28.8*	*0.0*	*17.1*	*0.0*
Meat, Fat & Skin, Raw	*1oz/28g*	*101*	*9.2*	*361*	*16.5*	*0.0*	*32.8*	*0.0*
Meat, Raw	*1 Portion/185g*	*298*	*12.9*	*161*	*23.0*	*0.0*	*7.0*	*0.0*
Meat, Roasted	*1 Portion/143g*	*340*	*18.6*	*238*	*29.0*	*0.0*	*13.0*	*0.0*
Meat & Skin, Roasted	*½ Goose/774g*	*2361*	*169.5*	*305*	*25.2*	*0.0*	*21.9*	*0.0*
GOOSEBERRIES								
Dessert, Raw	*1oz/28g*	*11*	*0.1*	*40*	*0.7*	*9.2*	*0.3*	*2.4*
Stewed with Sugar	*1 Serving/25g*	*13*	*0.1*	*54*	*0.7*	*12.9*	*0.3*	*4.2*
Stewed without Sugar	*1 Serving/25g*	*4*	*0.1*	*16*	*0.9*	*2.5*	*0.3*	*4.4*
GOULASH								
Beef, Bistro Range, Tesco*	1 Pack/450g	544	15.3	121	7.9	14.6	3.4	0.6
Beef, Finest, Tesco*	½ Pack/300g	297	9.3	99	11.6	6.2	3.1	0.6
Beef, Weight Watchers*	1 Pack/330g	241	5.6	73	4.8	9.5	1.7	0.6
Beef, with Tagliatelle, COU, M & S*	1 Pack/360g	414	8.3	115	8.5	14.5	2.3	1.0
GRANOLA								
Nibbles, Apple Crumbles, We Are Bear*	1 Serving/30g	98	1.5	329	13.0	76.0	4.9	14.0
Nibbles, Coco Berry Crumbles, We Are Bear*	1 Bag/30g	99	1.5	332	13.0	73.0	5.0	15.5
Nibbles, Coconut Crumbles, We Are Bear*	1 Bag/30g	98	1.5	329	13.0	76.0	4.9	14.0
Nibbles, Tropical Crunch, We Are Bear*	1 Pack/30g	99	1.5	329	13.0	76.0	4.9	15.5
GRAPEFRUIT								
in Juice, Average	*1oz/28g*	*13*	*0.0*	*46*	*0.5*	*10.6*	*0.0*	*0.4*
in Syrup, Average	*1oz/28g*	*19*	*0.0*	*69*	*0.5*	*16.8*	*0.1*	*0.5*
Raw, Flesh Only, Average	*½ Fruit/160g*	*34*	*0.1*	*21*	*0.5*	*4.8*	*0.1*	*0.9*
Raw, Weighed with Skin & Seeds, Average	*1 Lge/340g*	*109*	*0.3*	*32*	*0.6*	*8.1*	*0.1*	*1.1*
Ruby Red, in Juice, Average	*1 Serving/135g*	*54*	*0.1*	*40*	*0.5*	*9.3*	*0.1*	*0.5*
GRAPES								
Green, without Stalk, Average	*1oz/28g*	*17*	*0.0*	*61*	*0.4*	*15.2*	*0.1*	*0.7*
Red, Average	*1 Serving/80g*	*53*	*0.1*	*67*	*0.4*	*16.5*	*0.1*	*0.7*
Red & Green Selection, Average	*1 Serving/80g*	*50*	*0.1*	*62*	*0.4*	*15.2*	*0.1*	*0.8*
Seedless, Black, Asda*	1 Serving/80g	51	0.1	64	0.4	15.4	0.1	0.7
GRATIN								
Cauliflower, Findus*	1 Pack/400g	340	20.0	85	3.5	7.0	5.0	0.0
Leek & Carrot, Findus*	1 Pack/400g	440	26.0	110	3.5	9.5	6.5	0.0
Potato, Creamy, M & S*	½ Pack/225g	360	25.0	160	2.2	11.9	11.1	0.9
Potato, HL, Tesco*	1 Serving/225g	169	4.9	75	2.3	11.4	2.2	0.6

G

	Measure INFO/WEIGHT	per Measure		Nutrition Values per 100g / 100ml				
		KCAL	FAT	KCAL	PROT	CARB	FAT	FIBRE
GRATIN								
Potato, Sainsbury's*	½ Pack/225g	448	34.0	199	4.4	11.4	15.1	1.0
GRAVY								
Beef, Aunt Bessie's*	1 Serving/100g	73	5.3	73	1.0	5.3	5.3	0.5
Beef, Free From, Sainsbury's*	½ Pack/151g	47	1.5	31	1.5	4.1	1.0	0.2
Beef, Fresh, Sainsbury's*	1 Serving/83ml	47	2.7	56	2.4	4.5	3.2	0.6
Beef, Heat & Serve, Morrisons*	1 Serving/150g	27	0.4	18	0.3	3.9	0.3	0.5
Beef, Home Style, Savoury, Heinz*	¼ Cup/60g	30	1.0	50	1.7	6.7	1.7	0.0
Beef, Rich, Ready to Heat, Schwartz*	½ Pack/100g	31	1.6	31	0.8	3.4	1.6	0.5
Beef, Winter Berry & Shallot, Made Up, Oxo*	1 Serving/105ml	24	0.3	23	0.6	4.3	0.3	0.1
Chicken, Granules For, Dry Weight, Bisto*	1 Serving/20g	80	3.2	400	1.9	62.5	15.8	0.2
Chicken, Rich, Ready to Heat, Schwartz*	½ Pack/100g	27	1.2	27	0.8	3.3	1.2	0.5
Chips & Onion, Asda*	1 Pack/358g	329	9.3	92	2.1	15.0	2.6	1.2
Favourite, Granules, Made Up, Bisto*	1 Serving/50ml	15	0.6	30	0.2	4.4	1.2	0.0
Granules, Beef, Dry, Tesco*	1 Serving/6g	29	2.1	480	5.5	36.4	34.7	1.5
Granules, Beef, Made Up, Tesco*	1 Serving/140ml	48	3.6	35	0.3	2.6	2.5	0.1
Granules, Chicken, Dry, Oxo*	1oz/28g	83	1.4	296	11.1	54.2	4.9	0.7
Granules, Chicken, Made Up, Oxo*	1 fl oz/30ml	5	0.1	18	0.7	3.3	0.3	0.0
Granules, Dry, Bisto*	1 Serving/10g	38	1.6	384	3.1	56.4	16.2	1.5
Granules, Instant, Dry	**1oz/28g**	**129**	**9.1**	**462**	**4.4**	**40.6**	**32.5**	**0.0**
Granules, Instant, Made Up	**1oz/28g**	**10**	**0.7**	**34**	**0.3**	**3.0**	**2.4**	**0.0**
Granules, Lamb, Hint of Mint, Made Up, Oxo*	1 Serving/100ml	25	0.5	25	0.7	4.3	0.5	0.0
Granules, Made Up, Bisto*	1 Serving/50ml	15	0.6	30	0.2	4.4	1.2	0.2
Granules, Made Up, Oxo*	1 Serving/150ml	28	0.4	19	0.6	3.4	0.3	0.0
Granules, Onion, Dry, Morrisons*	1 Serving/25g	124	8.7	495	3.4	44.0	34.7	0.0
Granules, Onion, Dry, Oxo*	1oz/28g	92	1.3	328	8.2	62.3	4.8	0.8
Granules, Onion, Made Up, Oxo*	1 fl oz/30ml	6	0.1	20	0.5	3.7	0.3	0.0
Granules, Original, Dry, Oxo*	1oz/28g	88	1.3	313	10.2	57.2	4.8	1.0
Granules, Vegetable, Dry, Oxo*	1oz/28g	88	1.4	316	8.4	59.5	4.9	0.9
Granules, Vegetable, Dry, Tesco*	½ Pint/20g	94	6.7	470	3.8	38.5	33.4	3.7
Granules for Meat, Made Up, Asda*	1 Serving/100ml	38	2.4	38	0.6	4.0	2.4	0.1
Granules for Vegetarian Dishes, Dry Weight, Bisto*	1 Serving/28g	100	3.7	356	2.7	56.0	13.3	4.5
Onion, Fresh, Asda*	1/6 Pot/77g	30	1.6	39	1.7	3.3	2.1	0.4
Onion, Granules, Made Up, Bisto*	1 Serving/50ml	14	0.3	28	0.2	5.6	0.6	0.0
Onion, Granules For, Dry Weight, Bisto*	4 Tsp/20g	78	2.9	391	2.4	62.3	14.7	2.3
Onion, Rich, M & S*	½ Pack/150g	60	1.8	40	2.0	5.9	1.2	0.3
Onion, Rich, Ready to Heat, Schwartz*	½ Sachet/100g	24	0.6	24	0.4	4.3	0.6	0.5
Paste, Beef, Antony Worrall Thompson's*	1 Portion/31g	104	5.7	334	11.8	30.3	18.4	0.6
Paste, Onion, Antony Worrall Thompson's*	1 Tsp/10g	26	0.4	262	7.0	48.7	4.4	1.4
Poultry, Concentrate, Bouillon, Made Up, Just*	1 Serving/200ml	124	4.0	62	1.8	9.2	2.0	0.6
Poultry, Fresh, Signature, TTD, Sainsbury's*	¼ Pot/126g	58	2.0	46	3.1	4.9	1.6	0.6
Poultry, TTD, Sainsbury's*	1 Portion/125g	76	5.6	61	1.8	3.5	4.5	0.8
Powder, Gluten Free, Dry, Allergycare*	1 Tbsp/10g	26	0.0	260	0.3	63.8	0.4	0.0
Powder, Made Up, Sainsbury's*	1 Serving/100ml	15	0.1	15	0.4	3.2	0.1	0.1
Powder, Vegetarian, Organic, Marigold*	1 Serving/22g	79	1.7	361	10.6	61.5	7.7	1.3
Roast Beef, Best, in Glass Jar, Made Up, Bisto*	1 Serving/70ml	21	0.3	30	0.3	6.1	0.4	0.0
Roast Lamb, Bisto*	1 Serving/20g	60	0.9	302	3.4	62.3	4.3	0.0
Roast Pork, Best, in Glass Jar, Dry Weight, Bisto*	4 Tsp/20g	63	0.9	314	4.3	64.1	4.5	0.0
Turkey, Granules, Made Up, Bisto*	1 Serving/50ml	14	0.6	28	0.2	4.0	1.2	0.2
Turkey, Granules For, Dry Weight, Bisto*	4 Tsp/20g	75	3.1	377	2.4	57.2	15.5	1.0
Turkey, Pour Over, Bisto*	1 Pack/100g	23	0.6	23	0.4	4.1	0.6	0.1
Turkey, Rich, Ready to Heat, Schwartz*	1 Pack/200g	62	2.4	31	1.9	3.1	1.2	0.5
Vegetable, Granules For, Dry Weight, Bisto*	1 Tsp/4g	15	0.5	380	2.1	63.0	13.3	4.5
Vegetable, Granules For, Made Up, Bisto*	1 Serving/50ml	14	0.2	28	0.2	5.6	0.4	0.2

G

	Measure INFO/WEIGHT	per Measure KCAL	FAT	Nutrition Values per 100g / 100ml KCAL	PROT	CARB	FAT	FIBRE
GRAVY MIX								
Instant, Dry Weight, BFY, Morrisons*	1 Serving/25g	80	0.1	320	3.5	77.0	0.3	1.2
Instant, Made Up, BGTY, Sainsbury's*	1 fl oz/30ml	10	0.0	32	0.3	7.4	0.1	0.1
Roast Beef, Classic, Schwartz*	1 Pack/27g	83	0.8	306	11.2	58.8	2.9	3.8
Roast Chicken, Classic, Schwartz*	1 Pack/26g	49	1.5	189	10.3	23.6	5.9	2.5
Roast Lamb, Classic, Schwartz*	1 Pack/26g	87	1.2	336	10.4	63.6	4.5	0.0
Roast Onion, Classic, Schwartz*	1 Pack/27g	85	1.1	315	8.8	61.0	4.0	4.6
Roast Pork & Sage, Classic, Schwartz*	1 Pack/25g	88	1.4	354	11.8	63.8	5.8	0.0
Roast Turkey, Classic, Schwartz*	1 Pack/25g	84	1.7	337	12.2	56.8	6.8	2.9
GREENGAGES								
Raw, Average	*1 Fruit/66g*	*26*	*0.1*	*39*	*0.7*	*9.4*	*0.1*	*2.0*
GREENS								
Spring, Boiled, Average	*1 Serving/80g*	*16*	*0.6*	*20*	*1.9*	*1.6*	*0.7*	*2.6*
Spring, Raw, Average	*1 Serving/80g*	*26*	*0.8*	*33*	*3.0*	*3.1*	*1.0*	*3.4*
Spring, Sliced, Fresh, Tesco*	1 Serving/100g	33	1.0	33	0.0	2.7	1.0	2.6
GRILLS								
Bacon & Cheese, Tesco*	1 Grill/78g	222	14.7	284	15.0	13.4	18.9	1.2
Cheese & Bacon, Danepak*	1 Grill/85g	241	16.0	284	15.0	13.4	18.9	1.2
Tikka, Organic, Waitrose*	1 Grill/100g	185	9.3	185	6.9	18.5	9.3	3.4
Vegetable, Dalepak*	1 Grill/83g	125	4.1	151	4.0	22.5	5.0	1.6
Vegetable, Mediterranean, Cauldron Foods*	1 Grill/88g	145	10.4	166	5.3	15.8	11.9	6.5
Vegetable, Ross*	1 Grill/114g	252	12.9	221	4.3	25.5	11.3	0.9
Vegetable, Tesco*	1 Grill/72g	129	7.2	179	4.2	18.0	10.0	2.2
Vegetarian, Mushroom & Oregano, Organic, Waitrose*	1 Grill/100g	200	10.0	200	7.9	19.5	10.0	4.3
GRITS								
Enriched White Hominy, Old Fashioned, Quaker Oats*	¼ Cup/41g	140	0.5	341	7.3	78.0	1.2	4.9
GROUSE								
Meat Only, Roasted	*1oz/28g*	*36*	*0.6*	*128*	*27.6*	*0.0*	*2.0*	*0.0*
GUACAMOLE								
Average	1 Tbsp/17g	22	2.2	128	1.4	2.2	12.7	2.5
Chunky, M & S*	1 Pot/170g	221	19.2	130	1.5	5.1	11.3	1.7
Chunky, Sainsbury's*	½ Pot/65g	120	11.9	185	1.6	3.2	18.4	3.8
Doritos, Walkers*	1 Tbsp/20g	32	3.2	159	1.2	2.6	16.0	0.1
Fresh, VLH Kitchens*	1 Tbsp/17g	26.9	2.5	158	1.5	3.0	14.6	2.5
Fresh, Waitrose*	½ Pack/100g	190	18.4	190	1.9	4.1	18.4	2.5
GFY, Asda*	1 Pack/113g	144	12.4	127	2.8	4.3	11.0	2.2
Mexican Style, Dip Selection, Morrisons*	½ Pack/50g	102	10.2	204	1.5	3.7	20.4	0.9
Reduced Fat Average	1 Serving/100g	129	10.8	129	2.4	5.2	10.8	3.0
GUAVA								
Canned, in Syrup	*1oz/28g*	*17*	*0.0*	*60*	*0.4*	*15.7*	*0.0*	*3.0*
Raw, Flesh Only, Average	*1 Fruit/55g*	*37*	*0.5*	*68*	*3.0*	*14.0*	*1.0*	*5.0*
GUINEA FOWL								
Boned & Stuffed, Fresh, Fayrefield Foods*	1 Serving/325g	650	39.3	200	19.1	3.3	12.1	0.5
Fresh, Free Range, Waitrose*	1 Portion/193g	258	11.9	134	19.5	0.0	6.2	0.3
GUMBO								
Cajun Vegetable, Sainsbury's*	1 Serving/450g	265	11.2	59	1.4	7.7	2.5	1.5
Louisiana Chicken, Perfectly Balanced, Waitrose*	1 Serving/235g	207	6.6	88	12.2	3.5	2.8	1.3
GUMS								
American, Hard, Tesco*	1 Serving/200g	646	0.0	323	0.0	80.8	0.0	0.0
American Hard, Sainsbury's*	1 Sweet/6g	22	0.0	360	0.1	90.0	0.1	0.0
Milk Bottles, Bassett's*	1 Pack/25g	88	0.4	353	6.2	78.3	1.6	0.0
Milk Bottles, Milk Flavour, Asda*	1 Pack/100g	369	2.3	369	7.0	80.0	2.3	0.4

G

	Measure INFO/WEIGHT	per Measure KCAL	per Measure FAT	Nutrition Values per 100g / 100ml KCAL	PROT	CARB	FAT	FIBRE
HADDOCK								
Fillet, Smoked, in Mustard & Dill, The Saucy Fish Co.*	2 Fillets/270g	262	9.7	97	15.5	0.1	3.6	0.0
Fillets, Battered, Average	1oz/28g	64	3.4	228	13.4	16.3	12.2	1.1
Fillets, in Breadcrumbs, Average	1oz/28g	57	2.8	203	13.5	14.9	9.9	1.2
Fillets, Raw, Average	*1oz/28g*	*22*	*0.2*	*80*	*18.0*	*0.2*	*0.8*	*0.0*
Fillets, Smoked, Cooked, Average	*1 Pack/300g*	*337*	*7.7*	*112*	*21.9*	*0.4*	*2.6*	*0.1*
Fillets, Smoked, Raw, Average	*1 Pack/227g*	*194*	*1.0*	*86*	*20.3*	*0.1*	*0.5*	*0.2*
Floured, Fried in Blended Oil	1oz/28g	39	1.1	138	21.1	4.5	4.1	0.2
Goujons, Batter, Crispy, M & S*	1 Serving/100g	250	14.1	250	11.7	18.5	14.1	0.8
Loins, Beer Battered, Chunky, TTD, Sainsbury's*	1 Fillet/93g	177	8.8	191	15.8	10.5	9.5	2.3
Loins, Skinless, Frozen, TTD, Sainsbury's*	1 Serving/100g	116	0.2	116	28.5	0.1	0.2	0.1
Loins, TTD, Sainsbury's*	1 Serving/100g	108	0.7	108	25.5	0.0	0.7	0.0
HADDOCK &								
Cauliflower Crunchies, Iceland*	1 Serving/111g	222	13.1	200	8.0	15.5	11.8	2.0
HADDOCK IN								
Butter Sauce, Steaks, Youngs*	1 Serving/150g	133	5.5	89	9.9	4.0	3.7	0.5
Cheese & Chive Sauce, Fillets, Go Cook, Asda*	1 Pack/360g	400	19.1	111	14.8	1.5	5.3	0.2
Cheese & Chive Sauce, Smoked Fillets, Seafresh*	1 Serving/170g	201	10.4	118	14.7	1.2	6.1	0.1
Fillets, in Cheese Sauce, Fresh Tastes, Asda*	½ Pack/180g	212	9.5	118	16.2	1.3	5.3	0.6
Smoked Leek & Cheese Sauce, Asda*	½ Pack/200g	232	10.0	116	14.0	3.7	5.0	1.5
Tomato Herb Sauce, Fillets, BGTY, Sainsbury's*	½ Pack/165g	150	4.6	91	12.9	3.6	2.8	0.1
Watercress Sauce, GFY, Asda*	1 Pack/400g	268	6.8	67	6.0	7.0	1.7	1.4
HADDOCK WITH								
a Rich Cheese Crust, Smoked, Sainsbury's*	1 Serving/199g	295	18.9	148	13.0	2.5	9.5	0.9
Cheese & Chive Sauce, Atlantic, Youngs*	½ Pack/180g	184	8.6	102	13.0	1.7	4.8	0.2
Creme Fraiche & Chive Sauce, Smoked, Tesco*	1 Serving/150g	154	4.6	103	16.8	2.1	3.1	0.3
HAGGIS								
Hall's*	1 Haggis/500g	1200	68.5	240	13.6	15.3	13.7	0.0
Neeps & Tatties, M & S*	1 Pack/300g	330	14.4	110	3.8	12.3	4.8	0.8
Traditional, Average	*1 Serving/454g*	*1119*	*66.5*	*246*	*12.3*	*17.2*	*14.6*	*1.0*
Traditional, Macsween*	1 Haggis/454g	1149	70.8	253	11.1	19.1	15.6	2.1
Vegetarian, Macsween*	1 Serving/100g	208	11.5	208	5.9	25.9	11.5	2.4
HAKE								
Fillets, in Breadcrumbs, Average	1oz/28g	66	3.7	234	12.9	15.9	13.3	1.0
Goujons, Average	1 Serving/150g	345	17.8	230	12.4	18.6	11.9	1.3
Raw, Average	*1oz/28g*	*29*	*0.6*	*102*	*20.4*	*0.0*	*2.2*	*0.0*
with Tomato & Chilli Salsa, Just Cook, Sainsbury's*	½ Pack/180g	112	1.6	62	11.4	2.2	0.9	0.0
HALIBUT								
Cooked, Average	*1oz/28g*	*38*	*1.1*	*135*	*24.6*	*0.4*	*4.0*	*0.0*
Raw	*1oz/28g*	*29*	*0.5*	*103*	*21.5*	*0.0*	*1.9*	*0.0*
with Roasted Pepper Sauce, Fillets, M & S*	1 Serving/145g	217	14.4	150	12.7	2.4	9.9	0.6
HALVA								
Average	*1oz/28g*	*107*	*3.7*	*381*	*1.8*	*68.0*	*13.2*	*0.0*
HAM								
Applewood Smoked, Average	*1 Slice/28g*	*31*	*0.8*	*112*	*21.2*	*0.5*	*2.7*	*0.2*
Baked, Average	*1 Slice/74g*	*106*	*4.3*	*143*	*21.1*	*1.8*	*5.8*	*0.3*
Boiled, Average	*1 Pack/113g*	*154*	*6.5*	*136*	*20.6*	*0.6*	*5.7*	*0.0*
Breaded, Average	*1 Slice/37g*	*57*	*2.3*	*155*	*23.1*	*1.8*	*6.3*	*1.6*
Breaded, Dry Cured, Average	*1 Slice/33g*	*47*	*1.8*	*142*	*22.1*	*1.4*	*5.4*	*0.0*
Brunswick, Average	*1 Slice/20g*	*32*	*1.8*	*160*	*19.5*	*0.6*	*8.8*	*0.0*
Cooked, Sliced, Average	*1 Serving/50g*	*57*	*1.9*	*115*	*19.1*	*0.9*	*3.9*	*0.1*
Crumbed, Sliced, Average	*1 Slice/28g*	*33*	*0.9*	*117*	*21.5*	*0.9*	*3.1*	*0.0*
Danish, Average	*1 Slice/11g*	*14*	*0.6*	*125*	*18.4*	*1.0*	*5.3*	*0.0*
Danish, Lean, Average	*1 Slice/15g*	*14*	*0.3*	*92*	*17.8*	*1.0*	*1.8*	*0.0*

H

INFO/WEIGHT	Measure	per Measure		Nutrition Values per 100g / 100ml				
		KCAL	FAT	KCAL	PROT	CARB	FAT	FIBRE
HAM								
Dry Cured, Average	1 Slice/18g	26	1.0	144	22.4	1.0	5.5	0.2
Extra Lean, Average	1 Slice/11g	10	0.2	90	18.0	1.4	1.4	0.0
Gammon, Breaded, Average	1 Serving/25g	31	0.8	122	22.0	1.5	3.1	0.0
Gammon, Dry Cured, Sliced, Average	1 Slice/33g	43	1.4	131	22.9	0.4	4.2	0.0
Gammon, Honey Roast, Average	1 Serving/60g	81	2.8	134	22.4	0.4	4.7	0.0
Gammon, Smoked, Average	1 Slice/43g	59	2.1	137	22.3	0.7	4.9	0.2
German Black Forest, Average	½ Pack/35g	93	5.9	267	27.2	1.3	17.0	0.5
Honey & Mustard, Average	1oz/28g	39	1.2	140	20.8	4.6	4.3	0.0
Honey Roast, Average	1 Slice/20g	25	0.8	123	20.3	1.5	3.8	0.1
Honey Roast, Dry Cured, Average	1 Slice/33g	46	1.5	140	22.7	2.3	4.4	0.2
Honey Roast, Lean, Average	1 Serving/25g	28	0.8	111	18.1	2.7	3.1	0.0
Honey Roast, Wafer Thin, Average	1 Slice/10g	11	0.3	113	17.4	3.7	3.2	0.3
Honey Roast, Wafer Thin, Premium, Average	1 Slice/10g	15	0.6	149	22.0	1.6	6.0	0.0
Lean, Average	1 Slice/18g	19	0.4	104	19.5	1.1	2.4	0.3
Maple Drycure, Asda*	1 Slice/37g	49	1.3	132	22.0	3.0	3.5	0.0
Oak Smoked, Average	1 Slice/20g	26	0.9	130	21.0	1.0	4.7	0.3
Parma, Average	1 Slice/10g	21	1.1	213	29.3	0.0	10.6	0.0
Parma, Premium, Average	1 Slice/14g	36	2.3	258	27.9	0.3	16.1	0.0
Peppered, Average	1 Slice/12g	13	0.3	109	18.5	2.0	2.7	0.0
Peppered, Dry Cured, Average	1 Slice/31g	43	1.5	140	23.1	1.3	4.7	0.2
Prosciutto, Average	1 Slice/12g	27	1.5	226	28.7	0.0	12.3	0.3
Serrano, Average	1 Slice/20g	46	2.4	230	30.5	0.4	11.8	0.0
Smoked, Average	1Slice/18g	21	0.7	117	19.7	0.9	3.7	0.0
Smoked, Dry Cured, Average	1 Slice/28g	38	1.2	137	23.0	1.4	4.4	0.1
Smoked, Wafer Thin, Average	1 Serving/40g	41	1.2	102	17.7	1.2	2.9	0.2
Thick Cut, Average	1 Slice/74g	94	2.9	127	22.4	0.6	3.9	0.1
Tinned, Average	½ Can/100g	136	8.7	136	12.2	2.0	8.7	0.0
Tinned, Lean, Average	½ Can/100g	94	2.3	94	18.1	0.2	2.3	0.4
Wafer Thin, Average	1 Slice/10g	10	0.3	101	17.9	1.4	2.6	0.1
Wiltshire, Average	1oz/28g	41	1.7	147	23.1	0.0	6.0	0.0
Wiltshire, Breaded, Average	1oz/28g	41	1.4	145	23.9	1.0	5.0	0.0
HARE								
Raw, Lean Only, Average	1oz/28g	35	1.0	125	23.5	0.2	3.5	0.0
Stewed, Lean Only, Average	1oz/28g	48	1.5	170	29.5	0.2	5.5	0.0
HARIBO*								
American Hard Gums, Haribo*	1 Pack/175g	630	3.3	360	0.3	85.5	1.9	0.2
Cola Bottles, Fizzy, Haribo*	1 Pack/175g	595	0.3	340	6.3	78.3	0.2	0.3
Cola Bottles, Haribo*	1 Pack/16g	56	0.0	348	7.7	78.9	0.2	0.3
Dolly Mixtures, Haribo*	1 Pack/175g	719	8.4	411	1.8	90.2	4.8	0.2
Fantasy Mix, Haribo*	1 Pack/100g	344	0.2	344	6.6	79.0	0.2	0.3
Gold Bears, Haribo*	1 Pack/100g	348	0.2	348	7.7	78.9	0.2	0.3
Horror Mix, Haribo*	1 Pack/100g	344	0.2	344	6.6	79.0	0.2	0.3
Kiddies Super Mix, Haribo*	1 Pack/100g	344	0.2	344	6.6	79.0	0.2	0.3
Maoam Stripes, Haribo*	1 Chew/7g	27	0.4	384	1.2	81.7	6.1	0.3
Milky Mix, Haribo*	1 Pack/175g	607	0.3	347	7.1	79.6	0.2	0.4
Mint Imperials, Haribo*	1 Pack/175g	695	0.9	397	0.4	98.8	0.5	0.1
Pontefract Cakes, Haribo*	1 Serving/40g	118	0.1	296	5.3	68.2	0.2	0.5
Snakes, Haribo*	1 Snake/8g	28	0.0	348	7.7	78.9	0.2	0.3
Starmix, Haribo*	1 Pack/100g	344	0.2	344	6.6	79.0	0.2	0.3
Tangfastics, Haribo*	1 Pack/100g	359	2.3	359	6.3	78.3	2.3	0.5
HARISSA PASTE								
Average	1 Tsp/5g	6	0.3	123	2.9	12.9	6.7	2.8
Barts*	1 Tbsp/15g	11	0.3	76	4.0	10.7	1.9	0.0

H

	Measure INFO/WEIGHT	per Measure		Nutrition Values per 100g / 100ml				
		KCAL	FAT	KCAL	PROT	CARB	FAT	FIBRE
HARISSA PASTE								
Easy, M & S*	1 Tbsp/15g	16	0.8	105	2.5	11.2	5.5	4.4
Moroccan Style, Al'fez*	1 Tsp/10g	19	1.1	190	4.0	18.2	11.2	3.4
HASH								
Barbecue Beef, COU, M & S*	1 Pack/400g	360	1.6	90	7.0	14.0	0.4	1.4
Corned Beef, Apetito*	1 Pack/380g	423	23.6	111	3.8	10.3	6.2	1.3
Corned Beef, Asda*	1 Pack/400g	416	14.4	104	6.0	12.0	3.6	1.1
Corned Beef, Chilled, Co-Op*	1 Pack/300g	345	18.0	115	9.0	5.0	6.0	1.0
Corned Beef, Frozen, Tesco*	1 Serving/400g	348	10.4	87	5.7	10.3	2.6	0.7
Corned Beef, M & S*	½ Pack/321g	385	20.2	120	8.1	7.4	6.3	1.3
Vegetable & Lentil, Asda*	1 Pack/289g	254	6.1	88	3.2	14.0	2.1	0.0
HASH BROWNS								
Aldi*	1 Serving/42g	61	2.9	146	1.7	19.3	6.9	1.8
Birds Eye*	1 Serving/63g	126	7.3	200	2.0	21.9	11.6	1.6
Oven Baked, Cooked, McCain*	1 Piece/38g	80	4.3	214	2.1	25.7	11.4	2.2
Oven Baked, Frozen, McCain*	1 Piece/40g	75	4.1	187	1.7	21.8	10.3	2.1
Potato, Iceland*	1 Piece/33g	75	4.0	227	2.2	27.1	12.2	2.6
Ross*	1 Piece/46g	84	4.0	183	2.0	23.9	8.7	2.0
HAZELNUTS								
Chopped, Average	*1 Serving/10g*	*67*	*6.4*	*665*	*16.7*	*5.6*	*64.0*	*6.5*
Whole, Average	*10 Whole/10g*	*65*	*6.3*	*655*	*15.3*	*5.8*	*63.5*	*6.5*
HEART								
Lambs, Average	*1 Heart/75g*	*91*	*4.5*	*122*	*16.0*	*1.0*	*6.0*	*0.0*
Ox, Raw	*1oz/28g*	*29*	*1.0*	*104*	*18.2*	*0.0*	*3.5*	*0.0*
Ox, Stewed	*1oz/28g*	*44*	*1.4*	*157*	*27.8*	*0.0*	*5.1*	*0.0*
Pig, Raw	*1oz/28g*	*27*	*0.9*	*97*	*17.1*	*0.0*	*3.2*	*0.0*
Pig, Stewed	*1oz/28g*	*45*	*1.9*	*162*	*25.1*	*0.0*	*6.8*	*0.0*
HERMESETAS								
Powdered, Hermes*	1 Tsp/0.78g	3	0.0	387	1.0	96.8	0.0	0.0
The Classic Sweetener, Hermes*	1 Tablet/0.5g	0	0.0	294	14.2	59.3	0.0	0.0
HEROES								
Dairy Milk, Whole Nut, Cadbury*	1 Chocolate/11g	60	3.9	545	9.1	48.2	35.2	0.0
Fudge, Cadbury*	1 Sweet/10g	43	1.5	435	2.5	72.7	14.9	0.0
HERRING								
Canned, in Tomato Sauce, Average	1oz/28g	57	4.3	204	11.9	4.1	15.5	0.1
Dried, Salted, Average	*1oz/28g*	*47*	*2.1*	*168*	*25.3*	*0.0*	*7.4*	*0.0*
Fillets, in Mustard & Dill Sauce, John West*	1 Can/190g	332	26.6	175	9.4	2.9	14.0	0.1
Fillets, in Olive Oil, Succulent, Princes*	1 Serving/50g	107	7.5	215	20.0	0.0	15.0	0.0
Fillets, Raw, Average	*1 Herring/100g*	*185*	*12.6*	*185*	*18.4*	*0.0*	*12.6*	*0.0*
Grilled, Average	*1oz/28g*	*51*	*3.1*	*181*	*20.1*	*0.0*	*11.2*	*0.0*
in Horseradish Sauce, John West*	1oz/28g	64	5.0	230	13.0	4.0	18.0	0.0
Pickled, Average	1oz/28g	73	5.0	262	14.2	9.6	18.0	0.0
Rollmop, Tesco*	1 Rollmop/65g	110	5.5	170	12.0	10.4	8.4	0.4
Rollmop, with Onion, Asda*	1 Rollmop/65g	89	3.1	137	13.2	10.3	4.8	0.8
Smoked, Pepper, in Oil, Glyngøre*	1 Can/130g	338	24.7	260	21.0	0.0	19.0	0.0
HIGH LIGHTS								
Choc Mint, Made Up, Cadbury*	1 Serving/200ml	40	1.4	20	1.0	2.5	0.7	0.3
Chocolate, Dairy Fudge, Dry Weight, Cadbury*	1 Serving/11g	40	1.1	363	17.0	50.0	10.0	0.0
Chocolate Orange, Made Up, Cadbury*	1 Serving/200ml	40	1.4	20	1.0	2.3	0.7	0.3
Dairy Fudge, Made Up, Cadbury*	1 Serving/200ml	40	1.0	20	1.0	2.8	0.5	0.2
Dark Chocolate, Cadbury*	1 Sachet/11g	35	0.9	315	23.1	37.3	8.1	0.0
Dark Chocolate, Made Up, Cadbury*	1 Serving/200ml	35	0.9	17	1.2	2.0	0.4	0.0
Espresso, Made Up, Cadbury*	1 Serving/200ml	35	0.9	17	1.2	1.9	0.4	0.0
Fudge, Made Up, Cadbury*	1 Serving/200ml	40	1.1	20	0.9	2.5	0.5	0.0

H

	Measure INFO/WEIGHT	per Measure KCAL	FAT	Nutrition Values per 100g / 100ml KCAL	PROT	CARB	FAT	FIBRE
HIGH LIGHTS								
Hot Chocolate Drink, Instant, Dry Weight, Cadbury*	1 Sachet/11g	38	1.4	350	16.6	42.0	12.8	3.0
Hot Chocolate Drink, Instant, Made Up, Cadbury*	1 Cup/200ml	40	1.4	20	1.0	2.5	0.7	0.3
Instant Hot Chocolate, Cadbury*	1 Sachet/22g	80	2.8	364	17.3	44.5	12.7	0.0
Mint, Cadbury*	1 Serving/200ml	40	1.4	20	1.0	2.5	0.7	0.0
Toffee Flavour, Made Up, Cadbury*	1 Serving/200ml	40	1.4	20	1.0	2.6	0.7	0.0
HOKI								
Grilled	*1oz/28g*	*34*	*0.8*	*121*	*24.1*	*0.0*	*2.7*	*0.0*
in Breadcrumbs, Average	1 Piece/156g	298	13.8	191	14.5	13.9	8.9	1.2
Raw	*1oz/28g*	*24*	*0.5*	*85*	*16.9*	*0.0*	*1.9*	*0.0*
Steaks, in Batter, Crispy, Birds Eye*	1 Steak/123g	320	17.1	260	12.4	21.3	13.9	0.8
HONEY								
Acacia, Tesco*	1 Tsp/4g	12	0.0	307	0.4	76.4	0.0	0.0
Acacia Blossom, Sainsbury's*	1 Serving/24g	81	0.0	339	0.1	84.7	0.1	0.3
Australian Eucalyptus, Finest, Tesco*	1 Tsp/4g	12	0.0	307	0.4	76.4	0.0	0.0
Bio Active, New Zealand Honey Co*	1 Serving/10g	32	0.0	325	1.0	80.0	0.0	0.0
Clover, Canadian, TTD, Sainsbury's*	1 Tbsp/15g	50	0.0	336	0.2	83.6	0.1	0.1
Florida Orange, Extra Special, Asda*	1 Tbsp/15g	50	0.0	334	0.5	83.0	0.0	0.0
Greek, Waitrose*	1 Tsp/6g	18	0.0	307	0.4	76.4	0.0	0.0
Pure, Clear, Average	*1 Tbsp/20g*	*63*	*0.0*	*314*	*0.3*	*79.1*	*0.0*	*0.0*
Pure, Clear, Squeezy, Oak Lane*	1 Tsp/5ml	16	0.0	330	0.5	81.0	0.0	0.0
Pure, Set, Average	*1 Tbsp/20g*	*62*	*0.0*	*312*	*0.4*	*77.6*	*0.0*	*0.0*
Scottish Heather, Waitrose*	1 Serving/20g	61	0.0	307	0.4	76.4	0.0	0.0
Spanish Orange Blossom, Sainsbury's*	1 Tbsp/15g	51	0.0	339	0.1	84.7	0.0	0.3
HONEYCOMB								
Natural, Epicure*	1 Serving/100g	290	4.6	290	0.4	74.4	4.6	0.0
HOOCH*								
Vodka, Calculated Estimate, Hooch*	1 Bottle/330ml	244	0.0	74	0.3	5.1	0.0	0.0
HORLICKS								
Malted Drink, Chocolate, Extra Light, Dry, Horlicks*	1 Serving/32g	95	2.5	296	9.2	47.0	7.8	17.3
Malted Drink, Extra Light, Instant, Dry Weight, Horlicks*	1 Serving/11g	35	0.7	319	8.4	57.4	6.2	10.5
Malted Drink, Light, Dry Weight, Horlicks*	1 Serving/32g	116	1.2	364	14.8	72.2	3.8	1.9
Malted Drink, Light, Made Up, Horlicks*	1 Mug/200ml	116	1.2	58	2.3	11.5	0.6	0.3
Powder, Made Up with Semi-Skimmed Milk	1 Mug/227ml	184	4.3	81	4.3	12.9	1.9	0.0
Powder, Made Up with Skimmed Milk	1 Mug/227ml	159	1.1	70	4.3	12.9	0.5	0.0
Powder, Made Up with Whole Milk	1 Mug/227ml	225	8.9	99	4.2	12.7	3.9	0.0
Snoozoo, Chocolate, Horlicks*	1 Sachet/20g	74	0.9	370	8.6	74.2	4.3	4.3
HORSE								
Meat, Raw, Average	*1 Serving/110g*	*146*	*5.1*	*133*	*21.4*	*0.0*	*4.6*	*0.0*
HORSERADISH								
Prepared, Average	*1 Tsp/5g*	*3*	*0.0*	*62*	*4.5*	*11.0*	*0.3*	*6.2*
HOT CHOCOLATE								
Cadbury*	1 Serving/12g	44	0.7	370	6.3	73.3	5.9	0.0
Caramel, Whittards of Chelsea*	1 Serving/20g	71	1.5	355	7.5	64.5	7.5	13.0
Chococino, Dulce Gusto, Nescafe*	1 Serving/34g	149	5.5	437	14.6	58.6	16.1	4.6
Chocolate Break, Dry, Tesco*	1 Serving/21g	110	6.0	524	7.9	58.9	28.5	1.7
Drink, Organic, Green & Black's*	1 Tsp/4g	13	0.3	374	9.1	63.5	9.3	0.1
Drink, Twinings*	3 Tbsp/21g	81	0.7	387	5.0	82.0	3.3	6.0
Dry Weight, Tassimo, Suchard*	1 Serving/27g	88	2.4	325	3.2	58.0	8.9	2.6
Fairtrade, Whittards of Chelsea*	5 Tsp/20g	68	0.8	342	7.8	69.0	3.9	10.9
Galaxy, Mars*	1 Sachet/28g	115	3.4	411	7.0	68.7	12.1	0.0
Horlicks*	1 Serving/32g	128	2.6	400	8.7	72.5	8.1	3.7
Instant, GFY, Asda*	1 Tsp/10g	32	1.3	321	13.2	37.0	13.4	7.7
Instant, Low Fat, Solo Slim, Rosemary Conley*	1 Sachet/18g	66	0.5	368	17.0	66.7	2.8	3.8

H

	Measure INFO/WEIGHT	per Measure KCAL	FAT	Nutrition Values per 100g / 100ml KCAL	PROT	CARB	FAT	FIBRE

HOT CHOCOLATE

	Measure INFO/WEIGHT	KCAL	FAT	KCAL	PROT	CARB	FAT	FIBRE
Instant, Skinny Cow*	1 Sachet/10g	37	1.5	370	19.7	39.3	14.6	0.0
Instant, Tesco*	1 Serving/32g	155	10.3	485	10.5	38.1	32.3	5.0
Luxury, Skinny, Whittards of Chelsea*	1 Serving/28g	92	0.8	328	12.9	67.1	2.8	13.5
Made Up, Tassimo, Suchard*	1 Serving/280ml	88	2.4	31	0.3	5.5	0.9	0.2
Maltesers, Malt Drink, Instant, Made Up, Mars*	1 Serving/220ml	104	3.0	47	0.9	7.7	1.4	0.0
Options, Belgian Chocolate, Double, Instant, Ovaltine*	1 Serving/11g	39	0.9	354	12.3	48.5	7.8	20.1
Orange Flavour, Solo Slim, Rosemary Conley*	1 Sachet/18g	66	0.5	368	17.1	66.7	2.8	3.9
Slim Fast*	1 Serving/59g	203	2.8	347	22.2	53.8	4.8	8.4
Velvet, Cadbury*	1 Serving/28g	136	6.9	487	8.6	57.8	24.6	2.0

HOT DOG

Sausage, American Style, Average	1 Sausage/75g	180	14.3	241	11.6	6.2	19.0	0.0
Sausage, Average	1 Sausage/23g	40	3.0	175	10.8	4.3	12.8	0.3

HOT DOG VEGETARIAN

Meat Free, Sainsbury's*	1 Sausage/30g	71	4.5	237	18.0	7.6	15.0	1.0
Tesco*	1 Sausage/30g	66	4.5	220	18.0	2.7	15.0	2.0

HOT POT

Beef, Classic, Weight Watchers*	1 Pack/321g	231	7.7	72	3.6	8.4	2.4	1.6
Beef, Healthy Options, Birds Eye*	1 Pack/350g	294	7.0	84	4.5	12.0	2.0	1.2
Beef, Minced, Sainsbury's*	1 Pack/450g	463	22.0	103	5.3	9.5	4.9	2.2
Beef, Ross*	1 Pack/322g	254	11.3	79	2.5	9.4	3.5	0.4
Beef, Weight Watchers*	1 Pack/320g	209	6.6	65	3.5	8.1	2.1	1.3
Chicken, Chunky, Weight Watchers*	1 Pack/320g	275	9.0	86	4.7	10.4	2.8	0.6
Chicken, Frozen, Asda*	1 Pack/400g	300	6.0	75	5.5	9.9	1.5	0.8
Chicken, Light Choices, Tesco*	1 Pack/450g	315	7.2	70	4.1	9.6	1.6	1.2
Chicken, Low Fat, Solo Slim, Rosemary Conley*	1 Serving/100g	81	2.9	81	6.7	7.1	2.9	2.5
Chicken, Sainsbury's*	1 Pack/400g	340	11.0	85	5.2	9.8	2.7	1.3
Chicken, Weight Watchers*	1 Pack/320g	275	9.0	86	4.7	10.4	2.8	0.6
Chicken & Cider, Ready Meals, Waitrose*	1 Pack/400g	500	20.4	125	6.8	12.9	5.1	1.1
Lamb, Diet Chef Ltd*	1 Pack/300g	276	5.4	92	8.9	10.1	1.8	3.0
Lamb, Heinz*	1 Pack/340g	337	10.5	99	4.9	12.7	3.1	1.7
Lamb, Low Fat, Solo Slim, Rosemary Conley*	1 Serving/100g	92	1.8	92	8.9	10.1	1.8	3.0
Lamb, Minced, Mini Classics, Asda*	1 Pack/300g	222	10.5	74	5.3	5.4	3.5	3.3
Lamb, Mini, Classics, Asda*	1 Pack/300g	223	10.5	74	5.3	5.4	3.5	3.3
Lamb, Organic, Great Stuff, Asda*	1 Pack/300g	327	10.2	109	8.0	11.6	3.4	1.1
Lancashire, M & S*	1 Pack/454g	431	15.0	95	10.1	6.7	3.3	1.0
Lancashire, Sainsbury's*	½ Pack/225g	220	8.8	98	6.1	9.5	3.9	1.0
Liver & Bacon, Tesco*	1 Pack/550g	693	31.4	126	6.4	12.3	5.7	1.5
Minced Beef, Asda*	1 Pack/375g	409	17.2	109	7.0	10.0	4.6	1.7
Minced Beef & Vegetable, COU, M & S*	1 Pack/400g	380	6.8	95	10.3	9.0	1.7	2.4
Minced Lamb & Vegetable, COU, M & S*	1 Pack/400g	340	10.8	85	5.7	12.5	2.7	1.8
Sausage, Aunt Bessie's*	¼ Pack/200g	212	9.2	106	3.6	12.6	4.6	1.9
Sausage with Baked Beans, Heinz*	1 Can/340g	354	10.9	104	4.6	14.3	3.2	2.4
Vegetable, Tesco*	1 Serving/450g	432	22.0	96	1.7	11.2	4.9	3.5
Vegetable, Vegetable Recipes, Ross*	1 Pack/300g	159	5.4	53	1.5	9.4	1.8	1.6
Vegetable, Weight Watchers*	1 Pack/335g	228	6.4	68	2.6	9.9	1.9	1.5

HOUMOUS

Balsamic Caramelised Red Onion, Extra Special, Asda*	½ Pack/50g	146	10.7	293	6.8	18.2	21.4	1.0
Caramelised Onion, Tesco*	¼ Pack/50g	125	9.7	250	5.5	13.0	19.4	4.2
Carrot with Lemon & Coriander, Shapers, Boots*	1 Pack/75g	64	1.9	85	3.0	11.0	2.5	3.4
Chilli & Red Pepper, Topped, Tesco*	½ Pack/100g	281	25.1	281	7.1	6.6	25.1	8.1
Feta, Fresh, Sainsbury's*	1 Serving/100g	292	27.4	292	8.0	3.5	27.4	6.7
Fresh, Sainsbury's*	1 Serving/50g	156	13.7	312	7.3	8.9	27.5	2.2
Fresh, Waitrose*	1 Serving/75g	219	19.8	292	7.2	6.3	26.4	7.6

H

HOUMOUS

	Measure INFO/WEIGHT	per Measure KCAL	FAT	Nutrition Values per 100g / 100ml KCAL	PROT	CARB	FAT	FIBRE
Garlic & Pesto, Asda*	1 Serving/34g	107	8.8	314	8.0	12.0	26.0	0.0
GFY, Asda*	1 Serving/50g	136	10.0	272	9.0	14.0	20.0	3.8
Indian Spiced, Glorious!*	1 Serving/100g	78	3.9	78	5.2	14.0	3.9	3.0
Jalapeno, Asda*	1 Serving/50g	165	14.5	331	7.0	10.6	29.0	4.5
Jalapeno, Sainsbury's*	¼ Pot/50g	148	13.4	296	6.4	7.2	26.8	5.7
Lemon & Coriander, BGTY, Sainsbury's*	½ Tub/100g	145	9.0	145	6.3	9.7	9.0	5.9
Lemon & Coriander, Reduced Fat, Tesco*	1 Pot/60g	135	9.2	225	7.4	13.8	15.3	4.7
Lemon & Coriander, Sainsbury's*	¼ Tub/50g	145	12.5	291	7.0	9.1	25.1	6.0
Light, Morrisons*	½ Pack/85g	200	15.3	235	7.4	10.9	18.0	0.0
Mediterranean Deli, M & S*	¼ Pack/70g	203	17.7	290	7.8	8.0	25.3	6.5
Mixed Olive, Sainsbury's*	¼ Pot/50g	134	11.5	268	6.7	8.4	23.1	7.7
Moroccan, Tesco*	¼ Pot/50g	144	12.7	289	6.8	8.1	25.5	7.3
Moroccan, with Coriander & Spices, Tesco*	¼ Pot/50g	131	9.9	262	9.4	11.6	19.8	5.2
Moroccan Style, Sainsbury's*	¼ Pot/50g	113	9.7	227	5.5	7.3	19.5	6.6
Moroccan Style Topped, M & S*	1 Serving/100g	220	15.3	220	6.5	13.2	15.3	9.2
Olive & Sundried Tomato, Tesco*	1 Serving/50g	117	9.7	235	6.5	8.0	19.5	7.4
Olive & Tomato, Mixed, Sainsbury's*	¼ Tub/50g	136	12.6	272	6.0	5.3	25.2	7.4
Organic, M & S*	¼ Pack/25g	82	7.4	330	6.9	9.1	29.7	3.3
Pesto Style Houmous, Sainsbury's*	1 Spread/25g	85	7.3	339	7.9	10.8	29.4	5.7
Red Pepper, Reduced Fat, Tesco*	1 Pot/60g	159	11.0	265	7.2	17.4	18.3	4.8
Red Pepper, Roasted, VLH Kitchens*	1 Tbsp/17g	31	1.4	183	6.5	15.6	8.4	6.2
Red Pepper Pesto, Tesco*	¼ Pot/50g	137	11.3	275	7.4	9.7	22.6	5.7
Reduced Fat, Average	1 Serving/30g	72	5.0	241	9.2	13.3	16.8	3.6
Reduced Fat, Mediterranean Deli, M & S*	1 Mini Pot/60g	126	9.7	210	7.5	8.3	16.2	9.3
Reduced Fat, Moroccan Style, Topped, M & S*	1 Tub/170g	374	26.0	220	6.6	13.2	15.3	9.2
Reduced Fat, Snack Pots, Mini, BGTY, Sainsbury's*	1 Mini Pot/60g	115	7.3	192	7.0	13.8	12.1	5.5
Roasted Aubergine, M & S*	½ Pot/85g	132	10.3	155	4.9	6.9	12.1	5.1
Roasted Red Pepper, 50% Less Fat, Tesco*	½ Pot/85g	156	10.5	184	7.3	10.9	12.4	9.5
Roasted Red Pepper, BGTY, Sainsbury's*	¼ Tub/50g	64	3.4	129	4.9	11.9	6.9	5.3
Roasted Red Pepper, Sainsbury's*	½ Pot/85g	253	22.7	297	7.0	7.4	26.6	3.5
Roasted Red Pepper, Tesco*	1 Serving/75g	255	22.3	340	7.1	11.1	29.7	2.4
Roasted Vegetable, Fresh, Sainsbury's*	¼ Pot/50g	144	13.6	287	5.9	4.9	27.1	7.8
Sea Salt & Cracked Black Pepper, Tesco*	¼ Pot/50g	147	13.6	295	7.0	4.8	27.2	9.5
Spicy Red Pepper, with Crudite Dippers, M & S*	1 Pack/130g	123	7.9	95	3.3	7.1	6.1	3.4
Sun Dried Tomato, Chunky, Tesco*	½ Pot/95g	322	27.0	339	6.7	14.0	28.4	3.3
Sweet Chilli, Tesco*	¼ Pot/50g	120	8.3	240	6.9	15.2	16.7	5.4
Tesco*	¼ Pot/51g	160	13.6	315	7.4	9.8	26.8	3.4
Three Bean, Reduced Fat, BGTY, Sainsbury's*	¼ Tub/50g	91	6.0	183	7.3	11.4	12.0	6.0
Zorba Delicacies Ltd*	1 Serving/50g	156	13.3	313	7.6	10.7	26.6	3.0

HULA HOOPS

	Measure INFO/WEIGHT	per Measure KCAL	FAT	Nutrition Values per 100g / 100ml KCAL	PROT	CARB	FAT	FIBRE
Bacon & Ketchup Flavour, KP Snacks*	1 Bag/27g	140	8.3	517	3.4	56.3	30.9	2.0
BBQ Beef, 55% Less Saturated Fat, KP Snacks*	1 Pack/34g	174	9.7	512	3.4	60.5	28.5	1.7
Cheese & Onion 55% Less Saturated Fat, KP Snacks*	1 Bag/34g	175	9.7	515	3.6	61.0	28.5	1.9
Chilli Salsa, Tortilla, KP Snacks*	1 Bag /25g	123	6.8	494	4.9	57.2	27.3	5.3
Minis, Original, KP Snacks*	1 Tub/140g	752	48.7	537	3.0	52.9	34.8	1.7
Multigrain, KP Snacks*	1 Pack/23g	113	5.9	491	5.6	60.0	25.6	4.3
Original, 55% Less Saturated Fat, KP Snacks*	1 Bag/34g	175	9.7	515	3.2	61.6	28.4	1.8
Original, KP Snacks*	1 Bag/25g	128	7.1	514	3.2	61.5	28.4	1.8
Roast Chicken, 50% Less Saturated Fat, KP Snacks*	1 Bag/34g	175	9.7	514	3.4	61.0	28.5	1.7
Salt & Vinegar, 50% Less Saturated Fat, KP Snacks*	1 Pack/25g	128	7.1	513	3.2	61.0	28.4	1.7
Sizzling Bacon, KP Snacks*	1 Bag/34g	175	9.7	514	3.4	60.9	28.5	1.7

ICE CREAM

	Measure INFO/WEIGHT	per Measure KCAL	FAT	Nutrition Values per 100g / 100ml KCAL	PROT	CARB	FAT	FIBRE
After Dinner, Mint, Dairy, Asda*	1 Serving/100g	182	8.0	182	3.4	24.0	8.0	0.4
After Dinner Bites, Vanilla, Magnum, Wall's Ice Cream*	1 Serving/29g	100	6.7	344	3.4	31.0	23.0	1.4
After Eight, Nestle*	1 Serving/55g	114	5.2	207	3.6	27.1	9.4	0.3
Almond Indulgence, Sainsbury's*	1 Serving/120g	286	18.8	238	2.8	21.4	15.7	0.6
Baked Alaska, Ben & Jerry's*	1 Serving/100g	260	15.0	260	4.0	29.0	15.0	0.1
Billionaire Shortcake, Chokablok*	1 Scoop/100ml	225	11.4	225	2.8	27.0	11.4	0.7
Bourbon Biscuit, Asda*	1 Dessert/37g	120	4.5	324	5.9	48.6	12.2	1.6
Brandy, Luxurious, M & S*	1 Serving/100g	228	13.3	228	3.8	19.1	13.3	0.2
Caramel, Carte d'Or*	2 Boules/50g	106	4.3	212	2.6	30.8	8.7	0.0
Caramel & Cinnamon Waffle, Carte d'Or*	2 Scoops/55g	121	6.0	220	3.0	27.0	11.0	0.0
Caramel Chew Chew, Ben & Jerry's*	1 Serving/100g	270	16.0	270	3.0	29.0	16.0	0.0
Caramel Craze, Organic, Tesco*	1 Serving/100g	253	15.3	253	3.3	25.5	15.3	0.0
Caramella, Tesco*	1 Serving/51g	120	5.5	235	2.6	32.0	10.7	1.1
Cheeky Choc, Brownie, Skinny Cow*	1 Tub/500ml	590	5.5	118	3.0	23.9	1.1	4.1
Cheesecake Brownie, Ben & Jerry's*	1 Serving 100g	260	16.0	260	4.0	26.0	16.0	0.0
Cherry Bomb Brownie, Chokablok*	1 Scoop/87g	191	8.3	220	3.3	29.9	9.5	1.4
Cherry Garcia, Ben & Jerry's*	1 Serving/100g	250	15.0	250	3.0	26.0	15.0	0.0
Chilli Red, Purbeck*	1 Serving/50g	99	5.7	198	4.8	18.7	11.5	0.0
Chocolate, COU, M & S*	1 Serving/140g	231	4.1	165	3.9	35.0	2.9	0.8
Chocolate, Haagen-Dazs*	1 Serving/120ml	269	18.0	224	4.0	19.0	15.0	0.0
Chocolate, Organic, Green & Black's*	1 Serving/125g	310	17.6	248	5.0	25.3	14.1	1.1
Chocolate, Rich, Organic, Sainsbury's*	1 Serving/100g	213	11.7	213	4.4	22.6	11.7	1.2
Chocolate, Soft Scoop, Asda*	1 Scoop/47g	84	3.8	179	3.7	23.0	8.0	0.0
Chocolate, Soft Scoop, Morrisons*	1 Serving/50g	99	5.3	199	3.3	22.3	10.6	1.1
Chocolate, Soft Scoop, Tesco*	1 Serving/50g	93	4.0	186	3.2	25.1	8.1	0.3
Chocolate, Swirl Pot, Skinny Cow*	1 Pot/100ml	98	0.6	98	2.9	20.2	0.6	2.7
Chocolate, Weight Watchers*	1 Serving/100ml	140	1.2	140	4.3	28.7	1.2	0.0
Chocolate & Orange, Organic, Green & Black's*	1 Serving/100g	248	14.1	248	5.0	25.3	14.1	0.1
Chocolate Brownie with Walnuts, Haagen-Dazs*	1 Cup/101g	223	16.4	221	4.4	21.0	16.2	0.0
Chocolate Chip, Baskin Robbins*	1 Serving/75g	170	10.0	227	4.0	24.0	13.3	0.0
Chocolate Flavour, Soft Scoop, Sainsbury's*	1 Serving/70g	122	5.2	174	3.1	23.6	7.5	0.3
Chocolate Fudge Brownie, Ben & Jerry's*	1 Serving/50g	125	6.5	250	4.0	32.0	13.0	1.5
Chocolate Honeycomb, COU, M & S*	1 Serving/100ml	150	2.6	150	3.5	31.5	2.6	0.7
Chocolate Macadamia, Ben & Jerry's*	1 Serving/100g	260	18.0	260	4.0	22.0	18.0	0.8
Chocolate Ripple, Perfectly Balanced, Waitrose*	1 Serving/125ml	205	3.1	164	4.8	30.5	2.5	4.1
Chocolate Sandwich, Skinny Cow*	1 Portion/36g	101	2.8	280	6.0	46.0	7.9	2.9
Chocolatino, Sundae, Tesco*	1 Tub/80g	160	5.9	200	4.4	29.0	7.4	2.4
Chocolatino, Tesco*	1 Serving/56g	115	3.8	205	3.4	31.4	6.8	1.8
Chunky Monkey, Ben & Jerry's*	1 Serving/100g	290	17.0	290	4.0	27.0	17.0	1.0
Chunky Monkey, Fairtrade, Ben & Jerry's*	1 Serving/100g	290	17.0	290	4.0	27.0	17.0	1.0
Coconut, Carte d'Or*	1 Serving/100ml	125	7.1	125	1.8	14.0	7.1	0.5
Coffee, Finest, Tesco*	¼ Pot/93g	236	14.9	254	4.9	22.5	16.0	0.0
Coffee, Haagen-Dazs*	1 Serving/120ml	271	18.4	226	4.1	17.9	15.3	0.0
Coffee, Waitrose*	¼ Tub/125ml	292	16.4	234	3.6	25.4	13.1	0.0
Cookie Dough, Ben & Jerry's*	1 Serving/100g	270	14.0	270	4.0	31.0	14.0	0.0
Cookies & Cream, Haagen-Dazs*	1 Pot/100ml	226	14.7	226	4.0	19.5	14.7	0.0
Cornetto Soft, Chocolate Chip, Wall's Ice Cream*	1 Serving/80g	256	13.6	320	3.5	37.0	17.0	1.5
Cornetto Soft, Mint Chocolate Chip, Wall's Ice Cream*	1 Serving/80g	240	13.6	300	4.0	33.0	17.0	1.0
Cornetto Soft, Strawberry, Wall's Ice Cream*	1 Serving/80g	208	8.0	260	2.5	38.0	10.0	1.0
Cornetto Soft, Vanilla, Wall's Ice Cream*	1 Serving/80g	264	16.0	330	4.5	33.0	20.0	0.0
Cornish, Full Fat, Asda*	1 Serving/100g	204	11.6	204	3.5	21.4	11.6	0.1
Cornish Clotted, M & S*	1 Pot/90g	207	13.0	230	2.8	21.8	14.5	0.1
Cornish Dairy, Waitrose*	1 Serving/125ml	121	6.6	97	1.7	10.7	5.3	0.1

ICE CREAM

	Measure INFO/WEIGHT	per Measure KCAL	per Measure FAT	Nutrition Values per 100g / 100ml KCAL	PROT	CARB	FAT	FIBRE
Crema Di Mascarpone, Carte d'Or*	1 Serving/100g	207	8.9	207	2.8	29.0	8.9	0.0
Dairy, Flavoured	1oz/28g	50	2.2	179	3.5	24.7	8.0	0.0
Dairy Cornish, Tesco*	1 Serving/49g	112	6.0	228	3.2	24.7	12.3	0.1
Dairy Milk, Orange, Cadbury*	1 Serving/120ml	259	13.9	216	3.5	26.0	11.6	0.0
Dark Toffee, Organic, Green & Black's*	¼ Pot/125ml	192	9.9	154	2.8	18.1	7.9	0.1
Date & Almond Cream, Haagen-Dazs*	1 Serving/120ml	254	15.6	212	5.0	19.0	13.0	0.0
Demon Chocolate, M & S*	1 Serving/79g	208	8.8	263	3.7	37.1	11.1	0.6
Double Chocolate, Nestle*	1 Serving/78g	248	14.3	320	4.8	33.7	18.4	0.0
Dreamy Creamy Cookie, Skinny Cow*	1 Serving/100ml	117	1.1	117	2.7	24.1	1.1	3.9
Farmhouse Toffee, TTD, Sainsbury's*	¼ Pot/100g	293	18.6	293	3.2	28.3	18.6	0.6
Fig & Orange Blossom Honey, Waitrose*	1 Serving/100g	219	11.8	219	3.9	24.3	11.8	0.4
French Toast Flavour, Baskin Robbins*	1 Scoop/71g	180	9.0	254	4.2	31.0	12.7	0.0
Fruit & Fresh Tropical, Carte d'Or*	1 Serving/83g	154	7.1	185	2.5	24.5	8.5	0.0
Fun-Illa, Skinny Cow*	1 Serving/100ml	97	1.6	97	3.1	17.6	1.6	2.4
Gelato, Vanilla	1 Serving/100g	162	7.2	162	2.4	22.6	7.2	0.3
Get Fruit, Tropical, Solero*	1 Serving/125ml	162	5.5	130	1.6	20.6	4.4	0.4
Gold Digger Dynamite, Chokablok*	¼ Tub/125ml	287	14.0	230	3.2	28.2	11.2	0.9
Greek Yoghurt & Honey, Carte d'Or*	1 Serving/55g	114	4.8	207	2.7	29.0	8.8	0.0
Half Baked, Ben & Jerry's*	1 Serving/100g	270	13.0	270	5.0	32.0	13.0	1.0
Heavenly Vanilla, Cadbury*	1 Serving/250ml	355	23.2	142	2.5	12.8	9.3	0.0
Honeycomb Harvest, Mackies*	1 Serving/100g	209	10.0	209	4.0	25.0	10.0	0.0
Knickerbocker Glory	1oz/28g	31	1.4	112	1.5	16.4	5.0	0.2
Lavazza, Carte d'Or*	1 Serving/55g	120	5.4	218	3.5	29.0	9.9	0.0
Lemon, Haagen-Dazs*	1 Serving/120ml	144	0.2	120	0.3	29.3	0.2	0.0
Lemon & White Chocolate, Crackpots, Iceland*	1 Serving/100g	202	8.4	202	1.7	29.9	8.4	0.3
Lemon Cream, Dairy, Sainsbury's*	1 Serving/100g	199	9.3	199	3.0	25.9	9.3	0.1
Lemon Curd Swirl, Duchy Originals*	¼ Pot/101g	247	14.2	245	3.7	25.8	14.1	0.0
Less Than 5% Fat, Asda*	1 Scoop/40g	56	1.8	139	2.7	22.0	4.5	0.0
Log, Mint Chocolate, Sainsbury's*	1 Serving/51g	100	5.1	197	3.0	23.8	10.0	0.2
Luscious Mint Choc Chip, Morrisons*	1 Serving/50g	99	5.2	198	2.9	23.1	10.5	0.7
Macadamia Night, Carte d'Or*	2 Scoops/56g	110	4.5	196	0.0	29.0	8.0	0.8
Macadamia Nut, Baskin Robbins*	1 Serving/113g	270	18.0	239	4.4	22.1	15.9	0.9
Madly Deeply, Skinny Cow*	1 Serving/100g	149	2.2	149	4.2	28.3	2.2	3.4
Magic Maple, M & S*	1 Serving/93g	259	11.4	278	2.9	39.0	12.3	0.6
Magic Stars, Milky Way*	1 Serving/53ml	67	3.3	127	2.1	15.5	6.2	0.0
Magnum Moments, Wall's Ice Cream*	1 Serving/18ml	58	3.7	323	4.0	30.0	20.8	0.0
Mango, 98% Fat Free, Bulla*	1 Serving/70g	94	1.1	134	4.2	25.4	1.6	0.0
Maple & Walnut, American, Sainsbury's*	1/8 Pot/68g	121	4.9	179	3.1	25.6	7.2	0.2
Mince Pie, Finest, Tesco*	¼ Pack/188g	476	22.1	254	3.9	33.0	11.8	1.1
Mini Chocolate Stick, Milk Chocolate, Weight Watchers*	1 Stick/32g	95	5.1	296	3.7	33.8	15.9	1.6
Mint, Majestic Luxury, Iceland*	1 Serving/80g	269	14.6	337	3.8	39.3	18.3	1.3
Mint & Chocolate, Sainsbury's*	1 Serving/71g	137	6.7	192	3.4	23.5	9.4	0.4
Mint Choc Chip Soft Scoop, Asda*	1 Serving/46g	86	4.1	187	2.9	24.0	9.0	0.3
Mint Chocolate Chip, Baskin Robbins*	1 Scoop/113g	270	16.0	239	4.4	24.8	14.2	0.9
Mint Crisp, Nestle*	1 Serving/75ml	232	16.4	309	2.9	25.5	21.9	0.0
Mint Crunch, Dairy Milk, Cadbury*	1 Serving/60ml	162	13.3	270	3.0	29.0	22.2	0.0
Mint Ripple, Good Choice, Iceland*	1 Scoop/50g	58	1.0	117	3.0	21.7	2.1	0.1
Mocha Coffee Indulgence, Sainsbury's*	¼ Pot/82g	178	10.6	217	3.2	22.1	12.9	0.1
Monster Mint, Sainsbury's*	1/8 Pot/67g	121	4.6	180	3.0	26.3	6.9	0.3
My Carte D'or, Caramel, Carte d'Or*	1 Tub/200ml	210	8.0	105	1.5	16.0	4.0	0.2
My Carte D'or, Chocolate, Carte d'Or*	1 Tub/200ml	220	11.0	110	1.7	12.5	5.5	0.4
Neapolitan, Brick, Tesco*	1 Serving/50g	81	3.4	163	3.3	21.9	6.9	0.4
Neapolitan, Soft Scoop, Asda*	1 Scoop/47g	82	3.8	175	2.8	23.0	8.0	0.2

ICE CREAM

	Measure INFO/WEIGHT	per Measure KCAL	per Measure FAT	Nutrition Values per 100g / 100ml KCAL	PROT	CARB	FAT	FIBRE
Neapolitan, Soft Scoop, M & S*	1/8 Tub/63g	100	4.6	160	2.7	21.3	7.4	0.3
Neapolitan, Soft Scoop, Sainsbury's*	1 Serving/75g	124	5.2	165	2.8	22.8	6.9	0.2
Neapolitan, Soft Scoop, Tesco*	1 Serving/43g	70	3.0	163	3.3	21.9	6.9	0.4
Neapolitan Sandwich, Gelatelli*	1 Serving/106g	233	9.5	220	4.9	29.0	9.0	1.9
Non-Dairy, Mixes	1oz/28g	51	2.2	182	4.1	25.1	7.9	0.0
Non-Dairy, Reduced Calorie	1oz/28g	33	1.7	119	3.4	13.7	6.0	0.0
Organic, Madagascan Vanilla, Yeo Valley*	1 Serving/40ml	45	2.5	112	2.4	11.4	6.3	0.1
Panna Cotta, Haagen-Dazs*	1 Serving/120ml	248	16.0	207	3.4	18.4	13.3	0.0
Phish Food, Ben & Jerry's*	1 Serving/100g	260	13.0	260	3.5	35.0	13.0	0.1
Pistachio, Haagen-Dazs*	1 Serving/120ml	276	18.8	230	4.4	17.7	15.7	0.0
Praline, Green & Black's*	1 Sm Pot/100g	191	10.8	191	3.5	20.0	10.8	0.9
Pralines & Cream, Baskin Robbins*	1 Serving/100g	252	13.6	252	4.5	27.7	13.6	0.3
Pralines & Cream, Haagen-Dazs*	1 Pot/500ml	1210	75.5	242	3.7	22.9	15.1	0.0
Raspberries, Clotted Cream, Waitrose*	1 Tub/500ml	790	39.5	158	2.9	18.9	7.9	0.1
Raspberry, Haagen-Dazs*	1 Serving/120ml	127	0.2	106	0.2	25.9	0.2	0.0
Raspberry, Swirl Pot, Skinny Cow*	1 Pot/100ml	86	0.3	86	2.5	18.4	0.3	2.2
Raspberry Ripple, Dairy, Waitrose*	1 Serving/186ml	195	10.0	105	1.9	12.3	5.4	0.0
Raspberry Ripple, Soft Scoop, Asda*	1 Scoop/46g	75	2.8	164	2.5	25.0	6.0	0.0
Raspberry Ripple, Soft Scoop, Sainsbury's*	1 Serving/75g	127	5.2	170	2.6	24.2	7.0	0.3
Raspberry Ripple, Soft Scoop, Tesco*	1 Scoop/25g	39	1.5	157	2.5	23.0	6.1	0.2
Raspberry Ripple Brick, Tesco*	1 Serving/48g	71	2.9	148	2.6	20.8	6.0	0.2
Really Creamy After Dinner Mint, Asda*	1 Serving/100g	191	9.0	191	3.4	24.0	9.0	0.4
Really Creamy Chocolate, Asda*	1 Serving/100g	227	11.0	227	4.1	28.0	11.0	0.4
Really Creamy Lemon Meringue, Asda*	1 Serving/100ml	100	5.0	100	1.8	12.0	5.0	0.1
Really Creamy Toffee, Asda*	1 Serving/120ml	146	6.0	122	1.7	17.5	5.0	0.1
Rocky Road, M & S*	1 Tub/500g	1475	88.5	295	4.2	29.5	17.7	1.2
Rocky Road, Sainsbury's*	1/8 Pot/67g	137	4.9	205	3.8	30.9	7.3	1.0
Rolo, Nestle*	½ Tub/500ml	1180	52.5	236	3.4	31.9	10.5	0.2
Rum & Raisin, Carte d'Or*	2 Scoops/50g	100	4.0	200	2.5	24.0	8.0	1.0
Rum & Raisin, Haagen-Dazs*	1 Serving/120ml	264	17.6	220	3.4	18.6	14.7	0.0
Rum & Raisin, TTD, Sainsbury's*	¼ Pot/100g	220	10.4	220	3.8	27.7	10.4	1.0
Sandwich, Vanilla, Skinny Cow*	1 Portion/36g	100	3.0	277	5.4	45.1	8.2	2.1
Screwball, Asda*	1 Screwball/60g	122	6.0	203	3.3	25.0	10.0	1.5
Smarties, Nestle*	1 Serving/50g	125	5.9	250	3.6	32.3	11.9	0.2
Smarties Ice Cream Pot, Nestle*	1 Pot/69g	151	5.7	218	4.4	33.6	8.2	0.0
Soft Scoop, Vanilla, Light, Wall's*	1 Serving/100g	140	6.0	140	3.0	19.0	6.0	2.0
Spagnola, Carte d'Or*	1 Serving/100g	187	5.7	187	2.0	32.0	5.7	0.0
Sticky Toffee, Cream O' Galloway*	1 Serving/30g	80	4.4	266	4.7	28.7	14.7	0.0
Strawberry, Soft Scoop, Tesco*	1 Serving/46g	78	3.4	170	2.8	23.1	7.4	0.1
Strawberry, Swirl Pot, Skinny Cow*	1 Pot/100ml	89	0.3	89	2.5	19.0	0.3	2.2
Strawberry, Weight Watchers*	1 Pot/57g	81	2.2	142	2.5	23.4	3.9	0.2
Strawberry & Cream, Mivvi, Nestle*	1 Serving/60g	118	4.6	196	2.6	29.4	7.6	0.1
Strawberry & Cream, Organic, Sainsbury's*	1 Serving/100g	193	9.8	193	3.6	22.6	9.8	0.4
Strawberry & Yoghurt Delice, Carte d'Or*	1 Portion/54g	95	2.0	175	1.5	34.0	3.6	0.0
Strawberry Cheesecake, Ben & Jerry's*	1 Serving 100g	240	14.0	240	3.0	27.0	14.0	0.0
Strawberry Cheesecake, Co-Op*	1/6 Pot/86g	163	6.0	190	3.0	29.0	7.0	0.2
Tantilising Toffee, COU, M & S*	¼ Pot/125ml	125	3.5	100	0.6	18.0	2.8	0.0
Taste Sensation, Mascarpone Forest Fruits, Aldi*	1 Pot/73g	159	7.4	217	1.8	29.6	10.1	0.6
Terry's Chocolate Orange, Carte d'Or*	1 Serving/100g	182	7.1	182	2.8	27.0	7.1	0.0
The Chocolate Extremist, Chokablok*	1 Serving/100g	255	11.7	255	4.7	32.2	11.7	1.2
Tiramisu, COU, M & S*	¼ Tub/86g	120	2.5	140	2.1	26.4	2.9	3.0
Toblerone, Carte d'Or*	1 Serving/100g	211	9.1	211	3.7	29.0	9.1	0.0
Toffee, Swirl Pot, Skinny Cow*	1 Pot/66g	92	0.4	140	3.8	29.8	0.6	4.5

ICE CREAM

	Measure INFO/WEIGHT	per Measure KCAL	FAT	Nutrition Values per 100g / 100ml KCAL	PROT	CARB	FAT	FIBRE
Toffee & Biscuit, Weight Watchers*	1 Pot/100ml	93	2.7	93	1.5	14.9	2.7	0.1
Toffee & Honeycomb Sundaes, Weight Watchers*	1 Pot/150g	222	4.6	148	2.1	32.7	3.1	1.6
Toffee & Vanilla, Sainsbury's*	1 Serving/71g	146	6.8	205	3.1	26.7	9.5	0.1
Toffee Fudge, Soft Scoop, Asda*	1 Serving/50g	92	3.5	185	2.6	28.0	7.0	0.0
Toffee Ripple, Tesco*	1 Serving/100g	173	7.2	173	2.7	24.4	7.2	0.1
Triple Chocolate, Brownie, Skinny Cow*	1 Serving/65g	93	1.7	144	3.5	24.1	2.6	5.3
Triple Chocolate, Carte d'Or*	1 Serving/58g	122	5.7	210	3.7	27.0	9.8	0.0
Triple Chocolate, Dairy, Morrisons*	1 Serving/100g	233	10.8	233	3.8	30.0	10.8	0.4
Triple Chocolate, Dairy, Sainsbury's*	1/8 Litre/67g	123	4.4	184	3.5	27.6	6.6	1.0
Truffle Berry Fling, Skinny Cow*	1 Serving/100g	156	2.0	156	4.0	30.5	2.0	3.3
Truly Lovin' Toffee, Skinny Cow*	1 Tub/352g	510	3.5	145	3.5	30.5	1.0	6.6
Vanilla, Ben & Jerry's*	1 Tub/116g	267	17.4	230	4.0	20.0	15.0	0.1
Vanilla, Carte d'Or*	1 Serving/50g	105	4.7	210	3.0	26.0	9.5	0.0
Vanilla, COU, M & S*	¼ Pot/79g	111	2.2	140	1.7	25.9	2.8	0.8
Vanilla, Dairy, Average	1 Scoop/40g	80	4.4	201	3.5	23.6	11.0	0.7
Vanilla, Dairy, Finest, Tesco*	1 Serving/92g	227	16.0	247	4.5	18.0	17.4	0.3
Vanilla, Dairy, Organic, Yeo Valley*	1 Serving/100g	206	11.2	206	4.9	21.3	11.2	0.0
Vanilla, Dairy Milk, Cadbury*	1 Serving/120g	259	13.9	216	3.5	26.0	11.6	0.1
Vanilla, Fairtrade, Ben & Jerry's*	1 Serving/100g	230	15.0	230	4.0	20.0	15.0	0.1
Vanilla, Light, Carte d'Or*	1 Serving/100g	136	4.4	136	2.4	22.0	4.4	4.0
Vanilla, Light Soft Scoop, 25% Less Fat, Morrisons*	1 Scoop/50g	75	2.5	150	2.9	23.2	5.0	0.2
Vanilla, Low Fat, Average	1 Scoop/50g	59	1.7	118	2.3	19.4	3.4	0.6
Vanilla, Low Fat, Weight Watchers*	1 Scoop/125ml	75	2.1	60	1.1	9.7	1.7	0.1
Vanilla, Mackies*	1 Serving/100g	193	11.0	193	4.0	18.0	11.0	0.0
Vanilla, Non-Dairy, Average	1 Serving/60g	107	5.2	178	3.2	23.1	8.7	0.0
Vanilla, Organic, Sainsbury's*	1 Serving/85g	176	10.2	207	4.3	20.5	12.0	0.1
Vanilla, Organic, Tesco*	1 Serving/100g	237	17.2	237	3.7	16.8	17.2	0.0
Vanilla, Organic, Waitrose*	1 Serving/125g	177	11.2	142	2.7	12.4	9.0	0.0
Vanilla, Really Creamy, Asda*	1 Serving/50g	98	5.0	196	3.5	23.0	10.0	0.1
Vanilla, Soft Scoop, BGTY, Sainsbury's*	1 Serving/75g	88	1.3	117	3.1	22.2	1.7	0.2
Vanilla, Soft Scoop, GFY, Asda*	1 Serving/100g	117	1.7	117	3.1	22.0	1.7	0.2
Vanilla, Soft Scoop, Light, Wall's*, Wall's Ice Cream*	1 Scoop/50ml	31	1.3	62	1.3	7.0	2.6	0.9
Vanilla, Strawberry Swirl, Mini Tub, Weight Watchers*	1 Tub/57g	81	2.2	142	2.5	23.4	3.9	0.2
Vanilla, Toffee Crunch, Ben & Jerry's*	1 Tub/407g	1099	65.1	270	4.0	29.0	16.0	0.5
Vanilla, Toffee Crunch, Fairtrade, Ben & Jerry's*	1 Serving/100g	280	16.0	280	4.0	29.0	16.0	0.5
Vanilla, Too Good to Be True, Wall's Ice Cream*	1 Serving/50ml	35	0.2	70	2.0	14.9	0.4	0.1
Vanilla, TTD, Sainsbury's*	¼ Pot/100g	246	16.9	246	5.2	18.2	16.9	0.0
Vanilla, with Vanilla Pods, Sainsbury's*	1 Serving/100g	195	10.1	195	3.5	22.5	10.1	0.1
Vanilla & Cinnamon, Finest, Tesco*	1 Serving/50g	114	7.3	229	3.9	20.2	14.7	0.4
Vanilla & Strawberry, Weight Watchers*	1 Serving/100ml	81	2.2	81	1.4	13.3	2.2	0.1
Vanilla Bean, Light, Deluxe*	1 Serving/64g	110	2.5	172	4.7	26.6	3.9	0.0
Vanilla Bean, Purbeck*	1 Serving/100g	198	11.5	198	4.8	18.7	11.5	0.0
Vanilla Caramel Brownie, Haagen-Dazs*	1 Serving/150g	410	24.7	273	4.5	26.8	16.5	0.0
Vanilla Chocolate, Taste Sensation, Frosty's, Aldi*	1 Pot/73g	164	7.0	224	2.1	32.4	9.6	0.7
Vanilla Flavour, Soft Scoop, Sainsbury's*	1 Serving/71g	96	3.9	136	2.9	18.8	5.5	0.2
Vanilla Flavour, Soft, VLH Kitchens*	1 Serving/100g	235	15.0	235	4.0	22.1	15.0	0.2
Vanilletta, Tesco*	1 Serving/47g	82	3.8	175	4.0	21.6	8.1	0.0
Viennetta, Biscuit Caramel, Wall's Ice Cream*	1/6 Serving/58g	183	12.1	315	3.3	27.8	20.9	0.0
Viennetta, Cappuccino, Wall's Ice Cream*	1 Serving/75g	191	12.7	255	3.5	22.0	17.0	0.0
Viennetta, Chocolate, Wall's Ice Cream*	¼ Pot/80g	200	12.2	250	4.1	24.0	15.2	0.0
Viennetta, Forest Fruit, Wall's Ice Cream*	1 Serving/98g	265	15.9	270	3.4	27.2	16.2	0.0
Viennetta, Mint, Wall's Ice Cream*	1 Serving/80g	204	13.3	255	3.4	23.0	16.6	0.0
Viennetta, Selection Brownie, Wall's Ice Cream*	1 Serving/70g	194	11.3	277	4.2	28.5	16.2	0.0

	Measure INFO/WEIGHT	per Measure KCAL	FAT	Nutrition Values per 100g / 100ml KCAL	PROT	CARB	FAT	FIBRE

ICE CREAM

	Measure INFO/WEIGHT	KCAL	FAT	KCAL	PROT	CARB	FAT	FIBRE
Viennetta, Strawberry, Wall's Ice Cream*	1 Serving/80g	204	13.4	255	3.4	22.1	16.8	0.0
Viennetta, Vanilla, Wall's Ice Cream*	¼ Bar/80g	204	13.4	255	3.3	23.0	16.7	0.0
Voluptuous Vanilla, COU, M & S*	1 Pot/400g	520	10.4	130	4.6	22.0	2.6	0.6
Walnut & Maple, Waitrose*	1 Serving/60g	68	2.3	114	1.8	18.2	3.8	0.0
with Cherry Sauce, Tesco*	1 Serving/58g	121	3.2	210	2.8	37.0	5.6	0.2
with Raspberry Sauce, Movenpick*	1 Serving/50g	130	7.0	260	4.0	27.0	14.0	0.2
Zesty Lemon Meringue, COU, M & S*	¼ Pot/73g	120	1.8	165	2.6	33.0	2.5	0.5

ICE CREAM BAR

	Measure INFO/WEIGHT	KCAL	FAT	KCAL	PROT	CARB	FAT	FIBRE
Chunky Chocolate, Co-Op*	1 Bar/60g	204	12.0	340	5.0	35.0	20.0	1.0
Chunky Toffee, Co-Op*	1 Bar/60g	204	12.6	340	4.0	34.0	21.0	1.0
Dairy Milk, Caramel, Cadbury*	1 Bar/60ml	175	10.3	290	3.6	30.2	17.1	0.0
Dairy Milk, Fruit & Nut, Cadbury*	1 Bar/90ml	243	15.3	270	3.5	26.1	17.0	0.0
Dairy Milk, Fudge, Cadbury*	1 Bar/60g	165	10.3	275	3.0	27.6	17.2	0.0
Dream, Cadbury*	1 Bar/118g	260	14.0	220	3.6	26.0	11.9	0.0
Galaxy, Mars*	1 Bar/54g	184	12.1	341	3.8	30.7	22.5	0.6
Lion, Nestle*	1 Bar/45g	166	9.9	370	4.2	39.1	21.9	1.0
Maltesers, Mars*	1 Bar/45ml	113	7.0	252	2.9	25.0	15.6	0.7
Mars, Mars*	1 Bar/63g	177	10.3	283	3.6	30.1	16.4	0.0
Rage, Chocolate with Caramel Sauce, Treats*	1 Bar/60g	177	10.5	295	3.3	30.9	17.5	0.0
Red Fruits, Solero*	1 Bar/80g	99	2.2	124	1.6	25.0	2.7	0.0
Snickers, Mars*	1 Bar/67g	250	15.0	373	6.0	37.3	22.4	0.0
Toffee Crunch, English, Weight Watchers*	1 Bar/40g	110	6.0	275	2.5	32.5	15.0	5.0
Twix, Mars*	1 Serving/44g	228	14.0	524	6.9	52.9	32.2	0.0
Vanilla & Raspberry, Weight Watchers*	1 Serving/100g	81	0.3	81	2.0	23.0	0.3	0.0
Yorkie, Nestle*	1 Bar	144	8.7	359	4.8	36.5	21.6	0.0

ICE CREAM CONE

	Measure INFO/WEIGHT	KCAL	FAT	KCAL	PROT	CARB	FAT	FIBRE
After Eight, Nestle*	1 Cone/100ml	174	8.0	174	2.4	23.0	8.0	0.9
Average	1 Cone/75g	139	6.4	186	3.5	25.5	8.5	0.0
Blackcurrant, GFY, Asda*	1 Cone/67g	162	6.0	241	3.0	37.0	9.0	0.1
Carousel Wafer Company*	1 Cone/5g	19	0.2	392	9.8	78.6	4.2	0.0
Chocolate, Mini, Cornetto, Wall's Ice Cream*	1 Cone/19g	69	4.4	363	4.2	34.2	23.2	0.0
Chocolate, Vanilla & Hazelnut, Sainsbury's*	1 Cone/62g	190	10.5	306	4.5	33.9	16.9	0.6
Chocolate & Caramel, Skinny Cow*	1 Cone/110ml	121	2.8	110	2.5	19.3	2.5	2.7
Chocolate & Nut, Co-Op*	1 Cone/110g	307	17.0	279	3.9	31.0	15.5	0.6
Chocolate & Vanilla, Good Choice, Iceland*	1 Cone/110ml	161	7.1	146	2.7	22.9	6.5	0.8
Cornet, Wafer Cone, Askeys*	1 Cone/4g	13	0.1	376	10.7	77.6	2.5	0.0
Cornetto, Classico, Mini, Wall's Ice Cream*	1 Cone/19g	67	4.4	353	4.2	32.6	23.2	0.0
Cornetto, Classico, Wall's Ice Cream*	1 Cone/98g	200	12.6	205	2.7	19.7	12.9	0.0
Cornetto, Frutti Disc, Wall's Ice Cream*	1 Cone/80g	200	8.8	250	2.5	35.0	11.0	0.0
Cornetto, GFY, Asda*	1 Cone/67g	162	6.0	241	3.0	37.0	9.0	0.1
Cornetto, Mint, Wall's Ice Cream*	1 Cone/75g	190	9.9	250	4.0	31.0	13.0	0.8
Cornetto, Wall's Ice Cream*	1 Cone/75g	195	9.7	260	3.7	34.5	12.9	0.0
Creme Egg, Cadbury*	1 Cone/115ml	270	13.3	235	2.9	29.3	11.6	0.0
Cup Cornet, Wafer Cone, Askeys*	1 Cone/4g	13	0.1	376	10.7	77.6	2.5	0.0
Dairy Milk, Mint, Cadbury*	1 Cone/115mll	190	8.9	165	2.4	21.5	7.7	0.0
Extreme Raspberry, Cornetto, Nestle*	1 Cone/88g	220	8.8	250	2.5	36.0	10.0	0.2
Flake 99, Cadbury*	1 Cone/125ml	244	12.5	195	2.6	23.2	10.0	0.0
Flake 99, Strawberry, Cadbury*	1 Cone/125g	250	10.9	200	2.6	27.3	8.7	0.0
Mini, Sainsbury's*	1 Cone/18g	66	3.8	366	4.4	39.8	21.0	3.4
Mini, Tesco*	1 Cone/48g	152	9.3	316	4.1	31.5	19.3	0.8
Mint Choc Chip, Iceland*	1 Cone/72g	210	9.4	292	3.3	40.4	13.0	1.0
Raspberry & Vanilla, Refreshing, Skinny Cow*	1 Cone/110ml	122	2.8	111	1.7	20.4	2.5	1.5
Smarties, Nestle*	1 Cone/100g	177	8.1	177	2.4	23.6	8.1	0.7

	Measure INFO/WEIGHT	per Measure		Nutrition Values per 100g / 100ml				
		KCAL	FAT	KCAL	PROT	CARB	FAT	FIBRE
ICE CREAM CONE								
Strawberry, BGTY, Sainsbury's*	1 Cone/69g	151	4.5	219	2.6	37.5	6.5	1.3
Strawberry, Co-Op*	1 Cone/110g	283	13.3	257	3.5	33.6	12.1	0.5
Strawberry & Vanilla, Asda*	1 Cone/115ml	193	9.0	168	1.8	22.6	7.8	0.1
Strawberry & Vanilla, HL, Tesco*	1 Cone/69g	149	4.3	216	3.4	36.4	6.3	1.4
Strawberry & Vanilla, Iceland*	1 Cone/70g	182	7.6	260	3.3	37.5	10.8	0.7
Strawberry & Vanilla, Sainsbury's*	1 Cone/70g	171	6.8	243	3.4	35.6	9.7	1.0
Strawberry & Vanilla, Tesco*	1 Cone/70g	194	9.4	277	3.0	35.9	13.5	0.3
Tropical, GFY, Asda*	1 Cone/100g	135	5.0	135	2.6	20.0	5.0	0.3
ICE CREAM ROLL								
Arctic, Average	1 Serving/70g	140	4.6	200	4.1	33.3	6.6	0.0
Mini, Cadbury*	1 Roll/45ml	99	5.9	220	3.4	24.3	13.1	0.0
Tesco*	¼ Roll/57g	131	4.9	230	3.7	34.5	8.6	0.4
ICE CREAM SANDWICH								
Mint, Skinny Cow*	1 Piece/71g	140	2.0	197	4.2	39.4	2.8	1.4
Wich, Ben & Jerry's*	1 Pack/117g	398	19.9	340	4.0	44.0	17.0	1.0
ICE CREAM STICK								
Berry Blast, Smoothie, Skinny Cow*	1 Stick/110ml	71	0.1	65	0.9	15.1	0.1	1.9
Chocolate Cookies, Haagen-Dazs*	1 Stick/43g	162	10.9	376	4.9	31.8	25.4	0.0
Cookies 'n' Cream, Skinny Cow*	1 Stick/67g	89	1.0	133	4.8	25.3	1.5	3.6
Mint Double Chocolate, Skinny Cow*	1 Stick/110ml	94	1.8	85	2.7	15.1	1.6	2.4
Strawberries & Cream, Skinny Cow*	1 Stick/110ml	82	1.0	75	2.8	13.6	0.9	2.3
Toffee, Skinny Cow*	1 Stick/72g	87	0.4	121	3.9	25.2	0.5	4.2
Triple Chocolate, Skinny Cow*	1 Stick/68g	87	1.5	128	4.3	22.8	2.2	2.8
Vanilla Macadamia, Haagen-Dazs*	1 Stick/42g	161	11.6	383	4.6	28.7	27.7	0.0
ICE LOLLY								
Assorted, De Roma*	1 Lolly/55ml	48	0.2	87	0.2	20.9	0.4	0.2
Assorted, Iceland*	1 Lolly/51g	33	0.0	65	0.0	16.2	0.0	0.0
Baby, Tesco*	1 Lolly/32g	26	0.0	80	0.1	20.0	0.0	0.1
Blackcurrant, Dairy Split, Sainsbury's*	1 Lolly/73ml	88	2.6	121	1.8	20.4	3.6	0.1
Blackcurrant, Ribena*	1 Lolly/55ml	43	0.0	79	0.0	19.2	0.0	0.0
Blackcurrant Split, Iceland*	1 Lolly/75g	61	2.4	81	1.1	12.0	3.2	0.1
Bournville, Cadbury*	1 Lolly/110g	269	17.2	245	2.5	23.2	15.6	0.0
Calippo, Lemon Lime, Mini, Wall's Ice Cream*	1 Lolly/80g	68	0.0	85	0.0	21.0	0.0	0.2
Calippo, Orange, Mini, Wall's Ice Cream*	1 Lolly/78g	70	0.0	90	0.0	21.9	0.0	0.2
Calippo, Strawberry Tropical, Wall's Ice Cream*	1 Lolly/105g	89	0.1	85	0.1	21.0	0.1	0.0
Choc & Almond, Mini, Tesco*	1 Lolly/31g	103	7.4	331	4.4	24.8	23.8	0.9
Choc Lime Split, Morrisons*	1 Lolly/73ml	120	6.1	164	1.6	20.4	8.4	0.1
Chocolate, Mini Milk, Milk Time, Wall's Ice Cream*	1 Lolly/23g	31	0.7	135	4.3	22.0	3.1	1.0
Chocolate, Plain, Mini, Tesco*	1 Lolly/31g	94	6.6	304	3.1	24.8	21.4	1.2
Chocolate, Pooh Stick, Nestle*	1 Lolly/40g	36	1.4	89	2.1	12.9	3.6	0.0
Chocolate & Vanilla, Sainsbury's*	1 Lolly/40g	143	10.1	357	3.7	28.7	25.3	2.2
Cider Refresher, Treats*	1 Lolly/70ml	54	0.0	77	0.0	19.2	0.0	0.0
Creamy Tropical Sorbet, Sticks, Waitrose*	1 Lolly/85g	100	1.8	118	1.9	22.9	2.1	0.8
Exotic Fruit, Mini, HL, Tesco*	1 Lolly/31g	41	0.6	131	1.0	26.4	2.0	1.0
Fab, Nestle*	1 Lolly/57g	78	2.7	136	0.5	22.8	4.7	0.2
Fab, Orange, Nestle*	1 Lolly/58g	81	2.7	140	0.6	24.0	4.7	0.0
Feast, Chocolate, Mini, Wall's Ice Cream*	1 Lolly/52g	165	11.9	318	3.3	24.0	23.0	0.0
Feast, Ice Cream, Original, Wall's Ice Cream*	1 Lolly/92ml	294	21.6	320	3.2	23.8	23.5	0.0
Feast, Toffee, Mini, Wall's Ice Cream*	1 Lolly/52g	163	12.0	313	3.0	24.0	23.0	0.0
Feast, Wall's Ice Cream*	1 Lolly/92ml	276	20.2	300	3.2	22.0	22.0	0.0
Fruit, Assorted, Waitrose*	1 Lolly/73g	59	0.0	81	0.0	20.0	0.0	0.1
Fruit, Red, Tesco*	1 Lolly/32g	40	0.6	128	1.8	25.6	2.0	0.6
Fruit Ices, Made with Orange Juice, Del Monte*	1 Lolly/75ml	79	0.0	105	0.5	25.7	0.0	0.0

	Measure INFO/WEIGHT	per Measure		Nutrition Values per 100g / 100ml				
		KCAL	FAT	KCAL	PROT	CARB	FAT	FIBRE
ICE LOLLY								
Fruit Luxury, Mini, Co-Op*	1 Lolly/45g	58	2.7	130	2.0	18.0	6.0	0.2
Fruit Pastilles, Rowntree's*	1 Lolly/65ml	61	0.0	94	0.1	23.2	0.0	0.0
Fruit Split, Asda*	1 Lolly/74g	85	2.7	115	1.7	19.0	3.6	0.0
Fruit Split, Assorted, Co-Op*	1 Lolly/73g	80	2.2	110	1.0	20.0	3.0	0.1
Fruit Split, BFY, Morrisons*	1 Lolly/73g	50	0.5	69	1.6	13.9	0.7	0.1
Fruit Split, Waitrose*	1 Lolly/73g	91	2.6	124	2.5	21.7	3.6	0.4
Fruit Splits, Treats*	1 Lolly/75ml	77	3.1	103	1.4	17.6	4.1	0.0
Fruity 'n' Freezy, Asda*	1 Lolly/30ml	24	0.0	80	0.1	20.0	0.0	0.0
Ice Lolly, Twister, Choc, Wall's Ice Cream*	1 Lolly/27g	40	1.6	150	3.5	22.0	6.0	0.9
Icicles, All Flavours, Freezepops, Calypso*	1 Lolly/50ml	1	0.0	1	0.0	0.3	0.0	0.0
Lemon & Lime, Mini Bar, M & S*	1 Lolly/50g	47	0.0	95	0.1	23.6	0.1	0.2
Lemon & Lime, Rocket Split, De Roma*	1 Lolly/60ml	65	2.6	108	1.0	16.0	4.3	0.2
Lemon Sorbet, Mercadona*	1 Lolly/63g	38	0.2	61	0.5	32.4	0.3	8.0
Lemonade & Cola, Morrisons*	1 Lolly/55ml	36	0.0	65	0.0	16.2	0.0	0.0
Lemonade Sparkle, Wall's Ice Cream*	1 Lolly/55g	40	0.0	73	0.0	18.2	0.0	0.0
Mango & Lemon, BGTY, Sainsbury's*	1 Lolly/72g	84	0.2	116	0.3	28.1	0.3	0.5
Mango & Passion Fruit Bursts, Sainsbury's*	1 Lolly/89ml	75	0.1	84	0.2	20.4	0.1	0.0
Mango & Passion Fruit Smoothie, Waitrose*	1 Lolly/73g	60	0.3	82	0.7	18.9	0.4	0.7
Milk, Blue Parrot Cafe, Sainsbury's*	1 Lolly/30ml	34	1.0	113	2.7	18.0	3.3	0.3
Milk Chocolate & Crisped Wheat, Co-Op*	1 Lolly/110g	258	13.2	235	3.0	28.0	12.0	0.7
Mint Chocolate, Tesco*	1 Lolly/70g	234	13.9	334	3.6	35.4	19.8	1.2
Morrisons*	1 Lolly/100g	30	0.0	30	0.0	7.4	0.0	0.0
Nobbly Bobbly, Nestle*	1 Lolly/70ml	158	8.2	226	2.3	27.6	11.7	0.3
Orange, Real Fruit Juice, Sainsbury's*	1 Lolly/73ml	49	0.1	67	0.2	16.5	0.1	0.1
Orange, Real Juice, Sainsbury's*	1 Lolly/72ml	63	0.1	88	0.7	21.0	0.1	0.1
Orange, Real Juice, Tesco*	1 Lolly/32g	25	0.0	78	0.6	18.7	0.0	0.3
Orange, Ribena*	1 Lolly/110ml	95	0.0	86	0.1	21.4	0.0	0.0
Orange, Tesco*	1 Lolly/77g	53	0.0	68	0.2	16.8	0.0	0.3
Orange, Water, Iceland*	1 Lolly/75g	73	0.0	98	0.2	24.4	0.0	0.2
Orange Juice, Asda*	1 Lolly/70g	58	0.0	83	0.7	20.0	0.0	0.0
Orange Juice, Bar, M & S*	1 Lolly/75g	64	0.0	86	0.5	21.0	0.0	0.1
Orange Juice, Co-Op*	1 Lolly/73g	51	0.1	70	0.4	17.0	0.1	0.1
Orange Juice, Freshly Squeezed, Finest, Tesco*	1 Lolly/80ml	89	0.0	111	0.7	27.0	0.0	0.0
Orange Juice, Freshly Squeezed, Waitrose*	1 Lolly/73g	88	0.1	120	0.6	29.7	0.1	0.0
Orange Juice, Milfina*	1 Lolly/79g	69	0.0	87	0.5	23.3	0.0	0.0
Orange Juice, Morrisons*	1 Lolly/55ml	46	0.0	84	0.0	20.0	0.0	0.0
Orange Juice, Tropicana*	1 Lolly/50g	42	0.0	85	0.5	20.7	0.0	0.0
Orange Maid, Nestle*	1 Lolly/73ml	66	0.0	91	0.5	21.6	0.0	0.0
Orange 'n' Cream, Tropicana*	1 Lolly/65g	83	2.9	129	1.4	20.5	4.5	0.3
Pineapple, Dairy Split, Sainsbury's*	1 Lolly/72ml	84	2.6	116	1.8	19.0	3.6	0.1
Pineapple, Real Fruit Juice, Sainsbury's*	1 Lolly/73ml	55	0.1	76	0.1	19.0	0.1	0.1
Pop Up, Chosen By You, Asda*	1 Lolly/80ml	65	0.0	81	0.0	20.1	0.0	0.3
Raspberry, Real Fruit Juice, Sainsbury's*	1 Lolly/72g	62	0.1	86	0.3	21.0	0.1	0.1
Raspberry, Smoothie, Iced, Del Monte*	1 Lolly/90ml	84	0.0	94	0.3	22.8	0.0	0.8
Raspberry & Apple, Sainsbury's*	1 Lolly/57ml	39	0.1	68	0.1	17.1	0.1	0.1
Real Fruit, Dairy Split, Sainsbury's*	1 Lolly/73ml	100	3.1	137	2.1	22.8	4.2	0.1
Real Fruit Juice, Rocket, Blue Parrot Cafe, Sainsbury's*	1 Lolly/58ml	45	0.0	77	0.2	19.1	0.0	0.1
Real Orange, Kids, Tesco*	1 Lolly/32g	25	0.0	78	0.6	18.7	0.0	0.3
Refresher, Bassett's*	1 Lolly/40g	47	0.9	117	2.2	22.2	2.2	0.3
Rocket, Co-Op*	1 Lolly/60g	42	0.0	70	0.0	17.0	0.0	0.0
Rocket, Sainsbury's*	1 Lolly/58g	42	0.1	72	0.1	17.8	0.1	0.1
Rolo, Nestle*	1 Lolly/75ml	243	14.1	324	3.8	36.5	18.8	0.0
Scooby-Doo, Freezepops, Calypso*	1 Lolly/50ml	14	0.0	28	0.0	7.0	0.0	0.0

	Measure INFO/WEIGHT	per Measure KCAL	FAT	Nutrition Values per 100g / 100ml KCAL	PROT	CARB	FAT	FIBRE
ICE LOLLY								
Solero, Exotic, Wall's Ice Cream*	1 Lolly/82g	99	2.3	121	1.6	21.9	2.8	0.5
Solero, Orange Fresh, Wall's Ice Cream*	1 Lolly/96g	78	0.0	81	0.2	20.0	0.0	0.0
Solero, Red Fruits, Wall's Ice Cream*	1 Lolly/95g	99	2.1	104	1.3	21.0	2.2	0.0
Strawberries & Cream, Cadbury*	1 Lolly/100ml	225	11.7	225	2.9	27.0	11.7	0.0
Strawberries 'n' Cream, Tropicana*	1 Lolly/50g	58	0.6	117	1.6	25.0	1.2	0.0
Strawberry, Dairy Split, Sainsbury's*	1 Lolly/73ml	86	2.6	118	1.7	19.8	3.6	0.1
Strawberry, Fruit Split, Iceland*	1 Lolly/73g	77	2.4	105	0.9	17.8	3.3	0.5
Strawberry, Mini Milk, Milk Time, Wall's Ice Cream*	1 Lolly/23g	30	0.7	131	4.0	22.0	2.9	0.5
Strawberry, Orange & Pineapple, Rocket, Iceland*	1 Lolly/47g	38	0.0	81	0.0	20.2	0.0	0.1
Strawberry, So-Lo, Good Choice, Iceland*	1 Lolly/66g	85	1.2	128	2.4	25.6	1.8	0.1
Strawberry & Banana, Smoothies, Sainsbury's*	1 Lolly/60g	100	3.2	166	1.5	28.0	5.3	0.2
Strawberry & Vanilla, 99% Fat Free, So-Lo, Iceland*	1 Lolly/92g	98	0.4	107	2.3	23.5	0.4	2.2
Strawberry Fruit, Double, Del Monte*	1 Lolly/76g	84	2.0	111	1.8	20.1	2.6	0.0
Strawberry Split, Co-Op*	1 Lolly/71ml	75	2.1	105	1.0	17.0	3.0	0.1
Tip Top, Calypso*	1 Lolly/20ml	6	0.0	30	0.1	7.1	0.1	0.0
Traffic Light, Co-Op*	1 Lolly/52g	55	0.4	105	0.4	25.0	0.8	0.0
Tropical, Mmmm, Tesco*	1 Lolly/73g	109	3.1	150	1.2	26.6	4.3	0.4
Tropical Fruit, Starburst, Mars*	1 Lolly/93ml	94	0.1	101	0.3	24.8	0.1	0.0
Tropical Fruit Sorbet, Waitrose*	1 Lolly/110g	90	2.2	82	1.5	14.5	2.0	0.2
Twister, Wall's Ice Cream*	1 Lolly/80ml	76	1.5	95	0.6	18.4	1.9	0.0
Vanilla, Mini Milk, Milk Time, Wall's Ice Cream*	1 Lolly/23g	29	0.7	127	3.8	21.0	2.9	0.3
Vimto Soft Drinks*	1 Lolly/73ml	84	3.0	115	1.3	18.2	4.1	0.1
Wonka Super Sour Tastic, Nestle*	1 Lolly/60ml	84	2.2	140	0.0	26.1	3.6	0.0
Zoom, Nestle*	1 Lolly/58ml	54	0.4	93	0.9	20.6	0.7	0.0
ICED DESSERT								
Cafe Latte, BGTY, Sainsbury's*	1 Serving/75g	104	2.7	139	2.9	23.7	3.6	3.3
Chocolate, Honeycomb Pieces, Weight Watchers*	1 Pot/58g	92	2.5	159	3.1	26.2	4.3	0.8
Chocolate & Mallow, GFY, Asda*	1 Pot/150ml	142	1.8	95	2.0	19.0	1.2	2.3
Chocolate Mint Crisp, COU, M & S*	¼ Pot/85g	115	2.5	135	5.4	21.9	2.9	1.0
Greek Style, Yoghurt, Tesco*	1 Serving/56g	90	1.8	160	2.6	29.7	3.3	1.4
Raspberry Swirl, Weight Watchers*	1 Scoop/60g	74	1.5	124	1.7	23.4	2.5	0.3
Strawberry Swirl, Weight Watchers*	1 Pot/100ml	92	1.7	92	1.1	18.1	1.7	0.5
Summer Fruits, Yoghurt, BGTY, Sainsbury's*	¼ Pot/85g	105	0.8	124	3.3	25.6	0.9	0.5
Toffee, 3% Fat, M & S*	1oz/28g	51	0.7	183	3.1	37.2	2.4	0.5
Toffee & Walnut, Free From, Sainsbury's*	¼ Tub/81g	203	10.0	251	3.3	31.6	12.4	0.3
Toffee Flavoured, Dairy, BGTY, Sainsbury's*	1 Serving/70g	103	3.1	147	2.7	24.0	4.5	0.2
Vanilla, Dairy, BGTY, Sainsbury's*	1 Serving/65g	78	1.0	120	3.0	23.6	1.5	0.6
Vanilla, Non Dairy, Soft, Swedish Glace*	1 Serving/100g	200	10.0	200	2.5	25.0	10.0	1.0
Vanilla & Chocolate, HL, Tesco*	1 Pot/73g	104	1.9	143	3.0	26.9	2.6	0.7
INDIAN MEAL								
Banquet, for One, COU, M & S*	1 Pack/500g	400	6.0	80	6.7	10.2	1.2	3.1
for One, Asda*	1 Pack/550g	834	25.3	152	6.7	20.9	4.6	1.4
for One, GFY, Asda*	1 Serving/495g	643	23.3	130	8.0	14.0	4.7	1.0
for One, Vegetarian, Asda*	1 Pack/499g	789	44.9	158	3.2	16.0	9.0	1.4
for Two, Hot, Takeaway, Tesco*	1 Pack/825g	1215	60.6	147	6.6	13.6	7.3	1.9
for Two, Menu, Tesco*	1 Serving/537g	811	34.4	151	6.3	17.0	6.4	0.8
for Two, Peshwari Naan, Finest, Tesco*	½ Pack/200g	612	17.8	306	8.3	48.3	8.9	5.2
INSTANT WHIP								
Chocolate Flavour, Dry, Bird's*	1oz/28g	109	1.7	390	3.8	80.5	5.9	0.7
Strawberry Flavour, Dry, Bird's*	1oz/28g	112	1.5	400	2.5	85.0	5.4	0.4
IRN BRU								
Diet, Barr's*	1 Can/330ml	2	0.0	1	0.1	0.1	0.0	0.0
Original, Barr's*	1 Bottle/498ml	214	0.0	43	0.0	10.5	0.0	0.0

	Measure INFO/WEIGHT	per Measure KCAL	per Measure FAT	Nutrition Values per 100g / 100ml KCAL	PROT	CARB	FAT	FIBRE
JACKFRUIT								
Raw, Average, Flesh Only	*1 Portion/162g*	*155*	*0.5*	*95*	*1.5*	*24.4*	*0.3*	*1.6*
JALFREZI								
Chicken, & Pilau Rice, Sainsbury's*	1 Pack/500g	600	20.5	120	6.9	13.9	4.1	1.5
Chicken, & Pilau Rice, Takeaway, Asda*	1 Pack/558g	792	23.4	142	7.0	19.0	4.2	1.3
Chicken, & Rice, Serves 1, Tesco*	1 Serving/475g	589	38.0	124	7.4	5.7	8.0	1.6
Chicken, Asda*	1 Pack/340g	415	20.4	122	10.0	7.0	6.0	1.6
Chicken, Finest, Tesco*	1 Pack/350g	402	16.4	115	10.4	6.9	4.7	1.2
Chicken, GFY, Asda*	1 Pack/350g	238	3.1	68	9.0	6.0	0.9	1.8
Chicken, Hot & Spicy, Sainsbury's*	½ Pack/200g	228	11.4	114	12.8	2.9	5.7	1.0
Chicken, Indian Takeaway, Tesco*	1 Serving/350g	245	8.7	70	7.4	4.3	2.5	1.8
Chicken, Medium, GFY, Asda*	1 Pack/644g	972	27.7	151	6.0	22.0	4.3	0.9
Chicken, with Basmati Rice, Weight Watchers*	1 Pack/330g	238	1.6	72	5.0	11.8	0.5	0.5
Chicken, with Lemon Pilau Rice, Finest, Tesco*	1 Pack/493g	665	21.7	135	6.9	16.4	4.4	1.8
Chicken, with Pilau Basmati Rice, Frozen, Patak's*	1 Pack/400g	556	18.4	139	9.8	14.7	4.6	0.9
Chicken, with Pilau Rice, Asda*	1 Pack/450g	568	13.5	126	7.1	16.1	3.0	3.2
Chicken, with Pilau Rice, BGTY, Sainsbury's*	1 Pack/400g	337	4.4	84	7.1	11.5	1.1	1.9
Chicken, with Pilau Rice, GFY, Asda*	1 Pack/446g	495	11.1	111	8.0	14.0	2.5	1.2
Chicken, with Pilau Rice, Perfectly Balanced, Waitrose*	1 Pack/400g	388	4.0	97	8.0	14.0	1.0	2.4
Chicken, with Pilau Rice, Tesco*	1 Pack/460g	506	17.5	110	5.3	13.6	3.8	0.9
Chicken, with Rice, COU, M & S*	1 Pack/400g	320	4.4	80	9.2	8.3	1.1	1.2
Chicken, with Rice, Morrisons*	1 Pack/400g	564	20.8	141	7.7	15.9	5.2	1.4
Chicken, with Rice, Tesco*	1 Pack/550g	731	26.4	133	5.5	17.0	4.8	1.0
Meal for One, M & S*	1 Serving/500g	700	35.0	140	6.1	13.4	7.0	3.0
Vegetable, Co-Op*	1 Pack/400g	320	16.0	80	1.0	9.0	4.0	2.0
Vegetable, Eastern Indian, Sainsbury's*	1 Pack/400g	208	13.6	52	3.4	2.0	3.4	1.7
Vegetable, Indian, Sainsbury's*	½ Pack/200g	156	9.0	78	2.0	5.3	4.5	4.2
Vegetable, Waitrose*	1 Pack/400g	256	16.0	64	2.2	4.7	4.0	3.7
Vegetable, with Rice, Birds Eye*	1 Pack/350g	353	3.9	101	2.5	20.2	1.1	1.0
JAM								
Apricot, Average	*1 Tbsp/15g*	*37*	*0.0*	*248*	*0.2*	*61.6*	*0.0*	*1.5*
Apricot, Reduced Sugar, Average	*1 Serving/20g*	*37*	*0.1*	*186*	*0.4*	*46.0*	*0.3*	*0.4*
Apricot, Reduced Sugar, Weight Watchers*	1 Tsp/15g	23	0.0	153	0.5	37.5	0.1	1.2
Black Cherry, Average	*1 Tsp/5g*	*12*	*0.0*	*247*	*0.4*	*61.2*	*0.3*	*0.4*
Blackberry, Extra Special, Asda*	1 Tbsp/15g	29	0.1	190	0.9	45.0	0.7	0.0
Blackcurrant, Average	*1 Tbsp/15g*	*38*	*0.0*	*250*	*0.2*	*62.3*	*0.0*	*1.0*
Blackcurrant, Reduced Sugar, Average	*1 Tsp/6g*	*10*	*0.0*	*178*	*0.4*	*44.4*	*0.1*	*1.0*
Blackcurrant, Reduced Sugar, Weight Watchers*	1 Tsp/15g	22	0.0	144	0.5	35.3	0.1	3.1
Blueberry, Best, Hartley's*	1 Tsp/20g	49	0.0	244	0.3	60.6	0.1	0.0
Blueberry & Blackberry, Baxters*	1 Tsp/15g	38	0.0	252	0.0	63.0	0.0	1.2
Country Berries, Luxury, Baxters*	1 Tsp/15g	38	0.0	252	0.0	63.0	0.0	1.1
Damson, Extra Fruit, Best, Hartley's*	1 Tsp/5g	12	0.0	244	0.2	60.8	0.0	0.0
Golden Peach, Rhapsodie De Fruit, St Dalfour*	1 Tsp/10g	23	0.0	227	0.5	56.0	0.1	1.3
Mixed Fruit, Average	*1 Tbsp/15g*	*38*	*0.0*	*252*	*0.3*	*63.5*	*0.0*	*0.5*
Raspberry, Average	*1 Tbsp/15g*	*36*	*0.0*	*239*	*0.6*	*58.6*	*0.1*	*0.9*
Raspberry, GFY, Asda*	1 Tbsp/19g	24	0.1	124	0.6	29.0	0.6	1.5
Raspberry, Reduced Sugar, Average	*1 Tsp/6g*	*10*	*0.0*	*160*	*0.5*	*39.3*	*0.2*	*0.6*
Raspberry, Reduced Sugar, Weight Watchers*	1 Tsp/15g	22	0.0	149	0.7	36.1	0.2	2.9
Raspberry, Seedless, Average	*1 Tsp/10g*	*26*	*0.0*	*257*	*0.4*	*63.6*	*0.0*	*0.3*
Rhubarb & Ginger, Baxters*	1 Tsp/15g	31	0.0	210	0.0	53.0	0.0	0.6
Strawberry, Average	*1 Tsp/10g*	*25*	*0.0*	*253*	*0.3*	*62.7*	*0.0*	*0.6*
Strawberry, Reduced Sugar, Average	*1 Tbsp/15g*	*28*	*0.0*	*187*	*0.4*	*45.8*	*0.3*	*0.2*
Strawberry & Redcurrant, Reduced Sugar, Streamline*	1 Tbsp/15g	29	0.0	192	0.4	46.8	0.3	0.0
Strawberry & Vanilla, Best, Hartley's*	1 Tsp/5g	12	0.0	244	0.4	60.6	0.0	0.0

J

	Measure INFO/WEIGHT	per Measure KCAL	FAT	Nutrition Values per 100g / 100ml KCAL	PROT	CARB	FAT	FIBRE
JAM								
Wild Blackberry Jelly, Baxters*	1 Tsp/15g	31	0.0	210	0.0	53.0	0.0	1.2
JAMBALAYA								
American Style, Tesco*	1 Serving/275g	432	19.2	157	7.7	16.0	7.0	0.5
Cajun Chicken, BGTY, Sainsbury's*	1 Pack/400g	364	5.6	91	7.7	11.9	1.4	1.1
COU, M & S*	1 Pack/400g	340	8.0	85	6.5	10.8	2.0	0.9
GFY, Asda*	1 Pack/450g	387	3.1	86	6.0	14.0	0.7	2.7
M & S*	1 Pack/480g	552	16.8	115	5.8	14.6	3.5	1.2
Tesco*	1 Pack/550g	764	36.3	139	6.9	13.1	6.6	1.1
JELLY								
Apple & Watermelon, Low Calorie, Hartley's*	1 Serving/175g	5	0.0	3	0.0	0.3	0.0	0.3
Blackberry, Unprepared, Morrisons*	1 Serving/20g	52	0.0	261	0.3	65.0	0.0	0.0
Blackcurrant, Made Up, Rowntree's*	¼ Jelly/140ml	100	0.1	71	1.4	16.4	0.1	0.0
Blackcurrant, Made Up, Sainsbury's*	¼ Jelly/150g	97	0.0	65	1.2	15.1	0.0	0.0
Blackcurrant, Sugar Free, Unprepared, Rowntree's*	1 Pack/24g	73	0.0	305	50.0	25.0	0.0	25.0
Blackcurrant, Tesco*	1 Serving/100g	84	0.1	84	0.2	20.5	0.1	0.4
Bramble, Tesco*	1 Serving/100g	257	0.1	257	0.3	63.7	0.1	1.3
Crystals, Orange, Sugar Free, Bird's*	1 Sachet/12g	39	0.1	335	62.5	6.4	0.9	0.0
Crystals, Strawberry, Made Up, Tesco*	1 Serving/145g	9	0.0	6	1.3	0.3	0.0	0.0
Crystals Apple & Blackcurrant, Weight Watchers*	1 Packet/204g	14	0.2	7	0.1	1.4	0.1	0.1
Exotic Fruit, M & S*	1 Pot/175g	140	0.3	80	0.1	18.9	0.2	0.9
Fresh Fruit, M & S*	1 Pot/175g	131	0.2	75	0.2	18.4	0.1	0.3
Fruitini, Del Monte*	1 Serving/120g	78	0.1	65	0.3	15.3	0.1	0.5
Lemon, Unprepared, Co-Op*	1 Pack/135g	412	0.0	305	5.0	71.0	0.0	0.0
Lime, Made Up, Rowntree's*	¼ Jelly/140ml	100	0.1	71	1.3	16.3	0.1	0.0
Lime, Unprepared, Co-Op*	1 Pack/135g	397	0.1	294	5.5	68.1	0.0	1.0
Lime Flavour, Unprepared, Waitrose*	1 Square/11g	33	0.0	296	4.5	69.5	0.0	0.0
Made Up with Water, Average	*1oz/28g*	*17*	*0.0*	*61*	*1.2*	*15.1*	*0.0*	*0.0*
Mandarin & Pineapple, Sainsbury's*	1 Pot/125g	95	0.1	76	0.2	18.9	0.1	1.2
Mixed Berry, WT5, Sainsbury's*	1 Serving/160g	112	0.3	70	0.7	16.3	0.2	1.5
Orange, Sugar Free, Crystals, Dry Weight, Hartley's*	1 Pack/26g	66	0.0	254	57.4	6.1	0.0	0.0
Orange, Sugar Free, Made Up, Hartley's*	1 Serving/140ml	8	0.0	6	1.4	0.1	0.0	0.0
Orange, Sugar Free, Rowntree's*	1 Serving/140ml	8	0.0	6	1.4	0.1	0.0	0.0
Orange, Sugar Free, Unprepared, Asda*	1 Serving/12g	36	0.0	303	63.6	12.0	0.1	0.2
Orange, Unprepared, Rowntree's*	1 Square/11g	33	0.0	296	4.4	69.6	0.0	0.0
Peach Melba, Eat Well, M & S*	1 Pot/175g	114	0.3	65	0.2	15.9	0.2	0.2
Pineapple, with Pineapple Pieces, Tesco*	1 Serving/120g	96	0.1	80	1.2	18.6	0.1	0.7
Raspberry, Crystals, Vegetarian, Just Wholefoods*	1 Packet/85g	293	0.0	345	0.5	85.7	0.0	0.0
Raspberry, Unprepared, Co-Op*	1 Pack/135g	402	0.1	298	5.5	68.9	0.0	0.0
Raspberry, Unprepared, Rowntree's*	1 Serving/135g	405	0.5	300	5.6	67.3	0.4	0.0
Raspberry Flavour, Sugar Free, Made Up, Rowntree's*	1 Serving/140ml	9	0.0	6	1.4	0.1	0.0	0.0
Raspberry Flavour, Tesco*	1 Serving/34g	22	0.0	64	1.0	15.0	0.0	0.1
Raspberry Flavoured, with Raspberries, M & S*	1 Sm Pot/175g	105	0.5	60	0.2	14.0	0.3	1.5
Redcurrant, Average	*1oz/28g*	*70*	*0.0*	*250*	*0.1*	*64.4*	*0.0*	*0.0*
Strawberry, No Added Sugar, Hartley's*	1 Pot/115g	3	0.0	3	0.0	0.4	0.0	0.3
Strawberry, Sugar Free, Crystals, Dry Weight, Hartley's*	1 Sachet/26g	73	0.0	280	56.8	13.1	0.0	0.0
Strawberry, Unprepared, Co-Op*	1 Pack/135g	402	0.1	298	5.5	69.1	0.0	0.0
Strawberry & Raspberry, Sainsbury's*	½ Pot/280g	230	0.0	82	0.2	20.2	0.0	1.2
Strawberry Flavour, Sugar Free, Made Up, Rowntree's*	1 Serving/140ml	10	0.0	7	1.5	0.1	0.0	0.0
Sugar Free, Dry, Tesco*	1 Pack/13g	36	0.0	285	55.4	15.6	0.0	0.2
Tangerine, Unprepared, Rowntree's*	1 Serving/33g	99	0.1	300	5.6	67.3	0.4	0.0
Tropical Fruit, Way to Five, Sainsbury's*	1 Serving/160g	144	1.6	90	0.3	19.9	1.0	0.9
Unprepared, Hartley's*	1 Serving/31g	92	0.0	296	5.1	68.9	0.0	0.0

J

	Measure INFO/WEIGHT	per Measure KCAL	FAT	Nutrition Values per 100g / 100ml KCAL	PROT	CARB	FAT	FIBRE
JELLY BABIES								
Bassett's*	1 Jelly/6g	20	0.0	335	4.0	79.5	0.0	0.0
M & S*	1 Pack/125g	417	0.0	334	5.2	78.0	0.0	0.0
Mini, Rowntree's*	1 Bag/35g	128	0.0	366	4.6	86.9	0.0	0.0
Mini, Waitrose*	1 Bag/125g	370	0.5	296	4.3	68.7	0.4	0.0
Sainsbury's*	1 Serving/70g	247	0.5	353	4.1	82.5	0.7	0.3
JELLY BEANS								
Asda*	1 Bag/100g	364	0.4	364	0.1	90.0	0.4	0.2
Jelly Belly*	35 Beans/40g	140	0.0	350	0.0	90.0	0.0	0.0
M & S*	1 Bag/113g	407	0.0	360	0.1	89.6	0.0	0.0
No Added Sugar, Jelly Belly*	1 Serving/40g	80	0.0	200	0.0	50.0	0.0	20.0
Rowntree's*	1 Pack/35g	128	0.0	367	0.0	91.8	0.0	0.0
JELLY BEARS								
Co-Op*	1 Sweet/3g	10	0.0	325	6.0	76.0	0.1	0.0
JELLY TOTS								
Rowntree's*	1 Pack/42g	145	0.0	346	0.1	86.5	0.0	0.0
JERKY								
Beef, Peppered, Jack Link's*	1 Serving/28g	80	0.5	286	53.6	14.3	1.8	0.0
Soy, Cajun Chick'n, Vegan, Tasty Eats*	1 Pack/28g	90	3.0	321	42.9	14.3	10.7	7.1
JUICE								
Apple, Concentrate, Average	*1 Tbsp/15ml*	*45*	*0.0*	*302*	*0.0*	*73.5*	*0.1*	*0.0*
Apple, Pure, Average	*1 Glass/100ml*	*47*	*0.0*	*47*	*0.1*	*11.2*	*0.0*	*0.0*
Apple, Pure, Organic, Average	*1 Glass/200ml*	*92*	*0.1*	*46*	*0.0*	*11.1*	*0.0*	*0.0*
Apple & Cranberry, Average	*1 Glass/250ml*	*114*	*0.0*	*45*	*0.1*	*10.1*	*0.0*	*0.0*
Apple & Elderflower, Copella*	1 Glass/250ml	107	0.2	43	0.4	10.2	0.1	0.0
Apple & Mango, Average	*1 Glass/200ml*	*108*	*0.1*	*54*	*0.3*	*12.6*	*0.0*	*0.1*
Apple & Raspberry, Average	*1 Serving/200ml*	*89*	*0.1*	*44*	*0.4*	*10.1*	*0.0*	*0.1*
Apple & Rhubarb, Pressed, Cawston Press*	1 Glass/200ml	92	0.8	46	0.2	9.7	0.4	0.0
Beetroot, Organic, James White*	1 Glass/250ml	105	0.2	42	0.9	9.3	0.1	0.0
Beetroot & Evesse Apple, Sunraysia*	1 Glass/200ml	262	0.0	131	0.4	7.3	0.0	0.0
Blackberry, Vita, Co-Op*	1 Glass/200ml	110	0.0	55	0.0	13.0	0.0	0.5
Breakfast, Ruby, Tropicana*	1 Glass/200ml	90	0.0	45	0.8	9.7	0.0	0.7
Breakfast, Sainsbury's*	1 Glass/200ml	94	0.2	47	0.7	11.3	0.1	0.3
Carrot, Average	*1 Glass/200ml*	*48*	*0.2*	*24*	*0.5*	*5.7*	*0.1*	*0.0*
Cherry, Original, Cherrygood*	1 Glass/250ml	112	0.2	45	0.0	10.5	0.1	0.0
Clementine, Morrisons*	1 Serving/100ml	48	0.1	48	0.5	10.9	0.1	0.1
Coconut, Foco*	1 Can/520ml	182	1.1	35	0.1	8.2	0.2	0.0
Cranberry, Average	*1 Bottle/250ml*	*139*	*0.2*	*56*	*0.1*	*13.4*	*0.1*	*0.3*
Cranberry, No Added Sugar, Average	*1 Glass/200ml*	*11*	*0.1*	*5*	*0.1*	*0.8*	*0.0*	*0.0*
Exotic Fruit, Pure, Del Monte*	1 Glass/200ml	96	0.0	48	0.3	11.3	0.0	0.0
Exotic Fruit, Waitrose*	1 Glass/175ml	87	0.0	50	0.4	11.6	0.0	0.0
Fibre, Tropicana*	1 Serving/200ml	130	0.0	65	0.4	15.8	0.0	3.4
Go!, Tropicana*	1 Bottle/200ml	80	0.0	40	0.3	9.7	0.0	0.0
Grape, Purple, Light, Welch's*	1 Serving/100ml	27	0.3	27	0.2	6.1	0.3	0.3
Grape, Purple, Welch's*	1 Serving/200ml	136	0.0	68	0.1	16.5	0.0	0.0
Grape, Red, Average	*1 Serving/100ml*	*62*	*0.0*	*62*	*0.1*	*15.1*	*0.0*	*0.0*
Grape, White, Average	*1 Can/160ml*	*95*	*0.1*	*59*	*0.2*	*14.3*	*0.1*	*0.1*
Grape & Peach, Don Simon*	1 Serving/200ml	94	0.0	47	0.4	11.3	0.0	0.0
Grape & Raspberry, Pressed, M & S*	1 Carton/330ml	181	0.3	55	0.4	12.9	0.1	0.1
Grapefruit, Pink, Average	*1 Glass/200ml*	*81*	*0.1*	*40*	*0.6*	*9.0*	*0.0*	*0.2*
Grapefruit, Pure, Average	*1 Glass/200ml*	*77*	*0.2*	*38*	*0.5*	*8.5*	*0.1*	*0.1*
Lemon, Fresh, Average	*1 Juiced/36ml*	*2*	*0.0*	*7*	*0.3*	*1.6*	*0.0*	*0.1*
Lime, Fresh, Average	*1 Tsp/5ml*	*0*	*0.0*	*9*	*0.4*	*1.6*	*0.1*	*0.1*
Mango, Peach, Papaya, Pure, Premium, Tropicana*	1 Glass/200ml	88	0.0	44	0.5	9.8	0.0	0.1

J

	Measure INFO/WEIGHT	per Measure KCAL	FAT	Nutrition Values per 100g / 100ml KCAL	PROT	CARB	FAT	FIBRE
JUICE								
Mango, Pure, Canned	**1 Glass/250ml**	**97**	**0.5**	**39**	**0.1**	**9.8**	**0.2**	**0.0**
Orange, Apple & Mango, Calypso*	1 Carton/200ml	92	0.4	46	0.0	11.0	0.2	0.1
Orange, C, No Added Sugar, Libby's*	1 Serving/250ml	32	0.0	13	0.1	2.7	0.0	0.1
Orange, Freshly Squeezed, Average	1 Serving/200ml	66	0.0	33	0.6	8.1	0.0	1.0
Orange, Pure, Smooth, Average	**1 Glass/200ml**	**88**	**0.1**	**44**	**0.7**	**9.8**	**0.0**	**0.2**
Orange, Pure, with Bits, Average	**1 Glass/200ml**	**90**	**0.1**	**45**	**0.6**	**10.2**	**0.1**	**0.1**
Orange, Red, Average	**1 Glass/250ml**	**115**	**0.1**	**46**	**0.4**	**10.7**	**0.0**	**0.2**
Orange & Banana, Pure, Average	**1 Glass/150ml**	**79**	**0.1**	**53**	**0.7**	**12.1**	**0.1**	**0.2**
Orange & Carrot, Love Life, Waitrose*	1 Serving/150ml	57	0.3	38	0.6	8.5	0.2	1.2
Orange & Grapefruit, Average	**1 Serving/200ml**	**84**	**0.2**	**42**	**0.7**	**9.2**	**0.1**	**0.4**
Orange & Kiwi Fruit, Tropicana*	1 Serving/175ml	90	0.0	51	0.5	12.0	0.0	0.0
Orange & Lime, Tropicana*	1 Serving/250ml	115	0.0	46	1.1	9.4	0.0	0.6
Orange & Mango, Average	**1 Bottle/375ml**	**176**	**0.4**	**47**	**0.5**	**10.7**	**0.1**	**0.2**
Orange & Passionfruit, Tropicana*	1 Serving/200ml	94	0.0	47	0.8	10.0	0.0	0.7
Orange & Pineapple, Average	**1 Glass/120ml**	**56**	**0.6**	**46**	**0.4**	**10.5**	**0.5**	**0.5**
Orange & Raspberry, Average	**1 fl oz/30ml**	**15**	**0.0**	**50**	**0.6**	**11.4**	**0.1**	**0.2**
Orange & Strawberry, Average	**1 Serving/125ml**	**64**	**0.5**	**51**	**0.6**	**10.9**	**0.4**	**0.8**
Passion Fruit, Average	**1 Glass/200ml**	**94**	**0.2**	**47**	**0.8**	**10.7**	**0.1**	**0.0**
Peach, Mango & Passion Fruit, Sainsbury's*	1 Glass/200ml	92	0.2	46	0.3	10.3	0.1	0.5
Pear, Pure, Heinz*	1 Serving/100ml	41	0.1	41	0.1	9.8	0.1	0.0
Pear, with a Hint of Ginger, Pressed, M & S*	1 Glass/250ml	125	0.2	50	0.3	11.7	0.1	0.0
Pineapple, Average	**1 Glass/200ml**	**100**	**0.1**	**50**	**0.3**	**11.7**	**0.1**	**0.1**
Pineapple & Coconut, Waitrose*	1 Serving/250ml	125	0.7	50	0.2	11.5	0.3	0.2
Pineapple & Guava, Tropicana*	1 Glass/200ml	106	0.0	53	0.3	12.3	0.0	1.2
Pomegranate, Grape & Apple, Tropicana*	1 Bottle/330ml	211	0.0	64	0.2	15.5	0.0	0.6
Pomegranate, Pomegreat*	1 Glass/200ml	88	0.0	44	0.1	11.1	0.0	0.0
Pomegranate with Cherry, Pomegreat*	1 Serving/200ml	75	0.0	37	0.1	8.8	0.0	0.1
Prune, Average	**1 Serving/200ml**	**123**	**0.1**	**61**	**0.6**	**15.3**	**0.1**	**1.8**
Simpleberry 100 Purple, Pressed, The Berry Company*	1 Glass/200ml	122	0.2	61	0.6	14.0	0.1	0.1
Tomato, Average	**1 Glass/200ml**	**40**	**0.1**	**20**	**0.7**	**4.0**	**0.0**	**0.4**
Tropical, Pure, Sainsbury's*	1 Glass/200ml	104	0.2	52	0.5	12.0	0.1	0.1
Vegetable, Organic, Evernat*	1 Glass/200ml	36	0.2	18	0.9	3.5	0.1	0.2
White Apple & Ginger, James White*	1 Glass/250ml	122	0.0	49	0.1	11.8	0.0	0.0
JUICE DRINK								
Apple, Cranberry, & Blueberry, Waitrose*	1 Serving/150ml	75	0.0	50	0.1	11.9	0.0	0.1
Apple, No Added Sugar, Asda*	1 Glass/200ml	10	0.0	5	0.0	1.0	0.0	0.0
Apple & Blueberry, The Feel Good Drinks Co*	1 Serving/375ml	163	0.4	43	0.1	10.6	0.1	0.0
Apple & Elderflower, Tesco*	1 Serving/200ml	76	0.0	38	0.0	9.4	0.0	0.0
Apple & Mango, Chosen By You, Asda*	1 Carton/250ml	115	0.0	46	0.0	11.0	0.0	0.0
Apple & Raspberry, Sainsbury's*	1 Serving/200ml	112	0.2	56	0.1	13.8	0.1	0.1
Apple & Strawberry, Sainsbury's*	1 Serving/250ml	13	0.1	5	0.0	1.0	0.0	0.0
Berry Blast, 5 Alive*	1 Glass/200ml	50	0.0	25	0.0	6.1	0.0	0.0
Blackcurrant, 45% High, No Added Sugar, Asda*	1 Serving/25ml	2	0.0	7	0.0	1.4	0.0	0.0
Blackcurrant, CVit*	1 Glass/200ml	4	0.0	2	0.0	0.2	0.0	0.0
Blackcurrant, Extra Light, Ribena*	1 Serving/200ml	8	0.0	4	0.0	0.5	0.0	0.0
Blackcurrant & Apple, Oasis*	1 Serving/500ml	90	0.0	18	0.0	4.1	0.0	0.0
Blueberry, BGTY, Sainsbury's*	1 Serving/250ml	15	0.0	6	0.1	1.0	0.0	0.0
Cherry, No Added Sugar, Sainsbury's*	1 Carton/250ml	25	0.1	10	0.2	1.9	0.0	0.0
Citrus Burst, 5 Alive*	1 Carton/250ml	125	0.0	50	0.0	12.8	0.0	0.0
Cranberry, Classic, Ocean Spray*	1 Bottle/500ml	245	0.5	49	0.1	11.7	0.1	0.1
Cranberry, Grape & Apple, Ocean Spray*	1 Glass/200ml	108	0.0	54	0.1	12.9	0.0	0.0
Cranberry, Light, Classic, Ocean Spray*	1 Glass/200ml	16	0.0	8	0.0	1.4	0.0	0.0
Cranberry, Original, Concentrated, Ocean Spray*	1 Serving/15ml	27	0.0	183	0.2	44.1	0.0	0.0

J

	Measure INFO/WEIGHT	per Measure KCAL	FAT	Nutrition Values per 100g / 100ml KCAL	PROT	CARB	FAT	FIBRE
JUICE DRINK								
Cranberry, Tropical, Ocean Spray*	1 Glass/200ml	96	0.0	48	0.1	11.5	0.0	0.0
Cranberry & Apple, Ocean Spray*	1 Glass/200ml	92	0.0	46	0.0	11.1	0.0	0.0
Cranberry & Blackberry, Ocean Spray*	1 Glass/250ml	120	0.2	48	0.1	11.3	0.1	0.2
Cranberry & Blackcurrant, Ocean Spray*	1 Bottle/500ml	265	0.0	53	0.2	12.7	0.0	0.0
Cranberry & Blueberry, Ocean Spray*	1 Serving/100ml	48	0.0	48	0.0	11.6	0.0	0.0
Cranberry & Mango, Light, Ocean Spray*	1 Glass/250ml	22	0.0	9	0.0	2.0	0.0	0.1
Cranberry & Orange, No Added Sugar, Sainsbury's*	1 Glass/250ml	15	0.2	6	0.1	1.2	0.1	0.1
Cranberry & Pomegranate, Ocean Spray*	1 Glass/250ml	120	0.0	48	0.0	11.5	0.0	0.0
Cranberry & Raspberry, BGTY, Sainsbury's*	1 Glass/250ml	10	0.2	4	0.1	0.7	0.1	0.1
Cranberry & Raspberry, Ocean Spray*	1 Glass/200ml	104	0.0	52	0.0	12.6	0.0	0.0
Exotic, Tesco*	1 Serving/250ml	127	0.0	51	0.1	12.3	0.0	0.0
Forest Fruits, Asda*	1 200ml/200ml	88	0.0	44	0.3	10.9	0.0	0.3
Fruit Cocktail, Sainsbury's*	1 Glass/200ml	90	0.0	45	0.2	10.6	0.0	0.1
Grape, Apple & Raspberry, Asda*	1 Glass/200ml	90	0.0	45	0.2	11.0	0.0	0.0
Grape, Red, Sparkling, Schloer*	1 Glass/200ml	84	0.0	42	0.0	10.4	0.0	0.0
Grape, White, Sparkling, Schloer*	1 Serving/120ml	59	0.0	49	0.0	11.6	0.0	0.0
Grape & Elderflower, White, Sparkling, Schloer*	1 Glass/200ml	74	0.0	37	0.0	9.2	0.0	0.0
Grapefruit & Cranberry, M & S*	1 Serving/250ml	125	0.2	50	0.2	11.9	0.1	0.0
Grapefruit & Lime, Quest, M & S*	1 Bottle/330ml	53	0.0	16	0.0	4.0	0.0	0.0
J20, Apple & Mango, Britvic*	1 Bottle/275ml	118	0.0	43	0.1	10.0	0.0	0.2
J20, Apple & Raspberry, Britvic*	1 Bottle/275ml	146	0.3	53	0.1	12.0	0.1	0.0
J20, Orange & Passion Fruit, Britvic*	1 Bottle/275ml	132	0.2	48	0.1	11.3	0.1	0.0
Lemon & Lime, Light, Oasis*	1 Bottle/250ml	6	0.0	3	0.0	0.2	0.0	0.0
Lemon & Mandarin, Diet, Quest, M & S*	1 Bottle/330ml	13	0.0	4	0.0	1.0	0.0	0.0
Mango, Rubicon*	1 Serving/100ml	54	0.1	54	0.1	13.1	0.1	0.0
Mango Madness, Snapple*	1 Bottle/227ml	104	0.0	46	0.0	12.0	0.0	0.0
Orange, Caprisun*	1 Pouch/200ml	89	0.0	45	0.0	10.8	0.0	0.0
Orange, Juice Burst, Purity*	1 Bottle/500ml	220	0.0	44	1.0	10.2	0.0	0.0
Orange, Mango & Lime, Fruit Crush, Shapers, Boots*	1 Bottle/330ml	150	0.6	45	0.4	10.6	0.2	0.4
Orange, Morrisons*	1 Serving/250ml	12	0.2	5	0.1	0.9	0.1	0.1
Passion Fruit, Exotic, Rubicon*	1 Serving/200ml	110	0.0	55	0.1	13.6	0.0	0.0
Peach, Passion Fruit, Extra Light, Oasis*	1 Bottle/500ml	17	0.0	3	0.0	0.6	0.0	0.0
Pear & Plum, Shapers, Boots*	1 Bottle/500ml	10	0.0	2	0.0	0.2	0.0	0.0
Pineapple, Mango & Passionfruit, Sainsbury's*	1 Serving/200ml	74	0.0	37	0.1	8.7	0.0	0.2
Pineapple & Grapefruit, Shapers, Boots*	1 Bottle/500ml	10	0.5	2	0.1	0.2	0.1	0.0
Pink Grapefruit, Juice Burst, Purity*	1 Bottle/500ml	210	0.0	42	0.4	10.0	0.0	0.0
Pomegranate, Rubicon*	1 Can/330mll	108	0.0	54	0.0	13.5	0.0	0.0
Pomegranate & Blueberry, Weight Watchers*	1 Bottle/500ml	15	0.0	3	0.0	0.5	0.0	0.0
Pomegranate & Raspberry, Still, Shapers, Boots*	1 Bottle/500ml	45	0.0	9	0.0	2.0	0.0	0.0
Raspberry & Pear, Tesco*	1 Serving/250ml	117	0.0	47	0.0	11.3	0.0	0.0
Summer Fruits, Fresh, Tesco*	1 Glass/250ml	112	0.2	45	0.1	10.8	0.1	0.3
Summer Fruits, Oasis*	1 Bottle/500ml	90	0.0	18	0.0	4.2	0.0	0.0
Tropical, No Added Sugar, Tesco*	1 Carton/250ml	12	0.0	5	0.0	1.1	0.0	0.0
Tropical Fruit, Tesco*	1 Glass/250ml	117	0.0	47	0.0	11.4	0.0	0.0
Tropical Hit, 5 Alive*	1 Carton/250ml	92	0.0	37	0.0	9.3	0.0	0.0
White Cranberry & Grape, Ocean Spray*	1 Serving/100ml	48	0.0	48	0.0	11.6	0.0	0.0
White Cranberry & Lychee, Ocean Spray*	1 Glass/200ml	86	0.0	43	0.0	11.5	0.0	0.0
White Grape & Peach, Sainsbury's*	1 Glass/250ml	95	0.2	38	0.2	9.0	0.1	0.1
JUNIPER								
Berries, Dried, Average	1 Tsp/2g	6	0.3	292	4.0	33.0	16.0	0.0

J

	Measure INFO/WEIGHT	per Measure KCAL	FAT	Nutrition Values per 100g / 100ml KCAL	PROT	CARB	FAT	FIBRE
KALE								
Curly, Boiled in Salted Water, Average	*1 Serving/60g*	*14*	*0.7*	*24*	*2.4*	*1.0*	*1.1*	*2.8*
Curly, Raw, Average	*1 Serving/90g*	*30*	*1.4*	*33*	*3.4*	*1.4*	*1.6*	*3.1*
KANGAROO								
Raw, Average	*1 Serving/200g*	*196*	*2.0*	*98*	*22.0*	*1.0*	*1.0*	*0.0*
Steak, Grilled, Average	*1 Fillet/150g*	*198*	*1.8*	*132*	*30.0*	*0.0*	*1.2*	*0.0*
KEBAB								
Beef, Hot & Spicy, Tesco*	1 Kebab/41g	111	8.4	270	15.7	4.4	20.6	1.6
Beef, Kofta, Uncooked, Tesco*	1 Kebab/73g	163	12.5	225	14.0	3.2	17.3	1.2
Beef & Pepper Kofta, Waitrose*	1 Kebab/138g	223	13.9	162	14.8	2.9	10.1	0.6
Beef with Sweet Chilli Seasoning, Sainsbury's*	1 Kebab/61g	151	8.0	248	24.1	8.5	13.1	0.8
Cajun Salmon, Tesco*	1 Kebab/75g	100	3.1	133	19.8	3.9	4.2	1.3
Chicken, Barbecue, Sainsbury's*	1 Pack/200g	238	3.4	119	24.4	1.5	1.7	1.8
Chicken, Breast, Mediterranean, Sainsbury's*	1 Kebab/65g	73	2.1	113	16.5	4.6	3.2	0.6
Chicken, Breast, Salsa, Sainsbury's*	1 Kebab/80g	94	0.9	117	20.1	6.5	1.1	0.6
Chicken, Breast, Sweet, Oriental, COU, M & S*	½ Pack/200g	220	2.0	110	20.8	4.3	1.0	0.1
Chicken, Caribbean, Iceland*	1 Kebab/44g	36	0.1	82	12.0	8.0	0.2	0.5
Chicken, Chilli & Lime, Breast Fillet, Sainsbury's*	1 Kebab/77g	120	0.7	156	29.9	6.2	0.9	0.3
Chicken, Red Pepper, Mini, Sainsbury's*	1 Kebab/52g	79	1.0	152	30.1	3.5	2.0	0.2
Chicken, Shish, Meat Only, Average	1 Kebab/250g	312	5.2	125	25.7	0.9	2.1	0.1
Chicken, Shish in Pitta Bread with Salad	1 Kebab/250g	387	10.2	155	13.5	17.2	4.1	1.0
Chicken, Sweet Chilli, Perfectly Balanced, Waitrose*	1 Kebab/83g	111	0.9	135	28.6	1.7	1.1	0.5
Chicken, Thigh, Sticky Barbecue, M & S*	1 Kebab/100g	160	7.5	160	15.6	7.4	7.5	0.8
Chicken Tikka, with Red Pepper & Pineapple, Tesco*	1 Kebab/80g	92	1.9	115	16.5	6.7	2.4	0.5
Doner, Heat 'n' Eat Thin Sliced, Asda*	1 Pack/100g	196	10.6	196	16.7	8.4	10.6	1.7
Green Thai Chicken, Waitrose*	1 Serving/180g	223	7.2	124	20.5	1.4	4.0	1.4
Halloumi & Vegetable, Waitrose*	1 Kebab/127g	235	21.6	185	5.6	2.2	17.0	2.4
Lamb, Greek Style, Sainsbury's*	1 Serving/70g	196	15.3	282	16.1	4.9	22.0	1.8
Lamb, Shish, Waitrose*	1 Kebab/56g	114	7.1	203	15.3	6.8	12.7	1.1
Lamb, Shoulder, M & S*	½ Pack/250g	312	10.7	125	20.4	0.9	4.3	1.7
Lamb, with Halloumi Cheese & Olives, Waitrose*	1 Kebab/75g	123	6.2	164	20.0	2.4	8.3	0.2
Lamb, with Mint, Tesco*	1 Serving/80g	192	13.4	240	16.0	5.5	16.7	0.4
Lamb Kofta, Indian Style, Waitrose*	1 Kebab/125g	266	19.7	213	12.3	5.5	15.8	1.6
Lamb Shami with a Mint Raita Dip, M & S*	½ Pack/90g	189	12.1	210	12.8	9.7	13.4	3.5
Lemon & Ginger Chicken, Delicatezze, Waitrose*	1 Kebab/25g	50	2.8	201	24.5	0.3	11.3	2.7
Pork & Pepper, BBQ, Sainsbury's*	1 Kebab/41g	65	2.2	158	24.1	3.1	5.4	1.9
Salmon, Hot & Spicy, Tesco*	1 Kebab/75g	88	2.2	118	22.0	1.1	2.9	0.0
Sweetcorn, Tesco*	1 Kebab/130g	74	1.3	57	2.0	9.9	1.0	0.9
Tikka, Mini, M & S*	1 Kebab/11g	23	1.4	205	18.4	4.0	12.7	0.6
Turkey, with Chinese Style Dressing, Sainsbury's*	1 Kebab/54g	84	2.7	157	21.4	6.4	5.1	1.7
Vegetable, Asda*	1 Kebab/40g	25	1.7	63	1.8	4.5	4.3	2.4
Vegetable, Sainsbury's*	1 Kebab/100g	36	0.5	36	1.5	6.4	0.5	1.2
KEDGEREE								
Average	1oz/28g	48	2.4	171	15.9	7.8	8.7	0.1
COU, M & S*	1 Pack/370g	388	8.1	105	7.6	13.7	2.2	2.1
Smoked Haddock, Big Dish, M & S*	1 Pack/450g	585	22.5	130	8.5	13.0	5.0	1.9
KETCHUP								
BBQ, Heinz*	1 Serving/10g	14	0.0	137	1.3	31.3	0.3	0.3
Mild Chilli, Twisted, Heinz*	1 Tbsp/15g	16	0.0	108	1.0	24.9	0.2	0.7
Tomato, Average	*1 Tsp/5g*	*6*	*0.0*	*120*	*1.5*	*28.1*	*0.2*	*0.8*
Tomato, Reduced Sugar, Average	*1 Tbsp/10g*	*9*	*0.1*	*87*	*2.0*	*16.9*	*1.2*	*0.9*
KIDNEY								
Lamb, Raw, Average	*1oz/28g*	*44*	*2.2*	*156*	*21.5*	*0.0*	*7.7*	*0.0*
Ox, Raw	*1oz/28g*	*25*	*0.6*	*88*	*17.2*	*0.0*	*2.1*	*0.0*

K

	Measure INFO/WEIGHT	per Measure KCAL	FAT	Nutrition Values per 100g / 100ml KCAL	PROT	CARB	FAT	FIBRE
KIDNEY								
Ox, Stewed	*1oz/28g*	*39*	*1.2*	*138*	*24.5*	*0.0*	*4.4*	*0.0*
Pig, Fried	*1oz/28g*	*57*	*2.7*	*202*	*29.2*	*0.0*	*9.5*	*0.0*
Pig, Raw	*1oz/28g*	*24*	*0.8*	*86*	*15.5*	*0.0*	*2.7*	*0.0*
Pig, Stewed	*1oz/28g*	*43*	*1.7*	*153*	*24.4*	*0.0*	*6.1*	*0.0*
Veal, Raw, Average	1 Serving/100g	99	3.1	99	15.8	0.8	3.1	0.0
KIEV								
Cheese & Herb, Mini, Bernard Matthews*	1 Kiev/23g	46	2.3	199	15.7	12.1	9.8	0.0
Chicken, Bernard Matthews*	1 Kiev/125g	374	27.9	299	10.6	13.9	22.3	2.7
Chicken, BFY, Morrisons*	1 Kiev/134g	304	17.4	227	16.1	11.5	13.0	1.0
Chicken, Cheesy Bean, Asda*	1 Kiev/94g	202	10.3	215	12.0	17.0	11.0	1.9
Chicken, COU, M & S*	1 Kiev/150g	187	2.7	125	15.8	10.8	1.8	0.5
Chicken, Creamy Garlic, Chilled, Tesco*	½ Pack/143g	285	17.1	200	12.9	9.7	12.0	1.3
Chicken, Creamy Peppercorn, Sun Valley*	1 Kiev/140g	382	25.9	273	13.3	13.5	18.5	0.0
Chicken, Creamy Peppercorn, Tesco*	1 Kiev/130g	312	20.5	240	11.5	12.0	15.8	1.4
Chicken, Finest, Tesco*	1 Kiev/237g	503	26.6	212	19.5	8.2	11.2	2.6
Chicken, Garlic, 25% Less Fat, GFY, Asda*	1 Kiev/134g	296	15.7	221	17.0	11.9	11.7	0.5
Chicken, Garlic, Fresh, Reduced Fat, Morrisons*	1 Kiev/141g	350	25.5	248	13.2	8.0	18.1	0.7
Chicken, Garlic, M & S*	1 Kiev/150g	370	24.8	247	15.6	8.2	16.5	2.9
Chicken, Garlic, Whole Breast, Asda*	1 Pack/290g	638	38.0	220	15.2	10.4	13.1	0.0
Chicken, Garlic & Herb, Reduced Fat, Sainsbury's*	1 Kiev/142g	317	18.0	223	15.1	12.1	12.7	0.6
Chicken, Garlic & Herb, Sainsbury's*	1 Kiev/134g	319	19.6	239	15.0	11.7	14.7	1.3
Chicken, Garlic & Mushroom, Sainsbury's*	1 Kiev/142g	346	19.1	243	16.2	14.5	13.4	1.4
Chicken, Garlic & Parsley, BGTY, Sainsbury's*	1 Kiev/126g	289	15.3	229	14.0	15.9	12.1	1.1
Chicken, Garlic & Parsley, Sainsbury's*	1 Kiev/120g	365	25.6	304	11.1	17.1	21.3	0.8
Chicken, Good Choice, Iceland*	1 Kiev/120g	366	27.2	305	12.7	12.6	22.7	0.8
Chicken, Ham & Cheese, BGTY, Sainsbury's*	1 Kiev/132g	264	10.2	200	13.2	19.5	7.7	0.8
Chicken, Italian Style, Sainsbury's*	1 Kiev/135g	341	21.7	253	14.3	12.8	16.1	1.3
Chicken, Maitre Jean-Pierre*	1 Kiev/140g	385	26.7	275	13.3	12.7	19.1	0.8
Chicken, Roast Garlic & Parsley, Sainsbury's*	1 Kiev/143g	369	21.3	258	14.5	16.5	14.9	0.8
Chicken, Tomato & Mozzarella, Tesco*	1 Kiev/143g	285	17.4	200	13.4	9.0	12.2	1.4
Chicken Tikka, Asda*	1 Kiev/134g	274	14.8	205	12.8	13.5	11.1	0.6
Garlic, Meat Free, Tesco*	1 Kiev/125g	244	11.2	195	15.0	12.5	9.0	2.6
Salmon, Fillet, Tesco*	1 Kiev/160g	376	19.5	235	13.3	18.0	12.2	2.5
KIEV VEGETARIAN								
Cheesy Garlic, Meat Free, Sainsbury's*	1 Kiev/123g	274	15.1	223	13.8	14.3	12.3	3.5
Garlic, Meat Free, Asda*	1 Kiev/125g	239	11.2	191	15.0	12.5	9.0	2.6
Garlic Butter, Tivall*	1 Kiev/125g	366	26.2	293	15.1	10.8	21.0	2.6
Vegetable, M & S*	1 Kiev/155g	325	20.8	210	4.6	17.8	13.4	2.5
KIPPER								
Baked, Average	*1oz/28g*	*57*	*3.2*	*205*	*25.5*	*0.0*	*11.4*	*0.0*
Fillets, in Brine, John West*	1 Can/140g	269	16.8	192	21.0	0.0	12.0	0.0
Fillets, in Sunflower Oil, John West*	1 Can/140g	321	23.8	229	19.0	0.0	17.0	0.0
Fillets, Raw, Average	*1 Serving/200g*	*451*	*34.3*	*226*	*17.0*	*0.0*	*17.1*	*0.0*
Grilled, Average	*1oz/28g*	*71*	*5.4*	*255*	*20.1*	*0.0*	*19.4*	*0.0*
Smoked, Average	*1 Serving/150g*	*322*	*23.0*	*214*	*18.9*	*0.0*	*15.3*	*0.0*
KIT KAT								
2 Finger, Nestle*	2 Fingers/21g	107	5.4	510	6.4	62.8	25.6	2.3
4 Finger, Nestle*	4 Fingers/46g	233	11.8	512	6.3	62.6	25.9	1.1
Caramac, 4 Finger, Nestle*	4 Fingers/49g	259	14.1	532	5.9	61.9	29.0	0.6
Chunky, Nestle*	1 Bar/50hg	259	14.1	518	5.2	60.9	28.2	1.0
Chunky, Peanut, Nestle*	1 Bar/50g	268	15.7	537	8.4	54.9	31.5	0.0
Chunky, Snack Size, Nestle*	1 Bar/26g	133	7.1	513	6.6	60.4	27.2	1.1
Editions, Mango & Passionfruit, Nestle*	1 Bar/45g	225	10.5	499	4.7	69.0	23.4	0.0

K

INFO/WEIGHT	Measure	per Measure		Nutrition Values per 100g / 100ml				
		KCAL	FAT	KCAL	PROT	CARB	FAT	FIBRE

KIT KAT

Editions, Seville Orange, Nestle*	1 Bar/45g	223	10.3	496	4.6	69.3	23.0	0.8
Kubes, Nestle*	1 Pack/50g	257	13.7	515	5.9	60.9	27.5	1.0
Kubes, Orange, Nestle*	4 Kubes/13g	66	3.5	514	5.7	61.1	27.4	1.0
Low Carb, 2 Finger, Nestle*	2 Fingers/21g	92	6.6	438	9.2	28.3	31.3	1.3
Low Carb, 4 Finger, Nestle*	1 Finger/11g	46	3.3	438	9.2	28.3	31.3	1.3
Mini, Nestle*	1 Bar/15g	75	3.9	502	7.5	59.4	26.0	0.0
Mint, 4 Finger, Nestle*	4 Fingers/48g	244	12.7	508	6.0	61.5	26.4	1.1
Orange, 2 Finger, Nestle*	2 Fingers/21g	107	5.6	507	5.5	61.7	26.5	0.0
Senses, Nestle*	1 Bar/31g	165	9.5	531	7.5	56.3	30.7	0.0
White, Chunky, Nestle*	1 Bar/53g	276	14.6	521	8.3	60.3	27.5	0.7

KIWI FRUIT

Fresh, Raw, Average	*1 Med Kiwi/60g*	*29*	*0.3*	*49*	*1.1*	*10.6*	*0.5*	*1.9*
Weighed with Skin, Average	*1 Kiwi/60g*	*25*	*0.2*	*42*	*1.0*	*9.1*	*0.4*	*1.6*

KOHLRABI

Boiled in Salted Water	*1oz/28g*	*5*	*0.1*	*18*	*1.2*	*3.1*	*0.2*	*1.9*
Raw	*1oz/28g*	*6*	*0.1*	*23*	*1.6*	*3.7*	*0.2*	*2.2*

KORMA

Chicken, & Basmati Rice, Tesco*	1 Pot/350g	588	32.6	168	4.3	16.9	9.3	2.3
Chicken, & Pilau Rice, BGTY, Sainsbury's*	1 Pack/400g	404	5.2	101	8.0	14.3	1.3	0.6
Chicken, & Pilau Rice, GFY, Asda*	1 Pack/400g	600	24.0	150	8.0	16.0	6.0	1.3
Chicken, & Pilau Rice, Tesco*	1 Serving/460g	722	45.1	157	5.6	11.5	9.8	1.3
Chicken, & Rice, 95% Fat Free, Birds Eye*	1 Pack/370g	444	7.0	120	6.2	19.6	1.9	1.1
Chicken, & Rice, Indian Meal for Two, Sainsbury's*	1 Pack/500g	785	40.5	157	6.8	14.3	8.1	3.1
Chicken, & Rice, Light Choices, Tesco*	1 Pack/450g	495	9.0	110	7.2	16.0	2.0	0.8
Chicken, & Rice, Organic, Tesco*	1 Pack/450g	922	47.7	205	6.0	21.5	10.6	0.4
Chicken, & White Rice, BGTY, Frozen, Sainsbury's*	1 Pack/375g	341	3.7	91	5.6	14.9	1.0	0.5
Chicken, Fresh, Chilled, Tesco*	1 Pack/350g	819	60.9	234	13.1	6.3	17.4	2.3
Chicken, HL, Tesco*	1 Pack/350g	371	4.2	106	7.7	15.9	1.2	0.8
Chicken, Indian Meal for 2, Finest, Tesco*	½ Pack/200g	348	24.0	174	10.3	6.2	12.0	2.5
Chicken, Indian Takeaway for One, Sainsbury's*	1 Serving/300g	498	30.9	166	13.0	5.3	10.3	1.6
Chicken, Less Than 3% Fat, Birds Eye*	1 Pack/358g	440	6.8	123	6.5	20.4	1.9	0.8
Chicken, Plumrose*	1 Can/392g	431	22.0	110	8.0	6.9	5.6	0.0
Chicken, Solo Slim, Rosemary Conley*	1 Pack/300g	315	12.9	105	8.7	7.9	4.3	0.8
Chicken, Tinned, Asda*	½ Can/197g	321	21.7	163	8.0	8.0	11.0	2.3
Chicken, Waitrose*	1 Pack/400g	680	46.8	170	13.7	2.4	11.7	1.9
Chicken, with Peshwari Coriander Rice, Finest, Tesco*	1 Pack/550g	907	48.4	165	7.5	13.9	8.8	0.9
Chicken, with Pilau Rice, Asda*	1 Serving/350g	735	49.0	210	12.0	9.0	14.0	2.0
Chicken, with Pilau Rice, Perfectly Balanced, Waitrose*	1 Pack/400g	452	6.8	113	8.9	15.4	1.7	1.3
Chicken, with Pilau Rice, Sharwood's*	1 Pack/375g	2186	80.2	583	21.1	76.5	21.4	4.1
Vegetable, Sainsbury's*	1 Serving/200g	302	25.2	151	2.7	6.6	12.6	2.2

KRISPROLLS

Cracked Wheat, Original, Pagen*	1 Krisproll/12g	47	0.9	380	12.0	67.0	7.0	9.0
Golden, Swedish Toasts, Pagen*	1 Krisproll/12g	48	1.0	400	11.0	69.0	8.5	5.0
Organic, Bio, Pagen*	1 Krisproll/12g	46	0.8	380	12.0	67.0	7.0	8.0
Swedish Toasts, Wholegrain, Pagen*	1 Toast/13g	51	0.8	390	11.0	67.0	6.5	8.5

KULFI

Average	*1oz/28g*	*119*	*11.2*	*424*	*5.4*	*11.8*	*39.9*	*0.6*

KUMQUATS

Raw	*1oz/28g*	*12*	*0.1*	*43*	*0.9*	*9.3*	*0.5*	*3.8*

INFO/WEIGHT	Measure		per Measure		Nutrition Values per 100g / 100ml				
			KCAL	FAT	KCAL	PROT	CARB	FAT	FIBRE
LACES									
Apple Flavour, Tesco*	5 Laces/15g		52	0.5	347	3.6	74.8	3.2	2.1
Strawberry, Sainsbury's*	1 Serving/25g		94	1.1	377	3.3	76.3	4.6	0.1
Strawberry, Tesco*	1 Serving/75g		260	2.4	347	3.6	74.8	3.2	2.1
LAGER									
Alcohol Free, Becks*	1 Serving/275ml		55	0.0	20	0.7	5.0	0.0	0.0
Amstel, Heineken*	1 Pint/568ml		227	0.0	40	0.5	3.0	0.0	0.0
Average	1 Pint/568ml		233	0.0	41	0.3	3.1	0.0	0.0
Becks*	1 Can/275ml		113	0.0	41	0.0	3.0	0.0	0.0
Blanc, Kronenbourg*	½ Pint/284ml		119	0.0	42	0.0	3.3	0.0	0.0
Boston, Samuel Adams*	1 Bottle/355ml		160	0.0	45	0.0	0.0	0.0	0.0
Bottled, Brahma*	1 Bottle/330ml		125	0.0	38	0.0	0.0	0.0	0.0
Can, Carlsberg*	1 Can/440ml		141	0.0	32	0.0	2.0	0.0	0.0
Draught, Carling*	1 Pint/568ml		189	0.0	33	0.0	1.4	0.0	0.0
Edge, Carlsberg*	1 Can/300ml		126	0.0	42	0.0	4.3	0.0	0.0
Export, Carlsberg*	1 Can/440ml		185	0.0	42	0.3	2.8	0.0	0.3
Export, Foster's*	1 Pint/568ml		210	0.0	37	0.0	2.2	0.0	0.0
Foster's*	1 Pint/568ml		227	0.0	40	0.0	3.1	0.0	0.0
Gold, Foster's, Heineken*	1 Can/440ml		145	0.0	33	0.3	1.2	0.0	0.0
Grolsch*	1 Can/330ml		145	0.0	44	0.0	2.2	0.0	0.0
Heineken*, 5%, Heineken*	1 Bottle/250ml		110	0.0	44	0.4	3.4	0.0	0.0
Kaliber, Guinness*	1 Can/440ml		110	0.0	25	0.2	6.0	0.0	0.0
Light, Coors*	1 Pint/500ml		160	0.0	32	0.3	1.7	0.0	0.0
Light, Michelob*	1 Glass/340ml		113	0.0	33	0.3	2.0	0.0	0.0
Lite, Carlsberg*	1 Bottle/330ml		89	0.0	27	0.1	0.5	0.0	0.0
Low Alcohol	1 Can/440ml		44	0.0	10	0.2	1.5	0.0	0.0
Pils, Holsten*	1 Can/440ml		167	0.0	38	0.3	2.4	0.0	0.0
Pilsner, Efes*	1 Can/500ml		226	0.0	45	0.0	7.6	0.0	0.0
Polish, Tyskie*	1 Can/549ml		236	0.0	43	0.0	0.0	0.0	0.0
Premier, Kronenbourg*	½ Pint/284ml		136	0.0	48	0.0	0.0	0.0	0.0
Premium	1 Can/440ml		260	0.0	59	0.3	2.4	0.0	0.0
Stella Artois*	1 Can/550ml		247	0.0	45	1.2	2.9	0.0	0.0
Tuborg Green, Carlsberg*	1 Serving/200ml		78	0.0	39	0.5	2.5	0.0	0.0
Ultra Low Carb, Michelob*	1 Bottle/275ml		88	0.0	32	0.2	0.9	0.0	0.0
LAKSA									
Chicken, COU, M & S*	1 Pack/450g		360	9.9	80	7.5	7.0	2.2	1.1
Thai Noodle, with Chicken, M & S*	1 Pack/400g		460	21.6	115	7.0	9.8	5.4	1.1
LAMB									
Chops, Average	*1oz/28g*		*65*	*4.6*	*231*	*20.5*	*0.4*	*16.3*	*0.0*
Chops, Minted, Average	*1 Chop/100g*		*260*	*15.1*	*260*	*25.9*	*5.1*	*15.1*	*0.3*
Cutlets, Neck, Raw, Lean & Fat, Weighed with Bone	*1 Pack 210g*		*485*	*42.8*	*231*	*11.9*	*0.0*	*20.4*	*0.0*
Diced, From Supermarket, Healthy Range, Average	*½ Pack/200g*		*277*	*8.9*	*138*	*24.6*	*0.1*	*4.5*	*0.0*
Escalope, Asda*	1 Serving/100g		173	5.0	173	32.0	0.0	5.0	0.0
Grill Steak, Average	*1oz/28g*		*70*	*4.7*	*250*	*20.2*	*4.4*	*16.9*	*0.4*
Grill Steak, Prime, Average	*1 Steak/63g*		*197*	*16.1*	*312*	*18.5*	*2.0*	*25.5*	*0.1*
Leg, Joint, Raw, Average	*1 Joint/510g*		*858*	*45.5*	*168*	*20.9*	*1.4*	*8.9*	*0.2*
Leg, Roasted, Lean, Average	*1oz/28g*		*58*	*2.7*	*206*	*29.9*	*0.0*	*9.6*	*0.0*
Leg, Roasted, Lean & Fat, Average	*1oz/28g*		*66*	*3.8*	*237*	*28.6*	*0.0*	*13.6*	*0.0*
Loin, Chop, Grilled, Lean & Fat, Weighed with Bone	1 Serving/100g		247	17.9	247	21.5	0.0	17.9	0.0
Loin, Chops, Grilled, Lean & Fat, Weighed with Bone	1 Serving/100g		247	17.9	247	21.5	0.0	17.9	0.0
Loin, Chops, Raw, Lean & Fat, Weighed with Bone	1 Serving/100g		216	17.9	216	13.7	0.0	17.9	0.0
Mince, Average	*1oz/28g*		*58*	*4.2*	*207*	*17.6*	*0.5*	*14.8*	*0.0*
Mince, Extra Lean, Sainsbury's*	1 Serving/225g		324	11.9	144	24.1	0.0	5.3	0.1
Neck Fillet, Lean, Raw	1 Serving/100g		184	9.3	184	19.6	0.3	9.3	0.0

L

	INFO/WEIGHT	KCAL	FAT	KCAL	PROT	CARB	FAT	FIBRE
LAMB								
Rack, Raw, Lean & Fat	1oz/28g	79	6.7	283	17.3	0.0	23.8	0.0
Rack, Raw, Lean Only, Weighed with Bone	1oz/28g	48	2.6	169	20.0	0.0	9.2	0.0
Rack, Roasted, Lean	1oz/28g	63	3.6	225	27.1	0.0	13.0	0.0
Rack, Roasted, Lean & Fat	1oz/28g	102	8.4	363	23.0	0.0	30.1	0.0
Shoulder, Cooked, Lean & Fat	1oz/28g	84	6.3	301	24.4	0.0	22.5	0.0
Shoulder, Fillet, Average	1oz/28g	66	5.1	235	17.6	0.0	18.3	0.0
Shoulder, Raw, Average	1oz/28g	70	5.7	248	16.7	0.0	20.2	0.0
Shoulder, Roasted, Whole, Lean	1oz/28g	61	3.4	218	27.2	0.0	12.1	0.0
Steak, Leg, Raw, Average	1 Steak/150g	169	5.5	112	20.0	0.0	3.6	0.0
Steak, Minted, Average	1 Steak/125g	212	9.0	170	22.7	3.4	7.2	0.9
Steak, Raw, Average	1 Steak/140g	190	7.6	136	21.7	0.2	5.4	0.0
Stewing, Raw, Lean & Fat	1oz/28g	57	3.5	203	22.5	0.0	12.6	0.0
Stewing, Stewed, Lean	1oz/28g	67	4.1	240	26.6	0.0	14.8	0.0
Stewing, Stewed, Lean & Fat	1oz/28g	78	5.6	279	24.4	0.0	20.1	0.0
Trimmed Fat, Raw, Average	1 Serving/100g	518	51.6	518	13.3	0.0	51.6	0.0
LAMB IN								
Garlic & Rosemary Gravy, Shank, Asda*	1 Shank/280g	451	23.2	161	19.8	1.7	8.3	0.5
Gravy, Minted, Roast, M & S*	1 Pack/200g	140	3.0	70	6.8	6.6	1.5	0.9
Gravy, Roast, Birds Eye*	1 Pack/239g	160	5.3	67	8.1	3.8	2.2	0.1
Mint Gravy, Sliced, Sainsbury's*	1 Pack/125g	134	4.7	107	15.3	2.9	3.8	0.8
Rich Minted Gravy, Shank, Morrisons*	1 Pack/400g	612	26.4	153	18.8	5.2	6.6	0.0
LAMB MEDITERRANEAN								
Shanks, Finest, Tesco*	1 Serving/404g	671	35.6	166	15.0	6.6	8.8	2.0
LAMB MOROCCAN								
with Cous Cous, Perfectly Balanced, Waitrose*	1 Pack/400g	390	5.2	97	7.7	13.6	1.3	2.2
LAMB TAGINE								
Moroccan Style, with Couscous, COU, M & S*	1 Pack/400g	340	5.6	85	8.9	8.3	1.4	1.6
LAMB WITH								
Gravy, Joint, Tesco*	1 Serving/225g	277	13.0	123	14.9	2.8	5.8	0.0
Honey Roast Vegetables, Extra Special, Asda*	1 Pack/400g	400	14.8	100	9.9	6.7	3.7	2.5
Mango & Mint, Shoulder Chops, Waitrose*	1 Chop/250g	555	40.5	222	16.7	2.3	16.2	0.5
Mango & Mint Sauce, Boneless Joint, Asda*	1 Serving/100g	302	22.0	302	26.0	0.0	22.0	1.4
Mint & Balsamic Vinegar Crust, Rump, Waitrose*	1 Serving/166g	259	11.8	156	18.1	5.0	7.1	0.0
Mint Butter, Leg Steaks, Waitrose*	1 Serving/155g	270	16.3	174	19.6	0.4	10.5	0.0
Mint Gravy, Joint, Tesco*	1 Serving/100g	88	1.7	88	16.6	1.8	1.7	0.1
Mint Gravy, Leg Chops, Tesco*	1 Serving/175g	213	9.8	122	15.0	3.2	5.6	1.7
Mint Gravy, Shanks, Frozen, Tesco*	1 Shank/200g	420	26.4	210	20.1	1.6	13.2	0.7
Redcurrant & Rosemary Sauce, Chops, Leg, Tesco*	1 Pack/325g	604	36.1	186	17.6	4.0	11.1	0.5
Roasted Vegetables, Shank, M & S*	½ Pack/420g	660	30.6	157	14.9	8.3	7.3	0.7
Rosemary, Joint, Tesco*	1 Serving/125g	250	17.6	200	17.5	0.8	14.1	0.5
Rosemary Gravy, Shank, Sainsbury's*	1 Serving/200g	204	8.2	102	13.2	3.1	4.1	0.3
Sticky Plum & Orange Glaze, Joint, Waitrose*	1 Serving/100g	164	7.9	164	13.4	9.8	7.9	3.1
LARD								
Average	1oz/28g	249	27.7	891	0.0	0.0	99.0	0.0
LASAGNE								
Al Forno, Beef, M & S*	1 Pack/400g	640	38.0	160	8.2	10.7	9.5	2.8
Al Forno, TTD, Sainsbury's*	1 Pack/383g	571	30.3	149	8.6	10.9	7.9	2.1
Alla Bolognese, Weight Watchers*	1 Pack/350g	416	8.7	119	8.0	16.0	2.5	0.0
Asda*	1 Pack/398g	502	23.9	126	7.3	10.6	6.0	1.1
Asparagus, M & S*	1 Pack/360g	432	22.0	120	4.3	11.9	6.1	1.1
Beef	1 Serving/400g	553	24.0	138	8.2	12.7	6.0	1.4
Beef, BGTY, Sainsbury's*	1 Pack/400g	352	8.0	88	7.8	9.8	2.0	1.4
Beef, Frozen, Tesco*	1 Pack/450g	607	25.2	135	7.5	12.6	5.6	0.8

	Measure INFO/WEIGHT	per Measure KCAL	per Measure FAT	Nutrition Values per 100g / 100ml KCAL	PROT	CARB	FAT	FIBRE
LASAGNE								
Beef, Frozen, Weight Watchers*	1 Pack/300g	252	7.2	84	5.4	10.2	2.4	0.3
Beef, GFY, Asda*	1 Pack/350g	385	7.0	110	9.0	14.0	2.0	1.0
Beef, Italian, Finest, Tesco*	½ Pack/310g	425	22.3	137	7.4	10.7	7.2	0.8
Beef, with Fresh Pasta, Birds Eye*	1 Pack/400g	396	9.2	99	7.3	12.2	2.3	0.5
Beef & Chunky Vegetable, HL, Tesco*	1 Pack/340g	354	9.5	104	5.9	13.8	2.8	1.2
Bolognese, & Vegetable, Weight Watchers*	1 Pack/300g	279	7.8	93	5.0	12.4	2.6	0.0
Chicken, Italian, Sainsbury's*	1 Pack/450g	549	18.9	122	8.4	12.6	4.2	0.5
Chicken, Light Choices, Tesco*	1 Pack/400g	344	6.8	86	7.1	10.5	1.7	1.8
Chicken, Mushroom & Asparagus, Finest, Tesco*	½ Pack/300g	360	16.2	120	7.6	10.2	5.4	0.8
Chicken, Ready Meals, Waitrose*	1 Pack/300g	411	19.8	137	6.3	13.0	6.6	0.9
Classic, Deep Filled, M & S*	1 Pack/400g	760	47.6	190	10.0	11.2	11.9	0.6
Creamy Ricotta & Vegetable, HL, Tesco*	1 Pack/384g	407	10.8	106	5.5	14.6	2.8	3.6
Diet Chef Ltd*	1 Pack/270g	288	13.8	107	5.6	9.6	5.1	1.9
Italian, Fresh, Chilled, Sainsbury's*	1 Pack/400g	480	22.0	120	10.1	7.5	5.5	1.4
Layered, Asda*	1 Pack/300g	444	24.0	148	5.0	14.0	8.0	0.3
Low Saturated Fat, Waitrose*	1 Pack/400g	312	6.0	78	4.7	11.4	1.5	0.4
Mediterranean Vegetable, COU, M & S*	1 Pack/360g	306	9.7	85	3.4	11.5	2.7	1.4
Mushroom & Spinach, Waitrose*	1 Pack/400g	373	14.0	93	3.1	12.3	3.5	1.3
Roasted Vegetable, M & S*	1 Pack/400g	440	20.4	110	3.4	12.8	5.1	1.7
Salmon, King Prawn & Spinach, Finest, Tesco*	1 Pack/400g	600	29.6	150	10.6	9.6	7.4	0.8
Sheets, Boiled, Average	*1 Sheet/20g*	*20*	*0.1*	*100*	*3.0*	*22.0*	*0.6*	*0.9*
Sheets, Dry, Average	*1 Sheet/20g*	*70*	*0.3*	*349*	*11.9*	*72.1*	*1.5*	*2.9*
Sheets, Fresh, Dry, Average	*1 Sheet/21g*	*56*	*0.4*	*271*	*10.9*	*52.7*	*2.1*	*1.9*
Sheets, Verdi, Dry, Average	*1 Sheet/20g*	*71*	*0.4*	*355*	*12.6*	*71.1*	*2.2*	*2.7*
Spinach & Cheese, Italian, Sainsbury's*	1 Pack/450g	666	30.6	148	6.0	15.5	6.8	0.5
Spinach & Ricotta, Giovanni Rana*	1 Pack/350g	728	39.6	208	7.4	19.2	11.3	0.0
Triangles with Chicken, COU, M & S*	1 Pack/360g	324	6.5	90	7.8	11.9	1.8	1.0
Vegetable, Average	1oz/28g	29	1.2	102	4.1	12.4	4.4	1.0
Vegetable, BGTY, Sainsbury's*	1 Pack/385g	339	7.7	88	3.5	13.9	2.0	2.3
Vegetable, Italian, Frozen, Cooked, Sainsbury's*	1 Pack/378g	442	18.9	117	4.6	13.5	5.0	1.1
Vegetable, Italian Roasted, Asda*	1 Serving/200g	234	14.0	117	2.6	11.0	7.0	0.7
Vegetable, Italian Three Layer, Sainsbury's*	1 Pack/450g	553	23.4	123	4.8	14.3	5.2	0.5
Vegetable, Low Saturated Fat, Waitrose*	1 Pack/400g	340	11.6	85	2.9	11.9	2.9	0.9
Vegetable, Morrisons*	1 Pack/400g	464	22.8	116	3.8	12.3	5.7	0.7
Vegetable, Weight Watchers*	1 Pack/330g	251	5.6	76	3.6	11.8	1.7	0.7
LASAGNE VEGETARIAN								
Linda McCartney*	1 Pack/360g	451	20.2	125	6.3	12.4	5.6	1.4
Tesco*	1 Pack/450g	630	34.6	140	6.0	11.6	7.7	1.6
LAVERBREAD								
Average	*1oz/28g*	*15*	*1.0*	*52*	*3.2*	*1.6*	*3.7*	*0.0*
LEEKS								
Boiled, Average	*1oz/28g*	*6*	*0.2*	*21*	*1.2*	*2.6*	*0.7*	*1.7*
Creamed, Frozen, Waitrose*	1 Serving/225g	115	5.4	51	1.8	5.5	2.4	0.0
Frozen, Sliced, Asda*	1 Serving/100g	27	0.5	27	1.6	2.9	0.5	2.2
Raw, Unprepared, Average	*1 Leek/166g*	*64*	*1.5*	*39*	*2.8*	*5.1*	*0.9*	*3.9*
LEMON								
Fresh, Raw, Average	*1 Slice/5g*	*0*	*0.0*	*7*	*0.3*	*1.6*	*0.0*	*1.7*
Peel, Raw, Average	*1 Tbsp/6g*	*3*	*0.0*	*47*	*1.5*	*16.0*	*0.3*	*10.6*
LEMON CURD								
Average	*1 Tbsp/15g*	*44*	*0.7*	*294*	*0.7*	*62.9*	*4.7*	*0.1*
Luxury, Average	*1 Tsp/7g*	*23*	*0.6*	*326*	*2.8*	*59.7*	*8.4*	*0.1*
LEMON SOLE								
Fillets, Raw, Average	*1 Serving/220g*	*180*	*2.8*	*82*	*17.3*	*0.2*	*1.3*	*0.3*

L

	Measure INFO/WEIGHT	per Measure KCAL	FAT	Nutrition Values per 100g / 100ml KCAL	PROT	CARB	FAT	FIBRE
LEMON SOLE								
Goujons, Average	1 Serving/150g	359	18.3	239	13.9	18.5	12.2	1.0
Grilled, Average	*1oz/28g*	*27*	*0.5*	*97*	*20.2*	*0.0*	*1.7*	*0.0*
in Breadcrumbs, Average	1 Fillet/142g	322	17.4	228	13.7	15.7	12.3	1.0
in White Wine, & Herb Butter, Fillets, M & S*	1 Pack/220g	385	27.7	175	15.1	0.1	12.6	0.0
Steamed, Average	*1oz/28g*	*25*	*0.3*	*91*	*20.6*	*0.0*	*0.9*	*0.0*
LEMONADE								
7-Up, Light, Britvic*	1 Can/330ml	4	0.0	1	0.1	0.2	0.0	0.0
7-Up, Zero, Britvic*	1 Can/330ml	6	0.0	2	0.1	0.1	0.0	0.0
Average	1 Glass/250ml	52	0.2	21	0.1	5.0	0.1	0.1
Cloudy, Gastropub, M & S*	1 Bottle/500ml	25	0.0	5	0.0	0.0	0.0	0.0
Cloudy, Waitrose*	1 Glass/250ml	125	0.0	50	0.0	12.2	0.0	0.0
Diet, Average	1 Glass/250ml	4	0.1	2	0.1	0.2	0.0	0.0
Organic, Tesco*	1 Can/142ml	61	0.0	43	0.0	10.6	0.0	0.0
Pink, Still, Pure Premium, Tropicana*	1 Serving/200ml	90	0.0	45	0.2	10.0	0.0	0.7
R White*	1 Glass/250ml	65	0.0	26	0.1	6.2	0.0	0.0
Schweppes*	1 Glass/250ml	45	0.0	18	0.0	4.2	0.0	0.0
Still, Freshly Squeezed, M & S*	½ Bottle/250ml	100	0.5	40	0.1	9.0	0.2	0.5
Still, Raspberry, M & S*	1 Glass/250ml	112	0.0	45	0.2	10.3	0.0	0.1
Victorian, Fentiman's*	1 Bottle/275ml	130	0.0	47	0.0	11.3	0.0	0.0
LEMONGRASS								
Easy, Asda*	1 Tsp/10g	5	0.1	52	0.4	7.4	1.2	5.2
Stalks, Tesco*	1 Stalk/13g	12	0.1	99	1.8	25.3	0.5	0.0
LEMSIP								
Beechams*	1 Sachet/3g	11	0.0	387	0.0	100.0	0.0	0.0
LENTILS								
Black Beluga, Ready to Eat, Merchant Gourmet*	1 Serving/63g	92	0.7	147	10.9	20.5	1.2	5.2
Campo Largo*	1 Jar/400g	304	2.4	76	6.0	8.0	0.6	0.0
Green & Brown, Dried, Boiled in Salted Water, Average	*1 Tbsp/30g*	*31*	*0.2*	*105*	*8.8*	*16.9*	*0.7*	*3.8*
Green Or Brown, Dried, Average	*1 Serving/50g*	*150*	*0.7*	*301*	*22.8*	*49.8*	*1.5*	*9.6*
Green Or Brown, in Water, Tinned, Average	*½ Can/132g*	*131*	*0.8*	*99*	*8.1*	*15.4*	*0.6*	*3.8*
Puy, Green, Dry, Average	1 Serving/100g	306	1.4	306	24.7	49.5	1.4	10.3
Red, Boiled in Unsalted Water, Average	*1oz/28g*	*28*	*0.1*	*101*	*7.6*	*17.5*	*0.4*	*2.6*
Red, Dried, Average	*1oz/28g*	*88*	*0.4*	*315*	*23.8*	*53.8*	*1.3*	*4.9*
LETTUCE								
Curly Leaf, Sainsbury's*	1 Serving/80g	11	0.4	14	0.8	1.7	0.5	0.0
Iceberg, Average	*1 Serving/80g*	*11*	*0.3*	*13*	*0.8*	*1.8*	*0.3*	*0.5*
Lamb's, Average	*1 Serving/80g*	*12*	*0.2*	*14*	*1.3*	*1.5*	*0.2*	*0.9*
Leafy, Tesco*	1 Serving/80g	11	0.3	14	1.2	1.5	0.4	1.9
Radicchio, Red, Raw, Average	*1 Head/220g*	*29*	*0.2*	*13*	*1.4*	*1.6*	*0.1*	*3.0*
Romaine, Average	*1 Serving/80g*	*12*	*0.4*	*15*	*0.9*	*1.7*	*0.5*	*0.7*
Romaine, Hearts, Average	*1 Serving/80g*	*12*	*0.4*	*15*	*0.9*	*1.7*	*0.5*	*1.0*
Romaine, Sweet, Average	*1 Serving/80g*	*12*	*0.4*	*15*	*0.9*	*1.6*	*0.5*	*0.8*
Sweet Gem, TTD, Sainsbury's*	1 Serving/100g	15	0.5	15	0.8	1.7	0.5	0.9
LILT								
Fruit Crush, Coca-Cola*	1 Can/330ml	66	0.0	20	0.0	4.6	0.0	0.0
Fruit Crush, Zero, Coca-Cola*	1 Can/330ml	12	0.0	3	0.0	0.3	0.0	0.0
Z, Coca-Cola*	1 Can/330ml	10	0.0	3	0.0	0.4	0.0	0.0
LIME								
Peel, Raw	*1 Tbsp/6g*	*3*	*0.0*	*47*	*1.5*	*16.0*	*0.3*	*10.6*
Raw, Flesh Only, Average	*1 Lime/71g*	*18*	*0.1*	*25*	*0.6*	*8.8*	*0.2*	*2.3*
Raw, Weighed with Peel & Seeds, Average	*1 Lime/85g*	*25*	*0.2*	*30*	*0.7*	*10.5*	*0.2*	*2.8*
LINGUINE								
Crab, Rocket & Chilli, Italian, Finest, Tesco*	1 Pack/350g	717	36.4	205	6.5	20.7	10.4	1.7

L

	Measure INFO/WEIGHT	per Measure KCAL	FAT	Nutrition Values per 100g / 100ml KCAL	PROT	CARB	FAT	FIBRE
LINGUINE								
Crab & Chilli, Waitrose*	1 Pack/350g	770	45.0	220	7.7	18.0	12.9	1.8
Dry, Average	*1 Serving/100g*	*352*	*2.2*	*352*	*13.1*	*70.0*	*2.2*	*2.8*
Fresh, Dry, Average	*1 Pack/250g*	*681*	*6.5*	*272*	*12.3*	*51.7*	*2.6*	*4.0*
Garlic & Basil, Asda*	1 Serving/75g	108	0.4	144	5.4	29.5	0.5	2.5
King Prawn, Meal for One, M & S*	1 Pack/400g	380	6.8	95	6.6	13.1	1.7	2.2
Pomodoro, M & S*	1 Pack/300g	360	10.5	120	4.1	17.6	3.5	1.2
Salmon & Prawn, Iceland*	1 Meal/450g	540	19.8	120	4.5	15.8	4.4	1.5
Smoked Salmon, Sainsbury's*	1 Serving/400g	586	28.8	146	6.2	14.2	7.2	1.2
Tomato & Mushroom, Perfectly Balanced, Waitrose*	1 Pack/350g	294	13.3	84	2.2	10.6	3.8	1.0
Vegetable & Ham, BGTY, Sainsbury's*	1 Pack/450g	409	13.5	91	4.4	11.7	3.0	0.9
with Chicken & Basil Dressing, HL, Tesco*	1 Pack/359g	503	15.4	140	8.6	16.6	4.3	2.2
with Prawns & Scallops, BGTY, Sainsbury's*	1 Pack/400g	320	2.0	80	6.2	12.7	0.5	0.8
with Salmon, Hot Smoked, GFY, Asda*	1 Pack/400g	348	9.2	87	6.0	10.6	2.3	1.6
LINSEEDS								
Average	*1 Tsp/5g*	*23*	*1.7*	*464*	*21.7*	*18.5*	*33.5*	*26.3*
LION BAR								
Mini, Nestle*	1 Bar/16g	80	3.6	486	4.6	67.7	21.7	0.0
Nestle*	1 Bar/43g	206	9.3	478	6.5	64.6	21.6	0.0
Peanut, Nestle*	1 Bar/49g	256	14.5	522	7.1	56.9	29.6	0.0
LIQUEURS								
Amaretto, Average	*1 Shot/25ml*	*97*	*0.0*	*388*	*0.0*	*60.0*	*0.0*	*0.0*
Cointreau, Specialite De France	*1 Serving/37ml*	*80*	*0.0*	*215*	*0.0*	*0.0*	*0.0*	*0.0*
Cream, Average	*1 Shot/25ml*	*81*	*4.0*	*325*	*0.0*	*22.8*	*16.1*	*0.0*
*Grand Marnier**	*1 Shot/35ml*	*94*	*0.0*	*268*	*0.0*	*22.9*	*0.0*	*0.0*
High Strength, Average	*1 Shot/25ml*	*78*	*0.0*	*314*	*0.0*	*24.4*	*0.0*	*0.0*
Kirsch, Average	*1 Shot/25ml*	*67*	*0.0*	*267*	*0.0*	*20.0*	*0.0*	*0.0*
Marula Fruit & Cream Cocktail, Amarula*	1 fl oz/30ml	103	0.0	343	0.0	36.7	0.0	0.0
LIQUORICE								
Allsorts, Average	1 Sm Bag/56g	195	2.9	349	3.7	76.7	5.2	2.0
Allsorts, Bassett's*	1 Pack/225g	855	11.0	380	5.6	77.8	4.9	1.6
Allsorts, Fruit, Bassett's*	1 Serving/50g	160	0.2	320	1.8	76.9	0.4	0.0
Assorted, Filled, Panda*	1 Sweet/4g	15	0.4	385	3.7	68.0	11.0	0.0
Bars, Panda*	1 Bar/32g	99	0.1	308	3.7	72.0	0.4	0.9
Catherine Wheels, Barratt*	1 Wheel/22g	65	0.1	290	3.8	67.2	0.3	0.7
Comfits, M & S*	1oz/28g	100	0.1	357	2.4	86.2	0.3	0.7
Organic, Laidback Liquorice*	1 Bar/28g	90	0.3	320	4.7	75.0	1.0	3.0
Piglets, Black, Old Fashioned, Route 29 Napa Inc*	1 Sweet/1.5g	5	0.0	325	2.5	70.0	2.5	0.0
Piglets, Red, Old Fashioned, Route 29 Napa Inc*	1 Sweet/1.5g	5	0.0	325	0.0	72.5	1.2	0.0
Red, Fresh, 98% Fat Free, RJ's Licorice Ltd*	1oz/28g	96	0.5	342	3.0	75.0	1.7	0.0
Shapes, Average	1oz/28g	78	0.4	278	5.5	65.0	1.4	1.9
Soft Eating, Australia, Darrell Lea*	1 Piece/20g	68	0.4	338	2.8	76.1	1.9	0.0
Sweets, Blackcurrant, Tesco*	1 Sweet/8g	32	0.3	410	0.0	92.3	3.8	0.0
Torpedos, Panda*	1 Serving/25g	91	0.0	366	1.9	88.0	0.2	1.4
LIVER								
Calves, Fried	*1oz/28g*	*49*	*2.7*	*176*	*22.3*	*0.0*	*9.6*	*0.0*
Calves, Raw	*1oz/28g*	*29*	*1.0*	*104*	*18.3*	*0.0*	*3.4*	*0.0*
Chicken, Cooked, Simmered, Average	*1 Serving/100g*	*167*	*6.5*	*167*	*24.5*	*0.9*	*6.5*	*0.0*
Chicken, Fried, Average	*1oz/28g*	*47*	*2.5*	*169*	*22.1*	*0.0*	*8.9*	*0.0*
Chicken, Raw, Average	*1oz/28g*	*26*	*0.6*	*92*	*17.7*	*0.0*	*2.3*	*0.0*
Lamb's, Braised, Average	*1 Serving/100g*	*220*	*8.8*	*220*	*30.6*	*2.5*	*8.8*	*0.0*
Lamb's, Fried, Average	*1oz/28g*	*66*	*3.6*	*237*	*30.1*	*0.0*	*12.9*	*0.0*
Lamb's, Raw, Average	*1 Serving/125g*	*171*	*7.7*	*137*	*20.3*	*0.0*	*6.2*	*0.0*
Ox, Raw	*1oz/28g*	*43*	*2.2*	*155*	*21.1*	*0.0*	*7.8*	*0.0*

L

	Measure INFO/WEIGHT	per Measure KCAL	per Measure FAT	Nutrition Values per 100g / 100ml KCAL	PROT	CARB	FAT	FIBRE
LIVER								
Ox, Stewed	*1oz/28g*	*55*	*2.7*	*198*	*24.8*	*3.6*	*9.5*	*0.0*
Pig's, Raw	*1oz/28g*	*32*	*0.9*	*113*	*21.3*	*0.0*	*3.1*	*0.0*
Pig's, Stewed	*1 Serving/70g*	*132*	*5.7*	*189*	*25.6*	*3.6*	*8.1*	*0.0*
LIVER & BACON								
Meal for One, M & S*	1 Pack/452g	430	16.7	95	7.0	8.0	3.7	1.2
with Fresh Mashed Potato, Waitrose*	1 Pack/400g	416	17.2	104	7.3	9.0	4.3	1.3
LIVER & ONIONS								
Finest, Tesco*	½ Pack/225g	349	18.7	155	15.6	3.7	8.3	1.6
M & S*	1 Serving/200g	250	12.0	125	7.6	10.5	6.0	0.9
LIVER SAUSAGE								
Average	*1 Slice/10g*	*22*	*1.5*	*216*	*15.3*	*4.4*	*15.2*	*0.2*
LOBSTER								
½, M & S*	1oz/28g	66	5.5	235	12.1	2.4	19.6	0.2
Boiled, Average	*1oz/28g*	*29*	*0.4*	*103*	*22.1*	*0.0*	*1.6*	*0.0*
Dressed, M & S*	1oz/28g	76	6.6	273	14.3	0.8	23.6	0.1
Squat, Tails, Youngs*	½ Pack/125g	246	10.7	197	9.8	20.1	8.6	1.1
Thermidor, M & S*	1 Serving/140g	287	19.2	205	10.7	9.7	13.7	0.0
LOGANBERRIES								
Raw	*1oz/28g*	*5*	*0.0*	*17*	*1.1*	*3.4*	*0.0*	*2.5*
LOLLIPOPS								
Assorted Flavours, Asda*	1 Lolly/7g	27	0.0	380	0.0	95.0	0.0	0.0
Blackcurrant, Sugar Free, Rowntree's*	1 Lolly/15g	35	0.0	233	0.1	89.4	0.0	0.0
Chocolate Lolly, M & S*	1 Lolly/45g	247	15.8	550	6.8	54.0	35.1	2.7
Chupa Chups*	1 Lolly/18g	44	0.2	247	0.0	96.5	1.3	0.0
Cremosa, Sugar Free, Chupa Chups*	1 Lolly/10g	27	0.5	275	0.2	92.5	5.4	0.0
No Added Sugar, Tesco*	1 Lolly/32g	26	0.0	80	0.1	20.0	0.0	0.1
Orange, Sugar Free, Rowntree's*	1 Lolly/15g	35	0.0	235	0.1	89.5	0.0	0.6
Refreshers, Bassett's*	1 Lolly/6g	25	0.0	417	0.0	108.3	0.0	0.0
Sugar Free, Simpkins*	1 Lolly/15g	51	0.0	340	0.0	88.0	0.0	0.0
Super Sour, Tesco*	1 Lolly/8g	32	0.0	385	0.1	95.6	0.2	0.5
LOQUATS								
Raw	*1oz/28g*	*8*	*0.1*	*28*	*0.7*	*6.3*	*0.2*	*0.0*
LOZENGES								
Fishermans Friend, Blackcurrant Flavour, Lofthouses*	1 Lozenge/1g	2	0.0	236	0.0	93.0	1.3	0.0
Original, Victory V*	1 Lozenge/3g	9	0.0	350	0.0	91.0	0.0	0.0
Original Extra Strong Lozenge, Fisherman's Friend*	1 Lozenge/1g	4	0.0	382	0.3	94.9	0.0	0.5
LUCOZADE								
Apple, Energy Drink, GlaxoSmithKline UK Limited*	1 Bottle/380ml	262	0.0	69	0.0	17.1	0.0	0.0
Citrus Clear, Energy, GlaxoSmithKline UK Limited*	1 Bottle/380ml	266	0.0	70	0.1	17.0	0.0	0.0
Citrus Fruits, Hydro Active, Sport, Lucozade*	1 Bottle/500ml	50	0.0	10	0.0	2.0	0.0	0.0
Orange Energy Drink, GlaxoSmithKline UK Limited*	1 Bottle/500ml	350	0.0	70	0.0	17.2	0.0	0.0
Original, GlaxoSmithKline UK Limited*	1 Bottle/345ml	241	0.0	70	0.0	17.2	0.0	0.0
Tropical, GlaxoSmithKline UK Limited*	1 Bottle/380ml	266	0.0	70	0.0	17.2	0.0	0.0
LUNCHEON MEAT								
Pork, Average	*1oz/28g*	*81*	*6.8*	*288*	*13.3*	*4.0*	*24.3*	*0.0*
LYCHEES								
Fresh, Raw, Flesh Only	*1oz/28g*	*16*	*0.0*	*58*	*0.9*	*14.3*	*0.1*	*0.7*
in Juice, Amoy*	1oz/28g	13	0.0	46	0.4	10.9	0.0	0.0
in Syrup, Average	*1oz/28g*	*19*	*0.0*	*69*	*0.4*	*17.7*	*0.0*	*0.4*
Raw, Weighed with Skin & Stone	*1oz/28g*	*10*	*0.0*	*36*	*0.5*	*8.9*	*0.1*	*0.4*

L

	Measure INFO/WEIGHT	per Measure KCAL	FAT	Nutrition Values per 100g / 100ml KCAL	PROT	CARB	FAT	FIBRE
M&M'S								
Mars*	1 Pack/20g	97	4.3	485	5.0	68.0	21.5	0.0
Mini, Mars*	1 Sm Pack/36g	176	8.4	489	6.3	63.6	23.2	0.0
Peanut, Mars*	1 Pack/45g	228	11.4	506	9.4	60.1	25.4	2.7
Peanut Butter, Mars*	1 Pack/42g	230	12.0	548	9.5	57.1	28.6	4.8
MACADAMIA NUTS								
Plain, Average	*1 Pack/100g*	*750*	*77.6*	*750*	*7.9*	*4.8*	*77.6*	*5.3*
Roasted, Salted, Average	*6 Nuts/10g*	*75*	*7.8*	*748*	*7.9*	*4.8*	*77.6*	*5.3*
MACARONI								
Dry, Average	*1oz/28g*	*99*	*0.5*	*354*	*11.9*	*73.5*	*1.7*	*2.6*
MACARONI CHEESE								
Average	1 Serving/300g	534	32.4	178	7.3	13.6	10.8	0.5
Canned	1oz/28g	39	1.8	138	4.5	16.4	6.5	0.4
Chilled, GFY, Asda*	1 Pack/443g	469	12.8	106	6.0	14.0	2.9	1.6
COU, M & S*	1 Pack/360g	360	8.6	100	5.8	13.9	2.4	1.2
Diet Chef Ltd*	1 Pouch/250g	247	7.7	99	7.3	12.7	3.1	0.4
Four Cheese, Extra Special, Asda*	1 Pack/400g	664	30.8	166	7.7	16.4	7.7	1.1
HL, Tesco*	1 Serving/385g	443	4.6	115	9.3	15.9	1.2	1.0
Italian, Sainsbury's*	½ Pack/225g	360	15.7	160	6.9	17.3	7.0	1.5
Light Choices, Tesco*	1 Pack/385g	465	7.3	121	7.0	18.7	1.9	1.5
Made with Fresh Pasta, Findus*	1 Pack/360g	360	7.2	100	5.0	16.0	2.0	0.5
Red Leicester, Heinz*	1 Can/400g	332	10.8	83	3.5	11.1	2.7	0.3
MACAROONS								
Butterscotch, Picard*	1 Macaroon/20g	85	3.6	424	9.7	55.1	18.2	0.0
Coconut, Sainsbury's*	1 Macaroon/33g	146	6.1	441	4.7	63.7	18.6	0.8
French, Average	1 Serving/60g	225	11.0	375	6.7	46.7	18.3	3.3
MACKEREL								
Atlantic, Raw, Average	*1 Fillet/75g*	*154*	*10.4*	*205*	*18.6*	*0.0*	*13.9*	*0.0*
Fillets, Honey Roast Smoked, Sainsbury's*	1 Serving/100g	349	27.3	349	21.5	4.5	27.3	12.4
Fillets, in a Hot Chilli Dressing, Princes*	1 Pack/125g	370	33.7	296	13.3	0.0	27.0	0.0
Fillets, in Brine, Average	*1 Can/88g*	*206*	*15.3*	*234*	*19.4*	*0.0*	*17.4*	*0.0*
Fillets, in Curry Sauce, John West*	1 Can/125g	275	20.7	220	14.2	3.5	16.6	0.2
Fillets, in Green Peppercorn Sauce, John West*	1 Can/125g	329	26.2	263	14.0	4.5	21.0	0.1
Fillets, in Hot Smoked Peppered, Asda*	1 Fillet/100g	341	28.0	341	19.0	3.3	28.0	0.6
Fillets, in Mustard Sauce, Average	1 Can/125g	274	19.4	219	14.1	5.4	15.5	0.0
Fillets, in Olive Oil, Average	1 Serving/50g	149	12.2	297	18.5	1.0	24.3	0.0
Fillets, in Spicy Tomato Sauce, Average	1oz/28g	56	3.9	199	14.3	3.8	14.0	0.0
Fillets, in Sunflower Oil, Average	1 Can/94g	262	20.6	279	20.2	0.2	21.9	0.2
Fillets, in Tomato Sauce, Average	1 Can/125g	251	18.3	200	14.3	2.7	14.7	0.0
Fillets, Red Pepper & Onion, Smoked, Asda*	1 Serving/90g	319	27.9	354	18.0	0.8	31.0	1.2
Fillets, Smoked, Average	*1oz/28g*	*94*	*7.9*	*335*	*19.7*	*0.5*	*28.2*	*0.3*
Fried in Blended Oil	*1oz/28g*	*76*	*5.5*	*272*	*24.0*	*0.0*	*19.5*	*0.0*
Grilled	*1oz/28g*	*67*	*4.8*	*239*	*20.8*	*0.0*	*17.3*	*0.0*
Raw, with Skin, Weighed with Bone, Average	*1oz/28g*	*67*	*4.9*	*238*	*19.9*	*0.0*	*17.6*	*0.0*
Roasted, with Piri-Piri, Tesco*	1 Fillet/80g	240	19.0	300	20.7	0.0	23.8	1.0
Smoked, Lemon & Parsley, Morrisons*	½ Pack/100g	282	20.0	282	20.9	4.6	20.0	1.0
Smoked, Peppered, Average	*1oz/28g*	*87*	*7.0*	*309*	*20.4*	*0.3*	*25.2*	*0.2*
MADRAS								
Beef, Canned, BGTY, Sainsbury's*	1 Can/400g	344	14.4	86	9.5	4.0	3.6	0.9
Beef, Tesco*	1 Pack/460g	616	37.7	134	10.6	4.5	8.2	1.2
Beef, Weight Watchers*	1 Pack/320g	317	4.8	99	5.6	15.8	1.5	0.3
Chicken, & Pilau Rice, Asda*	1 Pack/400g	588	28.0	147	8.0	13.0	7.0	1.7
Chicken, & Rice, Hot & Spicy, Sainsbury's*	1 Pack/500g	670	25.5	134	7.1	14.9	5.1	2.2
Chicken, Asda*	1 Serving/350g	430	31.5	123	7.0	3.6	9.0	2.3

	Measure INFO/WEIGHT	per Measure KCAL	FAT	Nutrition Values per 100g / 100ml KCAL	PROT	CARB	FAT	FIBRE
MADRAS								
Chicken, Frozen, GFY, Asda*	1 Pack/400g	448	5.2	112	5.6	19.4	1.3	1.2
Chicken, Indian, Tesco*	1 Pack/350g	518	31.1	148	11.3	5.6	8.9	1.9
Chicken, Sainsbury's*	1 Pack/400g	468	27.2	117	11.7	2.2	6.8	2.8
Chicken, Waitrose*	1 Pack/400g	672	42.0	168	14.6	3.7	10.5	1.8
MAGNUM								
Almond, Wall's Ice Cream*	1 Bar/86g	275	18.1	320	5.0	30.0	21.0	0.0
Caramel & Almond, Temptation, Wall's Ice Cream*	1 Lolly/68g	239	15.0	351	5.4	34.0	22.0	0.0
Caramel & Nuts Bar, Wall's Ice Cream*	1 Bar/60g	132	9.0	220	4.0	19.0	15.0	0.0
Classic, Mini, Wall's*	1 Lolly/50g	170	11.0	340	4.0	30.0	22.0	0.0
Classic, Wall's Ice Cream*	1 Lolly/86g	261	16.4	303	3.8	29.0	19.0	0.0
Double Chocolate, Wall's Ice Cream*	1 Bar/92g	346	22.0	378	4.5	36.0	24.0	0.0
Gluttony, Wall's Ice Cream*	1 Lolly/110ml	425	29.0	386	4.5	32.7	26.4	0.0
Greed, Wall's Ice Cream*	1 Bar/110ml	307	18.0	279	3.6	29.1	16.4	0.0
White, Wall's Ice Cream*	1 Lolly/87g	256	14.7	296	3.8	32.0	17.0	0.0
MAKHANI								
Chicken, Sainsbury's*	½ Pack/199g	313	21.3	157	12.2	2.9	10.7	2.5
Chicken Tikka, BGTY, Sainsbury's*	1 Pack/251g	186	4.8	74	11.3	3.0	1.9	1.7
Chicken Tikka, Waitrose*	1 Pack/400g	560	30.4	140	14.0	3.8	7.6	2.1
Chicken Tikka & Pilau Rice, BGTY, Sainsbury's*	1 Pack/400g	448	4.0	112	8.3	17.5	1.0	1.9
King Prawns, Finest, Tesco*	1 Pack/350g	514	38.8	147	6.0	6.0	11.1	1.3
Paneer, Ashoka*	½ Pouch/150g	283	23.0	189	4.7	8.0	15.3	1.0
MALT DRINK								
Non-alcoholic, Supermalt*	1 Bottle/330g	210	0.0	64	0.8	15.1	0.0	0.0
MALTESERS								
MaltEaster, Chocolate Bunny, Mars*	1 Bunny/29g	157	9.2	541	6.9	57.0	31.7	0.0
Mars*	1 Reg Bag/37g	187	9.1	505	7.9	62.8	24.6	0.9
White Chocolate, Mars*	1 Pack/37g	186	9.4	504	7.9	61.0	25.4	0.0
MANDARIN ORANGES								
in Juice, Average	*1oz/28g*	*11*	*0.0*	*39*	*0.7*	*9.0*	*0.0*	*0.5*
in Light Syrup, Average	*1 Can/298g*	*201*	*0.1*	*67*	*0.5*	*15.9*	*0.0*	*0.1*
in Orange Gel, Del Monte*	1 Can/128g	60	0.0	47	0.0	10.9	0.0	0.0
Weighed with Peel, Average	*1 Sm/50g*	*18*	*0.0*	*36*	*0.9*	*8.3*	*0.1*	*1.2*
MANGE TOUT								
Boiled in Salted Water	*1oz/28g*	*7*	*0.0*	*26*	*3.2*	*3.3*	*0.1*	*2.2*
Raw, Average	*1 Serving/80g*	*26*	*0.2*	*32*	*3.6*	*4.2*	*0.2*	*1.1*
Stir-Fried in Blended Oil	*1oz/28g*	*20*	*1.3*	*71*	*3.8*	*3.5*	*4.8*	*2.4*
MANGO								
& Melon, Sliced, Shapers, Boots*	1 Pack/80g	33	0.2	41	0.7	9.2	0.2	1.8
Dried, Average	*1 Serving/50g*	*173*	*0.5*	*347*	*1.4*	*83.1*	*1.0*	*4.9*
Dried, with Chilli, King Henry's*	1 Bag /120g	300	0.0	250	0.0	62.5	0.0	1.0
in Syrup, Average	*1oz/28g*	*22*	*0.0*	*80*	*0.3*	*20.5*	*0.0*	*0.9*
Pieces in Juice, Natures Finest*	1 Pot/220g	123	0.4	56	0.5	12.3	0.2	1.5
Pineapple & Passionfruit, M & S*	1 Pack/400g	200	0.8	50	0.6	10.9	0.2	1.7
Ripe, Raw, Weighed with Skin & Stone, Average	*1 Mango/225g*	*88*	*0.2*	*39*	*0.5*	*9.6*	*0.1*	*1.8*
Ripe, Raw, without Peel & Stone, Flesh Only, Average	*1 Mango/207g*	*81*	*1.0*	*39*	*0.5*	*9.6*	*0.5*	*1.8*
MANGOSTEEN								
Raw, Fresh, Average	*1 Serving/80g*	*50*	*0.5*	*63*	*0.6*	*15.6*	*0.6*	*5.1*
MARBLE								
Cadbury*	1 Bar/46g	246	14.4	535	8.4	54.8	31.2	0.0
MARGARINE								
Average	*1 Thin Spread/7g*	*51*	*5.7*	*726*	*0.1*	*0.5*	*81.0*	*0.0*
Butter Style, Average	*1 Thin Spread/7g*	*44*	*4.8*	*627*	*0.7*	*1.1*	*68.9*	*0.0*
for Baking, Average	*1 Thin Spread/7g*	*42*	*4.7*	*607*	*0.2*	*0.4*	*67.2*	*0.0*

INFO/WEIGHT	per Measure KCAL	FAT	Nutrition Values per 100g / 100ml KCAL	PROT	CARB	FAT	FIBRE

MARGARINE
	INFO/WEIGHT	KCAL	FAT	KCAL	PROT	CARB	FAT	FIBRE
No Salt, Flora*	1 Thin Spread/7g	37	4.1	531	0.0	0.0	59.0	0.0
Omega 3 Plus, Flora*	1 Thin Spread/7g	24	2.7	350	0.1	3.0	38.0	0.0
Pro Activ, Extra Light, Flora*	1 Thin Spread/7g	15	1.6	218	0.1	2.9	23.0	0.2
Pro Activ, Light, Flora*	1 Thin Spread/7g	23	2.4	331	0.1	4.0	35.0	0.0
Pro Activ, with Olive Oil, Flora*	1 Thin Spread/7g	23	2.4	331	0.1	4.0	35.0	0.0
Pro Active, Becel*	1 Serving/7g	22	1.7	320	0.0	0.0	25.0	0.0
Reduced Fat, Average	*1 Thin Spread/7g*	*25*	*2.7*	*356*	*0.5*	*3.0*	*38.0*	*0.0*
Soya, Granose*	1 Thin Spread/7g	52	5.7	745	0.1	0.1	82.0	0.0
Utterly Butterly*	1 Thin Spread/7g	32	3.4	452	0.3	2.5	49.0	0.0
White, Flora*	1 Thin Spread/7g	60	6.6	855	0.0	0.0	95.0	0.0

MARGARITA
	INFO/WEIGHT	KCAL	FAT	KCAL	PROT	CARB	FAT	FIBRE
Sainsbury's*	1 Serving/100ml	53	0.1	53	0.1	12.8	0.1	0.1

MARINADE
	INFO/WEIGHT	KCAL	FAT	KCAL	PROT	CARB	FAT	FIBRE
Barbecue, COU, M & S*	1 Serving/35g	52	0.1	150	1.2	35.5	0.2	1.0
Barbeque, Sticky, Sainsbury's*	¼ Jar/77g	112	2.8	145	0.8	26.7	3.6	1.0
Cajun Spice, The English Provender Co.*	1 Serving/50g	93	6.7	187	1.3	15.3	13.4	1.6
Chinese, Classic, Sharwood's*	1oz/28g	32	1.3	113	1.8	16.1	4.8	1.0
Hickory Dickory Smokey, Ainsley Harriott*	1 Pot/300ml	360	0.3	120	0.6	28.1	0.1	0.0
Hot & Spicy Barbecue, M & S*	1 Serving/18g	23	0.1	130	1.0	31.1	0.3	0.8
Lemon & Rosemary, Nando's*	1 fl oz/30ml	44	3.9	147	1.0	11.8	13.0	0.2
Lime & Coriander with Peri Peri, Nando's*	1 Tsp/5g	9	0.8	182	0.0	13.1	16.6	0.2
Peri Peri, Hot, Nando's*	1 Serving/40g	36	1.9	89	0.0	10.9	4.8	0.1
Sticky Barbecue, Tesco*	¼ Jar/70g	80	0.1	115	0.7	26.7	0.2	0.6
Sticky BBQ, Eat Well, M & S*	1 Bottle/250ml	400	1.2	160	0.7	37.8	0.5	1.0
Sun Dried Tomato & Basil with Peri-Peri, Nando's*	1 Bottle/270g	319	25.6	118	0.1	15.3	9.5	0.8
Tequila Chilli Lime, M & S*	1 Serving/75ml	116	1.2	155	0.6	34.0	1.6	0.5

MARJORAM
	INFO/WEIGHT	KCAL	FAT	KCAL	PROT	CARB	FAT	FIBRE
Dried	*1 Tsp/1g*	*2*	*0.0*	*271*	*12.7*	*42.5*	*7.0*	*0.0*

MARLIN
	INFO/WEIGHT	KCAL	FAT	KCAL	PROT	CARB	FAT	FIBRE
Smoked, H. Forman & Son*	1 Pack/200g	240	0.2	120	29.8	0.0	0.1	0.0
Steaks, Chargrilled, Sainsbury's*	1 Steak/240g	367	14.6	153	23.6	0.8	6.1	0.6
Steaks, Raw, Sainsbury's*	1 Steak/110g	109	0.2	99	24.3	0.0	0.2	0.0

MARMALADE
	INFO/WEIGHT	KCAL	FAT	KCAL	PROT	CARB	FAT	FIBRE
3 Fruit, Thick Cut, Waitrose*	1 Tsp/15g	39	0.0	262	0.4	64.8	0.1	0.7
Blood Orange, TTD, Sainsbury's*	1 Tbsp/15g	40	0.0	264	0.3	65.7	0.0	0.8
Citrus Shred, Robertson*	1 Tsp/5g	13	0.0	253	0.2	63.0	0.0	0.0
Five Fruit, Tesco*	1 Serving/10g	28	0.0	278	0.2	68.2	0.1	0.9
Grapefruit, Fine Cut, Duerr's*	1 Tsp/15g	39	0.0	261	0.2	65.0	0.0	0.0
Grapefruit & Cranberry, M & S*	1 Tsp/15g	36	0.0	240	0.3	60.3	0.0	1.5
Lemon, with Shred, Average	*1 Serving/20g*	*49*	*0.0*	*247*	*0.1*	*61.6*	*0.0*	*0.6*
Lemon & Lime, Average	*1 Tbsp/20g*	*53*	*0.0*	*267*	*0.1*	*66.3*	*0.1*	*0.4*
Lime, with Shred, Average	*1 Tbsp/15g*	*39*	*0.0*	*261*	*0.1*	*65.0*	*0.1*	*0.3*
Onion, Organic, Antony Worrall Thompson's*	1 Serving/11g	20	0.1	191	1.1	44.9	0.8	1.8
Onion, Organic, Duchy Originals*	1 Serving/40g	103	1.0	257	1.0	57.8	2.4	2.6
Orange, Lemon & Grapefruit, Baxters*	1 Tsp/15g	38	0.0	252	0.0	63.0	0.0	0.1
Orange, Reduced Sugar, Average	*1 Tbsp/15g*	*26*	*0.0*	*170*	*0.4*	*42.0*	*0.1*	*0.6*
Orange, Shredless, Average	*1 Tsp/10g*	*26*	*0.0*	*261*	*0.2*	*65.0*	*0.0*	*0.1*
Orange, with Drambuie, Finest, Tesco*	1 Serving/10g	33	0.0	329	0.3	82.0	0.0	0.7
Orange, with Shred, Average	*1 Tbsp/15g*	*39*	*0.0*	*263*	*0.2*	*65.2*	*0.0*	*0.3*
Orange & Ginger, Average	*1 Tbsp/15g*	*40*	*0.0*	*264*	*0.2*	*65.7*	*0.1*	*0.3*
Orange & Lemon, Reduced Sugar, Zest*	1 Tsp/6g	12	0.0	195	0.3	47.1	0.2	0.0
Orange & Tangerine, Tiptree, Wilkin & Sons*	1 Tsp/15g	40	0.0	268	0.0	67.0	0.0	0.0
Pink Grapefruit, Thin Cut, Waitrose*	1 Serving/10g	26	0.0	261	0.2	65.0	0.0	0.4

M

	Measure INFO/WEIGHT	per Measure		Nutrition Values per 100g / 100ml				
		KCAL	FAT	KCAL	PROT	CARB	FAT	FIBRE
MARMALADE								
Three Fruit, Diabetic, Thursday Cottage*	1 Serving/5g	8	0.0	154	0.4	38.0	0.0	1.0
MARMITE*								
Xo, Marmite*	1 Serving/4g	10	0.0	250	37.5	25.0	0.2	0.2
Yeast Extract, Marmite*	1 Tsp/9g	23	0.0	252	38.7	24.1	0.1	3.4
MARROW								
Boiled, Average	*1oz/28g*	*3*	*0.1*	*9*	*0.4*	*1.6*	*0.2*	*0.6*
Raw	*1oz/28g*	*3*	*0.1*	*12*	*0.5*	*2.2*	*0.2*	*0.5*
MARS								
Bar, 5 Little Ones, Mars*	1 Piece/8g	38	1.5	477	4.5	73.6	18.3	0.0
Bar, Duo, Mars*	1 Bar/42g	191	7.6	450	4.4	67.5	18.0	1.2
Bar, Funsize, Mars*	1 Bar/18g	80	3.0	446	3.5	70.1	16.8	1.1
Bar, Mars*	1 Std Bar/58	260	10.2	448	4.1	68.1	17.6	1.1
Bar, Medium, 58g, Mars*	1 Serving/58g	263	10.5	453	4.6	67.9	18.1	0.0
Delight, Mars*	1 Bar/20g	110	6.7	552	4.5	57.8	33.6	1.3
Triple Choc, Bar, Limited Edition, Mars*	1 Bar/52g	233	9.0	448	4.5	67.7	17.3	2.0
MARSHMALLOWS								
Average	1 Mallow/5g	16	0.0	327	3.9	83.1	0.0	0.0
Chocolate Mallows, Cadbury*	1 Mallow/13g	56	2.2	435	4.7	64.7	17.4	0.8
Raspberry & Cream, Sainsbury's*	1 Mallow/7g	23	0.0	330	4.1	78.5	0.0	0.5
MARZIPAN								
Bar, Chocolate, Plain, Thorntons*	1 Bar/46g	206	8.0	448	5.2	69.1	17.4	2.0
Dark Chocolate, Thorntons*	1 Serving/46g	207	8.0	451	5.2	69.4	17.4	2.1
Plain, Average	*1oz/28g*	*115*	*4.0*	*412*	*5.8*	*67.5*	*14.1*	*1.7*
MASALA								
Chicken, Tandoori, M & S*	½ Pack/175g	210	11.5	120	11.3	4.3	6.6	4.5
Dal with Channa & Toor Lentils, Waitrose*	½ Pack/150g	166	6.1	111	6.6	12.0	4.1	5.0
Prawn, & Rice, Tesco*	1 Pack/475g	655	24.7	138	5.2	17.9	5.2	1.2
Prawn, King, Waitrose*	1 Pack/350g	385	25.9	110	7.1	3.8	7.4	1.8
Vegetable, Waitrose*	1 Serving/400g	288	19.2	72	2.2	4.9	4.8	2.5
MASH								
Carrot, Parsnip & Turnip, Mash Direct*	1 Serving/100g	63	2.0	63	1.0	10.2	2.0	2.8
Carrot & Parsnip, Direct Foods*	1 Pack/380g	201	8.7	53	1.0	7.6	2.3	3.2
Creamy Carrot & Swede, Weight Watchers*	1 Pack/250g	182	4.2	73	1.4	11.8	1.7	2.4
Davidstow Cheddar, Extra Special, Asda*	1 Serving/225g	292	16.9	130	5.3	10.4	7.5	2.6
Parsnip & Parmesan, Finest, Tesco*	½ Packet/250g	245	12.2	98	1.6	11.9	4.9	2.4
Potato, Carrot, Swede, Parsnip, Cream & Butter, Asda*	½ Pack/200g	94	3.0	47	1.0	7.2	1.5	3.3
Root, Asda*	½ Pack/200g	142	8.0	71	0.7	8.0	4.0	3.1
Root Vegetable, Finest, Tesco*	½ Pack/250g	225	12.5	90	1.1	9.1	5.0	3.4
Winter Root, Sainsbury's*	1 Serving/140g	157	2.1	112	2.7	22.0	1.5	0.9
MAYONNAISE								
Aioli, Finest, Tesco*	1 Tsp/5g	20	2.1	408	0.8	8.5	41.2	0.0
Average	*1 Tsp/11g*	*80*	*8.7*	*724*	*1.9*	*0.2*	*79.3*	*0.0*
Beolive Roasted Garlic Flavour, Vandemooetele*	1 Serving/15ml	46	4.2	305	1.3	11.3	28.2	0.0
Bramwells, Extra Light, Specially Selected, Aldi*	1 Tbsp/33g	40	3.2	121	1.1	7.2	9.7	2.4
Deli, Caramelised Onion, Heinz*	1 Serving/20g	110	11.5	548	1.4	5.9	57.5	0.1
Deli, Moroccan, Heinz*	1 Tbsp/15g	80	8.5	532	0.9	4.6	56.5	0.1
Deli, Roasted Garlic, Heinz*	1 Tbsp/15g	81	8.5	537	1.1	5.5	56.6	0.0
Deli, Sundried Tomato, Heinz*	1 Tbsp/15g	88	9.4	589	1.3	4.9	62.5	0.0
Egg & Dairy Free, Life Free From*	1 Serving/15g	76	8.0	508	0.9	5.6	53.3	0.2
Extra Light, Heinz*	1 Tbsp/12ml	9	0.4	75	0.6	11.4	3.0	0.6
Extra Light, Now Only 3% Fat, Hellmann's*	1 Serving/16g	12	0.5	73	0.6	11.0	3.0	0.6
Extra Light, Weight Watchers*	1 Serving/15g	15	0.9	97	1.1	9.6	5.9	3.2
French, Light, Sainsbury's*	1 Serving/15ml	46	4.7	307	0.4	6.1	31.1	0.2

MAYONNAISE

	Measure INFO/WEIGHT	per Measure KCAL	FAT	per 100g / 100ml KCAL	PROT	CARB	FAT	FIBRE
French Style, BGTY, Sainsbury's*	1 Tbsp/15ml	55	5.5	366	0.6	7.5	36.9	0.0
Garlic, Waitrose*	1 Tsp/6g	21	2.1	346	0.6	8.6	34.3	0.0
Garlic & Herb, M & S*	1 Tsp/6g	43	4.6	712	3.4	2.4	76.9	0.9
Garlic & Herb, Reduced Calorie, Hellmann's*	1 Serving/25ml	58	4.8	233	0.7	13.1	19.3	0.4
Garlic Flavoured, Frank Cooper*	1 Tsp/6g	28	2.8	460	2.2	8.8	46.2	0.1
Lemon, Waitrose*	1 Tsp/8ml	56	6.1	694	1.2	1.3	76.0	5.4
Light, Hellmann's*	1 Serving/10g	30	3.0	298	0.7	6.5	29.8	0.1
Light, Knorr*	1 Tbsp/15g	50	5.0	333	0.0	6.7	33.3	0.0
Light, Kraft*	1 Serving/25g	61	5.0	245	0.6	15.0	20.0	0.0
Light, Reduced Fat, Heinz*	1 Tbsp/15g	42	4.0	279	1.1	7.7	26.8	0.5
Light Dijon, Benedicta*	1 Tbsp/15g	44	4.4	292	0.7	6.7	29.2	0.0
Made with Free Range Eggs, M & S*	1 Tbsp/15g	108	11.8	720	1.1	1.2	78.5	0.0
Mild Dijon Mustard, Frank Cooper*	1 Pot/28g	114	11.1	406	3.3	9.3	39.5	0.1
Organic, Evernat*	1 Tsp/11g	83	8.9	752	1.3	2.8	81.0	0.0
Original, Egg, Dairy & Gluten Free, Tiger Tiger*	1 Tbsp/15g	66	6.8	440	1.4	5.8	45.6	0.3
Reduced Calorie, Average	*1 Tsp/11g*	*32*	*3.1*	*288*	*1.0*	*8.2*	*28.1*	*0.0*
Vegetarian, Tesco*	1 Tsp/12g	89	9.7	738	1.5	0.8	81.0	0.0
with a Twist of Lemon & Roast Garlic, Branston*	1 Tbsp/15ml	64	6.1	428	0.9	13.8	41.0	0.3
with a Twist of Lime & Chilli, Branston*	1 Serving/15ml	65	6.2	436	1.0	15.6	41.1	0.2
with a Twist of Pesto, Branston*	1 Tbsp/30ml	124	11.6	412	1.2	14.1	38.6	0.2
with Coarse Ground Mustard, French, Sainsbury's*	1 Serving/15ml	93	10.1	618	0.8	1.7	67.3	0.3
with Dijon Mustard, Hellmann's*	1 Tbsp/15ml	31	3.0	210	2.9	5.1	19.7	0.0

MEAL REPLACEMENT

	Measure INFO/WEIGHT	per Measure KCAL	FAT	per 100g / 100ml KCAL	PROT	CARB	FAT	FIBRE
Banana Flavour Shake, Celebrity Slim*	1 Sachet/55g	214	2.4	389	34.5	51.5	4.4	0.6
Banana Flavoured, Shake, Mealpak, All About Weight*	1 Pack/32g	120	3.3	375	37.5	30.3	10.3	8.1
Bars, Chocolate, Slim Fast*	1 Bar/39g	107	3.5	274	20.6	35.3	9.0	5.5
Bars, Chocolate & Hazelnut, Tesco*	1 Bar/65g	250	7.1	385	24.2	41.0	11.0	6.3
Bars, Toffee Delight, Slim Fast*	1 Bar/78g	248	7.5	318	20.6	45.3	9.6	5.9
Caffe Latte Flavour, Shake, Mealpak, All About Weight*	1 Pack/32g	120	3.4	375	37.5	31.3	10.6	8.1
Caramel Flavour Shake, Celebrity Slim*	1 Pack/55g	212	2.4	385	34.2	50.9	4.4	0.6
Chocolate Flavour Shake, Celebrity Slim*	1 Sachet/55g	211	2.5	383	34.0	49.1	4.5	2.2
Crispy, Raspberry, Meal Bar, Tesco*	1 Bar/60g	216	6.7	360	22.3	42.1	11.2	7.6
Milk Shake, Rich Chocolate Flavour, Slim Fast*	1 Bottle/325ml	227	4.9	70	4.5	8.0	1.5	1.0
Powder, Cafe Latte, Ultra Slim, Tesco*	2 Scoops/29g	110	2.2	379	22.1	48.1	7.7	14.6
Shake, Chocolate, Advantage, Atkins*	1 Serving/34g	121	4.2	361	49.0	8.1	12.5	15.5
Shake, Chocolate, Ready to Drink, Advantage, Atkins*	1 Carton/330ml	172	9.2	52	6.0	0.6	2.8	1.2
Shake, Herbalife*	1 Serving/250ml	245	6.4	98	10.0	8.8	2.6	1.0
Shake, Neways*	1 Serving/39g	142	3.5	364	46.0	34.0	9.0	15.4
Shake, Vanilla, Ready to Drink, Advantage, Atkins*	1 Carton/330ml	175	8.9	53	6.2	0.6	2.7	0.9
Strawberry, High Protein, Energy Meal, Spiru-tein*	1 Serving/34g	99	0.0	291	41.2	32.3	0.0	2.9
Strawberry Flavour, Shake, Meal Pack, All About Weight*	1 Pack/5g	2	0.0	40	0.0	3.5	0.0	45.0
Strawberry Flavour Shake, Celebrity Slim*	1 Sachet/55g	214	2.4	389	34.4	51.6	4.4	0.6
Toffee Flavoured, Shake, Mealpak, All About Weight*	1 Sachet/36g	149	7.0	413	35.2	24.4	19.4	6.9
Ultimate Meal, The Ultimate Meal*	1/3 Cup/40g	170	4.0	425	37.5	75.0	10.0	20.0
Ultra Slim, Chocolate, Meal Bar, Tesco*	1 Bar/60g	219	6.7	365	28.5	37.3	11.1	8.2
Ultra Slim, Ready to Drink, Strawberry, Tesco*	1 Carton/330ml	231	3.0	70	4.2	10.5	0.9	1.5
Ultra Slim, Ready to Drink, Vanilla, Tesco*	1 Carton/330ml	224	3.0	68	4.2	10.5	0.9	1.5
Ultra-Slim, Ready to Drink, Chocolate, Tesco*	1 Carton/330ml	214	3.6	65	4.0	9.8	1.1	1.3
Vanilla Flavour Shake, Celebrity Slim*	1 Sachet/55g	215	2.4	391	34.2	52.0	4.4	0.6
Vanilla Flavoured, Shake, Mealpak, All About Weight*	1 Shake/32g	120	3.3	375	37.5	30.6	10.3	8.1

MEAT LOAF

	Measure INFO/WEIGHT	per Measure KCAL	FAT	per 100g / 100ml KCAL	PROT	CARB	FAT	FIBRE
Beef & Pork, Co-Op*	¼ Loaf/114g	313	25.1	275	13.0	7.0	22.0	1.0
Iceland*	1 Serving/150g	331	23.5	221	10.8	9.3	15.7	0.9

MEAT LOAF

	Measure INFO/WEIGHT	per Measure KCAL	FAT	Nutrition Values per 100g / 100ml KCAL	PROT	CARB	FAT	FIBRE
in Onion Gravy, M & S*	¼ Pack/140g	203	11.9	145	11.3	6.3	8.5	1.2
Turkey & Bacon, Tesco*	1 Serving/225g	400	22.3	178	14.7	7.4	9.9	1.1

MEATBALLS

	Measure INFO/WEIGHT	per Measure KCAL	FAT	Nutrition Values per 100g / 100ml KCAL	PROT	CARB	FAT	FIBRE
& Mashed Potato, Tesco*	1 Pack/450g	526	29.7	117	4.0	10.4	6.6	1.0
& Pasta, Sainsbury's*	1 Serving/300g	333	9.3	111	5.3	15.5	3.1	1.9
& Pasta in Tomato Sauce, Wayfayrer*	1 Pack/300g	375	17.4	125	9.0	9.2	5.8	1.0
Beef, Aberdeen Angus, 12 Pack, Waitrose*	1 Meatball/36g	93	7.1	259	18.0	2.3	19.8	0.1
Beef, British, with Italian Herbs, Finest, Tesco*	1oz/28g	63	4.7	225	15.4	2.1	16.8	1.7
Beef, in Tomato Sauce, Diet Chef Ltd*	1 Pack/300g	408	18.6	136	11.3	8.7	6.2	2.7
Beef, Sainsbury's*	1 Meatball/29g	75	5.1	257	21.7	3.4	17.4	0.8
Beef, TTD, Sainsbury's*	1 Meatball/35g	73	5.2	208	16.7	1.5	15.0	0.1
Chicken, in Tomato Sauce, Average	1 Can/392g	580	32.9	148	7.7	10.4	8.4	0.0
Greek, M & S*	1 Serving/350g	402	18.9	115	7.7	9.1	5.4	1.5
in Bolognese Sauce, Fray Bentos*	½ Can/204g	188	5.9	92	4.8	11.6	2.9	0.7
in Gravy, Campbell's*	½ Can/205g	164	5.3	80	5.6	8.6	2.6	0.0
in Gravy, Fray Bentos*	1 Meatball/21g	17	0.6	79	4.6	8.7	2.9	0.6
in Onion Gravy, Tesco*	½ Pack/200g	310	17.0	155	8.4	11.3	8.5	0.8
in Rich Gravy, Westlers*	½ Can/200g	170	6.8	85	4.1	9.5	3.4	0.4
in Sherry Sauce, Tapas, Waitrose*	1 Serving/185g	272	7.4	147	18.8	5.9	4.0	1.2
in Tomato & Basil Sauce, Go Cook, Asda*	½ Pack/270g	526	38.3	195	12.4	4.4	14.2	2.4
in Tomato Sauce, Canned, Average	1 Can/410g	387	15.1	94	5.6	9.8	3.7	0.0
in Tomato Sauce, Tapas, Waitrose*	1 Pack/185g	285	16.8	154	10.8	7.2	9.1	1.3
Italian Pork, Al Forno, Sainsbury's*	1 Pack/450g	643	23.8	143	6.1	17.6	5.3	1.4
Lamb, Asda*	1 Pack/340g	928	71.4	273	16.0	5.1	21.0	0.6
Lemon Chicken, with Rice, BGTY, Sainsbury's*	1 Pack/400g	388	8.4	97	6.8	12.8	2.1	1.4
Lion's Head, M & S*	1 Serving/300g	435	27.9	145	10.4	5.1	9.3	1.0
Pork, Diet Chef Ltd*	1 Pack/300g	273	5.1	91	9.4	9.4	1.7	3.2
Pork & Beef, Swedish Style, Tesco*	1 Meatball/14g	34	2.5	245	14.3	6.5	17.7	2.0
Pork & Chorizo with Paprika Potatoes, Finest, Tesco*	½ Pack/425g	527	25.9	124	7.5	9.8	6.1	2.8
Roman-Style with Basil Mash, COU, M & S*	1 Pack/430g	344	9.5	80	3.7	10.9	2.2	1.9
Spaghetti, Tesco*	1 Pack/385g	377	16.0	98	5.4	9.8	4.2	1.2
Spiced Lamb, Feta with Paprika Potatoes, Finest, Tesco*	1 Pack/400g	460	20.0	115	6.4	7.5	5.0	6.5
Spicy, Deli Melt, Sainsbury's*	1 Pack/200g	338	21.4	169	12.7	5.5	10.7	2.9
Spicy, M & S*	1 Pack/400g	540	24.0	135	8.8	12.0	6.0	1.4
Swedish, Average	¼ Pack/88g	198	13.8	224	14.0	7.4	15.7	1.3
Turkey, GFY, Asda*	½ Pack/330g	333	12.2	101	10.0	7.0	3.7	0.0
with Paprika-Spiced Potatoes, Extra Special, Asda*	1 Pack/450g	589	23.8	131	6.5	13.4	5.3	2.0
with Spicy Tomato Sauce, Just Cook, Sainsbury's*	½ Pack/170g	246	11.9	145	14.8	5.7	7.0	0.9

MEATBALLS VEGETARIAN

	Measure INFO/WEIGHT	per Measure KCAL	FAT	Nutrition Values per 100g / 100ml KCAL	PROT	CARB	FAT	FIBRE
Swedish Style, Sainsbury's*	1 Ball/27g	53	2.6	194	21.5	5.5	9.5	4.0
with Penne, Tesco*	1 Serving/460g	414	10.6	90	5.9	11.4	2.3	2.1

MEDLAR

	Measure INFO/WEIGHT	per Measure KCAL	FAT	Nutrition Values per 100g / 100ml KCAL	PROT	CARB	FAT	FIBRE
Raw, Flesh Only	*1 Fruit/28g*	*11*	*0.1*	*40*	*0.5*	*10.6*	*0.4*	*10.0*

MELBA TOAST

	Measure INFO/WEIGHT	per Measure KCAL	FAT	Nutrition Values per 100g / 100ml KCAL	PROT	CARB	FAT	FIBRE
Average	1 Serving/3g	13	0.2	396	12.0	76.0	4.9	4.6
Dutch, Light Choices, Tesco*	1 Pack/20g	75	0.5	375	13.1	75.0	2.4	4.6
Organic, Trimlyne*	2 Toasts/7g	28	0.5	407	13.7	71.6	6.8	5.3
Organic Spelt, Demeter*	2 Biscuits/25g	99	2.0	395	12.4	68.5	7.9	0.0
Original, Van Der Meulen*	1 Slice/3g	12	0.1	399	12.8	80.5	2.9	3.9
Tomato & Basil, Morrisons*	1 Pack/20g	77	0.6	383	13.6	75.7	2.9	2.4
Wholegrain, HL, Tesco*	1 Pack/20g	74	1.0	370	16.8	63.8	4.9	8.9
Wholegrain, Morrisons*	6 Toasts/20g	73	1.0	367	16.8	63.8	4.9	8.9
with Sesame, Tesco*	1 Slice/3g	11	0.2	370	12.8	61.7	8.0	3.8

INFO/WEIGHT	Measure	per Measure		Nutrition Values per 100g / 100ml				
		KCAL	FAT	KCAL	PROT	CARB	FAT	FIBRE
MELON								
Cantaloupe, Flesh Only, Average	*½ Melon/255g*	*87*	*0.5*	*34*	*0.8*	*8.2*	*0.2*	*0.9*
Cantaloupe, Weighed with Rind, Average	*1 Slice/100g*	*35*	*0.3*	*35*	*0.8*	*8.3*	*0.3*	*0.8*
Galia, Average	*1 Serving/240g*	*60*	*0.1*	*25*	*0.7*	*5.7*	*0.0*	*0.2*
Honeydew, Raw, Flesh Only, Average	*1oz/28g*	*8*	*0.0*	*29*	*0.7*	*6.9*	*0.1*	*0.5*
MELT								
Cheese, Chilli, Fresh, Asda*	1 Melt/29g	87	4.9	301	6.0	31.0	17.0	0.0
Cheesy Fish, Youngs*	1 Pack/340g	418	22.4	123	7.6	8.3	6.6	0.9
Chilli with Spicy Potato Wedges, Asda*	1 Pack/450g	540	19.8	120	8.0	12.0	4.4	1.2
Sausage & Bean, Iceland*	1 Pack/400g	588	23.2	147	6.5	17.1	5.8	1.6
Tuna, Go Large, Asda*	1 Melt/175g	509	26.2	291	12.0	27.0	15.0	0.0
Tuna, M & S*	1 Pack/218g	621	37.1	285	13.0	20.1	17.0	1.0
MENTOS								
Cola, Mentos*	1 Packet/38g	146	0.7	390	0.0	93.0	2.0	0.0
MERINGUE								
Average	*1 Meringue/8g*	*30*	*0.0*	*379*	*5.3*	*95.4*	*0.0*	*0.0*
Belgian Chocolate, Mini, Extra Special, Asda*	1 Meringue/6g	28	0.9	459	6.0	75.0	15.0	0.7
Bombe, Raspberry & Vanilla, M & S*	1 Bombe/100g	155	1.8	155	3.4	33.3	1.8	2.6
Chocolate, Waitrose*	1 Meringue/77g	341	11.3	444	2.6	75.3	14.7	0.5
Coffee Fresh Cream, Asda*	1 Meringue/28g	109	4.7	396	3.8	57.0	17.0	0.3
Cream, Fresh, Sainsbury's*	1 Meringue/35g	142	5.1	407	3.5	65.4	14.6	0.5
Cream, M & S*	1 Meringue/34g	145	7.6	425	4.1	52.6	22.2	1.4
Lemon, Morrisons*	1 Serving/120g	295	14.4	246	2.5	32.0	12.0	0.5
Nests, Average	1 Nest/16g	63	0.0	397	4.7	93.3	0.1	0.1
Nests, Tropical Fruit, Sainsbury's*	1 Nest/95g	234	7.4	246	2.0	42.0	7.8	2.4
Raspberry, M & S*	1 Serving/105g	215	13.8	205	1.8	20.6	13.1	3.1
Shells, Sainsbury's*	2 Shells/24g	93	0.0	387	3.9	92.8	0.0	0.0
Strawberry, COU, M & S*	1 Meringue/5g	20	0.0	385	6.4	90.0	0.1	1.4
Strawberry, Mini, Extra Special, Asda*	1 Meringue/4g	15	0.0	387	5.0	91.0	0.3	0.5
Toffee, COU, M & S*	1 Mini/5g	20	0.1	395	5.0	95.3	1.7	0.7
Toffee, M & S*	1 Meringue/30g	124	6.3	415	4.1	52.2	20.9	0.8
Tropical, M & S*	1 Serving/53g	212	14.3	400	3.1	37.0	26.9	0.0
MIDGET GEMS								
M & S*	1 Bag/113g	367	0.1	325	6.3	75.1	0.1	0.0
MILK								
Condensed, Caramel, Carnation, Nestle*	1 Serving/50g	148	3.0	296	5.5	55.1	6.0	0.0
Condensed, Semi Skimmed, Sweetened	*1oz/28g*	*75*	*0.1*	*267*	*10.0*	*60.0*	*0.2*	*0.0*
Condensed, Skimmed, Unsweetened, Average	*1oz/28g*	*30*	*1.1*	*108*	*7.5*	*10.5*	*4.0*	*0.0*
Condensed, Whole, Sweetened, Average	*1oz/28g*	*93*	*2.8*	*333*	*8.5*	*55.5*	*10.1*	*0.0*
Dried, Skimmed, Average	*1oz/28g*	*99*	*0.3*	*355*	*35.4*	*52.3*	*0.9*	*0.0*
Dried, Whole, Average	*1oz/28g*	*137*	*7.4*	*490*	*26.3*	*39.4*	*26.3*	*0.0*
Evaporated, Average	*1 Serving/85g*	*136*	*7.6*	*160*	*8.2*	*11.6*	*9.0*	*0.0*
Evaporated, Reduced Fat, Average	*1oz/28g*	*33*	*1.5*	*118*	*7.4*	*10.5*	*5.2*	*0.0*
Goats, Pasteurised	*1 fl oz/30ml*	*18*	*1.0*	*60*	*3.1*	*4.4*	*3.5*	*0.0*
Low Fat, Calcia Extra Calcium, Unigate*	1 fl oz/30ml	13	0.1	45	4.3	6.3	0.5	0.0
Semi Skimmed, Average	*1 fl oz/30ml*	*15*	*0.5*	*49*	*3.4*	*5.0*	*1.7*	*0.0*
Semi Skimmed, Lactose Free, Arla*	1 Serving/100ml	40	1.5	40	3.9	2.8	1.5	0.0
Semi Skimmed, Long Life, Average	*1 fl oz/30ml*	*15*	*0.5*	*49*	*3.4*	*5.0*	*1.7*	*0.0*
Semi Skimmed, Organic, Country Life*	1 fl oz/30ml	15	0.5	49	3.4	5.0	1.7	0.0
Skimmed, Average	*1 fl oz/30ml*	*10*	*0.0*	*34*	*3.3*	*5.0*	*0.1*	*0.0*
Skimmed, Uht, Average	*1 fl oz/30ml*	*10*	*0.0*	*34*	*3.3*	*5.0*	*0.1*	*0.0*
Soya, Vitasoy*	1 Serving/250ml	130	3.7	52	3.0	5.5	1.5	2.0
Super Milk Low Fat 1%, Avonmore*	1 Litre/1000ml	420	10.0	42	3.4	5.0	1.0	0.0
Whole, Average	*1 Serving/200ml*	*134*	*7.8*	*67*	*3.3*	*4.7*	*3.9*	*0.0*

	Measure INFO/WEIGHT	per Measure KCAL	FAT	Nutrition Values per 100g / 100ml KCAL	PROT	CARB	FAT	FIBRE
MILK								
Whole, Lactose Free, Lactofree, Arla*	1 Serving/200ml	116	7.0	58	3.9	2.7	3.5	0.0
MILK DRINK								
Family Fuel, Mars*	1 Serving/200ml	172	4.0	86	3.1	13.7	2.0	0.0
Mocalatte, Cafe Met*	1 Bottle/290ml	159	3.8	55	2.9	8.0	1.3	0.0
No Added Sugar, Mars*	1 Serving/200ml	108	3.4	54	3.4	6.2	1.7	0.5
Original, Mars*	1 Serving/330g	284	6.9	86	3.1	13.7	2.1	0.0
Refuel, Mars*	1 Bottle/388ml	299	5.8	77	3.1	13.5	1.5	0.0
Semi Skimmed, Cholesterol Lowering, Pro Activ, Flora*	1 Serving/250ml	125	4.5	50	3.6	4.8	1.8	0.0
Strawberry, Probiotic, WellYou, Kaufland*	1 Bottle/125g	77	0.1	62	2.5	11.9	0.1	0.1
Strawberry Flavoured, Goodness for Kids, Tesco*	1 Bottle/330ml	247	5.6	75	4.0	9.9	1.7	0.4
MILK SHAKE								
Banana, Diet Chef Ltd*	1 Drink/330ml	225	3.0	68	4.2	10.5	0.9	1.5
Banana, Yazoo, Campina*	1 Bottle/200ml	130	2.6	65	3.1	10.3	1.3	0.0
Banana Flavour, Frijj*	1 Bottle/500ml	325	4.5	65	3.7	10.5	0.9	0.0
Banana Flavour, Shapers, Boots*	1 Bottle/250ml	201	1.9	80	5.6	12.8	0.8	1.9
Cafe Latte, Diet Chef Ltd*	1 Carton/330ml	209	2.8	63	4.4	10.4	0.8	1.4
Chocolate, Asda*	1 Serving/250ml	197	9.2	79	4.4	7.0	3.7	0.4
Chocolate, Diet Chef Ltd*	1 Carton/330ml	214	3.6	65	3.9	9.8	1.1	1.3
Chocolate, Extreme, Frijj*	1 Bottle/500g	425	10.5	85	3.9	12.7	2.1	0.0
Chocolate Flavour, BGTY, Sainsbury's*	1 Bottle/500ml	290	2.5	58	5.3	8.0	0.5	0.9
Chocolate Flavoured, Fresh, Thick, Frijj*	1 Bottle/500ml	350	5.0	70	3.5	11.7	1.0	0.0
Honeycomb Choc Swirl Flavour, The Incredible, Frijj*	1 Bottle/500ml	450	12.5	90	4.0	13.0	2.5	0.2
Latte Coffee, Diet Chef Ltd*	1 Drink/330ml	225	3.0	68	4.2	10.5	0.9	1.5
Measure Up, Asda*	1 Glass/250ml	200	2.4	80	6.0	12.0	1.0	2.4
Mount Caramel, Frijj*	1 Bottle/500ml	360	4.5	72	3.4	12.7	0.9	0.0
Peachy Banana, Syrup, Robinson's*	1 Serving/50ml	79	0.0	158	0.0	39.0	0.0	0.0
Powder, Made Up with Semi-Skimmed Milk	1 Serving/250ml	172	4.0	69	3.2	11.3	1.6	0.0
Powder, Made Up with Whole Milk	1 Serving/250ml	217	9.2	87	3.1	11.1	3.7	0.0
Sticky Toffee Pudding Flavour, The Incredible, Frijj*	1 Bottle/500ml	445	10.0	89	4.0	13.7	2.0	0.1
Strawberry, Diet Chef Ltd*	1 Drink/330g	225	3.0	68	4.2	10.5	0.9	1.5
Strawberry, Yazoo, Campina*	1 Bottle/500ml	325	6.0	65	3.1	10.3	1.2	0.0
Strawberry & Raspberry, Syrup, Robinson's*	1 Serving/50ml	20	0.7	39	2.9	4.0	1.4	0.0
Strawberry Flavour, Thick, Low Fat, Frijj*	1 Bottle/250ml	155	2.0	62	3.4	10.1	0.8	0.0
Thick, Milky Way, Mars*	1 Bottle/440ml	282	4.8	64	3.4	10.0	1.1	0.7
Vanilla, Diet Chef Ltd*	1 Pack/330ml	225	3.0	68	4.2	10.5	0.9	1.5
Vanilla, Frijj*	1 Bottle/500ml	320	4.0	64	3.4	10.7	0.8	0.0
Vanilla Flavour, BGTY, Sainsbury's*	1 Bottle/500ml	230	0.5	46	5.3	5.9	0.1	0.4
MILKY BAR								
Buttons, Nestle*	1 Std Pack/30g	164	9.5	547	7.3	58.4	31.7	0.0
Choo, Nestle*	1 Bar/25g	116	4.3	464	4.2	73.1	17.2	0.0
Chunky, Nestle*	¼ Bar/38g	207	12.0	547	7.3	58.4	31.7	0.0
Crunchies, Nestle*	1 Pack/30g	168	10.4	560	7.0	54.9	34.7	0.0
Eggs, Mini, Nestle*	1 Pack/100g	500	23.3	500	4.2	68.4	23.3	0.0
Funsize, Mars*	1 Bar/17g	75	2.7	449	3.8	71.8	16.3	0.6
Munchies, Nestle*	1 Serving/70g	392	24.3	560	7.0	54.9	34.7	0.1
Nestle*	1 Sm Bar/13g	68	4.0	547	7.3	58.4	31.7	0.0
MILKY WAY								
Funsize, Mars*	1 Bar/16g	70	2.5	450	3.9	71.6	16.3	0.6
Magic Stars, Mars*	1 Bag/33g	183	11.5	555	6.2	54.1	34.9	1.8
Mars*	1 Bar/26g	118	4.1	455	3.7	72.4	15.9	0.6
MINCEMEAT								
Average	**1oz/28g**	**77**	**1.2**	**274**	**0.6**	**62.1**	**4.3**	**1.3**
Organic, Waitrose*	1oz/28g	81	0.7	290	0.9	65.8	2.6	2.0

	Measure INFO/WEIGHT	per Measure KCAL	FAT	Nutrition Values per 100g / 100ml KCAL	PROT	CARB	FAT	FIBRE
MINCEMEAT								
with Cherries, Almonds & Brandy, Tesco*	¼ Jar/103g	295	5.0	287	1.4	58.8	4.9	1.4
MINIS								
Cream Cheese & Chives, Ryvita*	1 Pack/30g	103	0.9	342	8.0	71.0	2.9	11.5
Salt & Vinegar, Ryvita*	1 Pack/24g	90	1.9	376	8.2	74.0	7.8	11.4
Sweet Chilli, Ryvita*	1 Pack/30g	100	0.8	335	7.0	71.0	2.6	11.9
MINSTRELS								
Galaxy, Mars*	1 Serving/100g	503	22.3	503	5.2	70.3	22.3	1.1
MINT								
Dried, Average	*1 Tsp/5g*	*14*	*0.2*	*279*	*24.8*	*34.6*	*4.6*	*0.0*
Fresh, Average	*2 Tbsp/3g*	*1*	*0.0*	*43*	*3.8*	*5.3*	*0.7*	*0.0*
MINTS								
After Dinner, Dark, Elizabeth Shaw*	1 Sweet/9g	42	2.1	469	2.8	62.5	23.1	0.0
After Dinner, Sainsbury's*	1 Mint/7g	32	1.5	456	4.1	62.1	21.2	4.1
After Dinner, Tesco*	1oz/28g	132	5.3	471	5.0	70.0	19.0	0.0
Butter Mintoes, M & S*	1 Sweet/9g	35	0.6	391	0.0	84.0	6.8	0.0
Butter Mintoes, Tesco*	1 Sweet/7g	24	0.5	349	0.0	71.3	7.1	0.0
Clear, Co-Op*	1 Sweet/6g	24	0.0	395	0.0	98.0	0.0	0.0
Cream, Luxury, Thorntons*	1 Sweet/13g	62	3.1	477	4.2	62.3	23.8	2.3
Creams, Bassett's*	1 Sweet/11g	40	0.0	365	0.0	91.8	0.0	0.0
Curiously Strong, M & S*	1 Sweet/1g	4	0.0	390	0.4	97.5	0.0	0.0
Everton, Co-Op*	1 Sweet/6g	25	0.2	410	0.6	92.0	4.0	0.0
Extra, Peppermint Coolburst, Wrigley's*	1 Pack/22g	53	0.2	240	0.0	98.0	1.0	0.0
Extra, Spearmint, Sugar Free, Wrigley's*	1 Sweet/1.1g	3	0.0	244	0.0	98.5	0.8	0.0
Extra, Wrigley's*	1 Sweet/1.1g	3	0.0	240	0.0	64.0	1.0	0.0
Extra Strong, Peppermint, Trebor*	1 Roll/46g	180	0.1	395	0.4	98.1	0.2	0.0
Extra Strong, Spearmint, Trebor*	1 Pack/44g	174	0.0	395	0.4	98.7	0.0	0.0
Glacier, Fox's*	1 Sweet/5g	19	0.0	386	0.0	96.4	0.0	0.0
Humbugs, M & S*	1 Sweet/9g	37	0.4	407	0.6	91.1	4.4	0.0
Humbugs, Thorntons*	1 Sweet/9g	31	0.4	340	1.0	87.8	4.4	0.0
Imperials, M & S*	1 Sweet/3g	12	0.0	391	0.0	97.8	0.0	0.0
Imperials, Sainsbury's*	1 Sweet/3g	10	0.0	374	0.0	92.1	0.0	0.0
Imperials, Tesco*	1 Sweet/3g	12	0.0	397	0.6	98.7	0.0	0.0
Mentos, Sugar Free, Mentos*	1 Sweet/2g	5	0.1	260	1.0	87.0	5.5	0.0
Mint Assortment, M & S*	1 Sweet/7g	26	0.5	375	0.4	78.2	6.9	0.0
Mint Favourites, Bassett's*	1 Sweet/6g	22	0.4	367	0.9	77.4	5.9	0.0
Smooth, Weight Watchers*	1 Tube/25g	58	0.0	231	0.2	61.6	0.0	0.0
Soft, Trebor*	1 Pack/48g	182	0.0	380	0.0	94.9	0.0	0.0
Softmints, Peppermint, Trebor*	1 Pack/48g	170	0.0	355	0.0	88.9	0.0	0.0
Softmints, Spearmint, Trebor*	1 Pack/45g	170	0.0	375	0.0	94.3	0.0	0.0
Thins, Chocolate, Waitrose*	1 Thin/5g	27	1.3	509	4.2	69.6	23.8	0.2
MIRIN								
Rice Wine, Sweetened, Average	*1 Tbsp/15ml*	*35*	*0.0*	*231*	*0.2*	*41.6*	*0.0*	*0.0*
MISO								
Average	*1oz/28g*	*57*	*1.7*	*203*	*13.3*	*23.5*	*6.2*	*0.0*
MIXED HERBS								
Average	*1 Tsp/5g*	*13*	*0.4*	*260*	*12.9*	*37.5*	*8.5*	*6.7*
Herbes De Provence, Dried, Schwartz*	1 Tsp/2g	7	0.1	364	12.9	65.0	5.8	0.0
MIXED SPICE								
Rub, Moroccan, Schwartz*	1 Serving/3g	9	0.3	309	15.0	36.4	11.4	19.5
Schwartz*	1 Tsp/2g	8	0.2	390	10.4	65.8	9.5	2.0
MIXED VEGETABLES								
Baby, Iceland*	1 Serving/100g	20	0.0	20	1.2	3.9	0.0	2.7
Baby, Steam, Fresh, Tesco*	1 Pack/160g	72	1.3	45	2.7	6.7	0.8	3.8

MIXED VEGETABLES

	Measure INFO/WEIGHT	per Measure KCAL	FAT	Nutrition Values per 100g / 100ml KCAL	PROT	CARB	FAT	FIBRE
Baby Corn, Mange Tout & Baby Carrots, Tesco*	1 Pack/220g	64	0.9	29	2.3	4.3	0.4	2.2
Bag, M & S*	1 Serving/200g	70	0.4	35	2.9	5.6	0.2	0.0
Broccoli & Cauliflower Florets, Baby Carrots, Asda*	1 Serving/113g	28	0.7	25	2.2	2.6	0.6	2.4
Canned, Re-Heated, Drained	1oz/28g	11	0.2	38	1.9	6.1	0.8	1.7
Carrot, Cauliflower, & Broccoli, Fresh, Tesco*	1 Serving/80g	26	0.2	32	2.6	3.9	0.2	2.8
Carrot, Swede, Leek & Onion for Casserole, M & S*	1 Serving/100g	35	0.4	35	0.8	5.6	0.4	2.6
Carrot Batons, Cauliflower & Broccoli, Steamed, Asda*	1 Bag/120g	28	0.7	23	1.8	2.6	0.6	3.1
Carrots, Broccoli & Sweetcorn, Steam Veg, Tesco*	1 Sachet/160g	80	1.8	50	2.5	7.5	1.1	3.0
Carrots, Cauliflower & Broccoli, Waitrose*	1 Serving/100g	35	0.6	35	2.4	4.9	0.6	2.9
Casserole, Co-Op*	1 Serving/100g	40	0.3	40	1.2	7.5	0.3	2.1
Casserole, Frozen, Tesco*	1 Serving/100g	26	0.4	26	0.8	4.8	0.4	2.0
Casserole, Ready to Cook, Sainsbury's*	½ Pack/240g	74	0.7	31	0.9	6.2	0.3	1.4
Casserole, Tesco*	1 Pack/440g	176	1.3	40	1.2	8.0	0.3	2.3
Casserole, with Baby Potatoes, Fresh, M & S*	½ Pack/350g	140	1.0	40	1.2	7.8	0.3	2.1
Chef's Style, Ready Prepared, M & S*	1 Pack/240g	72	1.2	30	2.6	4.5	0.5	2.9
Chinese, Stir Fry, Amoy*	1 Serving/110g	27	0.3	25	1.8	3.7	0.3	0.0
Chunky, Frozen, Sainsbury's*	1 Serving/85g	31	0.6	37	2.9	4.7	0.7	3.1
Corn Baby, Fine Beans & Baby Carrots, Tesco*	1 Pack/250g	67	1.2	27	1.7	4.0	0.5	2.2
Crunchy, Tesco*	1 Pack/210g	63	0.8	30	1.7	5.0	0.4	2.4
Farmhouse, Four Seasons*	1 Serving/100g	26	0.7	26	2.2	2.7	0.7	0.0
Farmhouse, Frozen, Waitrose*	1 Serving/90g	22	0.5	25	1.9	3.1	0.6	2.4
Freshly Frozen, Asda*	1 Serving/80g	42	0.6	52	3.2	8.0	0.8	3.0
Frozen, Aldi*	1 Serving/100g	34	0.7	34	2.8	4.3	0.7	0.0
Frozen, Boiled in Salted Water	1oz/28g	12	0.1	42	3.3	6.6	0.5	0.0
Frozen, Waitrose*	1 Serving/80g	43	0.6	54	3.1	8.7	0.8	3.5
Green, Microwave, Aldi*	1 Serving/300g	189	9.0	63	3.5	5.6	3.0	4.1
in Salt Water, Tesco*	1/3 Can/65g	34	0.4	53	2.6	9.2	0.6	2.7
in Salted Water, Canned, Asda*	1 Serving/65g	31	0.1	48	2.6	9.0	0.2	1.7
in Salted Water, Nisa Heritage*	1 Serving/100g	39	0.8	39	1.9	6.1	0.8	1.7
Layered, Classics, M & S*	½ Pack/160g	112	6.2	70	1.2	7.3	3.9	1.2
Oriental, M & S*	1 Serving/250g	50	0.7	20	1.6	3.4	0.3	1.6
Peas, Carrots, & Baby Leeks, Prepared, Tesco*	½ Pack/130g	57	1.2	44	3.1	5.8	0.9	3.5
Peas & Carrots Crinkle Cut, D'Aucy*	1 Serving/265g	138	1.3	52	3.2	6.5	0.5	4.3
Potatoes, Broad Beans & Peas, M & S*	1 Pack/245g	147	3.2	60	2.9	12.9	1.3	3.4
Ready to Roast, Asda*	½ Pack/362g	315	11.6	87	1.6	13.0	3.2	2.4
Red Peppers & Courgette, Tesco*	1 Pack/250g	67	1.2	27	1.7	3.8	0.5	2.0
Roast, Four Seasons*	1 Serving/187g	79	0.4	42	1.2	8.8	0.2	0.0
Sainsbury's*	1 Serving/230g	55	1.4	24	2.1	2.5	0.6	0.0
Seasonal Selection, Tesco*	1 Serving/100g	37	0.4	37	1.1	7.2	0.4	2.2
Special, Freshly Frozen, Morrisons*	1 Serving/100g	48	0.8	48	3.2	7.2	0.8	0.0
Special, Sainsbury's*	1 Serving/120g	68	1.2	57	3.2	8.9	1.0	2.9
Summer, Tesco*	1 Pack/167g	55	0.8	33	2.6	4.5	0.5	2.8
Tenderstem Broccoli, Carrots & Mange Tout, M & S*	½ Pack/100g	35	0.2	35	2.9	5.6	0.2	2.1
Thai Style, in a Herb Marinade, Straight to Wok, Amoy*	1 Pouch/400g	74	0.8	19	0.7	3.5	0.2	0.0

MOLASSES

	Measure INFO/WEIGHT	per Measure KCAL	FAT	KCAL	PROT	CARB	FAT	FIBRE
Average	1 Tsp/5g	13	0.0	266	0.0	68.8	0.1	0.0

MONKEY NUTS

	Measure INFO/WEIGHT	per Measure KCAL	FAT	KCAL	PROT	CARB	FAT	FIBRE
Average	1oz/28g	158	13.4	565	25.5	8.2	47.9	6.3

MONKFISH

	Measure INFO/WEIGHT	per Measure KCAL	FAT	KCAL	PROT	CARB	FAT	FIBRE
Grilled	1oz/28g	27	0.2	96	22.7	0.0	0.6	0.0
Raw	1oz/28g	18	0.1	66	15.7	0.0	0.4	0.0

MONSTER MUNCH

	Measure INFO/WEIGHT	per Measure KCAL	FAT	KCAL	PROT	CARB	FAT	FIBRE
Flamin' Hot, Walkers*	1 Std Bag/22g	108	5.5	490	7.0	59.0	25.0	1.5

INFO/WEIGHT	Measure	per Measure		Nutrition Values per 100g / 100ml				
		KCAL	FAT	KCAL	PROT	CARB	FAT	FIBRE

MONSTER MUNCH
Pickled Onion, Walkers*	1 Std Bag/22g	108	5.5	490	6.0	60.0	25.0	1.7
Roast Beef, Walkers*	1 Std Bag/22g	108	5.5	490	7.0	59.0	25.0	1.7
Spicy, Walkers*	1 Std Bag/25g	125	7.2	500	5.0	55.0	29.0	1.3

MORNAY
Cod, Fillets, Sainsbury's*	1 Serving/153g	236	14.4	154	15.2	2.2	9.4	0.9
Cod, Nutritionally Balanced, M & S*	1 Pack/400g	320	10.4	80	6.8	7.2	2.6	1.6
Cod, Sainsbury's*	1 Serving/180g	277	16.9	154	15.2	2.2	9.4	0.9
Haddock, COU, M & S*	½ Pack/194g	165	3.9	85	14.5	2.6	2.0	0.6
Haddock, Perfectly Balanced, Waitrose*	1 Pack/360g	310	5.4	86	16.6	1.6	1.5	0.5
Haddock, Youngs*	½ Pack/190g	236	14.8	124	12.1	1.3	7.8	0.6
Salmon, with Broccoli, Weight Watchers*	1 Pack/320g	231	9.6	72	4.5	6.5	3.0	0.5
Smoked Haddock, Fresh Ideas, Morrisons*	½ Pack/170g	201	9.3	118	13.6	3.2	5.5	0.1
Spinach, Waitrose*	½ Pack/125g	112	8.6	90	3.3	3.6	6.9	1.6

MOUSSAKA
Aubergine & Lentil, Asda*	1 Pack/451g	370	17.1	82	3.9	8.1	3.8	2.9
Beef, BGTY, Sainsbury's*	1 Pack/400g	300	10.4	75	6.1	6.8	2.6	1.2
Beef, HL, Tesco*	1 Pack/450g	396	12.1	88	5.0	10.9	2.7	0.8
Cafe Culture, M & S*	1 Serving/375g	619	39.4	165	9.2	7.8	10.5	0.8
COU, M & S*	1 Pack/340g	272	9.9	80	5.3	8.5	2.9	1.4
Lamb, Finest, Tesco*	1 Pack/349g	510	38.1	146	5.8	6.2	10.9	3.4
Lamb, Light Choices, Tesco*	1 Pack/350g	280	10.5	80	4.3	8.7	3.0	1.3
Lamb, Sainsbury's*	1 Pack/329g	497	32.3	151	8.4	7.2	9.8	1.0
Low Saturated Fat, Waitrose*	1 Pack/350g	304	10.8	87	6.3	8.4	3.1	3.1
TTD, Sainsbury's*	1 Pack/399g	546	35.9	137	8.1	5.8	9.0	0.6
Vegetable, BGTY, Sainsbury's*	1 Pack/333g	253	6.0	76	2.6	11.5	1.8	1.6
Vegetable, COU, M & S*	1 Pack/400g	280	10.8	70	2.7	9.1	2.7	2.4
Vegetarian, Tesco*	1 Pack/300g	489	31.2	163	6.4	11.0	10.4	0.9

MOUSSE
Aero Chocolate, Nestle*	1 Pot/58g	101	3.0	174	4.8	27.3	5.1	1.1
Aero Twist Cappuccino & Chocolate, Nestle*	1 Pot/75g	135	8.1	180	4.2	16.8	10.8	0.2
Apricot, Lite, Onken*	1 Pot/150g	156	2.2	104	4.6	18.0	1.5	0.3
Banoffee, COU, M & S*	1 Pot/70g	101	1.5	145	2.9	28.8	2.1	1.5
Belgian Chocolate, Finest, Tesco*	1 Pot/120g	360	22.7	300	5.1	26.6	18.9	1.1
Belgian Chocolate & Vanilla, Weight Watchers*	1 Pot/80g	106	2.2	132	4.4	22.2	2.8	0.9
Black Cherry, Lite, Onken*	1 Pot/150g	156	2.2	104	4.6	17.9	1.5	0.2
Blackcurrant, HL, Tesco*	1 Pot/113g	80	2.9	71	3.7	8.3	2.6	1.8
Blackcurrant, Onken*	1 Pot/150g	210	10.2	140	5.2	14.6	6.8	0.0
Cadbury's Light Chocolate, St Ivel*	1 Pot/64g	79	2.0	123	6.2	17.3	3.2	0.0
Caramel, Meringue, Cadbury*	1 Pot/65g	181	6.7	277	4.6	42.4	10.3	1.0
Caramelised Orange, COU, M & S*	1 Pot/70g	91	1.2	130	2.8	26.3	1.7	3.4
Chocolate	1 Pot/60g	83	3.2	139	4.0	19.9	5.4	0.0
Chocolate, BGTY, Sainsbury's*	1 Pot/63g	83	1.8	133	4.9	21.8	2.9	0.5
Chocolate, Cadbury*	1 Pot/55g	107	4.5	195	6.1	24.6	8.2	0.0
Chocolate, COU, M & S*	1 Pot/70g	84	1.9	120	5.2	20.3	2.7	1.0
Chocolate, Finest, Tesco*	1 Pot/82g	321	26.4	391	3.7	21.7	32.2	0.0
Chocolate, Italian Style, Tesco*	1 Pot/90g	243	11.9	270	5.0	32.8	13.2	2.4
Chocolate, Light, Cadbury*	1 Pot/55g	60	1.9	110	4.6	14.2	3.4	0.0
Chocolate, Light Choices, Light Choices, Tesco*	1 Pot/63g	91	1.7	145	4.3	25.3	2.7	0.5
Chocolate, Low Fat, Danette, Danone*	1 Pot/60g	73	1.1	121	5.1	20.8	1.9	1.5
Chocolate, Minty, Bubbly, Dessert, Aero, Nestle*	1 Pot/58g	108	5.9	186	4.6	18.9	10.2	0.3
Chocolate, Shapers, Boots*	1 Pot/70g	97	1.9	138	5.3	23.0	2.7	1.7
Chocolate, White, Bubbly, Dessert, Aero, Nestle*	1 Pot/58g	108	5.8	187	4.5	19.1	10.1	0.3
Chocolate, with Mini Chunks of, Dairy Milk, Cadbury*	1 Pot/100g	215	9.9	215	6.1	25.7	9.9	0.0

MOUSSE

	Measure INFO/WEIGHT	per Measure KCAL	FAT	Nutrition Values per 100g / 100ml KCAL	PROT	CARB	FAT	FIBRE
Chocolate & Hazelnut, Creamy, Dr Oetker*	1 Pot/115g	158	6.9	137	3.3	17.6	6.0	0.6
Chocolate & Hazelnut, Onken*	1 Pot/125g	171	7.5	137	3.3	17.8	6.0	0.0
Chocolate & Mint, COU, M & S*	1 Pot/70g	84	1.7	120	6.2	18.7	2.5	1.0
Chocolate & Orange, COU, M & S*	1 Pot/70g	77	1.8	110	5.9	16.0	2.6	0.9
Chocolate Orange, Low Fat, Cadbury*	1 Pot/100g	110	3.0	110	5.6	15.1	3.0	0.0
Chocolate with Vanilla Layer, Cadbury*	1 Pot/100g	162	6.1	162	4.8	21.9	6.1	0.0
Creamy Strawberry, Boots*	1 Pot/90g	59	2.5	66	3.9	6.4	2.8	0.3
Dream, Cadbury*	1 Pot/53g	100	4.2	189	6.0	22.0	8.0	0.0
Fruit Juice, Shape, Danone*	1 Pot/100g	115	2.8	115	3.5	18.5	2.8	0.0
Layered Lemon, Co-Op*	1 Pot/100g	140	3.0	140	3.0	24.0	3.0	0.2
Layered Strawberry, Co-Op*	1 Pot/100g	120	3.0	120	3.0	19.0	3.0	0.2
Lemon, Classic, Onken*	1 Pot/150g	210	9.4	140	5.1	15.8	6.3	0.0
Lemon, COU, M & S*	1 Pot/70g	80	2.4	115	2.9	19.4	3.5	3.5
Lemon, Dessert, Sainsbury's*	1 Pot/63g	114	5.9	182	3.6	20.7	9.4	0.6
Lemon, GFY, Asda*	1 Pot/63g	57	1.7	92	3.6	13.0	2.8	1.7
Lemon, Less Than 3% Fat, BGTY, Sainsbury's*	1 Pot/62g	70	1.7	113	4.5	17.6	2.8	0.3
Lemon, Lite, Onken*	1 Pot/150g	156	2.2	104	4.6	17.2	1.5	0.1
Lemon, Low Fat, Morrisons*	1 Pot/63g	99	5.8	158	3.7	15.4	9.3	0.3
Lemon, Perfectly Balanced, Waitrose*	1 Pot/95g	150	2.6	158	3.1	30.2	2.7	0.1
Lemon, Tesco*	1 Pot/60g	67	1.6	111	3.4	18.2	2.7	0.0
Lemon Fruit Juice, Shape, Danone*	1 Pot/100g	116	2.8	116	3.5	18.6	2.8	0.0
Milk Chocolate, M & S*	1 Pot/90g	180	7.8	200	5.3	24.8	8.7	1.5
Orange, Mango & Lime, Onken*	1 Pot/150g	207	9.4	138	5.1	15.3	6.3	0.1
Orange & Nectarine, Shape, Danone*	1 Pot/100g	47	1.9	47	3.0	4.9	1.9	0.0
Peach, Onken*	1 Pot/150g	204	9.4	136	5.1	15.1	6.3	0.2
Peach, Shape, Danone*	1 Pot/100g	43	1.8	43	3.0	3.9	1.8	0.1
Peach & Passion Fruit, Perfectly Balanced, Waitrose*	1 Pot/95g	118	2.7	124	3.5	21.2	2.8	0.5
Pineapple, COU, M & S*	1 Pot/70g	84	1.7	120	3.3	20.7	2.4	3.5
Plain Chocolate, Low Fat, Nestle*	1 Pot/120g	71	0.9	59	2.4	10.4	0.7	0.0
Raspberry, Lite, Onken*	1 Pot/150g	156	2.2	104	4.6	17.3	1.5	0.1
Raspberry & Cranberry, Luxury, Weight Watchers*	1 Pot/80g	62	1.0	78	3.8	13.0	1.2	1.0
Rhubarb, COU, M & S*	1 Pot/70g	87	1.5	125	2.9	25.7	2.1	4.2
Rhubarb, Lite, Onken*	1 Pot/150g	154	2.2	103	4.6	17.8	1.5	0.3
Rhubarb & Vanilla, Onken*	1 Pot/150g	210	9.4	140	5.0	15.8	6.3	0.2
Strawberry, Asda*	1 Pot/64g	107	5.8	167	3.5	18.0	9.0	0.2
Strawberry, HL, Tesco*	1 Pot/114g	90	3.0	79	3.8	10.2	2.6	0.8
Strawberry, Light, Muller*	1 Pot/150g	147	0.6	98	4.3	19.4	0.4	0.0
Strawberry, Lite, Onken*	1 Pot/150g	151	2.2	101	4.6	17.2	1.5	0.1
Strawberry, Low Fat, Waitrose*	1 Pot/95g	112	2.7	118	3.2	20.0	2.8	0.6
Strawberry, Sainsbury's*	1 Pot/63g	106	5.9	168	3.4	17.5	9.4	0.1
Strawberry, Shape, Danone*	1 Pot/100g	44	1.8	44	3.0	4.0	1.8	0.0
Strawberry & Vanilla, Weight Watchers*	1 Pot/80g	87	1.9	109	3.7	18.1	2.4	0.4
Strawberry Fruity, Organic, Sainsbury's*	1 Pot/125g	129	3.7	103	6.2	15.7	3.0	3.6
Summer Fruits, Light, Muller*	1 Pot/149g	143	0.6	96	4.3	18.7	0.4	0.0
Toffee, M & S*	1 Pot/90g	180	7.2	200	4.5	27.6	8.0	0.6
Vanilla, Finesse, Aero, Rowntree's*	1 Pot/57g	127	8.3	223	3.7	18.8	14.6	0.0
White Chocolate, Finest, Tesco*	1 Pot/92g	436	34.5	474	3.9	30.2	37.5	0.0

MUFFIN

	Measure INFO/WEIGHT	per Measure KCAL	FAT	Nutrition Values per 100g / 100ml KCAL	PROT	CARB	FAT	FIBRE
All Butter, M & S*	1 Muffin/65g	175	4.7	270	10.3	40.8	7.3	2.1
Apple, Sultana & Cinnamon, GFY, Asda*	1 Muffin/50g	134	1.7	268	6.0	53.0	3.5	3.9
Banana & Walnut, The Handmade Flapjack Company*	1 Muffin/135g	520	30.6	385	5.3	40.5	22.7	0.0
Banana Pecan, Organic, Honeyrose Bakery*	1 Muffin/110g	300	12.6	273	4.1	38.3	11.5	4.3
Berry Burst, Asda*	1 Muffin/60g	139	1.4	232	6.2	46.7	2.3	1.7

MUFFIN

	Measure INFO/WEIGHT	per Measure KCAL	FAT	Nutrition Values per 100g / 100ml KCAL	PROT	CARB	FAT	FIBRE
Blueberry, & Redcurrant, BGTY, Sainsbury's*	1 Muffin/65g	159	1.6	245	5.0	50.0	2.5	3.1
Blueberry, American Style, Sainsbury's*	1 Muffin/72g	256	13.1	355	5.1	42.7	18.2	1.9
Blueberry, GFY, Asda*	1 Muffin/59g	146	1.3	249	6.0	51.0	2.3	3.0
Blueberry, M & S*	1 Muffin/75g	255	12.6	340	4.9	41.9	16.8	1.3
Blueberry, Mini, Sainsbury's*	1 Muffin/28g	82	2.3	293	6.3	48.9	8.1	1.9
Blueberry, Perfectly Balanced, Waitrose*	1 Muffin/100g	225	2.2	225	4.6	46.5	2.2	1.8
Blueberry, Tesco*	1 Muffin/73g	248	12.5	340	4.7	41.0	17.1	1.9
Blueberry, The Handmade Flapjack Company*	1 Muffin/135g	479	26.6	355	4.7	39.9	19.7	0.0
Blueberry, Waitrose*	1 Muffin/65g	239	9.2	367	4.7	55.2	14.2	1.7
Blueberry, Weight Watchers*	1 Muffin/63g	156	2.0	247	4.8	46.4	3.1	7.0
Blueberry Buster, McVitie's*	1 Muffin/95g	408	22.4	429	4.3	49.9	23.6	1.1
Bran, Average	1 Muffin/57g	155	4.4	272	7.8	45.6	7.7	7.7
Caramel, Cadbury*	1 Muffin/116g	535	30.3	461	5.9	50.8	26.1	0.0
Carrot, Asda*	1 Muffin/59g	138	1.4	233	6.0	47.0	2.3	1.6
Carrot Cake, Entenmann's*	1 Muffin/105g	344	15.9	328	5.1	45.8	15.1	3.0
Carrot Cakelet, The Handmade Flapjack Company*	1 Muffin/135g	479	23.9	355	4.0	45.1	17.7	0.0
Cheese, Tesco*	1 Muffin/67g	150	1.9	224	13.0	36.4	2.9	3.0
Cherry, Cheeky, Fabulous Bakin' Boys*	1 Muffin/118g	446	21.0	378	5.5	51.0	17.8	0.7
Cherry, The Handmade Flapjack Company*	1 Muffin/135g	499	26.6	370	4.6	43.8	19.7	0.0
Cherry Bakewell, Mr Kipling*	1 Muffin/100g	355	19.6	355	5.0	55.0	19.6	1.4
Cherry Mega, The Handmade Flapjack Company*	1 Muffin/135g	506	26.7	375	4.4	44.8	19.8	0.0
Choc Chip, Mini, Weight Watchers*	1 Muffin/15g	47	1.3	312	6.6	52.1	8.6	3.1
Chocolate, Galaxy, McVitie's*	1 Muffin/88g	319	17.1	364	5.0	44.5	19.5	0.0
Chocolate, HL, Tesco*	1 Muffin/71g	204	6.2	288	5.5	46.9	8.7	5.5
Chocolate Chip, American Style, Sainsbury's*	1 Muffin/72g	284	14.4	395	5.0	48.8	20.0	2.1
Chocolate Chip, BGTY, Sainsbury's*	1 Muffin/75g	282	12.3	376	5.2	51.8	16.4	1.6
Chocolate Chip, Blackfriars*	1 Muffin/50g	217	11.5	435	6.0	51.0	23.0	4.0
Chocolate Chip, Gluten Free, Antoinette Savill*	1 Muffin/100g	472	31.9	472	5.3	44.9	31.9	3.3
Chocolate Chip, Mini, Asda*	1 Muffin/22g	77	2.9	349	7.0	51.0	13.0	2.1
Chocolate Chip, Plain, Tesco*	1 Muffin/72g	270	12.7	375	5.0	48.1	17.6	1.4
Chocolate Indulgence, McVitie's*	1 Muffin/75g	253	6.9	338	5.8	57.9	9.2	1.3
Chunky Chocolate Chip, McVitie's*	1 Muffin/94g	393	20.3	418	5.3	50.6	21.6	0.8
Cinnamon & Sultana, Morrisons*	1 Muffin/75g	169	1.2	226	8.7	44.1	1.6	4.5
Cranberry & White Chocolate, Sainsbury's*	1 Muffin/72g	253	13.3	352	5.7	40.7	18.5	1.5
Double Berry Burst, Entenmann's*	1 Muffin/59g	140	1.2	238	4.6	50.1	2.1	1.6
Double Choc Chip, Weight Watchers*	1 Muffin/65g	189	5.4	291	6.8	47.2	8.3	3.6
Double Chocolate, 95% Fat Free, Entenmann's*	1 Muffin/58g	152	2.7	262	2.6	52.3	4.7	1.8
Double Chocolate, Free From, Tesco*	1 Muffin/70g	281	12.7	402	4.7	54.8	18.2	1.7
Double Chocolate, Mini, M & S*	1 Muffin/32g	133	6.9	416	5.4	49.8	21.7	1.1
Double Chocolate Chip, American Style, Sainsbury's*	1 Muffin/72g	276	14.6	384	5.2	45.0	20.3	2.9
Double Chocolate Chip, Mini, Asda*	1 Muffin/19g	76	3.7	400	7.4	48.5	19.6	2.7
Double Chocolate Chip, Mini, Weight Watchers*	1 Muffin/15g	45	1.3	300	7.0	48.5	8.7	3.5
Double Chocolate Chip, Tesco*	1 Muffin/100g	360	17.9	360	6.1	44.9	17.9	5.4
English	1 Muffin/57g	120	1.0	211	7.0	43.9	1.8	1.8
English, Butter, Tesco*	1 Muffin/67g	170	3.6	253	11.2	39.8	5.4	2.0
English, Gluten, Wheat & Milk Free, Free From, Livwell*	1 Muffin/50g	160	4.9	320	4.6	52.8	9.8	3.2
Family, Irwin's Bakery*	1 Muffin/40g	116	2.5	291	8.9	50.0	6.2	0.0
Finger, Double Chocolate, Bakers Delight*	1 Muffin/25g	104	4.6	416	5.8	56.9	18.4	1.7
Fruit, Spiced, TTD, Sainsbury's*	1 Muffin/70g	181	3.6	259	10.1	43.1	5.1	2.1
Iceland*	1 Muffin/76g	173	1.3	228	8.6	44.5	1.7	2.0
Lemon, Boots*	1 Muffin/110g	423	20.9	385	3.6	50.0	19.0	1.3
Lemon & Blueberry, Tesco*	1 Muffin/110g	411	23.0	374	4.0	42.4	20.9	1.1
Lemon & Poppy Seed, Entenmann's*	1 Muffin/105g	417	20.3	397	5.6	52.8	19.3	2.5

MUFFIN	Measure INFO/WEIGHT	per Measure KCAL	FAT	Nutrition Values per 100g / 100ml KCAL	PROT	CARB	FAT	FIBRE
Lemon & Poppy Seed, M & S*	1 Muffin/72g	281	14.3	390	6.3	46.1	19.8	1.5
Lemon & Sultana, BGTY, Sainsbury's*	1 Muffin/75g	211	3.4	281	4.5	55.6	4.5	1.4
Mini, Tesco*	1 Muffin/28g	120	6.3	428	6.4	50.0	22.6	1.2
Mixed Fruit, Low Fat, Abbey Bakery*	1 Muffin/35g	93	1.6	267	4.5	55.6	4.5	1.4
Morning Sunrise, Ryvita*	1 Muffin/110g	330	10.0	300	4.5	49.1	9.1	1.8
Muesli, Sainsbury's*	1 Muffin/113g	447	25.7	396	6.5	41.5	22.7	1.4
Oven Bottom, Asda*	1 Muffin/68g	173	1.0	255	10.0	50.4	1.5	2.2
Oven Bottom, Warburton's*	1 Muffin/69g	175	2.0	253	10.9	45.8	2.9	0.0
Plain, Morrisons*	1 Muffin/70g	140	0.8	200	8.0	41.4	1.1	0.0
Plain, Prepared From Recipe, Average	1 Muffin/57g	169	6.5	296	6.9	41.4	11.4	2.7
Raspberry Cream, Sainsbury's*	1 Muffin/90g	314	19.8	349	3.9	33.8	22.0	1.3
Rolo, Nestle*	1 Muffin/80g	289	14.4	361	5.4	44.3	18.0	0.8
Spiced Fruit, Co-Op*	1 Muffin/60g	159	1.2	265	11.0	52.0	2.0	3.0
Spicy Fruit, Quality Bakers*	1 Muffin/65g	146	1.0	225	9.4	38.0	1.5	3.3
Strawberry Cakelet, The Handmade Flapjack Company*	1 Muffin/135g	526	29.6	390	4.5	43.6	21.9	0.0
Sultana, The Handmade Flapjack Company*	1 Muffin/135g	499	26.1	370	4.7	44.8	19.3	0.0
Sunblest*	1 Muffin/72g	166	1.3	230	9.6	43.9	1.8	2.2
Toasting, Warburton's*	1 Muffin/64g	138	1.0	216	8.9	41.4	1.6	2.9
Toffee, GFY, Asda*	1 Muffin/90g	151	2.3	168	2.1	34.0	2.6	0.0
Toffee, The Handmade Flapjack Company*	1 Muffin/135g	533	31.6	395	4.4	41.2	23.4	0.0
Toffee & Pecan, Finest, Tesco*	1 Muffin/127g	551	29.0	434	5.4	51.8	22.8	0.9
Toffee Choo Choo, Tesco*	1 Muffin/95g	402	21.3	423	6.4	49.1	22.4	1.0
Toffee Mega, The Handmade Flapjack Company*	1 Muffin/135g	567	34.7	420	4.5	43.2	25.7	0.0
Toffee Temptation, McVitie's*	1 Muffin/86g	297	8.1	347	4.7	60.8	9.5	0.8
Triple Chocolate, Triumph, Fabulous Bakin' Boys*	1 Muffin/40g	160	9.6	400	4.5	42.0	24.0	0.0
Truly Madly Chocolate, Fabulous Bakin' Boys*	1 Muffin/105g	405	23.1	386	5.0	41.0	22.0	2.0
Vanilla & Choc Chip, GFY, Asda*	1 Muffin/59g	152	1.3	260	7.0	53.0	2.2	1.6
White, All Butter, Sainsbury's*	1 Muffin/67g	173	4.2	258	10.6	39.6	6.3	3.6
White, Asda*	1 Muffin/67g	148	1.3	222	11.0	40.0	2.0	2.5
White, Finest, Tesco*	1 Muffin/70g	159	0.8	227	8.4	45.7	1.2	2.1
White, M & S*	1 Muffin/60g	135	1.1	225	11.2	43.7	1.9	2.9
White, Tesco*	1 Muffin/72g	173	2.3	240	11.3	41.6	3.2	2.8
White Chocolate & Strawberry Filled, Tesco*	1 Muffin/103g	415	20.3	405	5.2	51.3	19.8	1.3
White Chocolate Chunk Lemon, Mini, M & S*	1 Muffin/28g	130	6.7	464	6.4	55.4	23.9	2.1
Wholemeal, Tesco*	1 Muffin/65g	130	1.3	200	12.6	32.9	2.0	5.7
MULBERRIES								
Raw	*1oz/28g*	*10*	*0.0*	*36*	*1.3*	*8.1*	*0.0*	*0.0*
MULLET								
Grey, Grilled	*1oz/28g*	*42*	*1.5*	*150*	*25.7*	*0.0*	*5.2*	*0.0*
Grey, Raw	*1oz/28g*	*32*	*1.1*	*115*	*19.8*	*0.0*	*4.0*	*0.0*
Red, Grilled	*1oz/28g*	*34*	*1.2*	*121*	*20.4*	*0.0*	*4.4*	*0.0*
Red, Raw, Weighed Whole	*1oz/28g*	*31*	*1.1*	*109*	*18.7*	*0.0*	*3.8*	*0.0*
MUNCHIES								
Mint, Nestle*	1 Pack/62g	267	10.1	432	3.8	67.5	16.4	0.0
Original, Tube, Nestle*	1 Pack/55g	272	13.3	498	4.1	65.6	24.4	0.5
MUSHROOMS								
Breaded, Average	*1oz/28g*	*42*	*1.6*	*151*	*4.3*	*20.8*	*5.7*	*0.6*
Breaded, Garlic, Average	1 Serving/50g	92	4.9	183	5.2	18.7	9.7	1.7
Button, Average	*1 Serving/50g*	*7*	*0.2*	*15*	*2.3*	*0.5*	*0.4*	*1.2*
Chestnut, Average	*1 Med/5g*	*1*	*0.0*	*13*	*1.8*	*0.4*	*0.5*	*0.5*
Chinese, Dried, Raw	*1oz/28g*	*80*	*0.5*	*284*	*10.0*	*59.9*	*1.8*	*0.0*
Closed Cup, Average	*1oz/28g*	*5*	*0.1*	*18*	*2.9*	*0.4*	*0.5*	*0.5*
Common, Boiled in Salted Water, Average	*1oz/28g*	*3*	*0.1*	*11*	*1.8*	*0.4*	*0.3*	*1.1*

	Measure INFO/WEIGHT	per Measure KCAL	FAT	Nutrition Values per 100g / 100ml KCAL	PROT	CARB	FAT	FIBRE

M

MUSHROOMS

	Measure INFO/WEIGHT	KCAL	FAT	KCAL	PROT	CARB	FAT	FIBRE
Common, Fried, Average	*1oz/28g*	*44*	*4.5*	*157*	*2.4*	*0.3*	*16.2*	*1.5*
Common, Raw, Average	*1 Serving/80g*	*10*	*0.4*	*13*	*1.9*	*0.3*	*0.5*	*1.1*
Creamed, Average	*1oz/28g*	*23*	*1.5*	*82*	*1.3*	*6.8*	*5.5*	*0.5*
Dried	*1oz/28g*	*45*	*1.7*	*159*	*21.8*	*4.8*	*6.0*	*13.3*
Enoki, Average	*1 Serving/80g*	*34*	*0.0*	*42*	*3.0*	*7.0*	*0.0*	*3.0*
Flat, Large, Average	*1 Mushroom/52g*	*10*	*0.3*	*19*	*3.3*	*0.5*	*0.5*	*0.7*
Frozen, Cooks' Ingredients, Waitrose*	1 Serving/75g	13	0.2	18	2.1	1.8	0.3	2.5
Garlic, Average	½ Pack/150g	159	14.0	106	2.1	3.7	9.3	1.7
Oyster, Average	*1 Serving/80g*	*12*	*0.2*	*15*	*1.6*	*1.6*	*0.2*	*1.3*
Porcini, Wild, Dried, Merchant Gourmet*	1 Pack/25g	66	0.8	265	27.9	30.6	3.4	18.7
Shiitake, Cooked	*1oz/28g*	*15*	*0.1*	*55*	*1.6*	*12.3*	*0.2*	*0.0*
Shiitake, Dried, Raw	*1oz/28g*	*83*	*0.3*	*296*	*9.6*	*63.9*	*1.0*	*0.0*
Sliced, Average	*1oz/28g*	*3*	*0.1*	*12*	*1.8*	*0.4*	*0.3*	*1.1*
Straw, Canned, Drained	*1oz/28g*	*4*	*0.1*	*15*	*2.1*	*1.2*	*0.2*	*0.0*

MUSSELS

	Measure INFO/WEIGHT	KCAL	FAT	KCAL	PROT	CARB	FAT	FIBRE
Boiled, Flesh Only, Average	1 Mussel/1.9g	2	0.1	104	16.7	3.5	2.7	0.0
Boiled, Weighed in Shell, Average	*1 Mussel/7g*	*7*	*0.2*	*104*	*16.7*	*3.5*	*2.7*	*0.0*
Cooked & Shelled, Meat, Tesco*	1 Pack/240g	216	5.0	90	13.9	3.8	2.1	0.0
Pickled, Drained, Average	*1oz/28g*	*31*	*0.6*	*112*	*20.0*	*1.5*	*2.2*	*0.0*
Raw, Weighed in Shell, Average	*1oz/28g*	*24*	*0.7*	*87*	*12.7*	*3.6*	*2.5*	*0.2*

MUSSELS IN

	Measure INFO/WEIGHT	KCAL	FAT	KCAL	PROT	CARB	FAT	FIBRE
Creamy Garlic Butter Sauce, Bantry Bay*	1 Serving/225g	198	7.9	88	9.0	5.2	3.5	0.6
Garlic Butter Sauce, Average	½ Pack/225g	179	11.5	79	6.3	1.9	5.1	0.1
Seasoned White Wine Sauce, Bantry Bay*	1 Serving/450g	270	9.0	60	6.3	4.1	2.0	0.1
Thai Sauce, Scottish, Waitrose*	1 Serving/250g	135	6.2	54	5.4	2.6	2.5	0.6
White Wine Cream Sauce, Cooked, Scottish, Morrisons*	½ Pack/250g	222	9.2	89	8.0	5.8	3.7	0.0
White Wine Sauce, Sainsbury's*	½ Pack/250g	221	9.2	88	8.0	5.8	3.7	0.0

MUSSELS WITH

	Measure INFO/WEIGHT	KCAL	FAT	KCAL	PROT	CARB	FAT	FIBRE
Tomato & Garlic, Fresh, M & S*	1 Serving/650g	455	10.4	70	7.9	6.5	1.6	0.1

MUSTARD

	Measure INFO/WEIGHT	KCAL	FAT	KCAL	PROT	CARB	FAT	FIBRE
American, Average	*1 Tsp/5g*	*5*	*0.2*	*102*	*4.4*	*10.5*	*5.0*	*2.5*
Cajun, Colman's*	1 Tsp/6g	11	0.4	187	7.0	23.0	6.5	2.7
Coarse Grain, Average	*1 Tsp/5g*	*7*	*0.4*	*141*	*7.7*	*8.4*	*8.3*	*5.9*
Dijon, Average	*1 Tsp/5g*	*8*	*0.6*	*163*	*7.4*	*7.7*	*11.3*	*1.1*
English, Average	*1 Tsp/5g*	*9*	*0.4*	*173*	*6.8*	*19.2*	*7.6*	*1.2*
English, with Chillies, Sainsbury's*	1 Tsp/5g	10	0.5	204	8.3	18.1	10.9	6.4
French, Average	*1 Tsp/5g*	*5*	*0.3*	*105*	*5.4*	*8.1*	*5.6*	*1.8*
German Style, Sainsbury's*	1 Serving/10g	9	0.6	92	5.5	2.8	6.5	0.0
Honey, Colman's*	1 Tsp/6g	12	0.5	208	7.4	24.0	8.2	0.0
Powder, Average	*1 Tsp/3g*	*15*	*0.9*	*452*	*28.9*	*20.7*	*28.7*	*0.0*
Powder, Made Up, Average	*1oz/28g*	*63*	*4.0*	*226*	*14.5*	*10.4*	*14.4*	*0.0*
Smooth, Average	*1 Tsp/8g*	*11*	*0.7*	*139*	*7.1*	*9.7*	*8.2*	*0.0*
Sweet Peppers, Colman's*	1 Tsp/6g	13	0.7	218	7.9	20.0	11.0	4.9
Whole Grain, Average	*1 Tsp/8g*	*11*	*0.8*	*140*	*8.2*	*4.2*	*10.2*	*4.9*
Whole Grain, with Green Peppercorns, Finest, Tesco*	1 Serving/20g	41	1.9	205	7.9	22.0	9.5	3.3
Wholegrain, Essential, Waitrose*	1 Serving/10g	16	1.0	161	7.4	10.6	9.9	2.5
Yellow, Prepared	*1 Tbsp/15ml*	*11*	*0.6*	*73*	*4.0*	*6.0*	*4.0*	*0.0*

MUSTARD CRESS

	Measure INFO/WEIGHT	KCAL	FAT	KCAL	PROT	CARB	FAT	FIBRE
Raw	*1oz/28g*	*4*	*0.2*	*13*	*1.6*	*0.4*	*0.6*	*1.1*

MUTTON

	Measure INFO/WEIGHT	KCAL	FAT	KCAL	PROT	CARB	FAT	FIBRE
Lean, Raw, Average	1 Serving/100g	236	13.4	236	17.9	0.1	13.4	0.0

N

	Measure INFO/WEIGHT	per Measure KCAL	FAT	Nutrition Values per 100g / 100ml KCAL	PROT	CARB	FAT	FIBRE
NACHOS								
American Chilli Beef, Asda*	1 Serving/200g	208	10.0	104	10.0	4.7	5.0	0.8
Cheesy, with Salsa & Soured Cream, Sainsbury's*	½ Pack/170g	449	26.9	264	8.8	21.5	15.8	1.4
Chilli, Sainsbury's*	½ Pack/250g	695	32.2	278	10.9	29.5	12.9	1.3
Kit, Old El Paso*	½ Pack/260g	598	26.0	230	4.0	31.0	10.0	0.0
NASI GORENG								
Indonesian, Asda*	1 Pack/360g	778	22.7	216	7.4	32.3	6.3	1.3
NECTARINES								
Weighed with Stone, Fresh, Raw, Average	*1 Med/140g*	*53*	*0.1*	*38*	*1.3*	*8.5*	*0.1*	*1.1*
NESQUIK								
Chocolate Flavour, Powder, Dry Weight, Nestle*	1 Serving/15g	56	0.5	372	3.0	82.9	3.1	6.5
Strawberry Flavour, Powder, Dry Weight, Nestle*	1 Serving/15g	59	0.0	393	0.0	98.1	0.0	0.0
Strawberry Milk, Fresh, Nesquik, Nestle*	1 Glass/250g	175	4.0	70	3.3	10.4	1.6	0.3
NIK NAKS								
Cream 'n' Cheesy, Golden Wonder*	1 Bag/34g	195	13.0	575	5.2	52.7	38.1	0.2
Nice 'n' Spicy, KP Snacks*	1 Bag/30g	171	11.5	571	4.6	51.6	38.4	1.6
Rib 'n' Saucy, Golden Wonder*	1 Bag/34g	194	12.8	571	4.5	53.7	37.6	0.5
Scampi 'n' Lemon, Golden Wonder*	1 Bag/34g	195	12.7	573	4.9	53.1	37.5	0.1
NOODLES								
Barbecue Beef, Instant, Asda*	1 Pack/333g	420	16.0	126	2.6	18.0	4.8	0.0
Beef, Oriental, GFY, Asda*	1 Pack/400g	372	6.8	93	7.4	12.1	1.7	1.7
Beef Flavour, Instant, Prepared, Heinz*	1 Pack/384g	257	0.4	67	2.1	14.4	0.1	0.6
Buckwheat, Cold, Famima*	1 Pack/295g	163	3.0	55	4.7	9.5	1.0	0.7
Cellophane, Glass, Dry Weight	1 Serving/100g	351	0.1	351	0.1	86.1	0.1	0.5
Char Sui, Cantonese, Sainsbury's*	1 Pack/450g	378	7.2	84	6.8	10.5	1.6	1.5
Chicken, Chinese, Asda*	1 Pot/302g	305	4.2	101	6.0	16.0	1.4	0.8
Chicken, Dry Weight, Heinz*	1 Pack/85g	257	0.3	302	9.5	65.3	0.4	2.7
Chicken, Instant, Less Than 1% Fat, Prepared, Heinz*	1 Pack/385g	258	0.4	67	2.1	14.4	0.1	0.6
Chicken, Instant, Weight Watchers*	1 Pack/385g	269	0.4	70	2.3	14.9	0.1	0.6
Chicken & Coconut & Lime, Simply Fuller Longer, M & S*	1 Pack/390g	448	17.5	115	8.7	10.0	4.5	1.6
Chicken & Red Thai, Easy Steam, Tesco*	1 Serving/400g	556	28.4	139	10.3	8.6	7.1	1.1
Chicken Curry Flavour, Instant, Sainsbury's*	1 Pack/85g	167	6.2	196	4.6	27.9	7.3	0.8
Chicken Flavour, 3 Minute, Dry, Blue Dragon*	1 Pack/85g	403	18.2	475	9.3	61.2	21.4	0.0
Chicken Flavour, Dry, Eldorado*	1 Pack/85g	360	12.7	423	14.0	61.0	15.0	0.0
Chicken Flavour, Dry, Princes*	1 Pack/85g	395	16.0	465	10.0	63.8	18.8	0.0
Chicken Flavour, Instant, Made Up, Tesco*	½ Pack/168g	285	10.6	170	4.1	23.7	6.3	1.5
Chicken Flavour, Instant, Sainsbury's*	1 Pack/335g	549	21.4	164	4.4	22.3	6.4	1.3
Chilli Beef, Finest, Tesco*	1 Pack/450g	486	8.5	108	7.7	15.2	1.9	0.9
Chilli Chicken, GFY, Asda*	1 Pack/415g	461	3.3	111	6.0	20.0	0.8	1.0
Chilli Chicken, Sweet, Sainsbury's*	1 Pack/200g	202	2.8	101	6.6	15.5	1.4	0.8
Chilli Infused, Blue Dragon*	1 Serving/150g	286	1.0	191	6.1	33.6	0.7	0.3
Chinese, Stir Fry, Sainsbury's*	1 Serving/100g	185	4.8	185	6.0	29.5	4.8	1.5
Chinese Pork, Chosen By You, Asda*	1 Pack/400g	380	6.4	95	6.7	12.6	1.6	1.8
Chow Mein, Dry Weight, Snack in a Pot, HL, Tesco*	1 Pot/56g	202	0.8	360	13.4	72.2	1.4	5.0
Chow Mein, Instant, Made Up, Tesco*	1 Pack/168g	255	8.4	152	3.8	23.0	5.0	1.2
Chow Mein, Sainsbury's*	1 Pack/125g	136	2.2	109	3.9	19.2	1.8	0.8
Chow Mein, Snack in a Pot, Light Choices, Tesco*	1 Pot/235g	235	1.2	100	3.7	19.4	0.5	1.8
Chow Mein, Stir Fry, Tesco*	1 Serving/200g	116	2.4	58	2.1	9.7	1.2	1.0
Chow Mein Flavour, Dry, Princes*	1 Pack/85g	396	15.8	466	10.1	64.6	18.6	0.0
Crab Flavour, Dry, 3 Minute, Blue Dragon*	1 Pack/85g	393	16.3	463	9.9	62.6	19.2	0.0
Crispy, Dry, Blue Dragon*	1 Box/125g	437	0.6	350	2.4	84.0	0.5	0.0
Curry, Instant, Dry, Heinz*	1 Serving/85g	261	0.3	307	9.5	66.4	0.4	2.7
Curry, Mealpack, All About Weight*	1 Pack/37g	152	7.5	416	35.0	22.4	20.6	5.0
Curry Flavour, Instant, From Heinz, Weight Watchers*	1 Pack/385g	266	0.4	69	2.2	14.8	0.1	0.6

NOODLES

	Measure INFO/WEIGHT	per Measure KCAL	FAT	Nutrition Values per 100g / 100ml KCAL	PROT	CARB	FAT	FIBRE
Curry Flavour, Instant, Sainsbury's*	1 Pack/335g	412	15.4	123	2.6	17.8	4.6	0.1
Curry Flavour, Instant, Value, Made Up, Tesco*	1 Pack/65g	83	2.4	127	3.1	20.3	3.7	0.8
Egg, & Bean Sprouts, Cooked, Tesco*	1 Pack/250g	237	5.2	95	4.4	14.6	2.1	1.5
Egg, Boiled	*1oz/28g*	*17*	*0.1*	*62*	*2.2*	*13.0*	*0.5*	*0.6*
Egg, Dry	*1 Block/63g*	*244*	*5.1*	*391*	*12.1*	*71.7*	*8.2*	*2.9*
Egg, Fine, Blue Dragon*	1 Serving/100g	171	0.9	171	5.5	35.0	0.9	0.0
Egg, Fine, Dry Weight, Sharwood's*	1 Block/63g	216	1.3	346	12.0	70.0	2.1	2.5
Egg, Fine, Fresh, M & S*	1 Pack/275g	330	6.0	120	4.4	20.7	2.2	1.5
Egg, Fine, Waitrose*	¼ Pack/63g	221	1.6	353	15.0	67.3	2.6	3.8
Egg, Fine Thread, Dry, M & S*	1 Serving/63g	220	0.6	350	14.3	71.6	0.9	5.1
Egg, Free Range, Asda*	1 Serving/125g	205	4.9	164	5.1	27.0	3.9	1.8
Egg, Free Range, Morrisons*	1 Pack/300g	372	8.7	124	4.9	19.7	2.9	1.3
Egg, Fresh, Just Stir Fry, Sainsbury's*	½ Pack/192g	314	6.5	163	5.0	28.1	3.4	1.8
Egg, Fresh, Tesco*	½ Pack/205g	287	3.9	140	4.9	25.3	1.9	2.0
Egg, Medium, Asda*	1 Serving/83g	125	0.7	150	4.8	31.0	0.8	1.3
Egg, Medium, Dry, Blue Dragon*	1 Serving/81g	288	1.4	356	13.8	70.0	1.7	3.4
Egg, Medium, Dry, Sharwood's*	1 Serving/63g	216	1.3	346	12.0	70.0	2.1	2.5
Egg, Medium, Sainsbury's*	1 Serving/122g	168	1.0	138	5.7	26.9	0.8	1.0
Egg, Ramen, Fresh, The Original Noodle Company*	1 Serving/63g	186	1.7	298	11.3	57.0	2.7	0.0
Egg, Raw, Medium, Waitrose*	¼ Pack/63g	221	1.6	353	15.0	67.3	2.6	3.8
Egg, Thick, Dry Weight, Sharwood's*	1 Serving/63g	214	1.1	342	10.8	71.0	1.7	2.5
Egg, Thread, Cooked Weight, Sharwood's*	1oz/28g	30	0.2	107	3.6	21.8	0.6	1.1
Egg, Tossed in Sesame Oil, Asda*	½ Pack/150g	174	10.5	116	2.3	11.0	7.0	0.6
Fried, Average	*1oz/28g*	*43*	*3.2*	*153*	*1.9*	*11.3*	*11.5*	*0.5*
Garlic, Chilli & Ginger, Tesco*	1 Serving/350g	507	11.2	145	4.8	24.1	3.2	2.6
Hoisin, Vegelicious, Tesco*	1 Pack/400g	440	6.8	110	4.4	18.1	1.7	1.9
Instant, Dry, Sainsbury's*	1 Pack/100g	392	14.0	392	9.4	57.0	14.0	0.2
Instant, Express, Dry, Blue Dragon*	1 Serving/75g	337	12.7	450	10.0	65.0	17.0	2.0
Instant, Fat Free, Koka*	1 Piece/80g	143	0.0	179	6.2	38.5	0.0	1.0
Instant, Vegetable Flavour, Made Up, Indo Mie*	1 Pack/349g	373	15.7	107	2.6	14.0	4.5	0.8
Japanese Udon, Sainsbury's*	1 Serving/150g	210	2.7	140	3.9	27.1	1.8	1.2
Medium, Traditional, Straight to Wok, Amoy*	1 Serving/150g	243	2.2	162	4.3	34.3	1.5	1.3
Nest, Medium, Cooked, Waitrose*	1 Nest/63g	88	0.3	139	5.0	28.6	0.5	0.6
Oriental, Chinese, Tesco*	1 Pack/200g	184	5.0	92	2.8	14.7	2.5	1.0
Oriental, Snack Pot, Dry, HL, Tesco*	1 Pot/57g	210	1.0	369	14.0	74.4	1.7	2.0
Oriental, Snack Pot, Made Up, HL, Tesco*	1 Serving/238g	221	0.7	93	3.1	19.4	0.3	0.6
Pasta, 100% Hard Durum Wheat, Dry, Goody*	1 Serving/100g	362	1.7	362	12.5	73.0	1.7	0.0
Peking Duck, Shapers, Boots*	1 Pack/280g	395	3.9	141	7.2	25.0	1.4	1.8
Plain, Boiled	*1oz/28g*	*17*	*0.1*	*62*	*2.4*	*13.0*	*0.4*	*0.7*
Plain, Dry	*1oz/28g*	*109*	*6.2*	*388*	*11.7*	*76.1*	*6.2*	*2.9*
Prawn, Instant, Made Up, Tesco*	1 Serving/168g	251	8.7	150	3.8	21.9	5.2	1.3
Ramen, with Chilli Beef, M & S*	1 Pack/484g	532	17.4	110	8.1	11.9	3.6	0.8
Ramen, with Wakame, The Original Noodle Company*	½ Pack/124g	304	1.0	245	7.4	51.8	0.8	1.8
Ribbon, Thai Style, Ready To Wok, Sharwood's*	1 Pack/150g	205	1.6	137	5.0	26.3	1.1	1.0
Rice, Brown, 100%, Organic, King Soba*	1 Pack/83g	252	2.0	303	6.0	64.4	2.4	0.0
Rice, Cooked	1 Cup/176g	192	0.4	109	0.9	24.9	0.2	1.0
Rice, Dry, Blue Dragon*	1 Serving/30g	113	0.0	376	7.0	84.0	0.0	0.0
Rice, Oriental, Thai, Stir Fry, Dry Weight, Sharwood's*	1 Serving/63g	226	0.6	361	6.5	86.8	1.0	2.4
Rice, Stir Fry, Tesco*	½ Pack/190g	304	10.8	160	2.0	24.8	5.7	1.0
Rice, Thai, Wheat & Gluten Free, King Soba Noodles*	1 Serving/55g	193	0.8	351	8.9	75.6	1.4	0.0
Rice, Thick, Thai, Dry, M & S*	1 Serving/100g	355	0.7	355	6.5	80.6	0.7	1.4
Savoury Vegetable, COU, M & S*	1 Pack/450g	270	2.7	60	2.9	11.5	0.6	1.2
Shanghai Beef, COU, M & S*	1 Pack/400g	380	6.4	95	6.8	13.1	1.6	1.5

	Measure INFO/WEIGHT	per Measure		Nutrition Values per 100g / 100ml				
		KCAL	FAT	KCAL	PROT	CARB	FAT	FIBRE
NOODLES								
Singapore, BGTY, Sainsbury's*	1 Pack/369g	317	10.0	86	7.2	8.2	2.7	2.1
Singapore, Light Choices, Tesco*	1 Pack/450g	337	7.6	75	4.8	9.8	1.7	1.2
Singapore, Sainsbury's*	1 Pack/400g	432	15.6	108	6.5	11.7	3.9	2.8
Singapore, Waitrose*	1 Pack/400g	476	17.6	119	7.3	12.6	4.4	2.1
Singapore Style, Asda*	1 Pack/400g	688	32.0	172	7.0	18.0	8.0	1.0
Spicy, Sainsbury's*	1 Serving/180g	182	8.3	101	10.4	4.5	4.6	0.9
Spicy Curry Flavour, Dry, Princes*	1 Pack/85g	395	16.0	465	9.6	64.1	18.8	0.0
Spicy Thai, Instant, Heinz*	1 Pack/385g	262	0.4	68	2.1	14.6	0.1	0.6
Stir Fry, Tesco*	1 Serving/150g	202	3.6	135	5.3	23.0	2.4	1.5
Straight to Wok, Medium, Amoy*	1 Pack/150g	240	2.2	160	5.8	31.7	1.5	0.0
Straight to Wok, Rice, Amoy*	1 Pack/150g	174	0.1	116	1.6	27.4	0.1	0.0
Straight to Wok, Singapore, Amoy*	1 Serving/150g	232	4.2	155	4.8	28.4	2.8	0.0
Straight to Wok, Thread, Fine, Amoy*	1 Pack/150g	237	3.9	158	5.0	28.7	2.6	0.0
Straight to Wok, Udon, Amoy*	1 Pack/150g	211	1.9	141	4.4	28.8	1.3	0.0
Super, Bacon Flavour, Dry Weight, Batchelors*	1 Packet/100g	526	23.6	526	9.4	69.2	23.6	1.6
Super, Barbecue Beef, Made Up, Batchelors*	1 Serving/100g	156	6.7	156	3.2	20.9	6.7	1.1
Super, Cheese & Ham, Made Up, Batchelors*	1 Serving/100g	171	7.3	171	3.4	22.9	7.3	0.6
Super, Chicken & Ham, Dry Weight, Batchelors*	1 Pack/100g	472	20.2	472	9.4	63.2	20.2	1.5
Super, Chicken & Herb, Low Fat, Made Up, Batchelors*	1 Pack/170g	322	1.6	189	6.1	39.2	0.9	1.2
Super, Chicken Flavour, Dry Weight, Batchelors*	1 Serving/100g	449	19.2	449	8.7	60.3	19.2	2.5
Super, Chicken Flavour, Made Up, Batchelors*	1 Serving/100g	170	7.3	170	3.3	22.9	7.3	0.9
Super, Chow Mein Flavour, Made Up, Batchelors*	½ Pack/150g	262	11.8	175	3.0	23.0	7.9	0.4
Super, Mild Curry, Dry Weight, Batchelors*	½ Pack/50g	260	11.7	520	9.4	67.8	23.4	1.4
Super, Mild Curry Flavour, Made Up, Batchelors*	1 Serving/100g	157	6.7	157	3.2	20.9	6.7	1.0
Super, Mushroom Flavour, Made Up, Batchelors*	1 Serving/100g	157	6.8	157	3.2	20.9	6.8	1.0
Super, Southern Fried Chicken, Made Up, Batchelors*	1 Serving/100g	171	7.2	171	3.3	23.2	7.2	0.5
Super, Spicy Salsa, Dry Weight, Batchelors*	1 Pack/105g	474	19.5	451	7.0	63.8	18.6	1.7
Super, Sweet Thai Chilli, Dry Weight, Batchelors*	1 Pack/85g	292	1.0	343	10.6	72.5	1.2	3.0
Sweet & Sour, BGTY, Sainsbury's*	1 Serving/100g	112	3.1	112	2.3	18.6	3.1	0.0
Sweet Chilli, Sainsbury's*	½ Pack/110g	172	6.0	156	4.0	24.6	5.5	1.0
Sweet Chilli, Wok, Findus*	1 Pack/300g	300	1.5	100	3.0	20.0	0.5	0.0
Thai, Spicy, Stir Fry, HL, Tesco*	½ Pack/250g	220	5.5	88	4.1	12.9	2.2	1.7
Thai, Waitrose*	1 Pack/300g	357	6.3	119	6.8	18.4	2.1	1.7
Thai Glass, Vermicelli, Wai Wai*	1oz/28g	112	0.3	400	7.3	89.1	0.9	1.8
Thai Style, Asda*	1 Pot/238g	226	0.7	95	3.0	20.0	0.3	0.8
Thai Style, Sainsbury's*	1 Pack/340g	381	7.8	112	3.3	19.4	2.3	0.7
Tiger Prawn, Stir Fry, Tesco*	1 Pack/400g	596	14.8	149	6.0	23.0	3.7	2.7
Tomato & Herb, in a Mug, Pot Noodle*	1 Serving/44g	28	0.1	64	2.0	13.4	0.2	0.7
Udon Japanese, & Dashi Soup Stock, Yutaka*	1 Pack/230g	290	1.1	126	3.0	26.8	0.5	0.0
Vermicelli Rice, Mama*	1 Serving/45g	166	0.4	370	7.0	81.0	1.0	0.0
Whole Wheat, Dry, Blue Dragon*	1 Serving/65g	208	1.3	320	12.5	63.0	2.0	8.0
Yaki Udan, Chicken & Prawn, M & S*	1 Pack/395g	434	14.2	110	8.1	11.9	3.6	0.8
Zero, Glow Nutrition Ltd*	1 Serving/100g	5	0.0	5	0.0	4.0	0.0	4.0
NOUGAT								
Almond & Cherry, M & S*	1 Sweet/7g	28	0.6	405	4.5	76.0	9.1	1.1
Average	1 Sm Bar/28g	108	2.4	384	4.4	77.3	8.5	0.9
Raspberry & Orange Hazelnut, Thorntons*	1 Sweet/9g	39	1.8	433	4.8	60.0	20.0	2.2
NUT CLUSTERS								
Almond, Sweet, Pecan, and Peanut, Red Sky*	1 Serving/30g	182	13.9	607	17.9	32.1	46.4	7.1
Peanut, Red Sky*	1 Serving/30g	182	13.9	607	21.4	32.1	46.4	7.1
NUT MIX								
Black Forest, Graze*	1 Pack/55g	258	13.8	470	6.6	54.4	25.1	0.0
Fiery Almonds, Graze*	1 Punnet/35g	206	18.1	588	21.9	8.2	51.6	11.4

	Measure INFO/WEIGHT	per Measure		Nutrition Values per 100g / 100ml				
		KCAL	FAT	KCAL	PROT	CARB	FAT	FIBRE
NUT MIX								
Honey Monster, Graze*	1 Pack/50g	279	20.4	559	10.8	45.2	40.8	0.0
Island, Graze*	1 Pack/55g	354	33.0	643	15.1	10.5	60.0	0.0
Sweet & Sour, Graze*	1 Pack/40g	222	17.4	556	19.1	23.7	43.4	0.0
NUT ROAST								
Average	1 Serving/200g	704	51.4	352	13.3	18.3	25.7	4.2
Courgette & Spiced Tomato, Cauldron Foods*	1 Serving/100g	208	12.3	208	11.7	12.5	12.3	4.9
Leek, Cheese & Mushroom, Organic, Cauldron Foods*	½ Pack/143g	343	21.3	240	13.2	13.2	14.9	4.1
Lentil, Average	*1oz/28g*	*62*	*3.4*	*222*	*10.6*	*18.8*	*12.1*	*3.8*
Tomato & Courgette, Vegetarian, Organic, Waitrose*	½ Pack/142g	295	17.5	208	11.7	12.5	12.3	4.9
NUTMEG								
Ground, Average	*1 Tsp/3g*	*16*	*1.1*	*525*	*5.8*	*45.3*	*36.3*	*0.0*
NUTS								
Assortment, Eat Well, M & S*	1 Pack/70g	441	41.2	630	16.7	8.5	58.9	5.3
Bento Box, Mix, Graze*	1 Portion/30g	141	6.6	469	17.9	50.1	22.1	3.7
Fire, Graze*	1 Pack /40g	220	16.3	549	17.9	28.4	40.7	7.1
Luxury Assortment, Tesco*	1 Serving/10g	68	6.5	676	17.5	6.1	64.6	5.0
Mixed	1 Pack/40g	243	21.6	607	22.9	7.9	54.1	6.0
Mixed, Americas, Graze*	1 Punnet/40g	263	25.6	658	15.5	5.2	64.0	5.6
Mixed, Ancient Forest, Graze*	1 Pack/35g	221	21.1	632	17.6	5.9	60.3	7.0
Mixed, Chopped, Julian Graves*	1 Pack/300g	1773	152.7	591	23.2	10.0	50.9	0.0
Mixed, Honey Roasted, Waitrose*	1 Serving/50g	291	22.5	583	17.1	27.5	45.0	5.3
Mixed, Roasted, Salted, Waitrose*	1 Pack/200g	1252	116.8	626	13.7	11.3	58.4	4.4
Mixed, Roasted, Waitrose*	1 Serving/25g	165	16.0	662	15.2	6.2	64.0	8.2
Mixed, Unsalted, Sainsbury's*	1 Serving/50g	311	28.8	622	18.5	7.2	57.7	8.7
Mixed, Wholesome, Love Life, Waitrose*	1 Serving/30g	205	19.6	685	14.6	5.0	65.2	5.4
Natural, Mixed, Love Life, Waitrose*	1 Serving/50g	314	25.8	628	17.4	24.9	51.6	12.1
Natural Assortment, Tesco*	1 Serving/50g	338	32.3	676	17.5	6.1	64.6	5.0
Oak Smoke Flavour Selection, Finest, Tesco*	1 Serving/25g	158	13.9	633	21.4	11.2	55.8	6.3
Omega Booster Seeds, Graze*	1 Punnet/35g	189	15.6	540	22.8	16.2	44.7	6.4
Peanuts & Cashews, Honey Roast, Tesco*	1 Serving/25g	145	10.7	579	21.6	26.6	42.9	4.2
Pecan, Wholesome, Love Life, Waitrose*	1 Serving/30g	207	21.0	691	9.2	5.8	70.1	9.6
Peri-Peri, Nando's*	1 Serving/100g	631	54.1	631	23.8	8.5	54.1	7.8
Pine, Tesco*	1 Pack/100g	699	68.6	699	16.5	4.0	68.6	1.9
Roasted, Salted, Assortment, Luxury, Tesco*	1 Serving/25g	161	14.5	643	21.1	9.4	57.9	8.1
Salted, Selection, Sainsbury's*	1 Serving/30g	190	17.1	634	20.6	9.7	56.9	8.2
Soya, Dry Roasted, The Food Doctor*	1 Serving/50g	203	10.7	406	37.5	15.9	21.4	16.1
Soya Beans, Roasted & Salted, Chinese Style, Tesco*	1 Serving/26g	100	5.0	385	46.1	6.9	19.2	21.8
Unsalted, Selection, Sainsbury's*	1 Serving/75g	491	48.0	655	14.7	5.0	64.0	6.7
NUTS & RAISINS								
Mixed, Average	1 Serving/30g	144	10.2	481	14.1	31.5	34.1	4.5
Peanuts, Mixed, Average	1 Pack/40g	174	10.4	435	15.3	37.5	26.0	4.4
Yoghurt Coated, Waitrose*	1 Serving/50g	263	18.3	527	10.9	38.2	36.7	3.0

	Measure INFO/WEIGHT	per Measure KCAL	FAT	Nutrition Values per 100g / 100ml KCAL	PROT	CARB	FAT	FIBRE
OAT BAKES								
Cheese, Nairn's*	1 Bag/30g	130	4.7	432	15.0	57.4	15.8	1.3
Mediterranean Tomato and Herb, Nairn's*	1 Bag/30g	129	4.7	431	8.1	64.2	15.8	8.3
Sweet Chilli, Nairn's*	1 Bag/30g	128	4.0	426	8.1	68.4	13.3	7.2
OAT CAKES								
Bran, Paterson's*	1 Cake/13g	52	2.0	416	10.0	58.5	15.8	9.5
Cheese, Nairn's*	1 Cake/9g	42	2.4	471	13.2	43.3	27.2	6.8
Fine Milled, Nairn's*	1 Cake/8g	35	1.7	449	10.5	52.6	21.8	8.6
Herb and Pumpkin Seed, Nairn's*	1 Cake/10g	43	2.1	426	12.2	46.8	21.1	13.0
Highland, Organic, Sainsbury's*	1 Cake/13g	57	2.4	456	10.2	59.8	19.5	5.5
Highland, Walkers*	1 Cake/12g	54	2.5	451	10.3	56.0	20.6	6.7
Oatmeal, Rough, Nairn's*	1 Cake/11g	45	2.0	421	10.6	52.8	18.6	10.5
Oatmeal, Rough, Organic, Nairn's*	1 Cake/10g	43	1.7	418	10.2	57.7	16.3	7.5
Organic, The Village Bakery*	1 Cake/13g	56	2.7	452	10.9	54.5	21.3	5.6
Orkney, Stockan's*	1 Cake/14g	63	3.2	453	11.1	50.3	23.0	6.0
Retail, Average	1 Cake/13g	57	2.4	441	10.0	63.0	18.3	0.0
Rough, Sainsbury's*	1 Cake/11g	45	1.8	426	11.7	65.2	16.9	8.6
Rough, Scottish, Tesco*	1 Cake/10g	45	1.9	435	11.4	55.3	18.4	8.0
Rough, with Olive Oil, Paterson's*	1 Cake/13g	54	2.1	431	10.6	58.4	17.2	8.1
Rough Scottish, Sainsbury's*	1 Cake/11g	51	2.1	462	12.3	59.9	19.3	6.5
Rough with Bran, Walkers*	1 Cake/13g	55	2.2	424	11.0	57.1	16.8	8.1
Scottish, Organic, Waitrose*	1 Cake/13g	58	2.5	447	11.2	57.0	19.4	6.6
Scottish, Rough, Waitrose*	1 Cake/13g	55	2.3	438	10.4	57.4	18.5	8.0
Traditional, M & S*	1 Cake/11g	49	2.0	445	11.0	59.3	18.3	6.6
with Cracked Black Pepper, Walkers*	1 Cake/10g	41	1.8	433	10.4	55.0	19.0	8.5
OAT DRINK								
Healthy Oat, Enriched, Oatly*	1 Glass/250ml	112	3.7	45	1.0	6.5	1.5	0.8
Healthy Oat Milk, Organic, Oatly*	1 Glass/250ml	87	1.7	35	1.0	6.5	0.7	0.8
OATBRAN								
Original Pure, Mornflake*	1 Serving/30g	103	2.9	345	14.8	49.7	9.7	15.2
OATMEAL								
Raw	*1oz/28g*	*112*	*2.4*	*401*	*12.4*	*72.8*	*8.7*	*6.8*
OCTOPUS								
Chunks, in Olive Oil, Palacio De Oriente*	1 Tin/111g	148	4.0	133	21.6	4.5	3.6	0.0
Raw	*1oz/28g*	*23*	*0.4*	*83*	*17.9*	*0.0*	*1.3*	*0.0*
OIL								
Avocado, Olivado*	1 Tsp/5ml	40	4.4	802	0.0	0.0	88.0	0.0
Chilli, Average	*1 Tsp/5ml*	*41*	*4.6*	*823*	*0.0*	*0.0*	*91.5*	*0.0*
Chinese Stir Fry, Asda*	1 Tbsp/15ml	123	13.7	823	0.0	0.0	91.4	0.0
Coconut, Average	*1 Tsp/5ml*	*45*	*5.0*	*899*	*0.0*	*0.0*	*99.9*	*0.0*
Cod Liver, Average	*1 Capsule/1g*	*9*	*1.0*	*900*	*0.0*	*0.0*	*100.0*	*0.0*
Corn, Average	*1 Tsp/5ml*	*43*	*4.8*	*864*	*0.0*	*0.0*	*95.9*	*0.0*
Cuisine, Flora*	1 Tsp/5ml	31	3.5	630	0.1	1.0	70.3	0.0
Evening Primrose, Average	*1 Serving/1g*	*9*	*1.0*	*900*	*0.0*	*0.0*	*100.0*	*0.0*
Fish, Average	*1 Serving/1g*	*9*	*1.0*	*900*	*0.0*	*0.0*	*100.0*	*0.0*
Flax Seed, Average	*1 Tbsp/15ml*	*124*	*13.9*	*829*	*0.0*	*0.0*	*92.5*	*0.0*
Fry Light, Bodyline*	1 Spray/0.25ml	1	0.1	522	0.0	0.0	55.2	0.0
Grapeseed, Average	*1 Tsp/5ml*	*43*	*4.8*	*865*	*0.0*	*0.0*	*96.1*	*0.0*
Groundnut, Average	*1 Tsp/5ml*	*41*	*4.6*	*824*	*0.0*	*0.0*	*91.8*	*0.0*
Hazelnut, Average	*1 Tsp/5ml*	*45*	*5.0*	*899*	*0.0*	*0.0*	*99.9*	*0.0*
Linseed, Organic, Biona*	1 Serving/10ml	84	9.3	837	0.0	0.0	93.0	0.0
Macadamia Nut, Oz Tukka*	1 Tsp/5ml	40	4.5	805	0.0	0.0	91.0	0.0
Olive, Average	*1 Tsp/5ml*	*43*	*4.7*	*855*	*0.0*	*0.0*	*94.9*	*0.0*
Olive, Basil Infused, Tesco*	1 Serving/20ml	180	20.0	900	0.0	0.0	100.0	0.0

	Measure INFO/WEIGHT	per Measure KCAL	FAT	Nutrition Values per 100g / 100ml KCAL	PROT	CARB	FAT	FIBRE
OIL								
Olive, Evo Filtered, Italian, Parioli, Cucina*	1 Serving/100ml	825	91.6	825	0.0	0.0	91.6	0.0
Olive, Extra Virgin, Average	*1 Tsp/5ml*	*42*	*4.7*	*848*	*0.0*	*0.0*	*94.5*	*0.0*
Olive, Extra Virgin, Mist Spray, Belolive*	1 Serving/5ml	25	2.7	500	0.0	0.0	55.0	0.0
Olive, Extra Virgin, Only 1 Cal, Spray, Fry Light*	1 Spray/0.2ml	1	0.1	498	0.0	0.0	55.2	0.0
Olive, Garlic, Average	*1 Tbsp/15ml*	*127*	*14.1*	*848*	*0.0*	*0.0*	*94.3*	*0.0*
Olive, Lemon Flavoured, Sainsbury's*	1 Tbsp/15ml	123	13.7	823	0.1	0.0	91.4	0.1
Olive, Mild, Average	*1 Tbsp/15mll*	*129*	*14.4*	*861*	*0.0*	*0.0*	*95.7*	*0.0*
Omega, Organic, Clearspring*	1 Tbsp/15ml	124	13.8	828	0.0	0.0	92.0	0.0
Palm, Average	*1 Tsp/5ml*	*45*	*5.0*	*899*	*0.0*	*0.0*	*99.9*	*0.0*
Peanut, Average	*1 Tsp/5ml*	*45*	*5.0*	*899*	*0.0*	*0.0*	*99.9*	*0.0*
Rapeseed, Average	*1 Tbsp/15ml*	*130*	*14.4*	*863*	*0.0*	*0.0*	*95.9*	*0.0*
Red Palm & Canola, Carotino*	1 Tsp/5ml	41	4.6	812	0.0	0.0	92.0	0.0
Rice Bran, Average	1 Tbsp/14g	120	13.6	884	0.0	0.0	100.0	0.0
Safflower, Average	*1 Tsp/5ml*	*45*	*5.0*	*899*	*0.0*	*0.0*	*99.9*	*0.0*
Sesame, Average	*1 Tsp/5ml*	*45*	*5.0*	*892*	*0.1*	*0.0*	*99.9*	*0.0*
Soya, Average	*1 Tsp/5ml*	*45*	*5.0*	*899*	*0.0*	*0.0*	*99.9*	*0.0*
Stir Fry, Sharwood's*	1 fl oz/30ml	269	29.9	897	0.0	0.0	99.7	0.0
Sunflower, Average	*1 Tsp/5ml*	*43*	*4.8*	*869*	*0.0*	*0.0*	*96.6*	*0.0*
Sunflower, Spray, Fry Light*	1 Spray/0.2ml	1	0.1	522	0.0	0.0	55.2	0.0
Ultimate Blend, Ugo's*	1 Capsule/1ml	9	1.0	900	1.3	0.0	96.8	0.0
Vegetable, Average	*1 Tbsp/15ml*	*129*	*14.3*	*858*	*0.0*	*0.0*	*95.3*	*0.0*
Walnut, Average	*1 Tsp/5ml*	*45*	*5.0*	*899*	*0.0*	*0.0*	*99.9*	*0.0*
Wheatgerm, Average	*1 Tsp/5ml*	*45*	*5.0*	*899*	*0.0*	*0.0*	*99.9*	*0.0*
OKRA								
Boiled in Unsalted Water, Average	*1 Serving/80g*	*22*	*0.7*	*28*	*2.5*	*2.7*	*0.9*	*3.6*
Canned, Drained, Average	*1 Serving/80g*	*17*	*0.6*	*21*	*1.4*	*2.5*	*0.7*	*2.6*
Raw, Average	*1 Serving/80g*	*25*	*0.8*	*31*	*2.8*	*3.0*	*1.0*	*4.0*
Stir-Fried in Corn Oil, Average	*1 Serving/80g*	*215*	*20.9*	*269*	*4.3*	*4.4*	*26.1*	*6.3*
OLIVES								
Black, Pitted, Average	*½ Jar/82g*	*135*	*13.3*	*164*	*1.0*	*3.5*	*16.2*	*3.1*
Black & Green, with Greek Feta Cheese, Tesco*	1 Pot/100g	200	20.1	200	3.4	0.3	20.1	4.6
Green, Garlic Stuffed, Asda*	1 Olive/3g	6	0.6	174	1.8	3.5	17.0	0.0
Green, Lightly Flavoured with Lemon & Garlic, Attis*	1 Serving/50g	82	8.2	164	1.7	2.2	16.5	0.0
Green, Pitted, Average	*1 Olive/3g*	*4*	*0.4*	*129*	*1.1*	*0.9*	*13.3*	*2.5*
Green, Pitted, Stuffed with Anchovies, Sainsbury's*	1 Serving/50g	77	8.0	155	1.8	0.6	16.1	3.2
Green, Stuffed with Almonds, Pitted, Waitrose*	1 Serving/50g	90	8.4	180	3.8	3.2	16.9	2.5
Green, Stuffed with Anchovy, Waitrose*	½ Can/40g	38	3.1	94	1.5	4.7	7.7	2.3
Green, with Chilli & Garlic, Delicious, Boots*	1 Pack/60g	97	9.0	161	1.3	4.4	15.0	2.0
Kalamata & Halkidiki with Chilli & Garlic, Graze*	1 Punnet/51g	144	14.8	281	0.7	1.5	28.8	3.0
*Kalamata**	*1 Olive/3g*	*9*	*0.9*	*300*	*1.0*	*6.7*	*30.0*	*0.0*
Marinated, Mixed, M & S*	1 Serving/20g	33	3.0	165	1.6	6.5	14.9	3.0
Marinated, Selection, M & S*	4 Olives/20g	44	4.4	225	1.4	3.9	22.6	2.1
Mixed, Chilli & Garlic, Asda*	1 Serving/30g	43	4.7	144	0.9	0.0	15.6	6.1
Mixed, Marinated, Anti Pasti, Asda*	1 Serving/100g	215	22.0	215	1.8	0.7	22.0	3.1
Mixed, Marinated, with Feta & Red Peppers, Asda*	1 Pot/120g	233	21.6	194	5.8	2.2	18.0	1.7
Pimento Stuffed, in Brine, Tesco*	1 Serving/25g	38	4.1	153	0.8	0.1	16.4	2.1
OMELETTE								
Cheese, 2 Egg, Average	1 Omelette/180g	479	40.7	266	15.9	0.0	22.6	0.0
Cheese, Asda*	1 Omelette/119g	268	22.6	225	12.0	1.5	19.0	0.0
Cheese, Findus*	1 Serving/200g	400	26.0	200	9.5	14.0	13.0	0.0
Cheese & Mushroom, Apetito*	1 Serving/320g	486	25.0	152	6.2	14.4	7.8	1.9
Mushroom & Cheese, Tesco*	1 Omelette/120g	248	21.5	207	9.8	1.6	17.9	0.2
Plain, 2 Egg	1 Omelette/120g	229	19.7	191	10.9	0.0	16.4	0.0

	Measure INFO/WEIGHT	per Measure KCAL	FAT	Nutrition Values per 100g / 100ml KCAL	PROT	CARB	FAT	FIBRE
OMELETTE								
Spanish	1oz/28g	34	2.3	120	5.7	6.2	8.3	1.4
ONION RINGS								
Battered, Asda*	1 Serving/100g	343	22.7	343	3.8	31.0	22.7	1.7
Battered, Oven Baked, Tesco*	1 Serving/50g	109	5.0	219	3.9	28.4	10.0	3.5
Battered, Sainsbury's*	1 Ring/12g	26	1.2	219	3.9	28.4	10.0	3.5
Breadcrumbs, Tesco*	1 Serving/100g	294	15.6	294	4.3	34.1	15.6	2.3
Breaded, Asda*	1 Serving/10g	29	1.5	289	4.4	34.0	15.0	2.7
Breaded, Iceland*	1 Ring/11g	33	1.7	293	4.4	34.2	15.4	2.7
Breaded, Sainsbury's*	1 Serving/100g	280	12.4	280	4.6	37.6	12.4	4.1
Oven Crisp Batter, Tesco*	1 Ring/17g	40	2.3	236	4.2	24.8	13.3	2.5
ONIONS								
Baked	**1oz/28g**	**29**	**0.2**	**103**	**3.5**	**22.3**	**0.6**	**3.9**
Boiled in Unsalted Water	**1oz/28g**	**5**	**0.0**	**17**	**0.6**	**3.7**	**0.1**	**0.7**
Borettane, Char-Grilled, Sacla*	1 Serving/100g	90	5.6	90	0.9	8.9	5.6	2.5
Dried, Raw, Average	**1oz/28g**	**88**	**0.5**	**313**	**10.2**	**68.6**	**1.7**	**12.1**
Fried, Average	**1oz/28g**	**46**	**3.1**	**164**	**2.3**	**14.1**	**11.2**	**3.1**
Pickled, Average	**1 Onion/15g**	**3**	**0.0**	**23**	**0.8**	**4.9**	**0.1**	**0.7**
Powder	1 Tsp/2g	7	0.0	341	10.4	79.1	1.0	15.2
Raw, Average	**1 Med/180g**	**55**	**0.3**	**31**	**1.3**	**6.0**	**0.2**	**1.4**
Red, Raw, Average	**1 Med/180g**	**66**	**0.4**	**37**	**1.2**	**7.9**	**0.2**	**1.5**
Spring Or Scallion, Raw, Average	**1 Med/15g**	**5**	**0.0**	**33**	**1.8**	**7.3**	**0.2**	**2.6**
Sweet, TTD, Sainsbury's*	1 Serving/100g	39	0.2	39	1.3	7.9	0.2	1.4
OPTIONS								
Choca Mocha Drink, Ovaltine*	1 Sachet/11g	39	1.3	359	14.1	50.1	11.4	7.0
Chocolate Au Lait, Ovaltine*	1 Sachet/10g	35	1.0	355	11.8	54.5	10.0	7.3
Coffee, Dreamy Cappuccion, Cafe, Ovaltine*	1 Sachet/25g	64	4.2	256	12.9	58.1	16.9	0.0
Cracking Hazelnut, Ovaltine*	1 Sachet/11g	40	1.2	361	16.0	57.0	11.0	0.0
Dreamy Caramel, Hot Chocolate, Ovaltine*	1 Sachet/11g	39	0.9	354	12.3	48.5	7.8	0.0
Irish Cream, Ovaltine*	1 Sachet/11g	39	1.2	357	13.9	50.0	11.3	8.1
Mint Madness, Ovaltine*	1 Serving/11g	38	0.8	348	12.3	49.2	6.9	20.0
Outrageous Orange, Ovaltine*	1 Serving/11g	32	0.8	289	11.7	43.3	7.7	18.0
Tempting Toffee, Ovaltine*	1 Sachet/11g	43	1.0	391	13.6	66.4	9.1	0.0
Wicked White Chocolate, Ovaltine*	1 Sachet/11g	46	1.2	414	10.3	68.1	11.1	0.5
ORANGES								
Blood, Average	**1 Orange/140g**	**82**	**0.0**	**58**	**0.8**	**13.3**	**0.0**	**2.5**
Fresh, Weighed with Peel, Average	**1 Med/185g**	**115**	**0.5**	**62**	**1.0**	**15.6**	**0.3**	**3.2**
Fresh, without Peel, Average	**1 Med/145g**	**90**	**0.4**	**62**	**1.0**	**15.6**	**0.3**	**3.2**
Peel Only, Raw, Average	**1 Tbsp/6g**	**6**	**0.0**	**97**	**1.5**	**25.0**	**0.2**	**10.6**
Ruby Red, Tesco*	1 Med/130g	51	0.1	39	1.1	8.5	0.1	1.7
OREGANO								
Dried,	**1 Tsp/1g**	**3**	**0.1**	**306**	**11.0**	**49.5**	**10.3**	**0.0**
Fresh	**1 Tsp/1.25g**	**1**	**0.0**	**66**	**2.2**	**9.7**	**2.0**	**0.0**
OVALTINE*								
Hi Malt, Light, Instant Drink, Ovaltine*	1 Sachet/20g	72	1.2	358	9.1	67.1	5.9	2.8
Powder, Made Up with Semi-Skimmed Milk, Ovaltine*	1 Mug/227ml	179	3.9	79	3.9	13.0	1.7	0.0
Powder, Made Up with Whole Milk, Ovaltine*	1 Mug/227ml	220	8.6	97	3.8	12.9	3.8	0.0
OXTAIL								
Raw	**1oz/28g**	**48**	**2.8**	**171**	**20.0**	**0.0**	**10.1**	**0.0**
Stewed	**1oz/28g**	**68**	**3.8**	**243**	**30.5**	**0.0**	**13.4**	**0.0**
OYSTERS								
in Vegetable Oil, Smoked, John West*	1oz/28g	64	3.9	230	16.0	10.0	14.0	0.0
Raw, Shucked	**1 Oyster/14g**	**9**	**0.2**	**65**	**10.8**	**2.7**	**1.3**	**0.0**

	Measure INFO/WEIGHT	per Measure KCAL	FAT	Nutrition Values per 100g / 100ml KCAL	PROT	CARB	FAT	FIBRE
PAELLA								
Bistro, Waitrose*	1 Serving/300g	534	19.8	178	7.4	22.2	6.6	0.7
Chicken, Chorizo & King Prawn, Finest, Tesco*	½ Pack/400g	520	19.6	130	7.0	14.2	4.9	1.2
Chicken, HL, Tesco*	1 Pack/400g	432	2.0	108	6.7	19.2	0.5	1.7
Chicken, King Prawns, British, Sainsbury's*	1 Pack/400g	380	4.8	95	7.6	13.3	1.2	0.9
Chicken, Tesco*	1 Serving/475g	575	14.2	121	7.9	15.7	3.0	1.6
Chicken & Chorizo, Asda*	1 Pack/390g	484	8.6	124	10.0	16.0	2.2	2.6
Chicken & Chorizo, Big Dish, M & S*	1 Pack/450g	630	17.5	140	7.9	18.4	3.9	1.6
Chicken & King Prawn, HL, Tesco*	1 Pack/385g	346	6.2	90	5.3	12.7	1.6	2.0
Chicken & Prawn, Asda*	1 Pack/400g	352	4.4	88	5.8	13.7	1.1	1.4
Chicken & Vegetable, HL, Tesco*	1 Pack/450g	441	5.8	98	9.7	11.8	1.3	1.1
Diet Chef Ltd*	1 Pack/250g	355	3.0	142	11.2	21.7	1.2	0.4
Seafood, COU, M & S*	1 Pack/400g	400	7.2	100	6.2	13.8	1.8	1.4
Seafood, M & S*	1 Pack/450g	517	17.1	115	6.4	13.7	3.8	3.2
Seafood, Sainsbury's*	1 Pack/400g	504	5.2	126	8.3	20.3	1.3	0.6
Tesco*	1 Serving/460g	584	17.0	127	4.6	18.9	3.7	1.0
TTD, Sainsbury's*	½ Pack/374g	475	20.9	127	9.4	9.9	5.6	4.8
Vegetable, Waitrose*	1 Serving/174g	202	3.1	116	2.2	22.7	1.8	1.5
PAIN AU CHOCOLAT								
All Butter, Tesco*	1 Serving/59g	242	11.6	410	8.2	49.4	19.7	2.3
Asda*	1 Serving/58g	244	13.9	420	8.0	43.0	24.0	3.3
Chocolate Filled, Chosen By You, Asda*	1 Pain/45g	198	11.3	441	7.1	44.9	25.2	2.9
M & S*	1 Pastry/60g	210	11.5	350	5.9	38.0	19.2	1.6
Mini, Asda*	1 Pastry/23g	96	5.5	420	8.0	43.0	24.0	3.3
Sainsbury's*	1 Serving/58g	241	13.8	415	7.9	42.5	23.7	3.3
Small, Asda*	1 Serving/23g	106	6.0	462	8.0	49.0	26.0	0.0
TTD, Sainsbury's*	1 Pain/80g	341	18.6	426	7.5	46.9	23.2	3.0
Waitrose*	1 Pastry/53g	230	12.6	435	8.8	45.5	23.9	3.7
PAIN AU RAISIN								
Twist, Extra Special, Asda*	1 Pastry/110g	421	20.9	383	7.0	46.0	19.0	2.5
PAK CHOI								
Raw, Average	*1 Leaf/14g*	*2*	*0.0*	*13*	*1.5*	*2.2*	*0.2*	*1.0*
PAKORA								
Bhaji, Onion, Fried in Vegetable Oil	1oz/28g	76	4.1	271	9.8	26.2	14.7	5.5
Bhajia, Potato Carrot & Pea, Fried in Vegetable Oil	1oz/28g	100	6.3	357	10.9	28.8	22.6	6.1
Bhajia, Vegetable, Retail	1oz/28g	66	4.1	235	6.4	21.4	14.7	3.6
Chicken, Tikka, Asda*	1 Pack/350g	696	38.5	199	16.0	9.0	11.0	1.1
Potato & Spinach, Waitrose*	1 Pakora/50g	120	8.2	240	5.5	17.3	16.5	4.7
Prawn, Indian Appetisers, Waitrose*	1 Pakora/21g	35	1.7	165	16.8	5.9	8.2	1.5
Sainsbury's*	1 Pakora/55g	166	10.1	302	7.3	26.8	18.3	1.1
Spinach, Sainsbury's*	1 Pakora/18g	35	1.9	195	5.1	19.4	10.8	3.8
Vegetable, Indian Selection, Party, Co-Op*	1 Pakora/23g	47	1.6	205	6.0	28.0	7.0	4.0
Vegetable, Indian Starter Selection, M & S*	1 Pakora/23g	61	4.2	265	6.3	19.6	18.1	2.9
Vegetable, Mini, Indian Snack Collection, Tesco*	1 Pakora/21g	36	1.9	173	6.0	16.8	9.1	4.9
PANCAKE								
Apple, GFY, Asda*	1 Pancake/74g	100	1.8	135	4.2	24.0	2.5	1.0
Apple & Sultana, M & S*	1 Serving/80g	160	6.3	200	2.2	30.2	7.9	1.2
Asda*	1 Pancake/23g	59	1.6	254	4.8	43.0	7.0	4.0
Big, Crafty, Genesis*	1 Pancake/71g	171	3.7	241	6.2	42.3	5.2	2.1
Bramley Apple, Sainsbury's*	1 Pancake/85g	114	2.1	134	4.2	23.6	2.5	1.0
Cherry, GFY, Asda*	1 Serving/206g	206	3.8	100	1.9	18.9	1.8	1.8
Chinese Style, Cherry Valley*	1 Pancake/8g	25	0.5	310	9.2	54.7	6.0	0.0
Chocolate, M & S*	1 Pancake/80g	125	4.9	156	3.1	22.1	6.1	0.2
for Duck, Sainsbury's*	1 Pancake/10g	33	0.9	333	10.9	51.7	9.3	2.4

	Measure INFO/WEIGHT	per Measure KCAL	FAT	Nutrition Values per 100g / 100ml KCAL	PROT	CARB	FAT	FIBRE
PANCAKE								
HL, Tesco*	1 Pancake/25g	60	0.5	240	5.8	48.8	2.0	1.9
Lemon, M & S*	1 Pancake/38g	90	2.8	235	4.5	38.5	7.2	2.8
Lemon & Raisin, Crafty, Genesis*	1 Pancake/56g	130	1.8	232	5.8	44.8	3.3	3.1
Lemon & Raisin, Morrisons*	1 Pancake/36g	55	0.4	153	5.3	30.4	1.2	0.9
Light Choices, Tesco*	1 Pancake/27g	66	0.7	243	6.9	47.7	2.6	0.0
Low Calorie, Eurodiet*	1 Serving/30g	112	2.9	373	57.5	9.2	9.8	8.4
Maple & Raisin, M & S*	1 Pancake/33g	88	1.8	269	6.5	49.7	5.4	2.2
Mini, for Kids, Tesco*	1 Pancake/16g	45	0.9	283	6.6	51.7	5.5	1.3
Mini, Scotch, Tesco*	1 Pancake/16g	44	0.9	277	6.7	50.0	5.6	1.4
Morrisons*	1 Pancake/60g	133	3.0	221	8.4	37.3	5.0	1.5
Perfect, Kingsmill*	1 Pancake/27g	71	1.2	264	6.2	49.7	4.5	1.2
Plain, Sainsbury's*	1 Pancake/46g	102	2.4	221	6.9	36.1	5.3	1.2
Raisin & Lemon, Sainsbury's*	1 Pancake/35g	95	1.5	272	6.3	51.8	4.4	2.2
Savoury, Made with Skimmed Milk, Average	1 6inch/77g	192	11.3	249	6.4	24.1	14.7	0.8
Savoury, Made with Whole Milk, Average	1 6inch/77g	210	13.5	273	6.3	24.0	17.5	0.8
Scotch	1 Pancake/50g	146	5.8	292	5.8	43.6	11.7	1.4
Scotch, BGTY, Sainsbury's*	1 Pancake/30g	76	1.2	252	5.3	48.5	4.1	1.3
Sultana & Syrup, Asda*	1 Pancake/34g	89	2.4	263	5.9	43.7	7.2	1.5
Sultana & Syrup Scotch, Sainsbury's*	1 Pancake/35g	113	2.9	322	6.7	55.2	8.3	1.7
Sweet, Made with Skimmed Milk	1oz/28g	78	3.9	280	6.0	35.1	13.8	0.8
Sweet, Made with Whole Milk	1oz/28g	84	4.5	301	5.9	35.0	16.2	0.8
Sweet, Raspberry Ripple Sauce, Findus*	1 Pancake/38g	80	1.8	210	3.9	37.1	4.7	0.9
Syrup, Gluten, Wheat & Dairy Free, Free From, Livwell*	1 Pancake/40g	108	2.9	270	2.5	49.0	7.2	0.7
Syrup, Tesco*	1 Pancake/30g	79	2.5	265	4.7	42.1	8.2	1.5
Traditional, Aunt Bessie's*	1 Pancake/60g	90	1.9	150	6.1	24.6	3.1	1.1
Traditional, Tesco*	1 Pancake/62g	137	3.1	221	8.4	35.6	5.0	1.5
Vegetable Roll	1 Roll/85g	185	10.6	218	6.6	21.0	12.5	0.0
Warburton's*	1 Pancake/35g	88	2.1	252	6.4	43.0	6.0	1.8
PANCAKE MIX								
4 Grain, Wheat & Gluten Free, Organic, Hale & Hearty*	½ Pack/180g	562	2.9	312	7.8	66.6	1.6	5.7
Fresh, M & S*	1 Pancake/38g	90	5.0	235	7.5	22.4	13.1	0.5
Glutano*	1 Tbs/15g	57	0.3	378	8.9	75.6	2.2	0.0
Traditional, Asda*	1 Pack/256g	545	23.0	213	6.0	27.0	9.0	1.8
PANCETTA								
Average	*½ Pack/65g*	*212*	*18.7*	*326*	*17.0*	*0.1*	*28.7*	*0.0*
PANINI								
Bacon, British Midland*	1 Serving/150g	273	9.9	182	9.1	21.6	6.6	0.0
Chargrilled Chicken, Mozzarella & Pesto, Ugo's*	1 Panini/170g	389	14.6	229	16.4	21.6	8.6	2.0
Cheese, Tesco*	1 Panini/100g	249	9.1	249	10.5	31.3	9.1	3.1
Chicken Arrabbiata, Ginsters*	1 Panini/200g	489	16.8	245	12.8	29.4	8.4	2.4
Ham & Cheese, Ginsters*	1 Panini/200g	567	25.6	283	13.3	28.7	12.8	1.6
Mozzarella & Tomato, Ginsters*	1 Panini/207g	536	21.9	259	12.3	28.5	10.6	2.1
Mozzarella & Tomato, M & S*	1 Serving/176g	484	28.5	275	11.3	21.3	16.2	2.1
Tuna & Sweetcorn, Tesco*	1 Serving/250g	559	16.4	224	12.0	29.3	6.6	1.4
Tuna Melt, Ginsters*	1 Panini/210g	479	15.8	228	13.1	26.9	7.5	1.9
PANNA COTTA								
BGTY, Sainsbury's*	1 Pot/150g	150	2.8	100	2.4	18.2	1.9	1.4
Caramel, Sainsbury's*	1 Pot/120g	335	15.7	279	2.5	34.6	13.1	3.3
Sainsbury's*	1 Pot/100g	304	15.7	304	3.0	41.5	15.7	4.0
Strawberry, COU, M & S*	1 Pot/145g	145	3.8	100	2.6	15.7	2.6	0.8
PAPAYA								
Dried, Pieces, Nature's Harvest*	1 Serving/50g	177	0.0	355	0.2	85.4	0.0	2.6
Dried, Strips, Tropical Wholefoods*	1 Strip/10g	31	0.1	310	3.9	71.4	0.9	1.5

P

	Measure INFO/WEIGHT	per Measure		Nutrition Values per 100g / 100ml				
		KCAL	FAT	KCAL	PROT	CARB	FAT	FIBRE
PAPAYA								
Dried, Sweetened, Tesco*	4 Pieces/25g	59	0.2	235	0.4	56.3	0.9	2.9
Raw, Flesh Only, Average	*1 Serving/140g*	*37*	*0.1*	*26*	*0.4*	*6.6*	*0.1*	*1.2*
Raw, Unripe, Flesh Only	1 Serving/100g	27	0.1	27	0.9	5.5	0.1	1.0
Raw, Weighed with Seeds & Skin	*1 Cup,/ 140g*	*55*	*0.2*	*39*	*0.6*	*9.8*	*0.1*	*1.8*
Unripe, Raw, Weighed with Seeds & Skin	*1oz/28g*	*8*	*0.0*	*27*	*0.9*	*5.5*	*0.1*	*1.5*
PAPPARDELLE								
Basil, Fresh, Sainsbury's*	1 Serving/240g	281	3.4	117	5.0	21.2	1.4	2.0
Buitoni*	1 Serving/65g	242	3.1	373	15.0	67.5	4.8	0.0
Chilli, Fresh, Sainsbury's*	1 Serving/250g	302	4.2	121	5.7	20.7	1.7	2.0
Egg, Dry, Average	*1 Serving/100g*	*364*	*3.7*	*364*	*14.1*	*68.5*	*3.7*	*2.1*
Egg, Fresh, Waitrose*	¼ Pack/125g	350	3.4	280	12.9	51.0	2.7	1.9
Egg & Spinach, Extra Special, Asda*	½ Pack/200g	328	3.6	164	6.5	30.5	1.8	1.4
Saffron, Eat Well, M & S*	1 Serving/100g	360	2.5	360	14.0	69.0	2.5	3.2
The Best Fresh, Morrisons*	¼ Pack/240g	353	3.8	147	6.3	26.9	1.6	1.9
with Salmon, COU, M & S*	1 Pack/358g	340	6.8	95	6.3	13.0	1.9	0.8
PAPRIKA								
Average	*1 Tsp/2g*	*6*	*0.3*	*289*	*14.8*	*34.9*	*13.0*	*0.0*
PARATHA								
Average	*1 Paratha/80g*	*258*	*11.4*	*322*	*8.0*	*43.2*	*14.3*	*4.0*
Lachha, Waitrose*	1 Paratha/75g	322	17.8	429	7.8	46.0	23.8	1.8
PARSLEY								
Dried	*1 Tsp/1g*	*2*	*0.1*	*181*	*15.8*	*14.5*	*7.0*	*26.9*
Fresh, Average	*1 Tbsp/4g*	*1*	*0.0*	*34*	*3.0*	*2.7*	*1.3*	*5.0*
PARSNIP								
Boiled, Average	*1 Serving/80g*	*53*	*1.0*	*66*	*1.6*	*12.9*	*1.2*	*4.7*
Honey Roasted, Tesco*	1 Serving/125g	202	10.2	162	1.9	20.0	8.2	2.2
Raw, Unprepared, Average	*1oz/28g*	*19*	*0.3*	*66*	*1.8*	*12.5*	*1.1*	*4.6*
Roast, Honey Glazed, Baked, Aunt Bessie's*	1 Serving/125g	162	9.4	130	1.7	14.0	7.5	4.1
Roasting, Freshly Frozen, Chosen By You, Asda*	1 Serving/110g	221	8.5	201	2.5	30.4	7.7	7.8
PARTRIDGE								
Breast, Fillets, Raw, Skinned, Abel & Cole*	1 Serving/100g	145	4.7	145	25.8	0.0	4.7	0.0
Meat Only, Roasted	*1oz/28g*	*59*	*2.0*	*212*	*36.7*	*0.0*	*7.2*	*0.0*
PASANDA								
Chicken, M & S*	½ Pack/150g	240	16.3	160	11.3	3.8	10.9	1.3
Chicken, Sainsbury's*	1 Serving/200g	368	24.8	184	14.7	3.4	12.4	2.3
Chicken, Waitrose*	1oz/28g	52	3.4	185	14.8	3.8	12.3	1.1
Chicken, with Pilau Rice, HL, Tesco*	1 Pack/440g	466	11.0	106	5.7	15.2	2.5	0.9
PASSATA								
Basil, Del Monte*	1 Jar/500g	160	1.0	32	1.4	5.9	0.2	0.0
Classic, Italian, with Onion & Garlic, Sainsbury's*	1oz/28g	10	0.0	37	1.4	7.7	0.1	1.3
Napolina*	1 Bottle/690g	172	0.7	25	1.4	4.5	0.1	0.0
Sieved Tomato, Valfrutta*	1 Pack/500g	110	0.5	22	1.2	4.0	0.1	0.0
So Organic, Sainsbury's*	¼ Jar/175g	38	0.7	22	0.9	3.8	0.4	0.9
with Fresh Leaf Basil, Waitrose*	¼ Jar/170g	44	0.2	26	1.0	5.2	0.1	0.8
with Garlic & Herbs, Roughly Chopped, Tesco*	1 Serving/200g	56	0.0	28	1.4	5.5	0.0	1.0
with Garlic & Italian Herbs, Tesco*	1 Serving/165g	53	0.3	32	1.2	6.4	0.2	1.1
PASSION FRUIT								
Raw, Fresh	*1 Fruit/30g*	*18*	*0.1*	*60*	*0.7*	*14.4*	*0.2*	*0.2*
Weighed with Skin	*1oz/28g*	*6*	*0.1*	*22*	*1.7*	*3.5*	*0.2*	*2.0*
PASTA								
Angel Hair, Konjac, Slim Pasta*	1 Serving/100g	8	0.0	8	0.6	0.6	0.0	5.6
Arrabbiata Nodini, Asda*	1 Serving/150g	301	8.7	201	7.8	29.3	5.8	2.7
Bean & Tuna, BGTY, Sainsbury's*	1 Serving/200g	176	1.8	88	7.3	12.6	0.9	2.8

P

PASTA

INFO/WEIGHT	Measure	per Measure KCAL	FAT	Nutrition Values per 100g / 100ml KCAL	PROT	CARB	FAT	FIBRE
Blue Cheese, Bacon & Spinach, M & S*	1 Pack/400g	640	34.0	160	6.5	13.8	8.5	0.7
Boccoletti, Dried, Sainsbury's*	1 Serving/90g	321	1.5	357	12.3	73.1	1.7	2.5
Bolognese, Diet Chef Ltd*	1 Pack/300g	255	10.2	85	7.9	5.8	3.4	4.4
Brown Rice, Fusilli, Gluten Free, Dove's Farm*	1 Serving/30g	101	0.4	338	7.9	70.3	1.5	4.1
Brown Rice & Maize, Ditalini, Organic, Dove's Farm*	1 Serving/100g	347	0.9	347	7.0	76.0	0.9	2.4
Cajun Chicken, GFY, Asda*	1 Serving/297g	312	8.3	105	8.0	12.0	2.8	2.1
Carbonara, with Cheese & Bacon, Slim Fast*	1 Serving/70g	240	4.4	343	22.7	48.9	6.3	5.7
Cheddar, Country, Bowl, Haribo*	1 Serving/269g	400	19.0	149	5.6	15.2	7.1	1.5
Cheese, Tomato, & Pesto, Boots*	1 Pack/250g	355	11.0	142	5.9	20.0	4.4	2.0
Cheese & Broccoli, Light Choices, Tesco*	1 Pack/348g	435	8.0	125	4.4	21.2	2.3	2.4
Cheese & Broccoli, Tubes, Tesco*	1 Serving/202g	319	13.9	158	5.0	19.1	6.9	2.3
Cheese & Ham, Shapers, Boots*	1 Pack/76g	220	4.9	289	23.7	34.2	6.4	6.4
Cheese & Tortellini in Tomato Sauce, Heinz*	1 Pack/250g	229	7.6	92	2.2	13.7	3.0	0.2
Cheesy Spirals, Curly Whirly, Asda*	1/3 Pack/200g	214	5.2	107	6.0	15.0	2.6	0.5
Chicken, Tomato, & Basil, Asda*	1 Pack/400g	474	10.0	118	6.5	17.5	2.5	1.2
Chicken, Tomato, & Mascarpone, Italiano, Tesco*	1 Pack/400g	572	24.8	143	7.4	14.3	6.2	1.3
Chicken, Tomato & Basil, GFY, Asda*	1 Pack/400g	404	9.2	101	6.4	13.6	2.3	1.4
Chicken, Tomato & Herb, Easy Steam, Tesco*	1 Serving/400g	528	24.8	132	8.9	10.2	6.2	1.3
Chicken, Tomato & Mascarpone, Easy Steam, Tesco*	1 Pack/400g	468	16.4	117	9.7	10.3	4.1	0.9
Chicken & Asparagus, GFY, Asda*	1 Pack/400g	388	8.8	97	10.9	8.5	2.2	1.5
Chicken & Green Pesto, HL, Tesco*	1 Serving/376g	440	4.5	117	8.3	18.5	1.2	1.4
Chicken & Ham, Easy Steam, Tesco*	1 Pack/400g	572	26.4	143	9.8	11.2	6.6	0.6
Chicken & Mushroom, Big Eat, Heinz*	1 Pot/350g	339	15.7	97	4.8	9.2	4.5	0.5
Chicken & Mushroom Flavour, Quick, Sainsbury's*	1 Pot/220g	235	6.2	107	3.3	16.1	2.8	1.9
Chicken & Pineapple, Shapers, Boots*	1 Pack/221g	210	3.3	95	5.4	15.0	1.5	0.9
Chicken & Roasted Tomato, HL, Tesco*	1 Serving/374g	426	7.1	114	7.4	16.7	1.9	1.3
Chicken & Vegetable, Mediterranean, Waitrose*	1 Serving/400g	375	9.2	94	7.5	10.5	2.3	2.2
Chicken Penne, Weight Watchers*	1 Pot/261g	248	3.7	95	5.0	14.6	1.4	2.1
Conchiglie, Dry weight, Parioli, Cucina*	1 Serving/75g	266	1.0	355	12.5	73.0	1.4	2.6
Courgette, Green Bean & Basil Pappardelle, M & S*	1 Pack/270g	324	15.9	120	4.7	11.8	5.9	1.6
Creamy Garlic Mushroom, HL, Tesco*	1 Serving/100g	106	3.7	106	3.6	14.6	3.7	1.1
Creamy Mushroom, Light Choices, Tesco*	1 Pack/350g	455	4.9	130	4.3	25.0	1.4	1.3
Creamy Mushroom, Sainsbury's*	1 Serving/63g	148	9.1	237	4.5	21.7	14.6	1.2
Creamy Tomato & Chicken, Great Stuff, Asda*	1 Pack/300g	351	11.7	117	7.0	13.5	3.9	2.3
Creamy Vegetable, Meal in 5, Ainsley Harriott*	1 Pot/387g	414	10.1	107	2.8	18.1	2.6	0.8
Cup A, Creamy Cheese, Batchelors*	1 Pack/250g	197	3.5	79	2.7	13.7	1.4	0.5
Dischi Volanti, Tesco*	1 Serving/50g	177	0.7	355	12.5	73.0	1.4	2.6
Elicoidali, Waitrose*	1 Serving/200g	682	2.6	341	11.5	70.7	1.3	3.7
Fagottini, Wild Mushroom, Sainsbury's*	½ Pack/125g	274	9.4	219	10.2	27.7	7.5	2.7
Feta & Black Olive Girasole, Extra Special, Asda*	½ Pack/150g	360	15.4	240	8.3	28.4	10.3	0.0
Filled, Tomato & Mozzarella Caramella, Jamie Oliver*	½ Pack/165g	294	9.2	178	8.9	24.9	5.6	2.0
Fiorelli, Egg, M & S*	1 Serving/100g	355	2.8	355	13.9	68.5	2.8	3.0
Fiorelli, Mozzarella, Tomato & Basil, Waitrose*	1 Serving/125g	352	11.6	282	10.8	38.9	9.3	1.7
Fusilli, Wholewheat, Cooked, Tesco*	1 Portion/75g	245	1.9	327	12.5	62.5	2.5	9.1
Fusilloni, TTD, Sainsbury's*	1 Serving/90g	321	1.5	357	12.3	73.1	1.7	2.5
Garlic Mushroom Filled, Extra Special, Asda*	1 Serving/125g	224	8.7	179	8.0	21.0	7.0	2.5
High Fibre, Uncooked, Fiber Gourmet*	1 Serving/56g	130	1.0	232	12.5	75.0	1.8	32.1
Honey & Mustard Chicken, Tesco*	1 Pack/375g	865	48.3	231	6.7	21.9	12.9	0.0
Hot Smoked Salmon, Tesco*	1 Pack/275g	426	17.0	155	7.1	16.6	6.2	4.1
King Prawn & Pesto, Asda*	1 Pack/400g	488	17.7	122	7.6	12.9	4.4	1.2
Linguine, Cooked	1 Serving/100g	133	0.7	133	5.1	26.3	0.7	1.1
Linguine, Dry, Parioli, Cucina*	1 Serving/75g	270	1.0	360	12.5	73.0	1.4	2.6
Linguine, Dry Weight, De Cecco*	1 Serving/100g	350	1.5	350	13.0	71.0	1.5	2.9

	Measure INFO/WEIGHT	per Measure KCAL	FAT	Nutrition Values per 100g / 100ml KCAL	PROT	CARB	FAT	FIBRE

PASTA

	Measure INFO/WEIGHT	KCAL	FAT	KCAL	PROT	CARB	FAT	FIBRE
Lumache, Tesco*	1 Serving/100g	345	2.0	345	13.2	68.5	2.0	2.9
Lumaconi, TTD, Sainsbury's*	1 Serving/90g	321	1.5	357	12.3	73.1	1.7	2.5
Margherite, Basil & Pinenut, TTD, Sainsbury's*	½ Pack/150g	309	10.5	206	12.6	23.2	7.0	2.7
Meat Feast, Italian, Sainsbury's*	1 Pack/450g	508	18.0	113	7.4	11.8	4.0	0.6
Medaglioni, Bolognese, Rich Red Wine, Waitrose*	½ Pack/125g	266	7.0	213	12.5	28.1	5.6	2.6
Mediterranean Vegetable, Weight Watchers*	1 Pack/400g	262	3.2	65	2.6	12.0	0.8	1.6
Mini Spirals, in Cheese Sauce, Heinz*	1 Can/154g	120	3.5	78	3.9	10.4	2.3	0.3
Organic, Gluten Free, Dove's Farm*	1 Serving/100g	338	1.5	338	7.9	70.3	1.5	4.1
Paccheri, Finest, Tesco*	1 Serving/100g	360	1.5	360	13.5	72.5	1.5	1.6
Parcels, Basil & Parmesan, Fresh, Sainsbury's*	1 Serving/162g	357	13.5	220	10.0	26.4	8.3	3.3
Penne, Creamy Mushroom, Prepared, Tesco*	½ Pack/200g	288	12.8	144	4.5	17.4	6.4	3.3
Penne, Dry Weight, Parioli, Cucina*	1 Serving/76g	270	1.1	355	12.5	73.0	1.4	2.6
Penne, Mediterranean, HL, Tesco*	1 Pack/400g	296	10.8	74	2.9	9.6	2.7	1.5
Pennoni, TTD, Sainsbury's*	1 Serving/90g	321	1.5	357	12.3	73.1	1.7	2.5
Pepper & Tomato, Asda*	1 Serving/250g	340	17.5	136	3.2	15.0	7.0	2.4
Pomodoro, with Tomato & Herbs, Slim Fast*	1 Serving/71g	235	3.1	331	21.5	51.5	4.3	6.0
Raviolini, Gorgonzola & Walnut, M & S*	½ Pack/125g	381	16.5	305	12.6	33.6	13.2	2.0
Riccioli, Dry Weight, Buitoni*	1 Serving/75g	264	1.4	352	11.2	72.6	1.9	0.0
Roasted Vegetable Arrabbiata, Weight Watchers*	1 Pack/362g	246	1.4	68	3.4	11.4	0.4	2.8
Sausage & Tomato, Italiano, Tesco*	1 Serving/450g	679	26.5	151	5.7	18.8	5.9	1.6
Seafood, Retail	1oz/28g	31	1.3	110	8.9	7.6	4.8	0.4
Sicilian Chicken, City Kitchen, Tesco*	1 Pack/385g	500	13.5	130	9.1	14.6	3.5	0.6
Spicy Tomato, Meal in 5, Ainsley Harriott*	1 Pot/387g	369	2.1	95	2.6	19.9	0.5	1.5
Spicy Tomato & Pepperoni Sauce with Fusilli, Heinz*	1 Pack/250g	318	13.8	127	4.4	14.8	5.5	0.6
Spinach & Pine Nut, Finest, Tesco*	1 Pack/195g	546	34.9	280	6.4	23.1	17.9	1.5
Stuffed Mushroom & Emmental, Sainsbury's*	1 Pack/250g	650	23.0	260	11.3	33.5	9.2	3.7
Sundried Tomato, Sainsbury's*	1 Serving/50g	196	17.8	393	4.5	13.4	35.7	6.2
Tomato & Basil Chicken, Boots*	1 Serving/320g	621	28.8	194	9.0	19.0	9.0	1.4
Tomato & Chicken Spiralli, HL, Tesco*	1 Pack/350g	402	5.2	115	7.8	17.3	1.5	1.6
Tomato & Mascarpone, GFY, Asda*	½ Can/200g	128	4.4	64	2.1	9.0	2.2	0.0
Tomato & Mascarpone, Tesco*	1 Pack/400g	468	16.4	117	9.7	10.3	4.1	0.9
Tomato & Onion, Shells, Tesco*	1 Serving/193g	643	3.1	333	12.5	67.1	1.6	6.3
Tomato & Pepper, GFY, Asda*	1 Pack/400g	344	7.6	86	3.1	14.0	1.9	1.1
Tomato & Vegetable, Diet Chef Ltd*	1 Pack/300g	216	6.0	72	2.6	10.9	2.0	1.8
Tomato & Vegetable, Solo Slim, Rosemary Conley*	1 Pack /300g	216	5.4	72	2.8	11.1	1.8	2.0
Tortelloni, Spinach & Ricotta, Emma Giordani*	1 Pack/250g	685	15.0	274	10.0	45.0	6.0	0.0
Tortelloni, Spinach & Ricotta, Giovanni Rana*	½ Pack/190g	376	12.3	198	7.8	27.0	6.5	3.1
Tuna Rigatoni, Diet Chef Ltd*	1 Pack/300g	336	13.2	112	5.9	12.2	4.4	1.0
Twists, Quick Cook, Morrisons*	1 Serving/75g	265	1.5	353	12.0	72.0	2.0	3.1
Twists, Tuna & Tomato, Canned, Be Light, Aldi*	1 Can/400g	264	6.8	66	4.8	7.8	1.7	1.7
Twists, with Tuna, Italian, Weight Watchers*	1 Can/385g	239	5.4	62	4.3	8.2	1.4	0.6
Vegetable, Creamy, BGTY, Sainsbury's*	1 Pack/400g	348	6.0	87	4.0	14.3	1.5	1.9
Vegetable, Mediterranean, Sainsbury's*	1 Pack/400g	504	11.6	126	4.0	20.9	2.9	1.8
Vegetable Rice, Dry Weight, Orgran*	1 Serving/66g	233	1.3	353	6.8	80.0	2.0	4.8
Wheat Free, Delverde*	1 Serving/63g	229	1.2	366	0.5	86.9	1.9	1.2
Whole Wheat, Bella Terra*	1 Serving/100g	375	1.7	375	12.5	78.5	1.7	10.7
Whole Wheat, Penne, Asda*	1 Serving/100g	333	2.1	333	12.1	66.3	2.1	6.9
Wholewheat, Cooked, Tesco*	1 Serving/200g	284	1.8	142	5.7	27.9	0.9	4.5

PASTA BAKE

	Measure INFO/WEIGHT	KCAL	FAT	KCAL	PROT	CARB	FAT	FIBRE
Aberdeen Angus Meatball, Waitrose*	½ Pack/350g	501	28.0	143	5.2	12.5	8.0	0.9
Bacon & Leek, Sainsbury's*	1 Pack/400g	660	27.6	165	7.3	18.5	6.9	1.8
Bacon & Leek, Tesco*	1 Pack/450g	774	37.3	172	8.1	16.1	8.3	2.0
Bolognese, Asda*	¼ Pack/375g	514	23.6	137	7.3	12.7	6.3	1.8

PASTA BAKE

	Measure INFO/WEIGHT	per Measure KCAL	FAT	Nutrition Values per 100g / 100ml KCAL	PROT	CARB	FAT	FIBRE
Bolognese, Finest, Tesco*	1 Serving/250g	375	15.7	150	7.3	16.1	6.3	1.1
Bolognese, GFY, Asda*	1 Pack/400g	376	8.4	94	5.8	13.1	2.1	0.9
Bolognese, Weight Watchers*	1 Pack/400g	324	8.0	81	6.1	9.6	2.0	1.3
Cheese & Bacon, Asda*	1 Serving/120g	168	14.4	140	2.9	5.2	12.0	0.3
Cheese & Tomato, Italiano, Tesco*	1 Bake/300g	354	12.6	118	3.9	16.1	4.2	1.0
Cheese & Tomato, Tesco*	1 Pack/400g	388	5.6	97	3.4	17.8	1.4	1.2
Chicken, BGTY, Sainsbury's*	1 Pack/400g	348	8.0	87	9.7	7.5	2.0	0.8
Chicken, Italiano, Tesco*	1 Serving/190g	218	7.8	115	8.4	11.2	4.1	3.1
Chicken, Mozzarella & Tomato, Birds Eye*	1 Pack/360g	468	6.8	130	7.1	14.3	1.9	0.3
Chicken, Tomato, & Mascarpone, Tesco*	1 Serving/400g	448	8.4	112	8.0	15.2	2.1	1.7
Chicken, Weight Watchers*	1 Pack/300g	249	2.7	83	6.0	12.1	0.9	1.1
Chicken & Bacon, Asda*	¼ Pack/374g	610	26.2	163	9.0	16.0	7.0	4.1
Chicken & Broccoli, Pasta Presto, Findus*	1 Pack/321g	449	22.5	140	7.5	12.0	7.0	0.0
Chicken & Broccoli, Weight Watchers*	1 Bake/305g	290	4.6	95	6.0	14.2	1.5	0.9
Chicken & Courgette, Asda*	½ Pack/387g	519	23.2	134	6.0	14.0	6.0	0.6
Chicken & Leek, HL, Tesco*	1 Pack/400g	460	7.6	115	10.8	13.1	1.9	1.6
Chicken & Mushroom, Waitrose*	1 Pack/400g	532	30.8	133	6.7	9.1	7.7	0.8
Chicken & Roast Mushroom, HL, Tesco*	1 Pack/390g	413	0.4	106	8.6	17.6	0.1	1.3
Chicken & Spinach, GFY, Asda*	1 Pack/400g	374	6.0	93	5.0	15.0	1.5	1.2
Chicken & Spinach, Sainsbury's*	1 Pack/340g	286	9.2	84	4.9	10.0	2.7	0.6
Chilli & Cheese, American Style, Tesco*	1 Pack/425g	637	16.6	150	6.8	21.8	3.9	1.5
Chilli Beef, Asda*	1 Pack/1500g	2010	90.0	134	7.0	13.0	6.0	1.2
Creamy Mushroom, Dolmio*	½ Jar/245g	267	22.5	109	1.1	5.5	9.2	0.0
Creamy Tomato, Dolmio*	1 Serving/125g	141	9.0	113	2.3	8.4	7.2	0.0
Findus*	1 Pack/320g	448	22.4	140	7.5	12.0	7.0	0.0
Ham & Broccoli, Asda*	1 Pack/340g	309	13.9	91	3.4	10.0	4.1	0.5
Ham & Mushroom, Italiano, Tesco*	1 Pack/425g	646	20.4	152	5.8	21.3	4.8	1.7
Italian Creamy Tomato & Bacon, Asda*	1 Serving/125g	131	11.2	105	2.0	3.9	9.0	0.6
King Prawn & Salmon, GFY, Asda*	1 Pack/400g	420	11.6	105	6.9	12.7	2.9	1.2
Leek & Bacon, Morrisons*	1 Pack/401g	553	36.1	138	4.8	9.9	9.0	0.2
Meatball, Tesco*	1 Pack/400g	576	19.2	144	5.9	19.3	4.8	0.5
Meatfeast, Italian, Tesco*	1 Serving/500g	675	19.0	135	6.4	17.8	3.8	2.3
Mediterranean, Weight Watchers*	1 Pack/397g	262	3.2	66	2.6	12.0	0.8	1.6
Mediterranean Style, Tesco*	1 Pack/450g	423	1.8	94	2.9	19.6	0.4	2.0
Mix, Tuna, Colman's*	1 Sachet/45g	145	2.3	323	9.2	60.0	5.2	4.7
Mozzarella & Tomato, Asda*	1 Pack/400g	532	19.2	133	4.4	18.1	4.8	1.8
Mushroom, Creamy, Asda*	¼ Jar/118g	204	20.1	173	1.8	3.3	17.0	0.5
Penne Mozzarella, Tesco*	1 Pack/340g	408	8.5	120	4.7	19.7	2.5	0.6
Pepperoni & Ham, Tesco*	½ Pack/425g	501	2.5	118	8.9	19.3	0.6	2.5
Roasted Mediterranean Vegetables, Dolmio*	1 Portion/125g	66	2.1	53	1.3	8.1	1.7	1.2
Spicy Tomato & Pepperoni, Asda*	1 Pack/440g	431	26.4	98	1.1	10.0	6.0	1.2
Tomato & Cheese, Light Choices, Tesco*	1 Pack/350g	385	4.5	110	3.2	20.9	1.3	1.5
Tomato & Herb, Asda*	1 Jar/436g	715	56.7	164	1.8	10.0	13.0	1.2
Tomato & Mozzarella, Italiano, Tesco*	1 Pack/340g	398	8.5	117	4.8	18.9	2.5	1.7
Tomato & Mozzarella, Light Choices, Tesco*	1 Pack/400g	368	8.0	92	3.7	14.8	2.0	1.5
Tuna, Co-Op*	1 Serving/340g	306	6.8	90	7.0	12.0	2.0	1.0
Tuna, COU, M & S*	1 Pack/360g	432	15.5	120	8.0	11.9	4.3	0.8
Tuna, Lean Cuisine*	1 Pack/346g	380	8.6	110	5.0	16.0	2.5	1.5
Tuna, Light Choices, Tesco*	1 Pack/400g	380	5.2	95	10.8	10.0	1.3	2.2
Tuna, Weight Watchers*	1 Pack/400g	292	3.2	73	7.0	9.4	0.8	1.4
Tuna & Sweetcorn, Asda*	1 Serving/250g	332	22.5	133	5.0	8.0	9.0	0.9
Tuna & Tomato, BGTY, Sainsbury's*	1 Pack/450g	553	18.9	123	8.7	12.6	4.2	0.4
Tuna Conchiglie, M & S*	1 Pack/400g	520	17.2	130	8.6	14.3	4.3	1.1

P

	Measure INFO/WEIGHT	per Measure KCAL	FAT	Nutrition Values per 100g / 100ml KCAL	PROT	CARB	FAT	FIBRE
PASTA BAKE								
Vegetable, Findus*	1 Pack/331g	430	21.5	130	6.0	13.0	6.5	0.0
Vegetable, M & S*	½ Pack/225g	292	12.8	130	4.8	14.6	5.7	1.6
Vegetable, Mediterranean, HL, Tesco*	1 Serving/450g	373	3.6	83	2.9	16.0	0.8	1.5
Vegetable, Mediterranean, Tesco*	1 Serving/450g	495	20.7	110	4.3	12.9	4.6	1.3
Vegetable, Ready Meals, Waitrose*	1oz/28g	44	2.4	157	5.9	14.4	8.6	1.0
PASTA IN								
Arrabiata Sauce, Pasta King*	1 Serving/100g	104	1.4	104	3.5	19.5	1.4	1.8
Basilico Sauce, Pasta King*	1 Serving/100g	123	3.3	123	3.8	19.5	3.3	2.1
Bolognese Sauce, Pasta King*	1 Serving/100g	121	2.6	121	5.1	19.3	2.6	1.9
Carbonara Sauce, Pasta King*	1 Serving/100g	122	2.9	122	5.1	19.3	2.9	1.2
Cheese Sauce, Pasta King*	1 Serving/100g	117	2.3	117	5.0	19.2	2.3	1.1
Chicken Italiano Sauce, Pasta King*	1 Serving/100g	125	3.2	125	5.5	18.9	3.2	1.9
Chilli Beef Sauce, Pasta King*	1 Serving/100g	125	2.6	125	5.4	20.5	2.6	2.2
Garlic & Herb, Asda*	1 Serving/120g	487	12.0	406	10.0	69.0	10.0	2.3
Herb Sauce, Sainsbury's*	1 Pack/420g	441	0.8	105	3.5	22.4	0.2	0.8
Peperonata Sauce, Pasta King*	1 Serving/100g	104	1.4	104	3.5	19.4	1.4	1.8
Pomodoro Sauce, Pasta King*	1 Serving/100g	109	1.8	109	3.6	19.6	1.8	1.8
Vegetable Chilli, Pasta King*	1 Serving/100g	121	2.1	121	5.2	20.9	2.1	2.3
Vegetarian Bolognese, Pasta King*	1 Serving/100g	117	2.1	117	4.9	19.7	2.1	1.9
Zingy Pepper Sauce, Pasta King*	1 Serving/100g	106	1.5	106	3.6	19.6	1.5	1.8
PASTA 'N' SAUCE								
Bolognese Flavour, Dry, Batchelors*	½ Pack/65g	228	1.7	353	15.1	67.2	2.6	3.9
Carbonara Flavour, Dry, Batchelors*	1 Pack/120g	463	6.0	386	14.3	71.0	5.0	3.1
Cheese, Leek & Ham, Batchelors*	1 Pack/120g	454	6.1	378	16.1	67.0	5.1	2.0
Cheese & Broccoli Sauce Mix, Made Up, Sainsbury's*	1 Pack/120g	164	6.8	137	4.2	17.2	5.7	1.1
Chicken & Mushroom, Batchelors*	½ Pack/63g	227	1.1	361	14.1	72.3	1.7	2.8
Chicken & Mushroom, Made Up, Morrisons*	1 Pack/110g	166	6.2	151	5.0	20.3	5.6	2.1
Chicken & Roasted Garlic Flavour, Dry, Batchelors*	½ Pack/60g	223	1.7	372	12.6	73.8	2.9	3.4
Creamy Tikka Masala, Dry, Batchelors*	1 Pack/122g	426	2.7	349	12.7	69.5	2.2	4.4
Creamy Tomato & Mushroom, Dry, Batchelors*	1 Pack/125g	457	4.1	366	13.0	71.0	3.3	3.2
Macaroni Cheese, Dry, Batchelors*	1 Pack/108g	402	5.1	372	17.2	65.2	4.7	2.7
Mild Cheese & Broccoli, Batchelors*	½ Pack/61g	221	2.4	363	15.0	67.0	3.9	4.0
Mushroom & Wine, Batchelors*	½ Pack/50g	242	2.8	483	18.5	89.9	5.5	4.4
Mushroom & Wine, Dry, Batchelors*	1 Pack/132g	498	6.5	377	12.0	71.3	4.9	2.5
Tomato, Onion & Herb, Made Up, Morrisons*	1 Serving/110g	141	4.9	128	3.2	18.7	4.5	2.3
Tomato, Onion & Herbs, Dry, Batchelors*	1 Pack/135g	455	1.8	337	12.8	68.5	1.3	5.8
Tomato & Bacon Flavour, Dry, Batchelors*	1 Pack/134g	476	3.5	355	13.0	70.0	2.6	3.0
Tomato & Mascarpone, BGTY, Sainsbury's*	1 Pack/380g	555	7.2	146	6.6	25.6	1.9	1.3
PASTA QUILLS								
Dry, Average	*1 Serving/75g*	*256*	*0.9*	*342*	*12.0*	*72.3*	*1.2*	*2.0*
Gluten Free, Salute*	1 Serving/75g	269	1.4	359	7.5	78.0	1.9	0.0
PASTA SALAD								
Basil & Parmesan, Tesco*	1 Serving/50g	65	1.8	130	4.3	20.2	3.6	0.6
BBQ Chicken, Positive Eating, Scottish Slimmers*	1 Serving/240g	223	4.3	93	6.4	14.0	1.8	1.3
Caesar, Chicken, Shapers, Boots*	1 Pack/218g	288	8.3	132	6.7	18.0	3.8	1.8
Caesar & Santa Tomatoes, M & S*	1 Serving/220g	495	33.7	225	5.2	15.9	15.3	0.8
Chargrilled Chicken, Italian Style, Fresh, Asda*	1 Pack/200g	318	14.0	159	7.0	17.0	7.0	0.4
Chargrilled Chicken, M & S*	1 Serving/190g	285	5.5	150	9.6	23.6	2.9	1.6
Chargrilled Chicken & Pesto Pasta, Sainsbury's*	1 Pack/240g	454	22.1	189	7.2	19.4	9.2	0.0
Chargrilled Chicken & Red Pepper, Tesco*	1 Pack/270g	553	24.0	205	9.8	20.3	8.9	3.1
Chargrilled Vegetables, Sainsbury's*	1 Serving/178g	192	4.8	108	2.7	15.9	2.7	4.7
Chargrilled Vegetables & Tomato, Shapers, Boots*	1 Pack/175g	187	5.4	107	2.8	17.0	3.1	1.5
Cheddar Cheese, Tesco*	1 Pot/215g	546	43.9	254	5.7	12.0	20.4	0.8

P

PASTA SALAD

INFO/WEIGHT	Measure	per Measure KCAL	FAT	Nutrition Values per 100g / 100ml KCAL	PROT	CARB	FAT	FIBRE
Cheese, Asda*	1 Serving/40g	118	9.0	296	6.5	16.6	22.6	0.5
Cheese, Layered, Asda*	1 Pack/440g	647	40.9	147	4.5	11.4	9.3	0.0
Chicken, Asda*	1 Pot/250g	322	12.2	129	5.8	15.5	4.9	1.3
Chicken & Bacon, Tesco*	½ Pack/200g	450	29.0	225	6.3	16.8	14.5	3.2
Chicken & Bacon Layered, Fresh Tastes, Asda*	1 Pack/375g	266	30.0	71	5.9	11.5	8.0	0.0
Chicken & Smoked Bacon, M & S*	1 Pack/380g	817	46.7	215	7.5	19.0	12.3	1.9
Chicken Caesar, Asda*	1 Pack/297g	683	41.3	230	9.6	16.6	13.9	2.5
Chicken Caesar, Ginsters*	1 Pack/220g	504	35.4	229	7.5	13.6	16.1	0.0
Chilli & Cheese, Sainsbury's*	1 Serving/300g	384	16.8	128	4.3	15.5	5.6	0.3
Crayfish, Rocket & Lemon, Finest, Tesco*	1 Serving/250g	727	39.7	291	8.9	28.0	15.9	4.2
Crayfish, Shapers, Boots*	1 Pack/280g	269	6.4	96	6.0	13.0	2.3	0.7
Farfalle, Prawns Tomatoes & Cucumber, Sainsbury's*	1 Serving/260g	270	12.2	104	4.5	10.9	4.7	0.7
Goats Cheese, & Mixed Pepper, Sainsbury's*	1 Pack/200g	366	18.8	183	6.4	18.2	9.4	1.5
Ham, Sainsbury's*	1 Pot/250g	610	48.2	244	4.1	13.4	19.3	0.8
Honey & Mustard Chicken, M & S*	1 Serving/190g	304	4.7	160	8.7	26.7	2.5	1.5
Honey & Mustard Chicken, Shapers, Boots*	1 Serving/252g	350	5.5	139	8.4	22.0	2.2	2.8
Hot Smoked Salmon, No Mayonnaise, Tesco*	1 Pack/275g	426	17.0	155	7.1	16.6	6.2	4.1
Italian, Bowl, Sainsbury's*	1 Serving/210g	309	15.5	147	3.1	16.9	7.4	1.9
Italian, Tesco*	½ Pack/225g	315	8.3	140	3.5	22.6	3.7	2.3
Italian Style, Sainsbury's*	1/3 Pot/84g	129	5.3	153	3.5	20.5	6.3	1.4
Italian Style, Snack, Asda*	1 Pack/150g	141	6.0	94	3.4	11.0	4.0	4.1
Kraft*	½ Cup/68g	183	11.0	269	4.0	26.5	16.2	0.0
Lime & Coriander Chicken, M & S*	1 Serving/190g	370	23.2	195	7.6	14.4	12.2	0.6
Mediterranean Chicken, Waitrose*	1 Serving/200g	314	13.6	157	7.0	16.9	6.8	2.1
Mediterranean Style, Layered, Waitrose*	1 Pot/275g	190	3.6	69	2.6	11.8	1.3	1.0
Mediterranean Tuna, Shapers, Boots*	1 Serving/239g	232	3.1	97	6.2	15.0	1.3	0.9
Mediterranean Vegetable & Bean, BGTY, Sainsbury's*	1 Serving/66g	53	1.3	80	3.2	12.5	1.9	2.8
Mexican Chicken, Weight Watchers*	1 Pack/249g	284	4.2	114	7.8	16.9	1.7	3.6
Mixed Bean, Diet Chef Ltd*	1 Packet/300g	300	3.6	100	4.7	17.5	1.2	2.8
Mozzarella & Plum Tomatoes, COU, M & S*	1 Bowl/255g	204	4.1	80	4.6	11.5	1.6	1.7
Mozzarella & Sun Dried Tomato, Waitrose*	1 Serving/150g	312	18.3	208	5.8	18.8	12.2	1.3
Pepper, Side, Tesco*	1 Serving/46g	56	3.0	122	2.4	13.0	6.5	1.3
Pepper & Tomato, Fire Roasted, Finest, Tesco*	1 Pack/200g	260	8.2	130	3.7	19.4	4.1	2.5
Poached Salmon, M & S*	1 Serving/200g	340	16.8	170	7.8	16.2	8.4	1.4
Poached Salmon, Sainsbury's*	1 Serving/200g	472	30.6	236	6.7	17.9	15.3	12.0
Prawn, Layered, Asda*	½ Pack/220g	279	11.4	127	5.2	14.2	5.2	2.0
Prawn, Shapers, Boots*	1 Pot/250g	250	7.7	100	4.1	14.0	3.1	0.4
Prawn, Tesco*	½ Pack/250g	487	27.7	195	4.9	18.9	11.1	2.0
Prawn Cocktail, Shapers, Boots*	1 Pack/248g	255	6.7	103	5.0	15.0	2.7	1.6
Prawns, King, & Juicy Fresh Tomatoes, COU, M & S*	1 Serving/270g	256	4.0	95	5.1	16.4	1.5	0.9
Roasted Mushroom, Spinach & Tarragon, Tesco*	1 Pot/200g	216	4.8	108	4.3	17.2	2.4	0.8
Roasted Vegetable, Waitrose*	1 Pack/190g	270	8.7	142	6.8	18.2	4.6	1.1
Sainsbury's*	½ Pack/160g	235	9.6	147	3.2	20.0	6.0	1.5
Salmon, M & S*	1 Serving/380g	817	57.8	215	6.8	12.7	15.2	0.7
Spicy Chicken, Geo Adams*	1 Pack/230g	580	43.9	252	5.1	14.9	19.1	2.9
Spicy Chilli Pesto, Sainsbury's*	¼ Pot/63g	170	12.2	272	3.8	20.1	19.6	1.6
Sun Dried Tomato Dressing, Sainsbury's*	1 Pack/320g	442	14.1	138	3.7	20.8	4.4	3.6
Sweetcorn & Pepper, GFY, Asda*	1 Serving/175g	68	0.7	39	1.9	7.0	0.4	0.0
Three Cheese, Tesco*	1 Serving/300g	633	41.1	211	7.5	14.4	13.7	2.8
Tiger Prawn, Waitrose*	1 Serving/225g	544	38.5	242	5.4	16.7	17.1	0.4
Tiger Prawn & Tomato, GFY, Asda*	1 Serving/200g	250	5.8	125	4.6	20.0	2.9	2.0
Tomato, Aldi*	1 Serving/50g	58	1.8	117	3.9	18.6	3.6	0.0
Tomato, Bacon & Cheese, Ginsters*	1 Pack/220g	381	19.8	173	7.4	15.6	9.0	0.0

Measure INFO/WEIGHT	per Measure		Nutrition Values per 100g / 100ml				
	KCAL	FAT	KCAL	PROT	CARB	FAT	FIBRE

PASTA SALAD

	Measure	KCAL	FAT	KCAL	PROT	CARB	FAT	FIBRE
Tomato, Diet Chef Ltd*	1 Pack/300g	264	5.4	88	2.3	15.6	1.8	1.2
Tomato & Basil, Chicken, Waitrose*	1 Pack/205g	434	24.6	212	8.3	17.7	12.0	1.1
Tomato & Basil, M & S*	1 Pot/225g	484	35.8	215	2.9	15.0	15.9	1.2
Tomato & Basil, Perfectly Balanced, Waitrose*	1 Serving/100g	97	1.7	97	3.7	16.8	1.7	0.0
Tomato & Basil, Pot, HL, Tesco*	1 Pot/200g	242	5.4	121	2.0	22.1	2.7	2.2
Tomato & Basil, Sainsbury's*	1 Serving/62g	87	4.3	141	3.2	16.4	6.9	3.8
Tomato & Basil Chicken, M & S*	1 Serving/279g	446	22.0	160	7.0	14.8	7.9	1.8
Tomato & Basil with Red & Green Pepper, Sainsbury's*	¼ Pot/63g	89	4.3	141	3.2	16.4	6.9	3.8
Tomato & Chargrilled Vegetable, Tesco*	1 Serving/200g	248	7.8	124	3.7	18.6	3.9	1.4
Tomato & Mozzarella, Leaf, Shapers, Boots*	1 Pack/185g	356	22.3	192	5.1	16.0	12.0	2.5
Tomato & Mozzarella, Sainsbury's*	1 Pack/200g	440	22.6	220	7.5	22.2	11.3	1.3
Tomato & Mozzarella, Waitrose*	1 Pack/225g	380	27.9	169	4.3	10.0	12.4	0.6
Tomato & Pepper, HL, Tesco*	1 Serving/200g	162	3.2	81	2.6	13.9	1.6	1.4
Tomato & Tuna, Snack, Sainsbury's*	1 Serving/200g	238	2.4	119	5.3	21.7	1.2	0.0
Tuna, Arrabbiata, BGTY, Sainsbury's*	1 Serving/200g	196	2.6	98	6.8	14.7	1.3	0.0
Tuna, Mediterranean, Johnsons*	1 Serving/225g	148	6.2	66	2.8	7.5	2.8	0.9
Tuna, Perfectly Balanced, Waitrose*	1 Tub/190g	180	4.4	95	7.0	11.5	2.3	1.1
Tuna, Tesco*	1 Pot/300g	399	21.9	133	6.2	10.5	7.3	0.0
Tuna & Spinach, COU, M & S*	1 Pack/270g	256	4.9	95	6.8	14.3	1.8	3.8
Tuna & Sweetcorn, COU, M & S*	1 Pack/200g	210	1.8	105	7.1	18.3	0.9	1.2
Tuna & Sweetcorn, Sainsbury's*	1 Serving/100g	111	1.2	111	7.1	18.3	1.2	1.2
Tuna Crunch, Shapers, Boots*	1 Pack/250g	352	6.7	141	9.8	19.0	2.7	2.8
Tuna Nicoise, Waitrose*	1 Pot/190g	306	17.1	161	5.1	14.9	9.0	1.1

PASTA SAUCE

	Measure	KCAL	FAT	KCAL	PROT	CARB	FAT	FIBRE
Amatriciana, Asda*	1 Jar/320g	496	41.6	155	4.4	5.0	13.0	1.0
Amatriciana, Italiano, Tesco*	½ Pot/175g	124	6.6	71	4.1	5.3	3.8	0.9
Amatriciana, M & S*	1 Jar/340g	425	32.3	125	3.4	6.3	9.5	2.9
Arrabbiata, Barilla*	1 Serving/100g	47	3.0	47	1.5	3.5	3.0	0.0
Arrabbiata, Fresh, Morrisons*	1 Pot/350g	139	5.2	40	1.9	5.4	1.5	0.0
Arrabbiata, GFY, Asda*	1 Serving/350g	133	3.9	38	1.1	6.0	1.1	0.0
Arrabbiata, Italian, Waitrose*	1 Jar/320g	115	3.2	36	1.5	6.7	1.0	1.4
Arrabbiata, M & S*	1 Jar/320g	240	17.0	75	1.2	6.2	5.3	0.8
Arrabbiata, Red Pepper, Sainsbury's*	½ Pot/175g	79	5.1	45	1.4	3.3	2.9	1.6
Arrabbiata, Romano*	1 Serving/100g	69	3.4	69	2.5	7.0	3.4	0.6
Arrabbiata, Stir in, BGTY, Sainsbury's*	1 Serving/75g	53	2.9	71	1.3	7.6	3.9	0.7
Aubergine & Pepper, Sacla*	½ Pot/95g	237	23.3	250	1.8	5.6	24.5	0.0
Basil & Oregano, Ragu, Knorr*	1 Jar/500g	215	0.0	43	1.3	9.4	0.0	1.1
Bolognese, Carb Check, Heinz*	1 Serving/150g	79	3.9	53	3.8	3.6	2.6	0.4
Bolognese, Dolmio*	1 Serving/100g	56	1.5	56	1.5	9.4	1.5	1.1
Bolognese, Finest, Tesco*	1 Serving/175g	170	10.7	97	7.0	3.8	6.1	0.5
Bolognese, Fresh, Sainsbury's*	½ Pot/150g	120	6.1	80	6.0	4.7	4.1	1.2
Bolognese, Italiano, Tesco*	1 Serving/175g	194	13.1	111	5.9	4.8	7.5	0.8
Bolognese, Light, Original, Ragu, Knorr*	1 Jar/515g	196	0.5	38	1.4	8.2	0.1	1.2
Bolognese, Mediterranean Vegetable, Chunky, Dolmio*	½ Jar/250g	137	4.0	55	1.3	8.8	1.6	1.1
Bolognese, Organic, Seeds of Change*	1 Jar/500g	290	6.0	58	1.3	10.4	1.2	0.8
Bolognese, Original, Light, Low Fat, Dolmio*	1 Serving/125g	44	0.2	35	1.5	6.0	0.2	1.2
Bolognese, Original, Sainsbury's*	¼ Jar/136g	90	2.9	66	1.9	9.9	2.1	1.3
Bolognese, Spicy, Ragu, Knorr*	1 Jar/500g	220	0.5	44	1.3	9.6	0.1	1.1
Bolognese, Tesco*	1 Serving/175g	100	4.5	57	4.2	4.0	2.6	0.8
Bolognese, Traditional, Ragu, Knorr*	1 Jar/320g	157	5.4	49	1.3	7.1	1.7	1.2
Bolognese, VLH Kitchens*	1 Portion/380g	316	15.6	83	6.0	4.7	4.1	1.2
Bolognese with Beef, Tesco*	½ Can/213g	179	10.0	84	4.9	5.5	4.7	0.0
Cacciatore, Fresh, Sainsbury's*	½ Pot/150g	151	8.8	101	5.4	8.1	5.9	1.5

	Measure INFO/WEIGHT	per Measure		Nutrition Values per 100g / 100ml				
		KCAL	FAT	KCAL	PROT	CARB	FAT	FIBRE
Carbonara, 50% Less Fat, Asda*	½ Pot/175g	170	10.5	97	4.8	6.0	6.0	0.6
Carbonara, Asda*	½ Pot/175g	359	29.7	205	7.0	6.0	17.0	0.1
Carbonara, Bottled, Tesco*	1 Jar/315g	504	41.6	160	3.2	6.8	13.2	0.1
Carbonara, Creamy, Stir in Sauce, Dolmio*	1 Serving/75g	98	8.0	130	3.3	5.2	10.6	0.2
Carbonara, Fresh, BGTY, Sainsbury's*	1 Tub/300g	255	10.8	85	5.4	7.8	3.6	0.5
Carbonara, Fresh, Chilled, Finest, Tesco*	½ Tub/175g	297	24.8	170	5.5	4.2	14.2	0.0
Carbonara, Fresh, Chilled, Italiano, Tesco*	½ Tub/175g	201	11.4	115	6.1	7.2	6.5	0.1
Carbonara, Italian, Asda*	½ Pack/175g	359	29.7	205	7.0	6.0	17.0	0.1
Carbonara, Italian, Fresh, Sainsbury's*	½ Pot/176g	209	16.3	119	5.4	3.4	9.3	0.9
Carbonara, Reduced Fat, BFY, Morrisons*	½ Pot/175g	135	5.8	77	6.6	5.1	3.3	0.5
Carbonara, with Pancetta, Loyd Grossman*	½ Pack/170g	209	15.5	123	2.8	7.5	9.1	0.1
Cheese, Fresh, Perfectly Balanced, Waitrose*	½ Pot/175g	143	5.1	82	6.1	7.9	2.9	0.5
Cherry Tomato & Basil, Sacla*	1 Serving/96g	90	7.1	94	1.2	5.3	7.4	0.0
Cherry Tomato & Roasted Pepper, Asda*	1 Jar/172g	91	5.2	53	1.5	5.0	3.0	2.4
Chilli with Jalapeno Peppers, Seeds of Change*	1 Jar/350g	322	5.2	92	3.6	16.0	1.5	2.2
Chunky Vegetable, Asda*	1 Serving/250g	122	4.2	49	1.4	7.0	1.7	1.2
Country Mushroom, for Bolognese, Ragu, Knorr*	1 Jar/510g	347	10.7	68	2.0	9.5	2.1	1.2
Creamy Mushroom, Dolmio*	1 Pack/150g	166	15.0	111	1.3	3.7	10.0	0.0
Creamy Tomato, Carb Check, Heinz*	1 Serving/150g	91	6.0	61	2.0	4.2	4.0	0.5
Creamy Tomato & Basil, BGTY, Sainsbury's*	½ Jar/250g	172	9.0	69	1.7	7.6	3.6	1.0
Fiorentina, Fresh, Sainsbury's*	½ Pot/157g	165	13.2	105	3.2	4.3	8.4	0.9
Five Cheese, Italiano, Tesco*	½ Tub/175g	271	20.1	155	6.8	6.0	11.5	0.0
for Bolognese, Extra Mushrooms, Dolmio*	1 Jar/500g	240	6.5	48	1.6	7.6	1.3	1.1
for Bolognese, Extra Onion & Garlic, Dolmio*	1 Serving/125g	66	1.2	53	1.7	9.0	1.0	0.0
for Bolognese, Extra Spicy, Dolmio*	1 Jar/500g	260	5.5	52	1.7	8.8	1.1	0.8
for Lasagne, Tomato, Red, Ragu, Knorr*	1 Jar/500g	215	0.0	43	1.1	9.7	0.0	1.1
for Lasagne, White, Light, Ragu, Knorr*	¼ Jar/122g	88	6.1	72	0.5	6.3	5.0	0.2
for Lasagne, White, Ragu, Knorr*	1 Jar/475g	755	72.2	159	0.5	5.1	15.2	0.3
Four Cheese, BGTY, Sainsbury's*	1 Serving/150g	103	6.0	69	2.9	5.5	4.0	0.1
Four Cheese, Fresh, Asda*	½ Pot/162g	309	28.8	191	5.4	2.2	17.8	0.5
Four Cheese, GFY, Asda*	½ Pot/175g	144	8.0	82	4.0	6.3	4.6	0.5
Four Cheese, Loyd Grossman*	1 Jar/350g	476	41.6	136	2.6	4.6	11.9	0.0
Four Cheese, Sainsbury's*	1 Serving/150g	295	25.5	197	6.6	4.5	17.0	0.8
Garlic, Perfectly Balanced, Waitrose*	1 Jar/440g	330	7.5	75	2.3	12.7	1.7	2.3
Garlic & Chilli, Slow Roasted, Seeds of Change*	½ Jar/175g	157	9.3	90	1.7	8.7	5.3	2.0
Garlic & Onion, Finest, Tesco*	1 Serving/126g	43	0.5	34	0.8	6.9	0.4	1.3
Grilled Vegetables, Bertolli*	1 Jar/400g	215	10.0	43	1.4	4.9	2.0	1.1
Ham & Mushroom, Creamy, Stir & Serve, Homepride*	1 Serving/92g	124	10.8	135	1.8	5.5	11.7	0.0
Hot & Spicy, Morrisons*	1 Serving/130g	81	3.1	62	1.4	8.5	2.4	1.1
Hot Pepper & Mozzarella, Stir Through, Sacla*	½ Jar/95g	229	20.4	241	4.7	7.2	21.5	0.0
Italian, Amatriciana, Sainsbury's*	½ Pot/175g	136	3.0	78	2.6	5.7	1.7	0.5
Italian, Tomato, Mushroom & Pancetta, Sainsbury's*	½ Jar/75g	125	11.2	167	2.2	6.1	14.9	1.3
Italian, Vongole, Waitrose*	1 Serving/175g	115	5.6	66	4.2	5.2	3.2	0.7
Italian Cheese, Finest, Tesco*	½ Pot/175g	171	8.9	98	4.8	8.4	5.1	0.0
Italian Mushroom, Sainsbury's*	1 Serving/85g	56	1.8	66	2.0	9.8	2.1	1.7
Italian Tomato & Herb, for Pasta, Sainsbury's*	½ Jar/146g	102	2.9	70	2.0	11.1	2.0	1.4
Mediterranean, Fresh, Waitrose*	1 Pot/350g	213	13.6	61	1.4	5.0	3.9	2.4
Mediterranean Tomato, Asda*	1 Jar/500g	285	6.0	57	1.5	10.0	1.2	0.0
Mediterranean Vegetable, Organic, Seeds of Change*	1 Jar/350g	245	12.2	70	1.5	8.3	3.5	1.1
Mediterranean Vegetable, Rustico, Bertolli*	½ Jar/160g	141	11.5	88	1.7	4.1	7.2	0.7
Mediterranean Vegetable Pasta, Tesco*	1 Serving/166g	95	2.8	57	1.4	9.0	1.7	1.2
Mushroom, Fresh, Waitrose*	1 Serving/175g	142	10.0	81	1.6	5.7	5.7	0.5
Mushroom, GFY, Asda*	1 Serving/175g	112	4.9	64	2.7	7.0	2.8	0.0

PASTA SAUCE

INFO/WEIGHT	Measure per Measure			Nutrition Values per 100g / 100ml				
		KCAL	FAT	KCAL	PROT	CARB	FAT	FIBRE
Mushroom, Microwaveable, Dolmio*	1 Serving/150g	160	14.4	107	1.4	3.8	9.6	0.0
Mushroom, Perfectly Balanced, Waitrose*	1 Jar/440g	330	8.4	75	2.6	11.8	1.9	2.2
Mushroom, Sainsbury's*	1 Serving/100g	66	2.1	66	2.0	9.8	2.1	1.7
Mushroom, Tesco*	¼ Jar/188g	90	3.2	48	1.4	6.8	1.7	1.0
Mushroom & Garlic, 98% Fat Free, Homepride*	1 Jar/450g	229	6.3	51	1.1	8.9	1.4	0.5
Mushroom & Garlic, Deliciously Good, Homepride*	1/3 Jar/147g	109	7.1	74	0.9	6.9	4.8	0.3
Mushroom & Marsala Wine, Sacla*	½ Pot/85g	165	16.0	194	2.2	3.9	18.8	0.0
Mushroom & Mascarpone, Morrisons*	½ Pot/175g	199	17.0	114	2.3	4.3	9.7	0.0
Napoletana, BGTY, Sainsbury's*	½ Pot/151g	71	3.8	47	1.2	5.0	2.5	1.3
Napoletana, Buitoni*	½ Jar/200g	146	8.2	73	1.6	7.3	4.1	2.2
Napoletana, Fresh, Waitrose*	1 Serving/175g	82	3.0	47	1.3	6.6	1.7	1.0
Napoletana, GFY, Asda*	1 Serving/175g	58	1.7	33	1.0	5.0	1.0	0.0
Napoletana, Sainsbury's*	½ Pot/150g	126	8.4	84	1.9	6.6	5.6	0.9
Olive, Barilla*	1 Serving/100g	92	5.0	92	1.5	10.3	5.0	0.0
Olive & Tomato, Sacla*	1 Serving/95g	87	7.6	92	1.3	3.6	8.0	0.0
Onion & Garlic, Tesco*	1 Serving/125g	35	0.1	28	1.2	5.6	0.1	2.6
Onion & Roasted Garlic, Knorr*	1 Jar/500g	210	0.0	42	1.3	9.2	0.0	1.1
Original, BFY, Morrisons*	1/3 Jar/200g	100	0.2	50	1.6	10.6	0.1	1.2
Original, Tesco*	1 Jar/300g	123	4.2	41	1.0	6.1	1.4	2.3
Original, with Tomato & Onions, BFY, Morrisons*	1 Serving/125g	51	1.4	41	1.4	6.3	1.1	1.2
Original, with Tomatoes & Onions, Morrisons*	1 Serving/100g	64	2.5	64	1.2	9.3	2.5	1.0
Parmesan & Pesto, Weight Watchers*	½ Jar/175g	86	2.8	49	1.8	6.7	1.6	1.0
Pepper & Tomato, M & S*	1 Jar/320g	224	13.4	70	1.6	6.1	4.2	0.9
Pomodoro, Cirio*	1 Serving/200g	116	4.6	58	1.4	8.4	2.3	0.0
Porcini Mushroom & Pepperoni, Asda*	½ Jar/140g	158	8.4	113	3.8	11.0	6.0	0.0
Porcini Mushroom Stir in, BGTY, Sainsbury's*	½ Jar/75g	57	3.1	76	3.8	5.7	4.2	1.9
Primavera, Fresh, Morrisons*	½ Pot/175g	152	10.3	87	2.4	6.1	5.9	0.0
Primavera, Loyd Grossman*	1 Jar/350g	343	25.9	98	1.4	6.3	7.4	0.9
Puttanesca, Italian, Waitrose*	1 Jar/350g	195	9.8	56	1.5	6.1	2.8	1.3
Puttanesca, Loyd Grossman*	1 Jar/350g	315	21.7	90	1.7	6.8	6.2	0.9
Puttanesca, M & S*	1 Jar/320g	256	17.6	80	1.5	6.2	5.5	1.9
Red Pepper & Italian Cheese, Stir Through, Asda*	½ Jar/95g	85	4.7	90	2.9	8.5	4.9	0.9
Red Pepper & Plum, Finest, Tesco*	1 Serving/63g	109	7.2	173	3.7	14.0	11.4	5.4
Rich Tomato with Basil Pesto, Express, Dolmio*	1 Pack/170g	146	10.0	86	2.0	6.2	5.9	0.0
Roasted Garlic, Weight Watchers*	½ Jar/177g	60	0.7	34	1.3	6.4	0.4	1.2
Roasted Red Pepper & Tomato, Finest, Tesco*	1 Serving/145g	117	7.8	81	1.2	6.8	5.4	2.2
Roasted Vegetable, GFY, Asda*	½ Pot/175g	84	2.8	48	1.3	7.0	1.6	0.5
Roasted Vegetable, Microwaveable, Dolmio*	½ Pack/190g	103	3.8	54	1.4	7.6	2.0	0.0
Roasted Vegetable, Sainsbury's*	½ Pot/151g	103	5.9	68	1.6	6.7	3.9	0.4
Roasted Vegetables & Tuna, BGTY, Sainsbury's*	½ Pot/150g	73	2.8	49	3.5	4.5	1.9	3.1
Romano*	1 Serving/235g	141	4.7	60	1.7	8.8	2.0	1.1
Rustico Mushroom, Garlic & Oregano, Bertolli*	1 Serving/100g	90	7.5	90	1.9	3.8	7.5	0.0
Rustico Sweet Chilli & Red Onion, Bertolli*	½ Jar/160g	146	11.5	91	1.7	4.9	7.2	0.7
Salsina with Onions & Garlic, Valfrutta*	1 Serving/150g	36	0.0	24	1.6	4.5	0.0	1.4
Seasonal, Bolognese, Dolmio*	1 Jar/500g	205	1.0	41	1.5	7.4	0.2	1.4
Siciliana, Sainsbury's*	1/3 Jar/113g	168	14.7	149	1.8	6.2	13.0	0.0
Sliced Mushroom, Tesco*	1 Jar/460g	161	0.9	35	1.3	7.0	0.2	0.8
Smoky Bacon, Loyd Grossman*	½ Jar/175g	142	8.4	81	3.0	6.1	4.8	0.8
Spicy Italian Chilli, Express, Dolmio*	1 Serving/170g	87	2.7	51	1.5	7.5	1.6	0.0
Spicy Pepper, Tesco*	1 Jar/500g	245	5.0	49	1.7	8.4	1.0	1.0
Spicy Pepper & Tomato, Sacla*	½ Jar/95g	132	11.2	139	1.4	6.8	11.8	0.0
Spicy Red Pepper & Roasted Vegetable, Asda*	1 Serving/175g	140	7.7	80	1.2	9.0	4.4	1.0
Spicy Roasted Garlic, Seeds of Change*	1 Serving/195g	123	3.9	63	1.5	9.7	2.0	1.2

P

PASTA SAUCE

	Measure INFO/WEIGHT	per Measure KCAL	FAT	Nutrition Values per 100g / 100ml KCAL	PROT	CARB	FAT	FIBRE
Spicy Tomato, Asda*	1 Serving/155g	76	1.9	49	1.5	8.0	1.2	1.0
Spinach & Ricotta, Asda*	½ Pot/175g	175	12.2	100	3.2	6.0	7.0	0.5
Spinach & Ricotta, BGTY, Sainsbury's*	1 Serving/150g	73	4.0	49	2.7	3.4	2.7	2.2
Spinach & Ricotta, Stir Through, Sacla*	½ Jar/95g	196	18.6	206	3.7	3.7	19.6	0.0
Stir & Serve, Homepride*	1 Jar/480g	187	5.8	39	1.2	6.0	1.2	0.0
Sun Dried Tomato, Asda*	½ Jar/159g	165	12.7	104	1.9	6.0	8.0	1.5
Sun Dried Tomato, Garlic & Basil, Finest, Tesco*	1 Jar/340g	493	39.1	145	1.8	7.7	11.5	2.3
Sun Dried Tomato, Stir In, Light, Dolmio*	1 Serving/75g	62	3.5	83	1.7	9.8	4.7	0.0
Sun Dried Tomato & Basil, Free From, Sainsbury's*	½ Jar/172g	124	4.8	72	2.9	8.7	2.8	1.5
Sun Dried Tomato & Garlic, Sacla*	1 Serving/95g	177	14.0	186	3.0	10.3	14.7	0.0
Sun Ripened Tomato & Basil, Dolmio*	1 Serving/150g	117	6.9	78	1.3	7.9	4.6	0.0
Sun Ripened Tomato & Basil, Express, Dolmio*	1 Pouch/170g	88	2.7	52	1.5	7.9	1.6	0.0
Sun Ripened Tomato & Basil, Microwaveable, Dolmio*	½ Pack/190g	106	4.0	56	1.4	7.9	2.1	0.0
Sundried Tomato, Heinz*	½ Jar/150g	55	0.3	37	1.5	7.3	0.2	1.1
Sundried Tomato & Basil, Organic, Seeds of Change*	½ Jar/100g	155	13.1	155	1.6	7.7	13.1	0.0
Sundried Tomato & Garlic, M & S*	½ Jar/95g	147	13.0	155	2.9	4.4	13.7	0.8
Sweet Pepper, Dolmio*	1 Serving/150g	238	20.1	159	1.6	8.8	13.4	0.0
Sweet Red Pepper, Loyd Grossman*	1 Jar/350g	304	19.6	87	1.7	7.3	5.6	1.2
Three Cheeses, Co-Op*	1 Pack/300g	405	27.0	135	6.0	6.0	9.0	0.1
Tomato, Bacon & Mushroom, Asda*	½ Pot/50g	33	1.8	66	2.5	6.0	3.6	0.0
Tomato, Basil & Parmesan Stir in, BGTY, Sainsbury's*	1 Serving/75g	69	4.1	92	2.9	7.8	5.5	1.0
Tomato, Black Olive, Caper, Finest, Tesco*	1 Serving/145g	146	11.2	101	1.5	6.4	7.7	3.3
Tomato, Chilli & Onion, Bertolli*	1 Serving/100g	49	1.7	49	1.8	6.7	1.7	1.8
Tomato, Garlic & Chilli, Finest, Tesco*	1 Serving/145g	199	16.2	137	2.0	7.1	11.2	3.4
Tomato, Ginger & Basil, Cranks*	½ Jar/175g	129	8.2	74	1.7	6.3	4.7	1.1
Tomato, Mushroom & Roasted Garlic, Bertolli*	1 Jar/500g	235	9.5	47	1.9	5.3	1.9	0.0
Tomato, Pecorino Romano Cheese & Garlic, Bertolli*	1 Serving/125g	76	3.5	61	2.3	6.5	2.8	0.9
Tomato, Red Wine, Shallots, Bertolli*	½ Jar/250g	112	4.2	45	1.7	7.2	1.7	1.5
Tomato, Sweet Cherry, Slow Cooked, Dress Italian*	½ Jar/175g	163	11.2	93	1.8	7.2	6.4	2.1
Tomato & Basil, Bertolli*	1 Jar/500g	215	5.0	43	1.2	7.3	1.0	0.4
Tomato & Basil, Carb Check, Heinz*	1 Serving/150g	84	5.4	56	1.5	4.4	3.6	0.6
Tomato & Basil, Classic, Sacla*	1 Serving/100g	137	11.1	137	2.0	7.2	11.1	2.8
Tomato & Basil, Dolmio*	1 Serving/170g	95	3.6	56	1.4	7.9	2.1	0.0
Tomato & Basil, Loyd Grossman*	½ Jar/175g	107	5.9	61	1.5	5.8	3.4	0.8
Tomato & Basil, M & S*	1 Jar/340g	119	7.1	35	2.0	2.1	2.1	0.9
Tomato & Basil, Morrisons*	1 Serving/175g	63	1.0	36	2.0	5.6	0.6	1.0
Tomato & Basil, Organic, Pasta Reale*	1 Pack/300g	216	15.9	72	1.0	5.1	5.3	0.4
Tomato & Black Olive, Carb Control, Tesco*	1 Serving/110g	74	4.7	67	1.3	6.0	4.3	2.3
Tomato & Chargrilled Vegetable, Loyd Grossman*	1 Serving/150g	133	8.4	89	1.8	7.9	5.6	0.9
Tomato & Chilli, Loyd Grossman*	½ Jar/175g	101	5.9	58	1.4	5.5	3.4	0.7
Tomato & Chilli, Pour Over, M & S*	1 Jar/330g	231	12.5	70	1.3	7.6	3.8	1.8
Tomato & Chunky Mushroom, Dolmio*	1 Pack/475g	323	17.6	68	1.2	7.6	3.7	0.0
Tomato & Garlic, Chosen By You, Asda*	½ Jar/160g	74	0.8	46	1.6	7.9	0.5	1.7
Tomato & Herb, M & S*	1 Jar/500g	400	15.5	80	2.6	10.1	3.1	1.7
Tomato & Herb, Organic, M & S*	1 Jar/550g	302	19.8	55	1.4	4.2	3.6	2.6
Tomato & Herb, Organic, Meridian Foods*	½ Jar/220g	141	6.2	64	1.6	8.1	2.8	1.1
Tomato & Herb, Organic, Sainsbury's*	1 Serving/75g	38	1.5	51	1.2	6.6	2.0	0.5
Tomato & Herb, Perfectly Balanced, Waitrose*	½ Tub/176g	65	2.1	37	1.3	5.3	1.2	2.3
Tomato & Herb, with Extra Garlic, Sainsbury's*	½ Pot/150g	61	1.6	41	1.4	6.3	1.1	1.6
Tomato & Mascarpone, BGTY, Sainsbury's*	1 Pot/300g	150	9.0	50	2.0	3.6	3.0	3.6
Tomato & Mascarpone, Finest, Tesco*	1 Serving/175g	135	8.7	77	2.7	5.4	5.0	0.8
Tomato & Mascarpone, Fresh, Sainsbury's*	1 Serving/150g	177	15.4	118	2.2	4.2	10.3	1.1
Tomato & Mascarpone, Italiano, Tesco*	½ Pot/175g	168	12.2	96	2.8	5.5	7.0	0.7

	Measure INFO/WEIGHT	per Measure KCAL	per Measure FAT	Nutrition Values per 100g / 100ml KCAL	PROT	CARB	FAT	FIBRE
PASTA SAUCE								
Tomato & Mascarpone, Sacla*	½ Jar/95g	161	14.2	169	2.2	6.2	15.0	0.0
Tomato & Mascarpone, Sainsbury's*	½ Pot/150g	137	9.9	91	2.1	5.9	6.6	1.2
Tomato & Mascarpone, So Organic, Sainsbury's*	1/3 Jar/146g	180	13.2	123	1.9	8.7	9.0	2.8
Tomato & Mascarpone, Waitrose*	½ Pot/175g	184	14.7	105	1.9	5.5	8.4	1.1
Tomato & Mushroom, Chosen By You, Asda*	½ Jar/160g	70	1.0	44	2.1	7.0	0.6	1.1
Tomato & Mushroom, Organic, Sainsbury's*	1 Serving/150g	87	3.9	58	1.6	7.1	2.6	1.5
Tomato & Olives, La Doria*	1 Jar/90g	76	5.9	84	1.2	5.0	6.6	0.0
Tomato & Parmesan, Seeds of Change*	1 Serving/150g	100	4.3	67	2.5	7.8	2.9	1.1
Tomato & Pesto, Planet Cook, Heinz*	1 Jar/300g	237	17.1	79	1.7	5.2	5.7	1.0
Tomato & Ricotta, Italian, Sainsbury's*	1 Pack/390g	238	11.7	61	2.5	6.1	3.0	1.2
Tomato & Roasted Garlic, Chosen By You, Asda*	1 Pot/350g	122	2.1	35	1.5	5.0	0.6	1.7
Tomato & Roasted Garlic, Loyd Grossman*	½ Jar/175g	107	5.4	61	1.5	6.3	3.1	0.8
Tomato & Smokey Bacon, Dolmio*	1 Pot/150g	240	19.6	160	5.5	5.8	13.1	0.0
Tomato & Spicy Sausages, M & S*	1 Jar/330g	214	9.9	65	4.0	5.5	3.0	0.8
Tomato & Tuna, Loyd Grossman*	½ Jar/175g	154	7.7	88	4.4	7.5	4.4	0.8
Tomato & Wild Mushroom, Loyd Grossman*	½ Jar/175g	154	9.8	88	2.1	7.4	5.6	1.5
Tomato & Wild Mushroom, Waitrose*	1 Serving/175g	65	1.2	37	1.7	6.0	0.7	0.9
Vegetable, Chunky, Tesco*	1 Jar/455g	223	5.9	49	0.7	8.6	1.3	1.1
Vegetable & Garlic, Dolmio*	1 Serving/150g	108	6.1	72	1.3	7.4	4.1	0.0
Veneziana, M & S*	½ Jar/140g	196	15.0	140	5.7	5.5	10.7	1.6
PASTA SHAPES								
Alphabetti, in Tomato Sauce, Heinz*	1 Can/200g	118	1.0	59	1.8	11.7	0.5	1.5
Bob The Builder, in Tomato Sauce, Heinz*	1 Can/205g	111	0.6	54	1.7	11.3	0.3	1.5
Cooked, Tesco*	1 Serving/260g	356	2.1	137	5.1	26.3	0.8	1.1
Disney Princess, in Tomato Sauce, Heinz*	1 Can/200g	114	0.6	57	1.8	11.9	0.3	1.5
Dried, Tesco*	1 Serving/100g	345	2.0	345	13.2	68.5	2.0	2.9
Postman Pat, HP*	1 Can/410g	279	1.6	68	1.8	14.3	0.4	0.7
Scooby Doo, HP*	1 Can/410g	279	1.6	68	1.8	14.3	0.4	0.7
Spiderman, in Tomato Sauce, Heinz*	½ Can/200g	114	1.0	57	1.7	11.4	0.5	1.5
Teletubbies, in Tomato Sauce, Heinz*	1 Can/400g	244	1.6	61	2.0	12.3	0.4	0.6
Thomas Tank Engine, in Tomato Sauce, Heinz*	1 Can/205g	109	0.4	53	1.7	11.0	0.2	0.5
Tweenies, in Tomato Sauce, Heinz*	1 Can/205g	121	1.0	59	1.8	11.7	0.5	1.5
PASTA SHELLS								
Dry, Average	*1 Serving/75g*	*265*	*1.5*	*353*	*11.1*	*71.8*	*2.0*	*2.0*
Egg, Fresh, Average	*1 Serving/125g*	*344*	*3.6*	*275*	*11.5*	*49.7*	*2.8*	*3.4*
Fresh, Dry, Average	*1 Serving/125g*	*216*	*2.1*	*173*	*7.4*	*32.0*	*1.6*	*1.5*
Wholewheat, Healthy Living, Co-Op*	1 Serving/75g	232	0.7	310	11.0	64.0	1.0	12.0
PASTA SNACK								
Cheese & Ham, Pot, Tesco*	1 Serving/208g	254	8.5	122	3.4	17.9	4.1	1.5
Cheese & Ham, Tubes, Made Up to Instructions, Tesco*	1 Serving/214g	312	11.6	146	4.9	19.5	5.4	2.6
Chicken, Morrisons*	1 Pack/250g	285	6.7	114	3.3	19.3	2.7	0.0
Chicken, with Sweetcorn & Mushroom, Pot, Tesco*	1 Pot/216g	238	5.8	110	3.0	18.5	2.7	0.7
Chicken & Smoked Bacon, Sainsbury's*	1 Pack/190g	490	36.5	258	7.2	14.1	19.2	0.0
Ham & Mushroom, Tesco*	1 Pack/300g	618	42.9	206	4.2	15.0	14.3	1.1
Mug Shot, Creamy Cheese, Symingtons*	1 Sachet/271g	301	6.0	111	3.7	19.1	2.2	1.0
Mug Shot, Roast Chicken, Symingtons*	1 Sachet/258g	204	2.6	79	1.4	16.2	1.0	0.8
Tomato & Herb, in a Pot, Dry, Tesco*	1 Pot/59g	207	1.4	352	11.8	70.7	2.4	2.6
Tomato & Herb, Morrisons*	1 Pot/247g	247	2.7	100	3.1	19.5	1.1	0.0
Tomato 'n' Herb, Mug Shot*	1 Sachet/257g	265	2.1	103	2.3	21.6	0.8	1.2
PASTA SPIRALS								
Co-Op*	1 Serving/100g	350	1.0	350	12.0	73.0	1.0	3.0
PASTA TWIRLS								
Dry, Asda*	1 Serving/50g	173	0.7	346	12.0	71.0	1.5	3.0

	Measure INFO/WEIGHT	per Measure		Nutrition Values per 100g / 100ml				
		KCAL	FAT	KCAL	PROT	CARB	FAT	FIBRE
PASTA TWIRLS								
Tri-Colour, Sainsbury's*	1 Serving/75g	268	1.3	357	12.3	73.1	1.7	2.5
PASTA TWISTS								
Dry, Average	*1oz/28g*	*99*	*0.4*	*354*	*12.2*	*71.8*	*1.5*	*2.2*
Wheat & Gluten Free, Glutafin*	1 Serving/75g	262	1.5	350	8.0	75.0	2.0	0.1
PASTA WITH								
Amigo Meatballs, Pasta King*	1 Serving/100g	127	3.4	127	4.7	19.5	3.4	1.8
Cheese & Tomato, Al Forno, Sainsbury's*	½ Pack/499g	749	29.0	150	5.5	18.9	5.8	1.8
Chicken Balti, Pasta King*	1 Serving/100g	114	2.1	114	4.7	19.4	2.1	1.8
Chicken Korma, Pasta King*	1 Serving/100g	119	2.8	119	5.3	18.5	2.8	1.2
Chicken Marrakech, Pasta King*	1 Serving/100g	118	2.2	118	5.3	19.4	2.2	1.8
Chicken Tikka, Pasta King*	1 Serving/100g	116	2.0	116	5.4	19.2	2.0	1.7
Chicken Torino, Pasta King*	1 Serving/100g	117	1.7	117	5.3	20.3	1.7	1.7
Feta Cheese & Slow Roasted Tomatoes, M & S*	1 Pack/190g	332	13.3	175	6.0	22.3	7.0	2.5
Firecracker Chicken, Pasta King*	1 Serving/100g	115	1.9	115	5.4	19.2	1.9	1.7
Firecracker Salmon, Pasta King*	1 Serving/100g	114	1.9	114	4.5	19.6	1.9	1.8
Garlic Mushrooms, Pasta King*	1 Serving/100g	113	2.3	113	4.4	18.9	2.3	0.1
Honey Mustard Chicken, COU, M & S*	1 Pack/300g	360	7.2	120	8.4	16.2	2.4	1.9
Louisiana Chicken, Pasta King*	1 Serving/100g	112	1.8	112	4.6	19.6	1.8	1.8
Maiale Meatballs, Pasta King*	1 Serving/100g	128	3.4	128	4.8	19.7	3.4	1.9
Meatballs, Sainsbury's*	1 Can/300g	339	14.7	113	6.6	10.6	4.9	1.6
Mediterranean Vegetables, Pasta King*	1 Serving/100g	121	3.2	121	3.7	19.3	3.2	2.1
Pesto, Spinach & Pine Nuts, Tesco*	1 Pack/300g	480	22.2	160	5.2	17.1	7.4	1.5
Salmon & Broccoli, Lemon Dressed, Sainsbury's*	1 Serving/300g	486	17.7	162	6.9	20.4	5.9	2.1
Spicy Beef, Light Choices, Tesco*	1 Pack/350g	490	5.2	140	6.3	24.7	1.5	2.5
Spicy Beef & Chipotle Chilli, HL, Tesco*	1 Pack/350g	367	7.0	105	4.8	17.0	2.0	2.7
Spicy Chicken, Sainsbury's*	1 Pot/300g	489	18.3	163	7.1	20.1	6.1	2.3
Spicy Sausage, Pasta King*	1 Serving/100g	117	2.2	117	4.8	19.7	2.2	1.7
Sweet & Sour Chicken, Pasta King*	1 Serving/100g	118	1.5	118	5.2	21.1	1.5	1.6
Sweet & Sour Vegetables, Pasta King*	1 Serving/100g	111	1.2	111	3.5	21.6	1.2	1.7
Sweet Chilli Chicken, Pasta King*	1 Serving/100g	113	1.8	113	5.3	19.2	1.8	1.7
Tomato & Basil Chicken, BGTY, Sainsbury's*	1 Pack/189g	250	2.1	132	9.2	21.2	1.1	2.7
Tuna & Roasted Peppers, M & S*	1 Serving/220g	308	8.6	140	9.1	17.7	3.9	0.9
Vegetable Balti, Pasta King*	1 Serving/100g	115	2.0	115	4.0	20.3	2.0	2.0
PASTE								
Bacon & Tomato, Tesco*	1 Serving/20g	46	3.6	232	14.0	3.4	18.0	0.1
Beef, Asda*	1 Serving/37g	72	5.2	194	17.0	0.1	14.0	0.0
Beef, Princes*	1 Serving/18g	40	2.8	220	14.4	5.2	15.8	0.0
Beef, Sainsbury's*	1 Jar/75g	142	9.9	189	16.0	1.5	13.2	1.4
Chicken, Asda*	1 Thin Spread/7g	13	0.9	184	16.0	0.8	13.0	0.0
Chicken, Princes*	1 Thin Spread/9g	22	1.7	240	12.6	5.6	18.5	0.0
Chicken, Tesco*	1 Serving/12g	30	2.4	248	14.8	2.3	20.0	0.1
Chicken & Ham, Asda*	½ Jar/38g	82	6.5	217	14.0	2.1	17.0	0.0
Chicken & Ham, Princes*	1 Jar/100g	233	18.6	233	13.6	2.8	18.6	0.0
Chicken & Mushroom, Princes*	1 Serving/50g	93	5.5	187	17.1	5.0	11.0	0.0
Chicken & Stuffing, Princes*	1 Jar/100g	229	17.0	229	15.7	3.3	17.0	0.0
Crab, Princes*	1 Pot/35g	36	1.2	104	13.4	4.8	3.5	0.0
Crab, Sainsbury's*	1 Thick Spread/5g	6	0.2	115	16.5	1.7	4.7	0.5
Fruit, Golden Quince, Lowry Peaks*	1 Tsp/5g	16	0.0	321	0.8	83.6	0.2	0.0
Salmon, Asda*	1 Serving/53g	76	3.7	143	15.0	5.0	7.0	0.0
Salmon, Princes*	1 Serving/30g	58	3.8	195	13.5	6.5	12.8	0.0
Salmon & Shrimp, Tesco*	1 Jar/75g	83	2.5	111	15.1	5.0	3.4	0.1
Sardine & Tomato, Asda*	1 Thin Spread/9g	11	0.5	123	14.0	3.3	6.0	0.0
Sardine & Tomato, Princes*	1 Jar/75g	109	5.4	146	15.4	5.0	7.2	0.0

INFO/WEIGHT	Measure		per Measure		Nutrition Values per 100g / 100ml				
			KCAL	FAT	KCAL	PROT	CARB	FAT	FIBRE
PASTE									
Sardine & Tomato, Sainsbury's*	1 Mini Pot/35g		59	3.8	170	16.9	1.2	10.8	1.3
Tagine, Lemon, Spicy, Al'fez*	1 Tsp/6g		13	0.9	216	3.1	17.6	14.8	4.6
Tuna & Mayonnaise, Princes*	1 Pot/75g		86	12.3	115	16.8	3.8	16.4	0.0
Tuna & Mayonnaise, Sainsbury's*	1 Tbsp/17g		41	3.1	242	19.2	0.6	18.1	1.6
PASTILLES									
Blackcurrant, Rowntree's*	1 Tube/53g		188	0.0	353	4.4	84.0	0.0	0.0
Fruit, Average	1 Tube/33g		108	0.0	327	2.8	84.2	0.0	0.0
Wine, Maynards*	1 Sweet/5g		15	0.0	325	6.1	75.0	0.0	0.0
PASTRAMI									
Beef, Average	**1 Serving/40g**		**51**	**1.4**	**128**	**23.1**	**1.1**	**3.6**	**0.2**
Turkey, Average	**½ Packet/35g**		**38**	**0.5**	**107**	**21.8**	**1.7**	**1.5**	**0.5**
PASTRY									
Case, From Supermarket, Average	**1 Case/230g**		**1081**	**58.9**	**470**	**5.8**	**55.9**	**25.6**	**1.2**
Choux, Cooked, Average	**1oz/28g**		**91**	**5.5**	**325**	**8.5**	**29.8**	**19.8**	**1.2**
Choux, Raw, Average	**1oz/28g**		**59**	**3.6**	**211**	**5.5**	**19.4**	**12.9**	**0.8**
Filo, Average	**1 Sheet/45g**		**137**	**1.2**	**304**	**9.0**	**61.4**	**2.7**	**0.9**
Filo, Frozen, Jus-Rol*	1 Sheet/45g		105	1.2	234	8.1	52.1	2.7	2.1
Flaky, Chinese, Average	**1oz/28g**		**110**	**4.6**	**392**	**5.4**	**59.3**	**16.4**	**0.0**
Flaky, Cooked, Average	**1oz/28g**		**157**	**11.4**	**560**	**5.6**	**45.9**	**40.6**	**1.8**
Flaky, Raw, Average	**1oz/28g**		**119**	**8.6**	**424**	**4.2**	**34.8**	**30.7**	**1.4**
Flan Case, Average	**1 Case/113g**		**615**	**38.0**	**544**	**7.1**	**56.7**	**33.6**	**1.8**
Greek, Average	**1oz/28g**		**90**	**4.8**	**322**	**4.7**	**40.0**	**17.0**	**0.0**
Puff, Fresh, Sainsbury's*	½ Pack/250g		1112	85.7	445	5.4	28.8	34.3	1.3
Puff, Frozen, Average	**1 Serving/47g**		**188**	**12.0**	**400**	**5.0**	**29.2**	**25.6**	**0.0**
Shortcrust, Cooked, Average	**1oz/28g**		**146**	**9.0**	**521**	**6.6**	**54.2**	**32.3**	**2.2**
Shortcrust, Raw, Average	**1oz/28g**		**127**	**8.1**	**453**	**5.6**	**44.0**	**29.1**	**1.3**
Wholemeal, Cooked, Average	**1oz/28g**		**140**	**9.2**	**499**	**8.9**	**44.6**	**32.9**	**6.3**
Wholemeal, Raw, Average	**1oz/28g**		**121**	**8.0**	**431**	**7.7**	**38.5**	**28.4**	**5.4**
PASTY									
Beef, Port Royal*	1 Pattie/130g		299	13.3	230	10.2	24.4	10.2	0.0
Bite Size Pasties, Food to Go, Sainsbury's*	1 Serving/60g		226	14.6	377	8.2	31.2	24.4	1.5
Cheddar & Onion, Hand Crimped, Waitrose*	1 Pasty/200g		546	42.2	273	8.8	22.5	21.1	2.2
Cheese & Onion, Geo Adams*	1 Pasty/150g		420	23.4	280	6.9	27.9	15.6	1.1
Cheese & Onion, Sainsbury's*	1 Serving/150g		486	32.7	324	7.4	24.5	21.8	1.3
Chicken, Port Royal*	1 Pattie/130g		289	10.9	222	5.5	31.2	8.4	0.0
Chicken & Bacon, Ginsters*	1 Pasty/180g		457	29.0	254	8.0	19.3	16.1	2.8
Chicken & Vegetable, Proper Cornish Ltd*	1 Pasty/255g		671	34.7	263	7.4	30.2	13.6	2.4
Chicken Balti Special Edition, Ginsters*	1 Pasty/180g		398	23.2	221	6.7	19.5	12.9	2.6
Cornish, Asda*	1 Pasty/100g		287	19.0	287	7.0	22.0	19.0	1.2
Cornish, BGTY, Sainsbury's*	1 Pasty/135g		308	12.7	228	7.7	28.2	9.4	1.6
Cornish, Cheese & Onion, Ginsters*	1 Pasty/130g		511	33.0	393	10.4	30.7	25.4	2.3
Cornish, Chicken & Bacon, Ginsters*	1 Pasty/227g		574	34.5	253	6.9	22.2	15.2	0.8
Cornish, Crimped, TTD, Sainsbury's*	1 Pasty/200g		515	28.7	258	8.3	23.7	14.4	1.2
Cornish, Mini, M & S*	1 Pasty/75g		244	17.5	325	7.3	21.9	23.4	1.8
Cornish, Original, Ginsters*	1 Pasty/227g		549	32.2	242	5.3	23.2	14.2	3.1
Cornish, Pork Farms*	1 Pasty/250g		672	40.7	269	7.7	22.8	16.3	0.0
Cornish, Sainsbury's*	1 Pasty/150g		489	32.1	326	6.7	26.6	21.4	2.0
Cornish, Snack Pack, Six, Ginsters*	1 Pasty/40g		116	8.0	289	7.2	20.3	19.9	2.8
Cornish, Traditional Style, Geo Adams*	1 Pasty/165g		488	30.4	296	7.1	25.4	18.4	1.3
Cornish Roaster, Ginsters*	1 Pasty/130g		417	24.2	321	8.5	29.9	18.6	1.3
Lamb, Port Royal*	1 Pattie/130g		352	17.4	271	7.2	30.5	13.4	0.0
Olive & Cheese, Tapas, Waitrose*	1 Pack/130g		455	25.2	350	8.1	35.8	19.4	1.3
Salt Fish, Port Royal*	1 Pattie/130g		300	13.4	231	6.8	27.8	10.3	0.0

P

	Measure INFO/WEIGHT	per Measure		Nutrition Values per 100g / 100ml				
		KCAL	FAT	KCAL	PROT	CARB	FAT	FIBRE
PASTY								
Tandoori & Vegetable, Holland & Barrett*	1 Pack/110g	232	9.3	211	4.3	29.4	8.5	1.8
Three Cheese & Onion, Ginsters*	1 Pasty/180g	531	36.9	295	8.0	19.7	20.5	3.1
Vegetable	1oz/28g	77	4.2	274	4.1	33.3	14.9	1.9
Vegetable, Hand Crimped, Waitrose*	1 Pasty/200g	454	22.6	227	4.5	26.8	11.3	2.2
Vegetarian, Country Slice, Linda McCartney*	1 Pasty/150g	373	20.2	249	5.6	26.5	13.5	2.9
Vegetarian, Port Royal*	1 Pattie/130g	315	13.8	242	12.5	24.1	10.6	0.0
PATE								
Apricot, Asda*	1 Serving/50g	156	14.0	312	12.0	3.0	28.0	0.0
Ardennes, Asda*	1 Serving/50g	143	12.0	286	13.9	3.6	24.0	1.3
Ardennes, BGTY, Sainsbury's*	¼ Pack/50g	90	5.7	180	16.6	2.9	11.4	0.0
Ardennes, HL, Tesco*	½ Pack/88g	154	11.0	176	12.1	3.6	12.6	1.8
Ardennes, Reduced Fat, Waitrose*	¼ Pack/42g	94	7.1	224	15.4	2.6	16.9	0.5
Ardennes, Tesco*	1 Tbsp/15g	53	5.0	354	13.3	0.5	33.2	1.2
Ardennes, with Bacon, Tesco*	½ Pack/85g	241	20.6	284	11.4	5.1	24.2	1.1
Bean Feast, The Redwood Co*	1 Serving/60g	161	10.2	268	7.3	21.1	17.0	3.8
Breton, Country, with Apricots, Coarse, Sainsbury's*	1 Serving/21g	60	4.7	285	13.5	7.0	22.5	0.5
Brussels, & Garlic, Reduced Fat, Tesco*	1 Serving/65g	135	8.0	208	16.2	8.1	12.3	0.6
Brussels, & Garlic, Tesco*	1 Serving/40g	145	13.5	363	8.7	6.0	33.8	0.0
Brussels, & Mushroom, Mini, GFY, Asda*	1 Pack/40g	67	4.4	167	14.7	2.3	11.0	3.9
Brussels, 25% Less Fat, Morrisons*	¼ Pack/43g	106	8.8	249	14.2	0.7	20.6	0.0
Brussels, BGTY, 50% Less Fat, Sainsbury's*	1 Serving/100g	223	16.0	223	14.6	5.1	16.0	0.1
Brussels, Finest, Tesco*	½ Pack/85g	306	28.7	360	8.6	5.2	33.8	0.8
Brussels, HL, Tesco*	1 Serving/29g	66	4.4	229	14.4	8.4	15.3	1.8
Brussels, M & S*	1 Pot/170g	518	45.2	305	13.3	2.8	26.6	1.0
Brussels, Reduced Fat, Waitrose*	1 Serving/40g	92	7.4	229	13.2	2.4	18.5	0.5
Brussels, Sainsbury's*	1 Pack/170g	663	64.9	390	10.6	1.1	38.2	0.1
Brussels, Sanpareil*	¼ Pack/37g	121	11.1	326	13.0	1.0	30.0	0.0
Brussels, Smooth, 50% Less Fat, Tesco*	1 Pack/175g	350	26.8	200	14.1	1.2	15.3	1.8
Brussels, Smooth, Reduced Fat, Tesco*	1 Serving/15g	30	2.3	200	14.1	1.2	15.3	1.8
Brussels, Smooth, Spreadable, Sainsbury's*	1 Serving/30g	97	8.7	323	10.7	4.7	29.0	0.0
Brussels, with Forest Mushroom, Co-Op*	1 Serving/57g	180	16.5	315	12.0	2.0	29.0	1.0
Brussels, with Garlic, Asda*	1 Serving/50g	170	15.6	340	10.7	4.0	31.3	2.5
Brussels, with Herbs, Tesco*	1 Serving/25g	87	8.1	347	8.4	6.4	32.6	1.5
Brussels Style, Organic, The Redwood Co*	¼ Pack/30g	82	6.1	273	15.2	8.0	20.4	1.3
Carrot, Ginger & Spring Onion, M & S*	1 Serving/50g	72	5.5	145	1.5	9.6	11.0	0.9
Celery, Stilton & Walnut, Waitrose*	1 Pot/115g	294	26.4	256	9.0	3.2	23.0	2.2
Chargrilled Vegetable, BGTY, Sainsbury's*	½ Pot/57g	43	0.7	75	4.9	10.8	1.3	2.7
Chick Pea & Black Olive, Cauldron Foods*	1 Pot/113g	193	11.9	171	7.6	11.4	10.5	6.6
Chicken, with Sauternes, TTD, Sainsbury's*	1 Serving/30g	114	11.1	381	6.5	5.3	37.1	0.6
Chicken & Brandy, Morrisons*	1 Serving/44g	133	11.8	303	10.8	4.3	26.9	0.8
Chicken Liver, & Brandy, Asda*	1 Serving/50g	176	16.4	353	9.0	5.5	32.8	3.2
Chicken Liver, & Garlic, Smooth, Asda*	1 Serving/31g	119	11.1	388	9.0	7.0	36.0	3.2
Chicken Liver, Asda*	1 Serving/65g	131	10.4	202	13.0	4.0	16.0	0.8
Chicken Liver, BGTY, Sainsbury's*	1 Serving/30g	64	4.8	214	11.5	6.0	16.0	0.5
Chicken Liver, Organic, Waitrose*	½ Tub/88g	204	16.1	233	12.6	1.8	18.4	1.4
Chicken Liver, with Madeira, Sainsbury's*	1 Serving/30g	84	7.3	279	13.1	1.9	24.3	0.0
Chickpea, Moroccan, Organic, Cauldron Foods*	½ Pot/58g	119	7.9	207	6.8	16.3	13.7	4.9
Coarse Farmhouse, Organic, Sainsbury's*	1 Serving/56g	138	11.0	246	13.3	3.7	19.7	0.8
Coarse Pork Liver with Garlic, Asda*	1 Pack/40g	130	12.0	326	13.0	1.0	30.0	0.0
Crab, M & S*	1oz/28g	63	4.8	225	12.1	5.9	17.3	0.0
Crab, Terrine, Orkney, Luxury, Castle MacLellan*	1 Tub/113g	250	21.4	221	7.3	5.5	18.9	0.9
Duck & Orange, Asda*	1 Serving/40g	94	7.2	235	16.0	2.2	18.0	0.0
Duck & Orange, Smooth, Tesco*	1 Serving/50g	188	17.7	377	10.5	4.0	35.4	0.5

PATE

	Measure INFO/WEIGHT	per Measure KCAL	FAT	Nutrition Values per 100g / 100ml KCAL	PROT	CARB	FAT	FIBRE
Duck & Truffle, Medallions, M & S*	1 Serving/25g	91	8.7	365	9.0	4.8	35.0	1.4
Farmhouse Mushroom, Asda*	1 Serving/50g	126	10.0	252	13.0	5.0	20.0	0.7
Farmhouse Style, Finest, Tesco*	1 Serving/28g	83	7.3	295	11.9	3.6	25.9	1.0
Farmhouse Style, M & S*	¼ Pack/42g	90	7.1	215	14.4	1.9	16.9	1.2
Farmhouse Style, Weight Watchers*	1 Serving/37g	49	2.1	133	14.8	5.5	5.7	0.5
Farmhouse with Herbes De Provence, Tesco*	1 Serving/50g	136	10.8	273	13.9	5.4	21.6	1.0
Farmhouse with Mushrooms & Garlic, Tesco*	1 Serving/90g	256	22.8	285	13.8	0.6	25.3	1.3
Forestiere, M & S*	1 Serving/20g	61	5.3	305	11.5	4.2	26.6	1.4
Kipper, Waitrose*	¼ Tub/28g	105	9.2	370	16.8	2.0	32.7	0.6
Liver & Bacon, Tesco*	1 Serving/10g	28	2.3	276	12.9	4.3	23.0	0.4
Mackerel, Smoked	1oz/28g	103	9.6	368	13.4	1.3	34.4	0.0
Mackerel, Tesco*	1 Serving/29g	102	9.5	353	14.3	0.5	32.6	0.0
Mediterranean Roast Vegetable, Tesco*	1 Serving/28g	31	2.6	112	2.4	4.3	9.4	1.2
Mousse De Canard, French, Weight Watchers*	1 Portion/50g	122	9.5	245	14.0	4.4	19.0	0.0
Mushroom, BGTY, Sainsbury's*	½ Pot/58g	29	0.3	50	4.6	6.7	0.5	3.0
Mushroom, M & S*	1 Pot/115g	224	20.1	195	4.2	4.8	17.5	1.5
Mushroom, Organic, Cauldron Foods*	1 Pot/113g	169	15.0	150	2.9	6.2	13.3	1.5
Mushroom, Roast, Tesco*	1 Serving/25g	36	3.2	145	3.6	3.6	12.9	4.5
Mushroom, Sainsbury's*	½ Pot/58g	89	7.0	153	3.3	7.8	12.1	2.1
Mushroom & Tarragon, Cauldron Foods*	1 Pot/113g	118	9.4	104	2.7	5.9	8.3	1.2
Mushroom & Tarragon, Waitrose*	1 Serving/30g	46	4.0	155	2.8	5.5	13.5	1.4
Poached Salmon & Watercress, Tesco*	1 Serving/25g	59	4.4	238	19.2	0.4	17.7	0.2
Pork, with Apple & Cider, Sainsbury's*	1 Serving/50g	151	12.6	303	12.5	6.3	25.3	1.1
Pork, with Peppercorns, Tesco*	1 Serving/28g	84	7.5	300	12.9	1.4	26.8	0.7
Pork with Port & Cranberry, Tesco*	1 Serving/28g	83	7.2	296	12.1	4.3	25.6	0.6
Ricotta, Sundried Tomato & Basil, Princes*	1 Jar/110g	343	31.6	312	5.2	8.3	28.7	0.0
Roasted Carrot, Ginger & Spring Onion, M & S*	1 Serving/50g	72	5.5	145	1.5	9.6	11.0	0.9
Roasted Parsnip & Carrot, Organic, Cauldron Foods*	1 Pot/115g	132	7.7	115	3.5	10.2	6.7	4.9
Roasted Red Pepper, Princes*	1 Serving/35g	47	1.7	135	4.8	17.6	5.0	0.0
Roasted Red Pepper & Houmous, Princes*	¼ Jar/27g	32	1.6	120	4.6	12.4	5.8	0.0
Roasted Vegetable, COU, M & S*	1 Pot/115g	86	1.7	75	6.2	9.1	1.5	1.4
Salmon, John West*	1 Serving/50g	136	11.7	272	14.9	0.0	23.5	0.2
Salmon, Organic, M & S*	1oz/28g	76	6.3	270	16.9	0.0	22.5	0.0
Salmon, Smoked, Isle of Skye, TTD, Sainsbury's*	½ Pot/58g	133	9.8	231	17.5	1.8	17.1	0.2
Salmon Dill, Princes*	1 Serving/70g	124	7.8	177	15.4	4.0	11.1	0.5
Smoked Mackerel, Sainsbury's*	½ Pot/57g	215	20.1	378	14.2	0.8	35.3	0.0
Smoked Mackerel, Scottish, M & S*	½ Pot/58g	158	13.3	275	15.9	0.6	23.2	0.1
Smoked Salmon, Luxury, Morrisons*	½ Pot/57g	150	12.4	266	16.0	0.9	22.0	0.5
Smoked Salmon, Waitrose*	½ Pot/57g	120	8.9	212	17.1	0.5	15.7	0.6
Smoked Trout, Waitrose*	½ Pot/56g	130	10.3	232	15.8	0.9	18.4	0.6
Soya & Mushroom, Cauldron Foods*	1 Pot/115g	199	10.8	173	8.8	6.4	9.4	6.5
Spiced Aubergine, Waitrose*	¼ Pack/38g	71	5.2	186	4.9	10.9	13.6	2.4
Spiced Parsnip & Carrot, Organic, Asda*	½ Pot/58g	63	3.5	109	3.7	10.0	6.0	2.6
Spicy Bean, BGTY, Sainsbury's*	½ Pot/58g	56	1.1	97	5.0	15.1	1.9	5.4
Spicy Bean, Princes*	½ Pot/55g	46	0.2	84	3.6	16.7	0.3	0.0
Spicy Bean, Weight Watchers*	1 Serving/37g	33	0.6	89	5.7	12.9	1.6	4.2
Spicy Mexican, Organic, Waitrose*	1 Serving/50g	57	3.1	115	6.2	8.6	6.2	3.5
Spinach, Cheese & Almond, Organic, Cauldron Foods*	½ Pot/58g	103	8.2	179	7.7	5.1	14.2	3.2
Sun-Dried Tomato & Basil, Cauldron Foods*	1 Pot/115g	189	11.7	164	6.9	11.1	10.2	4.6
Tofu, Spicy Mexican, Organic, GranoVita*	1 Serving/50g	108	10.0	216	6.0	3.0	20.0	0.0
Tomato, Lentil & Basil, Cauldron Foods*	1 Pot/115g	161	7.8	140	6.8	14.0	6.8	3.2
Tuna, Tesco*	1 Pack/115g	332	26.7	289	19.8	0.3	23.2	0.2
Tuna with Butter & Lemon Juice, Sainsbury's*	½ Pot/58g	209	18.3	360	19.0	0.1	31.6	0.3

P

	Measure INFO/WEIGHT	per Measure		Nutrition Values per 100g / 100ml				
		KCAL	FAT	KCAL	PROT	CARB	FAT	FIBRE
PATE								
Vegetable, Cauldron Foods*	1 Pack/113g	220	12.7	195	9.2	14.1	11.3	4.4
Vegetarian, with Mushrooms, Organic, Tartex*	¼ Tube/50g	101	8.0	203	7.7	7.0	16.0	0.0
Yeast, Garlic & Herb, Tartex*	1 Serving/30g	69	5.4	230	7.0	10.0	18.0	0.0
Yeast, Pateole, GranoVita*	1 Portion/30g	66	5.3	219	10.2	4.5	17.8	0.0
PAVLOVA								
Mandarin, Mini, Iceland*	1 Pavlova/22g	59	2.6	268	2.1	37.9	12.0	1.7
Raspberry, Individual, M & S*	1 Pavlova/65g	133	1.6	205	4.0	41.8	2.4	0.2
Raspberry, M & S*	1 Serving/84g	193	8.1	230	2.3	33.3	9.6	0.3
Raspberry, Mini, Co-Op*	1 Pavlova/19g	61	1.7	320	3.0	56.0	9.0	0.6
Raspberry, Sara Lee*	1/6 Pavlova/55g	168	8.5	303	2.7	38.5	15.3	1.1
Raspberry, Tesco*	1 Serving/65g	191	8.4	294	2.7	41.8	12.9	1.1
Raspberry & Lemon, Asda*	1 Serving/43g	102	1.9	235	2.8	46.0	4.4	0.5
Sticky Toffee, Sainsbury's*	1/6 Pavlova/60g	249	9.8	415	3.7	63.1	16.4	0.9
Strawberry, Co-Op*	1 Serving/52g	177	7.3	340	3.0	50.0	14.0	0.4
Strawberry, COU, M & S*	1 Pot/95g	147	2.3	155	2.4	30.5	2.4	0.8
Strawberry & Champagne, Mini, Co-Op*	1 Pavlova/19g	65	3.6	340	3.0	40.0	19.0	0.8
Toffee, Co-Op*	1/6 Pavlova/53g	193	8.5	365	3.0	52.0	16.0	0.6
Toffee, Mini, Iceland*	1 Pavlova/19g	68	2.9	353	3.0	51.5	15.0	1.9
Toffee Pecan, M & S*	1oz/28g	118	7.4	420	3.9	41.5	26.6	0.4
PAW-PAW								
Raw, Fresh	*1oz/28g*	*10*	*0.0*	*36*	*0.5*	*8.8*	*0.1*	*2.2*
Raw, Weighed with Skin & Pips	*1oz/28g*	*8*	*0.0*	*27*	*0.4*	*6.6*	*0.1*	*1.7*
PEACH								
Dried, Average	*1 Pack/250g*	*472*	*1.6*	*189*	*2.5*	*44.9*	*0.6*	*6.9*
in Fruit Juice, Average	*1oz/28g*	*13*	*0.0*	*47*	*0.5*	*11.2*	*0.0*	*0.7*
in Syrup, Average	*1oz/28g*	*19*	*0.0*	*67*	*0.4*	*16.3*	*0.1*	*0.4*
Pieces in Strawberry Jelly, Fruitini, Del Monte*	1 Can/140g	91	0.1	65	0.3	15.3	0.1	0.0
Raw, Average	*1 Peach/125g*	*39*	*0.1*	*31*	*0.9*	*7.2*	*0.1*	*1.4*
Raw, Stoned	1oz/28g	11	0.1	39	0.9	9.5	0.2	1.5
Slices, in Fruit Juice, Average	1 Serving/100g	49	0.0	49	0.6	11.5	0.0	0.5
PEANUT BRITTLE								
Thorntons*	2 Pieces/32g	163	8.6	509	12.4	54.3	26.9	2.6
PEANUT BUTTER								
& Grape Jelly Stripes in Jar, Goober*	1 Tsp/15g	67	3.4	450	13.2	65.0	22.6	3.8
25% Less Fat, Tesco*	1 Tbsp/16g	85	5.6	529	22.6	30.7	35.1	6.7
Creamy, Smooth, Sun Pat*	1 Serving/15g	93	7.5	620	24.0	17.5	50.2	6.1
Crunchy, Chosen By You, Asda*	1 Serving/10g	60	4.9	603	24.5	15.5	49.2	6.6
Crunchy, Harvest Spread*	1 Serving/25g	148	12.4	592	23.6	12.5	49.7	6.9
Crunchy, No Added Sugar, Organic, Whole Earth*	1 Serving/25g	148	12.5	592	24.9	10.1	50.2	7.3
Crunchy, Organic, Evernat*	1 Tsp/10g	64	5.3	641	29.0	13.0	53.0	7.0
Crunchy, Organic, No Added Sugar, Waitrose*	1 Serving/12g	71	6.0	592	24.9	10.1	50.2	7.3
Crunchy, Original Style, No Added Sugar, Whole Earth*	1 Serving/20g	127	10.2	637	25.7	16.8	51.1	8.7
Crunchy, Route 66*	1 Serving/10g	65	5.8	648	20.0	13.0	58.0	5.4
Crunchy, Sainsbury's*	1 Serving/10g	59	5.0	594	23.2	12.4	50.2	6.7
Crunchy, Sun Pat*	1 Serving/50g	307	24.4	615	25.3	15.1	48.9	6.8
Crunchy, Whole Nut, Organic, Meridian Foods*	1 Serving/28g	171	13.6	612	31.2	12.2	48.7	6.5
Extra Crunch, Skippy*	2 Tbsps/40g	252	20.0	630	22.7	22.9	50.0	7.7
Extra Crunchy, Sun Pat*	1 Serving/20g	119	10.2	597	21.9	12.6	51.0	7.3
GFY, Asda*	1 Serving/15g	80	5.2	531	28.0	31.0	35.0	0.0
Organic, Rapunzel*	1 Serving/5g	31	2.6	613	29.0	4.5	53.0	0.0
Smooth, 30% Reduced Fat, Duerr's*	1 Serving/20g	107	7.0	533	22.6	31.7	35.1	6.7
Smooth, 33% Less Fat, BGTY, Sainsbury's*	1 Serving/10g	53	3.5	533	22.6	31.7	35.1	6.7
Smooth, Average	1 Serving/20g	125	10.7	623	22.6	13.1	53.7	5.4

	Measure INFO/WEIGHT	per Measure KCAL	FAT	Nutrition Values per 100g / 100ml KCAL	PROT	CARB	FAT	FIBRE
PEANUT BUTTER								
Smooth, No Added Sugar, Organic, Whole Earth*	1 Serving/20g	119	10.2	595	24.5	9.9	50.8	7.1
Smooth, Organic, Meridian Foods*	1 Serving/10g	61	4.9	612	31.2	12.2	48.7	6.5
Smooth, Organic, Waitrose*	1 Serving/20g	125	10.2	623	28.0	13.0	51.0	0.0
Smooth, Sun Pat*	1 Serving/20g	123	9.8	614	25.0	15.2	48.9	6.7
Smooth Original, No Added Sugar, Whole Earth*	1 Serving/10g	59	5.1	595	24.6	9.9	50.8	7.1
Stripy, Sun Pat*	1 Tsp/10g	62	4.7	617	13.0	35.0	47.0	3.0
Wholenut, Crunchy, Average	1 Tsp/10g	61	5.3	606	24.9	7.7	53.1	6.0
Wholenut, Sainsbury's*	1 Serving/15g	90	7.7	598	24.2	9.8	51.3	7.0
Wholenut, Waitrose*	1 Serving/12g	70	6.0	587	24.9	9.3	50.0	6.3
PEANUT SHOOTS								
Cooked with Oil, Sainsbury's*	1 Pack/80g	177	13.5	221	10.6	4.1	16.9	2.5
PEANUTS								
Chilli, Average	½ Pack/50g	303	25.3	605	28.2	9.3	50.6	6.8
Dry Roasted, Average	1 Serving/20g	117	9.8	587	25.7	11.5	48.8	6.5
Honey Roasted, Average	1oz/28g	169	13.2	605	26.8	23.5	47.0	5.5
Hot Chilli, Holland & Barrett*	1 Pack/100g	523	31.0	523	14.0	47.0	31.0	5.5
Milk Chocolate Coated, Graze*	1 Pack/35g	187	13.1	533	14.6	34.9	37.3	0.0
Plain, Average	*10 Whole/10g*	*59*	*5.0*	*592*	*24.7*	*11.0*	*50.0*	*6.3*
Roast, Salted, Average	10 Whole/12g	74	6.3	614	27.8	7.9	52.4	4.9
Salted, Average	10 Whole/6g	37	3.1	609	27.0	8.3	52.0	5.4
White Chocolate Coated, Graze*	1 Pack/30g	166	11.8	553	14.7	37.8	39.3	0.0
Yoghurt Coated, Graze*	1 Pack/35g	189	12.3	540	9.9	48.1	35.1	0.0
PEARL BARLEY								
Boiled	*1oz/28g*	*34*	*0.1*	*123*	*2.3*	*28.2*	*0.4*	*0.0*
Raw, Average	*1oz/28g*	*99*	*0.3*	*352*	*9.9*	*77.7*	*1.2*	*15.6*
PEARS								
Abate Fetel, Average	*1 Med/133g*	*48*	*0.1*	*36*	*0.4*	*8.3*	*0.1*	*2.2*
Asian, Nashi, Raw, Average	*1 Lge/209g*	*88*	*0.5*	*42*	*0.5*	*10.6*	*0.2*	*3.6*
Blush, Morrisons*	1 Sm/148g	86	0.2	58	0.4	15.5	0.1	3.1
Cape, Quartered, Tesco*	1 Serving/100g	35	0.0	35	0.3	8.5	0.0	1.4
Comice, Raw, Weighed with Core	*1 Med/170g*	*56*	*0.0*	*33*	*0.3*	*8.5*	*0.0*	*2.0*
Conference, Average	*1 Lge/209g*	*88*	*0.2*	*42*	*0.3*	*10.1*	*0.1*	*2.0*
Dried, Average	*1 Pear Half/16g*	*33*	*0.1*	*204*	*1.9*	*48.4*	*0.5*	*9.7*
Frozen, Diced, Asda*	1 Serving/50g	23	0.0	47	0.3	10.4	0.1	1.7
in Fruit Juice, Average	*1 Serving/225g*	*102*	*0.1*	*45*	*0.3*	*10.9*	*0.0*	*1.2*
in Syrup, Average	*1oz/28g*	*16*	*0.0*	*58*	*0.2*	*14.4*	*0.1*	*1.4*
Prickly, Raw, Fresh	*1oz/28g*	*14*	*0.1*	*49*	*0.7*	*11.5*	*0.3*	*0.0*
Raw, Weighed with Core, Average	*1 Lge/209g*	*78*	*0.2*	*37*	*0.3*	*9.1*	*0.1*	*1.4*
Red, Tesco*	1 Med/180g	65	0.2	36	0.4	8.3	0.1	2.2
William, Raw, Average	*1 Med/170g*	*58*	*0.2*	*34*	*0.4*	*8.3*	*0.1*	*2.2*
PEAS								
Dried, Boiled in Unsalted Water, Average	*1oz/28g*	*31*	*0.2*	*109*	*6.9*	*19.9*	*0.8*	*5.5*
Dried, Raw, Average	*1oz/28g*	*85*	*0.7*	*303*	*21.6*	*52.0*	*2.4*	*13.0*
Edible Podded, Raw	*1 Cup/63g*	*26*	*0.1*	*42*	*2.8*	*7.6*	*0.2*	*2.6*
Frozen, Average	*1 Serving/85g*	*55*	*0.7*	*64*	*5.4*	*9.0*	*0.8*	*4.9*
Frozen, Boiled, Average	*1 Serving/75g*	*51*	*0.7*	*68*	*6.0*	*9.4*	*0.9*	*5.1*
Garden, Canned, No Sugar Or Salt, Average	*1 Can/80g*	*36*	*0.3*	*45*	*4.4*	*6.0*	*0.4*	*2.8*
Garden, Canned, with Sugar & Salt, Average	*1 Serving/90g*	*59*	*0.6*	*66*	*5.3*	*9.3*	*0.7*	*5.1*
Garden, Frozen, Average	*1 Serving/90g*	*66*	*1.0*	*74*	*6.3*	*9.7*	*1.1*	*3.3*
Garden, Minted, Average	*1 Serving/80g*	*59*	*0.9*	*74*	*6.3*	*9.7*	*1.1*	*5.9*
Marrowfat, Average	*1 Sm Can/160g*	*140*	*0.9*	*88*	*6.4*	*14.3*	*0.6*	*3.9*
Mushy, Average	*1 Can/200g*	*173*	*1.0*	*86*	*6.2*	*14.3*	*0.5*	*2.2*
Processed, Canned, Average	*1 Sm Can/220g*	*176*	*1.8*	*80*	*6.1*	*12.3*	*0.8*	*3.6*

P

	Measure INFO/WEIGHT	per Measure KCAL	FAT	Nutrition Values per 100g / 100ml KCAL	PROT	CARB	FAT	FIBRE
PEAS								
Snow	**1 Serving/80g**	**24**	**0.2**	**29**	**3.3**	**3.9**	**0.2**	**2.1**
Sugar Snap, Average	**1 Serving/80g**	**27**	**0.2**	**34**	**3.3**	**4.9**	**0.2**	**1.4**
Wasabi, Average	1 Serving/28g	114	3.8	406	15.2	54.0	13.7	8.6
PEASE PUDDING								
Canned, Re-Heated, Drained	1oz/28g	26	0.2	93	6.8	16.1	0.6	1.8
PECAN NUTS								
Average	**3 Nuts/6g**	**42**	**4.2**	**692**	**10.0**	**5.6**	**70.1**	**4.7**
Honey, Golden, Graze*	1 Pack/26g	168	15.4	647	7.6	23.4	59.4	0.0
PENNE								
Arrabbiata, BGTY, Sainsbury's*	1 Pack/450g	414	7.2	92	2.9	16.5	1.6	1.9
Chicken & Red Wine, Italiana, Weight Watchers*	1 Pack/395g	249	2.8	63	3.7	10.1	0.7	0.6
Chicken & Tomato, Italian, Sainsbury's*	½ Pack/350g	472	11.2	135	7.6	19.0	3.2	1.6
Chilli, Asda*	1 Serving/100g	148	0.7	148	5.1	30.2	0.7	2.4
Chilli & Garlic, Asda*	1 Serving/75g	259	1.1	346	12.0	71.0	1.5	3.0
Cooked, Average	**1 Serving/185g**	**244**	**1.3**	**132**	**4.7**	**26.7**	**0.7**	**1.1**
Corn, Free From, Dry Weight, Sainsbury's*	1 Serving/100g	348	2.3	348	7.6	74.2	2.3	5.2
Dry, Average	**1 Serving/100g**	**352**	**1.9**	**352**	**12.4**	**71.3**	**1.9**	**2.7**
Egg, Fresh, Average	**1 Serving/125g**	**352**	**4.0**	**282**	**11.1**	**52.2**	**3.2**	**2.0**
Free From, Tesco*	1 Serving/100g	340	2.0	340	8.0	72.5	2.0	2.5
Fresh, Dry, Average	**1 Serving/125g**	**222**	**2.4**	**178**	**7.3**	**32.2**	**1.9**	**1.6**
Hickory Steak, M & S*	1 Pack/400g	540	12.4	135	6.9	19.3	3.1	1.3
in Tomato & Basil Sauce, Sainsbury's*	½ Pack/110g	118	0.7	107	3.6	21.8	0.6	1.1
Leek & Bacon, Al Forno, Asda*	½ Pack/300g	531	39.0	177	5.0	10.0	13.0	0.5
Napoletana Chicken, BFY, Morrisons*	1 Pack/350g	252	5.6	72	6.4	7.2	1.6	0.2
Organic, Dry, Average	**1 Serving/100g**	**352**	**1.8**	**352**	**12.4**	**71.6**	**1.8**	**1.9**
Rigate, Dry Weight, Average	**1 Serving/90g**	**318**	**1.6**	**353**	**12.3**	**72.1**	**1.8**	**1.8**
Roasted Red Pepper, GFY, Asda*	1 Pack/400g	212	2.4	53	1.9	10.0	0.6	0.8
Tomato & Basil Sauce, Asda*	½ Pack/314g	185	11.0	59	0.8	6.0	3.5	2.0
Tomato & Roasted Vegetable, Big Eat, Heinz*	1 Pot/351g	281	10.5	80	2.5	10.7	3.0	4.6
Tuna, Tomato & Olive, Asda*	1 Pack/340g	173	6.5	51	4.2	4.2	1.9	0.6
with Chicken & Vegetables, Eat Positive, Birds Eye*	1 Meal/396g	325	5.2	82	7.7	9.8	1.3	1.2
with Roasted Vegetables, Waitrose*	1 Pack/400g	424	15.6	106	2.8	15.0	3.9	0.8
PENNETTE								
Tricolore, Sainsbury's*	1 Serving/100g	357	1.7	357	12.3	73.1	1.7	2.5
PEPERAMI*								
Firestick, Peperami*	1 Stick/25g	127	11.0	508	24.5	3.5	44.0	1.2
Hot, Peperami*	1 Stick/25g	126	11.0	504	24.5	2.5	44.0	1.2
Mini, 30% Less Fat, Peperami*	1 Stick/10g	38	3.0	379	25.0	1.5	30.0	3.0
Mini, Peperami*	1 Sausage/10g	38	2.0	379	25.0	1.5	20.0	3.0
Original, Peperami*	1 Stick/25g	126	11.0	504	24.0	2.5	44.0	0.1
PEPPER								
Black, Freshly Ground, Average	**1 Tsp/2g**	**5**	**0.1**	**255**	**10.9**	**64.8**	**3.3**	**26.5**
Cayenne, Ground	**1 Tsp/2g**	**6**	**0.3**	**318**	**12.0**	**31.7**	**17.3**	**0.0**
White	**½ Tsp/1g**	**3**	**0.0**	**296**	**10.4**	**68.6**	**2.1**	**26.2**
PEPPERS								
Capsicum, Green, Boiled in Salted Water	**1oz/28g**	**5**	**0.1**	**18**	**1.0**	**2.6**	**0.5**	**1.8**
Capsicum, Green, Raw, Unprepared, Average	**1 Med/160g**	**24**	**0.5**	**15**	**0.8**	**2.6**	**0.3**	**1.6**
Capsicum, Red, Boiled in Salted Water	**1oz/28g**	**10**	**0.1**	**34**	**1.1**	**7.0**	**0.4**	**1.6**
Capsicum, Red, Raw, Unprepared, Average	**1 Med/160g**	**51**	**0.6**	**32**	**1.0**	**6.4**	**0.4**	**1.6**
Capsicum, Sweet, Raw, Average	**1 Serving/100g**	**16**	**0.3**	**16**	**0.8**	**2.6**	**0.3**	**1.6**
Capsicum, Yellow, Raw, Unprepared, Average	**1 Med/160g**	**42**	**0.3**	**26**	**1.2**	**5.3**	**0.2**	**1.7**
Chilli, Chopped, Stir Fry, Schwartz*	1 Tbsp/19g	24	1.2	130	2.2	15.6	6.5	0.0
Chilli, Crushed, Schwartz*	1 Tsp/0.5g	2	0.1	321	12.0	29.0	17.0	27.0

P

	Measure INFO/WEIGHT	per Measure		Nutrition Values per 100g / 100ml				
		KCAL	FAT	KCAL	PROT	CARB	FAT	FIBRE
PEPPERS								
Chilli, Dried, Whole, Red, Schwartz*	1 Tsp/0.5g	2	0.1	425	15.9	56.4	15.1	0.0
Chilli, Green, Raw, Unprepared, Average	*1 Med/13g*	*5*	*0.0*	*40*	*2.0*	*9.5*	*0.2*	*1.5*
Chilli, Green, Very Lazy, The English Provender Co.*	1 Serving/10g	11	0.4	114	4.2	15.3	4.0	0.5
Chilli, Red, Chopped, in Marinade, Chef Kuo*	1 Tbsp/15g	10	0.6	69	1.6	11.5	4.2	5.3
Chilli, Red, Raw, Unprepared, Average	*1 Pepper/13g*	*5*	*0.0*	*40*	*2.0*	*9.5*	*0.2*	*1.5*
Chilli, Red, Very Lazy, The English Provender Co.*	1 Serving/15g	17	0.6	114	4.2	15.3	4.0	0.5
Italian Style, Sainsbury's*	1 Serving/150g	160	7.5	107	3.5	14.1	5.0	2.1
Jalapeno, Crushed, Schwartz*	1 Tsp/0.5g	1	0.1	136	15.9	56.4	15.1	0.0
Jalapeno, Raw	*1 Cup/ 90g*	*27*	*0.6*	*30*	*1.3*	*5.9*	*0.6*	*2.8*
Mixed Bag, From Supermarket, Average	*1oz/28g*	*7*	*0.1*	*25*	*1.0*	*4.4*	*0.4*	*1.7*
Stuffed, Fresh, Asda*	1 Pepper/150g	144	7.5	96	3.8	9.0	5.0	1.2
Stuffed, Perfectly Balanced, Waitrose*	1 Pack/300g	243	7.2	81	3.0	11.8	2.4	1.3
Stuffed, Sainsbury's*	1 Serving/137g	169	9.5	123	3.3	11.8	6.9	1.0
Stuffed with Rice Based Filling, Average	1oz/28g	24	0.7	85	1.5	15.4	2.4	1.3
Stuffed with Vegetables, Cheese Topping, Average	1oz/28g	31	1.9	111	3.4	9.8	6.7	1.5
Sweet, Tinned, Sainsbury's*	½ Can/125g	45	0.5	36	1.1	7.0	0.4	1.7
Yellow, Italian, Ready to Roast, Stuffed, Sainsbury's*	1 Pack/136g	144	6.8	106	5.3	9.9	5.0	1.3
PERCH								
Raw, Atlantic	*1oz/28g*	*26*	*0.5*	*94*	*18.6*	*0.0*	*1.6*	*0.0*
PERNOD*								
*19% Volume, Pernod**	*1 Shot/35ml*	*45*	*0.0*	*130*	*0.0*	*0.0*	*0.0*	*0.0*
PESTO								
Sauce, Average	1oz/28g	145	13.3	517	20.4	2.0	47.5	0.0
Sauce, Fiery Chilli, Sacla*	½ Jar/95g	342	29.3	360	4.8	16.0	30.8	3.4
Sauce, Green, Alla Genovese, TTD, Sainsbury's*	1 Serving/30g	192	19.8	640	6.2	5.4	65.9	3.1
Sauce, Green, Classic, Sacla*	1 Serving/40g	185	18.6	462	5.2	7.6	46.5	0.0
Sauce, Green, GFY, Asda*	1 Jar/190g	338	29.6	178	5.0	4.3	15.6	3.3
Sauce, Green, Verde, Bertolli*	¼ Jar/46g	266	27.5	575	5.7	4.3	59.5	0.0
Sauce, Italian Style, Stir, Thru, Asda*	1 Serving/15g	55	5.2	369	4.4	9.0	35.0	0.9
Sauce, Mary Berry*	1 Serving/100g	528	49.3	528	1.1	19.4	49.3	1.1
Sauce, Red, Garlic & Chilli, Jamie Oliver*	1 Jar/190g	494	48.8	260	1.1	5.6	25.7	1.1
Sauce, Red, Rosso, Bertolli*	1 Jar/185g	703	64.7	380	6.8	9.5	35.0	2.0
Sauce, Ricotta & Red Pepper, Chosen By You, Asda*	1 Jar/190g	486	37.2	256	4.2	14.4	19.6	2.4
Sauce, Roasted Red Pepper, Sacla*	1 Serving/30g	72	6.8	241	4.3	4.6	22.8	5.3
Sauce, Spinach & Parmesan, Sainsbury's*	¼ Jar/46g	162	16.0	349	4.6	5.3	34.4	2.5
Sauce, Sun Dried Tomato, Sacla*	1 Serving/30g	87	8.4	289	4.2	5.2	27.9	0.0
Sauce, Verde, Traditional Italian, Sacla*	1 Serving/100g	454	45.4	454	5.3	6.0	45.4	0.0
Sauce & Balsamic Vinegar, Extra Special, Asda*	1 Tbsp/15g	33	3.0	213	0.3	8.6	19.7	0.0
PETIT POIS								
Average	*1 Serving/65g*	*34*	*0.5*	*53*	*5.0*	*6.8*	*0.7*	*3.5*
Freshly Frozen, Boiled, Asda*	1 Serving/80g	39	0.7	49	5.0	5.5	0.9	4.5
Frozen, M & S*	1 Serving/80g	56	0.7	70	5.0	5.5	0.9	4.5
in Water, Sugar & Salt Added, Sainsbury's*	½ Tin/140g	81	0.7	58	4.0	9.4	0.5	2.0
PHEASANT								
Meat Only, Roasted	*1oz/28g*	*62*	*3.4*	*220*	*27.9*	*0.0*	*12.0*	*0.0*
Meat Only, Roasted, Weighed with Bone	*1oz/28g*	*61*	*3.3*	*219*	*27.9*	*0.0*	*11.9*	*0.0*
Stuffed, Easy Carve, Finest, Tesco*	1 Serving/200g	540	37.4	270	23.2	2.2	18.7	0.9
PHYSALIS								
Raw, without Husk, Average	*5 Fruits/30g*	*16*	*0.2*	*53*	*1.9*	*11.2*	*0.7*	*0.4*
PICCALILLI								
Dijon, Sainsbury's*	1 Dtsp/15g	14	0.1	91	1.8	19.0	0.9	0.7
Haywards*	1 Serving/28g	18	0.1	66	1.4	13.9	0.5	0.0
Heinz*	1 Serving/10g	10	0.1	99	1.0	20.5	0.6	0.6

P

	Measure INFO/WEIGHT	per Measure		Nutrition Values per 100g / 100ml				
		KCAL	FAT	KCAL	PROT	CARB	FAT	FIBRE
PICCALILLI								
Morrisons*	1 Serving/50g	37	0.3	75	1.6	15.0	0.7	0.6
Sainsbury's*	1 Dtsp/15g	9	0.1	60	1.8	11.9	0.6	0.7
Sandwich, Tesco*	1 Serving/20g	16	0.0	80	0.4	18.5	0.0	1.6
Spicy, Sainsbury's*	1 Serving/15g	12	0.1	80	0.7	15.3	0.5	1.0
Sweet, Asda*	1 Tbsp/15g	17	0.0	112	0.5	27.0	0.2	0.6
Tesco*	1 Serving/50g	51	1.8	102	0.5	17.8	3.6	2.0
Three Mustard, Finest, Tesco*	1 Serving/30g	40	0.2	134	1.3	30.7	0.7	1.0
TTD, Sainsbury's*	1 Serving/19g	13	0.2	67	0.7	13.9	0.9	1.8
PICKLE								
Beetroot, Branston*	1 Tsp/20g	25	0.1	123	1.2	28.2	0.3	1.6
Branston, Crosse & Blackwell*	1 Tsp/10g	11	0.0	109	0.8	26.1	0.2	1.1
Brinjal, Patak's*	1 Tsp/16g	59	3.9	367	2.2	34.6	24.4	0.9
Chilli, Branston*	1 Tsp/16g	21	0.1	130	0.7	30.0	0.7	1.5
Chilli, Patak's*	1 Tsp/16g	52	5.4	325	4.3	1.3	33.7	0.0
Cornichons, in Sweet & Sour Vinegar, Waitrose*	1 Serving/10g	3	0.0	28	0.6	6.1	0.1	0.6
Garlic, Patak's*	1 Tsp/16g	42	3.0	261	3.6	20.0	18.5	1.6
Ginger, Priya*	1 Tsp/10g	27	1.7	270	3.3	26.7	16.7	0.0
Green Chilli, Priya*	1 Tsp/10g	19	1.7	190	3.3	6.7	16.7	4.8
Lime, Hot, Asda*	1 Dtsp/10g	12	1.0	123	2.2	6.0	10.0	1.0
Lime, Hot, Patak's*	1 Tsp/16g	31	3.0	194	2.2	4.0	18.7	0.4
Lime, M & S*	1 Tsp/16g	34	0.8	215	0.8	42.5	4.8	2.4
Lime, Oily	*1 Tbsp/39g*	*70*	*6.1*	*178*	*1.9*	*8.3*	*15.5*	*0.0*
Lime, Sharwood's*	1 Tsp/16g	24	1.5	152	2.2	15.0	9.3	2.9
Mango, Hot, Patak's*	1 Tsp/16g	43	4.1	270	2.3	7.4	25.7	1.9
Mild Mustard, Heinz*	1 Tbsp/10g	13	0.1	129	2.2	25.7	1.3	0.9
Mixed, Haywards*	½ Jar/120g	22	0.4	18	1.4	2.4	0.3	0.0
Mixed, Patak's*	1 Serving/30g	78	7.7	259	2.3	4.7	25.7	0.8
Mixed, Salad Bar, Asda*	1oz/28g	11	0.0	40	0.5	9.2	0.1	0.0
Mustard, Squeezy, Branston*	1 Serving/10g	11	0.1	108	0.9	24.7	0.6	0.8
Onion, Priya*	1 Tsp/10g	20	1.5	203	3.3	13.3	15.0	0.0
Red Cabbage, Asda*	1 Serving/50g	16	0.0	32	1.6	6.0	0.1	0.0
Red Chilli, Priya*	1 Tsp/10g	22	1.7	217	3.3	13.3	16.7	0.0
Sandwich, Branston*	1 Tsp/10g	14	0.0	140	0.7	34.2	0.3	1.3
Sandwich, Tesco*	1 Serving/5g	7	0.0	138	1.0	33.1	0.2	1.0
Small Chunk, Branston*	1 Serving/20g	22	0.0	109	0.8	26.1	0.2	1.1
Spicy, Branston*	1 Tsp/15g	21	0.0	140	0.7	34.7	0.3	1.3
Sweet	*1 Tsp/10g*	*14*	*0.0*	*141*	*0.6*	*36.0*	*0.1*	*1.2*
Sweet, Branston*	1 Serving/30g	33	0.1	109	0.8	26.1	0.2	1.1
Tomato, Tangy, Heinz*	1 Tsp/10g	10	0.0	102	2.0	22.0	0.3	1.5
PICNIC								
Cadbury*	1 Bar/48g	228	11.3	475	7.5	58.3	23.6	0.0
PIE								
2 Mini Pork, Ploughmans, Ginsters*	1 Pie/50g	190	12.6	380	8.9	29.2	25.3	2.0
Admiral's, Light & Easy, Youngs*	1 Pack/360g	342	14.0	95	4.1	10.9	3.9	0.8
Admiral's, Ross*	1 Pie/340g	357	15.6	105	4.8	10.9	4.6	0.7
All Steak, Pukka Pies Ltd*	1 Pie/233g	538	32.9	231	9.9	16.2	14.1	1.6
Apple, & Blackberry, Fruit, Finest, Tesco*	1 Pie/95g	265	11.3	279	13.7	29.3	11.9	2.8
Apple, American, Iceland*	1 Serving/92g	258	10.7	280	4.8	39.2	11.6	2.2
Apple, Asda*	¼ Pack/107g	287	11.7	269	3.6	39.0	11.0	1.7
Apple, Bramley, Aunt Bessie's*	¼ Pie/138g	351	15.1	255	2.8	36.2	11.0	1.2
Apple, Bramley, Free From, Tesco*	1 Pie/60g	185	7.5	309	2.5	55.4	8.6	1.4
Apple, Bramley, Large, Tesco*	1/8 Pie/87g	311	13.0	358	3.9	51.9	15.0	1.9
Apple, Bramley, Tesco*	1 Serving/106g	284	11.6	268	3.6	38.8	10.9	1.7

PIE

INFO/WEIGHT	Measure	per Measure KCAL	FAT	Nutrition Values per 100g / 100ml KCAL	PROT	CARB	FAT	FIBRE
Apple, Deep Filled, Amanda Smith*	1/5 Pie/150g	420	19.8	280	2.8	37.4	13.2	1.2
Apple, Deep Filled, Sainsbury's*	¼ Pie/137g	374	17.5	273	3.8	35.6	12.8	1.6
Apple, Family, Asda*	1/6 Pie/119g	314	13.0	265	3.6	38.0	11.0	2.9
Apple, Lattice, Tesco*	1 Serving/145g	325	13.3	224	2.2	33.2	9.2	1.4
Apple, McVitie's*	1 Serving/117g	316	12.9	270	3.0	39.0	11.0	2.0
Apple, Pastry Top & Bottom	1oz/28g	74	3.7	266	2.9	35.8	13.3	1.7
Apple, Puff Pastry, M & S*	1 Pie/135g	337	17.1	250	2.4	31.3	12.7	1.0
Apple, Ready Baked, Sara Lee*	1/6 Pie/90g	249	12.4	277	2.8	35.4	13.8	1.2
Apple, Sainsbury's*	1/6 Pie/118g	314	13.6	266	3.4	37.1	11.5	0.6
Apple, Sultana & Cinnamon, Finest, Tesco*	1 Slice/83g	193	7.3	233	2.8	35.6	8.8	5.0
Apple, VLH Kitchens*	1 Slice/50g	136	5.6	272	3.7	40.0	11.2	1.7
Apple & Blackberry, Co-Op*	1 Serving/138g	338	15.2	245	3.0	33.0	11.0	2.0
Apple & Blackberry, Shortcrust, M & S*	1 Serving/142g	469	17.7	330	4.3	50.2	12.5	1.1
Apple & Blackberry, Tesco*	1 Serving/106g	287	11.9	271	4.2	38.4	11.2	1.7
Apple & Blackcurrant, Mr Kipling*	1 Pie/66g	211	8.4	320	3.3	47.9	12.8	1.2
Apple Meringue, Frozen, Sara Lee*	1/6 Pie/74g	179	6.5	242	2.7	37.9	8.8	1.5
Apricot Fruit, GFY, Asda*	1 Serving/52g	162	5.2	311	3.3	52.0	10.0	0.0
Banoffee, Individual, Sainsbury's*	1 Pie/104g	365	21.0	351	3.2	39.2	20.2	2.2
Banoffee, Tesco*	1/6 Pie/94g	365	19.7	390	3.9	45.8	21.1	1.5
Banoffee Cream, American Dream, Heinz*	1/6 Pie/70g	239	15.0	342	3.7	33.7	21.4	3.9
Banoffee Cream, American Dream, McVitie's*	1 Serving/70g	277	17.8	396	4.3	36.7	25.5	0.8
Beef, Lean, BGTY, Sainsbury's*	1 Serving/212g	280	12.7	132	7.3	12.2	6.0	1.5
Beef, Minced, Aberdeen Angus, Shortcrust, M & S*	1 Pie/171g	435	26.6	255	9.3	19.3	15.6	3.0
Beef, Sainsbury's*	1 Pie/210g	535	30.0	255	10.3	21.2	14.3	2.0
Beef, Shamrock, Pieminister*	1 Pie/270g	648	30.8	240	8.8	24.5	11.4	1.8
Beef & Onion, Pukka Pies Ltd*	1 1/231g	529	32.6	229	7.6	17.9	14.1	3.0
Beef & Vegetable, McDougalls*	¼ Pie/114g	292	19.3	256	5.3	20.6	16.9	0.3
Beef Steak, Aberdeen Angus, Top Crust, Waitrose*	½ Pie/280g	476	24.1	170	10.0	13.4	8.6	4.1
Blackberry & Apple, Sara Lee*	1 Serving/100g	272	13.9	272	2.9	34.0	13.9	0.0
Blackcurrant, Deep Filled, Sainsbury's*	1 Slice/137g	440	19.3	321	5.8	42.6	14.1	2.2
Blackcurrant, Shortcrust, M & S*	1 Pie/142g	412	14.3	290	3.9	45.6	10.1	1.3
Cheese & Onion, Hollands*	1 Pie/200g	516	24.4	258	6.3	30.9	12.2	0.0
Cheese & Onion, Oven Baked, Average	1 Serving/200g	654	40.0	327	8.2	30.4	20.0	1.2
Cheese & Potato	1oz/28g	39	2.3	139	4.8	12.6	8.1	0.7
Cheese & Potato, Aunt Bessie's*	¼ Serving/200g	288	18.8	144	4.6	11.7	9.4	1.5
Cherry, Asda*	1/6 Pie/117g	337	14.5	289	3.1	41.2	12.4	1.8
Cherry, Sainsbury's*	1 Serving/117g	325	13.6	278	3.9	39.6	11.6	1.7
Chicken, Aunt Bessie's*	¼ Pie/200g	474	24.2	237	10.6	21.4	12.1	2.1
Chicken, Bacon & Cheddar Cheese, Lattice, Birds Eye*	1 Pie/155g	454	26.8	293	13.4	21.0	17.3	1.5
Chicken, Broccoli & White Wine, Waitrose*	1 Serving/200g	605	40.5	302	12.5	17.7	20.2	2.3
Chicken, Cheese & Bacon, HL, Tesco*	1 Pack/450g	382	9.9	85	5.9	9.4	2.2	1.6
Chicken, Cheese & Broccoli Lattice, Birds Eye*	1 Pie/155g	446	25.3	288	12.6	22.7	16.3	1.1
Chicken, Cheese & Leek Lattice, Sun Valley*	1 Lattice/125g	315	21.9	252	15.2	8.6	17.5	1.0
Chicken, Cottage, Frozen, Tesco*	1 Pack/450g	292	2.2	65	2.8	11.7	0.5	1.0
Chicken, Deep Filled, Puff Pastry, Sainsbury's*	1 Pie/210g	538	31.9	256	10.0	19.9	15.2	3.1
Chicken, Finest, Tesco*	1 Pie/250g	615	32.2	246	10.7	21.9	12.9	1.2
Chicken, Ginsters*	¼ Pie/136g	374	23.7	275	10.0	19.0	17.4	1.0
Chicken, Individual, Made with 100% Breast, Birds Eye*	1 Pie/154g	455	28.1	296	7.9	25.0	18.3	1.0
Chicken, Individual Shortcrust, Asda*	1 Pie/175g	534	29.7	305	10.0	28.0	17.0	1.0
Chicken, Leek & Ham, Morrisons*	1 Serving/113g	305	16.6	270	8.8	25.7	14.7	1.1
Chicken, Newgate*	1 Pie/142g	358	23.6	252	6.1	23.1	16.6	1.0
Chicken, Puff Pastry, Tesco*	¼ Pie/114g	250	12.7	220	8.6	21.3	11.2	1.4
Chicken, Roast, in Gravy, Deep Fill, Tesco*	1 Pie/800g	1640	77.6	205	9.3	20.2	9.7	3.0

PIE

	Measure INFO/WEIGHT	per Measure KCAL	FAT	Nutrition Values per 100g / 100ml KCAL	PROT	CARB	FAT	FIBRE
Chicken, Roast, Puff Pastry, Deep Fill, Asda*	½ Pie/259g	739	44.1	285	10.0	23.0	17.0	0.8
Chicken, Roast, Sainsbury's*	1/3 Pie/173g	538	30.8	311	10.5	27.2	17.8	0.9
Chicken, Roast, Shortcrust, Sainsbury's*	1 Pie/200g	1012	56.0	506	19.2	44.4	28.0	2.4
Chicken, Short Crust, M & S*	1 Pie/170g	510	29.6	300	9.7	26.2	17.4	1.7
Chicken, Tomato & Basil Lattice, Birds Eye*	1 Serving/155g	340	19.6	220	10.8	15.7	12.7	1.4
Chicken & Asparagus, Lattice, Waitrose*	1 Serving/100g	295	19.6	295	7.4	22.3	19.6	1.8
Chicken & Asparagus, McDougalls*	1 Serving/170g	394	21.9	232	7.4	21.6	12.9	1.5
Chicken & Asparagus, Puff Pasty, John Bullers*	1 Pie/174g	477	29.6	274	11.0	19.0	17.0	2.0
Chicken & Bacon, Filo Pastry, Finest, Tesco*	1 Serving/160g	362	18.7	226	11.3	18.9	11.7	1.7
Chicken & Bacon, Puff Pastry, Deep Fill, Sainsbury's*	1/3 Pie/200g	532	34.0	266	9.1	19.1	17.0	1.3
Chicken & Bacon, with Cheese Sauce, Tesco*	1 Serving/200g	540	33.6	270	12.0	17.6	16.8	0.8
Chicken & Basil, M & S*	1oz/28g	59	3.3	210	8.9	17.0	11.9	1.1
Chicken & Broccoli, BGTY, Sainsbury's*	1 Pack/450g	297	3.6	66	5.9	8.9	0.8	1.8
Chicken & Broccoli, COU, M & S*	1 Serving/320g	272	6.1	85	8.1	8.8	1.9	1.3
Chicken & Broccoli, Lattice, Tesco*	½ Pie/200g	496	30.8	248	8.5	18.9	15.4	2.1
Chicken & Broccoli, Light Choices, Tesco*	1 Pack/450g	382	7.2	85	7.0	10.3	1.6	0.8
Chicken & Broccoli Lattice, Sainsbury's*	½ Pie/192g	520	30.7	271	9.3	22.4	16.0	0.9
Chicken & Broccoli Potato, Top, Asda*	1 Pack/400g	319	7.0	80	5.2	10.7	1.7	0.6
Chicken & Gravy, Deep Fill, Asda*	1 Serving/130g	370	22.1	285	10.0	23.0	17.0	0.8
Chicken & Gravy, Light Choices, Tesco*	1 Pack/450g	405	10.8	90	5.9	10.6	2.4	1.4
Chicken & Gravy, Shortcrust Pastry, Sainsbury's*	1 Serving/250g	637	35.2	255	8.0	24.1	14.1	1.0
Chicken & Gravy, Shortcrust Pastry, Tesco*	1 Pie/250g	617	34.5	247	6.8	23.9	13.8	1.0
Chicken & Ham, Deep Filled, Sainsbury's*	1 Pie/210g	594	37.2	283	8.0	23.0	17.7	1.0
Chicken & Ham, Sainsbury's*	1 Pie/128g	461	28.7	360	11.0	28.5	22.4	2.0
Chicken & Leek, Deep Filled, Puff Pastry, Sainsbury's*	1/3 Pie/451g	1109	65.4	246	10.1	18.7	14.5	1.5
Chicken & Leek, Light Choices, Tesco*	1 Pie/350g	297	5.6	85	6.6	10.3	1.6	1.3
Chicken & Leek, M & S*	1oz/28g	70	4.2	250	10.1	18.8	15.1	1.1
Chicken & Leek, Shortcrust, TTD, Sainsbury's*	½ Pie/300g	824	48.8	275	12.2	19.8	16.3	1.1
Chicken & Mushroom, Asda*	1 Pie/ 150g	384	24.0	256	9.0	19.0	16.0	1.0
Chicken & Mushroom, Deep Filled, Frozen, Tesco*	¼ Pie/198g	465	22.2	235	9.0	23.8	11.2	1.2
Chicken & Mushroom, Dietary Specials*	1 Pie/140g	300	14.0	214	6.3	24.7	10.0	0.9
Chicken & Mushroom, Finest, Tesco*	1 Pie/250g	742	46.7	297	9.3	21.1	18.7	0.9
Chicken & Mushroom, Fray Bentos*	1 Pie/425g	684	40.4	161	6.7	11.5	9.5	0.0
Chicken & Mushroom, Ginsters*	1 Pie/180g	486	31.1	270	8.3	20.2	17.3	1.3
Chicken & Mushroom, Individual, Frozen, Tesco*	1 Pie/142ml	347	17.9	245	8.9	23.5	12.6	1.2
Chicken & Mushroom, Luxury, M & S*	½ Pie/275g	880	61.9	320	9.9	20.0	22.5	1.0
Chicken & Mushroom, Puff Pastry, Birds Eye*	1 Pie/152g	415	21.3	273	11.9	24.9	14.0	1.6
Chicken & Mushroom, Pukka Pies Ltd*	1 Pie/226g	475	29.2	210	7.6	15.7	12.9	3.5
Chicken & Mushroom, Weight Watchers*	1 Pie/136g	317	15.1	233	8.0	25.1	11.1	1.5
Chicken & Vegetable, Freshbake*	1 Pie/125g	319	19.6	255	6.5	21.8	15.7	2.7
Chicken & Vegetable, Kids, Tesco*	1 Serving/235g	235	10.6	100	5.9	9.1	4.5	0.7
Chicken & Vegetable, Perfectly Balanced, Waitrose*	1 Serving/375g	285	5.2	76	5.1	10.8	1.4	1.3
Chicken & Wiltshire Ham, Finest, Tesco*	1 Pie/250g	687	37.2	275	11.6	22.7	14.9	1.1
Chicken Balti, Ginsters*	1 Pie/180g	416	25.0	231	7.3	19.2	13.9	1.9
Chicken Curry, Iceland*	1 Pie/156g	440	23.7	282	10.2	26.2	15.2	2.0
Chicken Leek & Sweetcorn, Love Life, Waitrose*	1 Pie/421g	358	14.3	85	5.2	8.6	3.4	1.7
Chicken Pot with Ham & Leek, Higgidy*	1 Pie/250g	710	33.5	284	13.1	19.1	13.4	1.1
Chocolate, Mini, Waitrose*	1 Pie/24g	109	6.1	455	5.3	51.4	25.3	1.7
Cod & Prawn, M & S*	1oz/28g	43	2.5	155	10.6	8.7	8.9	0.7
Cod & Smoked Haddock, COU, M & S*	1 Pack/400g	320	9.6	80	6.1	9.0	2.4	1.2
Cottage, Aberdeen Angus, Waitrose*	1 Pie/350g	339	12.2	97	5.3	11.0	3.5	0.9
Cottage, Asda*	1 Pack/400g	360	9.6	90	6.5	10.6	2.4	1.0
Cottage, Aunt Bessie's*	1 Pack/350g	413	18.2	118	4.8	12.1	5.2	1.0

	Measure INFO/WEIGHT	per Measure		Nutrition Values per 100g / 100ml				
		KCAL	FAT	KCAL	PROT	CARB	FAT	FIBRE
PIE								
Cottage, British Pies, Chilled, Tesco*	1 Pack/500g	450	14.0	90	4.6	10.3	2.8	1.5
Cottage, Chicken, Tesco*	1 Pack/400g	340	2.8	85	6.0	12.8	0.7	1.7
Cottage, Classic British, Sainsbury's*	1 Pack/450g	499	20.7	111	6.3	11.1	4.6	0.6
Cottage, Classics, Asda*	½ Pack/450g	531	27.0	118	7.0	9.0	6.0	1.0
Cottage, COU, M & S*	1 Pack/400g	340	8.0	85	6.0	11.0	2.0	1.5
Cottage, Diet Chef Ltd*	1 Pack/270g	235	9.7	87	3.7	9.8	3.6	1.7
Cottage, Disney, Tesco*	1 Pack/281g	250	7.0	89	4.9	11.8	2.5	1.9
Cottage, Family, Iceland*	¼ Pack/259g	262	10.6	101	4.2	11.8	4.1	0.8
Cottage, Fresh, M & S*	1 Pie/400g	460	22.4	115	6.8	9.9	5.6	0.6
Cottage, Frozen, Asda*	1 Serving/121g	146	7.3	121	4.8	12.0	6.0	0.6
Cottage, Healthy Living, Co-Op*	1 Pack/400g	320	6.4	80	5.0	11.0	1.6	2.0
Cottage, Healthy Options, Birds Eye*	1oz/28g	23	0.5	83	4.9	11.9	1.8	1.0
Cottage, Light Choices, Tesco*	1 Pack/500g	400	8.5	80	4.5	11.4	1.7	1.7
Cottage, Luxury, M & S*	½ Pack/310g	403	21.7	130	7.9	8.3	7.0	1.8
Cottage, Meal for One, M & S*	1 Pack/445g	356	16.0	80	5.4	6.2	3.6	1.7
Cottage, Meatfree, Sainsbury's*	1 Pack/400g	364	12.0	91	4.4	11.7	3.0	0.7
Cottage, Mini, Waitrose*	1 Pack/250g	267	10.5	107	6.4	11.1	4.2	1.4
Cottage, Salmon, Sainsbury's*	1 Serving/299g	218	4.2	73	4.6	10.4	1.4	1.3
Cottage, The Best, Morrisons*	½ Pack/400g	424	16.4	106	7.7	9.5	4.1	1.2
Cottage, TTD, Sainsbury's*	1 Pack/387g	545	34.0	141	8.5	6.9	8.8	2.1
Cottage, Vegetarian, Sainsbury's*	1 Pack/450g	328	9.9	73	3.0	10.2	2.2	1.8
Cottage, Waitrose*	1 Pack/400g	424	19.6	106	3.4	12.1	4.9	1.2
Cottage, Weight Watchers*	1 Pack/300g	186	3.9	62	3.6	9.0	1.3	0.3
Cumberland, Asda*	1 Pack/400g	504	22.4	126	6.3	12.7	5.6	1.5
Cumberland, Beef, HL, Tesco*	1 Pack/500g	460	13.5	92	5.0	11.8	2.7	0.9
Cumberland, BGTY, Sainsbury's*	1 Pack/450g	360	9.0	80	5.3	10.1	2.0	1.6
Cumberland, Cod & Prawn, Tesco*	1 Pack/450g	427	11.2	95	7.9	9.5	2.5	1.3
Cumberland, GFY, Asda*	1 Pack/451g	469	9.9	104	11.4	11.4	2.2	2.1
Cumberland, HL, Tesco*	1 Pie/500g	430	13.5	86	4.5	10.8	2.7	1.2
Cumberland, M & S*	1 Pie/195g	312	20.3	160	6.9	10.1	10.4	1.1
Fish	1 Serving/250g	262	7.5	105	8.0	12.3	3.0	0.7
Fish, Chilled, GFY, Asda*	1 Pie/450g	405	12.6	90	6.8	9.3	2.8	1.4
Fish, Creamy, Classics, Large, Tesco*	½ Pack/350g	472	28.0	135	7.5	7.7	8.0	0.7
Fish, Cumberland, BGTY, Sainsbury's*	1 Serving/450g	342	8.5	76	7.3	7.3	1.9	1.8
Fish, Extra Special, Asda*	1 Pack/400g	540	30.8	135	9.8	6.5	7.7	1.1
Fish, Healthy Options, Birds Eye*	1 Pack/350g	238	2.8	68	3.7	11.6	0.8	0.7
Fish, Large, Extra Special, Asda*	1 Serving/350g	525	30.8	150	9.9	7.8	8.8	0.6
Fish, Mariner's, Frozen, Youngs*	1 Pack/360g	382	16.2	106	5.3	11.0	4.5	1.0
Fish, Mix, Tesco*	1 Pack/320g	480	25.6	150	19.3	0.0	8.0	0.0
Fish, Ocean Crumble, Low Fat, Light & Easy, Youngs*	1 Pack/300g	261	5.7	87	4.6	12.9	1.9	1.4
Fish, Seasonal, Mix, Sainsbury's*	1 Pack/320g	480	28.2	150	17.7	0.0	8.8	0.0
Fish, with Cheddar & Parsley Sauce, Go Cook, Asda*	½ Pack/450g	427	16.2	95	7.8	7.9	3.6	0.8
Fish, with Grated Cheddar, Asda*	¼ Pie/250g	262	12.5	105	7.0	8.0	5.0	1.0
Fish, Yummy Pollock, Jamie Oliver, Youngs*	1 Pie/217g	204	7.2	94	6.8	8.6	3.3	1.5
Fish, Yummy Salmon, Jamie Oliver, Youngs*	1 Pie/207g	224	8.5	108	8.1	9.3	4.1	0.9
Fish, Yummy Salmon & Broccoli, Jamie Oliver, Youngs*	1 Pie/220g	211	7.5	96	6.5	9.3	3.4	1.3
Fish & Prawn, Perfectly Balanced, Waitrose*	1 Serving/375g	379	13.5	101	6.8	10.4	3.6	0.7
Fish with Cheese, Ross*	1 Pack/300g	321	13.5	107	4.7	12.0	4.5	0.8
Fish with Vegetables, Ross*	1 Pack/300g	255	8.7	85	4.4	10.2	2.9	1.3
Fishermans, British Recipe, Waitrose*	1 Pack/400g	408	16.4	102	7.7	8.5	4.1	1.2
Fisherman's, Famous, Chilled, Youngs*	1 Pack/400g	448	22.8	112	7.6	7.6	5.7	0.9
Fisherman's, Healthy Options, Asda*	1 Pie/406g	337	10.1	83	5.0	10.0	2.5	0.9
Fisherman's, M & S*	1 Pie/248g	335	15.9	135	9.3	9.8	6.4	0.3

PIE

	INFO/WEIGHT	per Measure KCAL	FAT	Nutrition Values per 100g / 100ml KCAL	PROT	CARB	FAT	FIBRE
Fisherman's, Perfectly Balanced, Waitrose*	1 Pack/376g	380	13.5	101	6.8	10.4	3.6	0.7
Fruit, Pastry Top & Bottom	1oz/28g	73	3.7	260	3.0	34.0	13.3	1.8
Fruit, Selection, Mr Kipling*	1 Pie/66g	232	9.0	350	3.5	53.5	13.6	1.3
Gala, Tesco*	1 Serving/70g	241	17.6	344	10.6	24.5	25.2	0.0
Haddock & Broccoli, M & S*	1 Serving/250g	262	10.0	105	8.1	9.3	4.0	0.5
Key Lime, Sainsbury's*	¼ Pie/80g	280	11.2	350	4.2	51.8	14.0	0.7
Lamb & Mint, Shortcrust Pasty, Tesco*	¼ Pack/150g	412	26.1	275	5.9	23.6	17.4	1.6
Lemon Meringue	1 Portion/120g	383	17.3	319	4.5	45.9	14.4	0.7
Lemon Meringue, Mini, Asda*	1 Pie/26g	101	3.3	396	3.7	66.0	13.0	1.8
Lemon Meringue, Mr Kipling*	1 Pie/51g	184	6.2	360	2.9	59.9	12.1	3.0
Lemon Meringue, Sara Lee*	1oz/28g	77	2.6	276	2.6	46.6	9.2	0.9
Lemon Meringue, Weight Watchers*	1 Serving/85g	161	0.4	189	2.4	43.1	0.5	0.6
Meat, Freshbake*	1 Pie/49g	152	10.5	313	6.6	23.2	21.6	1.0
Meat & Potato, Hollands*	1 Pie/175g	409	19.2	234	6.1	27.5	11.0	0.0
Meat & Potato, Shortcrust, Co-Op*	¼ Pie/137g	403	26.2	294	7.3	23.3	19.1	1.4
Meat & Potato, Tesco*	1 Serving/150g	414	26.8	276	5.1	23.6	17.9	1.6
Mediterranean Vegetable, Cheesy, COU, M & S*	1 Pack/400g	280	8.4	70	2.1	10.6	2.1	2.1
Mince, Christmas, Finest, Tesco*	1 Pie/66g	257	8.8	390	4.6	62.4	13.3	2.6
Mince, Christmas, Sainsbury's*	1 Pie/37g	147	6.0	397	4.5	58.0	16.3	2.6
Mince, Dusted, Mini, Finest, Tesco*	1 Pie/20g	76	2.4	379	7.3	62.9	12.2	5.0
Mince, Extra Special, Asda*	1 Pie/60g	225	8.3	378	3.9	59.0	14.0	2.2
Mince, Iced Top, Asda*	1 Pie/57g	215	7.1	378	2.8	63.7	12.4	1.1
Mince, Iced Top, Tesco*	1 Pie/55g	209	6.3	380	3.1	65.7	11.4	2.1
Mince, Individual, Average	1 Pie/48g	203	9.8	423	4.3	59.0	20.4	2.1
Mince, Lattice, Classics, M & S*	1 Pie/53g	210	8.0	400	4.0	61.7	15.2	2.4
Mince, Luxury, Deep Filled, M & S*	1 Pie/65g	234	9.0	360	4.3	55.0	13.8	3.8
Mince, Mini, M & S*	1 Pie/28g	105	4.0	380	4.3	57.8	14.6	4.0
Mince, Mini, Waitrose*	1 Pie/30g	150	9.1	501	5.7	51.3	30.3	1.7
Mince, Organic, Sainsbury's*	1 Pie/46g	177	7.5	384	5.0	54.5	16.2	5.6
Mince, Shortcrust, Waitrose*	1 Pie/55g	210	8.0	385	3.6	60.0	14.6	20.9
Mince, Star Motif, Mini, Finest, Tesco*	1 Pie/17g	62	2.1	365	3.8	59.9	12.1	3.8
Mince Puff, Tesco*	1 Pie/25g	105	4.4	420	3.3	62.0	17.6	2.0
Minced Beef, Plate, M & S*	1oz/28g	71	4.5	253	7.6	20.7	16.0	2.0
Minced Beef & Onion, Birds Eye*	1 Pie/145g	419	25.1	289	7.1	26.3	17.3	0.7
Minced Beef & Onion, Denny*	1 Sm Pie/140g	288	19.7	206	6.1	17.3	14.1	0.0
Minced Beef & Onion, Tesco*	1 Pie/150g	454	28.5	303	5.7	27.4	19.0	1.7
Minced Beef & Potato, Weight Watchers*	1 Pie/200g	328	12.4	164	6.7	20.2	6.2	3.6
Minced Beef & Vegetable, Pot, M & S*	1/3 Pie/183g	366	26.5	200	7.8	9.1	14.5	7.1
Mississippi Mud, Tesco*	1 Serving/104g	399	26.6	384	5.3	33.1	25.6	1.8
Moroccan Vegetable & Feta, Little, Higgidy*	1 Pie/180g	418	22.5	232	5.1	24.7	12.5	0.6
Mushroom & Leaf Spinach, Little, Higgidy*	1 Pie/180g	441	25.9	245	6.6	22.3	14.4	0.7
Mushroom & Parsley Potato, Waitrose*	1 Pack/350g	346	17.5	99	2.5	10.9	5.0	1.2
Ocean, BGTY, Sainsbury's*	1 Pack/350g	285	4.7	81	6.3	11.1	1.3	0.8
Ocean, Frozen, BGTY, Sainsbury's*	1 Pack/350g	318	5.2	91	7.0	12.4	1.5	0.9
Ocean, M & S*	1 Pie/650g	617	22.7	95	8.2	7.6	3.5	0.9
Ocean, Original, Frozen, Youngs*	1 Pack/375g	420	21.4	112	7.6	7.6	5.7	0.9
Ocean, The Original, Light & Easy, Youngs*	1 Pack/415g	432	18.7	104	6.4	9.5	4.5	1.0
Ocean, Weight Watchers*	1 Pack/300g	204	3.9	68	4.5	9.5	1.3	0.2
Pork, & Egg, M & S*	¼ Pie/108g	379	28.0	351	9.7	19.8	25.9	0.8
Pork, & Pickle, Bowyers*	1 Pie/150g	576	40.9	384	10.0	26.3	27.3	0.0
Pork, Buffet, Bowyers*	1 Pie/60g	217	14.7	362	10.4	24.9	24.5	0.0
Pork, Cheese & Pickle, Mini, Tesco*	1 Pie/49g	191	12.8	389	9.2	29.3	26.1	1.2
Pork, Crusty Bake, Mini, Sainsbury's*	1 Pie/43g	165	11.2	384	11.5	26.0	26.0	1.5

PIE

	Measure INFO/WEIGHT	per Measure KCAL	FAT	Nutrition Values per 100g / 100ml KCAL	PROT	CARB	FAT	FIBRE
Pork, Crusty Bake, Sainsbury's*	1 Pie/75g	292	20.0	390	10.5	27.0	26.7	1.0
Pork, Geo Adams*	1 Pie/125g	487	34.7	390	11.8	23.1	27.8	0.9
Pork, Medium, Pork Farms*	1 Pie/200g	744	53.0	372	9.5	23.6	26.5	1.7
Pork, Melton, Mini, Pork Farms*	1 Pie/50g	199	14.6	399	8.9	26.2	29.2	0.0
Pork, Melton Mowbray, Cured, M & S*	1 Pie/290g	1044	71.0	360	10.1	25.9	24.5	1.0
Pork, Melton Mowbray, Cured, Mini, M & S*	1 Pie/50g	192	12.2	385	9.8	32.6	24.4	1.0
Pork, Melton Mowbray, Individual, Sainsbury's*	1 Pie/75g	296	20.8	395	10.2	26.1	27.7	2.4
Pork, Melton Mowbray, Large, Co-Op*	¼ Pie/110g	418	35.2	380	11.0	12.0	32.0	5.0
Pork, Melton Mowbray, Lattice, Sainsbury's*	1 Serving/100g	342	23.6	342	10.8	21.7	23.6	1.2
Pork, Melton Mowbray, Mini, Morrisons*	1 Pie/50g	197	12.5	393	10.9	31.3	24.9	0.9
Pork, Melton Mowbray, Mini, Tesco*	1 Pie/50g	196	14.3	392	12.6	20.8	28.7	2.9
Pork, Melton Mowbray, Uncured, Small, Tesco*	1 Pie/140g	465	29.5	332	11.2	24.4	21.1	2.4
Pork, Mini, Christmas, Tesco*	1 Pie/50g	195	13.5	390	10.6	25.7	27.0	1.4
Pork, Mini, Pack of 2, Ginsters*	2 Pies/100g	386	26.1	386	11.2	26.7	26.1	1.7
Pork, VLH Kitchens*	1 Pie/36g	168	13.0	466	11.0	26.0	36.0	0.0
Pork, with Cheese & Pickle, Waitrose*	1 Pack/150g	568	36.9	379	10.3	29.1	24.6	2.7
Quorn, Cottage, Tesco*	½ Pack/250g	167	5.1	67	5.1	22.4	2.0	3.7
Rhubarb, Sara Lee*	1 Serving/90g	224	12.4	250	2.9	28.7	13.8	1.3
Roast Chicken, COU, M & S*	1 Pack/320g	272	3.2	85	9.4	9.7	1.0	0.8
Roast Chicken, M & S*	1/3 Pie/182g	465	24.1	255	7.8	26.4	13.2	2.2
Roast Chicken & Vegetable, Pot, M & S*	1/3 Pie/183g	366	22.9	200	7.7	13.5	12.5	4.5
Salmon, Crumble, Light & Easy, Youngs*	1 Pack/320g	282	6.4	88	5.7	11.8	2.0	1.0
Salmon & Broccoli, Birds Eye*	1 Pie/351g	449	21.8	128	6.6	11.4	6.2	0.7
Salmon & Broccoli, Filo Pastry, Finest, Tesco*	1 Pie/170g	386	22.6	227	7.9	18.9	13.3	2.1
Salmon & Broccoli, Light Choices, Tesco*	1 Pack/400g	350	7.2	87	7.0	10.2	1.8	1.7
Salmon & Broccoli, Premium, Tesco*	1 Serving/170g	425	29.2	250	6.1	17.7	17.2	0.7
Salmon & Broccoli Lattice Bar, Asda*	1/3 Bar/133g	360	19.9	271	6.0	28.0	15.0	0.8
Sausage & Onion, Lattice, Puff Pastry, Tesco*	1/3 Pie/133g	480	22.5	361	9.1	20.6	16.9	4.6
Sausage & Onion, Tesco*	1 Pack/300g	333	18.3	111	2.3	11.7	6.1	0.5
Scotch, Co-Op*	1 Pie/132g	408	24.9	309	7.3	27.3	18.9	1.5
Shepherd's, Average	1oz/28g	31	1.7	112	6.0	9.3	5.9	0.7
Shepherd's, Baked Bean Cuisine, Heinz*	1 Pie/340g	299	9.5	88	4.1	11.6	2.8	1.5
Shepherd's, BGTY, Sainsbury's*	1 Pack/300g	225	6.6	75	3.6	10.2	2.2	1.7
Shepherd's, Chilled, Finest, Tesco*	½ Pack/400g	460	16.4	115	6.9	8.0	4.1	1.9
Shepherd's, COU, M & S*	1 Pack/300g	210	3.9	70	5.2	8.6	1.3	1.6
Shepherd's, Diet Chef Ltd*	1 Serving/270g	235	10.5	87	3.2	9.8	3.9	1.9
Shepherd's, Weight Watchers*	1 Pack/320g	221	7.4	69	3.2	8.8	2.3	0.3
Shepherd's, Welsh Hill Lamb, Gastropub, M & S*	½ Pack/330g	313	11.5	95	5.4	10.2	3.5	1.5
Steak, Braised, Shortcrust Pastry, Asda*	½ Pack/260g	785	46.8	302	9.0	26.0	18.0	0.9
Steak, Deep Fill, Tesco*	¼ Pie/195g	468	25.5	240	9.7	20.0	13.1	1.5
Steak, Dietary Specials*	1 Pie/140g	328	14.4	234	9.8	25.7	10.3	0.4
Steak, in Rich Gravy, Aunt Bessie's*	¼ Pie/200g	440	20.6	220	9.6	22.0	10.3	1.5
Steak, Individual, British Classics, Tesco*	1 Pie/150g	450	27.6	300	9.1	23.3	18.4	2.5
Steak, Large, Glenfell*	¼ Pie/170g	445	27.9	262	6.8	21.8	16.4	1.0
Steak, M & S*	1oz/28g	64	3.6	230	10.0	19.0	12.7	1.2
Steak, Mini, Asda*	1 Serving/67g	117	5.3	176	9.0	17.0	8.0	0.9
Steak, Mushroom & Ale, Topcrust, Waitrose*	1 Pie/250g	500	29.5	200	11.1	12.2	11.8	1.1
Steak, Puff Pastry, Deep Filled, Sainsbury's*	1 Pie/210g	535	30.0	255	10.3	21.2	14.3	2.0
Steak, Scotch, Bell's Bakery*	1 Serving/150g	378	20.2	252	13.6	18.6	13.5	0.7
Steak, Short Crust, Sainsbury's*	½ Pie/118g	314	24.1	267	10.9	22.2	20.5	1.7
Steak, Shortcrust Pastry, Finest, Tesco*	1 Pie/250g	660	37.7	264	10.9	21.2	15.1	0.8
Steak, Tesco*	1 Serving/205g	556	33.8	271	7.2	23.3	16.5	1.4
Steak, Top Crust, TTD, Sainsbury's*	½ Pie/299g	530	23.1	177	15.4	11.4	7.7	0.5

PIE	Measure INFO/WEIGHT	per Measure KCAL	FAT	Nutrition Values per 100g / 100ml KCAL	PROT	CARB	FAT	FIBRE
Steak, TTD, Sainsbury's*	½ Pie/300g	713	35.4	238	12.6	20.3	11.8	1.0
Steak & Ale, Deep Fill, Puff Pastry, Tesco*	¼ Pie/150g	324	19.6	216	8.0	16.6	13.1	2.3
Steak & Ale, Fray Bentos*	1 Pie/425g	697	38.7	164	7.6	13.0	9.1	0.0
Steak & Ale, Pub Style, Co-Op*	1 Pie/250g	537	30.0	215	9.0	17.0	12.0	2.0
Steak & Ale, Puff Pastry, Asda*	1/3 Pie/200g	520	30.2	260	10.6	20.4	15.1	1.6
Steak & Ale, Sainsbury's*	1 Serving/190g	445	23.4	234	8.3	22.6	12.3	0.9
Steak & Ale, TTD, Sainsbury's*	1 Pie/250g	681	35.6	272	11.6	24.4	14.2	1.4
Steak & Ale with Chips & Gravy	1 Serving/400g	825	42.2	206	7.2	20.5	10.6	0.5
Steak & Dorset Ale, Mini, Finest, Tesco*	1 Pie/30g	91	4.9	305	7.9	31.4	16.4	1.9
Steak & Guinness, Sainsbury's*	¼ Pie/137g	399	25.5	291	8.7	22.2	18.6	1.0
Steak & Kidney, Birds Eye*	1 Pie/146g	447	28.5	306	9.0	23.7	19.5	2.3
Steak & Kidney, Deep Fill, Sainsbury's*	½ Pie/125g	314	18.6	251	8.4	21.0	14.9	2.0
Steak & Kidney, Individual	1 Pie/200g	646	42.4	323	9.1	25.6	21.2	0.9
Steak & Kidney, Princes*	½ Pack/212g	379	19.9	179	8.8	14.8	9.4	0.0
Steak & Kidney, Puff Pastry, Sainsbury's*	1 Pie/150g	423	23.5	282	8.2	26.9	15.7	0.9
Steak & Kidney, Tinned, Fray Bentos*	½ Pie/212g	346	18.7	163	8.2	12.9	8.8	0.0
Steak & Mushroom, Asda*	1 Pie/130g	350	18.1	270	9.0	27.0	14.0	1.4
Steak & Mushroom, Deep Fill, Asda*	1/3 Pie/175g	476	28.0	272	11.0	21.0	16.0	1.1
Steak & Mushroom, Deep Fill, Puff Pastry, Tesco*	1 Slice/150g	339	20.7	226	9.1	16.3	13.8	1.9
Steak & Mushroom, Finest, Tesco*	1 Pie/250g	640	36.5	256	9.2	21.9	14.6	1.1
Steak & Mushroom, Home Comforts, Weight Watchers*	1 Pie/136g	322	15.9	237	5.8	26.9	11.7	1.4
Steak & Mushroom, Individual, Birds Eye*	1 Pie/142g	389	24.1	274	7.5	22.7	17.0	2.0
Steak & Mushroom, McDougalls*	1 Pack/340g	779	57.8	229	9.0	10.0	17.0	0.9
Steak & Mushroom, Sainsbury's*	¼ Pie/130g	372	21.3	286	8.6	26.0	16.4	1.0
Steak & Onion, Ginsters*	1 Pie/180g	481	30.8	267	8.0	20.3	17.1	1.3
Steak & Onion, Minced, Aberdeen Angus, Tesco*	½ Pie/300g	897	57.6	299	9.4	22.1	19.2	0.7
Steak & Peppered Sauce, Gastro Style, McDougalls*	1 Pie/192g	495	28.8	258	8.9	21.4	15.0	0.9
Steak & Potato, Asda*	1/3 Pie/173g	442	26.0	255	6.9	23.1	15.0	0.9
Steak & Red Wine, Puff Pastry, Pub, Sainsbury's*	1 Pie/240g	497	29.5	207	7.2	16.8	12.3	2.1
Summer Fruits, Orchard Tree*	1/8 Pie/75g	242	10.3	323	3.0	46.6	13.8	1.2
Teviot, Minced Beef, Morrisons*	½ Pie/250g	382	17.2	153	8.0	14.5	6.9	1.6
Tuna & Sweetcorn, HL, Tesco*	1 Pack/450g	391	12.1	87	7.1	8.6	2.7	2.0
Turkey & Ham, Shortcrust, M & S*	1/3 Pie/183g	494	29.1	270	11.9	19.5	15.9	1.0
Vegetable	1oz/28g	42	2.1	151	3.0	18.9	7.6	1.5
Vegetable & Cheddar Cheese, Waitrose*	1 Pie/210g	475	31.5	226	4.9	17.8	15.0	1.2
Vegetable & Cheese, Asda*	1 Pie/141g	330	16.2	234	5.8	26.9	11.5	1.0
Vegetarian, Cottage, Mealpak, All About Weight*	1 Sachet/32g	120	2.8	375	28.6	36.0	8.6	10.0
Vegetarian, Deep Country, Linda McCartney*	1 Pie/166g	412	22.8	248	5.1	26.1	13.7	1.4
Vegetarian, Shepherd's, Linda McCartney*	1 Pack/340g	286	7.5	84	3.7	12.3	2.2	2.3
Vegetarian, Vegetable Cumberland, M & S*	½ Pack/211g	190	5.5	90	2.8	13.4	2.6	1.6
Welsh Lamb, Sainsbury's*	¼ Pie/120g	290	17.2	242	9.1	19.2	14.3	0.8
West Country Chicken, Sainsbury's*	1 Serving/240g	614	37.4	256	11.9	17.1	15.6	2.1
PIE FILLING								
Apple, Sainsbury's*	1 Serving/75g	67	0.1	89	0.1	22.1	0.1	1.0
Black Cherry, Fruit, Sainsbury's*	1 Serving/100g	73	0.1	73	0.3	17.7	0.1	0.3
Blackcurrant, Fruit, Sainsbury's*	1 Serving/100g	82	0.1	82	0.4	20.0	0.1	1.6
Cherry	1oz/28g	23	0.0	82	0.4	21.5	0.0	0.4
Fruit	1oz/28g	22	0.0	77	0.4	20.1	0.0	1.0
PIGEON								
Meat Only, Roasted, Average	**1 Pigeon/115g**	**215**	**9.1**	**187**	**29.0**	**0.0**	**7.9**	**0.0**
Meat Only, Roasted, Weighed with Bone, Average	**1oz/28g**	**25**	**1.0**	**88**	**13.6**	**0.0**	**3.7**	**0.0**
PIKELETS								
Classics, M & S*	1 Pikelet/35g	70	0.5	200	7.3	39.1	1.3	1.6

	Measure INFO/WEIGHT	per Measure		Nutrition Values per 100g / 100ml				
		KCAL	FAT	KCAL	PROT	CARB	FAT	FIBRE
PIKELETS								
Free From, Tesco*	1 Pikelet/30g	58	1.3	194	2.8	36.2	4.3	1.4
Tesco*	1 Pikelet/35g	68	0.2	193	5.8	40.9	0.7	1.7
PILAF								
Bulgar Wheat, Sainsbury's*	1 Pack/381g	347	11.1	91	3.9	12.3	2.9	6.3
Forest Mushroom & Pine Nut, Bistro, Waitrose*	1 Serving/225g	337	14.6	150	7.0	15.8	6.5	1.5
with Tomato, Average	1oz/28g	40	0.9	144	2.5	28.0	3.3	0.4
PILCHARDS								
Fillets, in Tomato Sauce, Average	1 Can/120g	158	7.8	132	16.2	2.2	6.5	0.1
Fillets, in Virgin Olive Oil, Glenryck*	1 Serving/92g	223	14.4	242	23.3	2.0	15.7	0.0
in Brine, Average	*½ Can/77g*	*114*	*5.6*	*148*	*20.8*	*0.0*	*7.3*	*0.0*
PIMMS*								
& Lemonade, Premixed, Canned, Pimms*	1 Can/250ml	160	0.0	64	0.0	84.0	0.0	0.0
25% Volume, Pimms￼*	*1 Serving/25ml*	*40*	*0.0*	*160*	*0.0*	*5.0*	*0.0*	*0.0*
PINE NUTS								
Average	*1oz/28g*	*195*	*19.2*	*695*	*15.7*	*3.9*	*68.6*	*1.9*
PINEAPPLE								
& Papaya, Dried, Garden Gang, Asda*	1 Pack/50g	141	0.8	283	2.8	64.0	1.7	8.0
Dried, Sweetened, Ready to Eat, Tesco*	1/5 Pack/50g	117	0.9	235	0.4	52.9	1.9	1.7
Dried, Tropical Wholefoods*	1 Slice/10g	30	0.0	305	2.9	73.9	0.2	5.2
Dried, Unsweetened, Sainsbury's*	1 Bag/75g	255	1.5	340	1.7	84.7	2.0	6.0
in Juice, Average	*1 Can/106g*	*57*	*0.0*	*53*	*0.3*	*12.9*	*0.0*	*0.6*
in Own Juice, Del Monte*	1 Can/432g	298	0.4	69	0.4	15.5	0.1	0.0
in Syrup, Average	*1 Can/240g*	*158*	*0.0*	*66*	*0.3*	*16.1*	*0.0*	*0.8*
Pieces, Yoghurt Coated, Holland & Barrett*	1 Pack/100g	344	19.3	344	2.1	46.8	19.3	0.6
Raw, Flesh Only, Average	*1 Fruit/472g*	*233*	*0.7*	*49*	*0.4*	*11.6*	*0.1*	*0.9*
PISTACHIO NUTS								
Raw, Average, without Shells	1 Serving/20g	111	8.9	557	20.6	28.0	44.4	10.3
Roasted, Graze*	1 Pack/50g	166	15.5	333	9.9	4.6	31.0	0.0
Roasted & Salted, Average	*1 Serving/25g*	*152*	*13.6*	*608*	*19.6*	*9.9*	*54.5*	*6.1*
Roasted & Salted, Love Life, Waitrose*	1 Serving/25g	144	13.0	576	18.5	8.2	52.1	6.1
Salted, Lemon, Graze*	1 Box/26g	148	12.0	568	21.4	26.8	46.0	0.0
Shelled, Kernels, Wholesome, Love Life, Waitrose*	1 Serving/30g	181	16.6	603	17.9	8.2	55.4	10.3
PIZZA								
American Hot, 8 Inch, Supermarket, Pizza Express*	1 Pizza/295g	652	22.4	221	11.0	27.3	7.6	3.5
American Hot, Chicago Town*	1 Pizza/170g	445	20.1	262	8.2	30.8	11.8	0.9
Bacon, Mushroom & Tomato, HL, Tesco*	1 Pizza/231g	395	6.2	171	10.6	25.9	2.7	1.5
Bacon, Mushroom & Tomato, Stonebaked, Tesco*	1 Serving/173g	351	12.8	203	9.9	24.1	7.4	2.0
Bacon & Mushroom, Stone Bake, M & S*	1 Pizza/375g	750	24.0	200	9.9	27.2	6.4	1.6
Bacon & Mushroom, Thin & Crispy, Sainsbury's*	½ Pizza/150g	396	15.9	264	12.9	29.2	10.6	1.7
Bacon & Mushroom Pizzeria, Sainsbury's*	1 Pizza/355g	880	24.8	248	11.7	34.5	7.0	3.7
BBQ Chicken, M & S*	½ Pizza/210g	430	11.8	205	11.6	27.5	5.6	1.8
BBQ Chicken, Stonebaked, Tesco*	½ Pizza/158g	285	9.5	180	10.5	20.9	6.0	3.9
BBQ Chicken, Thin & Crispy, Sainsbury's*	½ Pizza/147g	384	12.1	261	13.8	33.1	8.2	1.6
BBQ Chicken, Thin & Crispy, Tesco*	1 Serving/165g	355	7.4	215	11.9	31.6	4.5	1.2
BBQ Chicken, Weight Watchers*	1 Pizza/224g	412	7.8	184	11.5	26.5	3.5	2.7
BBQ Chicken Stuffed Crust, Asda*	½ Pizza/245g	612	24.5	250	13.0	27.0	10.0	2.7
Bianca, Bistro, Waitrose*	½ Pizza/207g	618	32.6	298	12.9	26.2	15.7	2.3
Cajun Chicken, BGTY, Sainsbury's*	½ Pizza/165g	363	5.9	220	11.0	36.0	3.6	1.7
Cajun Chicken, Pizzatilla, M & S*	½ Pizza/240g	636	36.2	265	10.5	21.8	15.1	1.3
Cajun Chicken, Sainsbury's*	½ Pizza/146g	285	2.6	195	12.9	31.8	1.8	2.6
Cajun Style Chicken, Stonebaked, Tesco*	1 Pizza/561g	1318	55.0	235	11.9	24.8	9.8	1.4
Calzone Speciale, Ristorante, Dr Oetker*	½ Pizza/145g	378	23.2	261	11.5	22.1	16.0	0.0
Charged Up Chilli Beef, Goodfella's*	½ Pizza/357g	857	32.8	240	12.8	26.4	9.2	1.6

P

PIZZA

	Measure INFO/WEIGHT	per Measure KCAL	FAT	Nutrition Values per 100g / 100ml KCAL	PROT	CARB	FAT	FIBRE
Chargrilled Chicken, Iceland*	1 Pizza/381g	804	25.5	211	12.3	25.4	6.7	2.0
Chargrilled Chicken, Thin & Crispy, Asda*	1 Pizza/373g	780	18.6	209	9.0	32.0	5.0	1.6
Chargrilled Chicken & Vegetable, GFY, Asda*	½ Pizza/166g	355	3.3	214	13.0	36.0	2.0	2.0
Chargrilled Chicken & Vegetable, Low Fat, Bertorelli*	1 Pizza/180g	439	7.9	244	14.2	39.3	4.4	2.3
Chargrilled Vegetable, Frozen, BGTY, Sainsbury's*	1 Pizza/290g	548	13.3	189	10.2	26.7	4.6	3.0
Chargrilled Vegetable, Thin & Crispy, GFY, Asda*	1 Serving/188g	290	3.8	154	6.0	28.0	2.0	3.1
Cheese, Deep Pan, Tesco*	½ Pizza/455g	990	26.4	218	11.4	29.8	5.8	3.1
Cheese, Onion & Garlic, Pizzeria, Waitrose*	½ Pizza/245g	684	28.9	279	10.8	29.8	11.8	2.5
Cheese, Stuffed, Crust, Sainsbury's*	1 Pizza/525g	1428	52.5	272	14.0	31.5	10.0	2.0
Cheese, Thin & Crispy, Goodfella's*	1 Serving/275g	729	27.8	265	15.7	27.6	10.1	1.8
Cheese, Three, Slice, Microwaveable, Tesco*	1 Slice/160g	486	18.7	304	13.3	36.7	11.7	1.6
Cheese & Onion, Tesco*	1 Serving/22g	56	2.0	255	10.5	32.7	9.1	2.7
Cheese & Tomato, Average	1 Serving/300g	711	35.4	237	9.1	25.2	11.8	1.4
Cheese & Tomato, Deep & Crispy, Tesco*	1 Serving/197g	455	13.4	231	10.8	31.7	6.8	1.2
Cheese & Tomato, Deep Pan, Goodfella's*	¼ Pizza/102g	259	10.8	253	11.5	29.6	10.5	3.7
Cheese & Tomato, French Bread, Co-Op*	1 Pizza/135g	270	8.1	200	9.0	27.0	6.0	2.0
Cheese & Tomato, Fresh, Tesco*	1/3 Pizza/160g	413	13.8	258	9.6	36.3	8.6	1.4
Cheese & Tomato, Micro, McCain*	1 Pizza/122g	319	12.2	262	13.4	29.7	10.0	2.4
Cheese & Tomato, Mini, Bruschetta, Iceland*	1 Pizza/34g	63	2.3	188	8.0	23.0	7.0	2.1
Cheese & Tomato, Mini, M & S*	1 Pizza/95g	233	5.5	245	10.0	38.7	5.8	1.6
Cheese & Tomato, Piccadella, Tesco*	1 Pizza/295g	684	31.4	232	9.1	24.8	10.6	1.5
Cheese & Tomato, Retail, Frozen	1oz/28g	70	3.0	250	7.5	32.9	10.7	1.4
Cheese & Tomato, Square, Sainsbury's*	1 Square/160g	435	11.7	272	14.0	37.6	7.3	2.1
Cheese & Tomato, Stonebaked, Co-Op*	1 Pizza/325g	699	26.0	215	11.0	26.0	8.0	3.0
Cheese & Tomato, Stonebaked, Organic, Co-Op*	1 Pizza/330g	676	23.1	205	9.0	26.0	7.0	4.0
Cheese & Tomato, Stonebaked, Thin & Crispy, Tesco*	½ Pizza/161g	388	13.8	241	11.6	29.4	8.6	2.1
Cheese & Tomato, Thin & Crispy, Waitrose*	1 Pizza/280g	658	28.3	235	12.3	23.6	10.1	2.3
Cheese & Tomato French Bread, Findus*	1 Serving/143g	322	11.6	225	9.4	29.0	8.1	0.0
Cheese & Tomato Range, Italiano, Tesco*	1 Pizza/380g	969	35.0	255	11.4	31.7	9.2	3.3
Cheese & Tomato Slice, Ross*	1 Slice/77g	148	6.6	192	6.5	22.2	8.6	2.0
Cheese Feast, Deep Pan, Asda*	½ Pizza/210g	422	18.9	201	13.0	17.0	9.0	2.3
Cheese Feast, Thin Crust, Chilled, Tesco*	½ Pizza/175g	467	22.4	267	14.7	23.4	12.8	2.5
Cheese Supreme, New Recipe, Goodfella's*	¼ Pizza/102g	269	10.2	264	12.3	31.2	10.0	2.2
Cheesefeast, Deep & Crispy 12", Takeaway, Iceland*	1 Slice/132g	342	11.1	259	13.1	32.8	8.4	1.5
Chicken, Thin & Crispy, Iceland*	½ Pizza/157g	469	19.9	299	13.0	33.2	12.7	3.1
Chicken & Bacon, Loaded, Tesco*	1 Serving/258g	622	25.3	241	12.8	25.4	9.8	1.9
Chicken & Bacon Carbonara, Thin Crust, Italian, Asda*	1 Pizza/492g	1156	34.4	235	12.0	31.0	7.0	3.4
Chicken & Chorizo, 12", TTD, Sainsbury's*	½ Pizza/290g	702	20.9	242	12.2	32.1	7.2	2.6
Chicken & Maple Bacon Carbonara, Asda*	½ Pizza/195g	484	15.6	248	11.0	33.0	8.0	2.2
Chicken & Pesto, Californian Style, Asda*	½ Pizza/235g	533	16.4	227	10.0	31.0	7.0	2.0
Chicken & Sweetcorn, Stonebaked, Tesco*	1 Serving/177g	354	9.6	200	11.9	26.0	5.4	2.0
Chicken & Vegetable, Chargrill, Italiano, Tesco*	½ Pizza/184g	383	14.7	208	10.6	23.3	8.0	2.4
Chicken & Vegetable, Stone Baked, GFY, Asda*	½ Pizza/161g	349	3.7	217	13.0	36.0	2.3	1.7
Chicken Alfredo, Chicago Town*	1 Pizza/265g	583	24.9	220	11.9	21.9	9.4	1.8
Chicken Arrabbiata, Italian Style, M & S*	½ Pizza/225g	495	15.7	220	12.3	26.3	7.0	2.0
Chicken Arrabiata, Sainsbury's*	½ Pizza/191g	444	12.2	232	12.1	31.4	6.4	1.7
Chicken Provencal, Goodfella's*	½ Pizza/143g	388	18.0	272	13.7	25.9	12.6	2.1
Chicken Tikka, Stonebaked, Tesco*	1 Serving/153g	326	10.4	213	10.7	27.3	6.8	1.3
Chilli Beef, Stone Bake, M & S*	1 Pizza/395g	790	22.9	200	9.6	26.7	5.8	1.9
Cream Cheese & Pepperonata, Calzone, Waitrose*	½ Pizza/165g	383	15.8	232	7.0	29.4	9.6	1.5
Deep South, Chicago Town*	1 Pizza/171g	363	12.1	212	6.9	30.0	7.1	0.0
Double Cheese, Chicago Town*	1 Pizza/405g	931	27.1	230	11.7	30.6	6.7	0.0
Easy Cheesy, Deep Pan, Chicago Town*	½ Pizza/547g	1455	59.1	266	11.4	30.9	10.8	1.7

PIZZA

PIZZA	Measure INFO/WEIGHT	per Measure KCAL	FAT	KCAL	PROT	CARB	FAT	FIBRE
Etruscan Pepperoni, TTD, Sainsbury's*	½ Pizza/252g	676	20.9	268	13.2	35.1	8.3	2.4
Fajita Chicken, COU, M & S*	1 Pizza/255g	433	6.1	170	9.9	25.5	2.4	1.2
Fajita Vegetable, BGTY, Sainsbury's*	1 Pizza/214g	366	3.0	171	8.9	30.8	1.4	2.9
Fingers, Oven Baked, McCain*	1 Finger/30g	78	2.4	261	12.6	34.8	7.9	2.4
Fingers & Curly Fries, M & S*	1 Pack/212g	360	10.4	170	7.9	22.9	4.9	1.6
Fire Roasted Pepper, Sainsbury's*	1 Pizza/344g	605	5.2	176	5.3	35.3	1.5	1.6
Fire Roasted Peppers & Vegetables, Waitrose*	½ Pizza/235g	442	16.7	188	9.8	21.3	7.1	2.7
Five Cheese & Pepperoni, Deep & Crispy, Waitrose*	1/3 Pizza/200g	560	23.2	280	11.7	32.3	11.6	1.3
Flamed Chicken & Vegetables, BGTY, Sainsbury's*	1 Pizza/260g	660	11.4	254	14.2	39.3	4.4	2.3
Flamin' Hot, Deep Dish, Chicago Town*	1 Pizza/170g	454	20.4	267	8.6	31.1	12.0	0.0
Four Cheese, Finest, Tesco*	½ Pizza/230g	575	21.2	250	12.1	29.8	9.2	1.3
Four Cheese, M & S*	1oz/28g	67	2.1	240	13.2	30.3	7.5	1.2
Four Cheese, Thin & Crispy, Sainsbury's*	1 Pizza/265g	729	32.6	275	11.8	29.3	12.3	3.5
Four Cheese, Thin Crust, Tesco*	½ Pizza/142g	386	13.6	272	14.5	31.8	9.6	1.8
Four Cheese, Weight Watchers*	1 Pizza/186g	400	7.0	215	10.7	34.9	3.8	1.6
Four Cheese & Tomato, Pizzatilla, M & S*	1 Serving/69g	225	13.8	324	10.5	26.0	19.9	1.5
Four Seasons, Waitrose*	1/3 Pizza/174g	382	14.6	220	9.9	26.2	8.4	2.6
French Bread, Blue Parrot Cafe, Sainsbury's*	1 Pizza/132g	271	5.7	205	10.7	30.8	4.3	1.3
Funghi, Ristorante, Dr Oetker*	1 Pizza/365g	865	43.4	237	7.9	22.5	11.9	0.0
Garlic & Mushroom, Asda*	½ Pizza/241g	696	41.0	289	10.0	24.0	17.0	1.6
Garlic & Mushroom, Thin & Crispy, Sainsbury's*	1 Pizza/260g	829	43.2	319	11.1	31.2	16.6	1.7
Garlic Bread, Stonebaked, Italiano, Tesco*	1 Serving/117g	403	18.2	346	7.8	43.6	15.6	1.5
Garlic Chicken, Deep Pan, Sainsbury's*	½ Pizza/214g	464	13.9	217	11.2	28.3	6.5	3.3
Garlic Chicken, Thin & Crispy, Stonebake, Sainsbury's*	½ Pizza/160g	386	17.3	241	10.7	25.2	10.8	3.5
Garlic Mushroom, BGTY, Sainsbury's*	½ Pizza/123g	262	2.5	213	11.6	37.2	2.0	2.7
Garlic Mushroom, Classico, Tesco*	½ Pizza/208g	415	13.9	200	10.0	24.9	6.7	2.6
Garlic Mushroom, Tesco*	1 Pizza/425g	829	34.0	195	9.3	21.6	8.0	5.3
Garlic Mushroom, Thin & Crispy, Weight Watchers*	1 Pizza/240g	410	3.1	171	11.2	28.8	1.3	3.0
Garlic Mushroom, Thin Crust, Tesco*	½ Pizza/163g	340	14.6	209	11.0	21.1	9.0	3.6
Giardiniera, From Supermarket, Pizza Express*	½ Pizza/144g	291	10.5	202	8.6	25.5	7.3	2.1
Grilled Pepper, Weight Watchers*	1 Pizza/220g	392	5.1	178	10.0	29.3	2.3	1.8
Ham, Mushroom & Gruyere, Sainsbury's*	¼ Pizza/169g	404	13.7	239	10.2	31.3	8.1	3.7
Ham, Mushroom & Mascarpone, Italian Style, M & S*	1 Pizza/224g	515	21.7	230	10.0	25.5	9.7	2.9
Ham, Mushroom & Tomato, BGTY, Sainsbury's*	½ Pizza/150g	309	6.1	206	11.8	30.4	4.1	1.2
Ham, Pepperoni & Milano, M & S*	1 Pizza/290g	696	28.4	240	14.0	23.3	9.8	1.1
Ham & Cheese, Chunky, Asda*	1 Serving/90g	211	3.0	234	12.0	39.0	3.3	4.7
Ham & Mushroom, BGTY, Sainsbury's*	1 Pizza/248g	526	3.5	212	12.1	37.8	1.4	2.9
Ham & Mushroom, Deep & Crispy, Tesco*	1 Serving/210g	420	10.3	200	9.7	29.2	4.9	1.1
Ham & Mushroom, Deep Pan, Waitrose*	½ Pizza/220g	453	13.6	206	10.9	26.6	6.2	1.0
Ham & Mushroom, Finest, Tesco*	½ Pizza/240g	576	26.4	240	9.5	25.9	11.0	2.2
Ham & Mushroom, New, BGTY, Sainsbury's*	1 Pizza/248g	526	3.5	212	12.1	37.8	1.4	2.9
Ham & Mushroom, Stone Baked, Goodfella's*	½ Pizza/175g	439	19.9	251	9.6	27.6	11.4	1.2
Ham & Mushroom, Tesco*	1/6 Pizza/57g	132	4.4	232	11.2	29.2	7.8	1.9
Ham & Mushroom, Thin & Crispy, Asda*	1 Pizza/360g	760	25.2	211	11.0	26.0	7.0	2.4
Ham & Mushroom Calzone, Waitrose*	½ Pizza/145g	362	13.5	250	10.0	31.6	9.3	1.6
Ham & Onion, Tesco*	1 Serving/181g	452	17.4	250	11.8	29.0	9.6	2.2
Ham & Pineapple, American Deep Pan, Sainsbury's*	1 Pizza/412g	1001	32.1	243	10.5	32.6	7.8	1.7
Ham & Pineapple, Chicago Town*	1 Pizza/435g	866	19.6	199	10.0	29.7	4.5	0.0
Ham & Pineapple, Deep & Loaded, Sainsbury's*	1 Pizza/515g	1102	26.8	214	10.2	31.7	5.2	3.5
Ham & Pineapple, Deep Dish, Individual, Chicago Town*	1 Pizza/170g	410	15.1	241	9.9	30.4	8.9	1.6
Ham & Pineapple, Deep Pan, Ciabatta, Iceland*	½ Pizza/185g	440	14.4	238	11.6	30.3	7.8	0.8
Ham & Pineapple, Deep Pan, Tesco*	1 Pizza/237g	437	6.9	184	9.8	29.8	2.9	1.9
Ham & Pineapple, HL, Tesco*	¼ Pizza/105g	170	2.2	162	10.0	25.9	2.1	2.4

PIZZA

INFO/WEIGHT	Measure		per Measure		Nutrition Values per 100g / 100ml				
			KCAL	FAT	KCAL	PROT	CARB	FAT	FIBRE
Ham & Pineapple, Loaded, Tesco*	½ Pizza/265g		556	14.6	210	11.3	28.7	5.5	1.4
Ham & Pineapple, Pizzerai, Simply Italian, Sainsbury's*	½ Pizza/178g		434	15.1	244	11.5	30.4	8.5	2.4
Ham & Pineapple, Stone Bake, M & S*	1 Pizza/345g		690	19.7	200	10.1	28.3	5.7	1.6
Ham & Pineapple, Stonebaked, Tesco*	1 Pizza/161g		293	9.2	182	9.2	23.5	5.7	3.5
Ham & Pineapple, Tesco*	1/6 Pizza/56g		134	4.6	240	10.4	30.9	8.3	2.1
Ham & Pineapple, Thin & Crispy, Waitrose*	1 Pizza/220g		616	21.1	280	12.8	33.3	9.6	2.2
Ham & Pineapple, Thin & Crispy Italian, Morrisons*	1 Pizza/375g		746	22.9	199	10.2	24.9	6.1	0.0
Ham & Pineapple, Thin Crust, Tesco*	½ Pizza/175g		385	10.0	220	12.3	29.6	5.7	2.5
Ham & Pineapple Deep, Asda*	1 Pizza/486g		1055	22.4	217	11.3	32.5	4.6	3.0
Hawaiian, San Marco*	¼ Pizza/90g		208	8.3	231	8.9	29.7	9.2	1.5
Hawaiian, Thin Crust, Tesco*	½ Pizza/192g		365	9.4	190	10.3	25.6	4.9	1.8
Hickory Steak, M & S*	1 Pizza/400g		820	26.8	205	9.9	25.7	6.7	1.4
Honey Roast Salmon & Broccoli, BGTY, Sainsbury's*	1 Serving/280g		613	12.6	219	10.2	34.4	4.5	3.5
Hot & Spicy, Deep Dish, Chicago Town*	1 Pizza/177g		434	17.5	245	8.6	30.4	9.9	0.9
Hot & Spicy, Pizzeria Style, Sainsbury's*	1 Pizza/376g		986	46.3	262	12.5	25.5	12.3	2.4
Hot & Spicy, Thin & Crispy, Morrisons*	½ Pizza/170g		393	15.8	231	10.5	26.5	9.3	3.2
Hot & Spicy Chicken, Deep Pan, Tesco*	½ Pizza/222g		423	7.3	191	10.5	30.0	3.3	2.1
Hot Chicken, Stone Bake, M & S*	1 Pizza/380g		798	25.8	210	11.5	25.1	6.8	1.3
Italian Cheese & Ham, The Little Big Food Company*	1 Pizza/95g		236	6.2	248	10.9	36.2	6.5	1.0
Italian Meat Feast, Thin & Crispy, Waitrose*	1 Pizza/182g		477	22.9	262	10.7	26.5	12.6	1.8
Italian Meats, Finest, Tesco*	½ Pizza/217g		449	8.5	207	13.6	29.4	3.9	1.3
Italian Mozzarella & Black Forest Ham, Asda*	¼ Pizza/110g		227	6.6	206	10.0	28.0	6.0	2.7
Italian Sausage & Roasted Peppers, Finest, Tesco*	1 Pizza/325g		650	13.6	200	7.8	31.7	4.2	1.9
Le Reine, 8 Inch, Supermarket, Pizza Express*	1 Pizza/283g		546	16.4	193	10.2	25.0	5.8	2.7
Leggera, Dr Oetker*	½ Pizza/175g		317	10.2	181	8.8	23.1	5.8	2.7
Loaded Cheese, Goodfella's*	1 Pizza/410g		1115	49.6	272	11.4	29.4	12.1	1.7
Margherita, Average	1 Slice/108g		239	8.6	239	11.0	30.5	8.6	1.2
Margherita, Cheese & Tomato, San Marco*	½ Pizza/200g		454	14.4	227	10.7	29.8	7.2	1.2
Margherita, HL, Tesco*	½ Pizza/125g		222	2.5	178	10.8	29.3	2.0	2.5
Margherita, Italian Stonebaked, Asda*	¼ Pizza/135g		323	10.8	240	11.0	31.0	8.0	1.8
Margherita, Stonebaked Ciabatta, Goodfella's*	½ Pizza/150g		404	17.2	270	11.3	32.8	11.5	2.6
Margherita, Thin & Crispy, Iceland*	½ Pizza/170g		391	14.4	230	12.7	25.9	8.5	2.8
Massive on Meat, Deep Pan, Goodfella's*	1 Serving/106g		259	9.4	244	10.4	30.6	8.9	3.0
Meat, Mediterranean Style, Pizzeria, Waitrose*	¼ Pizza/174g		395	15.3	227	11.1	25.8	8.8	2.0
Meat Feast, American Style, Sainsbury's*	½ Pizza/263g		642	26.0	244	12.6	26.2	9.9	2.9
Meat Feast, Deep & Crispy, Iceland*	1/6 Pizza/136g		345	11.3	254	11.2	33.7	8.3	2.0
Meat Feast, Deep & Loaded, Sainsbury's*	½ Pizza/298g		818	30.0	275	13.2	32.7	10.1	2.6
Meat Feast, Deep Pan, Co-Op*	1 Pizza/450g		1102	45.0	245	11.0	28.0	10.0	2.0
Meat Feast, Hot & Spicy, Thin & Crispy, Sainsbury's*	½ Pizza/170g		462	21.6	272	13.0	26.5	12.7	3.2
Meat Feast, Large, Tesco*	1 Pizza/735g		1904	69.1	259	10.9	32.6	9.4	2.0
Meat Feast, Loaded, Deep Pan, Large, Tesco*	½ Pizza/282g		775	38.4	275	12.0	26.1	13.6	1.9
Meat Feast, Mega, Asda*	½ Pizza/428g		1044	33.8	244	9.5	33.6	7.9	3.2
Meat Feast, Stuffed Crust, Asda*	½ Pizza/238g		597	24.0	251	14.6	25.5	10.1	3.1
Meat Feast, Thin & Crispy, Asda*	½ Pizza/183g		410	14.6	224	11.0	27.0	8.0	1.4
Meat Feast, Thin Crust, Tesco*	½ Pizza/178g		430	20.2	242	13.6	21.3	11.4	2.3
Meat Mayhem, Goodfella's*	1 Pizza/437g		1100	41.9	252	10.6	30.9	9.6	2.5
Mediterranean Madness, Goodfella's*	¼ Pizza/109g		235	8.7	216	9.1	27.0	8.0	3.9
Mediterranean Vegetable, Pizzeria, Sainsbury's*	1 Serving/211g		397	13.5	188	8.0	24.7	6.4	3.2
Mediterranean Vegetable, Stonebaked, Sainsbury's*	½ Pizza/260g		622	16.4	239	9.8	35.7	6.3	3.1
Mexican Style, Morrisons*	½ Pizza/180g		437	16.9	243	13.7	26.0	9.4	2.0
Mini, Party, Tesco*	1 Pizza/11g		26	1.1	248	11.4	28.6	10.5	1.9
Mozzarella, Ristorante, Dr Oetker*	1 Pizza/335g		890	13.6	266	10.5	24.2	4.1	0.5
Mozzarella & Sunblush Tomato, 12", TTD, Sainsbury's*	½ Pizza/251g		638	17.8	254	12.4	35.0	7.1	2.6

PIZZA

INFO/WEIGHT	Measure	per Measure		Nutrition Values per 100g / 100ml				
		KCAL	FAT	KCAL	PROT	CARB	FAT	FIBRE
Mozzarella & Tomato, Asda*	1 Pizza/360g	824	32.4	229	12.0	25.0	9.0	2.4
Mozzarella E Provolone, La Bottega, Goodfella's*	½ Pizza/156g	372	15.0	238	10.1	27.9	9.6	2.4
Mushroom & Ham, COU, M & S*	1 Pizza/245g	355	4.4	145	8.8	24.0	1.8	2.2
Mushroom & Mascarpone, 12", TTD, Sainsbury's*	½ Pizza/255g	638	18.6	250	12.1	34.0	7.3	2.4
Mushroom & Roasted Onion, Waitrose*	½ Pizza/187g	403	12.6	215	9.8	28.9	6.7	1.3
Napoletana, Sainsbury's*	½ Pizza/186g	424	14.3	228	9.7	29.9	7.7	3.1
Napoli, Tesco*	½ Pizza/184g	431	11.6	235	11.9	32.6	6.3	1.4
Napoli Ham & Mushroom, San Marco*	½ Pizza/219g	449	13.4	205	10.0	27.5	6.1	2.8
Oval, Ham & Pineapple, Weight Watchers*	1 Pizza/130g	220	2.3	169	11.6	26.7	1.8	3.0
Pasta, Ristorante, Dr Oetker*	½ Pizza/205g	449	18.2	219	8.0	26.6	8.9	0.0
Pepperonata, Delicata, Sainsbury's*	1 Pizza/330g	917	47.5	278	12.9	24.3	14.4	2.6
Pepperoni, American Style Deep Pan, Co-Op*	1 Pizza/395g	987	39.5	250	12.0	28.0	10.0	1.0
Pepperoni, Asda*	½ Pizza/150g	385	13.5	257	10.0	34.0	9.0	2.7
Pepperoni, Deep & Crispy, Iceland*	1 Serving/175g	490	21.0	280	11.9	31.1	12.0	1.8
Pepperoni, Deep Filled, Chicago Town*	1 Serving/202g	621	33.6	307	11.5	28.0	16.6	1.3
Pepperoni, Deep Pan, Frozen, Tesco*	½ Pizza/215g	527	17.4	245	11.9	31.1	8.1	2.6
Pepperoni, Deluxe, American Deep Pan, Sainsbury's*	1 Pizza/424g	1077	40.3	254	13.3	28.7	9.5	2.7
Pepperoni, Double, Italian, Chilled, Tesco*	½ Pizza/160g	455	23.3	285	12.4	25.6	14.6	2.4
Pepperoni, Extra, Chicago Town*	1 Pizza/460g	994	34.0	216	9.6	27.7	7.4	0.0
Pepperoni, Feast, Deep Dish, Schwan's*	1 Pizza/435g	1188	61.8	273	9.9	26.3	14.2	0.0
Pepperoni, Goodfella's*	1 Pizza/337g	900	43.5	267	13.2	26.3	12.9	1.7
Pepperoni, Hot & Spicy, Stuffed Crust, Asda*	1 Pizza/245g	666	30.0	272	13.9	26.5	12.2	2.4
Pepperoni, Hot & Spicy, Thin Crust, Chilled, Tesco*	½ Pizza/174g	486	25.5	280	12.4	24.0	14.7	2.2
Pepperoni, Italian Stonebaked, Asda*	¼ Pizza/132g	329	13.2	250	12.0	28.0	10.0	2.8
Pepperoni, Mini, Tesco*	1 Serving/22g	71	3.7	323	11.8	30.5	16.8	2.7
Pepperoni, Pizzeria, Sainsbury's*	½ Pizza/197g	559	25.8	284	13.4	28.3	13.1	2.4
Pepperoni, Stonebaked, American Hot, Sainsbury's*	½ Pizza/276g	674	30.9	244	11.6	24.1	11.2	2.9
Pepperoni, Stonebaked Ciabatta, Goodfella's*	½ Pizza/181g	503	26.1	278	11.9	27.4	14.4	2.4
Pepperoni, Thin & Crispy, Essential, Waitrose*	½ Pizza/133g	380	18.0	286	12.3	28.8	13.5	1.0
Pepperoni, Thin & Crispy, Goodfella's*	1 Pizza/593g	1595	70.0	269	13.8	26.9	11.8	2.3
Pepperoni, Weight Watchers*	1 Pizza/300g	501	9.3	167	8.0	25.4	3.1	2.8
Pepperoni, Xxx Hot, Deep & Crispy, Chilled, Tesco*	½ Pizza/263ml	656	27.0	250	9.1	30.1	10.3	2.0
Pepperoni, Zingy, Asda*	1 Serving/90g	255	6.3	283	12.0	43.0	7.0	4.0
Pepperoni & Cheese, Asda*	½ Pizza/150g	385	13.5	257	10.0	34.0	9.0	2.7
Pepperoni & Jalapeno Chill, Asda*	1 Pizza/277g	742	22.2	268	10.0	39.0	8.0	1.8
Pepperoni & Onion, 9", Sainsbury's*	½ Pizza/207g	615	26.9	297	13.4	31.7	13.0	1.9
Pepperoni Bacon, Primo*	½ Pizza/111g	360	14.5	324	10.5	42.5	13.1	0.0
Pollo, Ristorante, Dr Oetker*	½ Pizza/178g	383	16.9	216	8.9	23.4	9.5	0.0
Pollo Pesto, Supermarket, Pizza Express*	1 Pizza/265g	500	10.1	189	9.2	25.0	3.8	2.0
Prosciutto, Classico, Tesco*	½ Pizza/205g	461	10.0	225	11.7	33.6	4.9	2.5
Prosciutto, Italian Style, Co-Op*	½ Pizza/183g	421	12.8	230	13.0	29.0	7.0	3.0
Prosciutto, Pizzaria, Sainsbury's*	1 Pizza/325g	806	23.1	248	11.4	34.7	7.1	3.2
Prosciutto, Ristorante, Dr Oetker*	1 Pizza/330g	752	32.3	228	10.3	24.6	9.8	0.0
Quattro Formaggi, 8 Inch, Supermarket, Pizza Express*	1 Pizza/266g	646	26.1	243	12.1	26.5	9.8	2.3
Quattro Formaggi, Ristorante, Dr Oetker*	½ Pizza/175g	472	25.0	270	11.4	23.9	14.3	0.0
Quattro Formaggi Pizzeria, Sainsbury's*	½ Pizza/175g	490	21.2	280	12.8	30.8	12.1	2.5
Roasted Tomato & Mozzarella, BGTY, Sainsbury's*	1 Pizza/204g	526	16.4	258	17.8	28.6	8.0	6.0
Roasted Vegetable, for One, GFY, Asda*	1 Pizza/96g	190	3.6	198	9.0	32.0	3.8	1.5
Salame, Ristorante, Dr Oetker*	½ Pizza/160g	455	24.5	285	10.4	26.3	15.3	0.0
Salami, Ultra Thin Italian, Tesco*	1 Serving/263g	692	25.5	263	12.0	31.9	9.7	1.0
Salami & Ham, Pizzeria, Waitrose*	½ Pizza/205g	443	13.7	216	10.1	28.7	6.7	1.8
Salami & Pepperoni, Waitrose*	½ Pizza/190g	578	30.8	304	13.4	23.9	16.2	2.1
Sicilian, Premium, Co-Op*	1 Pizza/600g	1320	48.0	220	9.0	27.0	8.0	2.0

P

PIZZA

INFO/WEIGHT	Measure KCAL	FAT	Nutrition Values per 100g / 100ml KCAL	PROT	CARB	FAT	FIBRE
Simply Cheese, Goodfella's*	¼ Pizza/82g	226	11.0	276	16.3	22.5	13.4	1.9
Slice Selection, M & S*	1 Serving/52g	120	4.1	230	9.4	30.3	7.8	1.9
Smoked Ham & Mushroom, Thin & Crispy, Co-Op*	1 Pizza/400g	792	18.0	198	9.0	30.3	4.5	1.7
Smoked Ham & Peppers, HL, Tesco*	1 Serving/282g	386	5.6	137	8.7	21.1	2.0	1.8
Smoked Ham & Pineapple, Deep Pan, Co-Op*	1 Pizza/395g	1142	41.9	289	11.6	36.7	10.6	1.7
Smoked Ham & Pineapple, Weight Watchers*	1 Pizza/241g	429	7.0	178	10.3	27.6	2.9	1.5
Smokey New York, Takeaway, Tesco*	½ Pizza/178g	479	16.5	270	12.7	31.7	9.3	2.3
Spicy Beef, Goodfella's*	½ Pizza/148g	391	17.8	265	12.4	26.5	12.1	2.2
Spicy Chicken, Anytime, McCain*	1 Pizza/150g	382	11.7	255	15.1	32.2	7.8	2.0
Spicy Chicken, BBQ, Deep Pan, Asda*	1 Pizza/476g	1033	25.2	217	10.9	31.4	5.3	0.0
Spicy Chicken, Focaccia, Sainsbury's*	½ Pizza/245g	581	18.6	237	12.0	30.3	7.6	2.5
Spicy Chicken, HL, Tesco*	1 Serving/252g	418	4.0	166	10.9	27.1	1.6	2.7
Spicy Chicken, Iceland*	1 Pizza/345g	797	22.8	231	13.4	29.9	6.6	1.5
Spicy Chicken, Micro, McCain*	1 Pizza/133g	388	19.9	292	12.4	26.9	15.0	0.0
Spicy Chorizo, Red Pepper & Chilli, Classico, Tesco*	1 Serving/218g	474	17.4	218	10.3	26.4	8.0	2.5
Spicy Vegetable, Low Fat, Bertorelli*	1 Pizza/180g	243	4.3	135	6.0	23.4	2.4	1.9
Spinach & Bacon, Thin & Crispy, M & S*	1 Pizza/290g	739	35.1	255	10.6	26.8	12.1	1.0
Spinach & Ricotta, BGTY, Sainsbury's*	1 Pizza/265g	535	6.6	202	10.4	34.4	2.5	2.6
Spinach & Ricotta, Extra Special, Asda*	1 Pizza/400g	940	28.0	235	9.0	34.0	7.0	1.9
Spinach & Ricotta, GFY, Asda*	1 Pizza/160g	375	7.0	234	8.7	40.0	4.4	1.8
Spinach & Ricotta, Italian, Chilled, Sainsbury's*	1 Pizza/361g	859	34.7	238	9.3	28.7	9.6	2.3
Spinach & Ricotta, Perfectly Balanced, Waitrose*	½ Pizza/165g	272	2.8	165	9.7	27.7	1.7	2.6
Spinach & Ricotta, Pizzaria, Waitrose*	½ Pizza/238g	501	21.1	211	10.7	21.9	8.9	2.6
Spinach & Ricotta, Thin Crust, Italian, Tesco*	½ Pizza/190g	365	16.7	192	9.6	18.7	8.8	1.9
Spinach with Bacon & Mushroom, GFY, Asda*	1 Serving/270g	618	12.1	229	13.0	34.0	4.5	2.6
Sunblushed Tomato & Mascarpone, Pizzadella, Tesco*	1 Serving/275g	894	44.0	325	8.5	36.7	16.0	1.5
Super Supreme, Family, Chicago Town*	¼ Pizza/225g	526	24.3	234	9.6	24.5	10.8	0.0
Supreme, Deep Dish, Individual, Chicago Town*	1 Pizza/170g	456	20.4	268	9.2	30.8	12.0	1.0
Supreme, McCain*	1 Serving/125g	267	8.6	214	10.9	27.0	6.9	0.0
Sweet & Sour Chicken, Thin Crust, Tesco*	½ Pizza/186g	366	12.8	197	11.9	21.9	6.9	2.3
Sweet Chilli Chicken, BGTY, Sainsbury's*	½ Pizza/138g	276	2.3	200	13.0	33.2	1.7	2.1
The Big Cheese, Deep Pan, Goodfella's*	1/6 Pizza/118g	295	12.7	250	12.2	25.9	10.8	1.1
The Big Eat Meat X-Treme, Deep Pan, Goodfella's*	½ Pizza/352g	806	28.9	229	11.6	27.1	8.2	3.6
Three Cheese, Ultra Thin, Sodebo*	1 Pizza/180g	450	18.4	250	10.9	28.5	10.2	1.8
Three Cheese & Cherry Tomato, Weight Watchers*	1 Pizza/256g	399	4.1	156	9.8	25.6	1.6	2.3
Three Cheese Calzone, Waitrose*	1 Pizza/265g	747	31.8	282	10.4	33.0	12.0	1.4
Three Cheeses & Tomato, Stonebaked, Co-Op*	1 Pizza/415g	888	33.6	214	10.0	25.2	8.1	1.5
Three Meat, Thin & Crispy, Sainsbury's*	½ Pizza/147g	344	15.7	234	12.5	23.4	10.7	1.3
Tomato, Aubergine & Spinach, Pizzeria, Waitrose*	½ Pizza/193g	403	7.7	209	7.8	35.4	4.0	3.6
Tomato, Basil & Garlic, Weight Watchers*	1 Serving/85g	169	2.9	199	12.3	29.8	3.4	1.6
Tomato, Mushroom & Bacon, Deep Pan, Co-Op*	1 Pizza/420g	882	33.6	210	9.0	25.0	8.0	2.0
Tomato & Cheese, Stone Bake, M & S*	1 Pizza/340g	782	28.6	230	10.8	30.1	8.4	1.6
Tomato & Cheese, Thin & Crispy, M & S*	1 Pizza/300g	705	28.2	235	11.0	27.7	9.4	1.2
Tomato & Pesto, Tesco*	1 Serving/176g	449	23.2	256	8.4	25.9	13.2	1.1
Tomato & Red Pepper, Perfectly Balanced, Waitrose*	½ Pizza/163g	313	2.4	192	6.6	38.1	1.5	1.9
Tomato & Ricotta, Waitrose*	½ Pizza/208g	444	18.5	214	7.8	25.7	8.9	2.2
Triple Cheese, Deep Dish, Chicago Town*	1 Serving/170g	418	18.2	246	9.9	27.6	10.7	0.0
Triple Cheese, Deep Pan, Morrisons*	1/6 Pizza/75g	198	9.2	265	10.4	28.2	12.3	1.9
Tuna & Caramelised Red Onion, COU, M & S*	1 Pizza/245g	429	5.6	175	9.6	26.7	2.3	1.2
Tuna Sweetcorn, BGTY, Sainsbury's*	1 Pizza/304g	602	5.8	198	13.5	31.7	1.9	2.7
Tuscana, Finest, Tesco*	1 Serving/255g	643	35.7	252	13.2	18.4	14.0	5.9
Ultimate Meat Feast, Sainsbury's*	1 Pizza/465g	1302	47.9	280	13.5	35.1	10.3	1.7
Vegetable, COU, M & S*	1 Pizza/294g	397	7.1	135	6.4	23.2	2.4	1.9

P

	Measure INFO/WEIGHT	per Measure KCAL	FAT	Nutrition Values per 100g / 100ml KCAL	PROT	CARB	FAT	FIBRE
PIZZA								
Vegetable, Deep Pan, Co-Op*	1 Pizza/425g	829	29.7	195	8.0	25.0	7.0	2.0
Vegetable, Frozen, HL, Tesco*	1 Pizza/400g	604	10.8	151	8.1	23.5	2.7	4.4
Vegetable, GFY, Asda*	¼ Pizza/94g	141	2.7	150	7.0	24.0	2.9	3.7
Vegetable, Stone Bake, M & S*	1 Serving/465g	837	26.0	180	7.8	25.0	5.6	1.5
Vegetable Feast, Thin & Crispy, Iceland*	1 Slice/63g	148	6.9	237	7.8	26.5	11.1	1.8
Vegetale, Ristorante, Dr Oetker*	½ Pizza/185g	386	16.6	209	8.1	23.9	9.0	0.0
Verona, Frozen, Finest, Tesco*	1 Serving/238g	541	23.3	228	11.6	23.2	9.8	2.7
PIZZA BASE								
Deep Pan, Italian, Sainsbury's*	1 Base/220g	684	11.0	311	7.0	59.5	5.0	1.4
Deep Pan, Napolina*	1 Base/260g	757	7.8	291	7.9	58.0	3.0	0.2
Garlic Bread, Sainsbury's*	¼ Base/59g	109	4.2	186	5.1	25.4	7.1	1.8
Gluten, Wheat & Dairy Free, Free From, Livwell*	1 Base/100g	237	2.6	237	5.2	48.3	2.6	4.7
Gluten & Wheat Free, Glutafin*	1 Base/110g	309	5.5	281	3.0	56.0	5.0	6.0
Gluten Free, Glutafin*	1 Base/110g	278	5.5	253	3.0	49.0	5.0	4.5
Italian, Classic, Sainsbury's*	1 Base/150g	451	7.2	301	7.6	57.0	4.8	1.5
Italian, The Pizza Company*	1 Base/260g	624	6.8	240	7.6	46.5	2.6	0.0
Italiana, Parmalat*	1 Base/150g	450	7.3	300	9.0	55.0	4.9	0.0
Light & Crispy, Napolina*	1 Base/150g	436	4.5	291	7.9	58.0	3.0	0.2
Mini, Napolina*	1 Base/75g	218	2.2	291	7.9	58.0	3.0	0.2
Thin & Crispy, Sainsbury's*	1 Base/150g	504	7.8	336	9.9	62.3	5.2	4.3
Thin & Crispy, Tesco*	1 Serving/110g	348	8.2	316	9.2	52.9	7.5	1.5
Trufree*	1 Base/110g	345	6.6	314	3.0	63.0	6.0	4.0
PIZZA BASE MIX								
Morrisons*	1 Serving/77g	313	3.8	407	12.7	77.9	5.0	3.6
Sainsbury's*	1 Pack/145g	486	5.5	335	12.8	62.3	3.8	2.9
Tesco*	1 Serving/36g	99	2.4	272	10.2	43.0	6.6	3.8
PLAICE								
Fillets, in Breadcrumbs, Average	1 Serving/150g	331	17.9	221	12.8	15.5	11.9	0.8
Fillets, Lightly Dusted, Average	1 Fillet/113g	188	9.2	166	12.9	10.4	8.1	0.6
Fillets, Raw, Average	*1oz/28g*	*24*	*0.4*	*87*	*18.2*	*0.0*	*1.5*	*0.0*
Goujons, Baked	1oz/28g	85	5.1	304	8.8	27.7	18.3	0.0
Goujons, Fried in Blended Oil	1oz/28g	119	9.0	426	8.5	27.0	32.3	0.0
Grilled	*1oz/28g*	*27*	*0.5*	*96*	*20.1*	*0.0*	*1.7*	*0.0*
in Batter, Fried in Blended Oil	1oz/28g	72	4.7	257	15.2	12.0	16.8	0.5
Steamed	*1oz/28g*	*26*	*0.5*	*93*	*18.9*	*0.0*	*1.9*	*0.0*
PLAICE &								
Prawns, in Breadcrumbs, Aldi*	1 Serving/100g	212	8.4	212	8.6	25.4	8.4	0.0
PLAICE WITH								
Mushrooms & Prawns, Sainsbury's*	1 Serving/170g	354	18.2	208	12.0	15.9	10.7	1.7
Prawns, Fillets, Asda*	1oz/28g	24	1.3	86	11.0	0.4	4.5	0.7
Spinach & Cheddar Cheese, Fillets, Sainsbury's*	1 Serving/154g	222	13.3	144	13.6	3.1	8.6	0.8
Spinach & Ricotta Cheese, Whole, Sainsbury's*	1 Serving/159g	334	16.7	210	11.6	17.2	10.5	0.8
PLANTAIN								
Boiled in Unsalted Water	*1oz/28g*	*31*	*0.1*	*112*	*0.8*	*28.5*	*0.2*	*1.2*
Raw, Average	*1 Med/179g*	*218*	*0.7*	*122*	*1.3*	*31.9*	*0.4*	*2.3*
Ripe, Fried in Vegetable Oil	*1oz/28g*	*75*	*2.6*	*267*	*1.5*	*47.5*	*9.2*	*2.3*
PLUMS								
Average, Stewed without Sugar	*1oz/28g*	*8*	*0.0*	*30*	*0.5*	*7.3*	*0.1*	*1.3*
Soft Dried, Blue Parrot Cafe, Sainsbury's*	1 Pack/50g	118	0.2	237	2.6	55.6	0.5	7.1
Weighed with Stone, Average	*1 Plum/90g*	*32*	*0.1*	*36*	*0.6*	*8.6*	*0.1*	*1.6*
Whole, Dried, Graze*	1 Pack/60g	143	0.3	239	2.6	56.0	0.5	0.0
Whole, Imperial, Graze*	1 Punnet/45g	124	0.0	275	2.6	56.0	0.1	7.1
Yellow, Waitrose*	1 Plum/50g	19	0.0	39	0.6	8.8	0.1	1.5

P

	Measure INFO/WEIGHT	per Measure KCAL	FAT	Nutrition Values per 100g / 100ml KCAL	PROT	CARB	FAT	FIBRE
POLENTA								
Merchant Gourmet*	1 Serving/65g	232	0.9	357	7.4	78.8	1.4	1.3
Organic, Kallo*	1 Serving/150g	543	2.7	362	8.5	78.0	1.8	0.0
POLLOCK								
Breaded, Asda*	1 Serving/97g	200	9.7	206	12.0	17.0	10.0	1.0
POLO								
Citrus Sharp, Nestle*	1 Tube/34g	134	0.3	393	0.0	96.6	1.0	0.0
Fruits, Nestle*	1 Tube/37g	142	0.0	383	0.0	96.0	0.0	0.0
Mints, Clear Ice, Nestle*	1 Sweet/4g	16	0.0	390	0.0	97.5	0.0	0.0
Mints, Original, Nestle*	1 Sweet/2g	8	0.0	404	0.0	98.9	1.1	0.0
Spearmint, Nestle*	1 Tube/35g	141	0.4	402	0.0	98.2	1.1	0.0
POMEGRANATE								
Raw, Fresh, Flesh Only, Average	*1 Sm Fruit/86g*	*59*	*0.3*	*68*	*0.9*	*17.2*	*0.3*	*0.6*
Raw, Weighed with Rind & Skin, Average	*1 Fruit/154g*	*105*	*0.5*	*68*	*0.9*	*17.2*	*0.3*	*0.1*
POMELO								
Fresh, Raw, Weighed with Skin & Seeds	*1 Serving/100g*	*18*	*0.1*	*18*	*0.4*	*4.1*	*0.1*	*0.0*
Raw, Flesh Only, Average	1 Fruit/340g	129	0.1	38	0.8	9.6	0.0	1.0
POP TARTS								
Bustin' Berry, Kellogg's*	1 Tart/50g	200	6.0	400	4.0	69.0	12.0	2.0
Chocolate, Kellogg's*	1 Tart/50g	198	8.5	396	5.0	136.0	17.0	2.0
Chocomallow, Kellogg's*	1 Tart/50g	198	6.0	396	6.0	66.0	12.0	2.5
Cookies 'n' Creme, Kellogg's*	1 Tart/50g	197	5.0	394	4.0	72.0	10.0	1.5
Cream Cheese & Cherry Swirl, Kellogg's*	1 Tart/62g	250	11.0	403	3.2	59.7	17.7	1.0
Frosted Brown Sugar Cinnamon, Kellogg's*	1 Tart/50g	210	7.0	420	6.0	68.0	14.0	2.0
Strawberry Sensation, Kellogg's*	1 Tart/50g	197	5.5	395	4.0	70.0	11.0	2.0
POPCORN								
94% Fat Free, Orville Redenbacher's*	1 Bag/76g	220	0.0	289	13.2	65.8	0.0	0.0
Air Popped, Plain, Average	1oz/28g	110	1.3	387	12.9	77.9	4.5	14.5
Butter, 6% Fat, Orville Redenbacher's*	1 Portion/21g	86	1.2	410	11.9	77.6	5.7	14.3
Butter, Microwave, 94% Fat Free, Act II*	½ Bag/41g	130	2.5	317	9.8	68.3	6.1	12.2
Butter, Microwave, Act II*	1 Bag/90g	425	16.2	472	9.0	69.0	18.0	9.0
Butter, Microwave, Butterkist*	1 Bag/100g	395	18.5	395	8.3	49.5	18.5	8.5
Butter Flavour, Microwave, Popz*	1 Serving/100g	480	27.5	480	7.5	51.1	27.5	9.2
Butter Toffee, Asda*	1 Serving/100g	364	8.0	364	2.1	71.0	8.0	4.1
Butter Toffee, Belgian Milk Chocolate Coated, M & S*	1 Pack/100g	495	26.3	495	5.7	59.0	26.3	2.3
Butter Toffee, Snack-A-Jacks, Quaker Oats*	1 Bag/35g	149	3.1	425	3.5	86.0	9.0	4.5
Butter Toffee, Tesco*	1 Pack/350g	1417	26.9	405	2.2	81.7	7.7	4.3
Butter Toffee, Yummies*	1 Serving/50g	227	6.4	455	2.5	82.4	12.8	3.1
Chocolate & Pecan, M & S*	1 Packet/27g	130	5.2	480	3.3	72.9	19.3	3.6
Kernels, Asda*	1 Portion/10g	50	3.3	502	6.2	44.9	33.1	11.5
Lightly Salted, Snack-A-Jack, Quaker Oats*	1 Bag/13g	48	1.3	370	12.1	58.0	9.9	14.6
Lite Toffee, Butterkist*	1 Bag/50g	130	1.3	260	2.0	49.4	2.6	39.8
Maize, Unpopped, Love Life, Waitrose*	1 Serving/33g	200	14.1	605	6.2	48.7	42.8	12.7
Maple, Shapers, Boots*	1 Bag/40g	188	7.2	469	12.0	59.0	18.0	10.0
Microwave, Salted, Sunsnacks*	1 Pack/100g	498	22.9	498	10.7	51.3	22.9	10.8
Organic Amaranth*	1 Serving/10g	36	0.9	365	14.6	26.8	8.8	0.0
Plain, Oil Popped, Average	1 Bag/74g	439	31.7	593	6.2	48.7	42.8	0.0
Ready Salted, Microwave, Popz*	1 Serving/20g	101	6.0	504	7.0	51.5	30.0	9.2
Salt & Vinegar, Diet Chef Ltd*	1 Serving/23g	106	3.6	461	10.4	69.8	15.8	13.0
Salt & Vinegar, Snack-A-Jacks, Quaker Oats*	1 Sm Pack/13g	47	1.3	360	12.0	55.0	9.9	14.0
Salted, Blockbuster*	1 Bowl/25g	99	2.9	397	10.6	62.2	11.7	8.6
Salted, Bop, Microwave, Zanuy*	1 Serving/25g	119	5.7	477	10.7	56.9	23.0	0.0
Salted, Diet Chef Ltd*	1 Pack/23g	107	3.8	465	10.5	68.6	16.6	14.0
Salted, Light, Microwave, Act II*	1 Pack/85g	336	6.5	395	10.6	71.0	7.6	15.8

	Measure INFO/WEIGHT	per Measure		Nutrition Values per 100g / 100ml				
		KCAL	FAT	KCAL	PROT	CARB	FAT	FIBRE
POPCORN								
Salted, M & S*	1 Pack/15g	82	4.7	545	9.4	56.8	31.1	6.3
Salted, Manhatten Peanuts Limited*	1 Bag/30g	135	4.3	450	10.0	70.0	14.3	13.7
Salted, Microwave, 93% Fat Free, Act II*	1 Pack/85g	345	5.9	406	10.0	76.0	7.0	13.0
Salted, Sold At Cinema, Playtime Popcorn*	1 Carton/74g	384	24.9	519	8.3	45.9	33.6	0.0
Sea Salt Flavour, Skinny, Topcorn, Metcalfe's Food Co*	1 Pack/23g	115	6.5	501	8.2	53.6	28.2	10.9
Sour Cream And Jalapeno Chilli, Tyrrells*	1 Serving/20g	97	5.2	484	6.4	49.9	26.0	12.5
Super, Perri*	1 Packet/30g	139	7.0	464	8.4	55.5	23.2	8.5
Sweet, Best-In*	1 Serving/34g	161	5.8	473	7.3	72.6	17.0	0.0
Sweet, Butterkist, Butterkist*	1 Pack/120g	612	29.8	510	2.8	68.5	24.8	5.6
Sweet, Cinema Style, Butterkist*	1 Bag/120g	612	29.8	510	2.8	68.5	24.8	5.6
Sweet, Microwave, Butterkist*	½ Pack/50g	205	8.8	410	7.7	54.6	17.7	7.9
Sweet, Microwave, Cinema, Popz*	1 Bag/85g	420	21.7	494	6.0	60.0	25.5	8.2
Sweet, Vanilla & Sugar, Microwave, Act II*	1 Pack75g	369	18.1	492	7.9	60.8	24.1	10.4
Sweet Maple, Diet Chef Ltd*	1 Pack/23g	111	3.6	483	9.7	75.2	15.7	13.0
Toffee, 90% Fat Free, Butterkist*	1 Pack/35g	142	3.3	406	2.8	77.7	9.3	0.0
Toffee, Best-In*	1 Bag/90g	356	3.2	396	5.0	85.9	3.6	0.0
Toffee, Butterkist*	1 Bag/30g	124	3.0	415	2.3	79.3	10.0	4.4
Toffee, Chicago Joes*	1 Serving/10g	31	0.5	314	3.1	84.6	4.8	0.0
Toffee, Milk Chocolate Coated, Butterkist*	1 Bag/50g	252	12.5	505	6.5	61.9	25.0	4.1
Toffee, Milk Chocolate Coated, Sainsbury's*	¼ Bag/25g	130	6.6	520	6.5	64.1	26.4	1.3
Toffee, Sainsbury's*	1 Serving/50g	207	6.3	415	1.8	73.8	12.7	3.3
Toffee, Snack Pack, Butterkist*	1 Bag/30g	124	3.0	415	2.3	79.3	10.0	4.4
Vanilla, Cinema Sweet Microwave, Act II*	½ Pack/50g	234	8.0	468	9.0	71.0	16.0	12.0
Wasabi Flavour, Skinny, Topcorn, Metcalfe's Food Co*	1 Bag/25g	121	6.5	484	8.4	54.1	26.2	9.7
White Cheddar Cheese, Manhatten Peanuts Limited*	1 Bag/30g	132	4.1	440	10.0	70.0	13.7	13.0
Yellow, Kernel, Unpopped, Jolly Time*	2 Tbsp/33g	110	1.0	333	12.1	78.8	3.0	21.2
POPPADOMS								
Fried in Vegetable Oil, Takeaway, Average	1 Poppadom/13g	65	5.0	501	11.5	28.3	38.8	5.8
Indian, Asda*	1 Pack/45g	232	15.7	516	14.5	36.2	34.8	7.8
Mercifully Mild, Phileas Fogg*	1 Serving/30g	150	9.8	499	14.8	36.8	32.6	6.0
Mini, Sainsbury's*	½ Pack/50g	249	16.1	498	14.9	36.9	32.3	7.6
Plain, Asda*	1 Poppadom/9g	44	2.5	484	18.0	40.0	28.0	0.0
Plain, Indian to Go, Sainsbury's*	1 Poppadom/8g	34	1.5	405	18.4	43.4	17.5	9.0
Plain, Tesco*	1 Serving/9ml	41	2.0	439	17.8	44.4	21.1	4.6
Plain, Waitrose*	1 Serving/9g	37	1.7	408	21.0	39.3	18.6	9.1
Spicy, COU, M & S*	1 Pack/26g	84	0.6	325	23.5	51.9	2.4	8.1
Tesco*	1 Poppadom/9g	39	1.9	440	17.8	44.4	21.1	4.6
POPPETS*								
Chocolate Raisins, Poppets*	1 Pack/35g	140	4.7	401	4.9	65.4	13.3	0.0
Mint Cream, Poppets*	1oz/28g	119	3.6	424	2.0	75.0	13.0	0.0
Peanut, Poppets*	1 Box/100g	544	37.0	544	16.4	37.0	37.0	0.0
Toffee, Milk Chocolate, Poppets*	1 Box/100g	491	23.0	491	5.3	68.0	23.0	0.0
POPPING CORN								
Average	1 Serving/30g	112	1.3	375	10.9	73.1	4.3	12.7
PORK								
Belly, Fresh, Raw, Weighed with Skin, Average	1 Serving/100g	518	53.0	518	9.3	0.0	53.0	0.0
Belly, Roasted, Lean & Fat	1oz/28g	82	6.0	293	25.1	0.0	21.4	0.0
Chop, Lean & Fat, Boneless, Raw, Average	*1oz/28g*	*67*	*3.8*	*240*	*29.2*	*0.0*	*13.7*	*0.0*
Diced, Lean, Average	*1oz/28g*	*31*	*0.5*	*109*	*22.0*	*0.0*	*1.7*	*0.0*
Escalope, Average	*1 Escalope/75g*	*108*	*1.7*	*144*	*31.0*	*0.0*	*2.2*	*0.0*
Escalope, Lean, Healthy Range, Average	*1 Escalope/75g*	*80*	*1.5*	*106*	*22.0*	*0.0*	*2.0*	*0.0*
Ham, Shank, Hock, Raw, Weight with Bone, Fat & Skin	1 Portion/100g	139	5.6	139	20.6	0.0	5.6	0.0
Joint, Ready to Roast, Average	*½ Joint/254g*	*375*	*18.0*	*147*	*19.2*	*2.3*	*7.1*	*0.1*

P

PORK

	Measure INFO/WEIGHT	per Measure KCAL	FAT	Nutrition Values per 100g / 100ml KCAL	PROT	CARB	FAT	FIBRE
Joint, with Crackling, Ready to Roast, Average	1 Joint/567g	1283	80.1	226	24.2	0.8	14.1	0.0
Leg, Joint, Healthy Range, Average	1 Serving/200g	206	4.4	103	20.0	0.6	2.2	0.0
Loin, Applewood Smoked, Asda*	1 Slice/15g	18	0.5	122	21.8	0.5	3.6	0.0
Loin, Chops, Boneless, Grilled, Average	1oz/28g	90	4.4	320	29.0	0.0	15.7	0.0
Loin, Chops, Grilled, Lean	1oz/28g	52	1.8	184	31.6	0.0	6.4	0.0
Loin, Joint, Roast, Lean	1oz/28g	51	1.9	182	30.1	0.0	6.8	0.0
Loin, Joint, Roasted, Lean & Fat	1oz/28g	71	4.3	253	26.3	0.0	15.3	0.0
Loin, Steak, Fried, Lean	1oz/28g	53	2.0	191	31.5	0.0	7.2	0.0
Loin, Steak, Fried, Lean & Fat	1oz/28g	77	5.2	276	27.5	0.0	18.4	0.0
Loin, Steak, Lean, Raw, Average	1 Serving/175g	345	19.6	197	22.7	1.8	11.2	0.4
Medallions, Average	1 Pack/220g	359	5.5	163	35.1	0.0	2.5	0.4
Mince, Lean, Healthy Range, Average	1 Pack/400g	504	20.2	126	19.7	0.4	5.0	0.3
Mince, Raw	1oz/28g	46	2.7	164	19.2	0.0	9.7	0.0
Mince, Stewed	1oz/28g	53	2.9	191	24.4	0.0	10.4	0.0
Raw, Lean, Average	1oz/28g	42	1.2	151	28.6	0.0	4.1	0.0
Roast, Lean Only, Average	1oz/28g	34	0.9	121	22.7	0.3	3.3	0.0
Roast, Slices, Average	1 Slice/30g	40	1.3	133	22.7	0.4	4.5	0.0
Shoulder, Slices, Cured	1oz/28g	29	1.0	103	16.9	0.9	3.6	0.0
Shoulder, Whole, Lean & Fat, Raw, Average	1 Serving/100g	236	18.0	236	17.2	0.0	18.0	0.0
Shoulder, Whole, Lean Only, Roasted	1 Serving/150g	345	20.3	230	25.3	0.0	13.5	0.0
Shoulder Steak, Boneless, Frozen, Grilled, Tesco*	1 Steak/125g	156	4.9	125	0.0	0.0	3.9	0.0
Slow Cooked, with Smoked Chilli Beans, HL, Tesco*	1 Pack/365g	255	4.7	70	6.6	8.0	1.3	2.5
Steak, Lean, Stewed	1oz/28g	49	1.3	176	33.6	0.0	4.6	0.0
Steak, Lean & Fat, Average	1oz/28g	61	3.8	219	23.8	0.0	13.7	0.1
Stir Fry Strips, Lean, Healthy Range, Average	¼ Pack/113g	118	2.3	104	21.3	0.0	2.0	0.0
Tenderloin, Lean, Boneless, Raw, Average	1 Serving/100g	109	2.2	109	20.9	0.0	2.2	0.0
Tenderloin, Separable Lean & Fat, Raw, Average	1 Loin/265g	318	9.4	120	20.6	0.0	3.5	0.0
PORK &								
Apricots, Aromatic, Cafe Culture, M & S*	½ Pack/420g	672	31.1	160	10.3	12.5	7.4	2.1
Chestnut Stuffing, M & S*	1oz/28g	64	4.8	230	5.3	12.6	17.1	3.7
PORK CHAR SUI								
Chinese, Tesco*	1 Pack/400g	520	17.2	130	7.2	15.7	4.3	0.6
Oriental, Finest, Tesco*	1 Pack/350g	245	5.2	70	6.8	6.2	1.5	2.1
Takeaway, Iceland*	1 Pack/400g	412	9.6	103	7.9	12.5	2.4	1.2
PORK CHINESE								
Sliced, M & S*	1 Serving/140g	224	4.3	160	26.4	6.1	3.1	0.0
Style, GFY, Asda*	1 Serving/170g	286	6.0	168	18.8	15.3	3.5	0.4
with Noodles, Tesco*	1 Serving/450g	612	25.6	136	7.0	14.2	5.7	1.1
PORK DINNER								
Roast, Birds Eye*	1 Pack/340g	410	12.0	121	7.6	14.7	3.5	1.6
PORK IN								
Light Mustard Sauce, Fillet, COU, M & S*	1 Pack/390g	312	9.4	80	10.9	3.5	2.4	0.7
Mustard & Cream, Chops	1oz/28g	73	6.0	261	14.5	2.4	21.6	0.3
Rich Sage & Onion Gravy, Steaks, Tesco*	1 Serving/160g	218	10.4	136	16.0	3.2	6.5	1.5
PORK SCRATCHINGS								
Crunch, Mr Porky*	1 Pack/30g	159	9.6	531	60.4	0.5	31.9	4.6
KP Snacks*	1 Pack/20g	125	9.6	624	47.3	0.5	48.1	0.5
Tavern Snacks*	1 Pack/30g	187	14.4	624	47.3	0.5	48.1	0.5
PORK WITH								
Apricot & Orange Stuffing, Joint, Sainsbury's*	¼ Joint/200g	566	36.2	283	29.0	0.9	18.1	1.4
Cheese & Pineapple, Loin Steaks, M & S*	1 Steak/141g	240	14.0	170	14.0	6.3	9.9	0.0
Herbes De Provence, Joint, Sainsbury's*	¼ Joint/200g	302	16.4	151	19.2	0.1	8.2	0.6
Honey & Mustard Sauce, Steaks, Tesco*	½ Pack/160g	258	11.8	161	16.3	8.7	7.4	1.4

	Measure INFO/WEIGHT	per Measure KCAL	per Measure FAT	Nutrition Values per 100g / 100ml KCAL	PROT	CARB	FAT	FIBRE
PORK WITH								
Honey & Soy, Sainsbury's*	1 Serving/260g	260	7.5	100	12.3	6.2	2.9	0.3
Leek & Bacon Stuffing, Roast, Shoulder, Sainsbury's*	1 Serving/150g	237	12.4	158	18.8	2.4	8.3	0.5
Leek & Cheese Stuffing, Joint, Sainsbury's*	1 Serving/100g	231	10.5	231	31.0	3.0	10.5	1.1
Medallions, with Bramley Apple, M & S*	1 Serving/380g	418	12.9	110	17.7	2.5	3.4	0.5
Noodles, Chinese, Tesco*	1 Serving/450g	463	13.5	103	5.3	13.7	3.0	1.4
Peppers, Marinated, Tapas, Waitrose*	1 Serving/105g	181	6.7	172	26.3	2.2	6.4	0.3
Rice & Beans, Jerk, Love Life, Waitrose*	1 Pack/380g	384	12.2	101	4.9	13.0	3.2	2.1
Roasted Rosemary Potatoes, Porchetta, Finest, Tesco*	½ Pack/370g	455	31.8	123	6.9	4.6	8.6	0.5
Sage, Onion & Lemon Stuffing, Joint, Sainsbury's*	1 Serving/260g	699	43.4	269	27.4	2.2	16.7	1.4
Sage & Onion Stuffing, Joint, BGTY, Sainsbury's*	1 Serving/150g	246	5.4	164	29.5	3.3	3.6	1.3
Sage & Onion Stuffing, Joint, Tesco*	1 Serving/200g	208	5.6	104	17.1	2.7	2.8	0.0
Sea Salt & Black Pepper, Tesco*	1 Serving/100g	225	15.5	225	21.4	0.0	15.5	0.0
Spiced Apple Stuffing, Steaks, Easy Cook, Waitrose*	1 Serving/190g	236	7.8	124	19.3	2.4	4.1	0.5
Stuffing, Belly, Norfolk Outdoor Reared, Finest, Tesco*	1 Serving/180g	524	44.8	291	14.9	1.7	24.9	0.0
Stroganoff Sauce, Sainsbury's*	½ Pack/180g	203	8.8	173	24.8	1.4	7.5	0.5
Thai Style Butter, Steaks, Asda*	4 Steaks/300g	810	54.0	270	26.0	1.0	18.0	0.0
Tomato & Apricot Sauce, Loin Steaks, Sainsbury's*	½ Pack/110g	216	10.6	196	24.4	3.1	9.6	0.6
PORT								
Average	*1 Serving/50ml*	*78*	*0.0*	*157*	*0.1*	*12.0*	*0.0*	*0.0*
POT NOODLE*								
Balti Curry, Made Up, Pot Noodle*	1 Pot/301g	268	1.5	89	3.1	17.8	0.5	0.5
Beef & Tomato, Made Up, Pot Noodle*	1 Pot/300g	378	14.1	126	3.1	18.1	4.7	1.1
Beef & Tomato, Mini, Pot Noodle*	1 Pot/190g	254	9.5	134	3.5	18.7	5.0	1.7
Beef & Tomato, Pot Noodle*	1 Pot/319g	424	14.7	133	3.4	19.4	4.6	1.3
Bombay Bad Boy, Made Up, Pot Noodle*	1 Pot/305g	384	14.0	126	3.1	17.9	4.6	1.1
Chicken & Mushroom, King, Pot Noodle*	1 Pack/401g	513	19.2	128	3.2	18.1	4.8	1.1
Chicken & Mushroom, Made Up, Pot Noodle*	1 Pot/300g	384	14.1	128	3.2	18.0	4.7	1.1
Chicken & Mushroom, Mini, Made Up, Pot Noodle*	1 Pot/190g	243	8.5	128	3.8	18.2	4.5	1.4
Chicken Curry, Hot, Made Up, Pot Noodle*	1 Pot/300g	384	14.1	128	2.8	18.7	4.7	1.1
Chow Mein Flavour, Made Up, Pot Noodle*	1 Pot/320g	416	14.7	130	3.2	19.0	4.6	1.3
Hot, Made Up, Pot Noodle*	1 Pot/300g	378	15.6	126	3.0	16.9	5.2	1.1
Korma Curry, Made Up, Pot Noodle*	1 Pot/300g	273	3.3	91	2.9	17.4	1.1	0.4
Nice & Spicy, Made Up, Pot Noodle*	1 Pot/300g	381	14.1	127	2.8	18.3	4.7	1.1
Roast Chicken, in a Mug, Made Up, Pot Noodle*	1 Mug/227g	141	1.8	62	2.1	11.5	0.8	0.4
Seedy Sanchez, Made Up, Pot Noodle*	1 Pot/300g	396	14.4	132	3.1	19.1	4.8	1.1
Spicy Chilli, Posh, Made Up, Pot Noodle*	1 Pot/301g	328	17.8	109	2.5	11.7	5.9	1.0
Spicy Curry, Made Up, Pot Noodle*	1 Pot/300g	393	14.4	131	2.9	19.1	4.8	1.1
Sweet & Sour, Dry, Pot Noodle*	1 Pot/86g	376	13.8	437	12.1	60.9	16.1	3.1
Sweet & Sour, King, Dry, Pot Noodle*	1 Pot/105g	473	20.1	450	8.8	60.0	19.1	4.8
Sweet & Sour, Oriental, Posh, Pot Noodle*	1 Pot/300g	375	13.8	125	1.7	19.2	4.6	0.5
POT RICE								
Chicken Curry, Dry, Pot Rice*	1 Pot/74g	253	1.7	342	11.0	67.2	2.3	3.3
POTATO BOMBAY								
Average	1oz/28g	33	1.9	117	2.0	13.7	6.8	1.2
Canned, Tesco*	1 Can/400g	380	11.6	95	2.5	13.5	2.9	2.3
Flavours of India, Canned, Sainsbury's*	½ Can/200g	160	3.8	80	2.4	13.3	1.9	1.8
Indian Meal for Two, Sainsbury's*	½ Pack/151g	154	8.5	102	1.6	11.4	5.6	3.1
Indian Takeaway for 1, Sainsbury's*	1 Serving/200g	202	10.4	101	1.8	11.8	5.2	1.7
POTATO CAKES								
Average	1 Cake/70g	127	1.2	180	3.8	37.5	1.7	2.4
Fried, Average	1oz/28g	66	2.5	237	4.9	35.0	9.0	0.8
POTATO CHIPS								
Beef & Horseradish, Tyrrells*	¼ Pack/37g	177	9.3	473	9.0	58.6	24.8	2.4

P

POTATO CHIPS

	Measure INFO/WEIGHT	per Measure KCAL	FAT	Nutrition Values per 100g / 100ml KCAL	PROT	CARB	FAT	FIBRE
Hand Fried Mature Cheddar, Burts*	1 Serving/40g	202	11.1	504	6.4	57.4	27.7	0.0
Lightly Sea Salted, Tyrrells*	1 Pack/150g	739	38.1	493	7.7	58.9	25.4	2.6
Mature Cheese & Chives, Tyrrells*	1 Bag/50g	261	13.9	522	6.1	56.5	27.9	0.0
Ready Salted, Sainsbury's*	¼ Pack/33g	174	10.9	526	5.6	51.7	33.0	3.8
Sweet Chilli & Red Pepper, Tyrrells*	¼ Pack/37g	180	9.2	481	7.9	59.7	24.5	2.4
Worcester Sauce, with Sun Dried Tomato, Tyrrells*	1 Bag/50g	241	12.4	482	7.6	60.1	24.8	2.5

POTATO CREAMED

with Cabbage, Asda*	1 Pack/350g	255	9.1	73	1.3	11.0	2.6	0.0

POTATO CRUNCHIES

Oven Crunchies, Ross*	1 Serving/100g	240	11.7	240	3.6	30.0	11.7	2.4

POTATO FRITTERS

Crispy, Oven Baked, Birds Eye*	1 Fritter/20g	29	1.6	145	2.0	16.3	8.0	1.2
with Sweetcorn, M & S*	1 Pack/135g	304	17.0	225	4.4	24.1	12.6	2.3

POTATO MASH

Bacon & Cheese, Tesco*	1 Serving/200g	252	12.8	126	3.1	13.9	6.4	1.3
Bacon & Spring Onion, Finest, Tesco*	½ Pack/200g	214	10.4	107	4.3	10.8	5.2	1.6
Carrot And Swede, Sainsbury's*	½ Pack/225g	101	3.8	45	0.7	6.8	1.7	2.8
Cheddar, Irish, Finest, Tesco*	½ Pack/250g	350	19.7	140	6.3	10.2	7.9	1.4
Cheese & Chive, Snack in a Pot, Tesco*	1 Pot/230g	304	21.6	132	2.2	9.6	9.4	0.9
Cheese & Onion, Tesco*	1 Serving/200g	210	9.4	105	3.2	12.6	4.7	1.0
Leek & Bacon, Tesco*	1 Serving/400g	356	14.4	89	3.0	11.1	3.6	1.9
Leek & Cheese, COU, M & S*	½ Pack/225g	180	4.7	80	3.0	12.0	2.1	1.3
Mustard, with Caramelised Onions, Finest, Tesco*	1 Serving/200g	232	9.2	116	2.6	16.0	4.6	1.8
Roast Onion, Snack in a Pot, Tesco*	1 Pot/218g	257	12.9	118	1.6	14.7	5.9	0.6
Savoy Cabbage & Spring Onion, M & S*	1 Serving/225g	250	15.5	111	2.0	10.2	6.9	1.3
Sun Dried Tomato & Basil, COU, M & S*	1 Serving/170g	127	2.5	75	1.0	14.4	1.5	1.2
with Cracked Pepper & Sea Salt, Luxury, Sainsbury's*	½ Pack/225g	389	28.3	173	1.6	13.2	12.6	1.0
with Sweetcorn & Flaked Tuna, Quick, Sainsbury's*	1 Pot/224g	240	9.2	107	2.4	15.0	4.1	2.1
with Vegetables, GFY, Asda*	1 Pack/290g	186	3.2	64	1.6	12.0	1.1	2.3
with Vegetables, Sainsbury's*	½ Pack/229g	142	2.3	62	1.8	11.4	1.0	3.1

POTATO RINGS

Mature Cheddar & Red Onion, GFY, Asda*	1 Pack/10g	36	0.1	360	5.2	81.6	1.5	2.9
Ready Salted, M & S*	1 Serving/75g	375	21.1	500	3.5	58.9	28.1	2.6
Ready Salted, Sainsbury's*	1 Serving/50g	257	14.2	514	3.2	61.5	28.4	1.8
Salt Vinegar, Sainsbury's*	1 Pack/25g	114	4.9	456	3.6	65.6	19.6	2.8

POTATO SALAD

baby, & Coleslaw, TTD, Sainsbury's*	1 Serving/100g	300	30.4	300	1.2	5.4	30.4	1.6

POTATO SKINS

¼ Cut, Deep Fried, McCain*	1oz/28g	52	1.7	186	3.0	30.1	6.0	0.0
¼ Cut, Oven Baked, McCain*	1oz/28g	53	1.3	190	3.6	33.1	4.8	0.0
American Style, Loaded, Asda*	1 Serving/78g	294	18.0	375	15.0	27.0	23.0	2.4
American Style, Loaded, Tesco*	1 Serving/340g	388	8.2	114	6.8	16.3	2.4	3.3
Cheese & Bacon, Loaded, Asda*	½ Pack/125g	275	15.0	220	13.0	15.0	12.0	3.3
Cheese & Bacon, Loaded, Tesco*	1 Skin/59g	150	9.1	255	9.2	19.5	15.5	3.0
Cheese & Bacon, Sainsbury's*	1 Serving/140g	349	21.6	249	10.3	17.3	15.4	2.5
Cheese & Bacon, Waitrose*	1 Serving/75g	146	9.4	195	7.3	13.1	12.6	3.5
Cheese & Chive, Sainsbury's*	2 Skins/150g	286	17.8	191	7.7	13.3	11.9	2.8
Cheese & Ham, Iceland*	2 Skins/108g	155	4.9	143	6.3	19.3	4.5	2.0
Soured Cream, Loaded, M & S*	½ Pack/150g	307	17.8	205	9.1	15.8	11.9	0.9
with Sour Cream	1 Serving/275g	541	34.6	197	7.2	13.8	12.6	2.1

POTATO SMILES

Weighed Baked, McCain*	1 Serving/100g	237	10.1	237	3.4	33.4	10.1	3.1
Weighed Frozen, McCain*	1 Serving/100g	191	8.0	191	2.6	27.0	8.0	2.7

	Measure INFO/WEIGHT	per Measure KCAL	FAT	Nutrition Values per 100g / 100ml KCAL	PROT	CARB	FAT	FIBRE
POTATO SUMTHINGS								
Weighed Baked, McCain*	1 Serving/100g	220	9.0	220	3.4	31.3	9.0	2.8
Weighed Frozen, McCain*	1 Serving/100g	187	7.9	187	2.9	26.2	7.9	2.4
POTATO TWIRLS								
Sainsbury's*	1 Serving/50g	217	7.3	435	3.0	72.8	14.6	3.1
POTATO WAFFLES								
Birds Eye*	1 Waffle/60g	105	5.2	175	2.5	21.6	8.7	1.5
Frozen, Cooked	1oz/28g	56	2.3	200	3.2	30.3	8.2	2.3
Frozen, Grilled, Asda*	1 Waffle/57g	104	5.8	183	2.0	21.0	10.1	1.7
Mini, Sainsbury's*	1 Waffle/11g	27	1.8	242	2.8	20.1	16.7	1.0
Oven Baked, Mini, McCain*	1oz/28g	62	2.4	221	3.9	32.0	8.6	0.0
Sainsbury's*	1 Waffle/56g	108	5.6	194	2.9	22.8	10.1	1.1
Southern Fried, Asda*	1 Waffle/51g	107	5.1	209	2.8	27.0	10.0	2.1
POTATO WEDGES								
& Dip, M & S*	1 Pack/450g	697	33.3	155	2.5	20.4	7.4	1.8
Aldi*	1 Serving/100g	150	6.8	150	2.1	20.2	6.8	0.0
Asda*	1 Wedge/40g	57	2.0	142	3.4	21.0	4.9	1.7
Baked, GFY, Asda*	1 Pack/450g	616	11.7	137	3.4	25.0	2.6	3.4
BBQ Flavour, Asda*	1 Serving/100g	185	9.0	185	2.9	23.0	9.0	1.7
BGTY, Sainsbury's*	½ Pack/190g	179	3.4	94	3.0	16.4	1.8	3.4
Bombay, with Yoghurt & Mint Dip, HL, Tesco*	1 Serving/170g	139	3.6	82	1.3	14.5	2.1	0.9
Co-Op*	1oz/28g	38	1.7	135	2.0	20.0	6.0	2.0
Crispy, M & S*	1 Serving/200g	340	14.2	170	1.3	25.3	7.1	1.7
Four Cheese & Red Onion, Chicago Town*	1 Serving/150g	210	7.9	140	2.1	21.0	5.3	2.4
Garlic & Herb, COU, M & S*	1 Pack/300g	300	7.8	100	2.3	16.4	2.6	3.2
Garlic & Herb, Kitchen Range Foods*	1oz/28g	42	2.2	151	1.6	18.5	7.8	0.0
Garlic & Herb Crusted, Chicago Town*	1 Serving/150g	216	6.4	144	1.9	24.4	4.3	2.2
Jacket, Spicy, American Style, Frozen, Sainsbury's*	1 Serving/125g	156	5.0	125	1.9	20.3	4.0	1.1
Jumbo, Finest, Tesco*	1 Serving/126g	145	2.6	115	1.4	22.7	2.1	1.7
Mexican, Inspire, Asda*	1 Pack/500g	525	17.0	105	2.2	16.5	3.4	1.8
Micro, Tesco*	1 Pack/100g	170	6.8	170	2.6	24.5	6.8	2.3
New York Style, HL, Tesco*	1 Serving/125g	129	3.0	103	2.0	18.3	2.4	2.3
Only 5% Fat, Weighed Baked, McCain*	1 Serving/100g	173	4.3	173	3.3	30.2	4.3	2.8
Only 5% Fat, Weighed Frozen, McCain*	1 Serving/100g	123	3.0	123	2.2	21.8	3.0	1.9
Oven Baked, Waitrose*	1oz/28g	46	1.2	165	2.4	29.2	4.3	2.1
Perfectly Balanced, Waitrose*	1 Serving/275g	278	4.7	101	2.5	19.0	1.7	3.5
Savoury, Waitrose*	1/3 Bag/250g	350	10.7	140	2.3	22.9	4.3	1.9
Slightly Spiced, Baked, Potato Winners, McCain*	1 Serving/100g	187	5.2	187	2.7	26.9	5.2	1.8
Slightly Spiced, Frozen, Potato Winners, McCain*	1 Serving/100g	144	5.9	144	2.0	20.8	5.9	1.7
Sour Cream & Chives, McCain*	1 Serving/100g	132	4.1	132	2.4	24.0	4.1	0.0
Southern Fried, Asda*	1 Serving/100g	157	4.5	157	3.0	26.0	4.5	3.5
Southern Fried Flavour, Champion*	1oz/28g	41	1.7	147	2.1	20.8	6.2	2.8
Southern Fried Style, Tesco*	1 Serving/155g	232	14.1	150	3.0	14.1	9.1	2.0
Spicy, & Garlic Dip, Linda McCartney*	1 Pack/300g	366	16.8	122	2.6	15.3	5.6	3.1
Spicy, Asda*	1 Serving/100g	145	5.7	145	1.8	21.8	5.7	2.1
Spicy, Deep Fried, McCain*	1oz/28g	52	2.3	187	3.6	27.3	8.1	0.0
Spicy, M & S*	½ Pack/225g	349	14.6	155	2.4	21.8	6.5	1.3
Spicy, Occasions, Sainsbury's*	1 Serving/100g	144	4.3	144	2.5	23.7	4.3	0.4
Spicy, Simple Solutions, Tesco*	1 Serving/150g	141	4.5	94	4.6	12.2	3.0	1.4
with a Parsley & Oil Dressing, Tesco*	½ Pack/280g	168	2.8	60	1.0	11.5	1.0	1.8
with Broccoli & Mozzarella Cheese, Weight Watchers*	1 Pack/320g	294	9.6	92	3.1	13.3	3.0	1.0
with Chilli, COU, M & S*	1 Pack/400g	380	10.8	95	5.2	13.7	2.7	2.3
with Olive Oil & Parsley Dressing, Inspire, Asda*	½ Pack/300g	219	7.2	73	0.1	12.7	2.4	2.1

P

POTATOES

	Measure INFO/WEIGHT	per Measure KCAL	FAT	Nutrition Values per 100g / 100ml KCAL	PROT	CARB	FAT	FIBRE
Alphabites, Captain Birds Eye, Birds Eye*	9 Bites/56g	75	3.0	134	2.0	19.5	5.3	1.4
Anya, Raw, TTD, Sainsbury's*	1 Serving/100g	75	0.3	75	1.5	17.8	0.3	1.1
Baby, Dressed with Garlic & Rosemary, M & S*	1 Serving/185g	129	5.2	70	2.0	9.0	2.8	2.4
Baby, Garlic & Sea Salt Roasted, Finest, Tesco*	1 Serving/200g	192	6.6	96	3.1	13.5	3.3	1.0
Baby, Oven Bake, Aunt Bessie's*	1 Serving/120g	103	1.7	86	2.2	16.3	1.4	3.0
Baby, with Butter & Herbs, Sainsbury's*	¼ Pack/148g	103	0.9	70	1.9	14.2	0.6	2.0
Baked, Flesh & Skin, Average	*1 Med/200g*	*218*	*0.2*	*109*	*2.3*	*25.2*	*0.1*	*2.4*
Baked, Flesh Only, Weighed with Skin, Average	*1oz/28g*	*26*	*0.0*	*93*	*2.0*	*21.6*	*0.1*	*1.5*
Baked, in Microwave, Flesh & Skin, Average	*1oz/28g*	*29*	*0.0*	*105*	*2.4*	*24.1*	*0.1*	*2.3*
Baked, in Microwave, Flesh Only, Average	*1oz/28g*	*28*	*0.0*	*100*	*2.1*	*23.3*	*0.1*	*1.6*
Baked, in Microwave, Skin Only, Average	*1oz/28g*	*37*	*0.0*	*132*	*4.4*	*29.6*	*0.1*	*5.5*
Baked, Jacket, Baby, Veg, COOK!, M & S*	1 Pack/675g	776	37.8	115	2.1	14.3	5.6	2.3
Baked, Jacket, Beef Chilli Filled, GFY, Asda*	1 Serving/300g	261	1.5	87	4.6	16.0	0.5	3.2
Baked, Jacket, Beef Chilli Filled, Mini, Classic, Asda*	1 Pack/300g	233	2.4	78	3.9	13.7	0.8	1.5
Baked, Jacket, Cheddar Cheese, COU, M & S*	1 Potato/164g	164	3.1	100	2.9	17.3	1.9	2.0
Baked, Jacket, Cheese, M & S*	1oz/28g	24	0.7	85	4.5	11.1	2.5	1.6
Baked, Jacket, Cheesy, GFY, Asda*	1 Serving/155g	129	1.5	83	2.6	16.0	1.0	2.1
Baked, Jacket, Chicken Tikka, COU, M & S*	1 Serving/300g	240	4.8	80	5.4	10.9	1.6	1.3
Baked, Jacket, Chilli, BGTY, Sainsbury's*	1 Pack/350g	318	4.9	91	5.3	14.3	1.4	1.2
Baked, Jacket, Chilli Con Carne, COU, M & S*	1 Pack/300g	270	6.3	90	6.0	11.1	2.1	1.2
Baked, Jacket, Chilli Con Carne, Pro Cuisine*	1 Pack/340g	347	3.4	102	4.6	18.7	1.0	0.0
Baked, Jacket, Creamy Mushroom, Asda*	1 Serving/100g	124	2.4	124	3.5	22.0	2.4	1.7
Baked, Jacket, Garlic, Mini, Asda*	1 Serving/65g	59	2.1	91	2.2	13.0	3.3	0.0
Baked, Jacket, Garlic Butter Filling, Morrisons*	1 Potato/210g	239	12.4	114	1.7	13.6	5.9	0.9
Baked, Jacket, Garlic Mushrooms, BGTY, Sainsbury's*	1 Pack/350g	262	3.1	75	2.3	14.4	0.9	1.2
Baked, Jacket, Halves, M & S*	1 Serving/250g	187	2.7	75	2.0	14.2	1.1	1.7
Baked, Jacket, Ham & Cheddar Cheese, Asda*	1 Pack/300g	435	11.1	145	7.0	21.0	3.7	1.6
Baked, Jacket, Leek & Cheese, M & S*	1 Serving/206g	206	6.4	100	3.8	13.4	3.1	3.2
Baked, Jacket, Mature Cheddar Cheese, Finest, Tesco*	1 Potato/245g	360	18.4	147	5.4	14.6	7.5	2.3
Baked, Jacket, Mature Cheddar Cheese, M & S*	½ Pack/206g	225	6.6	109	3.6	16.9	3.2	1.0
Baked, Jacket, Mature Cheddar Cheese, Morrisons*	1 Serving/400g	520	20.4	130	4.4	16.6	5.1	1.5
Baked, Jacket, Stuffed, Garlic & Herb Butter, Tesco*	1 Pack/435g	570	32.6	131	1.3	14.6	7.5	1.0
Baked, Jacket, Tuna & Sweetcorn, Average	1 Serving/300g	273	6.7	91	5.0	12.5	2.2	0.9
Baked, Jacket, Tuna & Sweetcorn, BGTY, Sainsbury's*	1 Pack/350g	360	9.5	103	6.5	13.2	2.7	1.3
Baked, Jacket, Tuna & Sweetcorn, COU, M & S*	1 Pack/300g	270	5.4	90	5.1	12.8	1.8	1.4
Baked, Jacket, Tuna & Sweetcorn, Morrisons*	1 Serving/300g	243	2.1	81	5.1	13.5	0.7	0.0
Baked, Jacket, with Baked Bean & Sausage, Asda*	1 Pack/300g	447	9.6	149	5.0	25.0	3.2	2.7
Baked, Jacket, with Baked Beans, Pro Cuisine*	1 Pack/340g	374	1.4	110	4.3	22.3	0.4	0.0
Baked, Jacket, with Beef Chilli, Asda*	1 Pack/300g	381	7.8	127	5.0	21.0	2.6	2.0
Baked, Jacket, with Beef Chilli, M & S*	1 Pack/360g	288	7.2	80	5.9	9.6	2.0	0.9
Baked, Jacket, with Cheese, Freshly Prepared, Tesco*	½ Pack/215g	150	3.0	70	3.9	9.7	1.4	2.8
Baked, Jacket, with Cheese, HL, Tesco*	1 Potato/225g	202	4.9	90	4.5	13.0	2.2	1.8
Baked, Jacket, with Cheese & Bacon, Finest, Tesco*	1 Potato/245g	360	19.6	147	6.0	12.6	8.0	2.5
Baked, Jacket, with Cheese Mash, GFY, Asda*	1 Potato/200g	192	5.6	96	4.8	13.0	2.8	2.2
Baked, Jacket, with Smoked Bacon, Finest, Tesco*	½ Pack/200g	165	6.4	85	3.0	9.9	3.3	1.3
Baked, Jackets, Stuffed, Mini, Tesco*	1 Serving/108g	130	6.3	120	2.3	14.6	5.8	2.3
Baked, Skin Only, Average	*1oz/28g*	*55*	*0.0*	*198*	*4.3*	*46.1*	*0.1*	*7.9*
Baking, Raw, Average	*1 Med/250g*	*197*	*0.2*	*79*	*2.1*	*18.0*	*0.1*	*1.6*
Boiled, Average	*1 Serving/120g*	*86*	*0.1*	*72*	*1.8*	*17.0*	*0.1*	*1.2*
Boiled, with Skin	*1 Potato/125g*	*97*	*0.1*	*78*	*2.9*	*17.2*	*0.1*	*3.3*
Boulangere, M & S*	½ Pack/225g	180	2.0	80	2.8	15.9	0.9	0.9
Charlotte, Average	*1 Serving/184g*	*139*	*0.5*	*76*	*1.6*	*17.4*	*0.2*	*3.3*
Crispy Bites, Weighed Frozen, McCain*	1 Serving/100g	141	4.4	141	2.5	20.4	4.4	1.5

POTATOES

	INFO/WEIGHT	KCAL	FAT	KCAL	PROT	CARB	FAT	FIBRE
Crispy Slices, M & S*	1/3 Pack/159g	231	8.3	145	2.9	22.2	5.2	1.9
Crispy Slices, Weighed Baked, McCain*	1 Serving/100g	240	11.0	240	3.2	32.1	11.0	2.1
Crispy Slices, Weighed Frozen, McCain*	1 Portion/100g	163	7.4	163	2.1	21.9	7.4	1.4
Dauphinoise, Average	*1 Serving/200g*	*335*	*23.9*	*167*	*2.2*	*12.7*	*11.9*	*1.5*
Dauphinoise, TTD, Sainsbury's*	½ Pack/174g	240	16.2	138	2.9	10.8	9.3	2.7
Desiree, Average	*1 Serving/200g*	*152*	*0.4*	*76*	*2.1*	*16.3*	*0.2*	*0.6*
Exquisa, Finest, Tesco*	¼ Pack/247g	185	0.7	75	1.7	16.1	0.3	1.0
Frites, Fries, Golden, Crunchy, M & S*	½ Pack/100g	158	6.2	158	2.2	23.4	6.2	1.0
Garlic, Tapas Selection, Sainsbury's*	1 Serving/22g	49	4.2	224	2.6	10.4	19.1	0.7
Hasselback, Average	*1 Serving/175g*	*182*	*1.6*	*104*	*1.9*	*22.0*	*0.9*	*2.9*
Jersey Royal, Canned, Average	*1 Can/186g*	*116*	*0.2*	*62*	*1.4*	*14.0*	*0.1*	*1.2*
Jersey Royal, New, Raw, Average	*1oz/28g*	*21*	*0.1*	*75*	*1.6*	*17.2*	*0.2*	*1.5*
Jersey Royal with Mint Butter, Extra Special, Asda*	½ Pack/172g	148	5.3	86	1.6	13.0	3.1	1.5
King Edward, Tesco*	1 Serving/100g	77	0.2	77	2.1	16.8	0.2	1.3
Maris Piper, Raw, Average	*1 Serving/200g*	*151*	*0.4*	*75*	*2.0*	*16.5*	*0.2*	*1.4*
Mashed, Buttery, Sainsbury's*	1 Pack /450g	454	25.6	101	1.3	11.1	5.7	3.0
Mashed, Chosen By You, Asda*	½ Pack/250g	177	5.5	71	1.0	10.3	2.2	2.8
Mashed, Colcannon, Co-Op*	1 Pack/500g	325	10.0	65	2.0	10.0	2.0	2.0
Mashed, Colcannon, Sainsbury's*	½ Pack/300g	192	12.0	64	0.4	6.7	4.0	1.4
Mashed, Colcannon, Tesco*	1 Serving/250g	225	13.5	90	1.6	8.4	5.4	1.8
Mashed, Colcannon, Waitrose*	½ Pack/225g	207	8.5	92	1.7	12.8	3.8	1.4
Mashed, Fresh Mash, Light Choices, Tesco*	1 Pack/450g	292	9.9	65	2.0	9.3	2.2	1.6
Mashed, From Supermarket, Average	½ Pack/200g	197	8.1	98	1.8	13.3	4.1	1.5
Mashed, From Supermarket, Healthy Range, Average	1 Serving/200g	160	3.1	80	1.8	14.6	1.6	1.3
Mashed, From Supermarket, Premium, Average	1 Serving/225g	305	17.8	136	1.7	14.4	7.9	1.1
Mashed, Home Prepared, with Whole Milk	1 Cup/210g	162	1.2	77	1.9	17.5	0.6	2.0
Mashed, Maris Piper, Tesco*	½ Pack/228g	182	3.9	80	1.5	14.0	1.7	0.9
Mashed, Maris Piper, with Cream & Butter, M & S*	½ Pack/200g	180	7.2	90	1.1	12.9	3.6	0.4
Mashed, Mash Direct*	½ Pack/200g	190	3.8	95	1.7	17.7	1.9	1.3
Mashed, Ready to Eat, Sainsbury's*	½ Pack/200g	142	3.8	71	1.4	12.1	1.9	2.0
Mashed, Vintage Cheddar Cheese, M & S*	½ Pack/225g	247	11.9	110	4.6	12.6	5.3	1.0
Mashed, with Carrot & Swede, COU, M & S*	1oz/28g	20	0.6	70	1.1	12.1	2.1	2.9
Mashed, with Carrot & Swede, M & S*	1 Serving/225g	214	14.4	95	1.6	8.3	6.4	1.4
Mashed, with Carrot & Swede, Morrisons*	1 Serving/100g	71	1.6	71	1.5	12.6	1.6	2.2
Mashed, with Carrot & Swede, Sainsbury's*	½ Pack/226g	230	12.0	102	1.9	11.7	5.3	1.5
Mashed, with Creme Fraiche & Seasoning, Waitrose*	½ Pack/225g	189	6.3	84	2.0	12.7	2.8	1.4
Mashed, with Leeks, Creamy, Birds Eye*	1 Pack/300g	300	21.0	100	2.0	7.3	7.0	0.8
Mashed, with Spring Onion, Weight Watchers*	1 Serving/100g	77	2.2	77	1.9	10.9	2.2	1.4
New, Average	*1 Serving/100g*	*75*	*0.3*	*75*	*1.5*	*17.8*	*0.3*	*1.1*
New, Baby, Average	*1 Serving/180g*	*135*	*0.5*	*75*	*1.7*	*17.1*	*0.3*	*1.6*
New, Baby, Canned, Average	*1 Can/120g*	*70*	*0.2*	*59*	*1.4*	*13.2*	*0.2*	*1.4*
New, Easy Steam, with Herbs & Butter, Tesco*	1 Serving/125g	94	3.5	75	1.8	9.6	2.8	1.7
New, Garlic, Herb & Parsley Butter, Co-Op*	1 Serving/100g	115	5.0	115	1.0	15.0	5.0	2.0
New, in a Herb Marinade, Tesco*	¼ Pack/150g	151	7.3	101	1.3	13.0	4.9	1.5
New, with Butter, Chives & Mint, M & S*	¼ Pack/145g	116	2.0	80	1.1	16.2	1.4	2.3
New, with English Churned Butter, M & S*	1 Pack/180g	261	4.0	145	1.3	29.5	2.2	2.1
New, with Herbs & Butter, Asda*	½ Pack/170g	146	2.9	86	1.7	16.0	1.7	1.5
New, with Herbs & Butter, Waitrose*	1 Serving/385g	443	22.7	115	1.7	13.8	5.9	1.2
New, with Sunblush Tomato, M & S*	1 Pack/385g	346	6.9	90	1.6	17.2	1.8	1.3
Organics, Boiled, Asda*	1 Serving/200g	152	0.2	76	1.8	16.0	0.1	1.2
Pan Fried, Aldi*	1 Serving/250g	182	2.0	73	2.7	13.7	0.8	0.0
Red, Flesh Only, Average	*1 Serving/300g*	*217*	*0.4*	*72*	*1.9*	*16.3*	*0.1*	*1.2*
Redskin, Roasted, Frozen, Lamb Weston *	½ Pack/200g	202	4.0	101	2.4	18.0	2.0	1.9

P

POTATOES

	Measure INFO/WEIGHT	per Measure KCAL	FAT	Nutrition Values per 100g / 100ml KCAL	PROT	CARB	FAT	FIBRE
Roast, Basted in Beef Dripping, Waitrose*	1 Serving/165g	213	8.9	129	2.2	18.0	5.4	1.9
Roast, Dry, No Oil, No Fat	1 Serving/100g	79	0.1	79	2.7	18.0	0.1	1.6
Roast, Extra Crispy, Oven Baked, Aunt Bessie's*	1 Serving/100g	223	11.8	223	2.9	26.1	11.8	3.6
Roast, Frozen, Average	1 Potato/70g	105	3.5	149	2.6	23.5	5.0	1.4
Roast, Frozen, Healthy Range, Average	1 Potato/70g	70	1.7	100	2.5	18.1	2.4	2.1
Roast, Garlic, Sainsbury's*	½ Pack/225g	358	21.8	159	3.2	14.6	9.7	1.4
Roast, in Lard, Average	*1oz/28g*	*42*	*1.3*	*149*	*2.9*	*25.9*	*4.5*	*1.8*
Roast, in Oil, Average	*1oz/28g*	*42*	*1.3*	*149*	*2.9*	*25.9*	*4.5*	*1.8*
Roast, New, Rosemary, Ainsley Harriott*	1 Serving/150g	133	4.0	89	2.0	16.0	2.7	1.3
Roast, Oven Baked, Aunt Bessie's*	1 Serving/165g	305	15.3	185	2.3	22.9	9.3	1.8
Roast, Seasoned, Butter Basted, Tesco*	½ Pack/225g	337	12.8	150	2.3	21.9	5.7	2.4
Roast, with Caramelised Onions, Finest, Tesco*	½ Pack/200g	500	16.4	250	5.5	38.6	8.2	2.9
Roasted with Goose Fat, TTD, Sainsbury's*	½ Pack/185g	216	4.4	117	2.7	21.1	2.4	3.0
Roasting, Average	*1 Serving/150g*	*202*	*5.2*	*135*	*2.5*	*23.3*	*3.5*	*1.6*
Sauté, Deep Fried, McCain*	1oz/28g	47	2.0	167	2.6	23.3	7.0	0.0
Sauté, Oven Baked, McCain*	1oz/28g	56	1.1	199	4.4	36.9	3.8	0.0
Slices, Garlic & Herb, Heinz*	1oz/28g	23	1.1	82	1.7	10.2	3.9	0.7
Slices, in Batter, Crispy, Ready To Bake, Waitrose*	1 Pack/475g	860	45.1	181	2.5	21.4	9.5	3.1
Spicy, with Chorizo, Tapas, Waitrose*	1 Serving/260g	512	35.6	197	6.7	11.8	13.7	1.1
Vivaldi, Boiled in Unsalted Water, Sainsbury's*	1 Serving/200g	144	0.2	72	1.8	17.0	0.1	1.2
Waves, Frozen, Lamb Weston *	1 Serving/100g	125	3.9	125	2.8	19.6	3.9	2.6
Wedges, Jumbo, TTD, Sainsbury's*	1 Serving/165g	279	6.8	169	2.4	30.7	4.1	3.1
White, Raw, Weighed with Skin, Flesh Only, Average	*1 Med/213g*	*160*	*0.3*	*75*	*2.0*	*16.8*	*0.2*	*1.3*
White, Vivaldi, TTD, Sainsbury's*	1 Serving/100g	76	0.1	76	1.8	17.0	0.1	1.2

POTATOES INSTANT

	Measure INFO/WEIGHT	per Measure KCAL	FAT	Nutrition Values per 100g / 100ml KCAL	PROT	CARB	FAT	FIBRE
Mashed, Butter Flavour, Premier Foods*	1 Serving/180g	288	4.1	160	1.4	9.1	2.3	0.8
Mashed, Dry, Tesco*	1 Serving/70g	225	0.1	321	7.7	72.0	0.2	7.1
Mashed, Made Up with Water, Average	1 Serving/180g	118	0.3	66	1.7	14.5	0.2	1.3
Mashed, Original, Dry Weight, Smash*	1 Serving/30g	107	1.4	358	10.7	68.1	4.8	3.4
Mashed, with Fried Onion, Smash*	½ Pack/269g	191	3.5	71	1.6	13.4	1.3	0.7
Mashed, with Smoked Bacon, Smash*	1 Serving/169g	137	3.7	81	1.7	13.6	2.2	0.6

POUSSIN

	Measure INFO/WEIGHT	per Measure KCAL	FAT	Nutrition Values per 100g / 100ml KCAL	PROT	CARB	FAT	FIBRE
Meat & Skin, Raw, Average	*1oz/28g*	*57*	*3.9*	*202*	*19.1*	*0.0*	*13.9*	*0.0*
Spatchcock, British, Waitrose*	½ Poussin/225g	364	20.2	162	19.0	1.2	9.0	0.0
Spatchcock, with Garlic & Herbs, Finest, Tesco*	½ Poussin/235g	348	17.2	148	19.7	1.0	7.3	0.5

POWERADE

	Measure INFO/WEIGHT	per Measure KCAL	FAT	Nutrition Values per 100g / 100ml KCAL	PROT	CARB	FAT	FIBRE
Berry & Tropical Fruit, Coca-Cola*	1 Bottle/500ml	120	0.0	24	0.0	5.6	0.0	0.0
Citrus Charge, Coca-Cola*	1 Bottle/500ml	120	0.0	24	0.0	6.0	0.0	0.0
Gold Rush, Coca-Cola*	1 Bottle/500ml	120	0.0	24	0.0	6.0	0.0	0.0
Ice Storm, Coca-Cola*	1 Bottle/500ml	120	0.0	24	0.0	6.0	0.0	0.0
Isotonic, Sports Drink, Coca-Cola*	1 Bottle/500ml	120	0.0	24	0.0	5.6	0.0	0.0
Zero, Coca-Cola*	1 Bottle/500ml	6	0.0	1	0.0	0.0	0.0	0.0

PRAWN COCKTAIL

	Measure INFO/WEIGHT	per Measure KCAL	FAT	Nutrition Values per 100g / 100ml KCAL	PROT	CARB	FAT	FIBRE
& Orkney Crab, M & S*	1 Serving/90g	180	13.8	200	14.2	1.8	15.3	0.6
20% More Prawns, M & S*	½ Pack/100g	330	31.6	330	8.9	2.2	31.6	0.2
Asda*	1oz/28g	124	12.2	443	8.6	3.3	43.6	0.0
BFY, Morrisons*	1 Serving/100g	149	10.3	149	4.7	9.7	10.3	0.1
BGTY, Sainsbury's*	1 Pack/200g	330	23.4	165	10.1	4.8	11.7	0.9
Delicious, Boots*	1 Pack/250g	285	6.5	114	5.5	17.0	2.6	1.2
HL, Tesco*	1 Serving/200g	276	22.6	138	6.8	2.3	11.3	0.6
King, Sainsbury's*	1 Pack/260g	328	15.1	126	5.8	12.7	5.8	2.3
Light, Asda*	1oz/28g	45	3.1	160	9.9	4.8	11.2	0.0
Light Choices, Tesco*	1 Pot/140g	210	16.0	150	7.5	4.3	11.4	1.3

	Measure INFO/WEIGHT	per Measure KCAL	per Measure FAT	Nutrition Values per 100g / 100ml KCAL	PROT	CARB	FAT	FIBRE
PRAWN COCKTAIL								
Reduced Fat, M & S*	1 Pack/200g	260	15.0	130	11.9	3.2	7.5	0.7
Reduced Fat, Tesco*	1 Serving/200g	304	21.2	152	7.6	6.5	10.6	0.4
Sainsbury's*	1 Pot/200g	604	55.8	302	9.4	3.2	27.9	0.8
Tesco*	1 Tub/200g	834	83.0	417	7.3	3.5	41.5	0.1
TTD, Sainsbury's*	1 Serving/100g	333	30.6	333	11.5	2.9	30.6	0.5
PRAWN CRACKERS								
Asda*	1 Serving/25g	134	8.7	535	2.0	53.0	35.0	0.0
Cooked in Sunflower Oil, Sharwood's*	1 Cracker/2g	10	0.5	479	0.7	68.3	22.6	0.8
Food to Go, Sainsbury's*	1 Bag/40g	214	12.5	534	2.9	60.2	31.3	0.4
Green Thai Curry, M & S*	1 Pack/50g	250	12.9	500	3.2	62.2	25.8	1.6
M & S*	1 Bag/50g	262	15.6	525	2.8	57.4	31.3	0.8
Ready to Eat, Sharwood's*	1 Bag/60g	316	18.5	527	0.5	62.0	30.8	1.2
Red Mill*	1 Bag/50g	281	18.8	563	2.8	53.1	37.7	0.7
Sainsbury's*	1 Cracker/3g	16	1.0	537	2.4	60.4	31.7	0.8
Tesco*	1/3 Pack/20g	114	7.4	570	2.5	56.5	37.1	0.9
Uncooked, Sharwood's*	1oz/28g	136	8.3	487	0.7	52.7	29.7	1.7
Waitrose*	1 Pack/50g	266	16.0	533	2.4	58.6	32.1	1.6
PRAWN CREOLE								
with Rice, Perfectly Balanced, Waitrose*	1 Serving/404g	275	4.4	68	4.2	10.3	1.1	2.9
PRAWN TOAST								
Chinese Selection, Tesco*	1 Toast/10g	36	2.7	362	8.2	20.7	27.5	1.7
Chinese Snack Selection, Morrisons*	1 Toast/13g	41	2.6	328	11.3	23.1	21.2	6.6
Dim Sum Selection, Sainsbury's*	1 Toast/8g	23	1.5	283	9.9	19.2	18.5	2.0
Mini, Oriental Selection, Party, Iceland*	1 Toast/15g	52	3.6	345	10.5	22.0	23.9	2.1
Oriental Selection, Waitrose*	1 Toast/14g	38	2.4	272	11.1	18.3	17.2	2.1
Sesame, Occasions, Sainsbury's*	1 Toast/12g	34	2.2	283	9.9	19.2	18.5	2.0
Sesame, Oriental Snack Selection, Sainsbury's*	1 Toast/12g	40	2.7	335	9.3	23.0	22.9	5.1
Sesame Prawn, Toasted Triangles, M & S*	1 Pack/220g	616	39.6	280	12.4	17.3	18.0	2.0
Waitrose*	1 Toast/21g	47	3.6	223	9.7	7.4	17.2	5.8
PRAWNS								
Atlantic, Extra Large, TTD, Sainsbury's*	1/4 Pack/100g	79	1.0	79	17.4	0.1	1.0	0.5
Batter Crisp, Lyons*	1 Pack/160g	350	20.3	219	8.0	18.2	12.7	1.1
Boiled	*1 Prawn/3g*	*3*	*0.0*	*99*	*22.6*	*0.0*	*0.9*	*0.0*
Brine, John West*	1/2 Can/60g	58	0.6	97	21.0	1.0	1.0	0.0
Cooked & Peeled, Average	*1oz/28g*	*21*	*0.2*	*77*	*17.6*	*0.2*	*0.6*	*0.0*
Crevettes, Asda*	1oz/28g	11	0.2	41	8.6	0.0	0.7	0.0
Dried, Average	*1 Prawn/3g*	*8*	*0.1*	*281*	*62.4*	*0.0*	*3.5*	*0.0*
Filo Wrapped & Breaded, M & S*	1 Serving/19g	45	2.5	235	9.5	20.4	13.0	1.4
Honduran, & Cocktail Sauce Dipper, M & S*	1 Pack/120g	258	21.6	215	13.6	0.0	18.0	1.1
Hot & Spicy, Average	1 Serving/170g	461	26.9	271	9.4	22.8	15.8	2.1
Hot & Spicy, Whitby*	1 Portion/125g	319	16.4	255	9.3	25.0	13.1	2.2
Icelandic, Raw, Average	*1oz/28g*	*30*	*0.4*	*105*	*22.7*	*0.0*	*1.5*	*0.0*
King, BBQ Favourites, Sweet Chilli, Skewers, Asda*	1 Skewer/48g	48	0.5	100	16.6	5.4	1.1	1.0
King, Crevettes, Sainsbury's*	1 Pack/225g	205	1.1	91	21.8	0.1	0.5	0.3
King, Frozen, Morrisons*	1/2 Bag/100g	62	0.6	62	14.0	0.2	0.6	0.6
King, in Filo, Finest, Tesco*	1 Prawn/20g	38	0.6	189	13.0	27.8	2.9	1.6
King, in Sweet Chilli Sauce, with Noodles, COU, M & S*	1 Pack/400g	260	1.6	65	4.8	10.3	0.4	1.5
King, Jumbo, TTD, Sainsbury's*	1/2 Pack/90g	63	0.6	70	15.7	0.1	0.7	0.5
King, Raw, Average	*1 Bag/200g*	*145*	*1.9*	*72*	*15.8*	*0.2*	*0.9*	*0.1*
King, Raw, Peeled, Sainsbury's*	1/2 Pack/90g	61	0.6	68	14.3	0.8	0.7	0.5
King, Shell On, TTD, Sainsbury's*	1 Serving/100g	67	0.7	67	14.3	0.8	0.7	0.5
King, Sizzler, with Rice Noodles, BGTY, Sainsbury's*	1 Pack/400g	276	5.2	69	3.8	10.6	1.3	1.6
King, Tandoori, Average	1 Prawn/59g	33	0.6	55	5.7	5.9	1.1	0.7

	Measure INFO/WEIGHT	per Measure		Nutrition Values per 100g / 100ml				
		KCAL	FAT	KCAL	PROT	CARB	FAT	FIBRE
PRAWNS								
King, with Chilli & Coriander, M & S*	1 Pack/140g	147	5.6	105	17.1	0.5	4.0	0.5
King, with Garlic Butter, M & S*	1 Serving/100g	165	9.0	165	12.5	9.1	9.0	0.5
King, with Ginger & Spring Onion, Waitrose*	1 Pack/300g	207	5.1	69	6.4	7.1	1.7	1.9
Large, Wrapped, Party Food, Party Food, M & S*	1 Wrap/26g	49	1.5	190	14.7	18.8	5.7	1.3
North Atlantic, Peeled, Cooked, Average	*1oz/28g*	*22*	*0.3*	*80*	*17.5*	*0.0*	*1.1*	*0.0*
North Atlantic, Raw, Average	*1oz/28g*	*17*	*0.1*	*61*	*14.4*	*0.0*	*0.4*	*0.0*
Peeled, TTD, Sainsbury's*	1 Serving/100g	65	0.9	65	14.1	0.1	0.9	0.5
Raw, Average	*1oz/28g*	*22*	*0.2*	*79*	*17.8*	*0.2*	*0.7*	*0.0*
Raw, Jumbo, TTD, Sainsbury's*	½ Pack/85g	115	2.4	135	25.5	2.0	2.8	0.5
Spirals, Shapers, Boots*	1 Pack/100g	468	22.0	468	3.1	64.0	22.0	2.8
Succulent King, with a Sweet Chilli Sauce, Birds Eye*	1 Serving/140g	251	17.2	179	10.5	6.5	12.3	0.1
Sweet Chilli, Skewers, Tesco*	1 Skewer/22g	26	0.2	120	20.4	6.9	0.9	0.5
Tempura, Finest, Tesco*	1 Prawn/18g	31	1.6	175	11.5	11.0	9.1	4.0
Thai, M & S*	1oz/28g	29	0.9	103	5.2	13.6	3.1	1.3
Tiger, Cooked & Peeled, Average	*1 Pack/180g*	*151*	*2.0*	*84*	*18.4*	*0.1*	*1.1*	*0.0*
Tiger, Jumbo, Average	*1 Serving/50g*	*39*	*0.2*	*78*	*18.2*	*0.3*	*0.5*	*0.0*
Tiger, Raw, Average	*1 Prawn/30g*	*19*	*0.2*	*64*	*14.2*	*0.0*	*0.7*	*0.0*
Tiger, Vegetarian, Crispy, Tkc*	½ Pack/150g	225	6.0	150	12.0	17.0	4.0	5.0
Tiger, Wrapped, M & S*	1 Pack/190g	477	25.8	251	11.3	20.7	13.6	1.3
PRAWNS CHILLI								
& Coriander, King, Honduran, M & S*	½ Pack/70g	70	2.2	100	17.2	0.1	3.2	0.4
& Coriander, King, Sainsbury's*	1 Pack/140g	112	1.8	80	16.6	0.4	1.3	0.5
Battered, M & S*	1oz/28g	63	3.2	225	7.2	23.8	11.5	0.5
Sweet, Crispy, Dipping Sauce, M & S*	1 Pack/240g	515	27.8	215	7.5	19.9	11.6	2.3
Sweet, Thai, King, Sainsbury's*	1 Serving/150g	177	6.1	118	6.4	13.9	4.1	1.9
with Spicy Chilli Dip, King, Sainsbury's*	½ Pack/150g	282	10.8	188	8.6	22.2	7.2	1.0
PRAWNS CREOLE								
Spicy, BGTY, Sainsbury's*	1 Pack/350g	357	8.4	102	4.8	15.6	2.4	0.4
with Vegetable Rice, King, COU, M & S*	1 Pack/400g	300	2.4	75	4.5	13.3	0.6	0.7
PRAWNS IN								
Creamy Garlic Sauce, Youngs*	1 Serving/158g	261	22.9	165	8.5	0.3	14.5	0.0
Sweet Chilli Sauce, Asda*	1 Pack/360g	500	24.8	139	4.1	15.0	6.9	0.3
PRAWNS ORIENTAL								
M & S*	1 Pack/200g	440	23.4	220	11.9	16.9	11.7	0.9
PRAWNS SZECHUAN								
Spicy, COU, M & S*	1 Pack/400g	380	3.6	95	4.5	16.9	0.9	1.5
PRAWNS WITH								
a Spicy Cajun Dip, King, Sainsbury's*	1 Pack/240g	254	4.3	106	14.8	9.1	1.8	1.4
Chilli, Coriander & Lime, King, Waitrose*	1 Pack/140g	143	3.2	102	19.9	0.5	2.3	0.6
Garlic & Herb Butter, King, Fresh, M & S*	1 Serving/200g	330	18.0	165	12.5	9.1	9.0	0.5
Ginger & Spring Onion, Sainsbury's*	1 Pack/300g	198	9.3	66	4.7	4.7	3.1	0.3
Green Thai Sauce, Tiger, Waitrose*	½ Pack/117g	108	2.7	92	16.1	0.8	2.3	0.1
Lemon & Pepper, Honduran, King, M & S*	1 Pack/140g	133	3.6	95	17.4	0.4	2.6	0.7
Rice, Sweet Chilli, Tesco*	1 Pack/460g	488	10.1	106	2.4	19.2	2.2	0.6
with Creamy Lime Dip, King, Waitrose*	1 Pot/230g	517	40.7	225	15.8	0.8	17.7	0.2
PRETZELS								
American Style, Salted, Sainsbury's*	1 Serving/50g	201	2.2	403	10.8	79.7	4.5	1.8
Cheddar Cheese, Penn State Pretzels*	1 Sm Bag/30g	124	2.8	412	10.0	71.6	9.3	3.8
Giant, Penn State Pretzels*	1 Pretzel/18g	66	0.7	374	10.5	74.7	3.7	4.1
Giant, Salted, Tesco*	1 Serving/25g	99	1.1	395	12.2	75.8	4.3	3.4
Jumbo, Tesco*	1 Serving/50g	194	3.4	388	9.7	71.9	6.8	5.4
Lightly Salted, Tesco*	1 Serving/25g	99	1.8	395	9.3	73.4	7.1	5.5
Mini, 99% Fat Free, Free Natural*	1 Serving/50g	188	0.5	376	10.1	81.7	1.0	0.0

P

	Measure INFO/WEIGHT	per Measure KCAL	per Measure FAT	Nutrition Values per 100g / 100ml KCAL	PROT	CARB	FAT	FIBRE
PRETZELS								
Mini, M & S*	1 Pack/45g	193	6.0	430	10.4	66.6	13.4	4.9
New York Style, Salted, Mini, Shapers, Boots*	1 Bag/25g	94	0.5	375	10.0	79.0	2.1	4.2
Salt & Cracked Black Pepper, COU, M & S*	1 Pack/25g	95	0.6	380	9.7	83.3	2.4	2.7
Salted, Average	1 Serving/30g	114	0.8	380	10.3	79.8	2.6	3.0
Salted, Mini, M & S*	1 Pack/25g	94	0.5	375	10.0	79.0	2.1	4.2
Salted, Sainsbury's*	1 Serving/50g	200	1.8	401	9.8	82.4	3.6	3.4
Salted, Stars, Tesco*	1oz/28g	104	1.3	371	8.2	73.7	4.8	3.1
Sea Salt & Black Pepper, Penn State Pretzels*	1 Serving/25g	94	1.0	375	10.4	73.7	4.2	4.7
Sea Salt & Black Pepper, Tesco*	1 Serving/50g	189	1.3	379	10.0	79.0	2.6	4.1
Selection Tray, M & S*	1oz/28g	112	1.9	401	9.7	75.5	6.7	3.4
Snacks, Fabulous Bakin' Boys*	1 Pack/24g	96	1.2	401	9.0	79.5	4.9	2.5
Soft, Almond, Auntie Anne's*	1 Pretzel/112g	350	2.0	312	7.1	66.1	1.8	1.8
Soft, Cinnamon Sugar, Auntie Anne's*	1 Pretzel/112g	380	1.0	339	7.1	75.0	0.9	1.8
Soft, Cinnamon Sugar, with Butter, Auntie Anne's*	1 Pretzel/112g	470	12.0	420	7.1	75.0	10.7	1.8
Soft, Garlic, with Butter, Auntie Anne's*	1 Pretzel/112g	350	5.0	312	7.1	58.0	4.5	1.8
Soft, Jalapeno, Auntie Anne's*	1 Pretzel/126g	300	1.0	238	6.3	50.0	0.8	1.6
Soft, Salted, Original, Auntie Anne's*	1 Pretzel/112g	310	1.0	277	7.1	58.0	0.9	1.8
Soft, Salted, with Butter, Original, Auntie Anne's*	1 Pretzel/112g	340	5.0	304	7.1	26.2	4.5	1.8
Soft, Sesame, Auntie Anne's*	1 Pretzel/112g	360	6.0	321	8.9	59.8	5.4	2.7
Soft, Sesame, with Butter, Auntie Anne's*	1 Pretzel/112g	400	10.0	357	8.9	59.8	8.9	2.7
Soft, Sour Cream & Onion, with Butter, Auntie Anne's*	1 Pretzel/112g	360	5.0	321	8.0	60.7	4.5	1.8
Sour Cream & Chive, Hoops, BGTY, Sainsbury's*	1 Bag/25g	98	0.6	391	10.4	80.9	2.3	1.6
Sour Cream & Chive, Mini, HL, Tesco*	1 Pack/25g	92	0.5	369	10.9	76.3	2.2	4.6
Sour Cream & Chive, Penn State Pretzels*	1 Serving/25g	102	2.2	410	9.8	72.8	8.8	3.9
Sour Cream & Chive Flavour, Mini, Shapers, Boots*	1 Packet/25g	93	0.7	371	11.0	74.0	2.7	7.3
Sour Cream & Onion, M & S*	1 Serving/30g	136	4.3	455	11.0	70.9	14.5	0.7
Sour Cream & Onion, Tesco*	1 Serving/25g	114	4.2	457	8.4	67.7	17.0	2.3
Spicy Salsa, Penn State Pretzels*	1 Serving/25g	105	2.6	420	9.5	72.4	10.4	1.3
Sweet Thai Chilli Twists, Penn State Pretzels*	1 Serving/25g	98	2.0	393	9.8	70.1	8.2	6.8
Wheat, Gluten Free, Trufree*	1 Bag/60g	282	12.0	470	0.5	72.0	20.0	0.7
with Sea Salt, Giant, M & S*	1 Pretzel/8g	31	0.5	390	9.7	77.3	6.8	5.4
PRINGLES*								
Barbecue, Pringles*	1 Serving/50g	266	18.0	533	4.9	48.0	36.0	5.1
BBQ Spare Rib, Rice Infusions, Pringles*	1 Pack/23g	108	5.3	469	5.1	60.0	23.0	2.6
Burger, Take Away, Pringles*	1 Serving/25g	129	8.0	516	4.2	52.0	32.0	2.5
Cheese & Onion, Pringles*	1 Serving/25g	132	8.5	528	4.1	50.0	34.0	3.4
Chip n Ketchup, Pringles*	1 Serving/25g	129	8.0	516	3.9	52.0	32.0	2.5
Curry, Masala, Take Away, Pringles*	1 Serving/25g	128	8.7	514	4.3	52.0	35.0	2.6
Hot & Spicy, Pringles*	1 Serving/25g	132	8.5	530	4.6	49.0	34.0	3.7
Light, Aromas, Greek Cheese & Avocado Oil, Pringles*	1 Serving/25g	122	6.2	488	4.6	57.0	25.0	3.6
Light, Original, Pringles*	1 Serving/25g	121	6.2	484	4.3	59.0	25.0	3.6
Light, Sour Cream & Onion, Pringles*	1 Serving/25g	122	6.2	487	4.7	57.0	25.0	3.6
Margarita Pizza, Classic Takeaways, Pringles*	1 Serving/25g	134	8.0	538	3.9	53.0	32.0	2.6
Minis, Original, Pringles*	1 Pack/23g	118	6.9	514	5.1	55.0	30.0	3.7
Minis, Salt & Vinegar, Pringles*	1 Pack/23g	115	6.4	502	4.5	55.0	28.0	3.6
Minis, Sour Cream & Onion, Pringles*	1 Pack/23g	118	6.7	511	5.2	56.0	29.0	3.5
Minis, Texas BBQ Sauce, Pringles*	1 Pack/23g	116	6.4	504	5.0	56.0	28.0	3.8
Original, Pringles*	1 Serving/25g	131	8.5	526	3.9	52.0	34.0	2.6
Paprika, Pringles*	1 Serving/25g	132	8.5	529	4.9	49.0	34.0	6.5
Salt & Vinegar, Pringles*	1 Serving/25g	132	8.5	527	3.9	50.0	34.0	3.4
Sour Cream & Onion, Pringles*	1 Serving/25g	133	8.7	531	4.5	49.0	35.0	3.6
Texas BBQ Sauce, Pringles*	1 Serving/25g	132	8.5	527	4.2	50.0	34.0	3.5

P

	Measure INFO/WEIGHT	per Measure KCAL	per Measure FAT	Nutrition Values per 100g / 100ml KCAL	PROT	CARB	FAT	FIBRE
PROBIOTIC DRINK								
Cranberry & Raspberry, Dairy, Asda*	1 Bottle/100ml	64	0.8	64	2.3	12.0	0.8	2.4
Orange, Health, Tesco*	1 Serving/100g	67	0.9	67	1.5	13.4	0.9	1.3
Peach, Dairy, Asda*	1 Bottle/100ml	68	0.8	68	2.3	13.0	0.8	2.3
Strawberry, Dairy, Asda*	1 Bottle/100ml	64	0.8	64	2.3	12.0	0.8	2.3
Yoghurt, Original, Tesco*	1 Bottle/100g	68	1.0	68	1.7	13.1	1.0	1.4
PROFITEROLES								
Asda*	1 Serving/64g	218	17.2	343	5.0	20.0	27.0	0.0
Chocolate, 8 Pack, Co-Op*	¼ Pack/112g	330	17.9	295	6.0	31.0	16.0	2.0
Chocolate, Co-Op*	1 Pot/91g	260	13.7	285	6.0	33.0	15.0	3.0
Chocolate, Sainsbury's*	1/6 Pot/95g	192	8.5	202	5.4	25.1	8.9	0.8
Chocolate, Stack, Sainsbury's*	¼ Pack/76g	311	19.5	409	5.3	39.3	25.6	2.0
Chocolate, Tesco*	1 Serving/76g	293	21.8	386	5.1	26.9	28.7	0.5
Chocolate Covered, Tesco*	1 Serving/72g	295	21.2	410	5.7	29.3	29.5	2.0
Choux & Chocolate Sauce, Tesco*	1 Serving/77g	295	22.0	386	5.1	26.9	28.7	0.5
Classic French, Sainsbury's*	1 Serving/90g	284	15.5	316	6.6	33.7	17.2	0.1
Dairy Cream, Co-Op*	¼ Pack/70g	241	17.5	345	6.0	24.0	25.0	0.5
Filled with Cream, Stack, Fresh, M & S*	1 Serving/75g	281	21.4	375	5.3	23.6	28.5	1.9
in a Pot, Waitrose*	1 Pot/80g	207	11.3	259	6.3	25.6	14.1	2.9
PROVENCALE								
Chicken, M & S*	1 Pack/430g	365	11.6	85	13.2	2.3	2.7	0.6
King Prawn & Mushroom, M & S*	½ Pack/185g	120	4.6	65	7.2	3.9	2.5	0.9
Mushroom, Fresh, COU, M & S*	½ Pack/150g	60	2.2	40	2.6	4.1	1.5	1.8
Prawn & Mushroom with Pasta, COU, M & S*	1 Pack/400g	360	2.0	90	5.9	15.7	0.5	0.0
Ratatouille, Asda*	½ Can/195g	97	3.9	50	1.0	7.0	2.0	1.0
PRUNES								
Dried, Average	*1 Serving/50g*	*79*	*0.2*	*157*	*2.5*	*36.4*	*0.4*	*5.8*
in Apple Juice, Average	*1 Serving/90g*	*76*	*0.1*	*84*	*0.8*	*19.8*	*0.1*	*1.4*
in Fruit Juice, Average	*1oz/28g*	*25*	*0.0*	*88*	*0.9*	*21.4*	*0.2*	*3.0*
in Syrup, Average	*1oz/28g*	*26*	*0.0*	*92*	*1.0*	*22.1*	*0.2*	*2.6*
Pitted, Californian, Sweetvine*	1 Serving/25g	40	0.1	161	2.5	34.0	0.4	5.7
Ready to Eat, Dried, Organic, Love Life, Waitrose*	1 Serving/30g	73	0.1	243	2.2	56.8	0.4	7.3
Ready To Eat, Wholefoods, Tesco*	1 Serving/100g	230	0.3	230	1.9	54.9	0.3	6.5
Stewed with Sugar	*1oz/28g*	*29*	*0.1*	*103*	*1.3*	*25.5*	*0.2*	*3.1*
Stewed without Sugar	*1oz/28g*	*23*	*0.1*	*81*	*1.4*	*19.5*	*0.3*	*3.3*
PSYLLIUM								
Husks, Pure, Lepicol*	1 Tsp/5g	0	0.0	0	0.0	0.0	0.0	98.0
PUDDING								
Apple & Custard, Sainsbury's*	1 Serving/115g	132	2.2	115	5.4	19.0	1.9	0.1
Banana Fudge Crunch, Bird's*	1oz/28g	125	3.9	445	5.4	75.0	14.0	0.8
Blackberry & Bramley Apple, M & S*	¼ Pudding/152g	365	12.5	240	3.3	38.2	8.2	2.0
Butterscotch, Instant, Fat Free, Jell-O*	1 Serving/8g	25	0.1	333	1.3	78.7	1.3	0.0
Cherry Cobbler, GFY, Asda*	1 Pudding/100g	158	2.0	158	2.1	33.0	2.0	0.9
Chocolate, Gu*	1 Pack/240g	780	27.4	325	3.9	51.8	11.4	1.6
Chocolate, M & S*	¼ Pudding/76g	265	12.0	350	4.1	48.0	15.8	2.1
Chocolate, Melting Middle, M & S*	1 Pudding/155g	510	27.8	330	5.8	36.2	18.0	3.1
Chocolate, Perfectly Balanced, Waitrose*	1 Pot/105g	196	3.3	187	3.8	36.0	3.1	0.8
Chocolate, Tesco*	1 Serving/110g	348	21.0	316	3.1	32.9	19.1	1.9
Chocolate & Vanilla Swirls, Sugar Free, Jell-O*	1 Pot/106g	60	1.5	57	0.9	12.3	1.4	0.0
Chocolate Bombe, Finest, Tesco*	¼ Pudding/100g	350	12.9	350	5.1	53.0	12.9	2.6
Chocolate with Cream, Delice, Campina*	1 Pot/100g	136	5.4	136	2.5	18.9	5.4	0.0
Christmas, Free From, Sainsbury's*	¼ Pudding/114g	346	7.8	305	1.8	58.9	6.9	4.7
Creamed Sago, Ambrosia*	1 Serving/200g	158	3.2	79	2.5	13.6	1.6	0.2
Creme Aux Oeufs a la Vanille, Weight Watchers*	1 Pot/100g	116	3.2	116	4.8	17.0	3.2	0.0

	Measure INFO/WEIGHT	per Measure		Nutrition Values per 100g / 100ml				
		KCAL	FAT	KCAL	PROT	CARB	FAT	FIBRE

PUDDING

	Measure INFO/WEIGHT	KCAL	FAT	KCAL	PROT	CARB	FAT	FIBRE
Eve's, Average	1oz/28g	67	3.7	241	3.5	28.9	13.1	1.4
Eve's, BGTY, Sainsbury's*	1 Pudding/145g	164	1.7	113	2.2	23.4	1.2	0.7
Eve's, with Custard, Less Than 5% Fat, M & S*	1 Pudding/205g	318	9.4	155	3.4	24.7	4.6	0.7
Jam Roly Poly & Custard, Co-Op*	1 Serving/105g	262	7.3	250	3.0	44.0	7.0	0.8
Lemon, BGTY, Sainsbury's*	1 Serving/100g	151	1.9	151	2.9	31.0	1.9	0.5
Lemon, M & S*	1 Pudding/105g	328	16.0	312	4.3	39.4	15.2	2.3
Lemon, Perfectly Balanced, Waitrose*	1 Serving/105g	212	2.5	202	3.4	41.7	2.4	0.6
Lemon Crunch, Bird's*	1oz/28g	125	3.9	445	5.5	74.0	14.0	0.7
Luxury, Christmas X2, Tesco*	1 Serving/100g	295	8.1	295	2.6	52.1	8.1	6.0
Matured, Christmas, Finest, Tesco*	1 Serving/100g	353	13.4	353	4.6	51.4	13.4	2.0
Melting Chocolate & Pecan, Brownie Pud, Gu*	1/6 Pudding/67g	290	17.6	436	5.3	45.1	26.4	3.1
Panettone, Finest, Tesco*	1oz/28g	94	4.2	335	3.8	45.7	14.9	5.3
Queen of Puddings	1oz/28g	60	2.2	213	4.8	33.1	7.8	0.2
Raspberry, Jam Sponge Puddings, M & S*	1 Pot/119g	400	14.0	335	4.0	53.1	11.7	1.4
Rhubarb & Custard, BGTY, Sainsbury's*	1 Pudding/140g	137	2.8	98	2.0	18.4	2.0	1.4
Sticky Toffee, Co-Op*	1/4 Pudding/100g	355	20.0	355	3.0	40.0	20.0	0.7
Sticky Toffee, Extra Special, Asda*	1/4 Pudding/100g	378	18.0	378	1.9	52.0	18.0	1.8
Sticky Toffee, HL, Tesco*	1 Pack/125g	245	5.6	196	4.0	34.9	4.5	0.6
Sticky Toffee, Tesco*	1 Serving/110g	287	14.7	261	3.3	31.8	13.4	0.7
Sticky Toffee, Tryton Foods*	1oz/28g	88	1.5	314	3.7	62.7	5.4	1.0
Sticky Toffee, Weight Watchers*	1 Pudding/100g	172	1.1	172	3.0	27.2	1.1	20.5
Strawberry, Jelly Pud with Devon Custard, Ambrosia*	1 Pot/150g	129	1.2	86	0.7	19.4	0.8	0.0
Summer Fruits, Co-Op*	1 Pack/260g	273	0.5	105	1.0	25.0	0.2	1.0
Summer Fruits, Eat Well, M & S*	1 Pudding/135g	128	0.7	95	1.7	20.8	0.5	3.0
Summer Pudding, BGTY, Sainsbury's*	1 Pot/110g	223	5.1	203	3.2	40.9	4.6	2.4
Summer Pudding, Waitrose*	1 Pot/120g	125	0.5	104	2.0	23.1	0.4	1.4
Syrup, Individual, Co-Op*	1 Pudding/170g	603	35.7	355	3.0	38.0	21.0	1.0
Syrup, M & S*	1 Serving/105g	370	10.5	352	3.9	61.7	10.0	0.8
Truffle, Chocolate, with Raspberry Compote, Gu*	1 Pot/80g	250	14.6	312	2.7	28.7	18.2	1.7
Truffle, Chocolate Amaretto, Gu*	1 Pot/80g	272	15.5	340	3.2	34.9	19.4	1.6
Truffle, Double Chocolate, Cheeky Chocolate, Gu*	1 Pot/50g	216	17.9	433	3.2	24.1	35.9	2.1
Ultimate Christmas, Finest, Tesco*	1 Serving/100g	285	7.0	285	3.7	51.6	7.0	4.7

PUDDINGS

	Measure INFO/WEIGHT	KCAL	FAT	KCAL	PROT	CARB	FAT	FIBRE
Chocolate, Raspberry & Chilli Puds	1 Pot/85g	212	12.8	249	3.2	25.0	15.1	1.3
Hot Chocolate Melting Middle Puds, Gu*	1 Pud/100g	409	26.9	409	6.0	36.0	26.9	2.7
Souffle, Hot Chocolate, Gu*	1 Pot/65g	298	23.5	458	6.0	24.1	36.2	2.5
Torte, Cheeky Little Chocolate, Gu*	1 Pud/50g	211	14.5	422	5.7	31.6	29.1	1.8

PUMPKIN

	Measure INFO/WEIGHT	KCAL	FAT	KCAL	PROT	CARB	FAT	FIBRE
Boiled in Salted Water	**1oz/28g**	**4**	**0.1**	**13**	**0.6**	**2.1**	**0.3**	**1.1**
Kabocha, Tesco*	1 Serving 50g	19	0.0	39	1.1	8.3	0.1	1.6
Solid Pack, 100% Pure, Canned, Libby's*	1 Can/425g	139	1.7	33	1.6	7.4	0.4	4.1

PUPPODUMS

	Measure INFO/WEIGHT	KCAL	FAT	KCAL	PROT	CARB	FAT	FIBRE
Cracked Black Pepper, Ready to Eat, Sharwood's*	1 Puppodum/9g	41	2.4	461	16.7	37.2	27.3	7.3
Extra Large, Cook to Eat, Sharwood's*	1oz/28g	78	0.5	279	21.3	44.7	1.7	10.3
Garlic & Coriander, Ready to Eat, Sharwood's*	1 Puppodum/9g	39	1.9	438	18.4	43.0	21.4	6.5
Plain, Cook to Eat, Sharwood's*	1 Puppodum/12g	32	0.1	273	21.9	45.7	1.0	10.1
Plain, Mini, Cook to Eat, Sharwood's*	1 Puppodum/4g	11	0.0	273	21.9	45.7	0.3	10.1
Plain, Ready to Eat, Sharwood's*	1 Puppodum/9g	41	2.3	461	17.0	40.6	25.6	5.6
Spicy, Cook to Eat, Sharwood's*	1 Puppodum/12g	30	0.1	257	20.2	43.0	0.5	13.0

P

QUAVERS

	Measure INFO/WEIGHT	per Measure KCAL	FAT	KCAL	PROT	CARB	FAT	FIBRE
Cheese, Walkers*	1 Std Bag/16g	88	4.9	534	2.7	62.5	30.1	1.1
Prawn Cocktail, Walkers*	1 Bag/16g	90	5.2	550	1.9	63.7	31.9	1.2
Salt & Vinegar, Walkers*	1 Bag/16g	86	4.9	525	1.9	62.0	30.0	1.2

QUICHE

	Measure INFO/WEIGHT	per Measure KCAL	FAT	KCAL	PROT	CARB	FAT	FIBRE
Asparagus & Feta, Little, Higgidy*	1 Portion/155g	369	23.4	238	8.1	17.3	15.1	1.4
Asparagus & Herby Summer Vegetable, Higgidy*	1 Quiche/400g	848	50.0	212	5.9	18.9	12.5	2.7
Asparagus & Mushroom, Tesco*	½ Quiche/200g	474	32.8	237	5.1	17.2	16.4	1.2
Baby Spinach & Gruyere, Sainsbury's*	¼ Quiche/93g	228	16.0	245	7.4	15.1	17.2	1.0
Bacon, Leek, & Cheese, Weight Watchers*	1 Quiche/165g	327	15.7	198	8.2	18.0	9.5	1.8
Bacon, Leek & Mushroom, M & S*	¼ Quiche/100g	245	16.4	245	6.9	17.2	16.4	1.3
Bacon, Smoked, & Mature Cheddar, Higgidy*	1 Quiche/400g	1096	74.0	274	8.4	18.6	18.5	1.5
Bacon & Cheese, Pork Farms*	1 Pack/120g	378	24.0	315	11.1	20.8	20.0	0.0
Bacon & Cheese, Sainsbury's*	¼ Quiche/100g	237	15.0	237	7.0	18.6	15.0	0.7
Bacon & Leek, Asda*	¼ Quiche/100g	252	15.9	252	8.4	18.9	15.9	1.5
Bacon & Leek, Individual, Tesco*	1 Quiche/175g	485	32.4	277	8.3	19.4	18.5	0.9
Bacon & Leek, Tesco*	¼ Quiche/100g	260	18.0	260	6.9	17.5	18.0	1.2
Bacon & Tomato, Asda*	1 Serving/107g	201	8.6	188	8.0	21.0	8.0	1.1
Brie & Smoked Bacon, Asda*	¼ Quiche/90g	249	17.0	277	8.9	17.8	18.9	1.0
Broccoli, Tesco*	1 Serving/100g	249	17.2	249	6.0	17.6	17.2	1.4
Broccoli, Tomato & Cheese, BGTY, Sainsbury's*	1 Quiche/390g	632	32.0	162	6.4	15.7	8.2	1.3
Broccoli, Tomato & Cheese, Deep Filled, Sainsbury's*	¼ Quiche/100g	203	12.9	203	5.2	16.9	12.9	2.3
Broccoli & Gruyere Cheese, Waitrose*	1 Serving/100g	241	17.8	241	7.3	13.0	17.8	2.9
Broccoli & Stilton, Mini, Sainsbury's*	1 Quiche/14g	52	3.0	369	8.8	35.2	21.4	3.3
Cheese, Broccoli & Tomato, Nisa Heritage*	1 Serving/85g	234	16.6	275	7.3	17.5	19.5	1.4
Cheese, Onion & Chive, Tesco*	1oz/28g	90	6.7	320	10.6	15.5	24.0	0.6
Cheese & Bacon, Crustless, Tesco*	1 Serving/85g	170	11.7	200	8.8	9.6	13.8	3.3
Cheese & Broccoli, Morrisons*	1 Serving/134g	338	22.4	253	7.1	18.4	16.8	1.7
Cheese & Egg	1oz/28g	88	6.2	314	12.5	17.3	22.2	0.6
Cheese & Ham, Sainsbury's*	1 Serving/100g	266	19.0	266	9.3	14.4	19.0	1.2
Cheese & Onion, 25% Reduced Fat, Asda*	½ Quiche/78g	163	7.0	209	11.0	21.0	9.0	2.4
Cheese & Onion, Crustless, Asda*	1 Quiche/160g	277	15.2	173	7.6	14.3	9.5	1.3
Cheese & Onion, Deep Filled, Sainsbury's*	¼ Quiche/100g	254	17.2	254	7.3	17.2	17.2	2.2
Cheese & Onion, Finest, Tesco*	1 Serving/130g	346	24.3	266	9.1	15.3	18.7	2.5
Cheese & Onion, HL, Tesco*	1 Quarter/100g	180	7.8	180	9.4	17.6	7.8	1.8
Cheese & Onion, M & S*	1 Slice/100g	250	17.2	250	8.2	16.1	17.2	1.5
Cheese & Onion, VLH Kitchens*	1 Slice/80g	133.6	4.8	167	9.6	18.1	6.0	1.8
Cheese & Onion, Weight Watchers*	1 Quiche/165g	325	15.3	197	7.0	21.2	9.3	1.6
Cheese & Tomato, M & S*	1 Serving/100g	230	15.6	230	7.7	15.1	15.6	1.6
Cheese & Tomato, Morrisons*	½ Quiche/64g	195	13.1	304	7.3	22.8	20.5	1.0
Chicken, Garlic & Herb, Asda*	1/8 Quiche/52g	137	8.3	264	10.0	20.0	16.0	1.2
Chicken & Basil, Finest, Tesco*	1 Serving/134g	381	24.9	284	9.3	19.8	18.6	1.3
Crustless, Green Vegetable, Light Choices, Tesco*	1 Quiche/160g	200	9.3	125	6.0	11.9	5.8	4.7
Cumberland Sausage & Onion, Sainsbury's*	1 Serving/180g	486	33.3	270	7.0	18.8	18.5	1.3
Farmhouse Cheddar & Onion, Waitrose*	¼ Quiche/100g	257	18.1	257	8.1	15.4	18.1	1.3
Gammon, Leek & Mustard, Weight Watchers*	1 Quiche/165g	305	14.5	185	5.7	20.7	8.8	3.4
Garlic Mushroom, Asda*	¼ Quiche/105g	273	16.8	260	7.0	22.0	16.0	0.7
Goats Cheese & Red Pepper, Finest, Tesco*	1 Serving/200g	600	45.0	300	5.9	18.5	22.5	1.5
Ham, Cheese & Chive, GFY, Asda*	1 Serving/78g	173	7.8	222	9.0	24.0	10.0	1.5
Ham & Mustard, GFY, Asda*	1 Quiche/155g	327	17.0	211	9.0	19.0	11.0	3.9
Ham & Soft Cheese, Tesco*	¼ Quiche/100g	280	20.1	280	7.4	17.5	20.1	1.9
Ham & Tomato, M & S*	½ Pack/200g	440	31.0	220	8.1	12.4	15.5	2.9
Leek & Sweet Potato, Waitrose*	½ Quiche/200g	440	29.0	220	5.3	17.0	14.5	2.3
Lorraine, Average	1oz/28g	109	7.9	391	16.1	19.8	28.1	0.7

	Measure INFO/WEIGHT	per Measure		Nutrition Values per 100g / 100ml				
		KCAL	FAT	KCAL	PROT	CARB	FAT	FIBRE
QUICHE								
Lorraine, Crustless, Asda*	1 Quiche/160g	259	12.6	162	9.3	13.5	7.9	1.1
Lorraine, Crustless, Light Choices, Tesco*	1 Pack/160g	280	13.4	175	12.6	11.8	8.4	2.5
Lorraine, Half Fat, Waitrose*	¼ Quiche/100g	189	8.9	189	8.1	19.0	8.9	1.4
Lorraine, Light Choices, Tesco*	¼ Pack/100g	170	6.4	170	12.3	15.5	6.4	3.2
Lorraine, Meat Free, Tesco*	1 Quiche/140g	335	19.3	240	9.4	19.1	13.8	2.8
Lorraine, Smoked Bacon & Cheese, M & S*	¼ Quiche/100g	270	18.4	270	9.7	16.4	18.4	1.6
Lorraine, Weight Watchers*	1 Quiche/165g	292	13.2	177	8.7	17.5	8.0	3.2
Meat Feast, Tesco*	¼ Quiche/100g	265	19.0	265	6.2	17.2	19.0	2.5
Mediterranean, GFY, Asda*	1 Serving/25g	54	2.2	217	9.0	25.0	9.0	2.4
Mediterranean, M & S*	1oz/28g	64	4.3	230	6.6	16.6	15.3	0.9
Mediterranean Vegetable, BGTY, Sainsbury's*	½ Quiche/90g	160	7.2	178	7.3	19.2	8.0	1.7
Mediterranean Vegetable, Mini, M & S*	1oz/28g	78	4.9	280	6.8	23.9	17.5	1.6
Mediterranean Vegetable, Weight Watchers*	1 Quiche/165g	285	13.5	173	3.8	21.1	8.2	4.0
Mushroom	1oz/28g	80	5.5	284	10.0	18.3	19.5	0.9
Red Pepper, Goats Cheese & Spinach, Waitrose*	1 Serving/100g	218	14.3	218	6.5	15.8	14.3	2.6
Red Pepper, Rocket & Parmesan, Waitrose*	1 Serving/100g	236	16.9	236	6.1	14.8	16.9	1.9
Salmon & Broccoli, Sainsbury's*	1 Serving	346	22.8	260	7.9	18.5	17.1	0.8
Salmon & Broccoli, Tesco*	1 Serving/133g	311	20.1	234	7.9	16.6	15.1	0.9
Sausage & Onion, Sainsbury's*	1 Serving/100g	287	20.0	287	7.1	19.7	20.0	1.2
Smoked Bacon & Cheddar, Little, Higgidy*	1 Quiche/155g	485	33.8	313	11.5	17.6	21.8	1.0
Spinach, Feta & Roasted Red Pepper, Higgidy*	1 Quiche/400g	888	53.2	222	5.8	19.9	13.3	2.2
Spinach & Gruyere, Sainsbury's*	¼ Quiche/100g	258	19.1	258	7.7	13.9	19.1	1.0
Spinach & Ricotta, M & S*	1oz/28g	73	5.3	260	8.0	14.9	18.8	1.7
Spinach & Roast Red Pepper, Little, Higgidy*	1 Quiche/155g	397	27.3	256	9.1	15.2	17.6	1.2
Sweet Cherry Pepper & Fontal Cheese, Finest, Tesco*	¼ Quiche/100g	293	22.1	293	6.7	16.9	22.1	0.9
Sweetfire Pepper, Feta & Olive, Waitrose*	¼ Quiche/100g	238	16.9	238	5.7	15.7	16.9	1.4
Three Cheese & Onion, GFY, Asda*	1 Serving/73g	188	10.2	258	10.0	23.0	14.0	3.1
Tomato, Cheese & Courgette, Asda*	1 Quiche/100g	333	17.0	333	11.0	34.0	17.0	5.0
Tomato, GFY, Asda*	¼ Quiche/50g	94	4.0	188	8.0	21.0	8.0	0.8
Tomato, Mozzarella, & Basil, Weight Watchers*	1 Quiche/165g	300	12.2	182	6.1	22.8	7.4	1.3
Tomato, Mushroom & Bacon, Sainsbury's*	1 Serving/187g	447	30.9	239	7.5	15.2	16.5	1.1
Tomato, VLH Kitchens*	1 Slice/100g	215	11.0	215	7.0	22.0	11.0	3.3
Tuna, Tomato & Basil, Asda*	1 Serving/125g	305	20.0	244	9.0	16.0	16.0	1.5
Vegetable, Tesco*	1 Serving/100g	257	17.7	257	6.9	17.5	17.7	1.5
QUINCE								
Average	*1 Fruit/209g*	*54*	*0.2*	*26*	*0.3*	*6.3*	*0.1*	*1.9*
QUINOA								
Dry Weight, Average	*1 Serving/70g*	*258*	*4.2*	*368*	*14.1*	*64.2*	*6.1*	*7.0*
Organic, Dry Weight, Love Life, Waitrose*	1 Serving/40g	154	2.3	384	13.1	68.9	5.8	5.9
Red	1 Serving/100g	358	6.0	358	12.9	62.2	6.0	9.7
QUORN*								
Bacon Style, Slices, Smoky, Frozen, Quorn*	¼ Pack/38g	75	5.8	199	11.8	3.0	15.5	5.0
Bacon Style Rashers, Deli, Quorn*	4 Rashers	85	3.7	141	13.5	8.1	6.1	4.2
Balls, Al Forno, Quorn*	1 Serving/400g	348	7.2	87	4.7	13.1	1.8	1.8
Balls, Swedish Style, Quorn*	1 Pack/300g	354	6.0	118	17.0	8.0	2.0	2.0
Beef Style Pieces, in Red Wine Sauce, Quorn*	1 Pack/275g	165	4.1	60	5.0	6.5	1.5	1.7
Beef Style Pieces, Quorn*	½ Pack/75g	69	1.6	92	13.5	4.5	2.2	5.0
Bites, BBQ, Quorn*	1 Pack/140g	147	3.5	105	13.5	7.0	2.5	5.5
Bites, Indian, Quorn*	1 Bite/15g	34	1.5	222	6.0	27.0	10.0	3.0
Bites, Lamb Style Kofta, Quorn*	1 Bite/25g	47	2.4	186	5.0	20.0	9.5	3.0
Bites, Quorn*	½ Pack/70g	77	1.7	110	13.8	8.0	2.5	5.0
Burgers, Chicken Style, Quorn*	1 Burger/70g	136	6.7	194	11.0	16.0	9.6	4.6
Burgers, Minted Lamb Style, Quorn*	1 Burger/80g	86	3.2	108	12.0	6.0	4.0	4.0

Q

QUORN*

	Measure INFO/WEIGHT	per Measure KCAL	per Measure FAT	KCAL	PROT	CARB	FAT	FIBRE
Burgers, Original, Quorn*	1 Burger/50g	73	2.4	146	18.9	6.7	4.8	3.0
Burgers, Premium, Quorn*	1 Burger/82g	88	3.3	107	11.3	6.5	4.0	3.5
Burgers, Quarter Pounder, Mexican Style, Quorn*	1 Burger/113g	180	6.3	159	18.3	8.9	5.6	3.8
Burgers, Quarter Pounder, Quorn*	1 Burger/113g	158	5.1	139	18.0	6.5	4.5	4.5
Burgers, Sizzling, Quorn*	1 Burger/80g	123	4.8	154	18.0	7.0	6.0	3.0
Burgers, Southern Style, Quorn*	1 Burger/63g	119	6.2	189	10.7	14.5	9.8	3.1
Chicken Style Dippers, Quorn*	1 Dipper/19g	32	2.0	167	11.0	7.2	10.5	4.0
Chicken Style Pieces, Frozen Or Chilled, Quorn*	1 Serving/87g	90	2.3	103	14.0	5.8	2.6	5.5
Chilli, Quorn*	1oz/28g	23	1.2	81	4.7	6.9	4.2	2.5
Chilli, Vegetarian, Tesco*	1 Pack/400g	340	3.2	85	4.4	15.0	0.8	2.1
Cottage Pie, Quorn*	1 Pack/500g	335	5.0	67	2.5	11.0	1.0	1.8
Curry, Red Thai, Quorn*	1 Pack/400g	464	15.6	116	4.6	15.5	3.9	4.0
Curry & Rice, Quorn*	1 Pack/400g	412	8.0	103	3.8	17.5	2.0	1.5
Eggs, Picnic, Quorn*	1 Egg/20g	50	2.3	248	15.0	21.0	11.5	4.6
En Croute, Cheddar Cheese & Ham Style, Quorn*	1 Pastry/200g	486	28.0	243	7.2	22.0	14.0	3.0
En Croute, Creamy Mushroom & Garlic, Quorn*	1 Pastry/200g	460	29.0	230	5.9	19.0	14.5	3.2
Enchiladas, Quorn*	1 Pack/401g	405	14.8	101	5.3	11.7	3.7	1.9
Escalopes, Creamy Garlic & Mushroom, Quorn*	1 Piece/120g	266	15.0	222	7.9	19.4	12.5	3.1
Escalopes, Creamy Peppercorn, Quorn*	2 Piece/120g	252	15.2	210	7.8	16.0	12.7	4.0
Escalopes, Feta & Tomato, Quorn*	3 Piece/120g	257	14.6	214	8.0	18.0	12.2	4.0
Escalopes, Garlic & Herb, Quorn*	1 Piece/140g	293	16.5	209	8.9	16.9	11.8	3.8
Escalopes, Goats Cheese & Cranberry, Quorn*	1 Piece/120g	281	16.8	234	10.0	17.0	14.0	4.0
Escalopes, Gruyere Cheese, Quorn*	1 Piece/110g	262	15.4	238	10.0	18.0	14.0	2.6
Escalopes, Korma, Quorn*	1 Piece/120g	270	15.6	225	7.0	20.0	13.0	3.0
Escalopes, Lemon & Black Pepper, Quorn*	1 Piece/110g	249	12.9	226	9.6	20.5	11.7	2.1
Escalopes, Mature Cheddar & Broccoli, Quorn*	1 Piece/120g	244	13.7	203	8.7	16.5	11.4	2.9
Escalopes, Spinach & Soft Cheese, Quorn*	1 Piece/120g	236	13.2	197	8.5	16.1	11.0	2.9
Escalopes, Sweet Pepper & Mozzarella, Quorn*	1 Piece120g	231	12.4	193	8.7	16.1	10.4	3.8
Escalopes, Wensleydale & Blueberry, Quorn*	1 Piece/120g	281	16.8	234	10.0	17.0	14.0	4.0
Fajita Meal Kit, Quorn*	½ Pack/214g	268	5.4	125	7.0	18.5	2.5	3.5
Fillets, Cajun Spice, Quorn*	1 Serving/100g	176	8.2	176	10.9	14.7	8.2	3.4
Fillets, Chargrilled Tikka Style, Mini, Quorn*	½ Pack/85g	110	2.0	129	12.5	14.4	2.4	5.0
Fillets, Chinese Style Chargrilled, Mini, Quorn*	1 Serving/85g	115	2.3	135	12.1	15.6	2.7	4.7
Fillets, Crispy, Quorn*	1 Fillet/100g	197	9.8	197	13.0	14.2	9.8	4.0
Fillets, Garlic & Herb, Quorn*	1 Fillet/100g	208	9.8	208	13.9	16.1	9.8	4.1
Fillets, Hot & Spicy, Quorn*	1 Fillet/100g	176	8.2	176	10.9	14.7	8.2	6.4
Fillets, in a Mediterranean Marinade, Quorn*	1 Fillet/80g	90	2.4	112	12.5	8.8	3.0	4.0
Fillets, Lemon & Pepper, Quorn*	1 Fillet/100g	195	8.5	195	13.3	16.2	8.5	3.5
Fillets, Mushroom & White Wine Sauce, Quorn*	1oz/28g	18	0.5	65	6.3	6.0	1.8	2.1
Fillets, Oriental, Sainsbury's*	1 Serving/294g	353	1.8	120	4.0	24.6	0.6	1.8
Fillets, Plain, Quorn*	1 Fillet/52g	47	0.9	90	12.6	5.9	1.8	4.7
Fillets, Provencale, Morrisons*	1 Serving/165g	94	2.3	57	5.4	5.8	1.4	1.1
Fillets, Thai, Quorn*	1 Serving/79g	96	3.6	121	11.0	9.0	4.5	4.0
Florentine, Deli, Quorn*	1 Slice/15g	21	0.9	140	15.0	5.8	6.3	3.0
Goujons, Quorn*	1 Goujon/31g	57	2.9	187	10.2	15.0	9.6	4.5
Goujons, with Chunky Salsa Dip, Quorn*	1oz/28g	57	2.9	204	10.4	17.0	10.5	3.0
Grills, Lamb Style, Quorn*	1 Grill/89g	97	3.3	109	11.2	7.6	3.7	4.3
Kievs, Mini, Quorn*	1 Kiev/20g	41	2.2	207	14.0	13.0	11.0	6.5
Lasagne, Quorn*	1 Pack/400g	332	11.6	83	3.7	10.6	2.9	1.8
Mini Savoury Eggs, Quorn*	1 Egg/20g	50	2.3	248	15.0	21.0	11.5	4.6
Moussaka, Quorn*	1 Pack/400g	364	16.4	91	3.6	9.8	4.1	1.2
Noodles, Sweet Chilli, Quorn*	1 Pack/400g	352	9.2	88	4.2	12.7	2.3	1.5
Nuggets, Chicken Style, Quorn*	1 Nugget/20g	41	2.2	207	10.3	16.7	11.0	3.8

	Measure INFO/WEIGHT	per Measure KCAL	FAT	Nutrition Values per 100g / 100ml KCAL	PROT	CARB	FAT	FIBRE
QUORN*								
Nuggets, Crispy, Chicken Style, Quorn*	1 Nugget/16g	29	1.7	182	12.0	9.9	10.5	4.0
Nuggets, Crispy Chicken Style, Quorn*	1 Nugget/16g	29	1.7	182	12.0	9.9	10.5	4.0
Pasty, Cornish Style, Quorn*	1 Pasty/150g	399	24.0	266	5.5	25.0	16.0	3.0
Pate, Brussels Style, Deli, Quorn*	1/3 Pack/43g	55	2.3	128	11.3	8.5	5.4	4.0
Pate, Country Style Coarse, Quorn*	½ Pot/65g	68	2.7	104	9.2	7.3	4.2	2.7
Pie, & Vegetable, Quorn*	1oz/28g	52	3.2	186	6.9	14.7	11.5	2.0
Pie, Creamy Mushroom, Quorn*	1 Pie/142g	359	20.6	253	4.5	26.0	14.5	2.0
Pie, Creamy Mushroom, Sainsbury's*	1 Pie/134g	355	21.7	265	5.1	24.7	16.2	1.9
Pie, Mince & Onion, Quorn*	1 Pie/142ml	360	19.8	254	5.0	27.0	14.0	1.5
Pie, Quorn & Mushroom, Tesco*	1 Pie/141g	378	23.7	268	5.3	23.8	16.8	1.3
Pork Style Ribsters, Quorn*	2 Ribsters/85g	105	3.3	124	15.9	6.3	3.9	2.1
Roast, Chicken Style, Quorn*	1/5 Roast/91g	87	1.8	96	15.0	4.5	2.0	4.9
Satay Sticks, Quorn*	½ Pack/90g	149	8.5	165	13.0	7.1	9.4	3.2
Sausage & Mash, Sainsbury's*	1 Pack/394g	339	11.8	86	3.8	11.0	3.0	0.7
Sausage & Mash, Tesco*	1 Pack/400g	292	9.6	73	4.1	8.8	2.4	1.3
Sausage Roll, Chilled, Quorn*	1 Roll/75g	194	9.6	258	12.0	24.0	12.7	4.0
Sausages, Bangers, Bramley Apple, Quorn*	1 Sausage/50g	59	2.3	117	11.5	7.5	4.6	3.0
Sausages, Bangers, Quorn*	1 Sausage/50g	58	2.4	116	11.7	6.6	4.8	3.0
Sausages, Bangers, Sizzling, Quorn*	1 Sausage/50g	86	5.5	171	13.0	5.0	11.0	5.0
Sausages, Cumberland, Quorn*	1 Sausage/50g	60	2.2	120	13.1	7.0	4.4	2.4
Sausages, Leek & Pork Style, Quorn*	1 Sausage/44g	56	2.2	127	15.1	5.5	4.9	4.3
Sausages, Pork & Apple Style, Quorn*	1 Sausage/50g	58	2.3	117	11.5	7.5	4.6	3.0
Sausages, Quorn*	1 Sausage/43g	70	2.9	165	12.6	11.6	6.8	3.5
Sausages, Red Leicester & Onion, Quorn*	1 Sausage/50g	72	2.9	144	13.0	10.0	5.8	3.0
Sausages, Sizzlers, BBQ, Quorn*	1 Sausage/50g	83	5.4	165	13.0	4.0	10.8	4.0
Sausages, Smoky Red Pepper Sizzlers, Quorn*	1 Sausage/50g	83	5.4	165	13.0	4.0	10.8	4.0
Sausages, Spinach & Cheese, Quorn*	1 Sausage/50g	60	2.0	120	15.1	6.0	4.0	2.8
Sausages, Sweet Chilli, Quorn*	1 Sausage/50g	63	2.3	125	14.0	7.0	4.5	3.0
Sausages, Tomato & Basil, Quorn*	1 Sausage/50g	51	1.1	102	14.3	6.0	2.3	2.8
Seasoned Steak, Strips, Quorn*	½ Pack/70g	76	0.9	109	14.0	7.5	1.3	5.5
Slices, Chicken Style, Deli, Quorn*	½ Pack/50g	53	1.3	107	16.3	4.5	2.6	6.0
Slices, Chicken Style, Wafer Thin, Deli, Quorn*	1/3 Pack/60g	64	1.6	107	16.3	4.5	2.6	5.9
Slices, Ham Style, Deli, Quorn*	½ Pack/50g	55	1.1	110	16.0	6.5	2.2	5.8
Slices, Ham Style, Smoky, Quorn*	½ Pack/50g	55	1.2	110	16.5	5.7	2.4	5.0
Slices, Ham Style, Wafer Thin, Deli, Quorn*	1/3 Pack/60g	66	1.3	110	16.0	6.5	2.2	5.8
Slices, Peppered Beef Style, Quorn*	½ Pack/50g	53	1.0	107	14.5	7.6	2.1	4.0
Slices, Roast Chicken Style, Quorn*	½ Pack/50g	54	1.1	109	16.0	6.4	2.2	5.6
Slices, Turkey Style, with Stuffing, Deli, Quorn*	½ Pack/50g	53	1.1	107	14.9	6.6	2.3	4.7
Slices, Turkey Style & Cranberry, Quorn*	½ Pack/50g	56	1.2	113	14.5	8.0	2.5	4.0
Southern Style, Strips, Quorn*	1 Strip/31g	62	2.9	200	9.5	19.0	9.5	3.5
Spaghetti Bolognese, Quorn*	1 Pack/400g	240	3.6	60	3.7	9.2	0.9	1.6
Spaghetti Bolognese, Sainsbury's*	1 Pack/450g	346	4.9	77	4.9	11.9	1.1	1.8
Spaghetti Carbonara, Quorn*	1 Pack/400g	460	26.0	115	5.0	9.1	6.5	1.1
Steaks, Peppered, Quorn*	1 Steak/98g	107	3.7	109	11.4	7.4	3.8	4.0
Stir Fry, Spicy Chilli with Vegetables & Rice, Quorn*	½ Pack/170g	161	1.7	95	5.9	15.6	1.0	1.8
Sweet & Sour, with Long Grain Rice, Quorn*	1 Pack/400g	380	4.0	95	4.0	17.5	1.0	2.0
Tandoori Pieces, Quorn*	½ Pack/70g	93	3.1	133	12.0	11.0	4.5	5.0
Tikka Masala, & Rice, Tesco*	1 Pack/400g	364	9.6	91	3.4	13.9	2.4	1.7
Tikka Masala, with Rice, Quorn*	1 Pack/300g	261	2.4	87	3.5	15.0	0.8	2.8

Q

	Measure INFO/WEIGHT	per Measure KCAL	FAT	Nutrition Values per 100g / 100ml KCAL	PROT	CARB	FAT	FIBRE
RABBIT								
Meat Only, Raw	*1oz/28g*	*38*	*1.5*	*137*	*21.9*	*0.0*	*5.5*	*0.0*
Meat Only, Stewed	*1oz/28g*	*32*	*0.9*	*114*	*21.2*	*0.0*	*3.2*	*0.0*
Meat Only, Stewed, Weighed with Bone	*1oz/28g*	*19*	*0.5*	*68*	*12.7*	*0.0*	*1.9*	*0.0*
RADDICCIO								
Raw	*1oz/28g*	*4*	*0.1*	*14*	*1.4*	*1.7*	*0.2*	*1.8*
RADISH								
Red, Unprepared, Average	*1 Radish/8g*	*1*	*0.0*	*12*	*0.7*	*1.9*	*0.2*	*0.9*
White, Mooli, Raw	*1oz/28g*	*4*	*0.0*	*15*	*0.8*	*2.9*	*0.1*	*0.0*
RAISINS								
& Apricot, The Fruit Factory*	1 Box/14g	41	0.1	290	3.5	67.9	0.5	6.3
& Cranberries, Waitrose*	1 Serving/30g	94	0.1	312	1.5	75.7	0.3	3.4
& Sultanas, Jumbo, M & S*	1 Serving/80g	212	0.4	265	2.4	62.4	0.5	2.6
& Sultanas, Little Herberts, Nature's Harvest*	1 Pack/40g	128	0.2	319	3.1	75.5	0.5	3.7
& Sultanas, The Fruit Factory*	1 Box/14g	43	0.1	305	3.0	72.3	0.5	4.0
Blueberry Yoghurt Covered Raisins, Boots*	1 Pack/75g	322	13.5	429	2.7	64.0	18.0	0.7
Cherry, Naturally Infused, Graze*	1 Pack/30g	90	0.0	299	3.0	79.0	0.0	0.0
Lemon Infused, Nak'd*	1 Serving/25g	75	0.0	299	3.0	79.0	0.0	4.0
Orange, Naturally Infused, Graze*	1 Pack/30g	90	0.0	299	3.0	79.0	0.0	0.0
Seedless, Average	*1 Serving/75g*	*215*	*0.4*	*287*	*2.2*	*68.5*	*0.5*	*3.1*
Sunny, Whitworths*	1 Box/43g	116	0.2	272	2.4	65.0	0.4	4.9
Very Cherry, Graze*	1 Punnet/40g	110	0.4	275	2.1	69.0	0.9	0.0
White Chocolate Coated, Graze*	1 Pack/30g	135	6.6	451	4.7	59.7	21.9	0.0
Yoghurt Coated, Graze*	1 Pack/40g	182	8.5	456	2.9	64.1	21.3	0.0
RAITA								
Cucumber & Mint, Patak's*	1oz/28g	18	0.5	64	3.4	8.4	1.8	0.0
Plain, Average	1oz/28g	16	0.6	57	4.2	5.8	2.2	0.0
RASPBERRIES								
Dried, Graze*	1 Pack/30g	85	0.8	284	3.2	62.0	2.6	0.0
Freeze Dried, Simply*	1 Serving/10g	37	0.0	370	10.0	80.0	0.0	20.0
Fresh, Raw, Average	*1 Serving/80g*	*20*	*0.2*	*25*	*1.3*	*4.7*	*0.3*	*6.5*
in Fruit Juice, Average	*1oz/28g*	*9*	*0.0*	*31*	*0.8*	*6.7*	*0.1*	*1.7*
In Fruit Juice, Canned, John West*	1 Can/290g	93	0.6	32	0.9	6.7	0.2	1.5
in Syrup, Canned	*1oz/28g*	*25*	*0.0*	*88*	*0.6*	*22.5*	*0.1*	*1.5*
RATATOUILLE								
Average	1oz/28g	23	2.0	82	1.3	3.8	7.0	1.8
Chicken, Finest, Tesco*	1 Pack/550g	407	11.5	74	7.8	5.9	2.1	0.0
Princes*	1 Can/360g	86	1.4	24	1.0	4.2	0.4	0.0
Provencale, French Style Mixed Vegetables, Tesco*	½ Can/195g	76	3.9	39	1.1	4.2	2.0	1.9
Roasted Vegetable, Sainsbury's*	1 Pack/300g	134	3.0	45	1.4	7.5	1.0	2.3
Sainsbury's*	1 Pack/300g	99	1.8	33	1.5	5.5	0.6	1.6
RAVIOLI								
Asparagus, Waitrose*	1 Serving/150g	303	9.0	202	10.5	26.4	6.0	2.0
Basil & Parmesan, Organic, Sainsbury's*	½ Pack/192g	290	10.0	151	7.4	21.1	5.2	2.1
Beef	1 Serving/300g	501	13.7	167	6.4	25.0	4.6	1.4
Beef, Chef Boyardee*	1 Can/100g	190	5.0	190	6.0	31.0	5.0	2.0
Beef, GFY, Asda*	½ Pack/150g	288	4.8	192	7.0	33.9	3.2	1.9
Beef, Tesco*	1 Serving/194g	175	5.0	90	4.3	12.3	2.6	1.5
Beef & Red Wine, Italiano, Tesco*	½ Pack/150g	315	9.7	210	7.3	30.0	6.5	2.3
Beef & Shiraz, Finest, Tesco*	½ Pack/200g	358	9.0	179	8.4	26.1	4.5	1.8
Beef in Tomato Sauce, Canned, Asda*	1 Can/400g	352	8.0	88	3.6	14.0	2.0	3.0
Cheese, Garlic, & Herb, Fresh, Organic, Tesco*	1 Serving/125g	382	19.5	306	11.3	30.1	15.6	0.9
Cheese, in Tomato Sauce, Canned, Tesco*	1 Can/410g	328	8.2	80	2.5	13.0	2.0	0.5
Cheese, Tomato & Basil, Italiano, Tesco*	½ Pack/125g	309	11.0	247	13.1	28.5	8.8	2.1

RAVIOLI

	Measure INFO/WEIGHT	per Measure KCAL	FAT	Nutrition Values per 100g / 100ml KCAL	PROT	CARB	FAT	FIBRE
Cheese & Asparagus, Waitrose*	1 Serving/100g	242	7.2	242	12.6	31.7	7.2	2.4
Cheese & Tomato, Fresh, Organic, Tesco*	1 Serving/125g	342	14.0	274	12.5	30.8	11.2	1.1
Cheese & Tomato, Heinz*	1 Can/400g	340	8.4	85	2.4	13.9	2.1	0.9
Chicken, Tomato & Basil, Finest, Tesco*	1 Serving/200g	358	12.0	179	9.6	21.7	6.0	1.0
Chicken & Mushroom, Finest, Tesco*	½ Pack/125g	267	8.9	214	11.6	25.8	7.1	1.1
Chicken & Rosemary, Perfectly Balanced, Waitrose*	½ Pack/125g	266	4.4	213	14.9	30.4	3.5	2.1
Chicken & Tomato, Perfectly Balanced, Waitrose*	1 Serving/125g	265	3.4	212	13.5	33.4	2.7	2.8
Feta Cheese, M & S*	1 Serving/100g	195	8.5	195	9.1	20.5	8.5	1.3
Five Cheese, Weight Watchers*	1 Pack/330g	271	9.2	82	3.2	11.1	2.8	0.8
Florentine, Weight Watchers*	1 Serving/241g	220	5.0	91	3.7	14.1	2.1	1.2
Four Cheese, Italian Choice, Asda*	1 Pack/449g	467	26.9	104	3.4	9.0	6.0	2.1
Fresh, Pasta Reale*	1 Serving/150g	459	8.8	306	13.1	53.3	5.9	0.0
Garlic & Herb, Italiano, Tesco*	1 Serving/100g	318	13.0	318	11.1	39.1	13.0	2.6
Garlic Mushroom, Finest, Tesco*	1 Serving/250g	552	18.2	221	8.9	30.0	7.3	2.0
Goat's Cheese & Pesto, Asda*	½ Pack/150g	204	5.4	136	6.0	20.0	3.6	0.0
Goats Cheese & Roasted Red Pepper, Finest, Tesco*	½ Pack/125g	307	9.6	246	11.4	32.8	7.7	1.8
Grana Padano & Rocket, Finest, Tesco*	½ Pack/150g	270	7.5	180	7.5	26.0	5.0	1.8
in Tomato Sauce, Canned, Carlini*	1 Can/400g	324	4.0	81	3.1	15.0	1.0	0.5
in Tomato Sauce, Canned, Sainsbury's*	½ Can/200g	166	2.0	83	3.1	15.5	1.0	0.5
in Tomato Sauce, Heinz*	1 Can/400g	308	6.8	77	2.4	13.2	1.7	0.9
in Tomato Sauce, Meat Free, Heinz*	1 Can/410g	307	3.3	75	2.4	14.4	0.8	0.5
Meat, Italian, Fresh, Asda*	½ Pack/150g	261	6.3	174	8.0	26.0	4.2	0.0
Mozzarella Tomato & Basil, Tesco*	1 Serving/125g	304	12.7	243	13.6	24.1	10.2	0.5
Mushroom, Fresh, Sainsbury's*	½ Pack/125g	196	5.1	157	7.4	22.6	4.1	1.9
Mushroom, Italiano, Tesco*	1 Serving/125g	332	16.1	266	10.4	27.0	12.9	3.0
Mushroom, Ready Meals, M & S*	1oz/28g	38	0.5	135	8.1	22.0	1.9	2.2
Mushroom, Wild, Finest, Tesco*	1 Serving/200g	472	12.2	236	10.8	34.4	6.1	1.9
Mushroomi, Tesco*	½ Pack/125g	332	16.1	266	10.4	27.0	12.9	3.0
Pancetta & Mozzarella, Finest, Tesco*	1 Serving/125g	344	13.2	275	12.2	32.8	10.6	1.8
Pork, in Tomato Sauce, Low Fat, Morrisons*	1oz/28g	23	0.3	81	2.7	15.5	0.9	1.3
Prosciuttoi, Ready Meal, M & S*	1 Pack/100g	195	8.1	195	13.3	17.0	8.1	1.0
Red Pepper, Basil & Chilli, Waitrose*	½ Pack/125g	312	10.5	250	11.6	32.0	8.4	1.7
Rich Beef & Red Wine, Morrisons*	1 Pack/300g	813	20.7	271	12.0	42.8	6.9	2.6
Roast Garlic & Herb, Tesco*	½ Pack/125g	342	13.6	274	12.8	31.1	10.9	1.1
Roasted Pepper, M & S*	1 Pack/400g	540	30.8	135	5.4	11.0	7.7	1.1
Roasted Vegetable, Asda*	½ Pack/150g	217	0.7	145	6.0	29.0	0.5	0.0
Salmon & Dill, Sainsbury's*	1 Pack/300g	615	21.3	205	8.7	26.5	7.1	3.0
Smoked Ham, Bacon & Tomato, Italiano, Tesco*	1 Can/125g	302	9.6	242	10.8	32.3	7.7	2.9
Smoked Salmon & Dill, Sainsbury's*	1 Serving/125g	256	8.9	205	8.7	26.5	7.1	0.7
Spinach & Ricotta, Waitrose*	1 Serving/125g	309	9.0	247	10.5	35.0	7.2	1.9
Sweet Pepper & Chilli, Tesco*	½ Pack/125g	324	14.0	259	12.5	27.1	11.2	2.7
Tomato, Cheese & Meat, Sainsbury's*	1 Serving/125g	314	16.1	251	12.4	21.4	12.9	2.2
Tomato, Cheese & Mortadella, Sainsbury's*	1 Serving/125g	272	13.2	218	10.3	20.3	10.6	2.4
Vegetable, Canned, Sainsbury's*	1 Can/400g	328	2.8	82	2.6	16.3	0.7	0.7
Vegetable, Morrisons*	1 Can/400g	276	1.6	69	2.4	13.9	0.4	0.0
Vegetable, Tesco*	½ Can/200g	164	1.4	82	2.6	16.3	0.7	0.7
Vegetable, with Omega 3, Heinz*	1 Can/200g	144	3.2	72	2.2	12.2	1.6	0.6
Vegetable in Tomato Sauce, Italiana, Weight Watchers*	1 Can/385g	266	8.1	69	1.7	11.0	2.1	0.5

RED BULL*

Energy Shot, Red Bull*	1 Can/60ml	27	0.0	45	0.0	10.7	0.0	0.0
Regular, Red Bull*	1 Can/250ml	112	0.0	45	0.0	11.3	0.0	0.0

REDCURRANTS

Raw, Average	*1oz/28g*	*6*	*0.0*	*21*	*1.1*	*4.4*	*0.0*	*3.4*

	Measure INFO/WEIGHT	per Measure KCAL	FAT	Nutrition Values per 100g / 100ml KCAL	PROT	CARB	FAT	FIBRE
REDCURRANTS								
Raw, Stalks Removed	1 Serving/100g	21	0.0	21	1.1	4.4	0.0	0.0
REEF*								
Orange & Passionfruit, Reef*	1 Bottle/275ml	179	0.0	65	0.0	9.5	0.0	0.0
REFRESHERS								
Bassett's*	1oz/28g	106	0.0	377	4.3	78.1	0.0	0.0
RELISH								
Barbeque, Sainsbury's*	1 Serving/50g	50	1.0	100	1.0	19.3	2.1	1.1
Burger, Juicy, Asda*	1 Tbsp/15g	17	0.1	113	1.2	25.4	0.7	0.7
Caramelised Onion & Chilli, M & S*	1 Serving/20g	47	0.2	235	1.4	55.1	1.1	1.0
Caramelised Red Onion, Tesco*	1 Serving/10g	28	0.0	280	0.6	69.1	0.1	0.7
Hamburger, Bick's*	1oz/28g	27	0.1	96	1.3	22.3	0.2	0.0
Mango & Chilli, Levi Roots*	1 Serving/100g	110	0.2	110	0.7	25.0	0.2	1.1
Onion, M & S*	1oz/28g	46	0.8	165	1.0	32.1	3.0	1.1
Onion, Sainsbury's*	1 Serving/15g	23	0.1	151	0.9	36.0	0.4	0.7
Onion, Sweet, Heinz*	1 Tbsp/38g	38	0.1	102	1.0	23.5	0.4	0.6
Onion & Garlic, Spicy, Waitrose*	1 Tbsp/15g	35	0.2	232	0.8	54.2	1.1	1.7
Sweet Onion, Branston*	1 Serving/10g	14	0.0	145	1.0	34.2	0.4	0.6
Sweetcorn, American Style, Maryland, Tesco*	1 Serving/15g	15	0.0	101	1.1	23.9	0.1	0.9
Sweetcorn, Bick's*	1 Tbsp/22g	23	0.0	103	1.3	24.3	0.2	0.0
Tomato, M & S*	1oz/28g	36	0.1	130	1.8	30.2	0.3	1.5
Tomato, Sweet, Heinz*	1 Serving/25g	34	0.0	136	0.9	32.6	0.2	0.9
Tomato & Chilli Texan Style, Tesco*	1 Tbsp/14g	20	0.0	140	1.7	32.0	0.1	1.1
Tomato Spicy, Bick's*	1 Serving/28g	28	0.1	99	1.3	23.2	0.2	0.0
REVELS								
Mars*	1 Packet/35g	168	7.3	480	5.1	68.0	20.9	0.0
RHUBARB								
Raw, Average	*1 Stalk/51g*	*11*	*0.1*	*21*	*0.9*	*4.5*	*0.2*	*1.8*
Stewed with Sugar, Average	*1oz/28g*	*32*	*0.0*	*116*	*0.4*	*31.2*	*0.0*	*2.0*
RIBENA*								
Apple Juice Drink, Ribena*	1 Carton/287ml	132	0.0	46	0.0	11.1	0.0	0.0
Blackcurrant, Diluted with Water, Ribena*	1 Serving/100ml	46	0.0	46	0.0	11.4	0.0	0.0
Blackcurrant, Original, Undiluted, Ribena*	1 Serving/20ml	46	0.0	230	0.0	57.0	0.0	0.0
Blackcurrant, Really Light, No Added Sugar, Ribena*	1 Carton/250ml	7	0.0	3	0.0	0.7	0.0	0.0
Blackcurrant & Cranberry, Ribena*	1 Bottle/500ml	205	0.0	41	0.0	9.9	0.0	0.0
Blackcurrant Juice Drink, Ribena*	1 Carton/288ml	147	0.0	51	0.0	12.6	0.0	0.0
Light, Ribena*	1 Carton/288ml	26	0.0	9	0.1	2.1	0.0	0.0
Orange, Juice Drink, Ribena*	1 Serving/288ml	98	0.0	34	0.1	8.1	0.0	0.0
Really Light, Undiluted, Ribena*	1 Serving/25ml	20	0.0	80	0.0	2.5	0.0	0.0
Strawberry Juice Drink, Ribena*	1 Carton/288ml	130	0.0	45	0.0	10.9	0.0	0.0
RIBS								
in a Chinese Style Coating, Tesco*	1 Serving/250g	420	21.8	168	19.5	5.3	8.7	2.5
Loin, BBQ, Sainsbury's*	1 Rib/42g	104	5.5	247	24.7	7.3	13.2	0.9
Loin, Chinese, Sainsbury's*	1 Rib/42g	103	5.0	246	27.2	7.2	12.0	0.9
Loin, Chinese, Taste Summer, Sainsbury's*	1 Serving/30g	38	2.3	128	11.7	2.8	7.8	0.1
Pork, Barbecue, Average	1 Serving/100g	275	17.9	275	21.4	7.2	17.9	0.3
Pork, Chinese Style, Average	1 Serving/300g	736	44.7	245	17.9	10.0	14.9	0.7
Pork, Full Rack, Sainsbury's*	1 Serving/225g	567	38.7	252	18.0	6.5	17.2	0.9
Pork, Raw, Average	1oz/28g	47	2.8	169	18.6	1.8	9.9	0.2
Spare, Cantonese, Mini, Sainsbury's*	1 Rib/38g	97	5.0	259	17.2	17.3	13.4	1.0
Spare, Chinese Style, Meal Solutions, Co-Op*	1 Serving/165g	214	14.8	130	8.0	4.0	9.0	0.2
Spare, Chinese Style, Summer Eating, Asda*	1 Serving/116g	334	18.6	288	32.0	4.1	16.0	0.8
Spare, Sweet, Sticky, Mini, M & S*	1 Pack/300g	615	34.5	205	16.6	8.6	11.5	0.2

INFO/WEIGHT	Measure	per Measure KCAL	FAT	Nutrition Values per 100g / 100ml KCAL	PROT	CARB	FAT	FIBRE

RICCOLI

	Measure INFO/WEIGHT	per Measure KCAL	FAT	KCAL	PROT	CARB	FAT	FIBRE
Egg, Fresh, Waitrose*	1oz/28g	81	1.0	289	11.4	53.1	3.4	2.1

RICE

	Measure INFO/WEIGHT	per Measure KCAL	FAT	KCAL	PROT	CARB	FAT	FIBRE
Arborio, Dry, Average	*1 Serving/80g*	*279*	*0.6*	*348*	*7.1*	*78.3*	*0.8*	*0.8*
Balti Style, Quick, Sainsbury's*	1 Serving/228g	192	1.1	84	4.3	15.7	0.5	2.0
Basmati, & Wild, Cooked, Sainsbury's*	½ Pack/125g	150	0.7	120	3.1	25.7	0.6	1.3
Basmati, & Wild, Dry Weight, Tilda*	1 Serving/70g	244	0.3	349	9.4	77.0	0.5	1.0
Basmati, Boil in the Bag, Dry, Average	1 Serving/50g	176	0.4	352	8.4	77.8	0.8	0.4
Basmati, Brown, Dry, Average	*1 Serving/50g*	*177*	*1.5*	*353*	*9.5*	*71.8*	*3.0*	*2.2*
Basmati, Cooked, Average	*1 Serving/140g*	*189*	*2.5*	*135*	*3.6*	*26.0*	*1.8*	*0.7*
Basmati, Cooked, Tilda*	1 Serving/200g	214	0.2	107	2.4	24.0	0.1	1.2
Basmati, Dry Weight, Average	*1 Serving/60g*	*212*	*0.6*	*353*	*8.1*	*77.9*	*1.0*	*0.6*
Basmati, Indian, Dry, Average	*1 Serving/75g*	*260*	*0.7*	*346*	*8.4*	*76.1*	*0.9*	*0.1*
Basmati, Microwave, Cooked, Average	1 Serving/125g	182	2.3	145	2.7	30.0	1.8	0.0
Basmati, Microwaveable, Tesco*	½ Pack/125g	212	2.2	170	4.0	34.1	1.8	0.5
Basmati, Uncooked, TTD, Sainsbury's*	1 Serving/50g	87	0.2	174	4.1	38.6	0.4	0.4
Basmati, White, Dry, Average	*1 Serving/75g*	*262*	*0.4*	*349*	*8.1*	*77.1*	*0.6*	*2.2*
Basmati, Wholegrain, Cooked, Tilda*	1 Serving/60g	68	0.5	113	3.3	23.0	0.9	3.2
BBQ & Spicy, M & S*	1 Pack/250g	462	18.0	185	6.1	23.7	7.2	1.2
Beef, Savoury, Batchelors*	1 Pack/120g	431	2.8	359	8.9	75.7	2.3	2.5
Black, Artemide, Eat Well, M & S*	1 Serving/75g	251	1.9	335	8.5	73.3	2.6	4.0
Brown, Cooked, Average	*1 Serving/140g*	*173*	*1.5*	*123*	*2.6*	*26.6*	*1.1*	*0.9*
Brown, Dry, Average	*1 Serving/75g*	*266*	*2.3*	*355*	*7.5*	*76.2*	*3.0*	*1.4*
Brown, Long Grain, Dry, Average	*1 Serving/50g*	*182*	*1.4*	*363*	*7.6*	*76.8*	*2.8*	*2.0*
Brown, Short Grain, Dry, Average	*1 Serving/50g*	*175*	*1.4*	*351*	*6.8*	*77.6*	*2.8*	*0.9*
Brown, Whole Grain, Cooked, Average	*1 Serving/170g*	*223*	*1.9*	*131*	*2.6*	*27.8*	*1.1*	*1.2*
Brown, Whole Grain, Dry, Average	*1 Serving/40g*	*138*	*1.2*	*344*	*7.4*	*71.6*	*2.9*	*3.0*
Brown Basmati, Butternut Squash, Tilda*	½ Pack/125g	164	5.1	131	3.3	20.3	4.1	1.2
Chicken, Savoury, Batchelors*	1 Pack/124g	455	1.9	367	8.9	79.4	1.5	2.6
Chicken, Savoury, Tesco*	1 Serving/87g	177	1.9	204	6.4	39.4	2.2	6.7
Chicken & Sweetcorn, Savoury, Asda*	½ Pack/60g	195	1.7	325	10.0	65.0	2.8	10.0
Chilli & Coriander, TTD, Sainsbury's*	1 Pack/446g	522	12.5	117	6.5	16.5	2.8	2.2
Chinese Five Spice, Special Recipe, Sainsbury's*	1oz/28g	37	0.1	133	2.9	29.9	0.3	0.9
Chinese Savoury, Batchelors*	1 Serving/50g	177	1.2	354	9.9	73.1	2.4	2.8
Chinese Style, Express, Uncle Ben's*	1 Pack/250g	392	5.5	157	3.4	30.9	2.2	0.4
Chinese Style Savoury Five Spice, Made Up, Tesco*	1 Serving/141g	217	4.4	154	3.2	28.2	3.1	2.2
Coconut, M & S*	½ Pack/124g	217	5.0	175	3.1	31.8	4.0	0.3
Coconut, Thai, Sainsbury's*	½ Pack/100g	178	9.1	178	2.6	21.3	9.1	1.9
Coconut & Lime, Asda*	1 Pack/360g	695	17.6	193	4.5	32.7	4.9	0.9
Coriander & Herb, Packet, Cooked, Sainsbury's*	¼ Pack/150g	204	0.7	136	2.5	30.4	0.5	1.5
Coriander & Herbs, Batchelors*	1/3 Pack/76g	280	2.7	369	7.9	79.6	3.5	5.0
Egg, Chinese Style, Morrisons*	1 Serving/250g	285	11.9	114	2.1	16.8	4.8	0.7
Egg, Fried, 2 Minute Meals, Sainsbury's*	1 Pack/250g	342	1.5	137	3.8	29.2	0.6	0.8
Egg Fried, Asda*	1 Pack/229g	286	5.7	125	3.6	22.0	2.5	2.3
Egg Fried, Average	1 Serving/300g	624	31.8	208	4.2	25.7	10.6	0.4
Egg Fried, Chinese Style, Tesco*	1 Portion/250g	417	10.5	167	4.4	27.9	4.2	0.7
Egg Fried, Chinese Takeaway, Iceland*	1 Pack/340g	374	7.8	110	4.2	18.1	2.3	1.1
Egg Fried, Chinese Takeaway, Tesco*	1 Serving/200g	250	3.0	125	4.7	23.3	1.5	1.8
Egg Fried, Express, Uncle Ben's*	½ Pack/125g	216	5.2	173	4.0	29.9	4.2	0.3
Egg Fried, HL, Tesco*	1 Serving/250g	285	3.2	114	3.5	22.2	1.3	1.8
Egg Fried, M & S*	½ Pack/150g	315	10.5	210	4.2	32.4	7.0	0.3
Egg Fried, Micro, Tesco*	1 Pack/250g	312	9.2	125	4.6	18.3	3.7	6.4
Egg Fried, Sainsbury's*	1 Pack/250g	432	9.5	173	4.5	30.3	3.8	0.8
Express Microwave, Uncle Ben's*	1 Serving/250g	370	4.2	148	3.2	30.0	1.7	0.0

R

RICE

	Measure INFO/WEIGHT	per Measure KCAL	FAT	Nutrition Values per 100g / 100ml KCAL	PROT	CARB	FAT	FIBRE
Fried, Chicken, Chinese Takeaway, Iceland*	1 Pack/340g	510	15.6	150	6.5	20.7	4.6	0.6
Fried, Duck, Chicken & Pork Celebration, Sainsbury's*	1 Pack/450g	544	16.2	121	7.9	14.2	3.6	1.5
Garlic & Butter Flavoured, Batchelors*	1 Serving/50g	175	1.4	350	8.0	79.8	2.8	5.0
Garlic & Coriander Flavoured, Patak's*	1 Serving/125g	186	2.7	149	2.6	28.9	2.2	0.0
Golden Savoury, Dry Weight, Batchelors*	1 Pack/120g	437	3.4	364	10.1	74.7	2.8	2.4
Golden Savoury, Nirvana*	1 Pack/120g	142	0.8	118	2.5	25.4	0.7	2.9
Golden Vegetable, Freshly Frozen, Asda*	1 Sachet/200g	238	2.6	119	3.2	23.6	1.3	1.3
Golden Vegetable, Savoury, Morrisons*	1 Serving/50g	70	0.4	141	3.4	30.1	0.8	1.1
Golden Vegetable, Savoury, Sainsbury's*	¼ Pack/100g	122	1.0	122	2.9	25.4	1.0	0.3
Ground, Whitworths*	1 Serving/28g	98	0.2	349	7.7	77.7	0.8	0.7
Imperial Red, Merchant Gourmet*	1oz/28g	85	0.7	305	8.6	61.2	2.5	8.6
Lemon Pepper, in 5, Crosse & Blackwell*	½ Pack/163g	201	2.1	123	2.7	25.2	1.3	4.0
Lemon Pepper Speciality, Asda*	1 Serving/52g	67	0.7	129	2.0	27.0	1.4	0.1
Long Grain, & Wild, Dry, Average	*1 Serving/75g*	*254*	*1.5*	*338*	*7.6*	*72.6*	*2.0*	*1.7*
Long Grain, American, Cooked, Average	*1 Serving/160g*	*229*	*2.8*	*143*	*3.0*	*28.7*	*1.7*	*0.2*
Long Grain, American, Dry, Average	*1 Serving/50g*	*175*	*0.5*	*350*	*7.1*	*77.8*	*1.1*	*0.6*
Long Grain, Dry, Average	*1 Serving/50g*	*169*	*0.5*	*337*	*7.4*	*75.5*	*1.0*	*1.7*
Long Grain, Microwavable, Cooked, Average	1 Serving/150g	180	0.9	120	2.7	25.8	0.6	0.7
Mexican, Ready Meals, Waitrose*	1 Pack/300g	432	7.5	144	2.6	27.8	2.5	0.5
Mexican Style, Ainsley Harriott*	1 Pack/170g	206	1.5	121	1.7	26.5	0.9	2.3
Mexican Style, Cooked, Express, Uncle Ben's*	1 Pack/250g	385	4.7	154	3.2	31.1	1.9	0.7
Mexican Style, Old El Paso*	1 Serving/75g	268	0.7	357	9.0	78.0	1.0	0.0
Mild Curry, Cooked, Tesco*	1 Serving/154g	217	1.7	141	3.1	29.7	1.1	2.1
Mild Curry, Savoury, Batchelors*	1 Pack/120g	426	2.5	355	8.0	76.1	2.1	1.6
Mixed Vegetable, Savoury, Dry Weight, Tesco*	1 Pack/120g	450	3.2	375	7.8	79.1	2.7	2.9
Mushroom & Coconut, Organic, Waitrose*	1 Pack/300g	474	15.0	158	3.7	24.5	5.0	1.4
Mushroom & Pepper, Savoury, Cooked, Morrisons*	1 Serving/200g	204	1.6	102	2.3	21.5	0.8	0.0
Mushroom Pilau, Bombay Brasserie, Sainsbury's*	1 Pack/400g	672	17.2	168	3.7	28.6	4.3	0.7
Mushroom Savoury, Batchelors*	½ Pack/61g	217	1.3	356	10.7	73.6	2.1	2.8
Nine Jewel, Chef's Special, Waitrose*	½ Pot/175g	257	4.7	147	4.4	26.3	2.7	4.2
Paella, Savoury, Tesco*	1 Serving/60g	220	2.8	367	8.4	72.7	4.7	4.5
Pilau, Cooked, Average	*1 Serving/140g*	*244*	*6.2*	*174*	*3.5*	*30.3*	*4.4*	*0.8*
Pilau, Dry, Average	*1oz/28g*	*101*	*0.7*	*361*	*8.4*	*78.2*	*2.3*	*3.4*
Pilau, Indian Mushroom, Sainsbury's*	1 Serving/100g	119	2.4	119	3.0	21.3	2.4	1.9
Pilau, Mushroom, Sainsbury's*	1 Pack/250g	400	13.7	160	3.4	24.1	5.5	2.4
Pilau, Spinach, Bombay Brasserie, Sainsbury's*	1 Pack/401g	642	17.3	160	3.5	26.9	4.3	0.8
Pilau, Spinach & Carrot, Waitrose*	1 Pack/350g	465	8.4	133	3.1	24.8	2.4	1.2
Pudding, Dry Weight, Average	1 Serving/100g	355	1.1	355	6.9	82.0	1.1	0.3
Risotto, Dry, Average	*1 Serving/50g*	*174*	*0.6*	*348*	*7.8*	*76.2*	*1.3*	*2.4*
Saffron, Cooked, Average	*1 Serving/150g*	*208*	*4.7*	*139*	*2.5*	*25.3*	*3.1*	*0.5*
Special Fried, Asda*	1oz/28g	42	1.4	149	5.4	21.0	4.9	1.5
Special Fried, Cantonese, Sainsbury's*	½ Pack/250g	442	10.0	177	4.9	30.4	4.0	1.2
Special Fried, Chinese, Tesco*	1 Serving/300g	618	33.3	206	6.5	19.9	11.1	0.8
Special Fried, Chinese Takeaway, Iceland*	1 Pack/350g	630	17.5	180	5.5	28.2	5.0	1.2
Special Fried, M & S*	1 Pack/450g	922	35.1	205	6.2	27.2	7.8	0.5
Special Fried, Sainsbury's*	1 Serving/166g	272	7.6	164	5.1	25.5	4.6	0.7
Special Fried, Waitrose*	1 Serving/350g	532	22.4	152	6.1	17.6	6.4	3.2
Spicy Mexican Style, Savoury, Made Up, Tesco*	1 Serving/164g	213	2.5	130	2.9	26.3	1.5	2.4
Spicy Mexican Style, Savoury, Tesco*	1 Serving/164g	584	7.4	356	9.0	69.9	4.5	6.0
Steam Rice, White, Tesco*	1 Sachet/200g	274	2.5	140	2.8	28.1	1.3	0.4
Stir Fry, Oriental Style, Oriental Express*	1 Serving/150g	216	5.1	144	4.2	24.1	3.4	1.9
Sweet & Sour, Rice Bowl, Uncle Ben's*	1 Pack/350g	364	2.1	104	5.2	19.5	0.6	0.0
Sweet & Sour, Savoury, Batchelors*	1 Serving/135g	418	2.8	310	9.4	75.6	2.1	3.1

	Measure INFO/WEIGHT	per Measure		Nutrition Values per 100g / 100ml				
		KCAL	FAT	KCAL	PROT	CARB	FAT	FIBRE
RICE								
Sweet & Sour, Savoury, Cooked, Tesco*	½ Pack/153g	214	2.1	140	2.7	29.1	1.4	2.3
Sweet & Sour, Savoury, Sainsbury's*	1 Serving/145g	198	0.7	137	2.4	30.8	0.5	1.0
Sweet & Sour Savoury, Cooked, Asda*	½ Pack/126g	154	1.1	122	2.5	26.0	0.9	3.0
Sweet & Spicy, Express, Uncle Ben's*	1 Pack/250g	417	10.0	167	2.7	30.1	4.0	0.0
Tandoori, Savoury, Batchelors*	1 Serving/120g	430	3.0	358	10.3	73.5	2.5	3.0
Thai, Cooked, Average	*1 Serving/100g*	*135*	*1.7*	*135*	*2.5*	*27.4*	*1.7*	*0.3*
Thai, Dry, Average	*1 Serving/50g*	*174*	*0.2*	*348*	*7.1*	*78.9*	*0.4*	*0.9*
Thai, Fragrant, Dry, Average	*1 Serving/75g*	*272*	*0.5*	*363*	*7.2*	*82.0*	*0.7*	*0.3*
Thai Sticky, Tesco*	1 Serving/250g	357	6.2	143	2.5	27.6	2.5	0.4
Thai Style, Lemon Chicken, Savoury, Tesco*	1 Pack/105g	382	5.1	364	9.3	70.6	4.9	5.0
Thai Style Lemon Chicken, Made Up, Tesco*	½ Pack/138g	192	2.3	139	3.4	27.5	1.7	2.1
Three Grain Mix, Wholefoods, Tesco*	1 Portion/75g	266	1.6	355	9.6	73.3	2.2	2.3
Valencia for Paella, Asda*	1 Serving/125g	435	1.0	348	6.0	79.0	0.8	0.0
Vegetable, Original, Birds Eye*	1oz/28g	29	0.2	105	4.0	20.8	0.6	1.1
Vegetable, Savoury, Co-Op*	½ Pack/60g	210	0.6	350	9.0	76.0	1.0	3.0
White, Cooked, Average	*1 Serving/140g*	*182*	*1.1*	*130*	*2.6*	*28.7*	*0.8*	*0.1*
White, Cooked, Frozen, Average	*1 Serving/150g*	*168*	*0.8*	*112*	*2.9*	*23.8*	*0.5*	*1.1*
White, Flaked, Dry Weight, Average	*1oz/28g*	*97*	*0.3*	*346*	*6.6*	*77.5*	*1.2*	*0.0*
White, Fried	1oz/28g	37	0.9	131	2.2	25.0	3.2	0.6
White, Long Grain, Dry Weight, Average	*1 Serving/50g*	*181*	*1.0*	*362*	*7.1*	*79.1*	*1.9*	*0.4*
White, Microwave, Cooked, Average	1 Serving/150g	157	0.7	105	2.7	22.4	0.5	1.1
Whole Grain, Dry, Average	*1 Serving/50g*	*171*	*1.1*	*341*	*8.2*	*72.0*	*2.3*	*4.0*
Wholegrain, Microwave, Eat Well, M & S*	½ Pack/125g	181	1.5	145	2.5	31.0	1.2	2.2
Wild, Coronation, Sainsbury's*	¼ Pot/75g	139	4.8	186	3.1	29.1	6.4	0.9
Wild, Giant Canadian, Dry Weight, Tilda*	1 Serving/75g	262	0.6	350	11.5	74.2	0.8	1.9
with Red Kidney Beans, Average	1oz/28g	49	1.0	175	5.6	32.4	3.5	2.5
Yellow, Ready Cooked, Tesco*	1oz/28g	32	0.4	113	2.7	27.1	1.3	0.1
RICE BOWL								
Beef with Black Bean Sauce, Uncle Ben's*	1 Pack/350g	367	4.9	105	5.6	17.4	1.4	0.0
Chicken Tikka Masala, Uncle Ben's*	1 Pack/350g	381	8.4	109	5.9	15.9	2.4	0.0
Honey BBQ Chicken, Uncle Ben's*	1 Pack/350g	420	2.1	120	5.4	23.1	0.6	0.0
Sweet 'n' Sour, Sharwood's*	1 Serving/350g	437	12.2	125	4.8	18.6	3.5	0.8
Thai Green, Sharwood's*	1 Bowl/350g	549	26.6	157	4.8	17.3	7.6	0.9
Thai Red, Sharwood's*	1 Bowl/350g	486	18.5	139	4.7	18.1	5.3	1.0
RICE CAKES								
& Corn, Salt & Vinegar Flavour, M & S*	1 Pack/22g	80	1.3	365	6.7	71.7	5.9	0.7
Apple & Cinnamon Flavour, Kallo*	1 Cake/11g	41	0.2	376	6.2	83.1	2.2	3.9
Asda*	1 Cake/8g	31	0.2	386	8.7	81.1	3.0	2.8
Bacon, Asda*	1 Cake/9g	42	1.6	462	8.0	67.0	18.0	0.0
Barbecue, Sainsbury's*	1 Pack/30g	121	2.6	403	7.9	73.5	8.6	2.7
Barbeque, Tesco*	1 Cake/9g	28	0.2	328	9.6	66.8	2.5	6.2
Black & White Sesame, Clearspring*	1 Cake/8g	31	0.2	385	7.4	82.2	2.9	0.0
Brink*	1 Cake/15g	55	0.3	370	8.8	78.8	2.2	0.0
Butter Popcorn, Snack-A-Jacks, Quaker Oats*	1 Cake/9g	35	0.0	389	11.1	88.9	0.0	0.0
Caramel, Jumbo, Tesco*	1 Cake/10g	34	0.3	340	7.0	74.0	3.0	5.0
Caramel, Large, Tesco*	1 Cake/10g	34	0.2	344	6.5	73.9	2.5	5.1
Caramel, Less Than 3% Fat, Sainsbury's*	1 Pack/35g	134	0.6	382	5.6	86.4	1.6	1.8
Caramel, Snack Size, Tesco*	1 Pack/35g	133	1.0	379	5.5	82.7	2.9	0.9
Caramel, Tesco*	1 Serving/2g	9	0.1	379	5.5	98.2	2.9	0.9
Caramel Flavour, Kallo*	1 Cake/10g	38	0.5	383	6.2	78.9	4.8	3.9
Cheese, Jumbo, Free From, Tesco*	1 Serving/10g	44	1.8	439	8.1	62.1	17.6	3.8
Cheese & Onion, Namchow*	1 Serving/38g	141	1.2	377	7.2	79.5	3.3	0.0
Chilli, Mini, M & S*	1 Pack/22g	88	1.7	400	6.9	74.9	7.9	3.5

R

RICE CAKES

Measure INFO/WEIGHT		per Measure KCAL	FAT	Nutrition Values per 100g / 100ml KCAL	PROT	CARB	FAT	FIBRE
Chocolate, Fabulous Bakin' Boys*	1 Biscuit/17g	83	3.7	490	6.4	66.7	22.0	1.6
Co-Op*	1 Cake/20g	80	0.6	402	8.0	84.0	3.1	0.0
Dark Chocolate, Organic, Kallo*	1 Cake/12g	57	2.9	471	6.8	57.2	24.1	7.4
Five Grain, Finn Crisp*	1 Cake/10g	36	0.2	356	9.8	73.9	1.7	9.7
High Fibre, Oat & Rice, Slightly Salted, Thick, Kallo*	1 Cake/8g	27	0.4	356	10.6	75.0	5.5	9.0
Honey, Kallo*	1 Cake/10g	40	0.2	388	5.4	86.6	2.2	1.6
Japanese, Black Sesame, Clearspring*	1 Cake/8g	29	0.2	385	7.4	82.2	2.9	0.0
Japanese, Miso, Clearspring*	1 Cake/7g	27	0.2	365	9.2	77.0	3.0	2.0
Lightly Salted, Perfectly Balanced, Waitrose*	1 Cake/8g	31	0.2	387	8.3	82.4	2.7	2.1
Lightly Salted, Thick Slice, Low Fat, Kallo*	1 Cake/8g	28	0.2	372	8.0	78.7	2.8	5.1
Low Fat, Kallo*	1 Cake/10g	37	0.2	375	6.2	83.1	2.2	3.9
Milk Chocolate, Organic, Kallo*	1 Cake/11g	57	3.2	509	6.5	56.2	28.7	3.5
Multigrain, Ryvita*	3 Cakes/11g	43	0.5	384	9.1	76.2	4.7	5.3
Organic, Tesco*	1 Cake/8g	29	0.2	380	7.2	80.7	2.9	3.4
Plain, Finger Foods, Organic, Organix*	3 Cakes/6g	22	0.1	370	6.5	82.9	1.4	3.2
Rice Bites, Asda*	1 Cake/9g	41	1.6	466	8.0	68.0	18.0	0.0
Rikarikas, The Positive Food Co*	1 Pack/25g	91	0.1	366	7.5	83.0	0.6	1.6
Salt & Vinegar, Jumbo, Tesco*	1 Cake/9g	31	0.2	347	8.4	72.7	2.5	6.0
Salt & Vinegar, Sainsbury's*	1 Pack/30g	121	2.5	403	8.3	73.3	8.3	2.7
Salt & Vinegar, Snack, Tesco*	1 Pack/35g	116	0.6	332	7.5	71.5	1.8	1.1
Salt & Vinegar Flavour, Morrisons*	1 Bag/30g	122	2.6	407	6.7	75.8	8.6	1.2
Savoury, Jumbo, HL, Tesco*	1 Cake/8g	31	0.2	369	11.9	75.0	2.4	3.6
Sea Salt & Balsamic Vinegar, Kallo*	1 Cake/9g	32	0.2	361	6.5	78.1	2.5	3.0
Sesame, No Added Salt, Thick Sliced, Organic, Kallo*	1 Cake/10g	37	0.3	373	8.0	78.0	3.2	5.4
Sesame, Slightly Salted, Thick Slice, Organic, Kallo*	1 Cake/8g	28	0.2	373	8.0	78.0	3.2	5.4
Sesame, Slightly Salted, Thin Slice, Organic, Kallo*	1 Cake/5g	17	0.1	373	8.0	78.0	3.2	5.4
Sesame Garlic, Clearspring*	1 Serving/8g	29	0.2	382	7.8	82.3	2.4	0.0
Sesame Teriyaki, Clearspring*	1 Cake/7g	28	0.2	377	6.5	82.8	2.2	0.0
Slightly Salted, Mrs Crimble's*	1 Slice/6g	21	0.2	380	7.6	80.4	3.1	3.2
Slightly Salted, Organic, Thin Slice, Kallo*	1 Cake/5g	17	0.1	372	8.0	78.7	2.8	5.1
Slightly Salted, Thick Slice, Organic, Kallo*	1 Cake/8g	28	0.2	372	8.0	78.7	2.8	5.1
Slightly Salted, with Cracked Pepper, Snack Size, Kallo*	1 Cake/2g	8	0.1	372	8.0	78.7	2.8	5.1
Sour Cream & Chive Flavour, Sainsbury's*	1 Pack/30g	119	2.5	396	7.9	72.0	8.5	2.9
Thin Slice, No Added Salt, Organic, Kallo*	1 Cake/5g	19	0.1	372	8.0	78.7	2.8	5.1
Thin Slice, Organic, Hawkwood*	1 Cake/6g	21	0.2	378	7.6	79.1	3.5	3.4
Thin Slice, Organic, Waitrose*	1 Serving/5g	17	0.1	340	8.0	70.0	2.0	4.0
Toasted Sesame, Ryvita*	1 Pack/11g	43	0.5	391	8.4	78.4	4.9	3.5
Whole Grain, No Added Salt, Thick Slice, Organic, Kallo*	1 Cake/9g	33	0.3	365	7.6	80.0	3.1	3.4
Wholegrain, Mild Chilli, Tesco*	1 Cake/10g	38	1.4	400	7.2	59.8	14.4	5.8
Wholegrain, No Added Salt, BGTY, Sainsbury's*	1 Cake/8g	30	0.2	372	8.0	78.7	2.8	5.1
Wholegrain, Salt & Vinegar, Tesco*	1 Cake/9g	28	0.2	314	8.4	61.9	2.6	6.0
with Sesame, Organic, Evernat*	1 Cake/4g	15	0.2	368	8.5	74.5	4.0	0.0
with Yeast Extract, Snack Size, Kallo*	1 Cake/2g	7	0.1	364	12.6	71.1	2.8	4.7

RICE CRACKERS

Authentic Thai Chilli, Tyrrells*	½ Pack/75g	389	20.2	519	5.0	64.0	27.0	1.0
Barbecue, Sakata*	½ Pack/50g	203	1.3	407	7.3	85.2	2.6	1.6
Barbecue Flavour, Tesco*	1 Pack/25g	102	1.8	409	6.7	78.8	7.4	1.7
Brown, Wakama*	1 Cracker/5g	19	0.0	375	8.0	84.8	0.4	0.0
Cheddar Gorge, Graze*	1 Punnet/24g	128	8.3	534	10.6	48.3	34.7	2.3
Cheese, Tesco*	1 Serving/25g	104	2.0	416	7.9	78.1	8.0	1.8
Chilli, Temptations, Tesco*	1 Serving/25g	128	7.2	512	4.4	58.0	28.8	0.0
Chilli, Whitworths*	½ Pack/50g	253	12.8	507	5.1	63.9	25.7	0.5
Cracked Pepper, Sakata*	½ Pack/50g	200	1.5	400	7.3	84.4	3.0	2.0

	INFO/WEIGHT	KCAL	FAT	KCAL	PROT	CARB	FAT	FIBRE
RICE CRACKERS								
Crispy, Chilli & Lime, Go Ahead, McVitie's*	1 Serving/25g	101	0.9	405	7.1	83.6	3.6	2.1
Crispy, Sea Salt & Vinegar, Go Ahead, McVitie's*	1 Serving/25g	102	1.3	408	6.6	80.6	5.4	1.8
Crispy, Sour Cream & Herbs, Go Ahead, McVitie's*	1 Serving/25g	105	2.0	422	7.1	78.2	8.0	1.8
Japanese, Apollo*	1 Pack/75g	297	3.5	396	9.6	78.8	4.7	0.9
Japanese, Graze*	1 Pack/40g	159	1.9	397	9.0	79.7	4.7	0.0
Japanese, Hider*	1 Pack/70g	303	12.1	433	11.3	61.7	17.3	0.0
Japanese, Julian Graves*	1 Serving/25g	92	0.4	369	8.8	79.5	1.7	3.8
Japanese, Mini, Sunrise*	1 Serving/50g	180	0.0	360	7.0	83.0	0.0	7.0
Japanese Seaweed, Very Nori-sh, Graze*	1 Punnet/11g	50	1.4	454	5.9	78.8	12.7	1.0
Japanese Style, Tesco*	1 Serving/25g	101	1.5	405	11.7	75.2	6.1	3.3
Korean Chilli, Graze*	1 Pack/20g	117	7.9	585	3.5	54.4	39.3	0.0
Mix, M & S*	½ Pack/63g	225	0.1	360	6.5	82.9	0.1	1.6
Paprika Flavour, Namchow*	1 Serving/38g	141	1.2	375	7.5	78.9	3.3	0.0
Sainsbury's*	1 Serving/20g	87	1.9	433	11.2	74.3	9.4	1.0
Salt & Pepper, Asda*	1 Cracker/5g	19	0.0	385	7.0	87.0	1.0	2.2
Salt & Vinegar, Namchow*	1 Serving/38g	139	1.4	370	6.7	77.5	3.7	0.0
Sour Cream & Chive, Sakata*	1 Serving/25g	107	2.0	430	7.8	80.6	7.9	0.0
Spicy Mix, Asda*	1 Serving/25g	115	4.2	461	6.4	71.2	16.7	0.2
Thai, M & S*	1 Serving/55g	209	1.8	380	7.0	80.2	3.3	1.2
Thai, Sesame & Soy Sauce, M & S*	1 Pack/55g	210	2.6	385	7.6	77.8	4.8	1.4
Thai, Wakama*	1 Cracker/2g	8	0.1	400	6.9	86.9	2.7	0.5
Thai Chilli, Nature's Harvest*	1 Pack/75g	401	22.3	535	4.6	61.5	29.7	4.2
Thin, Blue Dragon*	3 Crackers/5g	20	0.2	395	6.1	84.4	3.7	0.0
Veggie Sushi Plate, Graze*	1 Punnet/24g	107	3.1	444	11.1	68.4	12.8	3.9
with Tamari, Clearspring*	1 Bag/50g	190	0.7	380	8.2	83.4	1.5	0.3
RICE MILK								
Organic, Provamel*	1 Serving/250ml	122	3.7	49	0.1	9.5	1.5	0.0
Original, Rice Dream*	1 Serving/150ml	70	1.5	47	0.1	9.4	1.0	0.1
RICE PUDDING								
& Conserve, M & S*	1oz/28g	53	3.5	190	2.3	17.4	12.5	0.3
50% Less Fat, Asda*	½ Can/212g	180	1.7	85	3.3	16.2	0.8	0.2
Apple, Mullerrice, Muller*	1 Pot/200g	224	4.4	112	3.2	19.8	2.2	0.4
Banana, Ambrosia*	1 Pot/150g	153	3.8	102	3.2	16.6	2.5	0.0
Canned, Average	1oz/28g	25	0.7	89	3.4	14.0	2.5	0.2
Canned, BGTY, Sainsbury's*	1 Can/425g	344	2.5	81	3.3	15.5	0.6	0.4
Canned, GFY, Asda*	½ Can/213g	168	1.3	79	2.8	15.5	0.6	0.1
Caramel, Ambrosia*	1 Pot/150g	149	3.8	99	3.1	16.1	2.5	0.0
Clotted Cream, Cornish, Waitrose*	1 Serving/150g	304	20.1	203	3.0	17.6	13.4	0.5
Clotted Cream, M & S*	1 Pudding/185g	431	30.7	233	3.0	19.2	16.6	0.2
Co-Op*	1oz/28g	49	2.5	175	5.0	20.0	9.0	2.0
COU, M & S*	1 Pot/171g	145	2.9	85	2.4	15.5	1.7	0.5
Creamed, Asda*	1 Serving/215g	196	3.4	91	3.2	16.0	1.6	0.0
Creamed, Canned, Ambrosia*	1 Can/425g	382	8.1	90	3.1	15.2	1.9	0.0
Creamed, Canned, Sainsbury's*	½ Can/212g	187	2.8	88	3.0	16.0	1.3	0.3
Creamed, Co-Op*	1 Can/170g	153	2.5	90	3.0	16.0	1.5	0.0
Creamed, HL, Tesco*	1 Can/425g	340	2.5	80	3.0	15.1	0.6	0.2
Creamed, Morrisons*	1 Can/212g	189	3.4	89	3.1	15.7	1.6	0.0
Creamed, Pot, Ambrosia*	1 Pot/150g	156	3.8	104	3.3	17.0	2.5	0.1
Creamed, Weight Watchers*	1 Pot/130g	108	0.9	83	3.2	16.0	0.7	0.3
Creamy, Ambrosia*	½ Can/212g	197	4.0	93	3.2	15.7	1.9	0.0
Creamy, Delicious, Taste of Home, Heinz*	½ Can/212g	225	4.0	106	3.4	18.6	1.9	0.2
Creamy Rice, Shape, Danone*	1 Serving/175g	149	1.7	85	3.5	15.4	1.0	0.4
Creamy Rice with Tropical Crunch, Ambrosia*	1 Pack/210g	307	8.8	146	3.6	23.4	4.2	0.6

R

	Measure INFO/WEIGHT	per Measure KCAL	FAT	Nutrition Values per 100g / 100ml KCAL	PROT	CARB	FAT	FIBRE
RICE PUDDING								
Creamy with Strawberry Crunch, Ambrosia*	1 Pack/205g	297	8.6	145	3.9	23.0	4.2	0.7
Light, Creamy, Delicious, Taste of Home, Heinz*	½ Can/213g	194	1.3	91	3.4	18.0	0.6	0.2
Low Fat, Co-Op*	1 Sm Can/170g	144	1.4	85	3.0	16.0	0.8	0.0
Low Fat, Devon, Creamed, Ambrosia*	½ Can/213g	193	2.8	91	3.2	16.5	1.3	0.0
Low Fat, No Added Sugar, Canned, Weight Watchers*	½ Can/212g	155	3.2	73	3.7	11.4	1.5	0.0
Low Fat, Tesco*	1 Can/425g	404	5.5	95	3.2	16.9	1.3	0.1
Luxury Rice, Llangadog Creamery*	1 Serving/220g	310	16.9	141	3.1	15.2	7.7	0.0
Organic, Ambrosia*	1 Can/425g	455	15.7	107	3.4	15.1	3.7	0.0
Organic, Co-Op*	1 Can/425g	446	12.7	105	3.0	16.0	3.0	0.2
Organic, Evernat*	1oz/28g	39	0.8	141	5.5	22.9	3.0	0.0
Original, Mullerrice, Muller*	1 Pot/190g	196	4.9	103	3.6	16.3	2.6	0.3
Perfectly Balanced, Waitrose*	1 Serving/154g	140	2.5	91	3.4	15.7	1.6	1.2
Raspberry, BGTY, Sainsbury's*	1 Pot/135g	126	1.6	93	3.2	17.2	1.2	1.3
Raspberry, Mullerice, Muller*	1 Std Pot/200g	218	4.4	109	3.2	19.1	2.2	0.6
Rhubarb, Muller*	1 Pot/200g	226	4.4	113	3.2	20.0	2.2	0.0
Strawberry, Mullerrice, Muller*	1 Pot/200g	220	4.4	110	3.2	19.3	2.2	0.4
Thick & Creamy, Co-Op*	1 Can/425g	531	25.5	125	3.0	16.0	6.0	0.0
Thick & Creamy, Nestle*	1 Can/425g	527	23.8	124	3.1	15.4	5.6	0.2
Vanilla Custard, Mullerrice, Muller*	1 Pot/200g	230	5.0	115	3.4	19.8	2.5	0.3
Venetian, Cafe Culture, M & S*	1 Serving/120g	300	19.7	250	3.4	21.8	16.4	0.2
with Jam, Kosy Shack, Costcutters*	1 Serving/150g	172	3.7	115	3.5	19.8	2.5	0.9
with Peach, Apricot & Passion Fruit, Onken*	1oz/28g	33	1.0	118	2.5	18.7	3.7	0.5
with Strawberry Compote, Onken*	1 Pot/160g	184	5.4	115	2.6	18.6	3.4	0.5
with Strawberry Sauce, Ambrosia*	1 Pot/160g	174	3.2	109	2.7	19.8	2.0	0.1
with Sultanas & Nutmeg, Ambrosia*	1 Pack/425g	446	12.3	105	3.2	16.6	2.9	0.1
with Sultanas & Nutmeg, Co-Op*	1 Can/425g	446	12.7	105	3.0	18.0	3.0	0.1
with Summer Fruit Compote, Onken*	1 Pot/160g	195	5.4	122	2.5	20.3	3.4	0.5
RICE SALAD								
Chicken Tikka, COU, M & S*	1 Pack/390g	409	3.9	105	5.1	18.7	1.0	0.6
Hot Smoked Salmon, Deli Meal, M & S*	1 Pack/380g	570	26.2	150	6.5	15.1	6.9	0.2
Mexican, with Beans, COU, M & S*	1 Serving/250g	250	3.5	100	6.0	15.6	1.4	1.2
Rainbow, M & S*	1 Serving/262g	340	8.4	130	2.5	23.3	3.2	1.5
Red, with Feta, M & S*	1 Pack/244g	440	20.8	180	4.8	21.0	8.5	1.3
Spanish Style, with Chicken, M & S*	1 Serving/220g	319	12.8	145	5.8	17.4	5.8	0.5
RICE STICKS								
Chakri, Cofresh*	1 Serving/100g	480	20.5	480	7.7	66.1	20.5	0.0
Salt & Vinegar, Weight Watchers*	1 Serving/20g	73	0.3	365	7.7	79.7	1.7	2.4
Thai Sweet Chilli Flavour, Weight Watchers*	1 Serving/20g	73	0.3	363	7.6	79.5	1.6	2.2
RICE WINE								
Sake, Average	*1oz/28g*	*38*	*0.0*	*134*	*0.5*	*5.0*	*0.0*	*0.0*
Shaoxing, Waitrose*	1 Tbsp/15ml	21	0.0	138	1.6	3.9	0.0	0.2
RIGATONI								
Carbonara, Tesco*	1 Serving/205g	236	11.9	115	5.2	10.6	5.8	1.2
Dry, Average	*1 Serving/80g*	*272*	*1.2*	*339*	*11.4*	*68.4*	*1.5*	*2.7*
Tomato & Cheese, Perfectly Balanced, Waitrose*	1 Pack/400g	664	9.2	166	7.6	28.6	2.3	2.3
Tuna, Diet Chef Ltd*	1 Pack/300g	336	13.2	112	5.9	12.2	4.4	1.0
RISOTTO								
Balls, Mushroom, Occasions, Sainsbury's*	1 Ball/25g	76	3.4	304	3.8	41.2	13.8	1.7
Balls, Sun Dried Tomato, Occasions, Sainsbury's*	1 Ball/25g	71	3.7	285	6.8	30.8	15.0	2.9
Beef, Vesta*	1 Serving/100g	346	5.9	346	15.3	57.8	5.9	5.6
Beetroot & Goats Cheese, Lovely Vegetables, M & S*	1 Pack/379g	530	17.0	140	4.4	20.7	4.5	3.6
Butternut, Pearl Barely, Veg Pot, Innocent*	1 Pot/390g	285	5.1	73	2.9	12.6	1.3	3.8
Caramelised Onion & Gruyere Cheese, M & S*	1 Pack/200g	350	20.6	175	3.0	17.8	10.3	1.7

	Measure INFO/WEIGHT	per Measure KCAL	FAT	Nutrition Values per 100g / 100ml KCAL	PROT	CARB	FAT	FIBRE
RISOTTO								
Chargrilled Chicken, Ready Meal, M & S*	1 Pack/365g	493	25.2	135	6.4	11.6	6.9	0.7
Cheese, Onion & Wine, Rice & Simple, Ainsley Harriott*	1 Pack/140g	253	7.0	181	3.1	31.0	5.0	1.6
Cheese Flavour, Made Up, Ainsley Harriott*	1 Sachet/140g	565	14.6	404	7.8	69.6	10.4	9.1
Cherry Tomato, COU, M & S*	1 Pack/360g	324	8.3	90	2.0	15.4	2.3	1.8
Chicken	1 Serving/380g	494	17.4	130	7.2	15.1	4.6	1.3
Chicken, BGTY, Sainsbury's*	1 Pack/327g	356	6.2	109	7.5	15.5	1.9	1.0
Chicken, Co-Op*	1 Pack/340g	442	17.0	130	6.0	16.0	5.0	2.0
Chicken, Enjoy, Birds Eye*	1 Pack/500g	735	31.5	147	8.5	14.0	6.3	0.5
Chicken, Lemon & Wild Rocket, Sainsbury's*	1 Pack/360g	683	41.0	190	16.2	5.6	11.4	0.1
Chicken, Ready Meal, M & S*	1 Pack/360g	450	15.8	125	6.7	14.4	4.4	0.9
Chicken, Tomato & Mozzarella, GFY, Asda*	1 Pack/400g	356	4.0	89	8.1	11.9	1.0	1.2
Chicken & Bacon, Italiano, Tesco*	1 Pack/450g	652	20.2	145	5.9	20.2	4.5	1.5
Chicken & Lemon, Weight Watchers*	1 Pack/330g	327	6.9	99	6.3	13.7	2.1	0.5
Chicken & Mushroom, Finest, Tesco*	1 Pack/400g	496	11.2	124	7.4	17.2	2.8	0.5
Chicken & Mushroom, Waitrose*	1 Pack/350g	364	16.1	104	6.0	9.7	4.6	0.8
Chicken & Mushroom, Weight Watchers*	1 Pack/320g	323	8.0	101	5.7	13.8	2.5	0.3
Chicken & Sun Dried Tomato, Waitrose*	1 Pack/350g	385	22.0	110	6.0	7.2	6.3	0.3
Green Bean, Asparagus & Pecorino, Finest, Tesco*	1 Pack/400g	460	15.6	115	4.4	15.0	3.9	1.5
Haddock & Mushroom, COU, M & S*	1 Pack/400g	320	3.2	80	6.4	12.1	0.8	2.0
Hot Smoked Salmon & Spinach, M & S*	½ Pack/300g	420	24.0	140	6.4	11.0	8.0	0.6
Italian, Smoked Haddock, Tesco*	½ Pack/350g	400	15.1	114	4.2	14.3	4.3	0.8
Italian Red Wine with Creamed Spinach, Sainsbury's*	1 Pack/400g	596	27.6	149	2.4	19.3	6.9	0.4
King Prawn, Pea & Mint, M & S*	½ Pack/300g	405	18.6	135	3.8	15.9	6.2	0.9
King Prawn & Snow Crab, M & S*	1 Pack/365g	401	16.4	110	4.1	12.7	4.5	0.5
Lemon & Mint, Perfectly Balanced, Waitrose*	1 Pack/350g	462	12.9	132	3.9	20.7	3.7	1.0
Mushroom	1 Serving/450g	456	12.8	101	2.7	16.2	2.8	1.3
Mushroom, Asda*	1 Pack/340g	340	11.6	100	2.3	15.0	3.4	0.6
Mushroom, BGTY, Sainsbury's*	1 Pack/400g	387	8.7	102	2.7	17.6	2.3	1.0
Mushroom, COU, M & S*	1 Pack/375g	337	5.6	90	3.0	16.1	1.5	1.5
Mushroom, Diet Chef Ltd*	1 Pack/250g	215	7.2	86	3.2	12.0	2.9	0.2
Mushroom, HL, Tesco*	1 Pack/400g	320	3.2	80	2.6	15.6	0.8	0.6
Mushroom, Italiano, Tesco*	1 Pack/340g	367	6.8	108	2.4	20.0	2.0	4.6
Mushroom, Low Saturated Fat, Waitrose*	1 Pack/400g	440	9.6	110	4.6	15.1	2.4	1.5
Mushroom, Perfectly Balanced, Waitrose*	1 Pack/400g	384	6.4	96	4.3	16.1	1.6	2.1
Mushroom & Chestnut, Waitrose*	1 Pack/400g	496	90.0	124	14.6	58.4	22.5	7.2
Roasted Red Pepper & Italian Cheese, M & S*	1 Pack/400g	500	13.2	125	2.9	20.4	3.3	1.0
Roasted Vegetable, Made Up, Ainsley Harriott*	1 Sachet/140g	766	18.2	547	11.0	96.5	13.0	15.5
Roasted Vegetable & Sunblush Tomato, Finest, Tesco*	½ Pack/200g	306	18.0	153	3.7	14.5	9.0	1.4
Roasted Vegetables, Stir-In, Uncle Ben's*	½ Pack/75g	86	7.3	115	1.7	5.0	9.7	0.0
Seafood, HL, Tesco*	1 Pack/365g	328	3.6	90	5.3	14.1	1.0	0.9
Seafood, Youngs*	1 Pack/350g	423	12.9	121	4.5	17.4	3.7	0.1
Spring Vegetable, M & S*	1 Serving/330g	330	13.2	100	2.0	14.2	4.0	0.9
Tomato & Cheese, GFY, Asda*	1 Pack/400g	428	12.0	107	3.1	17.0	3.0	0.7
Tomato & Chilli, Solo Slim, Rosemary Conley*	1 Pack/300g	240	8.7	80	6.8	6.7	2.9	3.5
Tomato & Mascarpone, Cooked, Ainsley Harriott*	1 Sachet/346g	553	18.7	160	2.5	25.3	5.4	1.6
Tomato & Mascarpone, M & S*	1 Pack/360g	468	19.1	130	2.7	17.5	5.3	0.9
Vegetable, Average	1oz/28g	41	1.8	147	4.2	19.2	6.5	2.2
Vegetable, Brown Rice, Average	1oz/28g	40	1.8	143	4.1	18.6	6.4	2.4
Vegetable, Great Stuff, Asda*	1 Pack/300g	315	5.7	105	4.3	17.6	1.9	1.3
Wild Mushroom, Made Up, Ainsley Harriott*	1 Sachet/140g	785	21.7	561	12.0	93.3	15.5	14.7
Wild Mushroom & Garlic, Tesco*	1 Pack/320g	522	14.1	163	3.6	27.2	4.4	1.6
RISSOLES								
Lentil, Fried in Vegetable Oil, Average	1oz/28g	59	2.9	211	8.9	22.0	10.5	3.6

R

	Measure INFO/WEIGHT	per Measure KCAL	FAT	Nutrition Values per 100g / 100ml KCAL	PROT	CARB	FAT	FIBRE
ROCK SALMON								
Raw, Flesh Only, Average	*1oz/28g*	*43*	*2.7*	*154*	*16.6*	*0.0*	*9.7*	*0.0*
ROCKET								
Fresh, Raw, Average	*1 Serving/80g*	*20*	*0.5*	*25*	*2.6*	*3.6*	*0.7*	*1.6*
Super Hot, Steve's Leaves*	1 Bag/30g	6	0.1	20	3.4	0.6	0.4	3.1
ROE								
Cod, Average	*1 Can/100g*	*96*	*2.8*	*96*	*17.1*	*0.5*	*2.8*	*0.0*
Cod, Hard, Coated in Batter, Fried	1oz/28g	53	3.3	189	12.4	8.9	11.8	0.2
Cod, Hard, Fried in Blended Oil	1oz/28g	57	3.3	202	20.9	3.0	11.9	0.1
Herring, Soft, Fried in Blended Oil	1oz/28g	74	4.4	265	26.3	4.7	15.8	0.2
Herring, Soft, Raw	*1oz/28g*	*25*	*0.7*	*91*	*16.8*	*0.0*	*2.6*	*0.0*
ROGAN JOSH								
Chicken & Rice, Sainsbury's*	1 Pack/500g	675	27.0	135	6.7	14.1	5.4	2.4
Chicken Breast, Chunks, Hot, Sainsbury's*	½ Pack/114g	143	2.0	126	23.6	3.9	1.8	1.0
King Prawn, with Rice, HL, Tesco*	1 Pack/400g	365	6.0	91	4.8	14.6	1.5	1.6
Lamb, & Pilau Rice, Indian Takeaway, Asda*	1 Pack/569g	888	27.9	156	7.0	21.0	4.9	1.7
Lamb, & Pilau Rice, Tesco*	1 Pack/550g	770	29.1	140	6.0	16.9	5.3	1.0
Lamb, Asda*	1 Pack/450g	688	40.5	153	13.0	5.0	9.0	3.1
Lamb, Sainsbury's*	1 Pack/400g	660	44.4	165	11.3	4.9	11.1	1.9
Lamb, Tesco*	1 Pack/350g	402	20.3	115	10.2	5.0	5.8	1.3
Lamb, Waitrose*	1 Serving/60g	79	4.7	131	12.3	3.0	7.8	1.3
Lamb, with Pilau Rice, Eastern Classics*	1 Pack/400g	604	21.6	151	5.6	19.9	5.4	1.0
Prawn, COU, M & S*	1 Pack/400g	360	2.4	90	4.9	16.2	0.6	0.8
Prawn & Pilau Rice, BGTY, Sainsbury's*	1 Pack/401g	353	3.2	88	4.8	15.3	0.8	1.9
ROLL								
All Day Breakfast, Asda*	1 Roll/220g	581	26.4	264	10.0	29.0	12.0	0.0
Bacon & Sausage, M & S*	1oz/28g	88	7.8	315	13.3	3.4	27.7	0.7
Beef, Weight Watchers*	1 Roll/174g	276	4.4	159	10.8	23.1	2.5	1.0
Brie & Grapes, M & S*	1 Roll/57g	174	10.4	306	11.1	24.5	18.2	1.4
Cheese, Tomato & Onion, Sainsbury's*	1 Pack/100g	518	28.1	518	18.4	47.9	28.1	0.0
Cheese & Chutney, M & S*	1 Roll/165g	256	1.2	155	13.9	23.1	0.7	1.2
Cheese & Onion, Asda*	1 Serving/67g	199	12.0	298	7.0	27.0	18.0	2.0
Cheese & Onion, Co-Op*	1 Roll/66g	195	11.9	295	7.0	26.0	18.0	2.0
Cheese & Onion, Iceland*	1 Roll/67g	222	13.6	332	7.5	29.6	20.4	1.5
Cheese & Onion, King Size, Pork Farms*	1 Serving/130g	443	28.6	341	7.4	28.4	22.0	0.0
Cheese & Onion, M & S*	1 Roll/25g	80	5.1	320	9.6	24.7	20.5	1.3
Cheese & Onion, Sainsbury's*	1 Roll/67g	205	13.6	306	8.0	22.9	20.3	1.9
Cheese & Onion, Tesco*	1 Roll/67g	203	12.1	305	7.3	28.0	18.1	1.9
Cheese & Pickle, Sainsbury's*	1 Roll/136g	359	13.6	264	10.6	35.1	10.0	0.0
Chicken, Salad, Mini, Selection Pack, British, M & S*	1 Roll/61g	134	4.1	220	11.9	28.1	6.8	2.1
Chicken & Beef Duo, M & S*	1 Serving/147g	235	3.8	160	12.0	22.1	2.6	2.7
Chicken & Herb, Shapers, Boots*	1 Roll/168g	290	4.7	173	12.0	25.0	2.8	1.7
Chicken & Stuffing, Tesco*	1 Roll/323g	1043	58.8	323	10.4	29.4	18.2	1.0
Chicken & Sun Dried Tomato, Weight Watchers*	1 Pack/170g	272	3.2	160	12.9	22.7	1.9	1.2
Chicken & Sweetcorn, Sainsbury's*	1 Serving/170g	462	23.6	272	12.5	24.2	13.9	0.0
Chicken Salad, HL, Tesco*	1 Serving/100g	149	2.0	149	10.6	22.3	2.0	1.2
Chunky Cheese & Mustard, Finest, Tesco*	1 Roll/88g	260	9.0	295	10.9	40.0	10.2	2.4
Cornish, in Pastry, Pork Farms*	1 Roll/75g	226	15.1	301	6.6	24.5	20.1	0.0
Egg & Bacon, Sub, Shapers, Boots*	1 Serving/169g	320	7.3	189	11.0	27.0	4.3	1.3
Egg & Cress, HL, Tesco*	1 Pack/175g	322	6.8	184	9.6	27.7	3.9	1.2
Egg & Tomato, Shapers, Boots*	1 Roll/166g	301	5.3	181	8.0	30.0	3.2	2.6
Egg Mayo & Cress, Fullfillers*	1 Roll/125g	266	11.8	213	10.0	25.7	9.4	0.0
Egg Mayonnaise & Cress, Sub, Delicious, Boots*	1 Pack/205g	399	14.1	195	10.0	23.0	6.9	2.4
Ham, Darwins Deli*	1 Serving/125g	298	7.5	238	11.0	37.4	6.0	0.0

	Measure INFO/WEIGHT	per Measure KCAL	FAT	Nutrition Values per 100g / 100ml KCAL	PROT	CARB	FAT	FIBRE
ROLL								
Ham & Cheese, in Pastry, Pork Farms*	1 Roll/70g	216	12.5	308	8.0	28.8	17.9	0.0
Ham & Tomato, Taste!*	1 Serving/112g	211	4.8	188	10.4	27.0	4.3	0.0
Ham Salad, BGTY, Sainsbury's*	1 Roll/178g	292	3.4	164	10.8	25.9	1.9	0.0
Ham Salad, HL, Tesco*	1 Roll/203g	284	5.3	140	9.8	19.3	2.6	0.0
Large Ploughmans, Ginsters*	1 Pack/140g	473	33.5	338	10.2	20.5	23.9	1.8
Leicester Ham & Cheese, Sub, Waitrose*	1 Pack/206ml	582	31.2	282	12.6	24.0	15.1	13.0
Lincolnshire Sausage, COU, M & S*	1 Roll/175g	280	4.7	160	10.0	23.2	2.7	2.6
Mushroom & Bacon, Crusty, M & S*	1 Roll/160g	424	20.2	265	8.7	29.0	12.6	2.3
Oak Smoked Salmon, M & S*	1 Roll/55g	139	6.2	252	14.6	23.1	11.3	1.2
Ploughmans 4 Pack, Ginsters*	1 Roll/60g	220	16.3	367	9.2	21.4	27.2	2.1
Roast Chicken & Mayonnaise, Big, Sainsbury's*	1 Pack/185g	479	27.4	259	9.6	21.8	14.8	0.0
Roast Chicken & Sweetcure Bacon, Boots*	1 Pack/245g	690	34.3	282	13.0	26.0	14.0	1.6
Roast Chicken Salad, Improved, Shapers, Boots*	1 Pack/188g	302	3.6	161	11.0	25.0	1.9	1.6
Roast Pork, Stuffing & Apple Sauce, Boots*	1 Roll/218g	602	26.2	276	10.0	32.0	12.0	1.8
Spicy Chicken, Crusty, M & S*	1 Roll/150g	382	16.6	255	12.8	25.8	11.1	2.0
Spicy Pork Large, Ginsters*	1 Roll/140g	511	38.9	365	9.0	19.8	27.8	4.1
Steak & Onion, M & S*	1 Serving/150g	307	10.5	205	11.0	24.5	7.0	3.8
Tomato & Basil, Sub, COU, M & S*	1 Roll/35g	93	0.9	265	11.0	48.7	2.7	2.4
Tuna & Sweetcorn with Mayonnaise, Shell*	1 Pack/180g	536	26.3	298	13.1	28.6	14.6	0.0
Tuna Cheese Melt, Boots*	1 Roll/199g	612	35.8	308	13.0	23.0	18.0	1.2
Tuna Mayo & Cucumber, Taste!*	1 Serving/111g	274	12.5	247	9.0	27.3	11.3	0.0
Tuna Mayonnaise, with Cucumber, Yummies*	1 Serving/132g	340	18.6	257	10.4	22.5	14.0	0.0
Turkey, Stuffed, GFY, Asda*	½ Pack/225g	319	9.4	142	14.0	12.0	4.2	0.8
Turkey Salad, Northern Bites*	1 Roll/231g	323	8.3	140	8.6	19.6	3.6	3.0
White, Cheese & Onion, Shell*	1 Roll/178g	554	26.3	311	14.5	30.2	14.8	0.0
ROLO								
Giant, Nestle*	1 Sweet/9g	42	1.8	470	3.1	70.1	19.7	0.3
Little, Nestle*	1 Pack/40g	196	9.4	491	4.0	65.5	23.5	0.5
Nestle*	1 Sweet/5g	24	1.0	471	3.2	68.5	20.5	0.3
ROLY POLY								
Jam, & Custard, Co-Op*	¼ Pack/100g	235	8.0	235	4.0	36.0	8.0	0.7
Jam, Aunt Bessie's*	1 Serving/75g	290	10.3	387	3.4	62.2	13.8	0.9
Jam, Sainsbury's*	¼ Pack/81g	291	11.5	359	4.4	53.3	14.2	0.5
Jam, Tesco*	1 Serving/90g	320	10.9	356	4.3	59.0	12.1	13.9
ROOT BAKES								
Herby, Red Sky*	1 Bag/30g	120	4.0	400	6.9	63.2	13.3	10.4
Spiced, Red Sky*	1 Bag/30g	122	4.1	408	8.0	62.9	13.8	9.2
ROOT BEER								
Average	1 Can/330ml	135	0.0	41	0.0	10.6	0.0	0.0
ROSE WATER								
English Provender*	1 Tsp/5g	0	0.0	2	0.1	0.6	0.1	0.1
ROSEMARY								
Dried	*1 Tsp/1g*	*3*	*0.2*	*331*	*4.9*	*46.4*	*15.2*	*0.0*
Fresh	*1 Tsp/0.7g*	*1*	*0.0*	*99*	*1.4*	*13.5*	*4.4*	*0.0*
ROSTI								
Garlic & Mushroom, Finest, Tesco*	1 Serving/200g	346	19.6	173	5.7	15.4	9.8	1.7
Honey & Parsnip, Tesco*	1 Rosti/75g	79	2.4	105	1.8	17.0	3.2	3.9
Oven Baked, McCain*	1 Rosti/100g	194	9.3	194	2.6	25.0	9.3	2.3
Peppered Steak, British Classics, Tesco*	1 Pack/450g	598	27.9	133	9.0	10.7	6.2	1.7
Potato, Chicken & Sweetcorn Bake, Asda*	1 Serving/400g	440	18.8	110	7.0	10.0	4.7	0.6
Potato, McCain*	1 Rosti/95g	161	8.6	169	2.2	19.6	9.1	0.0
Potato, Mini, Party Bites, Sainsbury's*	1 Serving/100g	218	11.5	218	2.5	26.2	11.5	3.0
Potato, Mini, Party Range, Tesco*	1 Rosti/17g	32	1.9	193	2.1	20.6	11.4	3.3

R

	Measure INFO/WEIGHT	per Measure		Nutrition Values per 100g / 100ml				
		KCAL	FAT	KCAL	PROT	CARB	FAT	FIBRE
ROSTI								
Potato, Onion & Gruyere, Finest, Tesco*	½ Pack/200g	206	10.6	103	3.2	10.5	5.3	2.0
Potato, Spinach & Mozzarella, Tesco*	1 Serving/140g	228	7.7	163	3.8	24.5	5.5	2.0
Potato & Leek, Sainsbury's*	½ Pack/190g	296	20.9	156	4.5	9.8	11.0	0.3
Potato & Root Vegetable, COU, M & S*	1 Rosti/100g	85	2.7	85	1.6	13.3	2.7	1.5
Potato Cakes, Baby, M & S*	1 Rosti/23g	40	1.5	175	3.5	25.1	6.7	1.6
Spinach & Mozzarella, Vegetarian, Tesco*	1 Rosti/140g	245	13.6	175	4.8	17.0	9.7	2.3
Vegetable, Waitrose*	1 Pack/400g	248	9.2	62	1.4	8.8	2.3	1.3
Waitrose*	1 Rosti/45g	112	7.2	248	3.8	22.5	15.9	2.7
ROULADE								
Chocolate, Finest, Tesco*	1 Serving/80g	222	4.5	277	3.4	53.2	5.6	2.3
Chocolate, Sainsbury's*	1 Serving/72g	264	15.7	367	5.7	36.9	21.8	1.8
Lemon, Asda*	1 Serving/100g	343	12.0	343	2.7	56.0	12.0	0.0
Mini, M & S*	1 Serving/63g	201	19.1	321	8.5	3.0	30.5	0.0
Orange & Lemon Meringue, Co-Op*	1 Serving/82g	287	9.8	350	3.0	57.0	12.0	0.3
Passion Fruit, M & S*	1oz/28g	83	2.6	295	2.8	50.0	9.2	0.2
Raspberry, Finest, Tesco*	1 Serving/67g	203	11.7	303	3.3	33.2	17.4	1.7
Raspberry, M & S*	1oz/28g	88	3.1	315	3.3	50.3	11.0	0.1
Smoked Salmon & Asparagus, Sainsbury's*	1 Serving/60g	122	9.6	204	13.0	2.2	16.0	0.3
Smoked Salmon & Spinach, Finest, Tesco*	1 Serving/60g	91	6.1	152	11.5	3.6	10.2	0.6
Toffee, M & S*	1oz/28g	104	4.1	371	4.1	56.0	14.5	0.3
Toffee Pecan, Finest, Tesco*	1 Serving/60g	218	8.9	363	3.6	53.8	14.8	0.5
RUM								
*21% Volume, Malibu**	*1 Shot/35ml*	*70*	*0.0*	*200*	*0.0*	*29.0*	*0.0*	*0.0*
37.5% Volume	*1 Shot/35ml*	*72*	*0.0*	*207*	*0.0*	*0.0*	*0.0*	*0.0*
40% Volume	*1 Shot/35ml*	*78*	*0.0*	*222*	*0.0*	*0.0*	*0.0*	*0.0*
Captain Morgans & Cola, Premixed, Canned, Diageo*	1 Can/250ml	180	0.0	72	0.0	91.0	0.0	0.0
White	*1 Shot/35ml*	*72*	*0.0*	*207*	*0.0*	*0.0*	*0.0*	*0.0*
RUSKS								
Banana, Farleys*	1 Serving/17g	70	1.5	409	7.3	75.1	8.8	2.9
Mini, Farleys*	1 Serving/30g	121	2.2	405	7.0	77.7	7.3	2.1
Original, Farleys*	1 Rusk/17g	69	1.2	406	7.1	77.6	7.1	2.3

R

	Measure INFO/WEIGHT	per Measure KCAL	FAT	Nutrition Values per 100g / 100ml KCAL	PROT	CARB	FAT	FIBRE
SAAG								
Aloo, Canned, Tesco*	½ Can/200g	124	3.8	62	1.8	9.3	1.9	2.0
Aloo, Fresh, Sainsbury's*	1 Pack/400g	388	13.2	97	2.0	14.7	3.3	4.8
Aloo, Jar, Sainsbury's*	½ Jar/135g	121	5.8	90	1.6	11.0	4.3	1.7
Aloo, North Indian, Sainsbury's*	1 Pack/300g	354	24.0	118	2.4	9.0	8.0	1.6
Aloo, Packet, Sainsbury's*	½ Pack/150g	184	12.4	123	2.1	9.9	8.3	2.7
Aloo, Sainsbury's*	1 Pack/300g	441	31.8	147	2.1	10.7	10.6	3.5
Aloo, Tesco*	1 Serving/200g	144	7.0	72	2.1	8.0	3.5	2.0
Aloo Gobi, M Kitchen, Morrisons*	1 Pack/225g	130	6.1	58	2.0	4.6	2.7	3.8
Aloo Gobi, Waitrose*	1 Pack/300g	240	13.8	80	2.6	7.1	4.6	2.9
Chicken, Masala, M & S*	½ Pack/175g	227	12.4	130	13.3	3.1	7.1	5.2
Chicken, Masala, Sainsbury's*	1oz/28g	36	2.0	127	13.2	2.4	7.2	2.3
Chicken, Masala, Waitrose*	1 Pack/400g	520	30.0	130	13.8	1.8	7.5	2.5
Gobi Aloo, Indian, Tesco*	1 Pack/225g	225	16.4	100	2.1	6.5	7.3	1.8
Gobi Aloo, Indian Takeaway, Sainsbury's*	1 Pack/334g	164	3.7	49	1.7	8.0	1.1	1.5
Gobi Aloo, M & S*	1 Pack/225g	270	19.1	120	1.9	9.3	8.5	2.4
Gobi Aloo, Tesco*	1 Serving/175g	166	8.9	95	2.1	9.5	5.1	1.9
Paneer, Sainsbury's*	1 Pack/300g	387	29.1	129	6.0	4.3	9.7	2.3
SAFFRON								
Average	*1 Tsp/1g*	*2*	*0.0*	*310*	*11.4*	*61.5*	*5.9*	*0.0*
SAGE								
Dried, Ground	*1 Tsp/1g*	*3*	*0.1*	*315*	*10.6*	*42.7*	*12.7*	*0.0*
Fresh	*1oz/28g*	*33*	*1.3*	*119*	*3.9*	*15.6*	*4.6*	*0.0*
SAGO								
Raw	*1oz/28g*	*99*	*0.1*	*355*	*0.2*	*94.0*	*0.2*	*0.5*
SALAD								
3 Bean, Sainsbury's*	1 Tub/270g	281	6.2	104	7.1	13.6	2.3	5.9
Alfresco Style, Tesco*	1 Serving/200g	40	0.6	20	0.9	3.3	0.3	2.1
All Seasons, Sainsbury's*	1oz/28g	3	0.1	12	1.0	1.5	0.2	1.2
American Ranch, Asda*	1 Serving/220g	253	19.8	115	2.5	6.0	9.0	2.0
American Style, Sweet & Crispy, Morrisons*	1 Serving/25g	7	0.1	28	1.2	4.2	0.3	2.0
Aromatic Herb, Waitrose*	¼ Pack/27g	4	0.1	15	0.9	1.7	0.5	1.0
Assorted, Asda*	1 Serving/100g	22	0.6	22	2.4	1.7	0.6	0.0
Avocado & Feta, Gourmet To Go, M & S*	1 Pack/320g	512	32.0	160	5.4	12.1	10.0	3.1
Baby Leaf, Aldi*	1 Serving/50g	11	0.0	22	3.5	1.0	0.1	1.5
Baby Leaf, Asda*	1 Serving/80g	10	0.2	12	2.1	0.2	0.3	1.7
Baby Leaf, Florette*	1 Serving/40g	5	0.1	12	2.0	0.4	0.3	1.0
Baby Leaf, Fully Prepared, Sainsbury's*	½ Bag/63g	10	0.3	16	1.3	1.9	0.4	1.5
Baby Leaf, Italian Style, M & S*	1 Serving/55g	11	0.3	20	1.3	2.3	0.5	1.3
Baby Leaf, M & S*	1 Pack/100g	20	0.2	20	3.0	1.7	0.2	0.5
Baby Leaf, Organic, Sainsbury's*	1 Serving/20g	3	0.1	14	1.5	1.4	0.3	1.1
Baby Leaf, Sainsbury's*	1 Serving/60g	12	1.1	20	2.8	1.1	1.9	1.9
Baby Leaf, Seasonal, Organic, Sainsbury's*	1 Serving/30g	3	0.1	10	1.6	0.4	0.3	1.2
Baby Leaf, Seasonal, Sainsbury's*	¼ Bag/63g	11	0.3	17	2.8	0.5	0.5	2.7
Baby Leaf, Seasonal, Tesco*	½ Pack/45g	9	0.3	20	1.8	1.6	0.7	2.1
Baby Leaf, Sweet, Seasonal, M & S*	½ Bag/60g	9	0.2	15	2.4	0.6	0.4	1.8
Baby Leaf, with Purple Basil, Finest, Tesco*	½ Pack/43g	7	0.1	17	2.9	0.9	0.2	1.8
Baby Leaf, with Watercress, Tesco*	1 Serving/30g	6	0.2	19	1.8	1.3	0.7	1.8
Baby Leaf & Herb, Asda*	1 Serving/50g	7	0.1	14	2.3	0.7	0.2	2.4
Baby Plum & Sundried Tomato Salad, Waitrose*	1 Serving/200g	226	17.8	113	1.3	6.8	8.9	0.8
Baby Spinach & Red Mustard, M & S*	1 Pack/170g	263	26.7	155	1.7	1.1	15.7	0.1
Baby Tomato, Tesco*	1 Pack/205g	35	0.6	17	0.8	2.8	0.3	0.9
Bacon Caesar, M & S*	1oz/28g	48	3.9	170	5.5	5.7	14.0	1.2
Bacon Caesar, Sainsbury's*	1 Pack/256g	415	32.5	162	4.7	12.0	12.7	1.4

SALAD

	Measure INFO/WEIGHT	per Measure KCAL	FAT	Nutrition Values per 100g / 100ml KCAL	PROT	CARB	FAT	FIBRE
Bag, Tesco*	1 Serving/200g	38	0.8	19	0.9	3.0	0.4	1.4
Basil, Pesto & Pine Nuts, Italian Style, Finest, Tesco*	½ Pack/90g	144	12.5	160	5.1	3.6	13.9	1.2
Bean, M & S*	1 Serving/80g	72	0.7	90	6.4	14.3	0.9	3.9
Bean, Mixed, Vinaigrette, Tesco*	1 Can/400g	280	2.0	70	3.2	13.1	0.5	1.9
Bean, Retail	1oz/28g	41	2.6	147	4.2	12.8	9.3	3.0
Bean, Three, M & S*	1 Pack/225g	225	3.0	100	5.8	16.7	1.3	3.9
Bean & Chorizo, Tapas Selection, Sainsbury's*	1 Serving/22g	29	1.4	132	8.1	10.7	6.3	1.9
Bean & Sweetcorn, Side, M & S*	1 Serving/125g	131	9.0	105	2.5	7.0	7.2	1.3
Beans, Mixed, Essential, Waitrose*	1 Serving/80g	87	1.8	109	8.7	13.6	2.2	3.1
Beetroot	1oz/28g	28	1.9	100	2.0	8.4	6.8	1.7
Beetroot, 1% Fat, M & S*	1 Serving/225g	130	6.1	58	1.1	7.7	2.7	1.7
Beetroot, Asda*	1 Carton/270g	119	1.1	44	1.3	8.8	0.4	2.4
Beetroot, Co-Op*	1 Pack/250g	100	0.7	40	0.9	8.0	0.3	2.0
Beetroot, Cous Cous & Quinoa, Tesco*	1 Serving/100g	70	0.6	70	2.3	12.9	0.6	2.3
Beetroot, Freshly Prepared, Tesco*	1 Pack/240g	58	0.7	24	1.9	3.3	0.3	2.7
Beetroot, GFY, Asda*	1 Pack/250g	130	1.0	52	1.1	11.0	0.4	2.3
Beetroot, M & S*	1 Serving/225g	124	0.7	55	1.0	12.0	0.3	3.0
Beetroot, Morrisons*	1 Pot/250g	137	1.0	55	1.2	11.6	0.4	1.6
Beetroot, Organic, M & S*	1oz/28g	20	1.0	73	1.5	9.1	3.4	1.9
Beetroot, Roast, with Quinoa & Feta, Tesco*	1 Pack/400g	452	19.6	113	4.8	12.4	4.9	2.3
Beetroot, Sainsbury's*	1 Tub/200g	148	2.4	74	1.7	14.1	1.2	1.7
Beetroot, with Balsamic Dressing, Finest, Tesco*	1 Portion/75g	49	1.1	65	1.1	11.9	1.5	2.4
Beetroot & Carrot, Continental, Iceland*	1 Serving/100g	24	0.2	24	1.2	4.3	0.2	2.1
Beetroot & Cherry Tomato, & Lemon Dressing, M & S*	1 Pack/215g	129	8.2	60	1.3	5.2	3.8	1.5
Beetroot & Lettuce, Asda*	1 Serving/30g	5	0.0	16	1.4	2.7	0.0	2.5
Bistro, Asda*	1 Serving/180g	29	0.0	16	1.4	2.7	0.0	2.5
Bistro, Morrisons*	1 Serving/20g	5	0.0	23	1.2	4.2	0.2	2.0
Bistro, Sainsbury's*	1 Pack/150g	25	0.3	17	1.9	2.0	0.2	2.0
Bistro, Washed Ready to Eat, Tesco*	1 Pack/140g	22	0.7	16	1.1	1.7	0.5	1.0
Bistro Style, Morrisons*	¼ Pack/45g	11	0.1	24	1.2	4.1	0.3	2.0
Black Bean Salsa, Salad Bar, Waitrose*	1 Serving/100g	118	5.8	118	0.0	0.0	5.8	0.0
British Ham & Free Range Egg, M & S*	1 Pack/280g	182	6.4	65	6.1	5.3	2.3	1.0
Brown Rice, Tossed UK*	1 Pack/200g	335	1.8	167	13.3	19.9	0.9	0.0
Bulgar Wheat, Lentil & Edamame Shaker, Waitrose*	1 Pack/190g	217	10.6	114	4.7	11.1	5.6	4.4
Bulgar Wheat & Carrot, Sainsbury's*	½ Pot/125g	167	6.7	134	2.8	16.1	5.4	4.8
Cabbage & Leek, Crunchy Mix, Sainsbury's*	½ Pack/126g	24	0.8	19	1.2	2.1	0.6	1.9
Caesar	1 Serving/200g	352	27.8	176	4.8	8.1	13.9	0.7
Caesar, & New Potatoes with Asparagus, M & S*	1 Pack/200g	270	15.2	135	3.1	13.8	7.6	1.7
Caesar, Bacon, M & S*	1 Serving/250g	400	31.2	160	7.1	4.1	12.5	1.3
Caesar, Chicken & Bacon, Gourmet, M & S*	1 Salad/250g	550	43.5	220	9.0	7.3	17.4	0.7
Caesar, Chicken & Bacon, Tesco*	1 Pack/200g	506	40.2	253	6.6	11.4	20.1	1.0
Caesar, Co-Op*	¼ Pack/50g	87	7.5	175	3.0	16.0	15.0	2.0
Caesar, Finest, Tesco*	1 Bowl/220g	374	30.6	170	4.9	5.1	13.9	1.6
Caesar, Florette*	1 Serving/100g	163	12.4	163	2.7	10.2	12.4	1.8
Caesar, GFY, Asda*	½ Pack/87g	76	2.6	87	8.0	7.0	3.0	1.5
Caesar, M & S*	1 Pack/268g	510	40.5	190	5.7	8.3	15.1	1.3
Caesar, Morrisons*	1 Serving/115g	194	18.1	169	3.6	5.9	15.7	0.3
Caesar, Sainsbury's*	½ Bag/128g	227	19.3	177	3.6	6.7	15.1	1.0
Caesar, with Dressing, Croutons & Parmesan, M & S*	1 Serving/115g	190	15.5	165	4.3	6.4	13.5	1.4
Caesar, with Parmigiano Reggiano, Tesco*	1 Bag/275g	552	49.0	201	4.1	5.8	17.8	1.3
Caesar, with Romaine Lettuce, Kit, BGTY, Sainsbury's*	½ Pack/130g	139	7.9	107	3.7	9.2	6.1	1.4
Caesar Pasta, Salad Bar, Waitrose*	1 Serving/100g	260	18.0	260	0.0	0.0	18.0	0.0
Cajun Chicken, David Lloyd Leisure*	1 Pack/300g	429	10.0	143	11.7	17.7	3.3	1.0

SALAD

INFO/WEIGHT		KCAL	FAT	KCAL	PROT	CARB	FAT	FIBRE
Cannellini Bean & Chicken, M & S*	1 Serving/225g	250	14.7	111	5.9	7.4	6.5	3.1
Cannellini Bean & Chorizo, Sainsbury's*	1 Pack/250g	227	8.0	91	5.3	10.2	3.2	1.6
Cannellini Bean & Tuna, M & S*	1 Serving/255g	215	11.6	84	5.3	5.4	4.5	2.1
Caponata, Organic, Florentin*	1 Serving/100g	111	12.3	111	1.5	3.7	12.3	0.0
Caribbean Chicken, Shapers, Boots*	1 Pack/220g	222	5.1	101	5.8	14.0	2.3	1.2
Carrot, Courgette & Coriander, Salad Bar, Waitrose*	1 Serving/100g	92	7.9	92	0.0	0.0	7.9	0.0
Carrot, M & S*	1 Pack/215g	280	7.3	130	3.1	22.4	3.4	2.7
Carrot, Peanut & Sultana, Asda*	1 Serving/20g	54	4.0	272	8.0	15.0	20.0	4.5
Carrot, with Fresh Coriander Vinaigrette, M & S*	½ Pack/105g	136	3.6	130	2.8	21.9	3.4	3.5
Carrot & Beetroot, Classic, Tesco*	½ Pack/83g	17	0.2	20	0.9	3.7	0.2	1.6
Carrot & Beetroot, with a Balsamic Dressing, Asda*	1 Pack/160g	101	6.6	63	0.9	5.6	4.1	1.0
Carrot & Nut, with French Dressing, Average	1oz/28g	61	4.9	218	2.1	13.7	17.6	2.4
Carrot & Sultana, BGTY, Sainsbury's*	½ Pack/100g	55	0.3	55	0.6	12.4	0.3	0.0
Carrot & Sultana, HL, Tesco*	1 Tub/225g	142	1.3	63	1.2	13.2	0.6	2.5
Celery, Nut & Sultana, Asda*	1oz/28g	76	6.7	272	2.9	11.2	23.9	1.9
Celery, Nut & Sultana, Waitrose*	1oz/28g	54	4.6	192	2.8	8.4	16.4	1.0
Celery & Apple, Salad Bar, Waitrose*	1 Serving/100g	136	12.9	136	0.0	0.0	12.9	0.0
Chargrilled Chicken, Tesco*	1 Serving/300g	384	14.4	128	6.1	15.0	4.8	2.4
Chargrilled Chicken, Weight Watchers*	1 Pack/182g	265	3.8	146	11.7	20.0	2.1	2.2
Chargrilled Chicken & Bacon, Tesco*	1 Pack/300g	657	37.8	219	7.8	18.7	12.6	0.9
Chargrilled Chicken & Pesto, Sainsbury's*	1 Pack/250g	375	15.2	150	7.9	15.8	6.1	1.3
Chargrilled Chicken & Quinoa, Shapers, Boots*	1 Pack/185g	139	1.8	75	6.2	10.0	1.0	1.8
Chargrilled Chicken Wholefood, M & S*	1 Pot/219g	230	4.2	105	10.1	11.6	1.9	4.8
Chargrilled Pepper with Cous Cous, Asda*	1 Pack/325g	426	10.7	131	4.3	21.0	3.3	0.0
Chargrilled Vegetable, M & S*	1 Tub/165g	91	5.4	55	1.4	5.3	3.3	2.6
Cheese, HL, Tesco*	1 Serving/30g	32	0.9	107	18.0	2.0	3.0	0.0
Cheese, Layered, Tesco*	1 Serving/225g	437	32.0	194	5.8	10.8	14.2	0.8
Cheese, Ploughmans, Asda*	1 Bowl/300g	246	10.8	82	3.6	8.9	3.6	1.0
Cheese & Coleslaw, Tesco*	1 Serving/125g	135	10.9	108	3.4	3.4	8.7	1.1
Cheese Layered, M & S*	½ Pack/230g	300	20.5	130	4.6	9.3	8.9	1.2
Cheesy Bean Pasta, Salad Bar, Waitrose*	1 Serving/100g	143	4.3	143	0.0	0.0	4.3	0.0
Cherry Tomato, All Good Things*	1 Pack/185g	31	0.6	17	0.8	2.8	0.3	1.4
Cherry Tomato, Salad Bar, Waitrose*	1 Serving/100g	77	5.3	77	0.0	0.0	5.3	0.0
Cherry Tomato, Tesco*	1 Pack/210g	136	9.4	65	0.9	4.2	4.5	1.1
Chick Pea & Cous Cous, Tesco*	1 Serving/250g	245	6.5	98	3.2	15.5	2.6	0.0
Chick Pea & Spinach, M & S*	1 Serving/260g	299	10.7	115	7.3	12.5	4.1	2.7
Chick Pea & Sweet Potato, Salad Bar, Sainsbury's*	1 Serving/100g	99	1.9	99	0.0	9.6	1.9	0.0
Chicken, Avocado & Bacon, M & S*	1 Serving/235g	235	13.6	100	8.5	2.8	5.8	2.8
Chicken, Caesar, Tesco*	1 Pack/300g	330	13.5	110	6.8	10.6	4.5	0.8
Chicken, Italian Style, Snack Pot, Carb Check, Heinz*	1 Pot/218g	131	4.4	60	5.9	4.3	2.0	1.0
Chicken, Roast, & Coleslaw, Boots*	1 Serving/245g	392	34.3	160	4.5	3.9	14.0	1.3
Chicken, Roast, 93 Cals, Shapers, Boots*	1 Pack/233g	93	0.9	40	8.6	0.6	0.4	1.8
Chicken, Sweet Chilli, BGTY, Sainsbury's*	1 Serving/200g	206	0.8	103	6.0	18.7	0.4	0.0
Chicken, Tesco*	1 Serving/300g	348	22.2	116	5.3	7.0	7.4	1.0
Chicken, Tomato Chilli, & Rice, COU, M & S*	1 Pack/340g	357	5.1	105	6.8	16.0	1.5	0.9
Chicken & Bacon, Asda*	1 Pack/381g	480	22.9	126	7.0	11.0	6.0	0.0
Chicken & Bacon, Carb Control, Tesco*	1 Serving/188g	244	14.7	130	13.2	1.7	7.8	0.5
Chicken & Bacon, Layered, Asda*	1 Serving/375g	472	22.5	126	7.0	11.0	6.0	1.6
Chicken & Bacon, Layered, Waitrose*	1 Serving/200g	246	14.8	123	6.7	7.4	7.4	2.1
Chicken & Bacon Layered, Tesco*	1 Pack/360g	600	39.6	167	4.6	12.1	11.0	1.8
Chicken & Bacon Ranch, Sainsbury's*	1 Pack/210g	315	15.7	150	8.4	12.1	7.5	0.9
Chicken & Moroccan Cous Cous, Tesco*	1 Pack/210g	252	4.2	120	7.8	16.9	2.0	3.5
Chicken Caesar, Asda*	1 Pack/273g	535	43.7	196	10.0	3.0	16.0	1.9

S

SALAD

INFO/WEIGHT	Measure	per Measure KCAL	FAT	Nutrition Values per 100g / 100ml KCAL	PROT	CARB	FAT	FIBRE
Chicken Caesar, Eat Well, M & S*	1 Pack/397g	595	24.6	150	9.9	18.7	6.2	2.1
Chicken Caesar, Fresh, Sainsbury's*	1 Serving/200g	278	20.0	139	6.0	6.2	10.0	1.2
Chicken Caesar, M & S*	½ Pack/140g	266	20.0	190	6.7	8.7	14.3	0.8
Chicken Caesar, Shapers, Boots*	1 Pack/200g	205	5.8	102	8.2	10.0	2.9	1.0
Chicken Caesar Bistro, M & S*	½ Pack/135g	189	14.3	140	5.0	6.5	10.6	0.6
Chicken Fajita, Shapers, Boots*	1 Pack/258g	181	3.4	70	7.0	7.4	1.3	2.7
Chicken Noodle, Thai Style, Sainsbury's*	1 Pack/260g	283	7.5	109	6.6	14.2	2.9	1.3
Chicken Noodle & Sweet Chilli, Shapers, Boots*	1 Pack/197g	266	5.1	135	12.0	16.0	2.6	0.9
Chicken Pesto Pasta, Royal London Hospital*	1oz/28g	37	1.0	132	10.4	15.3	3.5	0.0
Chicken with Mayonnaise, Waitrose*	1 Pack/208g	406	19.8	195	10.3	17.1	9.5	2.5
Chicken with Tomato & Basil Cous Cous, Tesco*	1 Pack/200g	270	4.2	135	8.3	19.7	2.1	1.5
Chickpea & Bean, Salad Bar, Waitrose*	1 Serving/100g	165	10.2	165	0.0	0.0	10.2	0.0
Chilli, Tomato, Chick Pea & Butterbean, Tesco*	1 Pack/130g	146	6.0	112	3.4	14.3	4.6	0.5
Chilli Chicken Noodle, Tesco*	1 Pack/230g	172	2.5	75	8.4	7.1	1.1	3.0
Classic, Complete Salad, Sainsbury's*	1 Pack/220g	112	8.4	51	1.0	3.3	3.8	1.4
Classic, Co-Op*	½ Pack/80g	16	0.2	20	0.8	2.9	0.3	2.2
Classic, with Chive Dressing, M & S*	½ Pack/138g	76	5.8	55	0.9	3.3	4.2	1.6
Classic Caesar, M & S*	½ Pack/112g	174	14.2	155	2.9	6.8	12.7	0.5
Classic Caesar, Reduced Fat, M & S*	1 Serving/115g	132	5.6	115	4.8	12.7	4.9	0.5
Classic with Green Herb Dressing, Co-Op*	1 Serving/90g	85	8.1	95	1.0	2.0	9.0	1.0
Classics, M & S*	1 Pack/255g	140	12.0	55	1.1	2.4	4.7	1.3
Coleslaw, Classics, M & S*	1 Pot/190g	123	4.4	65	1.9	8.8	2.3	1.3
Coleslaw, Layered, Fresh Tastes, Asda*	1oz/28g	17	1.3	59	1.1	3.4	4.5	1.6
Coleslaw & Potato, 3% Fat, M & S*	1oz/28g	20	1.0	72	2.7	7.7	3.4	1.5
Coleslaw Layered, Fresh, Asda*	1 Tub/197g	209	17.7	106	1.2	5.0	9.0	1.5
Complete Hot Greek, Sainsbury's*	1 Pack/299g	287	22.4	96	4.3	2.9	7.5	1.7
Continental, Co-Op*	1 Serving/80g	12	0.3	15	1.0	2.0	0.4	1.0
Continental Four Leaf, Sainsbury's*	½ Pack/100g	13	0.2	13	1.2	1.7	0.2	1.9
Continental Leaf, Asda*	1oz/28g	4	0.1	16	1.4	1.4	0.5	1.4
Continental Style, Co-Op*	1 Bag/100g	15	0.3	15	1.0	2.0	0.3	0.5
Co-op Crunchy Mini Salad, Co-Op*	1 Pack/80g	16	0.4	20	1.0	2.5	0.5	1.7
Coronation Chicken, Salad Bar, Asda*	1oz/28g	82	6.4	293	5.7	16.4	22.7	0.7
Coronation Chicken & Rice, Asda*	1oz/28g	67	4.8	241	6.7	15.2	17.0	0.4
Coronation Rice, Tesco*	1 Serving/50g	103	7.5	207	2.0	15.9	15.1	0.8
Cosmopolitan, Fresh, Sainsbury's*	1 Bag/135g	20	0.5	15	1.2	1.6	0.4	1.9
Cous Cous, & Roasted Vegetable, Waitrose*	1 Pack/220g	396	13.4	180	5.1	26.1	6.1	1.2
Cous Cous, BFY, Morrisons*	½ Pot/113g	164	4.0	145	4.6	23.8	3.5	0.5
Cous Cous, BGTY, Sainsbury's*	1 Pot/200g	236	4.4	118	4.7	19.7	2.2	2.8
Cous Cous, Tesco*	1 Serving/25g	35	0.4	141	4.8	26.9	1.6	0.6
Cous Cous, Waitrose*	1 Pot/200g	344	10.0	172	4.9	26.9	5.0	1.4
Cous Cous & Roast Vegetable, GFY, Asda*	1 Serving/100g	120	1.6	120	3.5	23.0	1.6	2.7
Cous Cous & Roasted Vegetable, Salad Bar, Waitrose*	1 Serving/100g	180	6.1	180	0.0	0.0	6.1	0.0
Cous Cous with Chargrilled Chicken, Sainsbury's*	1 Pack/240g	446	20.9	186	7.4	19.6	8.7	0.0
Crisp, Mixed, Morrisons*	1 Pack/230g	39	0.7	17	1.0	2.8	0.3	0.0
Crisp & Crunchy, Asda*	1 Pack/250g	55	1.5	22	0.8	3.3	0.6	1.4
Crisp & Crunchy with French Dressing, GFY, Asda*	1/3 Pack/116g	26	0.7	22	0.8	3.3	0.6	1.4
Crisp & Light, M & S*	1 Serving/170g	51	1.4	30	0.5	5.4	0.8	1.0
Crisp & Sweet Lettuce Leaves, Florette*	¼ Pack/70g	10	0.3	14	0.8	1.7	0.5	0.9
Crisp Mixed, Tesco*	1 Pack/200g	40	0.6	20	1.1	3.2	0.3	2.0
Crispy, Co-Op*	1 Serving/80g	13	0.2	16	0.8	3.0	0.3	1.0
Crispy, Florette*	1 Portion/100g	22	0.3	22	1.5	3.4	0.3	3.0
Crispy, Tesco*	1oz/28g	6	0.1	20	1.2	3.0	0.3	1.6
Crispy Crunch, Lasting Leaf*	1 Serving/75g	13	0.3	18	1.1	1.5	0.4	1.9

SALAD

INFO/WEIGHT	Measure KCAL	FAT	KCAL	PROT	CARB	FAT	FIBRE
Crispy Duck & Herb, M & S*	½ Pack/140g	378	25.6	270	20.7	3.7	18.3	1.4
Crispy Green, Sainsbury's*	1 Serving/70g	8	0.1	12	0.9	1.6	0.2	0.8
Crispy Leaf, Sainsbury's*	½ Pack/68g	9	0.3	14	1.0	1.7	0.4	1.7
Crispy Medley, Waitrose*	1 Serving/50g	7	0.2	15	0.8	1.7	0.5	0.9
Crunchy, Fully Prepared, Sainsbury's*	½ Pack/150g	24	0.1	16	1.1	3.0	0.1	1.7
Crunchy, Simple, M & S*	1 Serving/50g	7	0.2	15	1.0	1.6	0.5	1.8
Crunchy, Tesco*	1 Serving/56g	11	0.2	19	1.2	2.8	0.3	2.1
Crunchy, Waitrose*	½ Pack100g	18	0.4	18	1.0	2.6	0.4	1.5
Crunchy Layered, Tesco*	1 Serving/54g	15	0.2	27	1.1	4.9	0.3	1.7
Crunchy Mix, Co-Op*	1 Bag/200g	10	0.2	10	0.9	1.7	0.2	1.5
Crunchy Oriental Slaw, Salad Bar, Waitrose*	1 Serving/100g	68	2.8	68	0.0	0.0	2.8	0.0
Crunchy Spring, Side, M & S*	1 Serving/160g	32	0.3	20	0.9	4.1	0.2	1.3
Cucumber & Cherry Tomato, Fresh Tastes, Asda*	1 Serving/100g	22	0.3	22	1.6	2.4	0.3	0.0
Eat Me Keep Me, Tesco*	1 Serving/80g	14	0.2	18	0.8	3.0	0.3	1.7
Edamame & Butterbean, TTD, Sainsbury's*	1/3 Pack/62g	70	2.5	113	6.6	9.9	4.1	4.9
Edamame Bean, Oriental Style, Asda*	1 Pack/220g	183	8.4	83	4.8	7.3	3.8	4.0
Edamame Beans & Peppers, Delicious, Boots*	1 Pack/87g	121	2.3	139	0.0	4.1	2.6	0.0
Egg, Fresh4you*	1 Pack/55g	139	12.2	252	8.3	4.6	22.2	0.0
Egg & Baby Spinach, Waitrose*	1 Pack/215g	167	13.5	78	3.5	1.8	6.3	1.0
Egg & Coleslaw, Boots*	1 Pot/233g	405	37.3	174	3.0	4.6	16.0	1.0
Egg & Ham, with Salad Cream Dressing, M & S*	1 Pack/240g	168	8.4	70	5.2	4.0	3.5	0.6
Egg & Potato, Fresh, M & S*	1 Serving/250g	150	7.2	60	3.0	4.6	2.9	0.9
English Garden, Tesco*	1 Serving/180g	22	0.4	12	0.7	1.8	0.2	0.7
Exotic, with Mango & Chilli Dressing, Co-Op*	½ Pack/65g	25	0.4	38	0.6	7.7	0.6	0.8
Family, Florette*	1 Serving/50g	14	0.1	29	1.1	5.5	0.2	3.0
Feta Cheese & Sunblushed Tomato, M & S*	1 Serving/190g	361	21.1	190	5.5	17.2	11.1	2.1
Fine Cut, Asda*	1oz/28g	7	0.1	24	1.2	4.1	0.3	2.1
Fine Noodle with Duck Breast, COU, M & S*	1 Pack/280g	294	3.1	105	5.5	18.9	1.1	1.1
Florida, Retail, Average	1oz/28g	63	5.7	224	0.9	9.7	20.5	1.0
Four Bean, Finest, Tesco*	1 Pack/225g	259	9.4	115	5.0	14.2	4.2	4.6
Four Bean, Sainsbury's*	½ Pot/113g	114	2.5	101	6.7	6.2	2.2	15.0
Four Bean & Buckwheat, Waitrose*	1/3 Pack/67g	79	1.9	117	4.9	17.9	2.8	5.0
Four Leaf, M & S*	1 Serving/130g	19	0.4	15	0.9	2.0	0.3	1.4
Four Leaf, Tesco*	1oz/28g	4	0.1	15	0.8	1.8	0.5	0.9
French Goat's Cheese, Extra Fine, Asda*	1 Pack/185g	462	35.1	250	8.4	11.4	19.0	0.8
French Style, M & S*	1 Pack/140g	140	13.6	100	1.0	2.5	9.7	0.9
French Style, Morrisons*	1 Pack/200g	28	1.0	14	0.8	1.7	0.5	0.0
French Style, Waitrose*	½ Pack/82g	149	12.1	182	5.1	7.2	14.8	1.8
Fresh & Crispy, Tesco*	1 Serving/230g	30	0.7	13	0.7	1.9	0.3	1.3
Fruity Moroccan Cous Cous, Waitrose*	1 Pack/90g	139	3.2	154	5.0	25.6	3.6	4.6
Fruity Tabbouleh, Salad Bar, Waitrose*	1 Serving/100g	184	6.6	184	0.0	0.0	6.6	0.0
Fusion, Fully Prepared, Sainsbury's*	½ Pack/63g	15	0.5	24	3.7	0.3	0.8	3.4
Garden, Classic, Morrisons*	1 Tray/175g	33	0.5	19	0.8	3.2	0.3	2.8
Garden, Side, Asda*	1 Pack/175g	31	0.5	18	0.9	2.8	0.3	1.3
Garden, Sweet & Crispy, Tesco*	1 Bag/225g	54	0.9	24	1.0	4.2	0.4	1.4
Garden, Sweet & Crunchy, Tesco*	1 Pack/225g	54	0.9	24	1.0	4.2	0.4	1.4
Garden, Tesco*	1 Serving/225g	34	0.7	15	1.0	2.0	0.3	0.9
Garden, Tray, Asda*	½ Pack/88g	16	0.3	18	0.7	3.1	0.3	1.6
Garden Side with Dressing, Waitrose*	1 Pack/184g	101	8.1	55	12.0	2.6	4.4	13.0
Garden with Watercress, M & S*	1 Salad/80g	10	0.1	12	1.5	1.4	0.1	1.4
Garden with Yoghurt & Mint Dressing, GFY, Asda*	1 Serving/195g	51	1.9	26	1.1	3.2	1.0	0.0
Goat's Cheese, Sainsbury's*	1 Pack/192g	242	12.9	126	5.0	10.6	6.7	1.7
Goat's Cheese & Cous Cous, Waitrose*	1 Pack/300g	372	14.4	124	4.8	15.3	4.8	2.2

S

SALAD

	Measure INFO/WEIGHT	per Measure KCAL	FAT	Nutrition Values per 100g / 100ml KCAL	PROT	CARB	FAT	FIBRE
Goji Berry, Graze*	1 Pack/45g	234	17.3	521	17.1	28.4	38.4	0.0
Gourmet Chargrilled Chicken & Bacon, Atkins*	1 Pack/245g	311	20.1	127	12.0	2.5	8.2	1.0
Gourmet Continental, Waitrose*	1 Serving/150g	22	0.7	15	0.8	1.7	0.5	0.9
Greek	1oz/28g	36	3.5	130	2.7	1.9	12.5	0.8
Greek, BGTY, Sainsbury's*	1 Serving/199g	133	5.0	67	2.0	9.0	2.5	0.8
Greek, Classic, Tesco*	1 Pack/255g	293	23.7	115	2.6	5.2	9.3	1.2
Greek, Salad Bar, Waitrose*	1 Serving/100g	103	7.8	103	0.0	0.0	7.8	0.0
Greek, Side, Waitrose*	1 Pack/150g	156	12.1	104	3.2	4.6	8.1	0.9
Greek, Tesco*	1 Serving/200g	188	14.2	94	3.2	4.3	7.1	0.9
Greek, with Basil and Mint Oil Dressing, M & S*	1 Pack/200g	220	19.6	110	3.6	2.2	9.8	1.5
Greek Feta & Pepper, with Cous Cous, Asda*	1 Pack /316g	262	10.4	83	3.2	10.2	3.3	0.0
Greek Style, Delphi*	1 Serving/220g	306	27.1	139	3.7	3.5	12.3	0.9
Greek Style, Fresh, Food Counter, Sainsbury's*	1 Serving/166g	247	23.2	149	1.9	2.7	14.0	0.0
Greek Style, Waitrose*	½ Pack/125g	54	2.7	43	1.9	4.0	2.2	1.2
Greek Style, with Herb Dressing, Tesco*	1 Pack/240g	305	28.3	127	3.2	2.0	11.8	1.0
Greek Style, with Houmous Dip, & Pitta, Sainsbury's*	1 Bowl/195g	296	17.4	152	5.4	12.5	8.9	2.6
Greek Style, with White Wine Vinaigrette, Tesco*	1 Pack/235g	256	22.3	109	3.5	2.3	9.5	1.5
Greek Style Feta, Tip & Mix, M & S*	1 Pack/195g	214	18.3	110	4.0	2.5	9.4	1.6
Greek Style Layered, Perfectly Balanced, Waitrose*	1 Pack/280g	134	7.8	48	2.4	3.2	2.8	0.7
Green, Average	1oz/28g	4	0.1	13	0.8	1.8	0.3	0.9
Green, Complete, Sainsbury's*	1/3 Pack/55g	92	6.7	168	4.2	10.3	12.2	1.4
Green, Crispy, Fresh, Sainsbury's*	1 Serving/40g	5	0.1	12	0.9	1.6	0.2	0.8
Green, M & S*	1oz/28g	4	0.1	13	0.8	1.7	0.3	0.9
Green, Mixed, Average	1oz/28g	3	0.1	12	0.7	1.8	0.3	1.0
Green Lentil, Red Pepper & Spinach, Waitrose*	1 Pack/250g	485	20.0	194	8.6	22.0	8.0	2.9
Green Side, M & S*	1 Serving/200g	30	0.4	15	0.9	2.5	0.2	0.0
Green Side, Sainsbury's*	1 Pack/200g	28	0.2	14	1.2	2.1	0.1	1.4
Green Side, Tesco*	1 Serving/100g	12	0.3	12	0.7	1.6	0.3	1.3
Green with Chives, Tesco*	½ Pack/90g	13	0.4	14	1.0	1.6	0.4	1.7
Green with Honey & Mustard Dressing, M & S*	1 Pack/200g	120	9.6	60	0.9	2.7	4.8	0.8
Ham, Antony Worrall Thompson's*	1 Pack/202g	257	2.6	127	9.8	19.1	1.3	2.7
Ham & Free Range Egg, Fresh Tastes, Asda*	1 Bowl/265g	167	9.3	63	5.7	2.2	3.5	0.8
Ham Hock, Waitrose*	1 Pack/350g	245	9.5	70	6.6	4.8	2.7	2.0
Herb, Asda*	1 Serving/20g	2	0.1	12	1.8	0.6	0.3	2.0
Herb, M & S*	1 Pack/100g	20	0.4	20	2.9	1.4	0.4	1.9
Herb, Organic, Sainsbury's*	1 Serving/100g	17	0.5	17	1.8	1.3	0.5	1.8
Herb, Sainsbury's*	1 Pack/120g	22	0.6	18	2.7	0.8	0.5	2.2
Herb, Tesco*	1oz/28g	4	0.1	16	1.1	1.8	0.5	0.9
Herb Garden, Morrisons*	1 Serving/28g	4	0.1	14	0.9	1.7	0.5	0.0
Honey Smoked Salmon & New Potato, M & S*	1 Pack/270g	270	14.3	100	5.5	7.5	5.3	1.5
Hot, Roasted Beetroot, Lentil & Goats Cheese, M & S*	1 Pack/295g	354	8.6	120	4.9	16.6	2.9	3.3
Houmous, Delicious, Boots*	1 Pack/230g	154	4.4	67	5.3	7.4	1.9	3.1
Iceberg & Cabbage, Asda*	½ Pack/125g	24	0.4	19	1.0	3.1	0.3	1.5
Indian Spiced Chicken, Waitrose*	1 Pack/280g	328	12.0	117	7.8	8.9	4.3	5.6
Italian, Complete, Sainsbury's*	1 Pack/160g	237	14.4	148	5.4	11.4	9.0	1.6
Italian Style, Asda*	1 Serving/20g	3	0.1	15	1.1	1.6	0.5	1.2
Italian Style, Organic, Waitrose*	½ Pack/45g	7	0.2	15	0.8	1.7	0.5	0.9
Italian Style, Tesco*	1/3 Pack/40g	6	0.2	16	1.0	1.9	0.5	1.2
Italian Style, with Rocket & Lambs Lettuce, M & S*	½ Bag/60g	12	0.3	20	1.3	2.3	0.5	1.3
Italian Wild Rocket & Parmesan, Sainsbury's*	1 Serving/50g	88	7.4	177	7.5	3.4	14.8	0.5
Jardin, Tesco*	1 Serving/50g	7	0.3	14	0.8	1.8	0.6	1.4
King Prawn, GFY, Asda*	1 Serving/175g	112	2.6	64	4.7	8.0	1.5	1.3
King Prawn, Thai Style, M & S*	1 Pack/295g	265	7.4	90	4.4	12.6	2.5	1.3

S

SALAD	INFO/WEIGHT	per Measure KCAL	FAT	Nutrition Values per 100g / 100ml KCAL	PROT	CARB	FAT	FIBRE
King Prawn & New Potato, COU, M & S*	1 Pack/300g	180	6.9	60	3.0	6.9	2.3	0.8
King Prawn & Pasta, COU, M & S*	1 Pack/270g	283	6.5	105	5.9	15.1	2.4	2.7
Layered, King Prawn & Mango, Love Life, Waitrose*	1 Pack/300g	195	4.2	65	3.9	9.2	1.4	1.7
Leaf, Crispy, Asda*	1 Serving/80g	11	0.4	14	0.8	1.6	0.5	0.9
Leafy, Organic, Sainsbury's*	½ Pack/50g	7	0.1	15	1.7	1.3	0.3	1.8
Leafy, Tesco*	1oz/28g	4	0.1	14	1.2	1.5	0.4	1.9
Leafy, with Tatsoi, Sainsbury's*	1 Bag/115g	17	0.4	15	1.0	1.6	0.3	1.7
Leafy Mixed, Co-Op*	1 Bag/200g	40	0.6	20	1.0	4.0	0.3	1.0
Leaves, Oriental Mix, Waitrose*	1 Bag/100g	18	0.6	18	1.5	1.7	0.6	1.9
Leek & Pork Deli, Continental, Aldi*	¼ Tub/63g	68	3.1	108	1.9	13.9	5.0	2.3
Lemon Cous Cous & Roasted Pepper, COU, M & S*	1 Pack/340g	306	7.8	90	3.2	14.6	2.3	1.8
Lovely Summer, Jamie Oliver*	½ Bag/60g	48	4.0	80	1.7	4.0	6.6	1.2
Mediterranean, Side, Sainsbury's*	1 Pack/170g	44	2.2	26	0.9	2.7	1.3	1.3
Mediterranean Pasta, Salad Bar, Waitrose*	1 Serving/100g	156	4.0	156	0.0	0.0	4.0	0.0
Mediterranean Style, Asda*	½ Pack/135g	22	0.0	16	1.0	3.0	0.0	0.0
Mediterranean Style, Morrisons*	1 Serving/90g	13	0.2	14	1.5	1.9	0.2	0.0
Mexican Style Bean & Cheese, M & S*	½ Pot/150g	150	5.2	100	6.1	11.2	3.5	4.8
Mix, Crisp & Sweet Lettuce Leaves, Florette*	1 Portion/67g	12	0.2	18	1.5	1.2	0.3	2.5
Mix with Cabbage, Beetroot & Carrot, Florette*	½ Pack/100g	30	0.2	30	1.3	4.4	0.2	0.0
Mixed, Crisp, Mild, Tesco*	½ Pack/145g	29	0.4	20	1.2	3.0	0.3	2.1
Mixed, Florette*	1 Serving/100g	20	0.2	20	1.3	3.4	0.2	3.0
Mixed, Green Leaf, Lasting Leaf*	1 Serving/69g	12	0.3	17	0.8	1.8	0.4	1.5
Mixed, Iceland*	1 Serving/50g	12	0.1	24	1.2	4.3	0.2	2.1
Mixed, Sainsbury's*	1 Serving/100g	21	0.2	21	1.4	3.4	0.2	2.1
Mixed, Sweet & Crispy, Tesco*	1 Serving/200g	48	0.6	24	1.0	4.2	0.3	2.0
Mixed, Sweet & Crunchy, Lasting Leaf*	1 Serving/62g	15	0.2	24	0.8	3.6	0.3	1.9
Mixed, Tesco*	1 Serving/100g	24	0.3	24	1.0	4.2	0.3	2.0
Mixed Bean, Asda*	½ Can/145g	126	3.6	87	5.0	11.0	2.5	6.0
Mixed Bean, Canned, Waitrose*	1 Can/270g	251	1.6	93	6.4	15.5	0.6	5.5
Mixed Bean, Morrisons*	1 Serving/145g	129	1.7	89	5.8	13.7	1.2	0.0
Mixed Bean, Sainsbury's*	1 Can/270g	227	2.4	84	5.4	13.5	0.9	3.8
Mixed Bean, Tesco*	1 Serving/70g	49	0.3	70	3.2	13.1	0.5	1.9
Mixed Fish & Leaves	1 Serving/250g	203	9.5	81	5.3	6.8	3.8	0.8
Mixed Leaf, Asda*	1 Serving/100g	21	0.2	21	1.5	3.2	0.2	2.1
Mixed Leaf, Tomato, Feta, Boots*	1 Pack/179g	218	17.0	122	3.7	5.4	9.5	1.0
Mixed Leaf, Tomato & Olive, Tesco*	1 Serving/170g	150	13.3	88	1.0	3.4	7.8	0.0
Mixed Leaf & Baby Basil, a Taste of Italy, Florette*	1 Pack/155g	143	8.2	92	2.7	8.5	5.3	1.0
Mixed Leaf Medley, Waitrose*	1 Serving/25g	4	0.1	15	0.8	1.7	0.5	1.4
Mixed Leaf Tomato & Olive, Tesco*	1 Serving/170g	150	13.3	88	1.0	3.4	7.8	2.0
Mixed Leaves, Bondelle*	1 Serving/50g	10	0.1	21	1.4	3.3	0.2	0.0
Mixed Leaves, Tesco*	1 Serving/20g	3	0.1	14	0.9	1.6	0.4	0.9
Mixed Leaves, with Beetroot, Earthy, Waitrose*	1 Bag/140g	34	0.6	24	1.5	3.6	0.4	2.1
Mixed Pepper, Asda*	½ Pack/100g	24	0.3	24	1.0	4.3	0.3	1.7
Mixed Vegetable, Aldi*	1 Serving/200g	120	4.0	60	0.6	10.0	2.0	0.0
Moroccan Style, Chicken, Shapers, Boots*	1 Pack/240g	230	4.3	96	5.6	13.0	1.8	1.6
Moroccan Styles, COU, M & S*	½ Pack/100g	160	1.2	160	5.0	32.8	1.2	4.8
Mozzarella & Cherry Tomato, Shapers, Boots*	1 Bowl/194g	184	14.2	95	4.1	3.3	7.3	0.9
Mozzarella & Rocket, Asda*	1 Serving/265g	435	31.8	164	7.0	7.0	12.0	1.5
Mozzarella & Sunkissed Tomato, Tesco*	1 Bag/160g	270	22.9	169	4.6	4.3	14.3	2.1
Mozzarella & Tomato, M & S*	1 Serving/310g	400	14.8	129	5.5	15.5	4.8	0.9
New Potato, Co-Op*	1 Serving/50g	97	8.0	195	1.0	10.0	16.0	2.0
New Potato, Less Than 5% Fat, M & S*	1 Serving/110g	88	3.4	80	1.3	12.1	3.1	1.5
New Potato, Luxury, Morrisons*	½ Tub/125g	341	30.7	273	1.7	11.2	24.6	0.0

SALAD

	Measure INFO/WEIGHT	per Measure KCAL	FAT	Nutrition Values per 100g / 100ml KCAL	PROT	CARB	FAT	FIBRE
New Potato, M & S*	1 Serving/60g	114	9.8	190	0.9	9.9	16.3	1.3
New Potato, Tomato & Egg with Salad Cream, M & S*	1 Pack/300g	165	7.2	55	2.9	5.4	2.4	1.3
New Potato, Tuna & Egg, M & S*	1 Pack/340g	255	12.9	75	3.8	6.7	3.8	0.7
New Potato & Free Range Egg, M & S*	1 Pack/305g	213	11.6	70	2.5	7.0	3.8	0.8
New Potato & Free Range Egg, Side, Sainsbury's*	1 Pack/290g	174	12.2	60	2.5	3.1	4.2	1.4
New Potato & King Prawn, M & S*	1 Pack/210g	220	9.4	105	5.6	10.2	4.5	1.7
New Potato & Sweet Chilli Prawn, M & S*	1 Pack/210g	147	1.0	70	2.8	14.0	0.5	0.7
New Potato & Tuna Sweetcorn, Eat Well, M & S*	1 Pack/190g	133	3.4	70	5.4	8.4	1.8	1.9
Nicoise, Tesco*	1 Pack/260g	286	21.8	110	3.2	5.3	8.4	1.4
Nicoise Style, Layered, Waitrose*	1 Bowl/275g	129	3.8	47	2.7	5.8	1.4	1.0
Noodle, Sweet Chilli Chicken, Shapers, Boots*	1 Serving/197g	256	4.1	130	11.0	17.0	2.1	1.1
Noodle, Thai Style, BGTY, Sainsbury's*	1 Pack/185g	150	3.5	81	2.7	13.5	1.9	0.0
Noodle & King Prawn, Perfectly Balanced, Waitrose*	1 Pack/225g	223	2.2	99	5.0	17.4	1.0	1.0
Noodle & Sesame, Salad Bar, Waitrose*	1 Serving/100g	178	11.5	178	0.0	0.0	11.5	0.0
Noodle with Thai Style Chicken, M & S*	½ Pot/145g	159	7.1	110	5.2	11.6	4.9	1.4
Nutty Rice, Love Life, Waitrose*	1 Portion/200g	368	14.4	184	4.5	25.3	7.2	3.1
Nutty Super Wholefood, M & S*	½ Pack/115g	149	5.9	130	5.3	12.8	5.1	6.1
Orzo & Sunbaked Tomato, BGTY, Sainsbury's*	1 Tub/276g	292	6.1	106	3.1	18.5	2.2	2.5
Pasta, Chicken & Sweetcorn, Morrisons*	1 Serving/220g	255	3.5	116	6.7	18.7	1.6	1.0
Pasta, Tomato, Morrisons*	1 Serving/50g	46	0.6	92	3.0	17.3	1.2	2.4
Pasta, Tuna & Sweetcorn, Morrisons*	1 Serving/100g	227	15.1	227	5.0	16.1	15.1	2.2
Pasta & Cheese, Asda*	1 Serving/125g	319	23.7	255	6.0	15.0	19.0	1.2
Pasta & Garlic, Iceland*	1 Serving/75g	149	10.7	199	2.2	15.4	14.3	1.6
Pasta & Mushroom, Waitrose*	1 Pack/200g	320	19.4	160	4.1	14.0	9.7	0.6
Pasta & Pepper Side, Tesco*	1 Pack/230g	278	15.2	121	2.4	13.0	6.6	1.3
Pasta & Sweetcorn, Less Than 3% Fat, M & S*	½ Pack/100g	85	1.4	85	2.8	14.7	1.4	1.5
Pasta & Tomato, GFY, Asda*	1 Pack/300g	348	9.3	116	3.0	19.0	3.1	1.6
Pasta with Roasted Vegetables, Salad Bar, Waitrose*	1 Serving/100g	148	4.0	148	0.0	0.0	4.0	0.0
Pea Shoots & Baby Leaves, Steve's Leaves*	1 Pack/60g	14	0.4	24	2.7	2.0	0.6	2.0
Pepper, Sweetcorn & Cucumber, Salad Bar, Waitrose*	1 Serving/100g	71	3.1	71	0.0	0.0	3.1	0.0
Potato, 30% Less Fat, BGTY, Sainsbury's*	1 Serving/60g	64	3.7	106	1.7	11.1	6.1	1.1
Potato, Asda*	¼ Pot/57g	67	4.0	117	0.9	12.5	7.0	1.1
Potato, Creamy, Asda*	1oz/28g	61	5.2	219	1.0	11.9	18.6	0.7
Potato, Creamy, Waitrose*	1 Serving/100g	163	11.9	163	1.3	12.7	11.9	1.1
Potato, Finest, Tesco*	1 Tub/250g	587	51.5	235	2.4	9.7	20.6	1.2
Potato, From Salad Selection, Sainsbury's*	1 Serving/50g	102	8.7	204	1.0	10.5	17.5	1.3
Potato, GFY, Asda*	½ Pack/125g	145	8.7	116	1.3	12.0	7.0	0.0
Potato, Heinz*	½ Can/97g	137	8.2	141	1.4	14.8	8.5	0.8
Potato, HL, Tesco*	1 Tub/250g	287	12.0	115	1.7	15.4	4.8	1.2
Potato, Iceland*	1 Serving/75g	162	14.7	216	1.1	8.9	19.6	0.6
Potato, Light Choices, Tesco*	1 Pack/100g	110	5.9	110	1.3	12.5	5.9	0.9
Potato, Luxury, Asda*	1 Serving/50g	118	10.5	237	1.0	11.0	21.0	0.0
Potato, M & S*	1oz/28g	55	4.8	195	1.2	8.5	17.3	1.3
Potato, Perfectly Balanced, Waitrose*	½ Pot/125g	99	3.7	79	2.4	10.5	3.0	1.0
Potato, Salad Bar, Asda*	1oz/28g	52	4.3	187	0.6	11.6	15.4	1.1
Potato, Side, Waitrose*	1 Pack/250g	181	11.0	72	3.0	5.2	4.4	1.0
Potato, Tesco*	1 Serving/100g	165	13.5	165	1.3	9.5	13.5	1.3
Potato, with Onions & Chives, Co-Op*	1 Serving/50g	80	6.0	160	1.0	12.0	12.0	1.0
Potato & Cheese, Pasta & Mixed Leaf, Waitrose*	1 Serving/205g	266	17.4	130	3.2	10.1	8.5	1.1
Potato & Cheese, Sainsbury's*	1 Serving/125g	200	16.4	160	2.7	7.9	13.1	3.4
Potato & Egg, with Mayonnaise, Tesco*	½ Tub/150g	115	8.5	77	2.9	3.1	5.7	1.2
Potato Layered, Tesco*	1 Pack/350g	283	17.2	81	1.3	7.8	4.9	1.3
Potato with Mayonnaise	1oz/28g	67	5.8	239	1.6	12.2	20.8	0.9

S

SALAD

INFO/WEIGHT	Measure		Nutrition Values per 100g / 100ml				
	KCAL	FAT	KCAL	PROT	CARB	FAT	FIBRE
Potato with Mayonnaise, Retail	1oz/28g	80	7.4	287	1.5	11.4	26.5	0.8
Potato with Reduced Calorie Dressing, Retail	1oz/28g	27	1.1	97	1.3	14.8	4.1	0.8
Prawn, King, with Noodles, Delicious, Boots*	1 Pack/228g	251	3.7	110	6.3	18.0	1.6	1.8
Prawn, King & Rice Noodle, M & S*	1 Pack/320g	208	2.6	65	2.9	11.6	0.8	0.9
Prawn, Layered, Asda*	1 Tub/380g	403	15.6	106	5.0	11.5	4.1	0.0
Prawn, Layered, Individual, Tesco*	1 Pack/180g	215	10.0	120	4.3	12.5	5.6	1.4
Prawn, Layered, Sainsbury's*	1 Pack/275g	355	21.2	129	3.6	11.2	7.7	1.1
Prawn, Layered, Single Size, Asda*	1 Serving/197g	217	9.8	110	4.3	12.0	5.0	1.0
Prawn, Layered, Tesco*	1 Pack/180g	243	13.0	135	4.2	13.1	7.2	2.0
Prawn, Tesco*	1 Pack/280g	314	14.0	112	4.7	12.0	5.0	0.9
Prawn & Avocado, M & S*	1 Serving/220g	176	15.0	80	3.0	2.0	6.8	3.1
Prawn & Egg, Leaf, Shapers, Boots*	1 Pack/182g	193	14.4	106	6.7	2.1	7.9	1.0
Prawn Cocktail, HL, Tesco*	1 Serving/300g	279	3.0	93	5.7	15.3	1.0	2.0
Prawn Cocktail, Shapers, Boots*	1 Pack/245g	120	5.9	49	4.7	2.2	2.4	0.7
Prawn Cocktail, Tesco*	1 Pack/300g	360	18.0	120	5.7	10.9	6.0	0.8
Prawn Layer, Eat Well, M & S*	1 Pack/220g	143	4.6	65	4.3	6.9	2.1	1.4
Prawn Layered, Co-Op*	1 Pack/300g	375	18.0	125	4.0	14.0	6.0	2.0
Prawn Layered, M & S*	1 Pack/455g	409	17.7	90	4.5	8.9	3.9	1.2
Prawn Satay & Noodle, Tesco*	1 Serving/250g	320	17.0	128	7.1	9.5	6.8	1.2
Primavera, Finest, Tesco*	1 Pack/100g	25	0.6	25	2.4	2.4	0.6	2.6
Rainbow, Sainsbury's*	1 Pack/215g	300	14.8	140	5.5	13.8	6.9	3.9
Red Cabbage & Sweetcorn, Crunchy, M & S*	1 Serving/80g	28	0.4	35	1.3	6.6	0.5	1.2
Red Skinned Potato, Salad Bar, Waitrose*	1 Serving/100g	136	9.0	136	0.0	0.0	9.0	0.0
Red Thai Chicken with Noodles, Tesco*	1 Pack/300g	342	1.5	114	7.2	20.2	0.5	1.4
Rice, Courgette & Pine Nut, BGTY, Sainsbury's*	1/3 Pot/65g	68	1.0	105	2.7	20.0	1.6	1.5
Rice, Lentil & Mushroom, Salad Bar, Waitrose*	1 Serving/100g	135	5.4	135	0.0	0.0	5.4	0.0
Richly Dressed Coleslaw, Salad Bar, Waitrose*	1 Serving/100g	134	11.8	134	0.0	0.0	11.8	0.0
Roast Butternut Squash & Fennel, TTD, Sainsbury's*	1 Pack/165g	214	7.6	130	3.4	15.2	4.6	6.9
Roast Chicken, Layered, HL, Tesco*	1 Salad/400g	268	4.4	67	5.8	8.4	1.1	2.1
Roast Chicken, Tesco*	1 Salad/300g	348	22.2	116	5.3	7.0	7.4	1.0
Roast Pepper Cous Cous, HL, Tesco*	1 Pot/220g	308	4.6	140	5.6	24.3	2.1	1.7
Roasted Artichoke & Pepper, M & S*	1 Serving/220g	638	53.9	290	4.1	12.8	24.5	5.1
Roasted Vegetables & Cous Cous, Sainsbury's*	1 Pot/225g	378	24.1	168	5.3	12.6	10.7	1.9
Rocket, Leafy, Asda*	1 Serving/75g	10	0.1	13	1.5	1.4	0.1	1.8
Rocket, Morrisons*	1 Serving/100g	14	0.5	14	0.8	1.7	0.5	0.0
Rocket, Tesco*	1oz/28g	4	0.1	14	0.8	1.7	0.5	0.9
Salmon, Hot Smoked with Potato Salad, M & S*	1 Pack/338g	270	7.4	80	4.5	10.3	2.2	1.3
Salmon & Roquette, M & S*	1 Serving/255g	306	20.4	120	3.9	8.5	8.0	1.0
Santa Plum Tomato & Avocado, M & S*	1 Pack/240g	348	32.2	145	1.7	4.1	13.4	0.2
Santa Plum Tomato with Dressing, M & S*	1 Pack/225g	135	10.8	60	0.9	3.1	4.8	0.9
Santa Tomato, Side, M & S*	1 Pack/225g	146	12.4	65	0.8	3.3	5.5	0.9
Santini, Side, M & S*	1 Pack/195g	127	11.1	65	1.0	3.0	5.7	2.0
Sea Food, Family Mart*	1 Serving/100g	29	0.6	29	1.6	4.1	0.6	0.0
Seafood, Marinated, M & S*	1 Serving/90g	108	5.8	120	13.4	2.3	6.4	0.8
Seafood, Marinated, Waitrose*	1 Tub/160g	235	10.6	147	16.3	5.5	6.6	0.0
Seafood, Sunkis*	1 Tub/100g	83	3.9	83	4.6	7.4	3.9	0.0
Seasonal, Organic, Waitrose*	1/4 Pack/25g	4	0.1	15	0.8	1.7	0.5	0.9
Seasonal Potato, Salad Bar, Waitrose*	1 Serving/100g	109	3.4	109	0.0	0.0	3.4	0.0
Selection, Fresh, M & S*	1 Pack/230g	32	0.7	14	0.7	2.1	0.3	0.9
Selection, Side, M & S*	1 Serving/255g	153	12.7	60	1.1	2.5	5.0	1.3
Shredded Beetroot, Asda*	1 Serving/140g	29	0.4	21	1.1	3.5	0.3	1.5
Side, Baby Potato And Free Range Egg, Asda*	1 Pack/305g	204	11.3	67	2.5	6.0	3.7	1.0
Side, Fresh & Crispy, Tesco*	1 Salad/230g	30	0.7	13	0.7	1.9	0.3	1.3

SALAD

INFO/WEIGHT	Measure	per Measure KCAL	FAT	Nutrition Values per 100g / 100ml KCAL	PROT	CARB	FAT	FIBRE
Side, Garden, with Cherry Tomatoes, Waitrose*	1 Pack/170g	25	0.7	15	0.8	2.0	0.4	1.3
Simply Chicken, Ginsters*	1 Pack/187g	317	6.9	170	11.4	22.7	3.7	0.0
Skipjack Tuna, John West*	1 Can/192g	190	11.7	99	7.3	3.7	6.1	0.0
Smoked Ham, Weight Watchers*	1 Pack/181g	233	3.6	129	11.0	16.6	2.0	3.0
Spiced Potato, Salad Bar, Waitrose*	1 Serving/100g	88	2.0	88	0.0	0.0	2.0	0.0
Spicy Bean, Tesco*	1 Serving/125g	111	2.9	89	4.9	12.1	2.3	2.5
Spicy Chicken Couscous, Fresh Tastes, Asda*	1 Pack/230g	230	7.6	100	5.9	11.6	3.3	0.0
Spicy Chickpea, BGTY, Sainsbury's*	½ Pack/125g	119	2.1	95	4.7	15.3	1.7	5.5
Spicy Chickpea & Halloumi, Cranks*	1 Pack/238g	295	11.2	124	5.0	15.5	4.7	2.6
Spicy Mexican Bean, Salad Bar, Waitrose*	1 Serving/100g	119	4.7	119	0.0	0.0	4.7	0.0
Spicy Rice, Waitrose*	1 Serving/200g	318	13.2	159	3.2	21.7	6.6	0.9
Spinach, Rocket, & Watercress, Asda*	1 Serving/100g	21	0.6	21	2.8	1.2	0.6	1.9
Spinach, Waitrose*	1 Pack/100g	25	0.8	25	2.8	1.6	0.8	2.1
Spring, American Style, M & S*	1 Serving/60g	9	0.1	15	1.9	1.4	0.2	1.3
Sprouted Pea & Bean, Mint Dressing, Eat Well, M & S*	1 Pot/165g	181	8.7	110	7.3	8.7	5.3	7.4
Summer, M & S*	1oz/28g	6	0.1	20	0.8	3.6	0.4	1.2
Super Wholefood, with Blueberries & Mango, M & S*	1 Pack/215g	260	7.7	121	4.4	17.0	3.6	8.7
Super Wholefood Shaker, M & S*	1 Shaker/229g	389	23.6	170	5.6	13.9	10.3	5.6
Sweet, Baby Leaf Mix, Co-Op*	1 Serving/50g	7	0.2	15	0.8	2.0	0.5	2.0
Sweet, Crunchy, Mixed, Co-Op*	1 Serving/100g	35	0.3	35	1.1	5.9	0.3	1.8
Sweet, Layered, Tesco*	1 Serving/285g	80	1.1	28	1.1	5.0	0.4	1.6
Sweet, Shredded, Tesco*	1 Serving/100g	20	0.4	20	1.1	2.9	0.4	1.9
Sweet & Crispy, M & S*	1 Serving/140g	49	1.4	35	1.7	4.7	1.0	1.6
Sweet & Crispy, Side, Sainsbury's*	¼ Bag/93g	23	0.2	25	1.3	4.4	0.2	2.2
Sweet & Crunchy, Morrisons*	1 Serving/100g	20	0.3	20	0.8	4.0	0.3	1.3
Sweet & Crunchy, Sainsbury's*	1 Pack/150g	22	0.1	15	0.9	2.6	0.1	1.8
Sweet & Crunchy, Tesco*	1 Pack/285g	57	1.0	20	0.8	3.3	0.3	1.9
Sweet Carrot, 3% Fat, M & S*	1oz/28g	21	0.3	75	1.3	16.7	1.2	1.4
Sweet Carrot & Sultana, M & S*	1 Serving/100g	55	0.7	55	0.8	11.4	0.7	2.6
Sweet Chilli Chicken Noodle, COU, M & S*	1 Pack/340g	408	7.8	120	6.8	17.4	2.3	1.2
Sweet Green, M & S*	1 Serving/150g	22	0.4	15	1.5	1.3	0.3	2.0
Sweet Leaf, Fully Prepared, Fresh, Sainsbury's*	¼ Pack/75g	12	0.1	16	0.8	3.0	0.1	2.1
Sweet Leaf, M & S*	1 Pack/110g	38	0.9	35	1.5	5.3	0.8	2.1
Sweet Leaf, Sainsbury's*	1 Serving/100g	21	0.5	21	0.8	3.2	0.5	1.5
Sweet Leaf & Carrot, Asda*	½ Pack/164g	34	0.5	21	0.9	3.6	0.3	1.4
Sweet Leaf & Carrot, Lasting Leaf*	1 Serving/70g	16	0.3	23	1.0	2.8	0.4	2.2
Sweet Leafy, Organic, Tesco*	1 Serving/250g	45	1.0	18	0.8	2.7	0.4	1.9
Sweet Pepper, Medley, Waitrose*	½ Pack/100g	22	0.4	22	0.9	3.8	0.4	1.5
Sweet Pepper Side, Tesco*	1 Serving/54g	22	0.2	41	1.3	8.0	0.4	2.1
Sweet Pepper with Corn, Tesco*	1 Pack/270g	103	1.3	38	1.3	7.2	0.5	1.5
Tabbouleh, HL, Tesco*	1 Serving/200g	194	3.6	97	3.5	16.8	1.8	1.3
Tabbouleh, Salad Bar, Waitrose*	1 Serving/100g	94	1.7	94	0.0	0.0	1.7	0.0
Tabbouleh & Feta, Tesco*	1 Pack/225g	301	11.2	134	5.4	16.7	5.0	0.6
Tabbouleh Feta, Finest, Tesco*	1 Pack/225g	265	11.7	118	4.2	13.7	5.2	0.6
Tabbouleh Style, Perfectly Balanced, Waitrose*	1 Pack/225g	234	8.8	104	2.8	14.3	3.9	2.6
Tender Leaf, with Mizuna, Tesco*	1 Serving/30g	4	0.1	15	1.6	1.4	0.3	1.7
Tenderleaf, Waitrose*	1 Serving/200g	30	1.0	15	0.9	1.6	0.5	1.1
Tenderleaf, with Mizuna, Sainsbury's*	1 Serving/50g	10	0.3	20	3.6	0.2	0.6	2.2
Thai Style Chicken, M & S*	1 Serving/195g	205	3.7	105	6.7	15.1	1.9	1.9
Three Bean, Pot, Tesco*	1 Pot/210g	204	9.2	97	4.1	10.2	4.4	2.3
Three Bean, Sainsbury's*	1 Serving/125g	108	6.3	86	4.2	6.0	5.0	0.0
Three Bean, Tinned, Tesco*	1 Tin/160g	176	1.6	110	7.7	17.6	1.0	5.3
Three Bean, with Mint Vinaigrette, M & S*	1 Pack/250g	175	6.0	70	5.9	6.4	2.4	13.0

INFO/WEIGHT	Measure	per Measure		Nutrition Values per 100g / 100ml				
		KCAL	FAT	KCAL	PROT	CARB	FAT	FIBRE
SALAD								
Three Bean & Mint, Finest, Tesco*	½ Pot/115g	150	6.0	130	7.9	12.6	5.2	5.0
Three Bean & Pesto, Italian Style, Boots*	1 Serving/290g	374	12.5	129	8.3	14.0	4.3	1.8
Three Leaf Blend, Sainsbury's*	1 Pack/50g	9	0.3	19	1.7	1.8	0.6	1.2
Tiger Prawn & Pasta, GFY, Asda*	1 Serving/200g	250	5.8	125	4.6	20.0	2.9	2.0
Tomato, Avocado & Rocket, M & S*	1 Pack/350g	507	46.9	145	1.7	4.1	13.4	0.2
Tomato, Lettuce & Cucumber, Classics, M & S*	1 Serving/275g	151	11.5	55	0.9	3.3	4.2	1.6
Tomato & Cucumber, Ready to Eat, Morrisons*	¼ Pack/81g	17	0.2	21	0.9	3.7	0.3	2.0
Tomato & Mozzarella, Finest, Tesco*	1 Pack/175g	254	21.3	145	5.6	3.3	12.2	0.7
Tomato & Mozzarella, M & S*	1 Pack/220g	264	16.5	120	9.8	2.8	7.5	1.1
Tomato & Onion	1oz/28g	20	1.7	72	0.8	4.0	6.1	1.0
Tortellini & Chargrilled Vegetable, Tesco*	1 Serving/300g	492	23.1	164	5.1	18.7	7.7	1.7
Tortellini & Pepper, TTD, Sainsbury's*	1/3 Pack/74g	98	4.3	133	4.3	15.7	5.9	1.5
Trio Leaf, Lettuce, Asda*	1 Portion/80g	12	0.4	15	0.8	1.7	0.5	0.9
Tuna, Breton Style, Snack Pot, Carb Check, Heinz*	1 Pot/219g	239	13.8	109	8.4	4.6	6.3	1.5
Tuna, Layered, Tesco*	1 Serving/370g	466	29.2	126	4.4	9.4	7.9	1.0
Tuna, Pasta, Layered, Asda*	1 Serving/100g	98	2.8	98	5.4	12.7	2.8	1.9
Tuna, with Lemon Dressing, Tesco*	1 Serving/300g	282	24.0	94	4.2	1.4	8.0	1.0
Tuna & Mixed Bean	1 Serving/220g	287	14.4	131	9.5	11.2	6.6	3.7
Tuna & Three Bean, Healthily Balanced, M & S*	1 Serving/350g	332	10.1	95	8.7	8.8	2.9	4.6
Tuna & Tomato, Boots*	1 Pack/171g	150	10.3	88	6.5	2.0	6.0	1.0
Tuna & Vegetable, Tesco*	½ Can/140g	189	10.1	135	9.0	8.5	7.2	3.3
Tuna Layer, COU, M & S*	1 Pack/340g	272	8.8	80	6.2	7.5	2.6	1.5
Tuna Layered, Waitrose*	1 Bowl/300g	636	58.8	212	4.0	4.8	19.6	1.0
Tuna Nicoise, BGTY, Sainsbury's*	1 Pack/300g	315	6.0	105	6.3	15.5	2.0	2.5
Tuna Nicoise, Finest, Tesco*	1 Serving/250g	430	23.5	172	8.5	13.3	9.4	0.8
Tuna Nicoise, No Mayonnaise, Shapers, Boots*	1 Pack/276g	133	3.6	48	4.0	5.0	1.3	0.8
Tuscan Style Bean & Sunblush Tomato, Waitrose*	1 Pot/225g	308	10.8	137	5.6	17.9	4.8	1.0
Vegetable, Canned	1oz/28g	40	2.7	143	1.6	13.0	9.8	1.2
Vegetable, Heinz*	1 Can/195g	259	16.6	133	1.5	12.6	8.5	1.3
Vegetable, Nutty Grain, Eat Well, M & S*	1 Pack/230g	299	11.7	130	5.3	12.8	5.1	6.1
Vegetable, Salad Bar, Waitrose*	1 Serving/100g	206	2.9	206	0.0	0.0	2.9	0.0
Waldorf, Average	1 Serving/100g	193	17.7	193	1.4	7.5	17.7	1.3
Waldorf, TTD, Sainsbury's*	¼ Pot/69g	203	19.5	296	1.9	8.1	28.4	4.7
Wasabi Rocket & Cooler Leaves, Steve's Leaves*	1 Bag/60g	16	0.2	26	3.0	1.2	0.4	3.0
Watercress, Morrisons*	1 Bag/100g	17	0.7	17	1.7	1.2	0.7	0.0
Watercress, Mustard Leaf & Mizuna, M & S*	½ Pack/60g	9	0.2	15	2.4	0.4	0.3	3.0
Watercress, Spinach & Rocket, Tesco*	1 Serving/30g	7	0.2	22	3.0	0.8	0.8	1.9
Watercress, Spinach & Rocket, Waitrose*	1 Bag/145g	30	1.2	21	2.2	1.2	0.8	1.5
Watercress & Spinach, Asda*	1 Serving/50g	10	0.3	21	2.8	1.2	0.6	1.9
Wheat with Roasted Vegetables, Sainsbury's*	1 Pack/220g	339	18.3	154	3.3	17.0	8.3	4.5
Wholefood, Super, Nutritionally Balanced, M & S*	1 Pack/285g	271	8.0	95	2.6	14.7	2.8	3.5
Wild Red Rocket & Milder Leaves, Steve's Leaves*	1 Bag/500g	9	0.2	19	2.8	0.8	0.5	2.6
Wild Rice, Salad Bar, Waitrose*	1 Serving/100g	159	6.6	159	0.0	0.0	6.6	0.0
Wild Rocket, Spinach & Watercress, Asda*	1 Serving/100g	21	0.6	21	2.8	1.2	0.6	1.9
Wild Rocket & Chard, Waitrose*	½ Bag/53g	8	0.3	15	0.8	1.7	0.5	1.4
Winter Roasted Vegetable, Salad Bar, Waitrose*	1 Serving/100g	139	10.3	139	0.0	0.0	10.3	0.0
with Sweetcorn, Side, Tesco*	1 Serving/135g	51	0.7	38	1.3	7.2	0.5	1.5
Young, Whole Leaf, Tesco*	1 Pack/200g	28	1.0	14	0.8	1.6	0.5	1.4
SALAD BOWL								
Crispy, M & S*	1 Serving/250g	87	1.2	35	1.3	6.6	0.5	1.2
Egg Layered, Tesco*	1 Pack/410g	726	57.8	177	4.2	8.4	14.1	1.3
French Style, Sainsbury's*	1oz/28g	15	1.0	55	1.0	4.8	3.5	1.5
French Style, Way to Five, Sainsbury's*	1 Pack/264g	103	5.8	39	0.7	4.2	2.2	2.2

	Measure INFO/WEIGHT	per Measure KCAL	FAT	Nutrition Values per 100g / 100ml KCAL	PROT	CARB	FAT	FIBRE
SALAD BOWL								
Frisee, Radicchio & Green Oak Leaf Lettuce, M & S*	1 Bowl/150g	30	0.6	20	1.1	2.6	0.4	1.1
Goats Cheese, Sainsbury's*	1 Serving/100g	161	11.9	161	5.8	7.6	11.9	1.3
Greek Style, M & S*	1 Bowl/255g	242	20.9	95	2.5	2.4	8.2	0.7
Honey & Mustard Chicken, Fresh, Sainsbury's*	1 Serving/300g	408	23.7	136	5.9	10.3	7.9	1.7
Italian Avocado & Tomato, Sainsbury's*	1 Bowl/180g	97	4.7	54	1.0	6.7	2.6	1.3
Large, Sainsbury's*	1/6 Pack/52g	12	0.2	23	0.9	4.3	0.3	1.1
Mixed, Medley, Waitrose*	¼ Pack/60g	9	0.3	15	0.9	1.7	0.5	1.0
Mixed, Waitrose*	¼ Pack/64g	9	0.3	14	0.8	1.6	0.5	1.4
Mushrooms in Tomato Sauce, Sainsbury's*	1 Serving/100g	72	4.8	72	2.5	3.3	4.8	0.5
Prawn, Sainsbury's*	1 Bowl/400g	632	46.8	158	3.7	9.4	11.7	1.2
Red Cheddar & Edam, Way to Five, Sainsbury's*	½ Pack/224g	240	9.4	107	4.4	12.8	4.2	1.1
Tomato, Sainsbury's*	½ Bowl/150g	93	6.7	62	0.9	4.4	4.5	1.6
Tomato, Way to Five, Sainsbury's*	1 Bowl/300g	174	12.3	58	0.8	4.5	4.1	2.8
Tomato & Basil, M & S*	1 Serving/225g	225	22.7	100	0.8	3.7	10.1	1.1
Tuna, BGTY, Sainsbury's*	½ Pack/175g	180	2.6	103	7.0	15.4	1.5	1.7
Tuna, Fresh, Asda*	1 Serving/160g	184	11.2	115	8.0	5.0	7.0	0.0
Tuna, Sainsbury's*	1 Serving/200g	336	21.4	168	6.1	11.7	10.7	1.5
with Crunchy Coleslaw, M & S*	1 Pack/325g	455	44.8	140	1.0	2.5	13.8	2.0
SALAD CREAM								
Average	*1 Tsp/5g*	*17*	*1.4*	*335*	*1.7*	*18.6*	*27.8*	*0.1*
Heinz*	1 Tbsp/15g	50	4.0	332	1.4	20.0	26.8	0.0
Reduced Calorie, Average	*1 Tsp/5g*	*6*	*0.4*	*130*	*1.0*	*12.9*	*7.9*	*0.1*
Weight Watchers*	1 Serving/14g	16	0.6	115	1.5	16.2	4.4	0.0
SALAD KIT								
Caesar, Asda*	½ Pack/113g	154	9.0	136	5.0	11.0	8.0	1.4
Caesar, HL, Tesco*	½ Pack/133g	148	11.0	112	3.3	5.9	8.3	1.4
Caesar, New Improved, Tesco*	½ Pack/138g	279	25.3	202	4.7	4.5	18.3	1.3
Caesar, Tesco*	½ Pack/150g	237	19.8	158	3.2	6.7	13.2	0.7
Caesar, Waitrose*	1 Bag/250g	445	39.2	178	5.0	4.2	15.7	1.1
Ranch, HL, Tesco*	1 Serving/115g	69	2.9	60	4.4	5.0	2.5	1.8
SALAD SEASONING								
Sesame Seed, Coriander & Cumin, Schwartz*	1 Tsp/4g	13	0.4	314	16.5	38.5	10.4	11.4
SALAD SNACK								
Chargrilled Chicken, Tesco*	1 Pot/300g	384	14.4	128	6.1	15.0	4.8	2.4
Cheese & Tomato, Tesco*	1 Pot/300g	519	20.4	173	6.3	21.7	6.8	2.2
Cheese Layered, Sainsbury's*	1 Pack/190g	397	29.1	209	5.4	12.4	15.3	0.0
Chicken & Bacon, Tesco*	1 Pack/300g	501	31.5	167	7.2	10.9	10.5	3.2
Chicken Caesar, Sainsbury's*	1 Pack/182g	164	9.1	90	5.9	5.3	5.0	1.0
Chicken Caesar, Tesco*	1 Serving/300g	420	20.4	140	8.2	11.4	6.8	1.7
Chicken Noodle, Sainsbury's*	1 Snack/240g	278	12.2	116	5.2	12.4	5.1	1.4
Greek Style, BGTY, Sainsbury's*	1 Pack/199g	133	5.0	67	2.0	9.0	2.5	0.8
Ham & Mushroom, Tesco*	1 Pot/300g	600	32.1	200	4.7	21.2	10.7	1.4
Pasta, Egg Mayo, Asda*	1 Serving/180g	364	27.0	202	4.0	12.8	15.0	0.3
Pasta, Tuna, Asda*	1 Serving/180g	196	6.8	109	5.5	13.2	3.8	0.9
Pasta & Tuna, BGTY, Sainsbury's*	1 Pack/260g	218	4.2	84	6.0	11.5	1.6	2.3
Roast Chicken, Tesco*	1 Pack/300g	324	21.6	108	6.0	4.8	7.2	1.3
Salmon & Dill, Tesco*	1 Pack/300g	600	38.4	200	7.7	13.4	12.8	0.8
Sausage & Tomato, Tesco*	1 Serving/300g	529	27.3	176	4.5	19.1	9.1	4.0
Tuna, HL, Tesco*	1 Serving/300g	237	3.3	79	7.2	10.1	1.1	1.7
Tuna & Pasta, BGTY, Sainsbury's*	1 Pack/260g	255	5.7	98	5.7	13.9	2.2	1.3
Tuna & Sweetcorn, Tesco*	1 Pack/300g	540	18.3	180	7.3	23.9	6.1	0.7
SALAMI								
Ardennes Pepper, Waitrose*	1 Serving/7g	30	2.7	429	18.6	1.9	38.5	1.1

	Measure INFO/WEIGHT	per Measure KCAL	FAT	Nutrition Values per 100g / 100ml KCAL	PROT	CARB	FAT	FIBRE
SALAMI								
Average	*1 Slice/5g*	*18*	*1.3*	*360*	*28.4*	*1.8*	*26.1*	*0.0*
Danish, Average	*1 Serving/17g*	*89*	*8.8*	*524*	*13.2*	*1.3*	*51.7*	*0.0*
Emiliano, Sainsbury's*	1 Serving/70g	209	14.2	298	28.8	0.1	20.3	0.0
German, Average	*1 Serving/60g*	*200*	*16.4*	*333*	*20.3*	*1.6*	*27.3*	*0.1*
German, Peppered, Average	*3 Slices/25g*	*86*	*6.8*	*342*	*22.2*	*2.5*	*27.1*	*0.2*
Healthy Range, Average	*4 Slices/25g*	*55*	*3.6*	*220*	*22.3*	*0.6*	*14.3*	*0.0*
Milano, Average	*1 Serving/70g*	*278*	*22.6*	*397*	*25.9*	*0.9*	*32.2*	*0.0*
Napoli, Average	*1 Slice/5g*	*17*	*1.3*	*341*	*27.1*	*0.7*	*25.5*	*0.0*
Pepperoni, Italian, Morrisons*	1 Slice/6g	23	1.9	406	24.0	0.9	34.0	0.0
Spanish, Wafer Thin, Tesco*	1 Pack/80g	273	18.8	341	25.5	6.8	23.5	0.0
Ungherese, Tesco*	1 Serving/35g	136	11.2	388	24.5	0.5	32.0	0.0
SALMON								
Alaskan, Wild, TTD, Sainsbury's*	1 Fillet/115g	173	8.3	150	21.2	0.1	7.2	0.1
Crunchies, Tesco*	1 Serving/112g	211	11.0	188	9.0	15.9	9.8	1.3
Fillet, Dinner, Light & Easy, Youngs*	1 Pack/375g	315	10.5	84	6.7	7.9	2.8	1.6
Fillet, Skin On, TTD, Sainsbury's*	1 Fillet/126g	249	14.3	197	23.5	0.2	11.3	0.0
Fillets, a Malted Wholegrain Crumb, Simply, Birds Eye*	1 Fillet/130g	195	8.2	150	16.8	6.4	6.3	0.5
Fillets, Cajun, Waitrose*	1 Serving/150g	214	9.7	143	20.6	0.4	6.5	0.0
Fillets, Chargrilled, Sainsbury's*	1 Serving/270g	270	19.5	243	20.9	0.2	17.6	0.0
Fillets, Chilli & Lemon Pink, Aldi*	1 Fillet/140g	260	10.4	186	16.9	12.9	7.4	0.7
Fillets, Honey Roast, Co-Op*	1 Fillet/100g	250	13.8	250	26.7	4.7	13.8	0.1
Fillets, Lightly Smoked, TTD, Sainsbury's*	1 Serving/100g	201	13.2	201	20.2	0.3	13.2	0.6
Fillets, Lime & Coriander, Tesco*	1 Pack/250g	282	5.2	113	18.2	5.4	2.1	0.0
Fillets, Raw, Average	*1 Fillet/79g*	*149*	*9.2*	*189*	*20.9*	*0.1*	*11.7*	*0.1*
Fillets, with Lemon & Herb Butter, Asda*	1 Fillet/125g	305	22.5	244	20.0	0.4	18.0	0.0
Fillets, with Orange & Dill Dressing, Tesco*	1 Serving/300g	540	30.9	180	17.7	4.1	10.3	0.7
Fillets, with Sicilian Citrus Glaze, Sainsbury's*	1 Fillet/145g	371	25.8	256	21.9	2.3	17.8	0.0
Flakes, Honey Roast, Average	*1oz/28g*	*56*	*3.0*	*198*	*24.0*	*1.9*	*10.7*	*0.2*
Goujons, Average	1 Pack/150g	321	16.4	214	16.4	12.4	10.9	1.1
Gravadlax, Finest, Tesco*	1 Serving/70g	125	6.9	178	22.1	0.2	9.9	0.0
Gravadlax, M & S*	1 Serving/140g	294	16.0	210	18.4	5.3	11.4	0.5
Gravadlax, Scottish, M & S*	1 Serving/70g	147	8.0	210	18.4	5.3	11.4	0.5
Gravadlax, with Mustard Sauce, Waitrose*	1 Serving/100g	191	11.1	191	21.8	1.0	11.1	0.4
Grilled	*1oz/28g*	*60*	*3.7*	*215*	*24.2*	*0.0*	*13.1*	*0.0*
Honey Roast Flakes, Sainsbury's*	½ Pack/68g	166	9.5	244	25.9	3.6	14.0	0.0
Hot Smoked, Average	*1 Serving/62g*	*103*	*4.4*	*166*	*24.0*	*0.9*	*7.2*	*0.1*
Hot Smoked, Kiln Baked, TTD, Sainsbury's*	½ Pack/63g	121	6.4	193	24.6	0.7	10.2	0.5
Juniper & Birch Smoked, TTD, Sainsbury's*	½ Pack/60g	132	8.4	220	23.3	0.3	14.0	0.1
Lemon & Rosemary, Easy Steam, BGTY, Sainsbury's*	1 Pack/350g	329	12.6	94	6.4	9.0	3.6	1.3
Lime & Coriander, Tesco*	1 Serving/120g	176	4.4	147	21.4	7.0	3.7	0.7
Mild Oak Smoked, Average	*1 Slice/25g*	*45*	*2.5*	*182*	*22.6*	*0.1*	*10.2*	*0.0*
Moroccan Style, Light Lunch, John West*	1 Pack/240g	199	1.4	83	5.5	14.0	0.6	3.1
Mousse, Tesco*	1 Mousse/57g	100	7.0	177	13.5	2.9	12.4	0.2
Pink, Average	*1 Serving/125g*	*162*	*7.2*	*130*	*19.5*	*0.1*	*5.8*	*0.1*
Pink, in Brine, Average	*1oz/28g*	*43*	*1.8*	*153*	*23.5*	*0.0*	*6.6*	*0.0*
Poached, Average	*1 Serving/90g*	*176*	*10.5*	*195*	*22.5*	*0.2*	*11.7*	*0.3*
Potted, M & S*	1 Serving/75g	184	14.5	245	17.1	0.5	19.4	1.2
Red, Average	*½ Can/90g*	*141*	*7.4*	*156*	*20.4*	*0.1*	*8.2*	*0.1*
Red, in Brine, Average	*1oz/28g*	*47*	*2.5*	*169*	*22.4*	*0.0*	*8.9*	*0.0*
Rillettes, John West*	½ Can/62g	169	14.6	272	14.9	0.1	23.5	0.0
Roasted. Slices, Tesco*	1 Slice/33g	71	3.5	215	26.7	2.7	10.5	1.9
Scottish Lochmuir Sashimi Smoked, M & S*	1 Pack/130g	214	11.0	165	18.6	3.3	8.5	0.5
Smoked, Appetisers, Tesco*	1/3 Pack/33g	80	6.2	240	16.3	1.1	18.5	0.0

S

SALMON

INFO/WEIGHT	Measure INFO/WEIGHT	per Measure KCAL	FAT	Nutrition Values per 100g / 100ml KCAL	PROT	CARB	FAT	FIBRE
Smoked, Average	**1 Serving/70g**	**126**	**7.0**	**179**	**21.9**	**0.5**	**10.0**	**0.1**
Smoked, Birch & Juniper, Sainsbury's*	½ Pack/30g	47	1.9	156	24.7	0.3	6.4	0.0
Smoked, Parcels, TTD, Sainsbury's*	1 Serving/58g	144	11.1	250	13.4	5.7	19.3	1.0
Smoked, Sockeye, Wild, TTD, Sainsbury's*	½ Pack/60g	82	1.9	137	26.3	0.7	3.2	0.6
Smoked, Trimmings, Average	**1 Serving/55g**	**101**	**5.7**	**184**	**22.8**	**0.2**	**10.3**	**0.0**
Steaks	**1 Serving/100g**	**180**	**11.0**	**180**	**20.2**	**0.0**	**11.0**	**0.0**
Steamed	**1oz/28g**	**55**	**3.6**	**197**	**20.1**	**0.0**	**13.0**	**0.0**
Tail Joint, Lemon & Herb Butter, M & S*	1 Pack/480g	864	54.7	180	18.8	0.8	11.4	0.2
Whole, Raw, Average	1 Serving/100g	228	13.9	228	25.6	0.0	13.9	0.0
Wild Alaskan, Keta, Fillets, Sainsbury's*	1 Fillet/115g	178	6.4	155	25.9	0.2	5.6	0.3
with Basil, Lean Cuisine*	1 Pack/353g	260	7.4	74	5.3	8.8	2.1	1.7
Zesty, with Baby New Potatoes, GFY, Asda*	1 Pack/400g	264	6.8	66	6.8	5.9	1.7	2.0

SALMON &

	Measure INFO/WEIGHT	per Measure KCAL	FAT	Nutrition Values per 100g / 100ml KCAL	PROT	CARB	FAT	FIBRE
Broccoli Potato Wedge Melt, Weight Watchers*	1 Pack/320g	298	10.6	93	5.1	10.6	3.3	1.1
Spinach, Roulade, Tesco*	1 Serving/60g	155	14.2	258	9.5	1.7	23.7	0.2
Vegetables, M & S*	1 Serving/200g	220	13.8	110	6.0	5.2	6.9	0.8

SALMON EN CROUTE

	Measure INFO/WEIGHT	per Measure KCAL	FAT	Nutrition Values per 100g / 100ml KCAL	PROT	CARB	FAT	FIBRE
Chilled, Youngs*	1 Pastry/200g	531	37.3	265	9.6	14.8	18.6	2.3
Frozen, Tesco*	1 Serving/166g	365	18.4	220	10.1	19.1	11.1	1.1
Frozen, Youngs*	1 Pastry/185g	542	38.3	293	10.2	16.5	20.7	1.0
Iceland*	1 Serving/170g	476	31.3	280	8.5	20.1	18.4	1.0
Luxury, M & S*	1oz/28g	59	3.8	210	11.9	9.4	13.7	2.2
M & S*	½ Pack/185g	573	40.5	310	10.4	17.3	21.9	0.6
Retail, Average	1oz/28g	81	5.3	288	11.8	18.0	19.1	0.0
Wild Alaskan, Inspired To Cook, Sainsbury's*	1 Parcel/173g	476	24.4	275	12.5	24.7	14.1	10.8

SALMON IN

	Measure INFO/WEIGHT	per Measure KCAL	FAT	Nutrition Values per 100g / 100ml KCAL	PROT	CARB	FAT	FIBRE
a Creamy Horseradish Sauce, Fillets, Wonnemeyer*	1 Serving/300g	459	31.5	153	9.4	5.3	10.5	0.0
Chilli Lime & Ginger Dressing, The Saucy Fish Co.*	1 Fillet /140g	273	15.8	195	16.7	5.5	11.3	0.0
Creamy Watercress Sauce, Fillets, Scottish, Seafresh*	1 Pack 300g	528	38.7	176	13.7	1.2	12.9	0.1
Dill Sauce, Youngs*	1 Pack/435g	265	10.0	61	6.1	4.2	2.3	0.1
Lime & Coriander, Fillets, Good Choice, Iceland*	½ Pack/150g	189	4.3	126	19.8	5.1	2.9	0.8
Pancetta, Wrapped, Finest, Tesco*	1 Serving/150g	328	25.8	219	14.9	1.0	17.2	0.1
Tomato & Mascarpone Sauce, Fillets, Asda*	½ Pack/181g	279	19.9	154	13.0	0.8	11.0	0.6
Watercress Sauce, Pink, Wild Alaskan, Sainsbury's*	½ Pack/180g	194	9.7	108	13.9	0.9	5.4	0.8
Watercress Sauce, Waitrose*	½ Pack/150g	264	19.3	176	13.7	1.2	12.9	0.1
White Wine & Cream Sauce, Tesco*	1 Serving/170g	279	19.2	164	13.5	2.0	11.3	1.2
White Wine & Parsley Dressing, Fillets, Tesco*	1 Fillet/150g	291	20.4	194	17.5	0.3	13.6	0.6

SALMON WITH

	Measure INFO/WEIGHT	per Measure KCAL	FAT	Nutrition Values per 100g / 100ml KCAL	PROT	CARB	FAT	FIBRE
a Cream Sauce, Scottish Fillets, M & S*	1 Serving/200g	360	26.0	180	13.8	1.0	13.0	0.1
Coriander & Lime, Pacific, Asda*	1 Serving/113g	154	3.4	137	27.0	0.5	3.0	0.0
Garlic & Herb Butter, Tesco*	1 Fillet/112g	291	23.1	260	17.6	0.0	20.6	0.0
Mozzarella & Tomato Crust, Just Cook, Sainsbury's*	½ Pack/171g	220	9.2	129	15.0	5.2	5.4	0.4
Pasta, Frozen, Youngs*	½ Bag/175g	234	7.7	134	7.4	16.3	4.4	1.2
Penne Pasta & Dill Sauce, Steamfresh, Birds Eye*	1 Pack/424g	335	6.4	79	6.4	9.9	1.5	1.1
Potatoes, Honey Roast, Light Choices, Tesco*	1 Pack/350g	332	12.2	95	6.6	8.5	3.5	2.4
Prawns, & Fusilli Pasta, Frozen, Youngs*	1 Pack/375g	439	27.7	117	5.6	7.0	7.4	1.1
Rice, Oriental Style, M & S*	1 Pot/210g	252	6.9	120	5.9	16.5	3.3	3.3
Sweet Chilli, Fillets, Roasted, Tesco*	1 Fillet/100g	210	10.6	210	26.1	1.7	10.6	0.6
Sweet Chilli, Hot Smoked, Scottish, Tesco*	1 Fillet/120g	252	12.7	210	26.1	1.7	10.6	0.6
Sweet Chilli Lime & Ginger, Simply Fish, Tesco*	½ Pack/98g	235	17.1	240	17.4	3.2	17.5	0.0

SALSA

	Measure INFO/WEIGHT	per Measure KCAL	FAT	Nutrition Values per 100g / 100ml KCAL	PROT	CARB	FAT	FIBRE
Bottled, M & S*	½ Jar/136g	95	3.3	70	1.2	12.0	2.4	1.5
Chunky, Sainsbury's*	½ Pot/84g	43	1.4	51	1.1	7.8	1.7	1.2

S

	Measure INFO/WEIGHT	per Measure KCAL	FAT	Nutrition Values per 100g / 100ml KCAL	PROT	CARB	FAT	FIBRE
SALSA								
Cool, Sainsbury's*	1 Serving/100g	31	0.3	31	1.0	6.1	0.3	1.2
Fresh, Asda*	1oz/28g	10	0.2	35	1.2	6.2	0.6	2.0
Fresh, Sainsbury's*	1oz/28g	15	0.6	54	1.7	7.0	2.1	0.9
GFY, Asda*	½ Pot/236g	85	0.9	36	1.1	7.0	0.4	0.7
Hot, Fresh, Chilled, Tesco*	1 Tub/200g	120	4.8	60	1.4	7.5	2.4	1.2
Hot, Primula*	1oz/28g	10	0.1	35	1.8	6.6	0.2	0.0
Medium Hot, Discovery*	1 Serving/30g	17	0.1	56	1.4	11.7	0.4	0.8
Mild, Heinz*	1 Serving/20g	16	0.0	79	1.2	17.9	0.1	0.8
Mild, Original, Old El Paso*	1 Sachet/144g	60	0.7	42	1.6	9.0	0.5	0.0
Original, From Dinner Kit, Old El Paso*	1 Jar/226g	71	0.7	32	1.2	6.0	0.3	0.0
Prawn & Tomato, Fresh, Anti Pasti, Asda*	1 Pot/150g	100	3.7	67	8.0	3.1	2.5	1.3
Red Onion & Tomato, Tapas Selection, Sainsbury's*	1 Serving/22g	17	1.0	77	3.0	6.0	4.5	0.9
Red Pepper, Sainsbury's*	1 Serving/85g	31	1.4	37	1.7	3.8	1.7	1.5
Smokey BBQ, Weight Watchers*	1 Serving/56g	20	0.1	36	1.1	7.6	0.1	2.3
Spiced Mango, Ginger & Chilli, Weight Watchers*	½ Pot/50g	42	0.1	85	1.0	19.9	0.2	2.6
Spicy, Less Than 3% Fat, M & S*	½ Pot/85g	30	0.7	35	1.3	5.6	0.8	0.8
Spicy Bean, Chosen By You, Asda*	½ Pot/100g	71	1.2	71	3.1	10.6	1.2	2.5
Spicy Mango & Lime, Morrisons*	½ Pot/85g	62	0.3	73	1.0	15.9	0.4	1.3
Spicy Red Pepper, Fresh, Waitrose*	½ Pot/85g	27	0.8	32	1.9	4.1	0.9	1.6
Spicy Red Pepper, Sainsbury's*	1 Pot/170g	54	2.4	32	1.4	3.2	1.4	1.3
Sweetcorn, Fresh, Sainsbury's*	¼ Pot/51g	32	0.9	63	1.1	10.5	1.8	1.3
Tomato, Chunky, Tesco*	1 Pot/170g	68	2.2	40	1.1	5.9	1.3	1.1
Tomato, Chunky, Tex Mex, Tesco*	1 Serving/50g	26	1.2	52	1.0	6.4	2.5	1.0
Tomato, Mexican Style, Dip, Morrisons*	½ Pack/50g	25	0.9	51	1.2	7.6	1.8	0.8
Tomato, Onion, Coriander & Chilli, Fresh, Waitrose*	1 Tub/170g	110	5.3	65	1.3	8.0	3.1	1.2
Tomato, Reduced Fat, Waitrose*	1 Serving/1g	0	0.0	27	1.5	4.7	0.2	1.4
Tomato, Spicy, Worldwide Sauces*	1 Serving/25g	7	0.0	30	1.2	5.9	0.2	1.2
Tomato, Sun Ripened, Tesco*	1 Serving/40g	46	1.7	115	5.0	14.2	4.2	4.6
Tomato, Vine Ripened, Tesco*	½ Tub/100g	47	1.8	47	1.0	6.7	1.8	1.1
Tomato & Avocado, Chunky, COU, M & S*	½ Pack/86g	30	1.2	35	0.8	5.4	1.4	1.4
Vine Ripened Tomato & Jalapeno, Sainsbury's*	¼ Tub/50g	34	1.7	68	1.1	8.0	3.5	1.2
SALT								
Alternative, Reduced Sodium, Losalt*	10g	0	0.0	0	0.0	0.0	0.0	0.0
Rock, Average	¼ Tsp/1g	0	0.0	0	0.0	0.0	0.0	0.0
Rock, for Grinding, Saxa*	1 Serving/100g	0	0.0	0	0.0	0.0	0.0	0.0
Rock, Natural, Tidmans*	1 Serving/100g	0	0.0	0	0.0	0.0	0.0	0.0
Table, Average	*1 Tsp/5g*	*0*	*0.0*	*0*	*0.0*	*0.0*	*0.0*	*0.0*
SAMBUCA								
Average	*1 Shot/35ml*	*122*	*0.0*	*348*	*0.0*	*37.2*	*0.0*	*0.0*
SAMOSAS								
Chicken, Mumtaz*	1 Serving/105g	177	8.3	169	19.6	4.9	7.9	0.0
Chicken Tikka, Sainsbury's*	1 Samosa/50g	119	6.4	239	8.3	22.5	12.9	3.1
Co-Op*	1oz/28g	70	2.8	250	6.0	34.0	10.0	2.0
Dim Sum Selection, Sainsbury's*	1 Samosa/12g	24	0.9	196	3.4	28.6	7.6	2.8
Indian Style Selection, Co-Op*	1 Samosa/21g	50	2.7	240	5.0	27.0	13.0	3.0
Lamb, Morrisons*	1 Samosa/50g	144	7.8	288	9.8	27.0	15.7	1.5
Lamb, Waitrose*	1oz/28g	87	6.3	310	8.5	18.1	22.6	0.8
Vegetable, Indian Starter Selection, M & S*	1 Samosa/21g	60	3.5	290	5.0	29.0	16.9	3.3
Vegetable, Large, Individual, Sainsbury's*	1 Samosa/110g	254	16.5	231	3.3	20.7	15.0	2.1
Vegetable, Large, Tesco*	1 Samosa/64g	148	7.9	231	4.8	25.2	12.4	3.4
Vegetable, M & S*	1 Samosa/45g	115	6.9	255	5.1	24.8	15.3	2.8
Vegetable, Mini, Asda*	1 Samosa/23g	52	2.0	233	6.0	32.0	9.0	2.6
Vegetable, Mini, Indian, Party Selection, Tesco*	1 Samosa/30g	58	1.5	195	3.6	33.9	5.0	2.2

S

	Measure INFO/WEIGHT	per Measure KCAL	FAT	Nutrition Values per 100g / 100ml KCAL	PROT	CARB	FAT	FIBRE
SAMOSAS								
Vegetable, Mini, Indian Snack Selection, Sainsbury's*	1 Samosa/25g	70	3.9	280	4.7	29.8	15.8	3.2
Vegetable, Mini, Indian Snack Selection, Tesco*	1 Samosa/32g	76	4.2	238	4.7	25.5	13.0	3.3
Vegetable, Mini, Waitrose*	1 Samosa/29g	70	3.8	242	3.6	27.1	13.2	3.1
Vegetable, Morrisons*	1 Samosa/60g	101	3.5	169	4.9	24.1	5.8	2.0
Vegetable, Northern Indian, Sainsbury's*	1 Samosa/50g	126	5.9	252	5.8	30.6	11.8	2.6
Vegetable, Retail, Average	1 Samosa/110g	239	10.2	217	5.1	30.0	9.3	2.5
Vegetable, Waitrose*	1 Samosa/50g	118	7.1	236	3.7	23.1	14.3	2.7
SAMPHIRE								
Raw, Fresh	1 Serving/80g	24	0.0	30	12.0	0.0	0.0	3.0
SANDWICH								
All Day Breakfast, Aramark*	1 Serving/206g	441	19.0	214	9.6	23.3	9.2	0.0
All Day Breakfast, BGTY, Sainsbury's*	1 Pack/188g	294	4.5	156	9.6	22.7	2.4	0.0
All Day Breakfast, Finest, Tesco*	1 Pack/275g	660	41.5	240	9.7	16.4	15.1	1.6
All Day Breakfast, HL, Tesco*	1 Pack/223g	328	8.0	147	11.9	16.8	3.6	2.7
All Day Breakfast, Shapers, Boots*	1 Pack/207g	323	5.2	156	11.0	23.0	2.5	2.2
All Day Breakfast, Wall's*	1 Pack/225g	610	34.7	271	9.2	24.3	15.4	1.4
All Day Breakfast, Weight Watchers*	1 Pack/158g	298	4.3	189	11.0	30.2	2.7	1.9
Avocado, & Spinach, M & S*	1 Pack/242g	580	27.3	240	4.0	21.0	11.3	4.8
Avocado, Mozzarella & Tomato, M & S*	1 Pack/273g	655	36.0	240	8.8	21.7	13.2	2.3
Bacon, & Brie, Asda*	1 Pack/181g	603	38.2	333	13.3	22.9	21.1	1.3
Bacon, & Brie, Finest, Tesco*	1 Pack/201g	571	33.6	284	14.1	19.4	16.7	2.1
Bacon, & Egg, Boots*	1 Pack/179g	480	28.6	268	12.0	19.0	16.0	1.4
Bacon, & Egg, Classic, Felix Van Den Berghe*	1 Pack/138g	335	14.9	243	12.9	23.4	10.8	0.0
Bacon, & Egg, Co-Op*	1 Pack/188g	536	32.0	285	13.0	20.0	17.0	2.0
Bacon, & Egg, Free Range, Daily Bread*	1 Serving/175g	425	22.9	243	10.1	21.5	13.1	0.0
Bacon, & Egg, HL, Tesco*	1 Serving/178g	328	9.3	184	11.5	22.7	5.2	1.7
Bacon, & Egg, Sainsbury's*	1 Pack/160g	384	17.8	240	13.0	22.0	11.1	1.8
Bacon, & Egg, Scottish Slimmers, Tesco*	1 Pack/139g	279	6.4	201	13.6	26.3	4.6	1.2
Bacon, & Egg, Shell*	1 Pack/191g	579	38.0	303	12.2	18.7	19.9	0.0
Bacon, & Egg, Taste!*	1 Pack/187g	495	28.6	265	12.8	19.1	15.3	0.0
Bacon, & Egg, Tesco*	1 Pack/188g	481	24.2	256	14.1	21.0	12.9	1.9
Bacon, & Tomato, COU, M & S*	1 Pack/169g	270	4.6	160	9.5	25.6	2.7	2.5
Bacon, Brie, & Mango Chutney, Daily Bread*	1 Serving/213g	555	22.7	261	12.7	28.6	10.7	0.0
Bacon, Cheese & Chicken, Triple, BGTY, Sainsbury's*	1 Serving/266g	506	16.8	190	12.7	20.7	6.3	2.6
Bacon, Lettuce & Tomato, Shapers, Boots*	1 Pack/175g	272	7.5	155	11.0	18.0	4.3	5.9
Bacon, Lettuce & Tomato, Weight Watchers*	1 Pack/153g	237	2.4	155	9.4	25.8	1.6	2.4
Bacon & Brown Sauce, Ashberry*	1 Pack/419g	1207	53.6	288	12.0	31.0	12.8	0.0
Bacon Lettuce & Tomato, Deep Fill, Ginsters*	1 Pack/1197g	439	18.1	223	10.3	24.7	9.2	2.7
Bap, Chicken, & Sweetcorn, Sainsbury's*	1 Serving/170g	462	23.6	272	12.5	24.2	13.9	0.0
Bap, Chicken, Chargrilled, Malted, Co-Op*	1 Bap/201g	492	26.1	245	9.0	23.0	13.0	2.0
Bap, Ham, & Salad, Co-Op*	1 Bap/164g	295	4.9	180	8.0	30.0	3.0	2.0
Bap, Tuna, & Sweetcorn, Malted, Co-Op*	1 Bap/212g	530	27.6	250	9.0	24.0	13.0	2.0
Beef, & English Mustard Mayonnaise, Roast, Oldfields*	1 Pack/150g	405	17.9	270	16.0	29.0	11.9	0.0
Beef, & Horseradish, Deep Filled, BGTY, Sainsbury's*	1 Pack/202g	313	4.8	155	11.4	22.0	2.4	2.4
Beef, & Horseradish, Sainsbury's*	1 Pack/187g	389	13.3	208	12.0	24.1	7.1	0.0
Beef, & Horseradish, Shapers, Boots*	1 Pack/156g	276	2.7	177	12.0	28.0	1.7	1.8
Beef, & Horseradish Mayonnaise, Shapers, Boots*	1 Pack/159g	266	3.3	167	12.0	25.0	2.1	2.6
Beef, & Onion, Co-Op*	1 Pack/221g	530	24.3	240	11.0	24.0	11.0	1.0
Beef, & Onion, Roast, Deep Filled, Asda*	1 Pack/258g	550	27.9	213	11.3	22.6	10.8	1.1
Beef, & Onion, Roast, HL, Tesco*	1 Pack/185g	278	3.5	150	13.3	20.0	1.9	2.7
Beef, & Pate, M & S*	1 Pack/188g	310	7.3	165	11.2	21.6	3.9	2.4
Beef, & Salad, Deep Fill, Iceland*	1 Pack/188g	317	9.2	169	11.1	20.1	4.9	2.7
Beef, & Salad, Gibsons*	1 Pack/185g	348	10.6	188	10.6	23.5	5.7	0.0

S

SANDWICH

INFO/WEIGHT	Measure	per Measure KCAL	FAT	Nutrition Values per 100g / 100ml KCAL	PROT	CARB	FAT	FIBRE
Beef, & Salad, Roast, Daily Bread*	1 Pack/202g	319	8.3	158	9.0	21.4	4.1	0.0
Beef, Peppered, Shell*	1 Pack/181g	400	15.2	221	7.3	29.0	8.4	1.3
Beef, Roast, Daily Bread*	1 Pack/199g	281	5.4	141	8.7	20.0	2.7	0.0
Beef, Roast, Feel Good, Shell*	1 Pack/153g	390	14.8	255	17.6	24.2	9.7	0.0
Beef, Roast, Handmade, Tesco*	1 Pack/223g	439	15.8	197	12.5	20.7	7.1	1.6
Beef, Roast, Sainsbury's*	1 Pack/174g	426	17.4	245	9.4	29.3	10.0	0.0
Beef, Tomato & Horseradish, Asda*	1 Pack/169g	255	4.4	151	10.0	22.0	2.6	2.7
Beef, Topside, Deli Continental*	1 Serving/191g	447	21.1	234	15.4	18.3	11.0	0.0
Bloomer, Egg & Watercress, Fresh, M & S*	1 Pack/221g	465	26.1	210	10.2	15.3	11.8	3.0
BLT, & Chicken Salad, Co-Op*	1 Pack/230g	471	20.7	205	10.0	21.0	9.0	2.0
BLT, Bacon, Lettuce & Tomato, Light Choices, Tesco*	1 Pack/149g	290	7.0	195	11.6	24.3	4.7	3.4
BLT, BGTY, Sainsbury's*	1 Pack/196g	331	4.4	169	10.4	27.0	2.2	0.0
BLT, Classic, Taste!*	1 Serving/150g	345	14.8	230	9.3	25.2	9.9	0.0
BLT, COU, M & S*	1 Pack/174g	278	4.7	160	9.5	25.6	2.7	2.5
BLT, Daily Bread*	1 Pack/171g	344	18.8	201	9.1	21.6	11.0	0.0
BLT, Deep Fill, Tesco*	1 Pack/231g	635	38.1	275	11.8	19.8	16.5	1.2
BLT, Deep Filled, Asda*	1 Pack/206g	606	35.0	294	13.3	21.8	17.0	3.0
BLT, GFY, Asda*	1 Pack/171g	294	6.0	172	9.0	26.0	3.5	1.6
BLT, HL, Tesco*	1 Pack/190g	287	2.7	151	10.1	24.5	1.4	1.6
BLT, Impress*	1 Pack/189g	381	13.4	202	11.5	22.8	7.1	0.0
BLT, M & S*	1 Serving/181g	381	14.7	210	10.7	23.8	8.1	1.8
BLT, Max, Shell*	1 Pack/249g	665	35.1	267	10.8	24.1	14.1	0.0
BLT, Salt Controlled, Shapers, Boots*	1 Pack/180g	290	6.1	161	9.3	23.0	3.4	3.0
BLT, Shapers, Boots*	1 Pack/169g	254	6.3	150	10.7	18.9	3.7	5.9
BLT, Sutherland*	1 Pack/216g	624	37.9	289	9.1	23.7	17.5	0.0
BLT, Taste!*	1 Pack/169g	353	16.0	209	8.5	22.4	9.5	0.0
BLT, Tesco*	1 Pack/203g	520	29.2	256	11.9	19.5	14.4	1.5
BLT, Waitrose*	1 Pack/184g	398	16.4	216	9.5	24.5	8.9	2.3
Breakfast, Mega Triple, Co-Op*	1 Pack/267g	750	40.0	281	11.6	25.5	15.0	3.4
Brie, & Grape, Finest, Tesco*	1 Pack/209g	527	31.6	252	8.5	20.6	15.1	1.5
Brie, with Apple & Grapes, Sainsbury's*	1 Pack/220g	473	24.2	215	8.2	20.8	11.0	0.0
British Chicken & Sweetcorn, Eat Well, M & S*	1 Pack/194g	340	10.5	175	11.4	19.6	5.4	3.1
Brunch, St Ivel*	1 Pack/225g	580	28.3	258	10.2	26.0	12.6	0.0
Chargrilled Vegetable & Houmous, HL, Tesco*	1 Pack/167g	250	4.0	150	5.9	25.3	2.4	2.0
Cheddar, & Celery, M & S*	1 Pack/200g	540	31.8	270	9.7	22.4	15.9	1.5
Cheddar, & Coleslaw, Simply, Boots*	1 Pack/185g	538	33.3	291	9.2	23.0	18.0	1.8
Cheddar, & Ham, British, M & S*	1 Serving/165g	395	18.6	240	15.1	20.0	11.3	1.7
Cheddar, & Ham, M & S*	1 Pack/165g	396	18.6	240	15.1	20.0	11.3	1.7
Cheddar, & Ham, Oldfields*	1 Pack/246g	674	39.6	274	11.7	20.5	16.1	2.0
Cheddar, & Ham, Smoked, Deep Filled, Tesco*	1 Serving/203g	573	33.1	282	14.3	19.5	16.3	1.2
Cheddar, & Ham, with Pickle, Smoked, Finest, Tesco*	1 Pack/217g	532	24.7	245	11.9	23.7	11.4	3.9
Cheddar, & Pickle, Mature, Sainsbury's*	1 Pack/171g	588	27.0	344	14.3	38.7	15.8	7.0
Cheddar, & Salad, Mature, Upper Crust*	1 Pack/225g	466	22.1	207	9.5	20.3	9.8	0.0
Cheddar, & Tomato, Mature, Big, Sainsbury's*	1 Pack/233g	596	25.6	256	12.9	26.3	11.0	0.0
Cheddar, & Tomato, Red, Tesco*	1 Pack/182g	526	31.7	289	9.2	24.0	17.4	1.1
Cheddar, Oldfields*	1 Pack/121g	384	17.3	317	12.8	33.2	14.3	1.5
Cheddar, Red Leicester, & Onion, Tesco*	1 Pack/182g	604	38.9	332	11.0	23.8	21.4	2.5
Cheddar & Bacon, Deep Fill, Ginsters*	1 Serving/170g	550	28.2	324	14.1	28.3	16.6	2.3
Cheese, & Apple, & Celery, Asda*	1 Pack/173g	244	4.8	141	8.0	21.0	2.8	2.7
Cheese, & Apple & Grape, COU, M & S*	1 Pack/186g	270	2.2	145	8.5	24.9	1.2	2.0
Cheese, & Celery, Shapers, Boots*	1 Pack/181g	288	4.2	159	11.0	24.0	2.3	3.0
Cheese, & Coleslaw, Asda*	1 Pack/262g	799	51.4	305	10.1	22.1	19.6	3.3
Cheese, & Coleslaw, M & S*	1 Pack/186g	498	32.4	268	10.2	17.6	17.4	3.2

S

SANDWICH

INFO/WEIGHT	Measure	per Measure KCAL	FAT	Nutrition Values per 100g / 100ml KCAL	PROT	CARB	FAT	FIBRE
Cheese, & Coleslaw, Shapers, Boots*	1 Pack/224g	338	4.7	151	11.0	22.0	2.1	3.2
Cheese, & Coleslaw, Sutherland*	1 Pack/185g	376	8.3	203	10.7	29.9	4.5	0.0
Cheese, & Ham, & Pickle, Co-Op*	1 Serving/185g	370	7.4	200	13.0	27.0	4.0	3.0
Cheese, & Ham, & Pickle, HL, Tesco*	1 Pack/201g	312	4.2	155	13.1	21.0	2.1	1.7
Cheese, & Ham, & Pickle, Shapers, Boots*	1 Pack/184g	318	8.5	173	13.0	20.0	4.6	2.5
Cheese, & Ham, & Pickle, Simply, Boots*	1 Pack/225g	551	29.2	245	11.0	21.0	13.0	2.4
Cheese, & Ham, & Pickle, Tesco*	1 Serving/215g	497	24.7	231	11.7	20.3	11.5	1.8
Cheese, & Ham, Baxter & Platts*	1 Pack/168g	408	21.8	243	11.3	20.5	13.0	1.7
Cheese, & Ham, Smoked, Co-Op*	1 Pack/167g	334	8.3	200	15.0	24.0	5.0	2.0
Cheese, & Marmite, No Mayonnaise, Boots*	1 Pack/156g	420	20.0	269	12.2	26.3	12.8	1.7
Cheese, & Onion, Deep Fill, Tesco*	1 Pack/212g	742	51.9	350	12.3	20.2	24.5	1.3
Cheese, & Onion, GFY, Asda*	1 Pack/156g	317	4.1	203	14.0	31.0	2.6	2.7
Cheese, & Onion, HL, Tesco*	1 Pack/168g	314	9.9	187	10.3	23.2	5.9	1.7
Cheese, & Onion, Light Choices, Tesco*	1 Pack/144g	310	9.4	215	12.7	26.5	6.5	3.6
Cheese, & Onion, M & S*	1 Serving/188g	460	24.2	245	11.2	21.3	12.9	2.9
Cheese, & Onion, Morrisons*	1 Pack/142g	260	2.4	183	14.1	27.8	1.7	2.9
Cheese, & Onion, Tesco*	1 Pack/178g	573	37.9	322	11.6	21.0	21.3	3.5
Cheese, & Onion, Triple, Tesco*	1 Pack/273g	906	58.4	332	11.0	23.8	21.4	2.5
Cheese, & Onion, Waitrose*	1 Pack/176g	579	38.7	329	12.5	20.2	22.0	2.8
Cheese, & Pickle, BHS*	1 Pack/178g	503	22.6	283	12.5	29.6	12.7	1.8
Cheese, & Pickle, Heinz*	1 Pack/178g	543	26.9	305	13.8	28.4	15.1	3.8
Cheese, & Pickle, Shapers, Boots*	1 Pack/165g	342	8.1	207	9.8	31.0	4.9	2.3
Cheese, & Pickle, Tesco*	1 Pack/140g	400	19.3	286	12.7	27.8	13.8	1.4
Cheese, & Pickle, Virgin Trains*	1 Pack/158g	444	19.6	281	11.5	31.1	12.4	0.0
Cheese, & Salad, COU, M & S*	1 Pack/188g	244	3.0	130	12.1	17.0	1.6	2.4
Cheese, & Salad, Shapers, Boots*	1 Pack/205g	307	5.1	150	9.7	22.0	2.5	2.2
Cheese, & Salad, Tesco*	1 Serving/188g	429	22.4	228	10.1	20.2	11.9	2.1
Cheese, & Spring Onion, Asda*	1 Pack/160g	576	39.9	361	13.0	21.0	25.0	1.9
Cheese, & Spring Onion, Co-Op*	1 Pack/164g	607	42.6	370	12.0	21.0	26.0	3.0
Cheese, & Spring Onion, Mixed, Scottish Slimmers*	1 Pack/139g	298	9.1	214	12.4	26.5	6.5	2.1
Cheese, & Spring Onion, Sainsbury's*	1 Serving/177g	605	39.5	342	11.4	24.0	22.3	1.1
Cheese, & Tomato, Asda*	1 Pack/154g	388	19.7	252	11.0	23.2	12.8	3.7
Cheese, & Tomato, Co-Op*	1 Pack/155g	365	18.5	235	10.6	21.8	11.9	1.9
Cheese, & Tomato, Freshmans*	1 Pack/111g	248	18.6	223	11.0	8.0	16.8	0.0
Cheese, & Tomato, Organic, M & S*	1 Pack/165g	559	35.3	339	11.8	24.8	21.4	1.9
Cheese, & Tomato, Sainsbury's*	1 Pack/216g	542	26.3	251	12.9	22.8	12.2	0.0
Cheese, & Tomato, Tesco*	1 Pack/182g	582	38.9	320	9.2	22.6	21.4	1.1
Cheese, Asda*	1 Pack/262g	618	31.4	236	12.2	20.3	12.0	3.0
Cheese, Crunch, Scottish Slimmers*	1 Pack/137g	292	9.0	213	11.0	27.6	6.6	2.3
Cheese, Ham, BLT, Triple Pack, Asda*	1 Pack/260g	614	31.2	236	12.2	20.3	12.0	3.0
Cheese, Savoury, Northern Bites*	1 Serving/210g	212	4.0	101	3.6	18.5	1.9	0.0
Cheese, Savoury, Sandwich King*	1 Pack/135g	328	11.2	243	11.6	30.2	8.3	0.0
Cheese, Three, & Onion, Boots*	1 Pack/169g	566	33.8	335	11.0	28.0	20.0	1.9
Cheese, Three, & Spring Onion, Shell*	1 Pack/168g	672	50.9	400	11.1	20.8	30.3	0.0
Cheese & Onion, Ginsters*	1 Packet/172g	491	26.8	286	11.1	25.4	15.6	1.8
Cheese Ploughman's, Deep Fill, Ginsters*	1 Pack/213g	491	24.2	231	8.4	23.8	11.4	2.2
Cheesy Coleslaw, Ginsters*	1 Pack/164g	481	27.7	293	9.9	25.4	16.9	2.4
Chicken, & Avocado, Tesco*	1 Serving/219g	559	31.6	255	11.9	19.5	14.4	2.4
Chicken, & Bacon, & Salad, Big, Sainsbury's*	1 Pack/249g	610	31.6	245	11.1	21.7	12.7	0.0
Chicken, & Bacon, & Salad, Dash*	1 Serving/217g	449	15.8	207	9.9	25.3	7.3	0.0
Chicken, & Bacon, Antony Worrall Thompson's*	1 Pack/191g	577	27.3	302	16.0	25.9	14.3	2.1
Chicken, & Bacon, Baton, Tesco*	1 Pack/201g	511	26.3	254	9.4	24.7	13.1	1.7
Chicken, & Bacon, BGTY, Sainsbury's*	1 Pack/211g	315	4.9	149	11.7	20.8	2.3	0.0

SANDWICH

INFO/WEIGHT	Measure		per Measure		Nutrition Values per 100g / 100ml				
			KCAL	FAT	KCAL	PROT	CARB	FAT	FIBRE
Chicken, & Bacon, COU, M & S*	1 Pack/179g		250	3.6	140	13.5	15.8	2.0	3.8
Chicken, & Bacon, Deep Fill, Ginsters*	1 Pack/200g		435	15.7	224	12.4	25.3	8.1	2.4
Chicken, & Bacon, Deep Filled, Co-Op*	1 Pack/166g		556	33.2	335	16.0	23.0	20.0	3.0
Chicken, & Bacon, Healthy Living, Co-Op*	1 Pack/179g		277	3.4	155	12.3	21.8	1.9	3.4
Chicken, & Bacon, HL, Tesco*	1 Pack/193g		318	6.2	165	13.5	19.5	3.2	2.7
Chicken, & Bacon, M & S*	1 Pack/185g		509	27.2	275	15.9	20.2	14.7	2.1
Chicken, & Bacon, on Pepper Bread, M & S*	1 Serving/177g		265	1.6	150	13.2	22.7	0.9	2.1
Chicken, & Bacon, Roast, Boots*	1 Pack/175g		413	14.0	236	15.4	26.3	8.0	2.2
Chicken, & Bacon, Shapers, Boots*	1 Pack/179g		317	8.9	177	14.0	19.0	5.0	3.1
Chicken, & Bacon, Sutherland Deli*	1 Pack/169g		453	20.1	268	14.6	25.7	11.9	2.7
Chicken, & Bacon, Tesco*	1 Pack/195g		486	24.2	249	14.3	20.0	12.4	2.7
Chicken, & Bacon, Waitrose*	1 Serving/191g		495	23.5	259	11.8	25.3	12.3	2.2
Chicken, & Bacon & Tomato, Paprika, Shapers, Boots*	1 Pack/184g		296	8.5	161	11.0	19.0	4.6	2.3
Chicken, & Balsamic Roasted Tomatoes, COU, M & S*	1 Pack/200g		280	4.6	140	11.6	18.1	2.3	2.6
Chicken, & Balsamic Roasted Tomatoes, HL, Tesco*	1 Pack/196g		275	2.4	140	13.6	18.8	1.2	2.9
Chicken, & Coleslaw, Tesco*	1 Pack/160g		305	7.1	191	12.0	25.7	4.4	2.4
Chicken, & Coriander, Taste!*	1 Serving/159g		228	4.6	143	5.6	23.3	2.9	0.0
Chicken, & Coriander, with Lime, BGTY, Sainsbury's*	1 Pack/168g		282	5.9	168	10.6	23.5	3.5	0.0
Chicken, & Ham, Healthy Living, Co-Op*	1 Pack/150g		285	6.0	190	12.0	28.0	4.0	3.0
Chicken, & Ham, HL, Tesco*	1 Serving/244g		327	2.7	134	13.2	17.9	1.1	1.3
Chicken, & Ham, Oak Smoked, Big, Sainsbury's*	1 Pack/244g		461	17.6	189	12.3	18.8	7.2	0.0
Chicken, & Ham, Roast, Ginsters*	1 Pack/180g		425	24.5	236	11.2	18.5	13.6	0.0
Chicken, & Ham, Roast, Tesco*	1 Pack/228g		561	31.9	246	13.3	16.6	14.0	1.2
Chicken, & Lemon, with Mint, Delilite*	1 Pack/179g		325	6.4	182	12.3	23.1	3.6	1.7
Chicken, & Mayo, The Sandwich Company*	1 Pack/72g		251	10.7	348	17.8	35.9	14.8	0.0
Chicken, & Mayo, Wholemeal, Sodhexo*	1 Pack/128g		346	17.4	270	13.1	24.0	13.6	3.6
Chicken, & Mayonnaise, Country Harvest*	1 Pack/120g		268	9.0	223	13.1	27.6	7.5	0.0
Chicken, & Mayonnaise, Simply, Oldfields*	1 Pack/128g		357	16.4	279	12.8	30.2	12.8	2.1
Chicken, & Pepperonata, COU, M & S*	1 Pack/171g		240	2.9	140	10.4	20.9	1.7	1.3
Chicken, & Pesto, Shapers, Boots*	1 Pack/181g		311	4.2	172	12.0	26.0	2.3	1.7
Chicken, & Pesto Salad, Bells*	1 Pack/196g		430	22.9	220	12.0	16.6	11.7	0.0
Chicken, & Roasted Peppers, Chargrilled, BHS*	1 Pack/183g		295	5.7	161	11.5	22.0	3.1	3.1
Chicken, & Salad, Bernard Matthews*	1 Pack/162g		269	8.4	166	7.0	22.7	5.2	0.0
Chicken, & Salad, Best for You, BHS*	1 Pack/315g		992	16.7	315	23.2	43.1	5.3	3.3
Chicken, & Salad, Co-Op*	1 Pack/195g		448	21.4	230	10.0	24.0	11.0	2.0
Chicken, & Salad, COU, M & S*	1 Pack/194g		262	3.7	135	9.8	19.0	1.9	1.6
Chicken, & Salad, Daily Bread*	1 Serving/187g		270	15.4	144	9.6	13.4	8.2	0.0
Chicken, & Salad, Deep Filled, Asda*	1 Pack/247g		551	18.3	223	18.1	22.2	7.4	1.3
Chicken, & Salad, Deep Filled, Co-Op*	1 Pack/213g		437	19.2	205	10.0	20.0	9.0	1.0
Chicken, & Salad, Deep Filled, Tesco*	1 Pack/238g		440	19.5	185	13.1	14.6	8.2	2.8
Chicken, & Salad, Deli-Lite, Brambles*	1 Pack/175g		268	2.3	153	11.7	23.7	1.3	2.0
Chicken, & Salad, GFY, Asda*	1 Pack/194g		252	2.9	130	12.0	17.0	1.5	2.6
Chicken, & Salad, Ham & Cheese, Twin, Tesco*	1 Pack/189g		434	21.5	230	10.8	21.1	11.4	2.3
Chicken, & Salad, Healthy Choice, Ginsters*	1 Serving/100g		257	4.7	257	18.3	33.8	4.7	0.0
Chicken, & Salad, Healthy Living, Co-Op*	1 Pack/196g		265	3.5	135	10.4	19.1	1.8	3.9
Chicken, & Salad, Heinz*	1 Pack/166g		331	15.9	200	8.6	19.9	9.6	2.0
Chicken, & Salad, HL, Tesco*	1 Pack/207g		290	3.9	140	13.9	16.8	1.9	2.7
Chicken, & Salad, Low Fat, Heinz*	1 Pack/166g		246	2.2	148	11.8	22.3	1.3	5.3
Chicken, & Salad, Low Fat, Waitrose*	1 Pack/188g		291	8.1	155	10.4	18.6	4.3	2.1
Chicken, & Salad, Roast, COU, M & S*	1 Pack/196g		265	4.5	135	8.9	19.6	2.3	2.2
Chicken, & Salad, Roast, Feel Good, Shell*	1 Pack/191g		326	9.0	171	9.8	22.4	4.7	0.0
Chicken, & Salad, Roast, Waitrose*	1 Pack/217g		482	24.1	222	9.4	21.1	11.1	2.0
Chicken, & Salad, Roast, Weight Watchers*	1 Pack/186g		266	8.0	143	10.3	15.8	4.3	2.8

S

SANDWICH	Measure INFO/WEIGHT	per Measure KCAL	per Measure FAT	Nutrition Values per 100g / 100ml KCAL	PROT	CARB	FAT	FIBRE
Chicken, & Salad, Sainsbury's*	1 Pack/240g	425	14.2	177	12.1	18.8	5.9	0.0
Chicken, & Salad, Scottish Slimmers*	1 Pack/169g	275	6.4	163	9.5	22.8	3.8	1.8
Chicken, & Salad, Shell*	1 Pack/201g	404	19.7	201	8.7	19.4	9.8	0.0
Chicken, & Salad, Sutherland*	1 Pack/181g	302	6.7	167	10.3	23.1	3.7	0.0
Chicken, & Salad, Tesco*	1 Pack/193g	386	17.6	200	11.9	17.6	9.1	1.5
Chicken, & Salad, Waitrose*	1 Pack/208g	406	19.8	195	10.3	17.1	9.5	2.5
Chicken, & Salad, Wild Bean Cafe*	1 Pack/210g	273	1.0	130	12.4	18.9	0.5	2.8
Chicken, & Salad, with Mayo, BGTY, Sainsbury's*	1 Serving/200g	314	4.8	157	12.0	21.9	2.4	0.0
Chicken, & Salad, with Mayo, Yummies*	1 Pack/154g	275	10.2	178	11.9	17.8	6.6	0.0
Chicken, & Salad with Mayo, Roast, Big, Sainsbury's*	1 Pack/269g	559	23.9	208	11.0	20.9	8.9	9.0
Chicken, & Stuffing, Antony Worrall Thompson's*	1 Pack/198g	485	28.3	245	16.0	13.1	14.3	2.8
Chicken, & Stuffing, Light Choices, Tesco*	1 Pack/172g	275	4.8	160	14.4	18.7	2.8	6.9
Chicken, & Stuffing, M & S*	1 Pack/166g	398	17.1	240	13.9	23.1	10.3	5.6
Chicken, & Stuffing, Roast, Boots*	1 Pack/235g	669	39.9	285	12.0	22.0	17.0	1.9
Chicken, & Stuffing, Roast, Deep Fill, Tesco*	1 Serving/220g	532	26.8	242	14.0	19.0	12.2	1.3
Chicken, & Stuffing, Roast, Shapers, Boots*	1 Pack/186g	324	3.9	174	14.0	25.0	2.1	3.1
Chicken, & Stuffing, Roast, Weight Watchers*	1 Pack/159g	283	4.5	178	14.1	24.2	2.8	3.1
Chicken, & Stuffing, Shapers, Boots*	1 Serving/185g	327	5.2	177	13.0	25.0	2.8	2.2
Chicken, & Stuffing, Sutherland*	1 Pack/201g	505	25.8	251	11.9	22.1	12.8	3.0
Chicken, & Stuffing, Tesco*	1 Pack/323g	1043	58.8	323	10.4	29.4	18.2	1.0
Chicken, & Stuffing, Waitrose*	1 Pack/183g	450	18.8	246	12.8	25.6	10.3	1.5
Chicken, & Sweet Chilli, Flora Light, Flora*	1 Pack/154g	296	5.7	192	13.1	27.0	3.7	1.9
Chicken, & Sweetcorn, Scottish Slimmers*	1 Pack/147g	289	7.2	197	11.1	27.4	4.9	2.2
Chicken, & Sweetcorn, Shapers, Boots*	1 Pack/180g	324	6.3	180	12.0	25.0	3.5	2.0
Chicken, & Sweetcorn, with Mayo, Benedicts*	1 Pack/185g	437	19.8	236	12.2	20.6	10.7	0.0
Chicken, & Tomato Relish, Chargrilled, Shapers, Boots*	1 Pack/190g	294	5.7	155	12.0	20.0	3.0	3.1
Chicken, & Watercress, Chargrilled, M & S*	1 Pack/173g	285	2.9	165	12.8	23.9	1.7	2.1
Chicken, & Watercress, COU, M & S*	1 Pack/164g	266	2.8	162	12.8	23.9	1.7	2.1
Chicken, Asian, Shapers, Boots*	1 Pack/190g	273	4.6	144	12.0	19.0	2.4	2.9
Chicken, Bacon, & Avocado, M & S*	1 Pack/242g	508	28.3	210	10.7	15.8	11.7	3.2
Chicken, Bacon, & Cheese, Club, M & S*	1 Pack/383g	805	37.2	210	11.9	18.5	9.7	1.9
Chicken, Bacon & Sweet Chilli, Feel Good, Shell*	1 Pack/174g	366	8.7	211	14.1	29.2	5.0	0.0
Chicken, Bacon & Tomato, BGTY, Sainsbury's*	1 Pack/190g	270	4.4	142	11.4	19.0	2.3	0.0
Chicken, Basil & Sunblush Tomato, Harry Mason*	1 Pack/164g	272	5.2	166	13.0	21.8	3.2	0.6
Chicken, Bechamel & Leek, Daily Bread*	1 Pack/210g	383	7.2	182	11.0	26.8	3.4	0.0
Chicken, Beef, & Ham, Triple Pack, Tesco*	1 Serving/272g	583	20.7	214	12.1	24.3	7.6	2.0
Chicken, BLT, Daily Bread*	1 Pack/187g	322	13.1	172	9.0	19.5	7.0	0.0
Chicken, BLT, Deli Continental*	1 Pack/224g	509	26.9	227	12.4	17.3	12.0	0.0
Chicken, BLT, Taste!*	1 Pack/239g	458	19.8	192	10.3	19.0	8.3	0.0
Chicken, Breast, BGTY, Sainsbury's*	1 Pack/165g	251	0.8	152	12.2	24.7	0.5	0.0
Chicken, Breast, Millers*	1 Pack/162g	343	14.4	212	13.8	19.3	8.9	0.0
Chicken, Breast, Oldfields*	1 Pack/193g	311	8.1	161	11.7	19.8	4.2	3.0
Chicken, Caesar, & Salad, GFY, Asda*	1 Pack/163g	289	4.6	177	11.0	27.0	2.8	2.1
Chicken, Caesar, & Salad, Sainsbury's*	1 Pack/186g	299	7.1	161	11.2	20.4	3.8	0.0
Chicken, Caesar, Boots*	1 Pack/226g	531	27.1	235	9.8	22.0	12.0	1.7
Chicken, Caesar, Chargrilled, Big, Sainsbury's*	1 Pack/216g	657	36.9	304	12.2	25.3	17.1	0.0
Chicken, Caesar, COU, M & S*	1 Pack/181g	244	4.3	135	12.2	19.9	2.4	4.3
Chicken, Caesar, Deli Continental*	1 Pack/169g	455	25.4	269	13.0	20.4	15.0	0.0
Chicken, Caesar, Finest, Tesco*	1 Pack/199g	454	19.9	228	15.4	19.2	10.0	1.4
Chicken, Chargrill, Choice*	1 Serving/161g	320	8.0	199	15.2	23.3	5.0	1.9
Chicken, Chargrilled, Ginsters*	1 Pack/209g	431	17.3	206	11.3	21.6	8.3	0.0
Chicken, Chargrilled, No Mayo, Rustlers*	1 Pack/150g	228	1.2	152	16.0	20.1	0.8	0.0
Chicken, Chargrilled, Pitta Pocket, M & S*	1 Pack/208g	279	7.3	134	11.2	14.5	3.5	1.6

SANDWICH

INFO/WEIGHT	Measure	per Measure		Nutrition Values per 100g / 100ml				
		KCAL	FAT	KCAL	PROT	CARB	FAT	FIBRE
Chicken, Chargrilled, with Salad, Weight Watchers*	1 Pack/181g	264	3.8	146	11.7	20.0	2.1	2.2
Chicken, Cheese, Bacon, Big, Sainsbury's*	1 Pack/254g	734	45.5	289	11.7	18.0	17.9	0.0
Chicken, Chilli, Fresh, Taste!*	1 Pack/155g	224	4.9	145	5.6	23.4	3.2	0.0
Chicken, Chilli, Taste!*	1 Pack/196g	317	5.7	162	11.5	22.6	2.9	0.0
Chicken, Chinese, Low Calorie, Tesco*	1 Pack/169g	270	4.2	160	11.8	22.6	2.5	2.0
Chicken, Chinese, Malted Brown Bread, Waitrose*	1 Pack/164g	333	11.2	203	13.5	21.9	6.8	3.3
Chicken, Chinese, Snack & Shop, Esso*	1 Pack/178g	409	16.0	230	13.0	22.8	9.0	4.0
Chicken, Chinese, Treat Yourself, Shell*	1 Pack/178g	409	17.1	230	13.0	22.8	9.6	0.0
Chicken, Coronation, Indulgence, Taste!*	1 Pack/159g	396	18.8	249	9.1	26.5	11.8	0.0
Chicken, Coronation, M & S*	1 Pack/210g	420	20.4	200	11.2	20.2	9.7	3.1
Chicken, Coronation, Taste!*	1 Pack/178g	367	13.4	206	10.6	24.0	7.5	0.0
Chicken, Creole, & Italian Leaves, Northern Bites*	1 Pack/190g	298	4.6	157	13.1	22.1	2.4	2.4
Chicken, Curry, Lifestyle*	1 Serving/160g	211	9.6	132	13.0	6.0	6.0	0.0
Chicken, Flame Grilled, Rustlers*	1 Pack/150g	346	14.2	231	16.3	20.1	9.5	0.0
Chicken, Ham, & Prawn, Triple, Weight Watchers*	1 Pack/250g	337	3.7	135	9.8	20.5	1.5	2.6
Chicken, Ham, Prawn, Triple Pack, HL, Tesco*	1 Pack/247g	350	5.2	142	10.7	20.2	2.1	2.2
Chicken, Ham & Pepperoni, Meat Feast, Tesco*	1 Pack/196g	470	22.5	240	14.7	19.4	11.5	1.5
Chicken, Harvester, Taste!*	1 Pack/200g	295	8.0	147	7.6	20.3	4.0	0.0
Chicken, Healthier Choice, Ginsters*	1 Pack/183g	247	2.6	135	10.2	20.5	1.4	0.0
Chicken, Honey & Mustard, BGTY, Sainsbury's*	1 Pack/171g	296	4.6	173	13.1	24.0	2.7	0.0
Chicken, Jalfrezi, Naan, Ready to Go, M & S*	1 Pack/288g	576	18.1	200	9.8	26.3	6.3	2.9
Chicken, Kashmir, French Cuisiniers*	1 Pack/145g	204	2.3	141	12.9	20.3	1.6	2.9
Chicken, Mexican, Healthy Choices, Shell*	1 Serving/168g	376	11.8	224	12.2	28.1	7.0	0.0
Chicken, No Mayo, Cafe Revive, M & S*	1 Pack/153g	229	3.7	150	14.1	17.9	2.4	3.1
Chicken, No Mayo, Daily Bread*	1 Pack/160g	279	7.1	174	8.6	23.8	4.4	0.0
Chicken, No Mayo, M & S*	1 Pack/142g	220	4.3	155	15.0	17.5	3.0	3.1
Chicken, No Mayonnaise, Waitrose*	1 Pack/173g	332	9.5	192	11.6	24.0	5.5	2.1
Chicken, Pesano Pesto, Brambles*	1 Pack/417g	826	26.3	198	10.8	24.0	6.3	1.5
Chicken, Red Thai, BGTY, Sainsbury's*	1 Pack/195g	326	3.7	167	11.3	26.4	1.9	0.0
Chicken, Red Thai, Foo-Go*	1 Pack/188g	358	14.9	190	10.2	19.4	7.9	4.4
Chicken, Red Thai, Taste!*	1 Pack/164g	335	9.8	204	11.5	26.1	6.0	0.0
Chicken, Roast, & Salad, Shapers, Boots*	1 Pack/183g	274	4.4	150	12.0	20.0	2.4	3.4
Chicken, Roast, Breast, BGTY, Sainsbury's*	1 Pack/174g	275	4.3	158	14.8	20.9	2.5	1.8
Chicken, Roast, HL, Tesco*	1 Pack/155g	288	5.3	186	13.5	25.4	3.4	1.4
Chicken, Roast, Salad, BGTY, Sainsbury's*	1 Pack/182g	268	4.0	147	11.9	19.9	2.2	2.7
Chicken, Roast, Shapers, Boots*	1 Pack/163g	259	2.1	159	16.0	21.0	1.3	2.5
Chicken, Roast, Tesco*	1 Pack/158g	412	19.7	261	13.1	23.9	12.5	1.5
Chicken, Roast, Triple, Perfectly Balanced, Waitrose*	1 Pack/254g	356	8.1	140	8.7	19.2	3.2	2.8
Chicken, Rustlers*	1 Pack/150g	346	14.2	231	16.3	20.1	9.5	0.0
Chicken, Salad, Aldi*	1 Pack/195g	338	4.5	173	11.5	23.8	2.3	2.0
Chicken, Salad, M & S*	1 Pack/226g	350	9.3	155	10.6	18.8	4.1	3.0
Chicken, Salad, On Malted Bread, BGTY, Sainsbury's*	1 Pack/216g	346	7.3	160	12.7	19.7	3.4	2.7
Chicken, Shell*	1 Pack/121g	334	15.7	276	13.9	25.9	13.0	0.0
Chicken, Smokey, BGTY, Sainsbury's*	1 Pack/178g	276	1.8	155	11.1	25.6	1.0	0.0
Chicken, Southern Fried, Rustlers*	1 Serving/145g	436	21.3	301	11.7	30.6	14.7	0.0
Chicken, Southern Fried Breast, Microwave, Tesco*	1 Burger/135g	381	17.1	282	13.0	28.9	12.7	1.6
Chicken, Southern Spiced, M & S*	1 Pack/179g	421	23.3	235	11.2	21.7	13.0	3.1
Chicken, Spicy, Deep Filled, Co-Op*	1 Pack/216g	421	15.1	195	10.0	24.0	7.0	3.0
Chicken, Sundried Tomato & Herb, Bells*	1 Pack/198g	400	18.8	202	10.2	18.9	9.5	0.0
Chicken, Tandoori, Finest, Tesco*	1 Pack/224g	421	16.8	188	10.8	19.2	7.5	1.4
Chicken, Tandoori, Waitrose*	1 Pack/181g	302	5.6	167	11.6	23.0	3.1	4.1
Chicken, Tangy Lime & Ginger, Shapers, Boots*	1 Pack/168g	319	10.8	190	12.0	21.0	6.4	5.1
Chicken, Thai, BGTY, Sainsbury's*	1 Pack/196g	280	5.1	143	10.2	19.6	2.6	0.6

S

SANDWICH

	Measure INFO/WEIGHT	per Measure KCAL	FAT	Nutrition Values per 100g / 100ml KCAL	PROT	CARB	FAT	FIBRE
Chicken, Thai, Tesco*	1 Pack/244g	634	38.3	260	8.5	21.1	15.7	1.5
Chicken, Tikka, & Yoghurt, Taste!*	1 Pack/215g	437	21.1	203	8.2	20.4	9.8	0.0
Chicken, Tikka, Asda*	1 Pack/186g	316	8.7	170	11.0	21.0	4.7	1.5
Chicken, Tikka, COU, M & S*	1 Pack/185g	268	3.3	145	12.1	20.5	1.8	3.2
Chicken, Tikka, M & S*	1 Pack/180g	391	19.6	217	10.4	19.5	10.9	2.0
Chicken, Tikka, on Pepper Chilli Bread, Shapers, Boots*	1 Pack/172g	296	4.5	172	13.0	25.0	2.6	2.5
Chicken, Tikka, Open, COU, M & S*	1 Pack/190g	260	2.2	137	9.6	21.8	1.2	2.2
Chicken, Tikka, Sayers Bakery*	1 Pack/203g	315	7.5	155	10.8	19.8	3.7	2.8
Chicken, Tikka, Taste!*	1 Pack/196g	368	11.7	188	11.7	21.7	6.0	0.0
Chicken, Tikka, Thai Style, Korma, Big, Sainsbury's*	1 Pack/268g	581	26.0	217	11.9	20.5	9.7	0.0
Chicken, Tikka, Weight Watchers*	1 Pack/158g	250	2.2	158	13.1	23.2	1.4	2.9
Chicken, Tikka Masala, Go Foods Wonderfill*	1 Pack/136g	343	17.4	252	11.4	23.5	12.8	0.0
Chicken, Tomato & Rocket, Light Choices, Tesco*	1 Pack/184g	285	3.9	155	10.3	23.4	2.1	2.6
Chicken, Triple, GFY, Asda*	1 Pack/230g	453	11.5	197	13.0	25.0	5.0	1.6
Chicken, Triple, Shapers, Boots*	1 Serving/228g	440	12.3	193	13.0	23.0	5.4	2.3
Chicken, with Fresh Herb Salad, Roast, British, Asda*	1 Pack/214g	447	19.3	209	11.0	21.0	9.0	2.0
Chicken, with Mayo, on Thick Softgrain, Tasties*	1 Pack/192g	338	15.2	176	9.5	16.1	7.9	0.0
Chicken, with Pork Sage & Onion Stuffing, Tesco*	1 Pack/136g	376	17.0	276	12.1	28.1	12.5	1.4
Chicken, Working Lunch*	1 Pack/169g	298	7.7	176	14.0	19.9	4.5	1.8
Classic Feast, M & S*	1 Serving/295g	841	51.6	285	10.6	21.3	17.5	4.7
Club, New York Style, Sainsbury's*	1 Serving/212g	608	33.5	287	13.3	22.8	15.8	2.7
Corned Beef, & Tomato, & Onion, Salad Garden*	1 Pack/137g	338	14.8	247	14.2	23.0	10.8	0.0
Corned Beef, on White, Simply, Brambles*	1 Pack/126g	325	10.8	258	14.2	30.8	8.6	1.4
Coronation Chicken, in Pitta Bread, COU, M & S*	1 Serving/207g	269	2.5	130	9.2	20.4	1.2	2.0
Crayfish, & Lemon Mayonnaise, Daily Bread*	1 Pack/173g	391	11.4	226	9.5	31.0	6.6	0.0
Crayfish, & Rocket, Bistro, Waitrose*	1 Pack/193g	422	19.5	219	11.5	20.4	10.1	2.4
Crayfish, & Rocket, Shapers, Boots*	1 Pack/172g	291	3.8	169	11.0	26.0	2.2	2.5
Crayfish & Rocket, Bells*	1 Pack/144g	276	11.8	192	11.2	18.4	8.2	2.0
Crayfish & Rocket, Finest, Tesco*	1 Pack/178g	365	10.5	205	9.8	27.5	5.9	2.1
Cream Cheese, & Ham, Tesco*	1 Pack/212g	655	36.7	309	11.0	27.2	17.3	1.2
Cream Cheese, & Peppers, Taste!*	1 Pack/154g	296	10.5	192	7.3	25.5	6.8	0.0
Cream Cheese, & Salad, Choice*	1 Serving/156g	294	7.4	188	7.8	28.1	4.7	0.0
Cream Cheese, & Salad, Sandwich Box*	1 Pack/138g	250	8.0	181	5.6	26.3	5.8	0.0
Cream Cheese, Red Pepper & Spinach, Daily Bread*	1 Pack/156g	273	8.1	175	7.4	24.0	5.2	0.0
Cumberland Sausage, Ginsters*	1 Pack/210g	564	29.5	268	9.3	26.0	14.0	2.4
Duck, Peking, No Mayo, Boots*	1 Pack/222g	399	10.2	180	7.7	27.0	4.6	1.7
Edam, & Tomato, & Spring Onion, BHS*	1 Serving/184g	313	9.4	170	8.6	22.5	5.1	3.2
Edam, & Tomato, Low Fat, Oldfields*	1 Pack/173g	306	6.4	177	9.6	26.3	3.7	2.7
Edam, Oldfields*	1 Pack/175g	326	9.9	186	9.8	23.9	5.7	0.0
Egg, & Bacon, & Lincolnshire Sausage, Waitrose*	1 Pack/249g	655	32.9	263	11.3	24.7	13.2	0.9
Egg, & Bacon, Weight Watchers*	1 Pack/139g	246	5.0	177	10.1	26.1	3.6	1.9
Egg, & Cress, Co-Op*	1 Pack/159g	397	23.8	250	9.0	21.0	15.0	2.0
Egg, & Cress, COU, M & S*	1 Pack/192g	240	5.2	125	9.8	15.5	2.7	2.8
Egg, & Cress, Free Range, Co-Op*	1 Pack/154g	370	18.5	240	8.0	25.0	12.0	3.0
Egg, & Cress, Free Range, M & S*	1 Pack/192g	307	9.0	160	10.7	17.8	4.7	3.0
Egg, & Cress, Free Range, Sainsbury's*	1 Pack/204g	404	16.9	198	10.5	20.3	8.3	3.3
Egg, & Cress, Heinz*	1 Pack/200g	610	21.6	305	14.4	37.5	10.8	4.0
Egg, & Cress, M & S*	1 Pack/182g	331	17.7	182	10.1	13.6	9.7	3.2
Egg, & Cress, on Wholemeal Bread, Refectory*	1 Pack/140g	323	14.7	231	9.8	24.7	10.5	0.0
Egg, & Cress, Organic, M & S*	1 Pack/185g	444	26.3	240	9.6	18.0	14.2	3.6
Egg, & Cress, Reduced Fat, Waitrose*	1 Pack/162g	262	10.4	162	9.7	16.5	6.4	6.4
Egg, & Cress, with Mayo, Oatmeal Bread, Heinz*	1 Pack/150g	304	10.8	203	9.6	25.0	7.2	2.7
Egg, & Ham, Asda*	1 Pack/262g	589	33.5	225	10.4	16.8	12.8	2.1

S

SANDWICH	Measure INFO/WEIGHT	per Measure KCAL	FAT	Nutrition Values per 100g / 100ml KCAL	PROT	CARB	FAT	FIBRE
Egg, & Salad, Co-Op*	1 Pack/190g	285	7.6	150	7.0	22.0	4.0	4.0
Egg, & Salad, Deep Filled, Asda*	1 Pack/231g	395	16.2	171	8.0	19.0	7.0	1.0
Egg, & Salad, Free Range, Sainsbury's*	1 Pack/225g	449	16.8	200	8.5	24.5	7.5	0.0
Egg, & Salad, Free Range, Waitrose*	1 Pack/180g	281	11.5	156	7.6	16.9	6.4	3.3
Egg, & Salad, GFY, Asda*	1 Pack/157g	229	4.5	146	8.0	22.0	2.9	2.9
Egg, & Salad, Shapers, Boots*	1 Pack/184g	304	8.5	165	6.9	24.0	4.6	1.1
Egg, & Salad, Weight Watchers*	1 Pack/172g	237	4.6	138	7.1	21.3	2.7	2.2
Egg, & Salad, with Mayonnaise, Wholemeal, Waitrose*	1 Pack/180g	257	8.8	143	8.3	16.5	4.9	3.6
Egg, & Tomato, on Softgrain Bread, Daily Bread*	1 Pack/160g	279	7.1	174	8.6	23.8	4.4	0.0
Egg, & Tomato, Organic, Waitrose*	1 Pack/192g	359	18.6	187	9.7	15.3	9.7	4.0
Egg, & Tomato, Tesco*	1 Pack/172g	311	10.8	181	8.5	22.6	6.3	2.3
Egg, & Tomato, with Salad Cream, Big, Sainsbury's*	1 Pack/266g	463	15.4	174	9.1	21.3	5.8	0.0
Egg, Co-Op*	1 Pack/190g	285	7.0	150	6.8	22.1	3.7	3.7
Egg, Delilite*	1 Pack/180g	336	12.9	187	8.0	22.0	7.2	3.0
Egg & Bacon, Deep Fill, Ginsters*	1 Pack/216g	503	21.8	233	14.5	21.0	10.1	2.3
Egg & Bacon Mayo, Delifresh*	1 Pack/129g	310	12.6	240	10.1	29.7	9.8	2.1
Egg & Cress, BGTY, Sainsbury's*	1 Pack/145g	268	7.5	185	9.1	25.4	5.2	2.7
Egg & Cress, No Mayo, Light Choices, Tesco*	1 Pack/160g	280	6.9	175	9.5	24.2	4.3	2.7
Egg & Cress, on Wheat Germ Bread, Tesco*	1 Pack/174g	365	15.8	210	11.0	20.5	9.1	2.1
Egg & Cress, Reduced Fat, Asda*	1 Pack/164g	290	8.7	177	9.8	22.4	5.3	0.0
Egg & Tomato, Delicious, Boots*	1 Pack/218g	362	10.0	166	8.2	22.0	4.6	2.0
Egg Mayonnaise, & Bacon, Boots*	1 Serving/200g	426	14.0	213	13.5	23.5	7.0	2.8
Egg Mayonnaise, & Cress, BHS*	1 Serving/188g	462	23.9	246	10.0	24.7	12.7	1.9
Egg Mayonnaise, & Cress, Co-Op*	1 Pack/159g	405	24.0	255	8.8	20.8	15.1	1.9
Egg Mayonnaise, & Cress, Go Simple, Asda*	1 Pack/169g	370	18.6	219	10.0	20.0	11.0	1.7
Egg Mayonnaise, & Cress, Millers*	1 Pack/166g	369	20.3	222	9.4	18.8	12.2	0.0
Egg Mayonnaise, & Cress, Reduced Fat, Waitrose*	1 Pack/162g	300	12.8	185	10.4	18.1	7.9	3.4
Egg Mayonnaise, & Cress, Shapers, Boots*	1 Pack/156g	292	7.6	187	11.0	25.0	4.9	2.6
Egg Mayonnaise, & Cress, Weight Watchers*	1 Pack/126g	238	4.2	189	8.8	31.1	3.3	3.3
Egg Mayonnaise, & Cress, Wheatgerm Bread, Asda*	1 Pack/158g	371	19.6	235	9.7	21.3	12.4	1.9
Egg Mayonnaise, & Cress, Wholemeal Bread, Oldfields*	1 Pack/128g	301	14.3	235	9.7	24.0	11.2	3.6
Egg Mayonnaise, & Cress, Yummies*	1 Serving/150g	427	30.0	285	8.4	17.8	20.0	0.0
Egg Mayonnaise, & Gammon Ham, Strollers*	1 Pack/170g	400	19.3	236	13.0	20.5	11.4	0.0
Egg Mayonnaise, & Iceburg Lettuce, Northern Bites*	1 Serving/152g	333	17.2	219	7.7	20.9	11.3	0.0
Egg Mayonnaise, & Salad, Superdrug*	1 Pack/169g	286	12.3	169	7.6	18.3	7.3	2.4
Egg Mayonnaise, Boots*	1 Pack/184g	448	23.9	244	9.7	22.0	13.0	2.3
Egg Mayonnaise, Deep Fill, Benedicts*	1 Pack/195g	560	21.6	287	9.6	36.3	11.1	0.0
Egg Mayonnaise, Free Range, Finest, Tesco*	1 Pack/217g	412	19.1	190	10.9	16.8	8.8	2.3
Egg Mayonnaise, HL, Tesco*	1 Pack/162g	253	6.0	156	9.3	21.4	3.7	2.8
Egg Mayonnaise, on Hi Bran Bread, Ginsters*	1 Pack/143g	343	21.7	240	10.7	17.6	15.2	0.0
Egg Mayonnaise, on Malted Wheatgrain, Taste!*	1 Serving/169g	394	20.8	233	10.6	20.0	12.3	0.0
Egg Mayonnaise, Shell*	1 Pack/189g	522	29.1	276	9.8	24.7	15.4	0.0
Egg Mayonnaise, Simply, Boots*	1 Pack/181g	449	27.1	248	9.2	19.0	15.0	2.9
Egg Mayonnaise, Simply, Ginsters*	1 Serving/163g	365	15.9	224	10.1	24.0	9.7	3.1
Egg Mayonnaise, Snack & Shop, Esso*	1 Pack/240g	624	32.2	260	9.4	25.5	13.4	0.0
Egg Mayonnaise, Waitrose*	1 Pack/180g	396	20.5	220	10.1	19.1	11.4	3.4
Eggstatic, On Malted Brown Bread, Cranks*	1 Pack/193g	388	16.4	201	8.7	1.2	8.5	1.6
Feta Cheese, & Salad, Tastte*	1 Pack/178g	367	13.4	206	10.6	24.0	7.5	0.0
Feta Cheese, Bells*	1 Pack/223g	468	26.3	210	7.1	18.8	11.8	0.0
Fish, Triple, Co-Op*	1 Serving/233g	420	9.3	180	10.0	26.0	4.0	3.0
Gammon, & Salad, Tasties*	1 Pack/172g	261	6.0	152	9.6	20.6	3.5	0.0
Goat's Cheese, & Cranberry, Shapers, Boots*	1 Pack/150g	323	6.3	216	8.4	36.0	4.2	2.6
Goat's Cheese, Sunblush Tomato, Deli Continental*	1 Pack/179g	480	29.4	268	9.5	20.5	16.4	0.0

S

SANDWICH

	Measure INFO/WEIGHT	KCAL	FAT	KCAL	PROT	CARB	FAT	FIBRE
Greek Salad, Classic, Cafe, Primo*	1 Serving/216g	513	26.9	238	8.6	23.1	12.5	1.8
Ham, & Cheese, Light Choices, Tesco*	1 Pack/158g	284	5.1	180	14.5	22.8	3.2	5.0
Ham, & Cheese, Morrisons*	1 Serving/183g	273	4.6	149	12.5	19.2	2.5	4.1
Ham, & Coleslaw, Smoked, Brambles*	1 Pack/166g	283	4.1	171	8.2	28.8	2.5	1.8
Ham, & Edam, Smoked, Shapers, Boots*	1 Pack/183g	315	11.9	172	9.3	19.0	6.5	2.7
Ham, & Mustard, Heinz*	1 Pack/180g	460	20.7	255	11.8	25.6	11.5	5.0
Ham, & Mustard, Salad, BGTY, Sainsbury's*	1 Pack/183g	261	3.8	143	8.7	22.4	2.1	2.6
Ham, & Mustard, Smoked, Tesco*	1 Pack/156g	385	19.5	247	11.1	22.4	12.5	1.0
Ham, & Mustard, Tesco*	1 Pack/147g	437	27.9	297	10.6	20.8	19.0	1.2
Ham, & Philadelphia Light, Dry Cured, Boots*	1 Pack/172g	339	9.3	197	12.8	24.4	5.4	2.5
Ham, & Pineapple Salsa, Maple Flavoured, Waitrose*	1 Pack/194g	329	8.9	170	8.4	23.8	4.6	3.1
Ham, & Salad, & Mustard, Darwins Deli*	1 Serving/180g	574	13.7	319	14.0	48.5	7.6	0.0
Ham, & Salad, Brambles*	1 Serving/173g	289	6.8	167	10.1	23.2	3.9	1.2
Ham, & Salad, British, COU, M & S*	1 Pack/204g	255	4.3	125	6.7	19.9	2.1	2.9
Ham, & Salad, Foo-Go*	1 Pack/178g	297	7.1	167	9.8	22.9	4.0	0.0
Ham, & Salad, Fulfilled*	1 Serving/183g	288	6.4	157	11.8	19.9	3.5	0.0
Ham, & Salad, Fullfillers*	1 Pack/180g	290	7.9	161	7.3	22.9	4.4	0.0
Ham, & Salad, Ginsters*	1 Pack/179g	287	6.2	160	8.8	23.5	3.4	0.0
Ham, & Salad, Healthy Options, Oldfields*	1 Pack/156g	229	3.0	147	8.7	24.0	1.9	0.0
Ham, & Salad, Leicester, Waitrose*	1 Serving/187g	325	9.0	174	8.6	24.0	4.8	1.6
Ham, & Salad, Select*	1 Serving/180g	266	4.7	148	8.0	23.2	2.6	0.0
Ham, & Salad, Shapers, Boots*	1 Pack/195g	269	2.7	138	9.4	22.0	1.4	1.8
Ham, & Salad, Smoked, Ainsley Harriott*	1 Pack/218g	307	6.3	141	8.9	19.9	2.9	0.0
Ham, & Salad, Smoked, Taste!*	1 Serving/188g	309	9.7	164	9.8	19.8	5.2	0.0
Ham, & Salad, Snack & Shop, Esso*	1 Pack/191g	304	6.5	159	9.2	22.9	3.4	5.0
Ham, & Salad, Wild Bean Cafe*	1 Pack/212g	301	5.5	142	10.7	18.8	2.6	2.0
Ham, & Salad, with Mustard, Finest, Tesco*	1 Pack/200g	466	21.0	233	15.3	19.3	10.5	1.3
Ham, & Soft Cheese, Tesco*	1 Serving/164g	333	12.1	203	11.6	22.5	7.4	2.2
Ham, & Swiss Cheese, Big, Sainsbury's*	1 Pack/218g	652	36.4	299	11.6	25.4	16.7	0.5
Ham, & Swiss Cheese, M & S*	1 Pack/159g	393	20.0	247	14.7	18.9	12.6	3.3
Ham, & Tomato, Brambles*	1 Pack/159g	288	7.3	181	11.1	24.1	4.6	3.3
Ham, & Tomato, GFY, Asda*	1 Pack/173g	254	2.9	147	10.0	23.0	1.7	1.4
Ham, & Tomato, Honey Roast, Feel Good, Shell*	1 Pack/171g	388	18.8	227	9.8	22.1	11.0	0.0
Ham, & Turkey, & Salad, Sutherland*	1 Pack/185g	303	4.8	164	9.8	25.2	2.6	0.0
Ham, & Turkey, Asda*	1 Pack/190g	393	19.4	207	12.9	15.8	10.2	2.3
Ham, & Turkey, Healthy, Felix Van Den Berghe*	1 Pack/149g	263	5.9	177	9.4	26.2	4.0	0.0
Ham, & Turkey, with Salad, Co-Op*	1 Pack/188g	263	5.6	140	9.0	21.0	3.0	2.0
Ham, & Turkey, with Salad, Healthy Living, Co-Op*	1 Serving/181g	290	5.4	160	10.0	24.0	3.0	3.0
Ham, Cheese, & Pickle, Healthy Choice, Sutherland*	1 Pack/185g	368	7.4	199	13.4	27.4	4.0	0.0
Ham, Cheese, & Pickle, Healthy Living, Co-Op*	1 Pack/185g	370	7.4	200	13.0	27.0	4.0	3.0
Ham, Cheese, & Pickle, Heinz*	1 Pack/188g	466	24.2	248	11.3	21.7	12.9	4.8
Ham, Cheese, & Pickle, Leicester, Waitrose*	1 Pack/205g	512	24.4	250	11.9	23.7	11.9	2.1
Ham, Cheese, & Pickle, Taste!*	1 Pack/174g	414	21.7	238	11.1	20.3	12.5	0.0
Ham, Cheese, Pickle & Lettuce, No Mayo, Tesco*	1 Pack/207g	435	16.2	210	12.2	23.0	7.8	2.7
Ham, Cheese & Pickle, Deep Fill, Tesco*	1 Pack/225g	495	20.7	220	14.6	19.4	9.2	2.4
Ham, Cheese & Pickle, in a Soft Wrap, Sainsbury's*	1 Pack/195g	503	23.2	258	10.9	26.8	11.9	0.9
Ham, Just Ham, Shoprite*	1 Pack/148g	286	7.1	193	12.4	25.0	4.8	0.0
Ham, M & S*	1 Pack/200g	220	5.2	110	17.2	3.2	2.6	0.0
Ham, Smoked, Fresh, Taste!*	1 Pack/187g	286	9.0	153	9.1	18.4	4.8	0.0
Ham, Tomato, & Lettuce, Oldfields*	1 Pack/216g	393	17.5	182	12.3	19.0	8.1	3.5
Ham & Mustard, Ginsters*	1 Pack/140g	307	9.4	219	11.8	28.0	6.7	2.5
Ham Salad, Light Choices, HL, Tesco*	1 Pack/190g	266	5.3	140	11.0	19.8	2.8	2.1
Ham Smoked, on a Roll, Cafe Life, Brambles*	1 Pack/211g	485	12.4	230	9.0	35.2	5.9	2.2

SANDWICH

Measure INFO/WEIGHT		per Measure		Nutrition Values per 100g / 100ml				
		KCAL	FAT	KCAL	PROT	CARB	FAT	FIBRE
Houmous, & Crunchy Salad, Oldfields*	1 Pack/180g	256	7.6	142	6.3	20.0	4.2	0.0
Houmous, & Grilled Vegetable, Deep Filled, Dd's*	1 Pack/200g	314	6.0	157	6.4	26.2	3.0	1.5
Houmous, & Olive Bread, Flora Light, Flora*	1 Pack/160g	258	9.2	161	5.0	22.4	5.7	1.9
Houmous, Tomato, & Red Onion, Daily Bread*	1 Serving/184g	367	17.7	199	6.9	22.7	9.6	0.0
Houmous & Carrot, Shapers, Boots*	1 Pack/204g	323	10.2	158	7.5	21.0	5.0	5.2
Indian Triple, Sainsbury's*	1 Serving/265g	549	16.2	207	12.8	25.2	6.1	0.0
Just Chicken, No Mayo, Tesco*	1 Pack/120g	246	3.8	205	15.9	28.1	3.2	3.8
Just Ham, No Mayo, Tesco*	1 Pack/122g	250	4.9	205	11.6	30.4	4.0	2.1
King Prawn, & Wild Rocket, Honduran, M & S*	1 Serving/196g	450	23.9	230	9.4	20.3	12.2	1.4
King Prawn, Sainsbury's*	1 Pack/204g	424	16.3	208	11.6	22.3	8.0	0.0
King Prawn & Avocado, Finest, Tesco*	1 Pack/185g	370	16.6	200	9.1	19.6	9.0	2.5
King Prawn & Harissa, Foo-Go*	1 Pack/180g	282	6.8	157	9.1	21.6	3.8	3.4
Lemon Chicken & Mangetout Salad, COU, M & S*	1 Pack/186g	260	5.0	140	10.6	19.0	2.7	3.7
Lemon Chicken with Herb Dressing, Ginsters*	1 Pack/170g	363	12.3	213	12.2	25.0	7.2	2.6
Mediterranean Style, Triple, GFY, Asda*	1 Pack/211g	352	4.4	167	11.0	26.0	2.1	2.3
Mozzarella, & Pepperoni, Sainsbury's*	1 Pack/171g	380	12.2	222	10.5	29.0	7.1	0.0
Mozzarella, & Tomato, Waitrose*	1 Pack/193g	359	18.1	186	9.7	15.7	9.4	2.3
Mozzarella, & Tomato Calzone, Waitrose*	1 Pack/175g	409	19.4	234	10.8	22.7	11.1	2.2
Mozzarella, Italian Style, Taste!*	1 Pack/183g	390	19.4	213	9.2	20.1	10.6	2.0
Mozzarella, Pesto & Pine Nuts, Sainsbury's*	1 Pack/180g	423	17.5	235	10.2	26.8	9.7	2.8
Mozzarella, Tomato, & Basil, Healthy Options, Oldfields*	1 Pack/175g	285	8.4	163	8.1	22.1	4.8	3.3
New York Deli, Boots*	1 Pack/245g	397	12.5	162	10.0	19.0	5.1	1.7
New York Deli, Extra Special, Asda*	1 Pack/201g	403	15.4	201	12.4	20.6	7.7	3.8
Philadelphia Salad, The Classic Sandwich Co*	1 Pack/135g	264	12.3	196	6.2	22.1	9.1	0.0
Pitta, Falafel, Houmous & Salad, Benedicts*	1 Pack/220g	405	13.0	184	6.8	26.1	5.9	0.0
Ploughman's, Cheddar, Heinz*	1 Pack/208g	552	27.7	265	9.3	27.1	13.3	2.4
Ploughman's, Cheddar, Mature Vintage, Sainsbury's*	1 Pack/204g	439	20.2	215	9.3	22.3	9.9	0.0
Ploughman's, Cheddar Cheese, Deep Fill, Asda*	1 Pack/229g	471	22.9	206	9.0	20.0	10.0	4.3
Ploughman's, Cheese, BGTY, Sainsbury's*	1 Pack/193g	326	8.1	169	9.8	22.8	4.2	3.6
Ploughman's, Cheese, Deep Fill, Sutherland*	1 Pack/220g	558	32.3	254	9.2	21.4	14.7	0.0
Ploughman's, Deep Fill, Ginsters*	1 Pack/232g	636	40.8	274	9.6	20.8	17.6	0.0
Ploughman's, Deep Fill, Tesco*	1 Pack/245g	551	27.4	225	10.9	20.2	11.2	1.4
Ploughman's, Deep Filled, Asda*	1 Pack/254g	650	36.8	256	10.3	21.3	14.5	2.9
Ploughmans, Light Choices, Tesco*	1 Pack/178g	320	7.5	180	12.2	22.9	4.2	3.3
Ploughman's, Taste!*	1 Pack/205g	492	27.3	240	9.5	20.6	13.3	0.0
Poached Salmon, & Watercress, Lochmuir, M & S*	1 Pack/192g	355	11.7	185	10.3	22.3	6.1	1.6
Pork, & Apple Sauce, Bells*	1 Pack/180g	341	8.1	190	11.5	26.1	4.5	0.0
Prawn, & Egg, Deep Filled, Asda*	1 Pack/250g	570	30.0	228	12.0	17.0	12.0	2.3
Prawn, & Salmon, Waitrose*	1 Pack/154g	345	14.6	224	12.5	22.0	9.5	2.8
Prawn, & Smoked Salmon, M & S*	1 Pack/445g	1135	63.6	255	11.7	19.3	14.3	1.4
Prawn, & Thai Dressing, Tiger, Waitrose*	1 Pack/200g	342	8.6	171	9.6	23.6	4.3	2.2
Prawn, Crayfish & Rocket, Tesco*	1 Pack/193g	425	17.4	220	11.4	22.3	9.0	2.0
Prawn, Creme Fraiche, on Oatmeal Bread, Choice*	1 Pack/153g	265	5.2	173	11.7	23.8	3.4	1.9
Prawn, Egg & Chicken, Triple, Weight Watchers*	1 Pack/224g	367	6.0	164	10.2	24.8	2.7	2.9
Prawn, Marie Rose, Felix Van Den Berghe*	1 Pack/163g	372	16.3	228	12.8	21.9	10.0	0.0
Prawn, Marie Rose, Fulfilled*	1 Pack/149g	292	6.1	196	13.4	26.3	4.1	0.0
Prawn, Marie Rose, Waitrose*	1 Pack/164g	226	5.6	138	8.8	18.0	3.4	1.9
Prawn, Mayo, Tomato & Lettuce, Deep Fill, Benedicts*	1 Pack/200g	330	7.8	165	10.2	21.9	3.9	0.0
Prawn, Roast Chicken, BLT, Triple, Waitrose*	1 Pack/241g	653	42.7	271	9.2	18.8	17.7	1.6
Prawn, Salad, COU, M & S*	1 Pack/200g	230	3.6	115	8.0	16.6	1.8	3.8
Prawn, Shell*	1 Serving/209g	523	27.4	250	9.4	23.7	13.1	0.0
Prawn, Thai Style, Ginsters*	1 Pack/183g	313	9.0	171	9.2	22.5	4.9	0.0
Prawn Cocktail, Classic, Heinz*	1 Pack/193g	409	16.8	212	8.4	25.0	8.7	2.5

S

SANDWICH

	Measure INFO/WEIGHT	per Measure KCAL	FAT	Nutrition Values per 100g / 100ml KCAL	PROT	CARB	FAT	FIBRE
Prawn Cocktail, Jumbo Tiger, Benedicts*	1 Serving/225g	349	10.8	155	7.4	20.4	4.8	0.0
Prawn Cocktail, Waitrose*	1 Pack/196g	300	8.0	153	8.3	20.7	4.1	2.5
Prawn Cocktail, Weight Watchers*	1 Pack/168g	252	7.7	150	8.9	18.1	4.6	2.8
Prawn Mayo, Ham Salad Triple Pack, Sutherland*	1 Pack/253g	620	30.1	245	9.8	24.8	11.9	0.3
Prawn Mayonnaise, Cafe Collection*	1 Pack/165g	454	27.7	275	11.6	20.7	16.8	1.7
Prawn Mayonnaise, Co-Op*	1 Pack/154g	285	6.0	185	9.7	27.3	3.9	3.2
Prawn Mayonnaise, COU, M & S*	1 Pack/155g	240	3.6	155	10.2	22.9	2.3	2.8
Prawn Mayonnaise, Daily Bread*	1 Pack/157g	374	17.2	239	11.9	23.0	11.0	0.0
Prawn Mayonnaise, GFY, Asda*	1 Pack/160g	251	4.5	157	10.0	23.0	2.8	2.8
Prawn Mayonnaise, Ginsters*	1 Pack/160g	397	21.1	248	9.1	23.3	13.2	2.4
Prawn Mayonnaise, Healthy Living, Co-Op*	1 Pack/154g	246	3.5	160	10.0	24.0	2.3	3.0
Prawn Mayonnaise, Heinz*	1 Pack/180g	493	28.4	274	8.9	24.0	15.8	2.5
Prawn Mayonnaise, Light Choices, HL, Tesco*	1 Pack/147g	250	6.8	170	10.0	21.7	4.6	2.1
Prawn Mayonnaise, M & S*	1 Pack/156g	328	12.0	210	10.0	24.7	7.7	2.2
Prawn Mayonnaise, Morrisons*	1 Pack/157g	234	3.9	149	9.0	22.7	2.5	3.0
Prawn Mayonnaise, Nutritionally Balanced, M & S*	1 Pack/162g	300	10.7	185	10.2	21.2	6.6	1.9
Prawn Mayonnaise, Oatmeal Bread, Co-Op*	1 Pack/159g	445	22.3	280	11.0	28.0	14.0	2.0
Prawn Mayonnaise, Oatmeal Bread, Waitrose*	1 Pack/180g	463	27.0	257	10.2	20.4	15.0	3.2
Prawn Mayonnaise, on Oatmeal Bread, Fulfilled*	1 Pack/144g	393	19.9	273	12.7	24.3	13.8	0.0
Prawn Mayonnaise, on Oatmeal Bread, Taste!*	1 Pack/144g	320	12.0	222	12.6	24.3	8.3	1.5
Prawn Mayonnaise, Sainsbury's*	1 Pack/151g	323	14.0	214	11.6	20.9	9.3	0.0
Prawn Mayonnaise, Sayers Bakery*	1 Pack/155g	449	27.7	290	9.7	22.5	17.9	2.1
Prawn Mayonnaise, Shapers, Boots*	1 Pack/160g	293	7.5	183	9.4	25.6	4.7	2.5
Prawn Mayonnaise, Simply, Boots*	1 Pack/261g	736	47.0	282	11.0	19.0	18.0	2.2
Prawn Mayonnaise, Tesco*	1 Pack/152g	350	16.3	230	10.2	22.2	10.7	2.6
Prawn Mayonnaise, Triple, Asda*	1 Pack/248g	635	39.7	256	9.0	19.0	16.0	3.4
Prawn Mayonnaise, Triple, Tesco*	1 Pack/231g	603	33.0	261	9.5	23.5	14.3	1.6
Prawn Mayonnaise, Upper Crust*	1 Pack/208g	343	10.4	165	9.2	20.9	5.0	0.0
Prawn Mayonnaise On Oatmeal Bread, Sainsbury's*	1 Pack/150g	285	9.3	190	10.1	22.3	6.2	2.4
Rare Roast Beef, & Horseradish, Eat Well, M & S*	1 Serving/200g	360	9.2	180	13.1	21.9	4.6	2.7
Rib, BBQ, Pork, Rustlers*	1 Pack/170g	459	22.1	270	14.3	22.9	13.0	2.0
Roast Chicken, Bells*	1 Pack/196g	257	3.7	131	8.2	19.7	1.9	1.9
Roast Chicken, Ginsters*	1 Pack/160g	313	10.1	196	13.6	21.2	6.3	2.6
Roast Chicken & Stuffing, Light Choices, Tesco*	1 Pack/169g	304	3.4	180	14.9	24.6	2.0	1.9
Salad, & Salad Cream, Fulfilled*	1 Pack/172g	244	7.1	142	4.9	21.5	4.1	0.0
Salad, Healthy, Cambridge University Catering*	1 Pack/156g	246	4.4	158	5.9	27.4	2.8	0.0
Salad, Northern Bites*	1 Pack/210g	193	4.2	92	4.1	15.3	2.0	3.0
Salad, Serious About Sandwiches*	1 Pack/237g	322	11.6	136	5.8	17.1	4.9	0.8
Salad, Simply, Brambles*	1 Serving/151g	242	6.1	160	5.8	25.2	4.0	3.6
Salad, Simply, Shapers, Boots*	1 Pack/216g	300	6.3	139	5.2	23.0	2.9	1.8
Salad, Taste!*	1 Serving/200g	246	6.5	123	4.4	18.9	3.2	0.0
Salmon, & Black Pepper, Smoked, Fulfilled*	1 Pack/120g	293	10.3	244	13.8	29.0	8.6	0.0
Salmon, & Cucumber, Brown Bread, Waitrose*	1 Pack/150g	295	10.6	197	10.5	22.7	7.1	1.4
Salmon, & Cucumber, Healthy Choice, Sutherland*	1 Pack/164g	321	9.2	196	9.8	26.6	5.6	0.0
Salmon, & Cucumber, Light Choices, Tesco*	1 Pack/155g	262	3.9	169	12.3	24.1	2.5	2.1
Salmon, & Cucumber, M & S*	1 Pack/168g	329	13.9	196	11.0	19.5	8.3	2.6
Salmon, & Cucumber, Red, BGTY, Sainsbury's*	1 Pack/192g	278	4.4	145	9.4	21.7	2.3	2.4
Salmon, & Cucumber, Red, Healthy Choice, Asda*	1 Pack/149g	285	11.5	191	10.6	19.9	7.7	2.1
Salmon, & Cucumber, Red, Tesco*	1 Pack/144g	284	9.2	197	11.1	23.8	6.4	1.9
Salmon, & Cucumber, White Bread, Waitrose*	1 Pack/161g	305	8.6	189	9.8	25.5	5.3	1.7
Salmon, & Rocket, Poached, M & S*	1 Pack/180g	495	26.8	275	13.5	21.2	14.9	2.1
Salmon, & Soft Cheese, Feel Good, Shell*	1 Pack/174g	404	12.9	232	13.5	28.0	7.4	1.0
Salmon, & Soft Cheese, Smoked, Waitrose*	1 Pack/154g	300	10.0	195	14.8	19.2	6.5	4.2

S

SANDWICH

	Measure INFO/WEIGHT	per Measure KCAL	FAT	Nutrition Values per 100g / 100ml KCAL	PROT	CARB	FAT	FIBRE
Salmon, & Spinach, Poached, Shapers, Boots*	1 Pack/168g	284	7.6	169	9.2	23.0	4.5	3.1
Salmon, Poached, Prawn & Rocket, Waitrose*	1 Pack/166g	308	8.6	186	11.2	23.5	5.2	2.1
Salmon, Red, Wild & Cucumber, Eat Well, M & S*	1 Pack/182g	337	13.1	185	11.2	18.6	7.2	8.0
Salmon, Smoked, Daily Bread*	1 Pack/122g	296	10.6	243	13.5	28.0	8.7	0.0
Salmon, Smoked & Cream Cheese, M & S*	1 Pack/184g	450	22.4	245	12.7	20.8	12.2	1.8
Salmon, Smoked & Soft Cheese, Sainsbury's*	1 Pack/165g	383	15.2	232	11.9	25.1	9.2	2.4
Salsa Chicken, HL, Tesco*	1 Pack/182g	300	3.3	165	13.4	23.6	1.8	1.9
Sausage, Egg & Bacon, Boots*	1 Pack/325g	887	52.0	273	9.3	23.0	16.0	2.2
Sausage, Speedy Snacks*	1 Serving/93g	258	9.4	279	11.6	35.2	10.2	0.0
Sausage, Triple Pack, GFY, Asda*	1 Pack/215g	424	9.7	197	9.0	30.0	4.5	2.3
Seafood, Mixed, Tesco*	1 Pack/184g	502	30.9	273	7.3	23.2	16.8	0.8
Seafood Cocktail, Asda*	1 Pack/190g	486	30.0	256	6.7	21.3	15.8	1.6
Seafood Cocktail, Daily Bread*	1 Pack/147g	292	6.9	199	8.3	31.0	4.7	0.0
Seafood Cocktail, Waitrose*	1 Pack/210g	267	6.3	127	7.3	17.6	3.0	8.1
Seafood Medley, M & S*	1 Pack/227g	468	28.1	206	7.2	16.3	12.4	3.5
Soft Cheese, & Roasted Pepper, Weight Watchers*	1 Pack/158g	289	6.0	183	9.4	27.7	3.8	1.5
Southern Fried Chicken, Tesco*	1 Pack/174g	365	13.9	210	9.8	24.2	8.0	1.6
Spicy Falafel, & Houmous Salad, Delifresh*	1 Pack/209g	429	19.7	205	6.1	24.0	9.4	2.6
Spinach, Feta & Rocket, Amy's Kitchen*	1 Serving/128g	260	9.0	203	8.6	26.6	7.0	2.3
Spinach Feta, Amy's Kitchen*	1 Roll/128g	262	9.0	205	8.6	27.0	7.0	2.3
Steak, Hot, M & S*	1 Roll/190g	513	15.2	270	11.9	37.0	8.0	3.2
Sub, Beef, & Onion, M & S*	1 Pack/207g	611	31.7	295	13.3	25.6	15.3	1.5
Sub, Beef, & Onion, Roast, Sainsbury's*	1 Serving/174g	426	17.4	245	9.4	29.3	10.0	0.0
Sub, Chicken, & Bacon, Compass Foods*	1 Pack/165g	450	20.1	273	12.2	28.7	12.2	0.0
Sub, Chicken, & Salad, Asda*	1 Sub/200g	460	27.2	230	9.4	17.4	13.6	0.9
Sub, Chicken, & Stuffing, Shell*	1 Serving/183g	437	11.7	239	13.3	32.0	6.4	0.0
Sub, Chicken, Caesar, Chargrilled, Sainsbury's*	1 Pack/216g	611	30.5	283	13.4	25.6	14.1	0.0
Sub, Chicken & Bacon, Sainsbury's*	1 Pack/190g	554	27.0	291	13.4	27.4	14.2	0.8
Sub, Chicken Caesar, Sainsbury's*	1 Roll/210g	590	34.4	281	11.3	22.1	16.4	1.9
Sub, Egg Mayonnaise, Daily Bread*	1 Pack/165g	441	22.3	267	9.6	29.6	13.5	0.0
Sub, Ham, & Tomato Salad, Shapers, Boots*	1 Pack/170g	286	3.9	168	9.2	28.0	2.3	1.4
Sweet Chilli Chicken, in Pitta Bread, Shapers, Boots*	1 Pack/178g	245	5.0	138	9.2	19.0	2.8	2.2
Sweet Chilli Chicken, Special Edition, Ginsters*	1 Pack/172g	351	9.5	204	12.5	26.3	5.5	2.3
Three Cheese & Celery on Malted Brown, COU, M & S*	1 Pack/161g	250	4.2	155	8.0	24.7	2.6	2.1
Three Cheese Salad, Shapers, Boots*	1 Pack/169g	248	2.2	147	11.0	23.0	1.3	2.7
Tuna, & Celery, Perfectly Balanced, Waitrose*	1 Pack/172g	272	5.5	158	11.7	20.5	3.2	3.9
Tuna, & Celery, Waitrose*	1 Pack/168g	254	6.1	151	10.2	19.5	3.6	3.0
Tuna, & Chargrilled Vegetables, BGTY, Sainsbury's*	1 Pack/196g	329	8.6	168	10.7	21.5	4.4	0.0
Tuna, & Cucumber, & Red Onion, Brambles*	1 Pack/161g	264	3.9	164	11.3	24.3	2.4	1.6
Tuna, & Cucumber, Antony Worrall Thompson's*	1 Pack/188g	284	4.3	151	11.6	21.0	2.3	2.9
Tuna, & Cucumber, BGTY, Sainsbury's*	1 Pack/178g	268	3.2	151	11.3	22.3	1.8	3.1
Tuna, & Cucumber, BHS*	1 Pack/210g	479	24.2	228	10.8	24.2	11.5	1.2
Tuna, & Cucumber, Choice*	1 Serving/190g	392	16.6	206	12.1	19.8	8.7	0.0
Tuna, & Cucumber, Co-Op*	1 Serving/268g	510	13.4	190	12.0	25.0	5.0	2.0
Tuna, & Cucumber, Feel Good, Shell*	1 Pack/214g	518	16.0	242	12.6	31.2	7.5	0.0
Tuna, & Cucumber, Good Choice, Iceland*	1 Pack/185g	244	2.9	132	11.6	17.7	1.6	4.3
Tuna, & Cucumber, Healthy Choice, Sutherland*	1 Pack/179g	249	4.1	139	9.7	19.7	2.3	2.4
Tuna, & Cucumber, Healthy Harry's*	1 Pack/187g	271	5.6	145	14.1	15.4	3.0	0.8
Tuna, & Cucumber, Healthy Living, Co-Op*	1 Pack/192g	250	3.5	130	10.9	17.9	1.8	3.0
Tuna, & Cucumber, Less Than 350 Cals, Ginsters*	1 Serving/193g	298	7.5	154	10.8	19.0	3.9	3.1
Tuna, & Cucumber, Low Fat, Heinz*	1 Serving/183g	277	2.9	151	12.3	21.6	1.6	6.8
Tuna, & Cucumber, on a Roll, M & S*	1 Roll/160g	320	12.0	200	11.8	21.6	7.5	3.2
Tuna, & Cucumber, on Malted Wheatgrain, Ginsters*	1 Pack/175g	318	7.5	182	14.1	21.8	4.3	0.0

S

SANDWICH

	Measure INFO/WEIGHT	per Measure KCAL	FAT	Nutrition Values per 100g / 100ml KCAL	PROT	CARB	FAT	FIBRE
Tuna, & Cucumber, Perfectly Balanced, Waitrose*	1 Pack/178g	240	3.6	135	11.0	18.3	2.0	3.6
Tuna, & Cucumber, Shapers, Boots*	1 Pack/167g	267	5.3	160	11.0	22.0	3.2	2.4
Tuna, & Cucumber, Shell*	1 Pack/188g	431	19.2	229	12.3	21.9	10.2	0.0
Tuna, & Cucumber, Weight Watchers*	1 Pack/173g	279	2.9	161	11.4	25.1	1.7	1.4
Tuna, & Green Pesto, BGTY, Sainsbury's*	1 Pack/211g	279	4.7	132	11.0	17.0	2.2	0.0
Tuna, & Lemon Mayo, Shapers, Boots*	1 Pack/206g	318	9.7	154	10.0	18.0	4.7	1.7
Tuna, & Pepper & Sweetcorn Salad, Shapers, Boots*	1 Pack/204g	345	8.2	169	9.2	24.0	4.0	1.9
Tuna, & Salad, Bloomer, M & S*	1 Pack/231g	600	36.9	260	11.8	17.8	16.0	2.6
Tuna, & Salad, Classic*	1 Pack/230g	449	15.9	195	8.7	27.3	6.9	2.1
Tuna, & Salad, M & S*	1 Pack/250g	575	31.5	230	12.5	16.8	12.6	2.1
Tuna, & Salad, Maxi, Greenhalgh's*	1 Serving/216g	390	19.0	181	8.3	17.4	8.8	1.0
Tuna, & Salad, on White, Tesco*	1 Pack/190g	351	13.3	185	9.8	20.8	7.0	1.1
Tuna, & Salad, Tesco*	1 Pack/197g	339	14.6	172	9.9	16.5	7.4	2.8
Tuna, & Sweetcorn, & Red Onion, Co-Op*	1 Pack/256g	614	28.2	240	11.0	23.0	11.0	4.0
Tuna, & Sweetcorn, BGTY, Sainsbury's*	1 Pack/187g	309	5.1	165	10.8	24.7	2.7	2.8
Tuna, & Sweetcorn, COU, M & S*	1 Pack/180g	270	4.3	150	12.6	19.0	2.4	3.8
Tuna, & Sweetcorn, Felix Van Den Berghe*	1 Pack/129g	372	16.0	289	10.4	29.3	12.4	0.0
Tuna, & Sweetcorn, Ginsters*	1 Pack/169g	348	11.4	205	9.6	26.4	6.7	2.4
Tuna, & Sweetcorn, Heinz*	1 Pack/208g	528	27.5	254	10.4	23.5	13.2	1.6
Tuna, & Sweetcorn, Light Choices, HL, Tesco*	1 Pack/168g	285	3.2	170	11.2	25.9	1.9	2.8
Tuna, & Sweetcorn, on Malt Bread, Tesco*	1 Pack/175g	350	8.2	200	11.6	27.5	4.7	2.2
Tuna, & Sweetcorn, Sainsbury's*	1 Pack/183g	392	15.6	214	12.1	22.3	8.5	0.0
Tuna, & Sweetcorn, Shapers, Boots*	1 Pack/170g	295	4.4	174	12.4	25.3	2.6	2.0
Tuna, & Tomato, & Onion, COU, M & S*	1 Pack/177g	250	4.2	141	11.1	18.8	2.4	2.2
Tuna, Crunch, HL, Tesco*	1 Pack/180g	261	4.3	145	11.0	19.9	2.4	0.5
Tuna, Crunch, Shapers, Boots*	1 Pack/200g	290	6.4	145	9.1	20.0	3.2	3.2
Tuna, Heinz*	1 Serving/183g	277	2.9	151	12.3	21.6	1.6	6.8
Tuna, Mayonnaise & Cucumber, Finest, Tesco*	1 Pack/225g	484	19.1	215	11.6	23.1	8.5	1.7
Tuna, Mediterranean, COU, M & S*	1 Pack/260g	364	5.7	140	10.3	19.6	2.2	1.6
Tuna, Melt, Swedish Bread, Shapers, Boots*	1 Pack/163g	254	3.6	156	14.0	20.0	2.2	2.1
Tuna, Nicoise, Taste!*	1 Pack/218g	404	14.4	185	11.3	20.1	6.6	0.0
Tuna, Simply, Ginsters*	1 Pack/167g	466	25.2	279	12.8	22.9	15.1	0.0
Tuna & Cucumber, Finest, Tesco*	1 Pack/169g	380	16.7	225	10.2	23.4	9.9	2.7
Tuna & Cucumber On Oatmeal Bread, Ginsters*	1 Pack/175g	290	7.2	166	11.7	20.7	4.1	2.4
Tuna Mayonnaise, & Cucumber, Classic*	1 Serving/185g	429	22.8	232	10.6	19.8	12.3	0.0
Tuna Mayonnaise, & Cucumber, Daily Bread*	1 Pack/190g	392	16.6	206	12.1	19.8	8.7	0.0
Tuna Mayonnaise, & Cucumber, Darwins Deli*	1 Pack/155g	370	14.6	239	9.6	21.9	9.4	0.0
Tuna Mayonnaise, & Cucumber, Simply, Boots*	1 Pack/200g	498	26.0	249	12.0	21.0	13.0	2.4
Tuna Mayonnaise, & Sweetcorn, Whistlestop*	1 Pack/140g	378	17.7	271	13.6	25.5	12.7	0.0
Tuna Mayonnaise, Menu, Boots*	1 Pack/182g	451	20.0	248	13.0	23.0	11.0	1.1
Tuna Mayonnaise, on White Bread, Oldfields*	1 Pack/142g	394	18.1	278	15.2	27.4	12.8	2.0
Tuna Mayonnaise, White Bread, Open Choice Foods*	1 Pack/120g	298	10.1	248	12.0	29.6	8.4	0.0
Tuna Savoury, Bells*	1 Pack/149g	295	10.0	198	11.8	22.5	6.7	1.0
Turkey, & Bacon, COU, M & S*	1 Pack/165g	256	4.0	155	12.0	21.0	2.4	1.7
Turkey, & Cranberry, COU, M & S*	1 Pack/180g	279	3.1	155	12.1	22.8	1.7	2.9
Turkey, & Cranberry Salad, Fullfillers*	1 Serving/180g	319	5.8	177	13.0	23.3	3.2	2.9
Turkey, & Lettuce & Tomato, Shapers, Boots*	1 Pack/217g	310	4.8	143	9.8	21.0	2.2	2.9
Turkey, & Sage, & Mayonnaise, Bells*	1 Pack/164g	414	22.1	253	11.6	21.2	13.5	0.0
Turkey, & Salad, Brambles*	1 Pack/170g	248	2.0	146	9.3	24.5	1.2	2.0
Turkey, & Salad, Fullfillers*	1 Serving/218g	320	7.0	147	10.3	18.6	3.2	0.0
Turkey, & Salad, Healthy Eating, Wild Bean Cafe*	1 Serving/230g	315	2.5	137	10.0	21.5	1.1	1.8
Turkey, & Stuffing, & Bacon, Bernard Matthews*	1 Pack/127g	250	8.7	196	12.0	21.6	6.8	2.0
Turkey, & Stuffing, M & S*	1 Pack/190g	351	9.3	185	12.3	23.1	4.9	1.9

S

	Measure INFO/WEIGHT	per Measure KCAL	FAT	Nutrition Values per 100g / 100ml KCAL	PROT	CARB	FAT	FIBRE
SANDWICH								
Turkey, & Sun Dried Tomato, Festive Feast, Taste!*	1 Pack/159g	401	22.1	252	8.8	23.0	13.9	0.0
Turkey, Gibsons*	1 Pack/138g	260	5.3	188	12.5	26.0	3.8	0.0
Turkey, Just Turkey, White Bread, Sandwich King*	1 Serving/135g	317	7.0	235	17.3	29.7	5.2	0.0
Turkey, Northern Bites*	1 Pack/200g	354	8.6	177	11.9	22.8	4.3	0.0
Turkey, Smoked, on Wholemeal, Sodhexo*	1 Pack/128g	259	6.1	202	16.1	23.8	4.8	3.6
Turkey, Stuffing, & Cranberry, Shapers, Boots*	1oz/28g	53	0.7	190	12.0	28.0	2.5	2.6
Turkey, Stuffing & Cranberry, Boots*	1 Pack/192g	328	2.1	171	12.0	28.0	1.1	2.5
Turkey, with All the Christmas Trimmings, Tesco*	1 Pack/189g	425	14.2	225	10.8	28.0	7.5	1.9
Vegetable, & Chilli Bean, Roasted, M & S*	1 Pack/200g	340	11.4	170	5.2	24.5	5.7	2.1
Vegetable, M & S*	1 Serving/180g	252	4.1	140	6.1	23.5	2.3	2.1
Vegetable, Roasted, Open, COU, M & S*	1 Pack/150g	260	2.2	173	8.4	31.3	1.5	4.4
Wedge, Sausage, & Egg, Tesco*	1 Pack/269g	699	38.7	260	9.1	23.6	14.4	1.1
Wedge, Tuna, & Salad, Tesco*	1 Pack/205g	291	3.1	142	8.1	23.9	1.5	0.8
Wensleydale, & Carmelised Carrot Chutney, Brambles*	1 Pack/181g	445	21.5	246	10.8	24.4	11.9	1.9
Wensleydale, & Carrot, M & S*	1 Pack/183g	430	22.5	235	9.9	21.4	12.3	2.8
SANDWICH FILLER								
Beef & Onion, Deli, Asda*	1 Serving/50g	78	6.5	157	10.0	0.1	13.0	1.1
Big Breakfast, Asda*	1 Serving/125g	314	26.2	251	12.0	3.5	21.0	0.5
Cajun Chicken, Sainsbury's*	1 Serving/60g	109	8.1	182	13.4	1.8	13.5	1.8
Chargrilled Vegetable, Sainsbury's*	½ Pot/85g	192	19.3	226	3.4	2.2	22.7	0.6
Cheese & Bacon, Tesco*	1 Serving/50g	199	18.8	398	12.2	2.6	37.6	1.2
Cheese & Ham, Sainsbury's*	1 Serving/25g	124	12.3	497	12.4	0.8	49.3	0.3
Cheese & Onion, Deli, Asda*	1 Serving/57g	217	21.1	381	10.0	2.0	37.0	2.0
Cheese & Onion, Sainsbury's*	1 Tub/200g	632	59.6	316	8.7	3.2	29.8	2.2
Cheese & Onion, Tesco*	1 Pack/170g	721	72.4	424	10.0	0.2	42.6	1.5
Cheese & Spring Onion, M & S*	1 Serving/56g	199	18.8	355	8.5	5.0	33.6	0.2
Chicken, Bacon & Sweetcorn, BGTY, Sainsbury's*	1 Tub/300g	399	18.3	133	14.0	5.5	6.1	0.5
Chicken, Stuffing & Bacon, COU, M & S*	1 Pack/170g	170	3.7	100	13.1	6.2	2.2	1.3
Chicken, Sweetcorn & Bacon, Tesco*	1 Serving/50g	167	14.8	334	12.3	4.3	29.7	1.6
Chicken, Tomato & Sweetcure Bacon, M & S*	1 Pot/170g	501	44.9	295	11.4	2.8	26.4	0.7
Chicken & Bacon with Sweetcorn, Sainsbury's*	1 Serving/60g	123	9.4	205	12.0	4.0	15.7	0.9
Chicken & Stuffing, Sainsbury's*	½ Tub/120g	397	37.8	331	6.5	5.3	31.5	1.7
Chicken & Sweetcorn, Sainsbury's*	1 Tub/170g	396	33.7	233	11.0	2.7	19.8	1.9
Chicken Caesar, BGTY, Sainsbury's*	½ Jar/85g	117	6.1	137	15.6	2.5	7.2	2.2
Chicken Fajita, Tesco*	1 Serving/50g	77	4.2	155	13.8	5.9	8.5	1.4
Chicken Tikka, BGTY, Sainsbury's*	½ Pot/85g	99	2.5	117	16.5	6.0	3.0	1.0
Chicken Tikka, Mild, Heinz*	1 Serving/52g	102	7.3	196	5.2	12.3	14.0	0.7
Chicken Tikka & Citrus Raita, COU, M & S*	½ Pot/85g	76	1.7	90	12.6	4.9	2.0	0.9
Chicken with Salad Vegetables, Heinz*	1 Serving/56g	114	8.5	203	5.1	11.7	15.1	0.5
Chickpea, Moroccan Style, Sainsbury's*	½ Tub/120g	160	9.4	133	4.1	11.7	7.8	4.2
Chunky Egg & Smoked Ham, Tesco*	1 Serving/100g	234	20.7	234	11.8	0.2	20.7	0.3
Chunky Seafood Cocktail, Tesco*	1 Serving/100g	308	27.8	308	6.0	8.3	27.8	2.0
Corned Beef & Onion, Deli, Asda*	1 Serving/50g	170	15.5	340	12.0	3.3	31.0	0.7
Coronation Chicken, 50 % Less Fat, Tesco*	1 Serving/50g	102	6.3	205	11.5	9.7	12.6	2.7
Coronation Chicken, BGTY, Sainsbury's*	1 Portion/50g	73	3.5	146	11.9	8.9	7.0	1.4
Coronation Chicken, Sainsbury's*	¼ Tub/60g	183	14.8	305	12.1	8.9	24.6	1.2
Coronation Chicken, Tesco*	1 Tbsp/30g	84	6.5	279	14.7	6.1	21.8	0.7
Coronation Chicken, Waitrose*	1 Pack/170g	554	43.2	326	11.1	13.2	25.4	2.0
Coronation Tuna, BGTY, Sainsbury's*	1 Can/80g	90	2.1	112	16.5	5.7	2.6	1.0
Egg & Bacon, Fresh, Tesco*	1 Serving/45g	112	9.0	248	12.7	4.2	20.1	0.6
Egg & Smoked Bacon, BGTY, Sainsbury's*	½ Pot/120g	187	13.6	156	9.7	3.8	11.3	0.5
Egg Mayonnaise, BGTY, Sainsbury's*	1 Serving/63g	75	4.4	119	10.9	3.1	7.0	0.5
Egg Mayonnaise, Chunky Free Range, Tesco*	1 Serving/50g	104	8.9	209	11.3	0.9	17.8	1.6

SANDWICH FILLER

	Measure INFO/WEIGHT	per Measure KCAL	FAT	Nutrition Values per 100g / 100ml KCAL	PROT	CARB	FAT	FIBRE
Egg Mayonnaise, Deli, Asda*	1 Serving/50g	113	10.0	227	11.0	0.8	20.0	0.3
Egg Mayonnaise, Free Range, Co-Op*	1 Pack/200g	260	17.6	130	10.1	2.4	8.8	0.5
Egg Mayonnaise, M & S*	1oz/28g	62	5.5	220	10.1	0.8	19.7	1.1
Egg Mayonnaise, Morrisons*	1 Serving/50g	71	5.3	142	10.0	1.7	10.6	0.0
Egg Mayonnaise, Sainsbury's*	1 Serving/60g	129	11.0	215	10.4	2.0	18.4	0.5
Egg Mayonnaise, Tesco*	1 Serving/50g	114	10.0	228	10.2	1.9	20.0	0.5
Egg Mayonnaise & Bacon, Free Range, Co-Op*	1 Pot/200g	500	44.0	250	13.0	0.9	22.0	0.6
Egg Mayonnaise 50% Less Fat, Tesco*	1 Serving/50g	65	3.8	130	10.2	3.8	7.6	0.5
Ham & Salad Vegetables, Heinz*	1oz/28g	57	4.5	204	5.3	10.0	15.9	0.4
Peppered Mackerel, Creamy, Shippam*	1 Serving/15g	27	2.8	177	7.8	6.5	18.6	0.0
Poached Salmon & Cucumber, Deli, M & S*	1 Pot/170g	348	27.7	205	14.0	1.0	16.3	0.5
Prawn Marie Rose, Sainsbury's*	1 Serving/60g	121	10.6	201	8.1	2.5	17.6	0.9
Prawn Mayonnaise, Deli, Asda*	1 Serving/50g	169	16.5	339	9.0	1.6	33.0	0.4
Prawn Mayonnaise, GFY, Asda*	1 Serving/57g	101	7.4	177	12.0	3.0	13.0	0.1
Prawn Mayonnaise, M & S*	½ Pack/170g	501	47.6	295	10.6	0.6	28.0	0.3
Prawn Mayonnaise, Waitrose*	1 Pot/170g	537	52.9	316	8.9	0.2	31.1	0.0
Roast Beef, Onion & Horseradish, Sainsbury's*	1 Serving/100g	372	36.8	372	6.4	3.7	36.8	1.2
Roast Chicken & Stuffing, Sainsbury's*	1 Serving/100g	424	41.5	424	10.8	1.9	41.5	1.2
Seafood, BGTY, Sainsbury's*	1oz/28g	36	2.0	128	8.7	7.6	7.0	0.5
Seafood Cocktail, M & S*	1oz/28g	76	6.7	272	6.4	8.2	23.8	0.2
Seafood Cocktail, Sainsbury's*	½ Tub/120g	314	27.6	262	5.7	8.1	23.0	1.0
Smoked Ham, Roasted Onion & Mustard, Sainsbury's*	1 Serving/100g	343	33.4	343	7.3	3.4	33.4	0.0
Smoked Salmon & Soft Cheese, M & S*	1 Pack/170g	450	40.6	265	11.1	4.9	23.9	0.0
Tex-Mex Chicken, Tesco*	1 Pack/250g	255	2.2	102	12.3	11.2	0.9	1.2
Three Cheese & Onion, Premier Deli*	1 Serving/100g	540	54.8	540	10.8	1.0	54.8	2.0
Tuna, Carb Check, Heinz*	1 Serving/52g	84	6.2	161	6.6	6.3	12.0	0.7
Tuna, Tomato & Black Olive, BGTY, Sainsbury's*	1 Pack/100g	88	1.6	88	12.6	5.9	1.6	1.2
Tuna & Sweetcorn, COU, M & S*	½ Pot/85g	76	1.7	90	11.6	5.7	2.0	1.3
Tuna & Sweetcorn, Deli, Asda*	1 Serving/50g	148	13.0	296	12.0	3.4	26.0	1.4
Tuna & Sweetcorn, Deli Filler, Sainsbury's*	¼ Pack/58g	105	7.5	183	9.7	6.1	13.1	1.2
Tuna & Sweetcorn, GFY, Asda*	1/3 Pot/57g	71	2.3	125	12.0	10.0	4.1	0.8
Tuna & Sweetcorn, HL, Tesco*	1 Serving/60g	69	3.2	115	11.2	5.0	5.3	1.4
Tuna & Sweetcorn, M & S*	1oz/28g	70	5.8	250	14.2	2.3	20.7	1.3
Tuna & Sweetcorn, Morrisons*	1 Tub/170g	382	28.4	225	15.3	7.0	16.7	3.4
Tuna & Sweetcorn with Salad Vegetables, Heinz*	1oz/28g	53	3.7	191	5.8	12.1	13.2	0.7
Tuna Mayonnaise, & Cucumber, Choice, Tesco*	1 Serving/200g	463	22.8	231	12.8	23.2	11.4	1.5
Tuna Mayonnaise, BGTY, Sainsbury's*	1 Serving/100g	114	3.4	114	17.6	3.5	3.4	0.1

SANDWICH FILLING

	Measure INFO/WEIGHT	per Measure KCAL	FAT	Nutrition Values per 100g / 100ml KCAL	PROT	CARB	FAT	FIBRE
Cheese & Onion, Asda*	1 Serving/56g	288	28.5	515	9.8	4.4	50.9	0.3
Cheese & Onion, Co-Op*	1 Serving/56g	269	26.3	480	10.0	4.0	47.0	0.5
Cheese & Onion, GFY, Asda*	1 Serving/80g	206	16.8	257	11.0	6.0	21.0	0.8
Chicken & Bacon, Asda*	1 Serving/100g	341	29.0	341	17.0	3.0	29.0	0.5
Chicken & Sweetcorn, Asda*	1 Serving/60g	187	16.8	312	11.0	4.0	28.0	2.0
Chicken Tikka, Asda*	1 Serving/28g	80	5.6	284	13.0	13.0	20.0	0.7
Chicken Tikka, Less Than 5% Fat, Asda*	1 Serving/56g	65	2.6	116	11.0	7.3	4.7	1.2
Crab, BGTY, Sainsbury's*	1oz/28g	36	2.0	128	8.7	7.6	7.0	0.5
Egg Mayonnaise, Asda*	1oz/28g	72	6.5	258	10.3	1.9	23.3	0.7
Egg Mayonnaise, Co-Op*	1oz/28g	66	5.9	235	10.0	1.0	21.0	1.0
Egg Mayonnaise with Chives, Asda*	1oz/28g	92	8.9	327	9.1	1.1	31.8	0.0
Houmous & Vegetable, Asda*	1/3 Tub/57g	133	9.7	233	8.0	12.0	17.0	3.5
Prawns with Seafood Sauce, Asda*	1oz/28g	107	10.3	382	11.7	1.4	36.8	0.0
Tuna & Sweetcorn, Asda*	1oz/28g	83	7.4	295	8.2	6.0	26.5	0.6
Tuna & Sweetcorn, Reduced Fat, Co-Op*	1 Serving/50g	102	7.0	205	13.0	7.0	14.0	0.9

	Measure INFO/WEIGHT	per Measure		Nutrition Values per 100g / 100ml				
		KCAL	FAT	KCAL	PROT	CARB	FAT	FIBRE
SANDWICH FILLING								
Tuna & Sweetcorn, Reduced Fat, Morrisons*	1oz/28g	48	2.9	172	13.2	6.9	10.2	0.0
SANDWICH SPREAD								
Beef, Classic, Shippam*	1 Pot/75g	133	8.8	177	15.5	2.2	11.8	0.0
Chicken, Classic, Shippam*	1 Serving/35g	64	4.4	182	15.5	1.8	12.5	0.0
Chicken & Bacon, Asda*	¼ Jar/43g	153	13.2	359	18.0	2.0	31.0	1.0
Chicken Tikka, Asda*	1 Serving/50g	77	5.0	154	7.0	9.0	10.0	0.2
Crab, Classic, Shippam*	1 Jar/35g	59	3.8	170	13.1	4.6	10.9	0.0
Heinz*	1 Tbsp/10ml	22	1.3	220	1.0	24.0	13.0	1.0
Light, Heinz*	1 Tbsp/10g	16	0.9	161	1.1	18.2	9.2	0.9
Salmon, Classic, Shippam*	1 Serving/35g	70	4.9	200	14.7	4.2	14.1	0.0
Tuna & Mayonnaise, Shippam*	1 Pot/75g	189	13.9	252	18.3	3.1	18.5	0.0
SARDINES								
Boneless, in Tomato Sauce, John West*	1 Can/120g	197	12.0	164	17.0	1.5	10.0	0.0
Grilled	*1oz/28g*	*55*	*2.9*	*195*	*25.3*	*0.0*	*10.4*	*0.0*
in BBQ Sauce, John West*	1 Tin/121g	177	7.7	146	16.1	6.2	6.4	0.0
in Brine, Canned, Drained	*1oz/28g*	*48*	*2.7*	*172*	*21.5*	*0.0*	*9.6*	*0.0*
in Oil, Canned, Drained	*1oz/28g*	*62*	*3.9*	*220*	*23.3*	*0.0*	*14.1*	*0.0*
in Olive Oil, Canned, Ambrosia*	1 Can/100g	320	13.7	320	22.3	0.7	13.7	0.0
in Spring Water, Portuguese, Sainsbury's*	1 Can/90g	165	9.3	183	22.4	0.0	10.3	0.0
in Tomato Sauce, Canned	1oz/28g	45	2.8	162	17.0	1.4	9.9	0.0
Raw	*1oz/28g*	*46*	*2.6*	*165*	*20.6*	*0.0*	*9.2*	*0.0*
SATAY								
Chicken, Breast, Party Bites, Sainsbury's*	1 Stick/10g	16	0.1	157	34.1	2.7	0.9	0.1
Chicken, GFY, Asda*	1 Serving/168g	242	6.1	144	22.0	6.0	3.6	0.8
Chicken, Indonesian, Bighams*	1 Serving/240g	314	15.4	131	12.2	6.2	6.4	0.6
Chicken, Indonesian, Mini, Sainsbury's*	1 Stick/10g	17	0.7	171	23.0	4.0	7.0	0.7
Chicken, Kebab, Waitrose*	½ Pack/125g	246	13.5	197	18.9	6.0	10.8	0.5
Chicken, M & S*	1 Satay/43g	90	5.5	210	19.1	4.4	12.7	0.7
Chicken, Occasions, Sainsbury's*	1 Satay/10g	15	0.6	150	22.0	2.0	6.0	0.7
Chicken, Oriental, Tesco*	1 Serving/100g	160	5.0	160	23.6	5.1	5.0	0.4
Chicken, Party, Mini, Tesco*	1 Satay/10g	13	0.3	133	23.7	3.4	2.8	1.0
Chicken, Taste Original*	1 Stick/20g	33	1.3	164	23.0	2.5	6.5	0.7
Chicken, with Peanut Sauce, Waitrose*	1 Pack/250g	492	27.0	197	18.9	6.0	10.8	0.5
Chicken & Turkey, Sainsbury's*	1 Stick/20g	44	2.8	222	20.0	4.0	14.0	1.9
SATSUMAS								
Fresh, Raw, Flesh Only, Average	*1 Sm/56g*	*20*	*0.2*	*36*	*0.8*	*13.3*	*0.3*	*1.8*
Weighed with Peel, Average	*1 Med/80g*	*21*	*0.1*	*26*	*0.6*	*6.0*	*0.1*	*0.9*
SAUCE								
All Seasons, Mary Berry*	1 Serving/100g	159	0.9	159	2.4	35.3	0.9	0.4
Apple, Baxters*	1 Tsp/15g	7	0.1	49	0.1	11.1	0.4	0.7
Apple, Bramley, M & S*	1 Tbsp/15g	21	0.0	140	0.2	32.6	0.3	0.4
Apple, Heinz*	1 Tsp/15g	8	0.0	56	0.3	13.4	0.2	1.5
Apple & Brandy, Asda*	1 Serving/125g	56	0.0	45	0.2	11.0	0.0	0.0
Apricot & Almond Tagine, Sainsbury's*	1/3 Jar/120g	98	1.9	82	2.0	17.9	1.6	2.5
Aromatic Cantonese, Express, Uncle Ben's*	1 Serving/170g	172	0.2	101	0.6	24.6	0.1	0.0
Arrabbiata, Fresh, Waitrose*	1 Serving/100g	52	2.5	52	1.4	5.9	2.5	2.0
Arrabbiata, Weight Watchers*	½ Pot/150g	43	0.7	29	1.1	5.0	0.5	1.7
Balti, 97% Fat Free, Homepride*	1 Serving/230g	133	4.4	58	1.1	9.1	1.9	1.8
Balti, Cooking, Organic, Perfectly Balanced, Waitrose*	1 Jar/450g	301	5.8	67	1.6	12.1	1.3	3.1
Balti, Cooking, Sharwood's*	¼ Jar/140g	120	8.3	86	1.2	7.1	5.9	1.4
Balti, Deliciously Good, Homepride*	1/3 Jar/153g	89	2.9	58	1.1	9.1	1.9	0.6
Balti, Tomato & Coriander, Canned, Patak's*	1 Can/283g	235	17.0	83	0.8	6.5	6.0	1.2
Balti, TTD, Sainsbury's*	½ Pack/175g	159	11.9	91	1.4	6.0	6.8	2.0

S

SAUCE

INFO/WEIGHT	Measure	per Measure KCAL	FAT	Nutrition Values per 100g / 100ml KCAL	PROT	CARB	FAT	FIBRE
Balti Cooking, Chosen By You, Asda*	1 Jar/570g	473	27.9	83	1.7	6.9	4.9	2.3
Balti Curry, Tesco*	1 Serving/200g	126	9.2	63	1.7	4.3	4.6	1.7
Barbecue, Asda*	1 Serving/135g	128	0.3	95	1.2	22.0	0.2	0.6
Barbecue, Chicken Tonight, Knorr*	¼ Jar/125g	76	0.5	61	2.0	12.4	0.4	0.9
Barbeque, Cook in, Homepride*	1 Can/500g	375	7.5	75	0.7	14.6	1.5	0.6
Barbeque, Simply Sausages Ranch, Colman's*	1 Serving/130g	96	0.1	74	1.8	16.6	0.1	1.1
BBQ, Heinz*	1 Serving/20g	28	0.1	139	1.1	31.7	0.3	0.5
BBQ, HP*	1 Serving/20ml	29	0.0	143	0.8	33.1	0.2	0.0
BBQ, Spicy Mayhem, HP*	1 Serving/2g	3	0.0	156	0.9	36.7	0.1	0.0
Bearnaise, Mary Berry*	1 Serving/100g	435	39.8	435	1.7	17.3	39.8	0.4
Bechamel, for Lasagne, Loyd Grossman*	1 Jar/400g	396	33.2	99	0.6	5.4	8.3	0.1
Beef Bolognese, Weight Watchers*	1 Pot/300g	171	8.4	57	4.3	3.6	2.8	1.4
Bhuna, Cooking, Sharwood's*	1/3 Jar/140g	116	7.6	83	1.2	7.6	5.4	1.6
Black Bean, Canton, Stir Fry, Blue Dragon*	½ Pack/60g	53	1.2	88	2.8	14.8	2.0	1.5
Black Bean, Crushed, Stir Fry Sensations, Amoy*	1 Pouch/150g	150	4.3	100	2.4	16.9	2.9	1.0
Black Bean, Loyd Grossman*	1 Serving/175g	177	7.9	101	2.4	12.6	4.5	0.7
Black Bean, Ready to Stir Fry, M & S*	1 Sachet/120g	78	1.1	65	2.5	11.5	0.9	1.4
Black Bean, Sharwood's*	1 Serving/98g	96	1.5	98	2.2	18.8	1.5	0.6
Black Bean, Stir Fry, Fresh, M & S*	1 Pot/120g	120	0.7	100	2.6	20.3	0.6	1.4
Black Bean, Stir Fry, Sharwood's*	1 Jar/195g	191	2.9	98	2.2	18.8	1.5	0.6
Black Bean, Stir Fry Additions, Tesco*	1 Sachet/50g	69	1.5	138	4.1	23.6	3.0	0.0
Black Bean, Uncle Ben's*	1 Serving/125g	89	1.6	71	2.0	12.8	1.3	0.0
Black Bean & Chilli, Stir Fry, Asda*	½ Jar/97g	158	11.6	163	3.7	10.0	12.0	0.8
Black Bean & Green Pepper, Stir Fry, Sharwood's*	1 Serving/150g	82	0.4	55	2.0	11.0	0.3	0.5
Black Bean & Red Pepper, Sharwood's*	½ Jar/213g	132	3.0	62	1.9	10.5	1.4	1.2
Black Bean Sauce Cantonese, Sharwood's*	1 Serving/140g	87	2.0	62	1.9	10.5	1.4	1.2
Black Pepper, Lee Kum Kee*	1 Serving/90g	107	3.0	119	3.2	19.0	3.3	1.3
Black Pepper, Stir Fry, Blue Dragon*	½ Sachet/60g	47	2.6	79	1.6	8.4	4.4	0.1
Bolognese, for Beef, Tesco*	½ Pack/175g	177	10.1	101	5.4	6.9	5.8	0.8
Bolognese, Loyd Grossman*	¼ Jar/106g	79	3.1	75	2.0	10.2	2.9	1.4
Bolognese, Original, Deliciously Good, Homepride*	¼ Jar/112g	39	0.2	35	1.3	7.1	0.2	0.8
Bolognese, Tinned, Sainsbury's*	1/3 Can/141g	86	3.1	61	4.5	5.7	2.2	1.0
Bolognese, Waitrose*	1 Serving/175g	150	8.6	86	5.4	5.3	4.9	2.0
Bourguignon, Beef Tonight, Knorr*	¼ Jar/125g	71	3.2	57	0.6	7.6	2.6	0.4
Bramley Apple, Colman's*	1 Tbsp/15ml	16	0.0	107	0.2	26.5	0.0	1.3
Branston Smooth, Crosse & Blackwell*	1 Serving/25g	35	0.0	139	0.6	34.0	0.1	1.4
Brazilian Chicken, Chicken Tonight, Knorr*	¼ Jar/125g	49	0.9	39	1.2	7.0	0.7	1.3
Bread, M & S*	1 Serving/85g	153	12.4	180	3.1	8.7	14.6	0.2
Bread, Made with Semi-Skimmed Milk	1 Serving/45g	42	1.4	93	4.3	12.8	3.1	0.3
Brown, Bottled	1 Tsp/6g	6	0.0	99	1.1	25.2	0.0	0.7
Brown, Chop, Hammonds of Yorkshire*	1 Tbsp/15g	10	0.0	66	0.3	16.1	0.1	0.3
Brown, Tiptree, Wilkin & Sons*	1 Serving/100g	104	0.0	104	1.1	42.0	0.0	0.0
Burger, Hellmann's*	1 Tbsp/15g	36	3.1	240	1.1	12.0	21.0	0.0
Butter & Tarragon, Chicken Tonight, Knorr*	¼ Jar/125g	132	13.0	106	1.0	2.1	10.4	0.0
Butter Chicken, Patak's*	1 Jar/500g	725	60.0	145	1.2	7.6	12.0	1.4
Butter Chicken, Simmer, Passage To India*	½ Pack/100g	188	11.7	188	2.2	18.9	11.7	3.2
Butter Chicken, TTD, Sainsbury's*	½ Pack/174g	272	23.5	156	1.8	6.7	13.5	0.9
Cantonese, Sizzling, Uncle Ben's*	½ Jar/270g	416	16.5	154	0.7	24.0	6.1	0.0
Cantonese Chow Mein Stir Fry, Sainsbury's*	½ Jar/100g	67	1.9	67	0.4	12.1	1.9	0.8
Caramelised Onion & Red Wine, M & S*	1 Serving/52g	31	1.6	60	1.9	6.7	3.1	0.6
Carbonara, Less Than 5% Fat, GFY, Asda*	½ Tub/150g	121	6.7	81	5.0	5.0	4.5	0.5
Carbonara, TTD, Sainsbury's*	½ Pot/175g	347	31.0	198	5.2	4.5	17.7	0.5
Caribbean Curry, Levi Roots*	½ Jar/175g	182	14.2	104	0.4	7.2	8.1	0.3

S

SAUCE

INFO/WEIGHT	Measure		per Measure		Nutrition Values per 100g / 100ml				
			KCAL	FAT	KCAL	PROT	CARB	FAT	FIBRE
Chasseur, Classic, Chicken Tonight, Knorr*	¼ Jar/125g		61	3.6	49	0.6	5.3	2.9	0.7
Chasseur, Cook in, Homepride*	1 Can/390g		160	0.4	41	0.7	9.2	0.1	0.4
Cheddar Cheese, Colman's*	1 Serving/85ml		348	13.1	410	19.2	48.5	15.4	1.9
Cheddar Cheese, Dry, Knorr*	1 Serving/10g		47	3.2	469	7.8	38.0	31.8	0.3
Cheese, Fresh, Waitrose*	1 Pot/350g		458	34.3	131	5.1	5.7	9.8	0.0
Cheese, Italian, Tesco*	½ Carton/175g		238	15.6	136	5.8	8.3	8.9	0.0
Cheese, Italian Style, Finest, Tesco*	½ Pot/175g		355	20.8	203	10.1	14.0	11.9	0.0
Cheese, Made with Semi-Skimmed Milk	1 Serving/60g		107	7.6	179	8.1	9.1	12.6	0.2
Cheese, Made with Whole Milk	1 Serving/60g		118	8.8	197	8.0	9.0	14.6	0.2
Cherry Tomato & Fresh Basil, M & S*	1 Serving/175g		131	9.3	75	1.2	5.5	5.3	1.1
Chickpea & Spinach, Asda*	1 Jar/500g		365	14.0	73	3.5	8.4	2.8	2.0
Chilli, Amoy*	1 Tsp/6g		1	0.0	25	1.0	5.2	0.0	1.0
Chilli, Barbeque, Encona*	1 Tbsp/15ml		19	0.0	129	1.3	30.7	0.1	0.0
Chilli, Hot, Blue Dragon*	1 Tbsp/15ml		14	0.0	96	0.5	23.0	0.2	0.0
Chilli, Hot, Heinz*	1 Portion/10g		8	0.0	80	1.4	18.0	0.0	0.0
Chilli, Hot, Mexican, Morrisons*	¼ Jar/125g		72	0.6	58	2.2	11.2	0.5	2.0
Chilli, HP*	1 Tsp/6g		8	0.0	134	1.2	32.3	0.0	0.0
Chilli, Medium, Deliciously Good, Homepride*	1 Jar/460g		258	2.3	56	2.3	10.4	0.5	1.2
Chilli, Mild, Tesco*	1 Jar/550g		302	1.6	55	2.3	10.0	0.3	3.4
Chilli, Seeds of Change*	1 Jar/400g		408	6.0	102	4.0	18.2	1.5	2.2
Chilli, Sweet, Thai, Dipping, Original, Blue Dragon*	1 Serving/30ml		69	0.2	229	0.6	55.1	0.7	1.6
Chilli, Tomato Based, Bottled, Average	**1 Tbsp/15g**		**16**	**0.0**	**104**	**2.5**	**19.8**	**0.3**	**5.9**
Chilli, with Kidney Beans, Old El Paso*	1 Serving/115g		92	0.5	80	4.3	14.8	0.4	0.0
Chilli & Garlic, Blue Dragon*	1 Serving/30ml		25	0.1	85	1.1	19.7	0.2	0.0
Chilli & Garlic, Lea & Perrins*	1 Tsp/6g		4	0.0	60	1.0	14.9	0.0	0.0
Chilli & Garlic, Stir Fry, M & S*	1 Serving/83g		120	1.0	145	0.7	32.4	1.2	1.1
Chilli Con Carne, Classic, Loyd Grossman*	1 Jar/350g		241	10.5	69	2.2	7.6	3.0	1.3
Chilli Con Carne, Cook in, BGTY, Sainsbury's*	¼ Jar/125g		69	0.6	55	1.7	11.0	0.5	2.5
Chilli Con Carne, Cook in, Homepride*	1 Can/390g		234	2.3	60	2.5	11.2	0.6	0.0
Chilli Con Carne, Sizzle & Stir, Knorr*	1 Jar/455g		505	32.3	111	2.7	9.1	7.1	2.7
Chilli Con Carne, Weight Watchers*	½ Jar/175g		84	0.3	48	1.8	9.7	0.2	2.0
Chinese, Stir Fry, Sachet, Fresh, Sainsbury's*	½ Sachet/51ml		83	5.7	163	1.7	14.1	11.1	1.8
Chinese Style, Curry, Cooking, Chosen By You, Asda*	1 Serving/140g		89	4.3	63	1.5	7.4	3.1	3.5
Chinese Style, Stir Fry, Fresh, Asda*	½ Sachet/50ml		93	6.0	186	1.5	18.0	12.0	0.0
Chocolate, Dry, Sainsbury's*	1 Serving/30g		108	3.5	360	1.3	62.8	11.6	0.9
Chocolate, Sainsbury's*	1 Serving/25g		81	1.6	323	1.8	64.7	6.3	2.7
Chocolate Flavour, Dry, Lyle's*	1 Serving/10g		30	0.0	305	1.0	74.0	0.5	0.0
Chop Suey, Blue Dragon*	½ Sachet/60g		34	1.4	57	0.5	8.3	2.4	0.5
Chop Suey, Stir Fry, Sharwood's*	1 Jar/160g		120	2.4	75	0.7	14.6	1.5	0.2
Chow Mein, Stir Fry, Blue Dragon*	1 Sachet/120g		110	3.5	92	1.1	15.4	2.9	0.4
Chow Mein, Stir Fry, Straight to Wok, Amoy*	1 Packet/120g		172	7.0	143	0.9	21.9	5.8	0.5
Coconut, Chilli & Lime, Cook-In, Homepride*	1 Serving/115g		110	8.6	96	1.1	5.9	7.5	0.0
Coconut, Ginger & Lemongrass, Stir Fry, Wagamama*	½ Jar/125g		144	7.1	115	1.2	14.7	5.7	0.4
Coconut, Lime & Coriander, Cooking, Nando's*	1 Serving/65g		88	6.5	135	1.5	12.1	10.0	1.2
Coconut, Thai Style, Stir Fry, Waitrose*	½ Pack/50ml		52	4.3	105	1.5	5.5	8.6	1.8
Coconut & Red Chilli, Noodle Sauce, Tesco*	1/3 Jar/110g		88	7.0	80	1.7	3.8	6.4	0.7
Coconut RunDown, Levi Roots*	½ Jar/175g		178	8.7	102	0.7	13.3	5.0	0.1
Cooking, Balti, Extra Special, Asda*	1 Jar/120g		180	9.6	150	2.0	17.0	8.0	1.0
Cooking, Korma, Light Choices, Tesco*	¼ Jar/125g		100	4.0	80	1.6	10.2	3.2	1.6
Coronation, Heinz*	1 Tbsp/10g		33	3.1	334	0.8	13.1	31.0	0.9
Coronation Chicken, Cook in, Homepride*	1 Serving/250g		232	10.5	93	0.8	13.2	4.2	0.0
Country French, Chicken Tonight, Knorr*	¼ Jar/125g		112	10.0	90	0.5	4.1	8.0	0.7
Country French, Low Fat, Chicken Tonight, Knorr*	¼ Jar/125g		56	3.6	45	0.4	4.4	2.9	0.7

S

SAUCE

INFO/WEIGHT	Measure	per Measure		Nutrition Values per 100g / 100ml				
		KCAL	FAT	KCAL	PROT	CARB	FAT	FIBRE
Cranberry, Waitrose*	1 Tbsp/20g	31	0.0	156	0.2	38.5	0.2	14.0
Cranberry, with Brandy & Orange Zest, Finest, Tesco*	1 Serving/10g	23	0.1	235	0.3	57.2	0.6	1.3
Cranberry & Port, M & S*	1 Serving/75g	71	0.3	95	2.3	20.2	0.4	2.1
Cranberry & Red Onion, Sizzling, Homepride*	1 Serving/100g	83	1.0	83	0.5	17.7	1.0	0.0
Creamy, Curry, BGTY, Sainsbury's*	¼ Jar/125g	84	4.7	67	1.4	6.8	3.8	0.5
Creamy Mushroom, Cooking, M & S*	1 Jar/510g	663	57.6	130	1.3	5.4	11.3	0.5
Creamy Mushroom, Homepride*	1 Portion/100g	76	5.6	76	1.1	5.2	5.6	0.3
Creamy Mushroom, Knorr*	1 Serving/125g	111	9.6	89	0.4	4.5	7.7	0.4
Creamy Peppercorn & Whisky, Baxters*	1 Pack/320g	422	34.6	132	1.9	6.7	10.8	0.2
Cumberland Sausage, Colman's*	¼ Jar/126g	43	0.3	34	0.7	7.4	0.2	0.8
Curry, Cook in, Homepride*	½ Can/250g	140	4.7	56	1.1	8.6	1.9	0.5
Curry, Creamy, Chicken Tonight, Knorr*	½ Jar/250g	207	18.5	83	0.6	3.6	7.4	0.8
Curry, Creamy, Cooking, BGTY, Sainsbury's*	¼ Jar/125g	94	3.7	75	1.8	10.1	3.0	1.0
Curry, Deliciously Good, Homepride*	1/3 Jar/149g	91	2.7	61	1.1	10.0	1.8	0.5
Curry, Green Thai, BGTY, Sainsbury's*	¼ Jar/125g	61	3.2	49	0.6	5.7	2.6	1.4
Curry, Green Thai, Cooking, TTD, Sainsbury's*	½ Pack/175g	152	11.9	87	0.9	5.5	6.8	1.0
Curry, Green Thai, Finest, Tesco*	1 Serving/350g	420	37.1	120	1.4	4.8	10.6	0.7
Curry, Green Thai, Sharwood's*	1 Serving/403g	431	30.6	107	1.1	8.4	7.6	0.1
Curry, Hot Madras, The Curry Sauce Company*	1 Serving/100g	162	12.5	162	2.2	10.2	12.5	1.5
Curry, Mild, Tesco*	1 Jar/500g	420	14.0	84	1.1	13.4	2.8	0.8
Curry, Red Thai, Worldwide Sauces*	1 Jar/450g	630	45.0	140	1.5	10.9	10.0	0.0
Curry, Sri Lanken, Seasoned Pioneers*	½ Pack/200g	194	16.8	97	1.8	3.4	8.4	0.8
Curry, Sweet	1 Serving/115g	105	6.4	91	1.2	9.6	5.6	1.4
Curry, Thai Coconut, Uncle Ben's*	1 Serving/125g	127	6.0	102	1.4	13.2	4.8	0.0
Curry, Yellow Thai, Cooking, Sainsbury's*	1 Jar/500g	785	70.0	157	2.3	5.4	14.0	2.3
Dark Soy, Sesame & Ginger, for Fish, Schwartz*	1 Pack/300g	279	4.2	93	1.3	18.8	1.4	0.5
Dhansak, Medium, Sharwood's*	1 Jar/420g	370	13.4	88	3.6	11.1	3.2	1.0
Dhansak, Sharwood's*	1 Jar/445g	667	34.7	150	4.7	15.2	7.8	1.4
Dill & Lemon, Delicate, for Fish, Schwartz*	1 Pack/300g	387	34.2	129	1.1	5.6	11.4	0.5
Dill & Mustard, for Gravadlax, Dry, Waitrose*	1 Sachet/35g	123	9.0	352	2.5	27.8	25.7	0.6
Dopiaza, Cooking, Tesco*	1 Serving/166g	176	11.0	106	2.2	9.4	6.6	1.9
Dopiaza, Medium, Cook in, Sharwood's*	½ Bottle/210g	193	10.7	92	1.4	10.2	5.1	0.6
Enchilada, Medium, Old El Paso*	1 Can/270g	92	4.6	34	0.0	5.0	1.7	0.0
Exotic Curry, Heinz*	1 Serving/15ml	41	3.4	271	0.7	15.3	22.8	0.6
Fajita, M & S*	1oz/28g	24	1.7	85	1.3	6.4	6.1	2.2
Fiery Guava, Dipping, Levi Roots*	1 Serving/20g	26	0.0	128	0.4	31.5	0.0	0.1
Fish, Nuoc Mam, Thai, Blue Dragon*	1 Tsp/5ml	7	0.0	145	5.9	30.9	0.1	0.0
Fish Pie, Fresh, The Saucy Fish Co.*	1 Pack/230g	179	12.9	78	2.4	4.6	5.6	0.0
for Fajitas, Original Smoky BBQ, Cooking, Old El Paso*	1 Jar/395g	222	5.1	56	1.5	9.6	1.3	0.0
for Lasagne, White, Tesco*	1 Jar/460g	506	41.4	110	1.9	5.3	9.0	0.6
Four Cheese, Reduced Fat, Morrisons*	½ Tub/175g	161	9.5	92	6.1	4.8	5.4	0.5
Fruit Squirt, Passionfruit, Topping, Easiyo*	1 Serving/20g	34	0.0	172	1.0	38.9	0.1	6.3
Fruity, HP*	1 Tsp/6g	8	0.0	141	1.2	35.1	0.1	0.0
Garlic, Heinz*	1 Serving/10ml	32	3.0	323	1.0	12.1	29.9	1.2
Garlic, Lea & Perrins*	1 Tsp/6g	20	1.7	337	1.8	17.8	29.0	0.0
Garlic & Chive, Heinz*	1 Serving/10ml	35	3.3	350	1.0	11.3	33.2	0.1
Green Peppercorn, Dry, Sainsbury's*	1 Tbsp/15ml	68	7.3	455	0.4	3.8	48.5	0.1
Green Thai, Cooking, Perfectly Balanced, Waitrose*	½ Jar/215g	112	6.9	52	0.8	4.9	3.2	1.5
Green Thai, Loyd Grossman*	½ Jar/175g	182	11.2	104	1.6	10.0	6.4	0.8
Green Thai, Stir Fry, Fresh Ideas, Tesco*	1 Pack/50g	91	8.3	182	2.1	6.2	16.6	0.1
Green Thai, Stir Fry, Sainsbury's*	½ Pack/75g	112	8.0	149	1.2	11.9	10.7	1.0
Ham & Mushroom for Pasta, Stir & Serve, Homepride*	1 Serving/100g	95	9.3	95	1.5	1.3	9.3	0.0
Hoi Sin, M & S*	½ Pot/50ml	80	1.0	160	3.2	31.8	2.0	2.2

SAUCE	Measure INFO/WEIGHT	per Measure KCAL	FAT	Nutrition Values per 100g / 100ml KCAL	PROT	CARB	FAT	FIBRE
Hoi Sin, Sharwood's*	1 Tbsp/15g	32	0.0	211	2.7	49.5	0.3	0.1
Hoi Sin, Stir Fry, Asda*	1 Serving/100g	165	0.8	165	2.6	36.9	0.8	1.0
Hoi Sin & Garlic, Blue Dragon*	1 Serving/60g	80	1.6	133	1.2	26.1	2.6	0.0
Hoi Sin & Plum, Chinatown, Knorr*	¼ Jar/131g	96	0.9	73	0.8	15.8	0.7	1.2
Hoi Sin & Plum, Sweet & Fruity, Stir Fry, Sharwood's*	1 Serving/136g	128	1.8	94	0.7	19.9	1.3	0.9
Hoi Sin & Spring Onion, Stir Fry, Sharwood's*	1 Jar/165g	196	1.5	119	1.3	26.5	0.9	0.8
Hollandaise, Classic, for Fish, Schwartz*	1 Sachet/300g	456	49.2	152	0.7	0.4	16.4	2.0
Hollandaise, Classic, Knorr*	1 Serving/100ml	202	20.5	202	0.6	3.9	20.5	0.4
Hollandaise, Dry, Maille*	1 Serving/30g	148	15.2	495	1.0	10.8	50.6	0.0
Hollandaise, Fresh, Average	1 Pack/150g	342	32.4	228	2.4	6.1	21.6	0.0
Hollandaise, Full Fat, Dry, M & S*	1 Tbsp/20g	67	7.0	336	1.1	4.5	34.9	0.1
Hollandaise, Homemade, Average	1oz/28g	198	21.3	707	4.8	0.0	76.2	0.0
Hollandaise, M & S*	1 Serving/10g	41	4.4	410	0.9	3.6	43.6	0.5
Hollandaise, Mary Berry*	1 Serving/100g	472	43.8	472	1.4	17.8	43.8	0.3
Honey & Coriander, Stir Fry, Blue Dragon*	1 Pack/120g	115	0.7	96	0.5	22.1	0.6	0.3
Honey & Mustard, Chicken Tonight, Knorr*	¼ Jar/131g	139	6.2	106	0.8	15.1	4.7	0.6
Honey & Mustard, COU, M & S*	½ Jar/160g	112	4.6	70	2.3	9.2	2.9	0.7
Honey & Mustard, for Cooking, Asda*	1 Serving/200g	234	14.0	117	0.6	13.0	7.0	0.0
Honey & Mustard, Low Fat, Chicken Tonight, Knorr*	¼ Jar/131g	105	3.0	80	1.0	13.8	2.3	0.8
Hong Kong Curry, Loyd Grossman*	1 Jar/350g	371	26.9	106	1.3	7.8	7.7	0.8
Horseradish, Colman's*	1 Tbsp/15ml	17	0.9	112	1.9	9.8	6.2	2.6
Horseradish, Creamed, Colman's*	1 Tsp/16g	37	2.1	229	4.3	21.4	13.3	0.0
Horseradish, Creamed, M & S*	1 Tsp/5g	16	1.5	325	2.4	12.1	29.3	2.5
Horseradish, Creamy, Sainsbury's*	1 Tsp/5g	11	0.6	223	2.8	28.9	11.8	1.6
Horseradish, Mustard, Sainsbury's*	1 Tsp/5g	8	0.3	163	7.9	18.2	6.6	3.5
Hot Chilli, Deliciously Good, Homepride*	1 Serving/120g	62	0.6	52	1.3	10.6	0.5	1.1
Hot Onion, Sainsbury's*	1 Serving/10g	17	0.0	167	0.2	41.0	0.1	0.1
Hot Pepper	1oz/28g	7	0.4	26	1.6	1.7	1.5	0.0
HP*	1 Tbsp/15g	18	0.0	119	1.1	27.1	0.2	1.3
Indian Tikka, Chicken Tonight, Knorr*	1 Serving/250g	320	23.0	128	1.3	10.0	9.2	1.2
Italian, Basil & Onion, Slow Cooked, Dolmio*	1 Jar/350g	322	24.5	92	1.8	5.6	7.0	1.3
Italian, Tomato & Mascarpone, Tesco*	½ Tub/175g	159	11.0	91	2.7	5.9	6.3	0.7
Italian Hot Chilli, Dolmio*	½ Pack/150g	103	5.8	69	1.3	7.1	3.9	0.0
Italian Onion & Garlic, Sainsbury's*	1 Jar/500g	375	10.0	75	2.2	12.1	2.0	1.7
Italian Tomato & Herb, Sainsbury's*	¼ Jar/126g	88	2.5	70	2.0	11.1	2.0	1.4
Italian Tomato & Mascarpone, Sainsbury's*	½ Tub/175g	157	10.1	90	2.6	6.8	5.8	1.2
Italian Tomato & Sweet Basil, Go Organic*	1 Serving/80g	51	3.8	64	1.2	4.3	4.7	0.9
Jalfrezi, Cooking, Asda*	1 Jar/570g	519	35.9	91	1.2	7.4	6.3	1.7
Jalfrezi, Cooking, Sainsbury's*	1 Serving/250g	160	6.0	64	1.0	9.6	2.4	1.7
Jalfrezi, Spice & Stir, Geeta's*	½ Jar/175g	156	11.2	89	1.4	6.5	6.4	1.4
Jalfrezi, Stir Fry, Patak's*	1 Jar/250g	260	18.7	104	1.4	7.6	7.5	1.4
Jalfrezi, Sweet Pepper & Coconut, in Glass Jar, Patak's*	1 Jar/540g	626	37.8	116	1.7	11.3	7.0	1.4
Jambalaya, Cajun, Seasoned Pioneers*	1 Pack/400g	248	20.4	62	0.8	3.2	5.1	1.0
Jeera & Tamarind, Daal, Indian, Seasoned Pioneers*	1 Pouch/400g	228	12.0	57	1.8	7.2	3.0	1.6
Jerk/BBQ, Levi Roots*	¼ Bottle/78g	94	0.1	121	1.1	28.8	0.1	0.5
Kaffir Lime Chilli & Basil, Stir Fry, Sainsbury's*	1 Serving/150g	157	9.6	105	1.2	10.6	6.4	1.0
Kashmiri, Chilli & Peppers, Patak's*	½ Jar/212g	159	9.3	75	1.3	7.7	4.4	1.1
Korma, Authentic, VLH Kitchens*	1 Pot/118g	180	15.3	153	1.9	6.7	13.0	0.8
Korma, Coconut & Coriander, Canned, Patak's*	1 Can/283g	487	37.9	172	3.4	9.2	13.4	1.7
Korma, Coconut & Cream, Mild, in Glass Jar, Patak's*	1 Jar/540g	940	79.4	174	1.3	9.1	14.7	0.8
Korma, Cooking, Loyd Grossman*	½ Jar/175g	254	16.8	145	2.3	12.3	9.6	1.7
Korma, Cooking, Patak's*	¼ Jar/125g	211	17.5	169	1.3	9.3	14.0	2.4
Korma, Cooking, Sharwood's*	1 Jar/420g	680	42.8	162	1.7	15.9	10.2	2.2

SAUCE

INFO/WEIGHT	Measure	per Measure KCAL	FAT	Nutrition Values per 100g / 100ml KCAL	PROT	CARB	FAT	FIBRE
Korma, Deliciously Good, Homepride*	1 Jar/450g	396	19.8	88	1.4	10.6	4.4	1.4
Korma, Homepride*	1 Serving/160g	110	3.2	69	1.3	11.6	2.0	0.0
Korma, Organic, Patak's*	¼ Jar/106g	148	12.7	140	1.9	5.9	12.0	0.9
Korma, Royal, TTD, Sainsbury's*	½ Pack/175g	207	12.3	118	2.4	11.4	7.0	3.9
Korma, Sizzle & Stir, Knorr*	1 Jar/455g	1092	96.5	240	1.2	11.2	21.2	2.7
Korma with Flaked Almonds, Weight Watchers*	1 Serving/175g	107	3.7	61	2.0	8.5	2.1	1.6
Laksa, Finest, Tesco*	1/3 Jar/111g	105	8.2	95	1.3	5.5	7.4	1.8
Lemon, Amoy*	1 Tsp/5ml	5	0.0	104	0.0	26.0	0.0	0.0
Lemon, Stir Fry, Straight to Wok, Amoy*	½ Sachet/50g	81	0.1	162	0.3	40.0	0.2	0.0
Lemon, Stir Fry, Tesco*	1 Jar/450g	369	0.9	82	0.1	19.3	0.2	0.1
Lemon & Ginger, Stir Fry, Finest, Tesco*	¼ Jar/85g	144	0.2	169	0.2	41.7	0.2	0.2
Lemon & Sesame, Stir Fry, Sharwood's*	1 Serving/100g	125	0.1	125	0.1	30.9	0.1	0.1
Lime & Coriander, Tangy, for Fish, Schwartz*	1 Pack/300g	381	37.2	127	1.1	2.7	12.4	1.3
Lime Honey & Ginger, Stir Fry, Sharwood's*	1 Serving/50g	34	0.0	69	0.3	16.6	0.1	0.2
Madras, Cooking, HL, Tesco*	1 Serving/128g	55	2.6	43	1.6	4.8	2.0	2.3
Mango, Kashmiri Style, Finest, Tesco*	½ Jar/175g	285	23.8	163	2.4	7.7	13.6	0.9
Marie Rose, Fresh, The Saucy Fish Co.*	1 Pack/150g	589	59.7	393	1.6	7.0	39.8	0.0
Mediterranean Tomato, Spread & Bake, Heinz*	¼ Jar/70g	56	1.7	80	1.3	13.8	2.5	1.9
Mediterranean Vegetable, Chargrilled, Italiano, Tesco*	1 Pot/350g	175	3.9	50	1.6	8.4	1.1	1.3
Mexican, Cooking, BGTY, Sainsbury's*	¼ Jar/124g	51	0.2	41	0.7	9.2	0.2	0.8
Mexican Mild Chilli, Asda*	1 Serving/100g	55	0.4	55	2.0	10.8	0.4	1.8
Mint, Sainsbury's*	1 Dtsp/10g	13	0.0	126	2.5	28.7	0.1	4.0
Mint Garden, Fresh, Tesco*	1 Tsp/5g	2	0.0	40	2.6	3.6	0.4	1.5
Moglai, Tomato & Fennel, Cooking, Patak's*	1 Jar/283g	374	25.2	132	3.1	9.7	8.9	1.8
Mornay, Cheese, Asda*	¼ Pot/71g	114	9.0	161	6.8	6.6	12.7	0.4
Moroccan Chicken, Chicken Tonight, Knorr*	¼ Jar/125g	91	1.6	73	0.4	14.7	1.3	1.4
Moroccan Seven Vegetable Cous Cous, Sainsbury's*	1 Serving/50g	89	8.0	178	2.6	5.9	16.0	0.0
Mushroom, Creamy, Chicken Tonight, Knorr*	¼ Jar/125g	101	7.9	81	0.8	5.4	6.3	0.3
Mushroom, Creamy, Low Fat, Chicken Tonight, Knorr*	¼ Jar/125g	59	3.6	47	0.8	7.3	2.9	0.4
Mushroom, Schwartz*	1 Pack/170g	207	19.2	122	1.2	3.9	11.3	0.5
Mushroom & Garlic, 95% Fat Free, Homepride*	1 Serving/220g	154	9.2	70	0.9	7.0	4.2	0.3
Mushroom & Herb, Cooking, BGTY, Sainsbury's*	¼ Jar/125g	67	2.9	54	1.8	6.6	2.3	0.5
Mushroom & White Wine, Knorr*	1 Serving/100ml	99	8.0	99	1.0	4.0	8.0	0.6
Napoletana, Fresh, Sainsbury's*	½ Pot/150g	94	4.5	63	1.7	7.3	3.0	2.3
Napoletana, Italian, Tesco*	1 Pot/350g	178	4.2	51	1.5	8.5	1.2	1.0
Napoletana, Waitrose*	1 Pot/600g	252	8.4	42	1.8	5.5	1.4	1.7
Onion, Made with Semi-Skimmed Milk	1 Serving/60g	52	3.0	86	2.9	8.4	5.0	0.4
Onion, Made with Skimmed Milk	1 Serving/60g	46	2.4	77	2.9	8.4	4.0	0.4
Orange & Dill Sauce, for Fish, Zesty, Schwartz*	1 Pack/300g	180	1.5	60	0.4	13.5	0.5	0.5
Orange & Green Ginger, Blue Dragon*	1 Pack/120g	118	1.9	98	0.5	20.4	1.6	0.5
Oriental, Cantonese, Uncle Ben's*	¼ Jar/125g	107	0.2	86	0.8	20.3	0.2	1.2
Oriental Orange & Ginger, Homepride*	1 Serving/100g	68	0.1	68	0.7	15.9	0.1	0.0
Oriental Sweet & Sour, Express, Uncle Ben's*	1 Serving/170g	221	3.2	130	0.8	27.5	1.9	0.0
Oyster, Blue Dragon*	1 Tsp/5ml	6	0.0	121	3.4	26.9	0.0	0.0
Oyster & Garlic, Stir Fry, Straight to Wok, Amoy*	½ Pack/50g	97	1.5	195	4.9	37.0	3.0	0.0
Oyster & Spring Onion, Stir Fry, Blue Dragon*	1 Sachet/120g	122	0.1	102	1.4	23.5	0.1	0.1
Oyster Flavoured, Amoy*	1 Tsp/5ml	5	0.0	108	2.0	25.0	0.0	0.0
Panang, Thai, Seasoned Pioneers*	1 Pouch/400g	384	30.4	96	1.3	5.8	7.6	1.0
Paprika Chicken, Chicken Tonight, Knorr*	½ Jar/250g	240	21.7	96	0.9	3.5	8.7	1.4
Parsley, Instant, Dry, Asda*	1 Serving/23g	82	1.6	355	7.0	66.0	7.0	4.4
Parsley, Instant, Made Up, Semi Skim Milk, Sainsbury's*	¼ Sachet/51ml	34	1.1	67	3.5	8.6	2.1	0.1
Parsley, Made Up, Bisto*	1 Serving/50ml	41	2.4	82	0.6	9.2	4.8	0.0
Parsley, Tesco*	½ Pack/89g	85	5.1	95	2.8	8.1	5.7	1.1

SAUCE

INFO/WEIGHT	Measure	per Measure KCAL	FAT	Nutrition Values per 100g / 100ml KCAL	PROT	CARB	FAT	FIBRE
Parsley Lemon Caper, New Covent Garden Food Co*	¼ Carton/65ml	137	12.1	211	2.5	8.7	18.6	0.8
Peanut, Sainsbury's*	1 Sachet/70g	185	9.2	264	1.9	34.7	13.1	1.6
Peking Lemon, Stir Fry, Blue Dragon*	1 Serving/35g	47	0.2	134	0.0	31.6	0.7	0.5
Pepper, Creamy, Schwartz*	1 Pack/170g	116	9.2	68	1.5	3.4	5.4	1.0
Pepper, Creamy, Tesco*	1 Serving/85ml	128	11.4	151	1.2	6.4	13.4	0.5
Pepper & Tomato, Spicy, Stir Through, M & S*	½ Jar/95g	166	14.6	175	1.6	7.5	15.4	0.0
Peppercorn, Creamy, Asda*	¼ Jar/137g	137	11.0	100	1.1	6.0	8.0	0.2
Peppercorn, Creamy, Chicken Tonight, Knorr*	¼ Jar/125g	110	9.7	88	0.3	3.8	7.8	0.4
Peri-Peri, Extra Hot, Nando's*	1 Serving/5g	3	0.2	58	0.0	5.6	3.8	0.2
Peri-Peri, Hot, Nando's*	1 Serving/5g	3	0.2	65	0.0	5.2	4.8	0.6
Peri-Peri, Sweet, Nando's*	1 Tbsp/25g	35	0.5	142	0.5	30.7	2.1	0.0
Pimenton Bravas, Spanish, Seasoned Pioneers*	1 Pouch/400g	196	12.4	49	1.0	4.1	3.1	0.8
Pineapple Juice & Sweet Chilli, Stir Fry, M & S*	1 Pot/120g	192	0.6	160	1.6	36.8	0.5	0.5
Plum, Spiced, Heinz*	1 Serving/25g	32	0.0	128	0.5	31.1	0.1	1.0
Plum & Sesame, Stir Fry, M & S*	½ Jar/115g	138	0.1	120	0.9	29.0	0.1	1.8
Prawn Cocktail, Frank Cooper*	1 Tbsp/15g	47	4.0	316	0.8	18.3	26.7	0.1
Puttanesca, Fresh, Waitrose*	½ Pot/176g	118	7.7	67	1.8	6.2	4.4	1.2
Red & Yellow Pepper, Roasted, Sacla*	1 Serving/290g	232	17.1	80	1.1	5.5	5.9	0.0
Red Pepper, Sainsbury's*	1 Serving/37g	118	11.6	320	4.3	5.0	31.4	0.0
Red Thai, Loyd Grossman*	1Jar/350g	437	22.7	125	2.8	13.7	6.5	1.5
Red Wine, Cook in, Homepride*	¼ Can/98g	47	0.6	48	0.5	10.1	0.6	0.0
Red Wine, Cooking, BGTY, Sainsbury's*	1 Serving/125g	52	0.6	42	0.5	8.8	0.5	0.8
Red Wine & Onion, Rich, Simply Sausages, Colman's*	¼ Jar/125g	49	0.2	39	0.9	8.5	0.2	1.3
Redcurrant, Colman's*	1 Tsp/12g	44	0.0	368	0.7	90.0	0.0	0.0
Reggae Reggae, Cooking, Levi Roots*	½ Jar/175g	215	0.9	123	1.3	28.5	0.5	0.7
Reggae Reggae, Jerk BBQ, Levi Roots*	1 Jar/310g	375	0.3	121	1.1	28.8	0.1	0.5
Rendang, Indonesian, Seasoned Pioneers*	1 Pouch/400g	500	46.8	125	1.3	3.5	11.7	1.8
Rich Hoi Sin, Stir Fry, Straight to Wok, Amoy*	½ Sachet/60g	68	1.4	114	1.8	21.4	2.3	0.7
Risotto, Mushroom & White Wine, Sacla*	1 Serving/95g	151	12.3	159	3.7	6.9	13.0	0.0
Roast Peanut Satay, Stir Fry, Straight to Wok, Amoy*	½ Pack/60g	106	6.4	176	4.0	16.3	10.6	1.3
Roast Vegetable with Basil & Tomato, M & S*	1 Serving/100g	85	4.1	85	2.0	9.5	4.1	1.2
Roasted Peanut Satay, Stir Fry Sensations, Amoy*	1 Pouch/160g	354	19.8	221	4.7	21.9	12.4	1.0
Rogan Josh, 99% Fat Free, Homepride*	1/3 Jar/153g	92	1.1	60	1.8	11.6	0.7	2.0
Rogan Josh, Cooking, Light Choices, Tesco*	¼ Jar/125g	57	3.0	46	1.4	4.8	2.4	2.5
Rogan Josh, Curry, The Curry Sauce Company*	1 Serving/235g	310	23.7	132	1.9	8.4	10.1	1.5
Rogan Josh, Medium, Sharwood's*	½ Jar/210g	151	7.6	72	1.4	8.6	3.6	0.5
Rogan Josh, Sharwood's*	½ Jar/210g	220	16.8	105	1.2	7.0	8.0	1.5
Rogan Josh, VLH Kitchens*	1 Jar/460g	374	24.4	81.5	1.4	6.1	5.3	1.4
Romesco with Red Peppers & Nuts, M & S*	1 Serving /25g	94	8.3	375	3.3	5.7	33.3	5.9
Royal Korma, Tilda*	1 Pack/400ml	824	73.2	206	1.9	8.4	18.3	0.7
Rum, with Lambs Navy* Rum, Finest, Tesco*	¼ Pot/125ml	377	31.4	302	2.1	13.1	25.1	1.5
Satay, Stir Fry & Dipping, Finest, Tesco*	1 Tsp/5g	22	1.7	432	9.0	20.7	34.8	2.7
Sauce Ginger Garlic & Chilli Linghams, Linghams*	1 Serving/200ml	522	0.6	261	0.7	58.7	0.3	0.0
Sausage Casserole, Cook in, Homepride*	½ Jar/250g	92	0.5	37	0.7	8.0	0.2	0.6
Seafood, Colman's*	1 Tbsp/15g	44	3.4	296	0.9	21.5	22.9	0.4
Seafood, Organic, Simply Delicious*	1 Serving/35g	192	18.9	549	2.3	13.6	53.9	0.3
Seafood, Sainsbury's*	1 Tbsp/15g	49	4.2	330	0.7	17.6	28.2	0.1
Sizzling Szechuan, Uncle Ben's*	1 Serving/260g	289	18.5	111	0.9	10.8	7.1	0.0
Smoked Bacon & Tomato, Stir in, Dolmio*	½ Tub/75g	73	4.2	98	4.6	7.2	5.6	1.3
Smoked Paprika & Tomato, M & S*	1 Serving/300g	135	5.1	45	1.3	6.1	1.7	0.9
Soy, Average	1 Tsp/5ml	3	0.0	64	8.7	8.3	0.0	0.0
Soy, Dark, Amoy*	1 Tsp/5ml	5	0.0	106	0.9	25.6	0.0	0.0
Soy, Light, Amoy*	1 Tsp/5ml	3	0.0	52	2.5	10.5	0.0	0.0

SAUCE

Measure INFO/WEIGHT		per Measure		Nutrition Values per 100g / 100ml				
		KCAL	FAT	KCAL	PROT	CARB	FAT	FIBRE
Soy, Wasabi & Lemon Grass, Stir Fry, Finest, Tesco*	1 Pack/125g	119	2.7	95	1.5	16.3	2.2	0.9
Soy & Garlic, Stir Fry, Fresh Tastes, Asda*	1 Pack/180g	175	6.7	97	1.7	14.1	3.7	0.5
Soy and Plum, Stir Fry Additions, M & S*	½ Sachet/60g	48	0.2	80	1.5	17.5	0.3	1.5
Soya, Japanese, Waitrose*	1 Tbsp/15ml	11	0.1	74	7.7	9.4	0.6	0.8
Spanish Chicken, Chicken Tonight, Knorr*	½ Jar/250g	115	3.5	46	1.5	7.0	1.4	0.6
Spanish Style, Cooking, Light Choices, Tesco*	1 Jar/485g	131	1.5	27	1.0	5.0	0.3	1.4
Spiced Tomato Tagine, Sainsbury's*	1 Jar/355g	227	5.7	64	1.7	10.6	1.6	4.3
Spicy Pepperoni & Tomato, Stir in, Dolmio*	½ Pack/75g	115	8.7	154	3.3	9.3	11.6	0.8
Spicy Red Pepper & Roasted Vegetable, Sainsbury's*	1 Pot/302g	220	10.3	73	1.5	8.9	3.4	1.0
Spicy Sweet & Sour, Sharwood's*	1 Serving/138g	142	0.7	103	0.7	23.8	0.5	0.4
Spicy Szechuan, Safe To Eat*	1 Pouch/400g	124	2.4	31	1.0	4.8	0.6	0.3
Spicy Tikka, Cooking, Sharwood's*	1oz/28g	27	1.7	95	1.3	9.4	5.9	0.8
Spicy Tomato & Pesto, COU, M & S*	1 Serving/100g	60	2.5	60	2.2	6.8	2.5	1.3
Sticky BBQ, Spread & Bake, Heinz*	¼ Jar/78g	131	0.5	168	1.0	39.6	0.6	1.2
Sticky Plum, Stir Fry, Blue Dragon*	1 Serving/60g	145	0.2	242	0.1	35.6	0.3	0.0
Stir Fry, Chinese, with Soy, Ginger & Garlic, Tesco*	1 Pack/150g	180	8.4	120	2.1	14.2	5.6	0.8
Stir Fry, Fragrant Sichuan, M & S*	1 Jar/155g	194	4.5	125	0.7	24.4	2.9	0.3
Stir Fry, Hoi Sin with Garlic & Spring Onion, Tesco*	¼ Pack/38g	46	0.4	120	2.2	25.2	1.1	0.5
Stir Fry, Laksa, Cook Asian, M & S*	½ Pack/75g	82	6.0	110	0.9	8.9	8.0	1.0
Stir Fry, Pad Thai, Amoy*	1 Pack/120g	179	5.4	149	2.5	24.7	4.5	1.3
Stir Fry, Pad Thai, Tesco*	1 Pack/125g	112	2.9	90	1.3	15.8	2.3	0.8
Stir Fry, Sweet Soy with Ginger & Garlic, Blue Dragon*	½ Pack/60g	52	0.0	87	0.8	20.6	0.0	0.1
Stir Fry, Sweet Thai Chilli, Straight to Wok, Amoy*	1 Serving/60g	68	1.1	113	0.3	23.8	1.8	0.3
Stir Fry, Wasabi Plum Shot, Blue Dragon*	1 Sachet/140g	344	1.8	246	1.7	35.3	1.3	1.7
Stroganoff, Asda*	1 Serving/285g	305	25.6	107	1.5	5.0	9.0	0.3
Stroganoff, Mushroom, Creamy, M & S*	1 Serving/75g	86	6.9	115	3.3	4.8	9.2	0.6
Stroganoff, Tesco*	1 Serving/100g	89	7.3	89	0.7	5.3	7.3	0.4
Sun Dried Tomato, Heinz*	1 Serving/10ml	7	0.1	73	1.5	14.9	0.6	0.9
Sun Dried Tomato & Basil, Free From, Sainsbury's*	1 Serving/175g	126	4.9	72	2.9	8.7	2.8	1.5
Sun Dried Tomato & Basil, Seeds of Change*	1 Serving/100g	169	13.2	169	1.8	9.3	13.2	0.0
Sundried Tomato for Pasta, Dress Italian, Siciliana *	½ Jar/175g	93	8.6	53	1.3	4.0	4.9	8.0
Sweet & Sour, Aromatic, Stir Fry Sensations, Amoy*	1 Pack/160g	312	0.5	195	0.4	46.8	0.3	0.8
Sweet & Sour, Cantonese, Loyd Grossman*	1 Serving/225g	306	4.7	136	1.2	28.0	2.1	0.5
Sweet & Sour, Chinese, Sainsbury's*	½ Jar/150g	222	0.1	148	0.2	36.6	0.1	0.1
Sweet & Sour, Classic, Canned, Homepride*	1 Can/500g	440	0.5	88	0.3	21.5	0.1	0.5
Sweet & Sour, Cook In, Glass Jar, Homepride*	1 Jar/500g	335	0.5	67	0.3	16.2	0.1	0.5
Sweet & Sour, Cooking, Chinese, Sainsbury's*	¼ Jar/125g	155	0.1	124	0.6	30.1	0.1	0.7
Sweet & Sour, Cooking, Light Choices, Tesco*	1 Jar/510g	138	1.0	27	1.1	5.1	0.2	3.9
Sweet & Sour, Cooking, Organic, Sainsbury's*	1/3 Jar/150g	150	1.3	100	0.8	22.1	0.9	0.5
Sweet & Sour, Extra Pineapple, Uncle Ben's*	1 Serving/165g	147	0.3	89	0.3	21.2	0.2	0.7
Sweet & Sour, La Choy*	1/8th Jar/36g	68	0.0	189	0.0	38.9	0.0	0.0
Sweet & Sour, Light, Uncle Ben's*	¼ Jar/125g	65	0.1	52	0.4	11.6	0.1	0.8
Sweet & Sour, Organic, Seeds of Change*	1 Jar/350g	350	0.3	100	0.4	24.4	0.1	0.6
Sweet & Sour, Oriental, Chicken Tonight, Knorr*	½ Jar/262g	217	2.6	83	0.4	20.8	1.0	0.5
Sweet & Sour, Original, Uncle Ben's*	1 Pack/300g	264	0.6	88	0.4	21.9	0.2	0.8
Sweet & Sour, Perfectly Balanced, Waitrose*	1 Serving/175g	140	0.3	80	0.6	18.9	0.2	1.1
Sweet & Sour, Rice Time, Uncle Ben's*	1 Pot/300g	393	2.4	131	1.9	28.4	0.8	0.7
Sweet & Sour, Seeds of Change*	1 Serving/200g	174	0.0	87	0.3	21.3	0.0	0.7
Sweet & Sour, Sizzling, Uncle Ben's*	½ Jar/270g	375	18.1	139	0.6	19.2	6.7	0.0
Sweet & Sour, Spicy, Stir Fry, Sainsbury's*	1 Jar/500g	430	0.5	86	0.7	20.0	0.1	0.7
Sweet & Sour, Spicy, Uncle Ben's*	1 Jar/400g	364	0.4	91	0.6	22.1	0.1	0.0
Sweet & Sour, Stir Fry, GFY, Asda*	½ Pack/51ml	43	2.1	85	0.9	11.0	4.1	3.4
Sweet & Sour, Stir Fry, M & S*	1 Pack/120g	150	0.5	125	0.7	29.8	0.4	1.3

SAUCE	Measure INFO/WEIGHT	per Measure KCAL	FAT	Nutrition Values per 100g / 100ml KCAL	PROT	CARB	FAT	FIBRE
Sweet & Sour, Stir Fry, Sachet, Blue Dragon*	1 Sachet/120g	100	1.2	84	0.4	17.8	1.0	0.4
Sweet & Sour, Stir Fry, Sharwood's*	1 Jar 160g	168	0.8	105	0.6	24.5	0.5	0.8
Sweet & Sour, Stir Fry, Waitrose*	1 Serving/50ml	93	2.2	187	1.2	35.6	4.4	1.8
Sweet & Sour, Take-Away	1oz/28g	44	1.0	157	0.2	32.8	3.4	0.0
Sweet & Sour, Weight Watchers*	½ Jar/125g	61	0.1	49	0.6	11.5	0.1	0.2
Sweet Chilli, Dipping, M & S*	1 Tbsp/15g	34	0.1	225	0.9	53.2	0.7	0.6
Sweet Chilli, Dipping, Thai, Amoy*	1 Serving/10g	14	0.3	142	0.5	34.2	2.8	0.3
Sweet Chilli, Garlic, Stir Fry, Blue Dragon*	1 Pack/120g	142	0.1	118	0.2	28.8	0.1	0.3
Sweet Chilli, Heinz*	1 Serving/25g	37	0.1	150	0.3	36.5	0.4	6.4
Sweet Chilli, Lee Kum Kee*	1 Jar/215g	518	0.4	241	0.4	59.4	0.2	0.6
Sweet Chilli, Sharwood's*	1 Bottle/150ml	325	0.6	217	0.7	52.8	0.4	1.7
Sweet Chilli, Stir Fry, Additions, Tesco*	1 Serving/50g	105	3.8	211	0.3	35.2	7.6	0.6
Sweet Chilli, Stir Fry, BGTY, Sainsbury's*	1 Pack/150ml	178	2.8	119	0.6	25.0	1.9	1.1
Sweet Chilli & Coriander, Sharwood's*	1 Pack/370g	407	4.4	110	0.3	24.4	1.2	0.1
Sweet Chilli & Coriander, Sizzling, Homepride*	1 Serving/100g	51	0.2	51	0.7	11.5	0.2	0.0
Sweet Chilli & Lime, Chinatown, Knorr*	1 Jar/525g	635	17.3	121	0.6	22.0	3.3	0.5
Sweet Curry, Eazy Squirt, Heinz*	1 Serving/10ml	12	0.0	124	0.7	29.0	0.3	0.5
Sweet Pepper, Stir in, Dolmio*	½ Pot/75g	103	7.7	137	1.5	9.7	10.3	0.0
Sweet Soy & Roasted Red Chilli, Stir Fry, Blue Dragon*	½ Pack/60g	49	0.0	81	0.4	19.5	0.0	0.2
Sweet Soy & Sesame, Uncle Ben's*	1 Serving/100g	110	1.7	110	0.7	23.0	1.7	0.0
Sweet Soy & Spring Onion, Stir Fry Sensations, Amoy*	1 Pouch/160g	312	10.4	195	2.0	31.5	6.5	0.6
Sweet Thai Chilli, Uncle Ben's*	¼ Jar/125g	131	0.4	105	0.8	23.6	0.3	1.1
Szechuan, Spicy Tomato, Stir Fry, Blue Dragon*	1 Sachet/120g	151	6.7	126	1.3	17.6	5.6	2.0
Szechuan, Stir Fry, Sharwood's*	1 Jar/150g	126	1.6	84	3.0	15.5	1.1	0.4
Szechuan Style, Stir Fry, Fresh Ideas, Tesco*	1 Sachet/50g	114	4.8	228	1.9	33.4	9.7	0.1
Tabasco, Tabasco*	1 Tsp/5ml	1	0.0	12	1.3	0.8	0.8	0.6
Tamarind & Lime, Stir Fry, Sainsbury's*	1 Serving/75g	88	5.5	117	1.1	11.4	7.4	0.8
Tartare	1oz/28g	84	6.9	299	1.3	17.9	24.6	0.0
Tartare, with Olives, The English Provender Co.*	1 Tbsp/15g	64	6.6	425	2.2	5.7	43.7	0.7
Teriyaki, Fresh, The Saucy Fish Co.*	1 Pack/150g	318	2.8	212	2.8	45.8	1.9	0.0
Teriyaki, Japanese Grill, Kikkoman*	1 Serving/15ml	24	0.0	158	4.5	30.8	0.1	0.0
Teriyaki, Stir Fry, Blue Dragon*	1 Sachet/120g	124	0.0	103	0.5	25.0	0.0	0.0
Teriyaki, Stir Fry, Sharwood's*	1 Jar/150g	144	0.4	96	0.9	22.5	0.3	0.3
Thai, Sweet Chilli, Blue Dragon*	1 Serving/15g	28	0.1	188	0.5	45.5	0.6	0.0
Thai Chilli, Dipping, Sainsbury's*	1 Tbsp/15g	30	0.0	201	0.2	49.8	0.0	5.0
Thai Curry, Yellow, Loyd Grossman*	1 Serving/100g	111	7.5	111	1.7	9.1	7.5	1.0
Thai Fish, Nuoc Mam, Amoy*	1 Tbsp/15ml	12	0.0	80	13.4	6.7	0.0	0.0
Thai Green, Barts*	½ Pack/150ml	210	18.0	140	2.0	6.0	12.0	0.0
Thai Kaffir Lime, Chilli & Basil, Stir Fry, Sainsbury's*	½ Jar/175g	166	10.3	95	1.3	9.2	5.9	1.1
Thai Panang, Sainsbury's*	1/3 Pack/166g	229	19.6	138	1.4	6.6	11.8	1.4
Thai Satay, Sharwood's*	1oz/28g	160	13.4	573	17.2	18.0	48.0	6.3
Thai Satay, Taylor's *	1 1serving/50ml	122	8.4	245	4.8	31.6	16.9	2.0
Three Pepper, Bottled, Heinz*	1 Tbsp/10g	33	3.2	329	1.5	8.7	32.0	0.0
Tikka, BFY, Morrisons*	½ Jar/238g	259	8.1	109	2.3	17.2	3.4	1.3
Tikka, Cooking, BGTY, Sainsbury's*	1 Jar/500g	370	9.5	74	1.2	12.9	1.9	0.3
Tikka Bhuna, Sizzle & Stir, Chicken Tonight, Knorr*	½ Jar/230g	267	21.6	116	1.2	6.7	9.4	1.1
Tikka Masala, 98% Fat Free, Homepride*	1oz/28g	14	0.5	49	1.4	7.9	1.7	0.8
Tikka Masala, Cooking, Sharwood's*	1 Tsp/2g	2	0.2	122	1.2	11.9	7.8	0.9
Tikka Masala, Deliciously Good, Homepride*	¼ Jar/149g	121	5.4	81	2.1	10.0	3.6	1.5
Tikka Masala, Hot & Spicy, in Glass Jar, Patak's*	1oz/28g	29	2.2	105	1.9	6.6	7.9	1.1
Tikka Masala, Jar, Sharwood's*	1 Jar/435g	492	33.1	113	1.4	9.6	7.6	1.4
Tikka Masala, Lemon & Coriander, Canned, Patak's*	1 Can/283g	487	36.8	172	2.5	11.0	13.0	1.1
Tikka Masala, Light Choices, Tesco*	¼ Jar/125g	100	3.4	80	2.0	11.1	2.7	1.2

S

SAUCE	Measure INFO/WEIGHT	per Measure KCAL	FAT	Nutrition Values per 100g / 100ml KCAL	PROT	CARB	FAT	FIBRE
Tikka Masala, Perfectly Balanced, Waitrose*	½ Jar/175g	107	1.4	61	2.7	10.7	0.8	1.5
Tikka Masala, Spicy, Sharwood's*	1 Jar/420g	449	29.8	107	1.2	9.6	7.1	0.1
Tikka Masala for One, Express, Uncle Ben's*	1 Sachet/170g	168	10.7	99	1.5	9.0	6.3	0.0
Tikka Masala with Coriander, Weight Watchers*	½ Jar/175g	129	3.7	74	2.6	11.2	2.1	0.7
Toffee, Luxury, Rowse*	1 Serving/20g	67	0.7	336	1.9	73.9	3.7	0.4
Toffee Fudge, Sainsbury's*	1 Serving/40g	134	1.5	336	1.9	73.9	3.7	0.4
Tomato, Heinz*	1 Tbsp/17g	18	0.0	103	0.9	24.1	0.1	0.7
Tomato, Indian, Sizzling, Homepride*	1 Serving/240g	82	0.5	34	0.9	7.0	0.2	0.0
Tomato, Organic, Heinz*	1 Tsp/5g	5	0.0	105	1.3	24.0	0.1	0.9
Tomato, Pizza Topping, Napolina*	1 Serving/70g	34	1.5	49	0.9	6.3	2.2	0.6
Tomato & Basil, Cooking, BGTY, Sainsbury's*	1 Jar/500g	335	6.5	67	2.6	11.3	1.3	0.7
Tomato & Basil, Cooking, M & S*	1 Serving/130g	78	4.4	60	1.4	5.7	3.4	1.2
Tomato & Basil, Fresh, Organic, Waitrose*	¼ Pot/175g	77	3.0	44	1.0	6.2	1.7	0.8
Tomato & Basil, Italian, Sainsbury's*	½ Pot/175g	80	3.7	46	1.6	5.1	2.1	2.5
Tomato & Basil, Sun-Ripened, Microwaveable, Dolmio*	1 Sachet/170g	95	3.6	56	1.4	7.9	2.1	0.0
Tomato & Chilli, Waitrose*	1 Pot/350g	182	9.1	52	10.0	6.2	2.6	3.2
Tomato & Creme Fraiche, Less Than 3% Fat, Asda*	1 Pot/300g	168	8.4	56	0.7	7.0	2.8	0.5
Tomato & Mascarpone, Finest, Tesco*	1 Serving/350g	269	17.5	77	2.7	5.4	5.0	0.8
Tomato & Mascarpone, Fresh, Sainsbury's*	1/3 Pot/100g	91	6.6	91	2.1	5.9	6.6	1.2
Tomato & Mascarpone, Fresh, Tesco*	½ Pot/175g	206	15.2	118	2.8	7.1	8.7	0.6
Tomato & Mascarpone, Italiano, Tesco*	1 Serving/175g	194	15.2	111	2.8	5.4	8.7	0.6
Tomato & Mozzarella, Finest, Tesco*	1 Serving/175g	89	5.6	51	1.6	4.1	3.2	0.6
Tomato & Onion, Cook in, Homepride*	1 Can/390g	183	1.9	47	0.9	9.8	0.5	0.0
Tomato & Roasted Garlic, Stir in, Dolmio*	½ Pack/75g	94	7.6	125	1.2	7.7	10.2	0.0
Tomato & Smoked Bacon, Italiano, Tesco*	½ Pot/175g	96	4.4	55	3.0	4.7	2.5	1.0
Tomato & Wild Mushroom, Organic, Fresh, Sainsbury's*	1 Serving/152g	102	7.4	67	1.9	3.9	4.9	1.7
Tomato & Worcester, Table, Lea & Perrins*	1 Serving/10g	10	0.0	102	0.8	23.0	0.5	0.7
Tomato Frito, Heinz*	1 Serving/16g	13	0.6	80	1.5	9.7	3.9	0.8
Vegetable, Chunky, Tesco*	1 Can/455g	155	0.9	34	1.2	7.0	0.2	1.0
Vegetables, Hoi Sin & Plum, Stir Fry, Sharwood's*	1 Pack/360g	367	4.7	102	1.1	21.4	1.3	0.2
Watercress, & Stilton, Creamy, for Fish, Schwartz*	1 Pack/300g	141	12.3	47	0.6	2.0	4.1	0.7
Watercress, Fresh, The Saucy Fish Co.*	1 Pack/150g	169	14.5	113	2.2	5.8	9.7	0.0
Watercress & Creme Fraiche, COU, M & S*	½ Pack/154g	100	2.8	65	3.2	9.2	1.8	0.5
White, for Lasagne, Dolmio*	1 Jar/470g	451	34.3	96	0.6	7.0	7.3	0.0
White, Savoury, Made with Semi-Skimmed Milk	1oz/28g	36	2.2	128	4.2	11.1	7.8	0.2
White, Savoury, Made with Whole Milk	1oz/28g	42	2.9	150	4.1	10.9	10.3	0.2
White Wine, Chardonnay, M & S*	1 Serving/160ml	184	16.0	115	1.4	4.6	10.0	0.9
White Wine & Mushroom, BGTY, Sainsbury's*	¼ Jar/125g	81	2.5	65	2.8	9.0	2.0	0.3
White Wine & Tarragon, French, for Fish, Schwartz*	1 Pack/300g	372	33.3	124	1.1	5.0	11.1	0.8
White Wine and Cream, Cook in, Classic, Homepride*	¼ Can/125g	101	5.1	81	1.0	8.0	4.1	0.4
White Wine Mushroom & Herb, 98% Fat Free, Homepride*	1 Jar/450g	180	5.4	40	0.8	7.0	1.2	0.5
Wild Mushroom, Finest, Tesco*	½ Pack/175g	157	11.9	90	1.9	5.2	6.8	0.4
Worcestershire, Average	*1 Tsp/5g*	*3*	*0.0*	*65*	*1.4*	*15.5*	*0.1*	*0.0*
Worcestershire, Lea & Perrins*	1 Tsp/5ml	4	0.0	88	1.1	22.0	0.0	0.0
Worcestershire, Special Edition, Lea & Perrins*	1 Serving/10ml	13	0.0	130	1.3	28.8	0.2	0.1
Yellow Bean & Cashew, Tesco*	½ Jar/210g	170	6.1	81	1.6	11.9	2.9	0.3
SAUCE MIX								
Bacon & Mushroom Tagliatelle, Schwartz*	1 Pack/33g	110	1.0	333	7.5	69.2	2.9	8.3
Beef Bourguignon, Colman's*	1 Pack/40g	123	0.6	308	4.9	68.6	1.6	2.2
Beef Stroganoff, Colman's*	1 Pack/40g	140	3.6	350	11.6	56.1	8.9	2.7
Bombay Potatoes, Schwartz*	1 Pack/33g	84	4.0	254	16.1	20.1	12.1	31.1
Bread, Colman's*	1 Pack/40g	131	0.4	327	11.4	67.9	1.1	3.2
Bread, Knorr*	½ Pint/40g	177	9.3	442	7.9	49.9	23.3	2.1

SAUCE MIX	Measure INFO/WEIGHT	per Measure KCAL	FAT	Nutrition Values per 100g / 100ml KCAL	PROT	CARB	FAT	FIBRE
SAUCE MIX								
Bread, Luxury, Schwartz*	1 Pack/40g	142	2.6	355	12.9	61.5	6.4	6.5
Bread, Made Up, Colman's*	1 Serving/80ml	66	1.3	82	0.0	5.4	1.6	0.0
Cajun Chicken, Schwartz*	1 Pack/38g	108	0.5	285	6.4	61.9	1.3	0.5
Chargrilled Chicken Pasta, Schwartz*	1 Pack/35g	119	3.1	341	8.6	56.8	8.8	6.1
Cheddar Cheese, Colman's*	1 Pack/40g	163	6.2	407	18.3	48.8	15.4	1.2
Cheddar Cheese, Schwartz*	1 Pack/40g	144	3.0	361	18.4	55.1	7.4	2.3
Cheese, Knorr*	1 Pack/58g	132	2.8	227	7.8	38.0	4.9	1.8
Cheese, Made Up with Skimmed Milk	1 Serving/60g	47	1.4	78	5.4	9.5	2.3	0.0
Chicken Chasseur, Colman's*	1 Pack/45g	128	0.7	284	8.0	59.2	1.6	3.8
Chicken Chasseur, Schwartz*	1 Pack/40g	126	1.8	316	9.6	59.1	4.6	6.8
Chicken Korma, Colman's*	½ Pack/50g	229	15.4	459	6.6	38.8	30.8	13.2
Chicken Supreme, Colman's*	1 Pack/40g	143	3.7	358	12.1	56.7	9.2	2.4
Chilli Con Carne, Hot, Colman's*	1 Pack/40g	127	1.2	317	10.4	62.4	2.9	7.0
Chilli Con Carne, Schwartz*	1 Pack/41g	120	1.5	293	7.9	57.2	3.6	9.5
Chip Shop Curry, Dry Weight, Bisto*	1 Dtsp/9g	38	1.6	427	3.4	63.5	17.7	1.3
Coq Au Vin, Colman's*	1 Pack/50g	150	0.9	301	5.6	65.6	1.8	3.3
Creamy Chicken Curry, Colman's*	1 Sachet/50g	192	8.6	385	11.0	46.4	17.3	7.9
Creamy Pepper & Mushroom, Colman's*	1 Pack/25g	83	0.9	332	9.6	64.6	3.8	3.0
Curry, Batchelors*	1 Serving/100g	359	8.3	359	7.1	63.9	8.3	3.9
Four Cheese, Colman's*	1 Pack/35g	127	3.9	362	17.1	48.4	11.1	1.8
Hollandaise, Colman's*	1 Pack/28g	104	3.1	372	6.4	61.6	11.1	1.8
Hollandaise, Schwartz*	1 Pack/25g	98	3.2	394	10.6	59.2	12.8	3.7
Lamb Hotpot, Colman's*	1 Pack/40g	119	0.7	297	6.9	63.3	1.7	2.1
Lasagne, Schwartz*	1 Pack/36g	106	0.5	294	7.0	63.4	1.4	7.0
Lemon Butter, for Fish, Schwartz*	1 Pack/38g	136	3.0	357	6.1	65.3	8.0	5.8
Mexican Chilli Chicken, Schwartz*	1 Pack/35g	105	2.0	299	7.0	55.1	5.6	12.0
Mixed Herbs for Chicken, So Juicy, Maggi*	1 Pack/34g	97	1.0	285	8.3	53.8	2.8	5.5
Onion, Colman's*	½ Pack/17g	55	0.2	325	9.1	69.4	1.3	4.8
Onion, Creamy, Schwartz*	1 Pack/25g	90	2.3	362	10.1	59.6	9.2	5.3
Paprika Chicken, Creamy, Schwartz*	1 Pack/34g	116	3.3	342	9.7	53.9	9.8	9.5
Paprika For Chicken, So Juicy, Maggi*	1 Pack/34g	91	1.4	267	8.8	45.5	4.0	7.1
Parsley, Colman's*	1 Pack/20g	63	0.3	314	7.2	67.9	1.5	3.7
Parsley, Creamy, Schwartz*	1 Pack/26g	96	2.8	371	11.5	57.2	10.7	3.8
Parsley, Knorr*	1 Sachet/48g	210	11.6	437	4.2	50.6	24.2	0.8
Parsley & Chive, for Fish, Schwartz*	1 Pack/38g	132	3.2	348	9.0	58.9	8.5	7.7
Pepper, Creamy, Colman's*	1 Pack/25g	88	2.7	352	13.0	50.0	11.0	0.0
Pepper, Creamy, Schwartz*	1 Pack/25g	85	1.7	342	17.9	52.0	6.9	7.0
Pork & Mushroom, Creamy, Schwartz*	1 Pack/40g	116	1.6	289	8.6	54.7	4.0	12.1
Savoury Mince, Schwartz*	1 Pack/35g	108	0.7	310	14.6	58.3	2.0	1.8
Spaghetti Bolognese, Colman's*	1 Pack/40g	120	0.4	300	8.9	64.1	0.9	5.2
Spaghetti Bolognese, Schwartz*	1 Pack/40g	114	0.6	285	9.2	59.0	1.6	7.0
Stroganoff, Beef, Schwartz*	1 Pack/35g	125	3.6	358	15.6	50.8	10.3	4.4
Stroganoff, Mushroom, Schwartz*	1 Pack/35g	113	1.9	324	10.0	59.2	5.3	9.6
Sweet & Sour, Colman's*	1 Pack/40g	133	0.2	333	2.6	79.9	0.4	2.2
Sweet & Sour for Chicken, So Juicy, Maggi*	½ Pack/15g	42	0.3	279	7.1	55.8	2.3	3.5
Thai Green Curry, Schwartz*	1 Pack/41g	137	3.3	333	7.6	57.6	8.1	13.0
Thai Red Curry, Schwartz*	1 Pack/35g	120	2.5	342	5.9	63.5	7.1	7.6
Three Cheese, for Vegetables, Schwartz*	1 Pack/40g	168	8.2	421	17.4	41.7	20.5	4.8
Tikka Masala, Creamy, Schwartz*	1 Pack/31g	100	3.5	324	11.9	43.5	11.4	18.1
Tuna Napoletana, Schwartz*	1 Pack/30g	107	3.9	357	10.3	49.6	13.1	0.5
White, Dry Weight, Bisto*	1 Dtsp/9g	45	2.5	496	3.2	57.4	28.2	0.4
White, Instant, Made Up, Sainsbury's*	1 Serving/90ml	65	2.5	72	0.8	10.9	2.8	0.1
White, Made Up with Semi-Skimmed Milk	1oz/28g	20	0.7	73	4.0	9.6	2.4	0.0

S

	Measure INFO/WEIGHT	per Measure KCAL	FAT	Nutrition Values per 100g / 100ml KCAL	PROT	CARB	FAT	FIBRE
SAUCE MIX								
White, Made Up with Skimmed Milk	1oz/28g	17	0.3	59	4.0	9.6	0.9	0.0
White, Savoury, Colman's*	1 Pack/25g	84	0.7	335	10.7	66.5	2.9	2.6
White, Savoury, Knorr*	½ Pack/16g	46	0.9	290	7.8	52.2	5.6	5.2
White, Savoury, Schwartz*	1 Pack/25g	108	5.7	434	11.5	45.6	22.9	5.9
White Wine, with Herbs, Creamy, Schwartz*	1 Pack/26g	86	1.7	330	8.0	60.0	6.5	9.1
Wholegrain Mustard, Creamy, Schwartz*	1 Pack/25g	92	2.8	370	12.9	54.4	11.2	7.5
SAUERKRAUT								
Average	*1oz/28g*	*4*	*0.0*	*13*	*1.3*	*1.9*	*0.0*	*1.1*
SAUSAGE								
BBQ Hotdog, M & S*	1 Sausage/100g	300	25.3	300	12.1	5.4	25.3	2.0
Beef, Average	*1 Sausage/60g*	*151*	*11.1*	*252*	*14.5*	*7.0*	*18.5*	*0.6*
Beef, with Onion & Red Wine, Finest, Tesco*	1 Sausage/63g	117	6.9	185	13.2	8.5	10.9	1.2
Billy Bear, Kids, Tesco*	1 Slice/20g	37	2.2	185	13.7	7.5	11.2	0.4
Bockwurst, Average	*1 Sausage/45g*	*114*	*10.3*	*253*	*10.7*	*0.7*	*23.0*	*0.0*
Cheese & Leek, Tesco*	1 Sausage/55g	135	7.9	245	6.6	21.3	14.4	3.9
Chicken, Manor Farm*	1 Sausage/65g	126	8.1	194	13.7	6.6	12.5	1.2
Chicken & Tarragon, Butchers Choice, Sainsbury's*	1 Sausage/47g	106	6.8	225	18.1	5.8	14.4	0.2
Chicken & Turkey, Morrisons*	1 Sausage/57g	86	4.1	152	16.0	5.8	7.2	1.1
Chilli & Coriander, TTD, Sainsbury's*	1 Sausage/44g	136	10.7	310	18.5	4.2	24.4	1.2
Chilli Beef, Boston Style, Waitrose*	1 Sausage/67g	135	9.7	203	14.7	3.4	14.6	0.9
Chipolata, Average	*1 Sausage/28g*	*81*	*6.5*	*291*	*12.1*	*8.7*	*23.1*	*0.7*
Chipolata, Lamb & Rosemary, Tesco*	1 Sausage/32g	69	4.9	218	11.3	8.3	15.5	0.0
Chipolata, Pork, Extra Lean, BGTY, Sainsbury's*	1 Sausage/24g	46	2.1	189	16.9	10.9	8.6	0.5
Chipolata, Pork & Tomato, Organic, Tesco*	1 Sausage/28g	79	6.7	283	12.2	4.3	24.1	0.9
Chipolata, Premium, Average	*1 Serving/80g*	*187*	*13.8*	*233*	*14.8*	*4.7*	*17.3*	*1.2*
Chorizo, & Jalapeño, Pizzadella, Tesco*	1 Pizza/600g	1272	40.8	212	9.9	27.9	6.8	1.7
Chorizo, Average	*1 Serving/80g*	*250*	*19.4*	*313*	*21.1*	*2.6*	*24.2*	*0.2*
Chorizo, Lean, Average	*1 Sausage/67g*	*131*	*9.2*	*195*	*15.7*	*2.3*	*13.7*	*0.8*
Cocktail, Average	*1oz/28g*	*90*	*7.5*	*323*	*12.1*	*8.6*	*26.7*	*0.9*
Cumberland, Average	*1 Sausage/57g*	*167*	*13.0*	*293*	*13.8*	*8.5*	*22.7*	*0.8*
Cumberland, Healthy Range, Average	*1 Sausage/53g*	*75*	*2.1*	*142*	*17.4*	*9.0*	*4.0*	*0.9*
Debrecziner, Spicy Smoked, Gebirgsjager*	1 Sausage/37g	118	10.4	320	16.0	1.0	28.0	0.0
Extrawurst, German, Waitrose*	1 Slice/28g	80	7.1	281	13.0	1.0	25.0	0.0
Garlic, Average	*1 Slice/11g*	*25*	*2.0*	*227*	*15.7*	*0.8*	*18.2*	*0.0*
Irish, Average	*1 Sausage/40g*	*119*	*8.3*	*297*	*10.7*	*17.2*	*20.7*	*0.7*
Lamb & Mint, M & S*	1oz/28g	63	4.6	225	13.3	6.6	16.3	1.7
Lincolnshire, Average	*1 Sausage/42g*	*122*	*9.1*	*291*	*14.6*	*9.2*	*21.8*	*0.6*
Lincolnshire, Healthy Range, Average	*1 Sausage/50g*	*89*	*4.3*	*177*	*15.8*	*9.0*	*8.6*	*0.8*
Lorne, Average	*1 Sausage/25g*	*78*	*5.8*	*312*	*10.8*	*16.0*	*23.1*	*0.6*
Mediterranean Style, 95% Fat Free, Bowyers*	1 Sausage/50g	60	1.6	120	13.9	8.9	3.2	0.0
Mediterranean Style Paprika, Waitrose*	1 Sausage/67g	190	16.1	283	12.1	4.6	24.0	1.9
Merguez	1 Merguez/55g	165	14.3	300	16.0	0.6	26.0	0.0
Mortadella, Sainsbury's*	1 Slice/13g	34	2.8	261	17.3	0.1	21.2	0.1
Polish Kabanos, Sainsbury's*	1 Sausage/25g	92	7.6	366	23.0	0.1	30.4	0.1
Polony Slicing, Asda*	1oz/28g	60	3.9	214	11.0	11.0	14.0	0.0
Pork, & Sweet Chilli, Waitrose*	1 Sausage/67g	151	10.1	226	15.5	6.9	15.1	2.7
Pork, 30% Less Fat, Butcher's Choice, Sainsbury's*	1 Sausage/50g	99	5.3	198	15.9	9.5	10.7	0.5
Pork, Apricot & Herb, Waitrose*	1 Sausage/67g	165	11.1	246	11.2	12.9	16.6	1.3
Pork, Average	*1 Sausage/50g*	*152*	*11.9*	*305*	*12.8*	*9.8*	*23.8*	*0.7*
Pork, Bacon & Cheese, Asda*	¼ Pack/114g	329	23.9	289	18.0	7.0	21.0	0.4
Pork, Battered, Thick, Average	1oz/28g	126	10.2	448	17.3	21.7	36.3	2.0
Pork, Casserole, Diet Chef Ltd*	1 Portion/300g	303	18.3	101	6.6	4.9	6.1	1.4
Pork, Cumberland, Grilled, Light Choices, Tesco*	2 Sausages/96g	155	3.6	161	19.0	10.1	3.7	1.8

S

INFO/WEIGHT	per Measure KCAL	FAT	Nutrition Values per 100g / 100ml KCAL	PROT	CARB	FAT	FIBRE

SAUSAGE

	Measure INFO/WEIGHT	KCAL	FAT	KCAL	PROT	CARB	FAT	FIBRE
Pork, Cumberland, TTD, Sainsbury's*	1 Sausage/46g	132	9.7	288	21.4	3.1	21.1	0.6
Pork, Extra Lean, Average	1 Sausage/54g	84	3.7	155	17.3	6.1	6.8	0.8
Pork, Frozen, Fried	1oz/28g	88	6.9	316	13.8	10.0	24.8	0.0
Pork, Frozen, Grilled	1oz/28g	81	5.9	289	14.8	10.5	21.2	0.0
Pork, Garlic & Herb, Average	1 Sausage/76g	203	16.5	268	12.0	5.9	21.8	1.1
Pork, Lincolnshire, Traditionally Made, TTD, Sainsbury's*	1 Sausage/47g	149	11.4	318	20.2	4.5	24.3	0.7
Pork, Pancetta & Parmesan, TTD, Sainsbury's*	1 Sausage/47g	167	13.4	354	19.8	4.9	28.4	0.9
Pork, Plum Tomato & Herb, Uncooked, Finest, Tesco*	1 Sausage/55g	121	9.1	220	12.5	5.5	16.5	0.7
Pork, Premium, Average	1 Sausage/74g	191	13.6	258	14.9	8.3	18.4	1.0
Pork, Reduced Fat, Chilled, Grilled	1oz/28g	64	3.9	230	16.2	10.8	13.8	1.5
Pork, Reduced Fat, Chilled, Raw	1oz/28g	50	3.0	180	13.0	8.7	10.6	1.2
Pork, Reduced Fat, Healthy Range, Average	1 Sausage/57g	86	3.4	151	15.6	9.0	6.0	0.9
Pork, Roasted Pepper & Chilli, COU, M & S*	1 Sausage/57g	57	1.1	100	15.2	7.1	2.0	2.1
Pork, Skinless, Average	1oz/28g	81	6.6	291	11.7	8.2	23.6	0.6
Pork, Skinless, Sizzling, Classics, Grilled, Wall's*	1 Sausage/24g	48	5.9	201	11.5	8.9	24.6	1.4
Pork, Smoked Bacon, & Garlic, Finest, Tesco*	1 Sausage/67g	115	8.4	173	14.7	0.2	12.6	0.4
Pork, Thick, Average	1 Sausage/39g	115	8.7	296	13.3	10.0	22.4	1.0
Pork, Thick, Reduced Fat, Healthy Range, Average	1 Sausage/52g	90	3.8	172	14.0	12.3	7.4	0.8
Pork & Apple, Average	1 Sausage/57g	146	10.7	255	14.5	7.5	18.8	1.9
Pork & Beef, Average	1 Sausage/45g	133	10.2	295	8.7	13.6	22.7	0.5
Pork & Chilli, Tesco*	1 Sausage/67g	124	8.0	186	16.4	3.2	12.0	1.1
Pork & Herb, Average	1 Sausage/75g	231	19.5	308	13.1	5.4	25.9	0.3
Pork & Herb, Healthy Range, Average	1 Sausage/59g	75	1.4	126	16.0	10.7	2.4	1.1
Pork & Leek, Average	1oz/28g	73	5.6	262	14.6	6.0	19.9	1.1
Pork & Onion, Gluten Free, Asda*	1 Sausage/41g	105	7.0	257	20.0	6.0	17.0	1.8
Pork & Red Onion, TTD, Sainsbury's*	1 Sausage/48g	138	8.8	288	18.5	12.4	18.3	1.4
Pork & Smoked Bacon, Finest, Tesco*	1oz/28g	76	6.1	271	13.9	4.8	21.8	0.2
Pork & Stilton, Average	1 Sausage/57g	180	15.2	316	13.2	5.8	26.7	0.3
Pork & Tomato, Grilled, Average	1 Sausage/47g	127	9.7	273	13.9	7.5	20.8	0.4
Pork with Mozzarella, Italian Style, Tesco*	1 Sausage/76g	205	15.3	271	12.0	10.1	20.3	1.0
Premium, Chilled, Fried	1oz/28g	77	5.8	275	15.8	6.7	20.7	0.0
Premium, Chilled, Grilled	1oz/28g	82	6.3	292	16.8	6.3	22.4	0.0
Premium, Pork, Weight Watchers*	1 Sausage/39g	60	1.6	155	20.0	7.8	4.2	1.7
Saucisson Montagne, Waitrose*	1 Slice/5g	21	1.8	421	20.7	1.9	36.7	0.0
Schinkenwurst, German, Waitrose*	1 Slice/13g	28	2.2	224	16.0	0.8	17.6	0.0
Sicilian Style, TTD, Sainsbury's*	1 Sausage/50g	146	12.2	293	17.6	0.7	24.4	0.9
Smoked, Average	1 Sausage/174g	588	52.2	338	13.0	4.0	30.0	0.0
Toulouse, M & S*	1 Sausage/57g	123	8.9	215	12.4	5.8	15.6	1.3
Turkey, Average	1 Sausage/57g	90	4.6	157	15.7	6.3	8.0	0.0
Turkey & Chicken, Average	1 Sausage/57g	126	8.2	221	14.4	8.2	14.5	1.7
Tuscan, M & S*	1 Sausage/66g	145	10.6	220	14.9	4.6	16.0	0.6
Venison, Grilled, Finest, Tesco*	1 Sausage/41g	86	5.5	215	16.6	6.3	13.7	0.6
Venison, Oisin, M & S*	1 Serving/25g	41	2.3	165	16.8	3.8	9.3	0.7
Venison & Pork, Waitrose*	1 Sausage/63g	101	5.2	160	16.7	4.8	8.2	0.9
Venison & Red Wine, TTD, Sainsbury's*	1 Sausage/58g	130	7.7	226	19.7	6.8	13.3	1.7
Wiejska, Polish, Sainsbury's*	1/8 Pack/50g	78	4.5	157	18.7	0.4	9.0	0.5
Wild Boar	1 Sausage/85g	220	17.0	259	16.5	1.2	20.0	0.0

SAUSAGE & MASH

	Measure INFO/WEIGHT	KCAL	FAT	KCAL	PROT	CARB	FAT	FIBRE
2 British Pork & Rich Onion Gravy, M & S*	1 Pack/400g	340	6.8	85	5.7	12.2	1.7	1.3
British Classic, Tesco*	1 Pack/450g	675	42.7	150	5.1	11.1	9.5	0.9
GFY, Asda*	1 Pack/400g	330	10.0	82	4.2	10.7	2.5	1.7
Onion, M & S*	1 Pack/300g	315	17.1	105	4.1	9.0	5.7	1.5
Vegetarian, GFY, Asda*	1 Pack/400g	292	8.8	73	4.2	9.0	2.2	2.1

S

SAUSAGE & MASH	Measure INFO/WEIGHT	per Measure KCAL	FAT	Nutrition Values per 100g / 100ml KCAL	PROT	CARB	FAT	FIBRE
SAUSAGE & MASH								
Vegetarian, Tesco*	1 Pack/410g	398	15.6	97	4.6	11.1	3.8	2.0
Waitrose*	1 Pack/420g	517	31.1	123	4.2	9.9	7.4	0.1
with Onion Gravy, Tesco*	1 Pack/500g	525	27.0	105	3.0	11.1	5.4	1.6
with Red Wine & Onion Gravy, BGTY, Sainsbury's*	1 Pack/380g	315	7.2	83	5.0	11.4	1.9	2.0
SAUSAGE MEAT								
Pork, Average	*1oz/28g*	*96*	*8.2*	*344*	*9.9*	*10.1*	*29.4*	*0.6*
SAUSAGE ROLL								
Asda*	1 Roll/64g	216	16.0	337	7.0	21.0	25.0	0.8
BGTY, Sainsbury's*	1 Roll/65g	200	11.4	308	9.6	27.9	17.6	1.4
Cocktail, M & S*	1 Roll/14g	50	3.2	350	10.4	26.4	22.3	2.2
Cumberland, Chosen By You, Asda*	1 Roll/66g	201	10.9	304	8.3	28.9	16.5	3.1
Jumbo, Sainsbury's*	1 Roll/145g	492	34.4	339	8.2	23.2	23.7	1.5
Large, Freshbake*	1 Roll/52g	153	9.5	294	6.6	25.9	18.3	4.6
Lincolnshire, Geo Adams*	1 Roll/130g	474	31.6	365	8.3	28.2	24.3	1.1
M & S*	1 Roll/32g	122	9.1	380	10.5	21.0	28.4	0.9
Mini, M & S*	1oz/28g	122	8.7	435	9.8	29.6	30.9	1.8
Mini, Waitrose*	1 Roll/35g	124	9.2	353	13.0	16.1	26.3	1.0
Party, Sainsbury's*	1 Roll/13g	54	4.0	422	8.7	26.7	31.1	1.2
Pork, 30% Less Fat, Chosen By You, Asda*	1 Roll/66g	207	12.3	313	9.8	26.4	18.7	1.2
Pork, Snack, 30% Less Fat, Chosen By You, Asda*	1 Serving/33g	85	4.2	258	11.1	22.5	12.8	4.0
Pork Farms*	1 Roll/54g	196	12.9	363	7.9	30.0	23.9	0.0
Puff Pastry	1oz/28g	107	7.7	383	9.9	25.4	27.6	1.0
Reduced Fat, Sainsbury's*	1 Roll/66g	191	9.4	289	10.5	29.8	14.2	1.8
Sainsbury's*	1 Roll/67g	244	16.1	367	9.5	27.8	24.2	2.7
Snack, GFY, Asda*	1 Roll/34g	112	7.0	329	9.4	26.5	20.6	0.9
Snack Size, Tesco*	1 Roll/32g	118	8.8	369	9.1	21.7	27.4	2.3
TTD, Sainsbury's*	1 Roll/115g	440	31.9	383	11.9	21.3	27.8	2.0
Waitrose*	1 Roll/75g	287	19.6	383	10.1	27.0	26.1	1.3
SAUSAGE ROLL VEGETARIAN								
Linda McCartney*	1 Roll/52g	142	7.0	273	9.7	28.2	13.5	2.5
SAUSAGE VEGETARIAN								
Cumberland, Waitrose*	1 Sausage/50g	80	3.3	160	12.6	12.3	6.7	2.4
Glamorgan, Leek & Cheese, Goodlife*	1 Sausage/50g	94	4.9	188	4.9	20.0	9.8	2.3
Glamorgan, Organic, Waitrose*	1 Sausage/42g	81	4.2	194	14.5	11.2	10.1	1.7
Glamorgan Leek & Cheese, Sainsbury's*	1 Sausage/50g	98	5.2	197	4.3	21.3	10.5	2.7
Leek & Cheese, Organic, Cauldron Foods*	1 Sausage/41g	80	4.1	194	14.4	11.3	10.1	1.7
Lincolnshire, Chilled, Cauldron Foods*	1 Sausage/50g	83	4.9	166	10.0	9.5	9.8	7.0
Lincolnshire, Frozen, Tesco*	1 Sausage/50g	77	2.5	155	15.5	10.8	5.0	3.0
Linda McCartney*	1 Sausage/50g	101	4.4	202	22.6	8.2	8.8	1.6
Mushroom & Herb, Waitrose*	1 Sausage/50g	61	2.7	123	10.2	8.1	5.4	0.5
Mushroom & Tarragon, Wicken Fen*	1 Sausage/47g	82	3.5	175	10.1	17.0	7.4	2.4
Realeat*	1 Sausage/40g	66	3.9	165	17.2	2.0	9.8	8.1
Roasted Garlic & Oregano, Cauldron Foods*	1 Sausage/50g	89	5.0	179	13.1	9.0	10.1	2.1
Smoked Paprika & Chilli, Cauldron Foods*	1 Sausage/50g	76	4.1	152	7.8	11.8	8.2	2.6
Spinach, Leek & Cheese, Gourmet, Wicken Fen*	1 Sausage/46g	92	4.7	201	10.3	17.0	10.2	1.9
Sun Dried Tomato & Black Olive, Cauldron Foods*	1 Sausage/50g	71	3.8	142	8.7	9.4	7.7	2.6
Sun Dried Tomato & Herb, Linda McCartney*	1 Sausage/35g	93	5.4	266	21.8	10.1	15.4	1.7
SAVOURY EGGS								
Bites, Sainsbury's*	1 Egg/20g	55	3.6	277	9.6	18.8	18.2	2.1
Mini, Tesco*	1 Egg/20g	55	3.5	274	9.2	20.2	17.4	2.3
SCALLOPS								
Canadian, Finest, Tesco*	½ Pack/100g	80	0.2	80	16.4	2.6	0.2	0.1
Hotbake Shells, Sainsbury's*	1 Serving/140g	241	15.7	172	9.5	8.4	11.2	0.8

	Measure INFO/WEIGHT	per Measure KCAL	FAT	Nutrition Values per 100g / 100ml KCAL	PROT	CARB	FAT	FIBRE
SCALLOPS								
Lemon Grass & Ginger, Tesco*	½ Pack/112g	90	1.1	80	15.2	2.5	1.0	0.6
Raw, Bay Or Sea, with Roe, Average	*1 Lge/15g*	*13*	*0.1*	*88*	*16.8*	*2.4*	*0.8*	*0.0*
Steamed, Average	1oz/28g	33	0.4	118	23.2	3.4	1.4	0.0
with Roasted Garlic Butter, Finest, Tesco*	1 Serving/100g	201	14.3	201	16.2	1.8	14.3	0.4
SCAMPI								
Breaded, Baked, Average	½ Pack/255g	565	27.4	222	10.7	20.5	10.7	1.0
Breaded, Fried in Oil, Average	1 Serving/100g	237	13.6	237	9.4	20.5	13.6	0.0
SCAMPI & CHIPS								
Chunky, Finest, Tesco*	1 Pack/280g	420	15.4	150	5.9	18.3	5.5	1.4
with Peas	1 Serving/490g	822	43.6	168	10.1	11.3	8.9	1.2
Youngs*	1oz/28g	42	1.5	150	5.0	20.3	5.4	1.7
SCHNAPPS								
Vodkat, Intercontinental Brands Ltd*	1 Serving/25ml	31	0.0	124	0.0	0.8	0.0	0.0
SCHNITZEL VEGETARIAN								
Breaded, Tivall*	1 Piece/100g	172	8.0	172	16.0	9.0	8.0	5.0
SCONE								
3% Fat, M & S*	1 Scone/65g	179	1.6	275	7.2	55.1	2.5	2.3
All Butter, Sultana, Duchy Originals*	1 Scone/78g	276	9.8	353	7.3	52.9	12.5	2.6
All Butter, Tesco*	1 Scone/41g	126	3.2	308	7.2	52.3	7.8	1.6
Cheese, Average	1 Scone/40g	145	7.1	363	10.1	43.2	17.8	1.6
Cheese & Black Pepper, Mini, M & S*	1 Scone/18g	67	3.3	370	10.2	41.1	18.3	1.7
Cherry, Double Butter, Genesis Crafty*	1 Scone/63g	198	4.8	314	6.8	54.5	7.6	1.4
Cherry, Genesis Crafty*	1 Scone/81g	226	5.8	279	4.9	50.5	7.1	0.0
Cherry, M & S*	1 Scone/60g	202	7.3	337	6.9	49.7	12.2	1.9
Clotted Cream, Cornish, TTD, Sainsbury's*	1 Scone/70g	269	12.7	384	8.4	46.6	18.2	2.1
Cream, Sainsbury's*	1 Scone/50g	172	8.7	345	4.6	42.5	17.4	3.1
Derby, Asda*	1 Scone/59g	202	5.9	342	7.0	56.0	10.0	0.0
Derby, Mother's Pride*	1 Scone/60g	208	8.4	347	5.2	49.8	14.0	1.5
Devon, Asda*	1 Scone/59g	208	6.3	353	7.3	55.5	10.6	3.0
Devon, M & S*	1 Scone/59g	225	9.6	380	7.1	50.8	16.2	1.5
Devon, Waitrose*	1 Scone/72g	268	9.5	373	7.5	56.0	13.2	2.3
Fruit, Average	1 Scone/40g	126	3.9	316	7.3	52.9	9.8	0.0
Luxury, Hovis*	1 Scone/85g	267	7.9	314	5.6	51.8	9.3	2.2
Plain, Average	1 Scone/40g	145	5.8	362	7.2	53.8	14.6	1.9
Potato, Average	1 Scone/40g	118	5.7	296	5.1	39.1	14.3	1.6
Strawberry, Fresh Cream, Sainsbury's*	1 Scone/60g	218	11.2	363	6.5	42.5	18.6	1.4
Sultana, BGTY, Sainsbury's*	1 Scone/63g	178	1.8	283	7.7	56.7	2.8	2.4
Sultana, GFY, Asda*	1 Scone/59g	192	2.6	324	7.0	64.0	4.4	2.0
Sultana, M & S*	1 Scone/66g	231	8.2	350	6.5	53.0	12.5	2.0
Sultana, Reduced Fat, Waitrose*	1 Scone/65g	187	3.4	287	6.6	53.2	5.3	2.6
Sultana, Sainsbury's*	1 Scone/54g	176	5.9	327	6.9	50.2	11.0	6.5
Sultana, Tesco*	1 Scone/60g	189	5.0	315	7.1	52.5	8.4	2.6
Sultana, TTD, Sainsbury's*	1 Scone/70g	239	8.1	341	6.5	52.9	11.5	2.6
Tattie, Scottish, Nick Nairn's*	1 Scone/21g	42	0.3	199	4.0	34.7	1.6	0.7
Wholemeal	1 Scone/40g	130	5.8	326	8.7	43.1	14.4	5.2
Wholemeal, Fruit	1 Scone/40g	130	5.1	324	8.1	47.2	12.8	4.9
SCONE MIX								
Fruit, Asda*	1 Scone/48g	143	2.4	301	7.0	57.0	5.0	3.7
SCOTCH EGGS								
Retail	1 Egg/120g	301	20.5	251	12.0	13.1	17.1	0.0
Savoury, M & S*	1 Egg/21g	63	4.5	305	11.0	15.7	21.8	1.3
Super Mini, Asda*	1 Egg/13g	38	2.6	305	10.0	19.0	21.0	2.1

S

SEA BASS
Cooked, Dry Heat, Average	**1 Fillet/101g**	**125**	**2.6**	**124**	**23.6**	**0.0**	**2.6**	**0.0**
Fillet, in Beurre Blanc & Dill Sauce, The Saucy Fish Co.*	2 Fillets/230g	354	21.2	154	17.8	0.0	9.2	0.0
Fillets, Chosen By You, Asda*	½ Pack/120g	277	22.7	231	15.1	0.0	18.9	0.0
Fillets, Skinless, Boneless, TTD, Sainsbury's*	1 Serving/100g	162	9.2	162	19.4	0.5	9.2	0.5
Raw, Average	**1oz/28g**	**32**	**1.0**	**113**	**20.3**	**0.0**	**3.5**	**0.1**

SEA BREAM
Fillets, Raw, Average	**1oz/28g**	**27**	**0.8**	**96**	**17.5**	**0.0**	**2.9**	**0.0**

SEAFOOD COCKTAIL
Average	1oz/28g	24	0.4	87	15.6	2.9	1.5	0.0

SEAFOOD SELECTION
Fresh, Tesco*	1 Pack/234g	187	2.3	80	17.7	0.1	1.0	0.0
M & S*	1 Serving/200g	170	2.0	85	17.4	1.6	1.0	0.5
Sainsbury's*	½ Pack/125g	85	1.2	68	14.6	0.8	1.0	2.5

SEAFOOD STICKS
Average	1 Stick/15g	16	0.0	106	8.0	18.4	0.2	0.2
with Cocktail Dip, Asda*	1 Pot/95g	126	4.7	133	6.0	16.0	5.0	0.1

SEASONING
Aromat, Knorr*	1oz/28g	45	1.0	161	11.7	15.1	3.7	0.9
Spicy Cajun, Bags Better Chicken*	1 Pack/30g	94	3.2	313	7.7	58.0	10.7	11.7
Sushi, Mitsukan*	2 Tbsp/30ml	50	1.0	167	0.0	36.7	3.3	0.0

SEASONING CUBES
for Potato, Mint, Perfect Potato, Knorr*	1 Cube/10g	56	5.0	560	5.1	21.2	50.5	1.8
for Rice, Pilau, Knorr*	1 Cube/10g	30	2.3	305	11.4	13.9	22.6	1.4
for Rice, Saffron, Knorr*	1 Cube/10g	29	1.8	291	13.8	17.5	18.4	2.2

SEASONING MIX
Beef Taco, Colman's*	1 Pack/30g	76	3.6	252	9.1	26.9	12.0	14.0
Cajun, Sizzle & Grill, Schwartz*	1 Tsp/4g	7	0.2	182	9.8	23.0	5.6	24.4
Chicken, Chargrilled, Grill & Sizzle, Schwartz*	1 Tsp/5g	12	0.2	232	8.2	40.8	4.0	13.1
Chicken, Simply Shake, Schwartz*	1 Serving/100g	273	8.1	273	12.3	67.9	8.1	29.1
Chicken Fajitas, Schwartz*	1 Pack/35g	99	0.9	283	10.9	54.1	2.5	10.8
Chilli, Old El Paso*	Pack/39g	117	1.9	301	7.0	57.0	5.0	0.0
Chinese Curry, Youngs*	1 Serving/22g	109	6.8	495	8.3	46.4	30.7	0.0
Fajita, Chicken, Colman's*	1 Pack/40g	138	2.5	344	9.4	62.5	6.3	4.8
Fish, Schwartz*	1 Tsp/4g	9	0.1	222	6.5	55.5	2.3	11.6
Italian Herb, Schwartz*	1 Tsp/1g	3	0.0	338	11.0	64.5	4.0	0.0
Jamaican Jerk Chicken, Recipe, Schwartz*	1 Pack/27g	75	0.8	276	9.8	69.8	3.0	17.2
Lemon & Herb, Cous Cous, Asda*	1 Tbsp/15g	46	1.0	305	10.6	52.0	6.5	10.2
Mediterranean, Season & Shake, Colman's*	1 Pack/33g	99	0.7	300	10.3	56.8	2.1	5.9
Mediterranean Roasted Vegetable, Schwartz*	1 Pack/30g	86	1.2	288	6.9	56.1	4.0	10.3
Potato Roasties, Rosemary & Garlic, Crispy, Schwartz*	1 Pack/33g	88	2.6	267	13.0	36.1	7.8	21.1
Potato Roasties, Southern Fried, Crispy, Schwartz*	1 Pack/35g	78	1.5	222	9.2	36.2	4.4	25.1
Potato Wedges, Cajun, Schwartz*	1 Pack/38g	112	2.9	295	9.1	47.6	7.6	14.3
Potato Wedges, Garlic & Herb, Schwartz*	1 Pack/38g	106	1.9	278	11.4	47.1	4.9	11.7
Potato Wedges, Nacho Cheese, Schwartz*	1 Pack/38g	114	3.7	299	13.6	39.3	9.7	7.7
Potato Wedges, Onion & Chive, Schwartz*	1 Pack/38g	113	0.7	297	10.9	59.4	1.8	6.5
Season-All, Schwartz*	1 Tsp/6g	4	0.1	72	2.3	11.6	1.8	0.0
Shepherd's Pie, Colman's*	1 Pack/50g	141	0.7	282	12.5	54.7	1.4	4.3
Shotz, Cajun Chicken Seasoning, Schwartz*	1 Pack/3g	8	0.2	268	9.9	45.6	5.2	0.0
Shotz, Chargrilled Chicken Seasoning, Schwartz*	1 Pack/3g	8	0.1	283	7.5	52.0	4.9	0.0
Shotz, Garlic Pepper Steak Seasoning, Schwartz*	1 Pack/3g	11	0.1	370	14.0	67.0	5.0	0.0
Shotz, Moroccan Chicken Seasoning, Schwartz*	1 Pack/3g	9	0.2	312	9.7	56.7	5.2	0.0
Shotz, Seven Pepper Steak Seasoning, Schwartz*	1 Pack/3g	7	0.1	246	8.2	47.8	2.4	0.0
Spanish Roasted Vegetables, Schwartz*	1 Pack/15g	22	0.9	147	9.1	14.1	6.0	22.6

S

	Measure INFO/WEIGHT	per Measure KCAL	FAT	Nutrition Values per 100g / 100ml KCAL	PROT	CARB	FAT	FIBRE
SEASONING MIX								
Taco, Old El Paso*	¼ Pack/9g	30	0.4	334	5.5	69.0	4.0	0.0
Thai Seven Spice, Schwartz*	1 Serving/10g	24	0.4	243	7.5	44.1	4.1	0.0
SEAWEED								
Crispy, Average	*1oz/28g*	*182*	*17.3*	*651*	*7.5*	*15.6*	*61.9*	*7.0*
Irish Moss, Raw	*1oz/28g*	*2*	*0.1*	*8*	*1.5*	*0.0*	*0.2*	*12.3*
Kombu, Dried, Raw	*1oz/28g*	*12*	*0.4*	*43*	*7.1*	*0.0*	*1.6*	*58.7*
Nori, Dried, Raw	*1oz/28g*	*38*	*0.4*	*136*	*30.7*	*0.0*	*1.5*	*44.4*
Wakame, Dried, Raw	*1oz/28g*	*20*	*0.7*	*71*	*12.4*	*0.0*	*2.4*	*47.1*
SEEDS								
Chia, Black, The Chia Company*	1 Tbsp/15g	69	4.6	458	20.4	37.0	30.4	36.0
Chia, White, The Chia Company*	1 Tbsp/15g	69	5.1	458	20.4	37.0	34.0	36.0
Fenugreek, Average	*1 Tsp/4g*	*12*	*0.2*	*323*	*23.0*	*58.3*	*6.4*	*24.6*
Fiery, Graze*	1 Pack/35g	205	16.6	585	22.9	17.7	47.5	5.0
Flaxseed, Sunflower & Pumpkin, Milled, Linwoods*	1 Scoop/10g	54	4.9	542	22.7	2.4	49.1	16.2
Hemp, Raw, Organic, Navitas Naturals*	1 Serving/15g	80	7.0	533	33.3	20.0	46.7	6.7
Hemp, Shelled, Linwoods*	2 Dsp/30g	178	14.8	593	35.1	7.6	49.5	5.9
Melon, Average	*1 Tbsp/15g*	*87*	*7.2*	*583*	*28.5*	*9.9*	*47.7*	*0.0*
Mixed, Wholesome, Love Life, Waitrose*	1 Serving/30g	166	13.6	554	21.3	15.5	45.2	8.0
Mustard, Average	*1 Tsp/3g*	*15*	*0.9*	*469*	*34.9*	*34.9*	*28.8*	*14.7*
Nigella, Average	*1 Tsp/5g*	*20*	*1.7*	*392*	*21.3*	*1.9*	*33.3*	*8.4*
Poppy, Average	*1 Tbsp/9g*	*47*	*3.9*	*533*	*18.0*	*23.7*	*44.7*	*10.0*
Pumpkin, Average	*1 Tbsp/10g*	*57*	*4.6*	*568*	*27.9*	*13.0*	*45.9*	*3.8*
Pumpkin, Whole, Roasted, Salted, Average	*1 Serving/50g*	*261*	*21.1*	*522*	*33.0*	*13.4*	*42.1*	*3.9*
Sesame, Average	*1oz/28g*	*171*	*15.8*	*610*	*22.3*	*3.6*	*56.4*	*7.7*
Sunflower, Average	*1 Tbsp/10g*	*59*	*4.9*	*585*	*23.4*	*15.0*	*48.7*	*5.7*
SEMOLINA								
Average	*1oz/28g*	*98*	*0.5*	*348*	*11.0*	*75.2*	*1.8*	*2.1*
Pudding, Creamed, Ambrosia*	1 Can/425g	344	7.2	81	3.3	13.1	1.7	0.2
SHALLOTS								
Raw, Average	*1 Serving/80g*	*16*	*0.2*	*20*	*1.5*	*3.3*	*0.2*	*1.4*
SHANDY								
Bitter, Original, Ben Shaws*	1 Can/330ml	89	0.0	27	0.0	6.0	0.0	0.0
Homemade, Average	1 Pint/568ml	148	0.0	26	0.2	2.9	0.0	0.0
Lemonade, Schweppes*	1 Can/330ml	76	0.0	23	0.0	5.1	0.0	0.0
SHARK								
Raw	*1oz/28g*	*29*	*0.3*	*102*	*23.0*	*0.0*	*1.1*	*0.0*
SHARON FRUIT								
Average	*1oz/28g*	*20*	*0.0*	*73*	*0.8*	*18.6*	*0.0*	*1.6*
SHERBET LEMONS								
M & S*	1oz/28g	107	0.0	382	0.0	93.9	0.0	0.0
SHERRY								
Dry, Average	*1 Glass/120ml*	*139*	*0.0*	*116*	*0.2*	*1.4*	*0.0*	*0.0*
Medium	*1 Serving/50ml*	*58*	*0.0*	*116*	*0.1*	*5.9*	*0.0*	*0.0*
Sweet	*1 Serving/50ml*	*68*	*0.0*	*136*	*0.3*	*6.9*	*0.0*	*0.0*
SHORTBREAD								
All Butter, Deans*	1 Biscuit/15g	77	3.8	511	4.9	65.7	25.4	1.2
All Butter, Petticoat Tails, Gardiners of Scotland*	1 Biscuit/12g	64	3.4	514	5.2	62.1	27.2	0.0
All Butter, Round, Luxury, M & S*	1 Biscuit/20g	105	5.8	525	6.2	60.0	29.0	2.0
All Butter, Scottish, M & S*	1 Biscuit/34g	173	9.5	510	5.7	58.9	27.8	2.3
All Butter, Thins, M & S*	1 Biscuit/10g	50	2.2	485	5.8	68.4	21.1	3.5
All Butter, Trufree*	1 Biscuit/11g	58	3.1	524	2.0	66.0	28.0	0.9
Average	1oz/28g	139	7.3	498	5.9	63.9	26.1	1.9
Belgian Chocolate Chunk, Asda*	1 Biscuit/20g	106	6.2	531	7.0	56.0	31.0	1.8

S

	Measure INFO/WEIGHT	per Measure KCAL	FAT	Nutrition Values per 100g / 100ml KCAL	PROT	CARB	FAT	FIBRE
SHORTBREAD								
Butter, Extra Special, Asda*	1 Serving/19g	101	5.9	531	7.0	56.0	31.0	1.8
Caramel, Millionaires, Fox's*	1 Serving/16g	75	3.9	483	6.1	57.9	25.3	0.1
Choc Chip, Fair Trade, Co-Op*	1 Biscuit/19g	100	6.0	526	5.3	57.9	31.6	2.6
Chocolate, Waitrose*	1oz/28g	144	7.8	516	5.5	61.2	27.7	1.8
Chocolate Chip, Jacob's*	1 Biscuit/17g	87	4.7	513	5.2	61.2	27.5	1.8
Chocolate Chip, Tesco*	1 Serving/20g	105	6.1	525	7.5	55.0	30.6	3.0
Chocolate Chunk, Belgian, TTD, Sainsbury's*	1 Biscuit/19g	101	5.7	521	5.1	59.1	29.4	2.0
Clotted Cream, Finest, Tesco*	1 Biscuit/20g	109	6.4	543	5.2	58.0	32.2	1.7
Crawfords*	1 Biscuit/13g	67	3.4	533	6.6	65.0	27.4	2.0
Demerara, Rounds, TTD, Sainsbury's*	1 Biscuit/22g	113	5.9	508	5.1	62.2	26.5	1.8
Double Choc Chip, Petit Four, Scottish, Tesco*	1 Serving/50g	265	15.0	531	5.1	60.4	30.0	1.7
Dutch, M & S*	1 Biscuit/17g	90	5.2	530	5.7	58.2	30.6	0.9
Free From, Sainsbury's*	1 Biscuit/20g	98	5.2	490	6.0	58.0	26.0	6.0
Hearts, with Milk Chocolate, M & S*	1 Biscuit/25g	125	6.4	500	7.2	59.5	25.8	3.0
Highland, Organic, Duchy Originals*	1 Biscuit/16g	80	4.2	515	5.2	61.8	27.4	1.7
Highland Demerara Rounds, Sainsbury's*	1 Biscuit/20g	113	5.8	565	5.5	70.5	29.0	2.0
Honey & Oatmeal, Walkers*	1 Biscuit/34g	158	7.6	465	6.7	64.1	22.4	3.8
Orange Marmalade & Oatflake, Deans*	1 Biscuit/20g	105	5.9	524	6.7	59.3	29.6	3.2
Organic, Waitrose*	1 Biscuit/13g	62	3.0	495	5.8	63.0	24.4	1.8
Pecan All Butter, Sainsbury's*	1 Biscuit/18g	99	6.5	548	5.3	49.9	36.3	2.5
Pure Butter, Jacob's*	1 Biscuit/20g	105	5.9	525	5.7	58.6	29.7	1.8
Raspberry & Oatmeal, Deans*	1 Biscuit/20g	103	5.7	514	4.7	63.1	28.6	1.4
Reduced Sugar, Tesco*	1 Biscuit/17g	86	4.9	519	6.7	57.1	29.4	2.1
Rings, Handbaked, Border*	1 Biscuit/17g	86	4.9	520	6.2	61.2	29.5	0.0
Royal Edinburgh*	1 Biscuit/11g	56	2.9	507	6.1	61.1	26.5	4.5
Stem Ginger, Waitrose*	1 Biscuit/15g	71	3.3	487	4.7	66.0	22.7	1.6
Wheat & Gluten Free, Free From Range, Tesco*	1 Biscuit/20g	98	5.2	490	6.0	58.0	26.0	6.0
SHRIMP								
Boiled, Average	*1 Serving/60g*	*70*	*1.4*	*117*	*23.8*	*0.0*	*2.4*	*0.0*
Dried, Average	*1oz/28g*	*69*	*0.7*	*245*	*55.8*	*0.0*	*2.4*	*0.0*
Frozen, Average	*1oz/28g*	*20*	*0.2*	*73*	*16.5*	*0.0*	*0.8*	*0.0*
in Brine, Canned, Drained, Average	*1oz/28g*	*26*	*0.3*	*94*	*20.8*	*0.0*	*1.2*	*0.0*
SILVERBEET								
Fresh, Raw	1 Serving/100g	17	0.0	17	1.6	1.1	0.0	1.9
Fresh, Steamed	1 Serving/100g	15	0.0	15	1.9	1.3	0.0	3.3
SKATE								
Grilled	*1oz/28g*	*22*	*0.1*	*79*	*18.9*	*0.0*	*0.5*	*0.0*
in Batter, Fried in Blended Oil	1oz/28g	47	2.8	168	14.7	4.9	10.1	0.2
Raw	*1oz/28g*	*18*	*0.1*	*64*	*15.1*	*0.0*	*0.4*	*0.0*
SKIPS								
Bacon, KP Snacks*	1 Bag/17g	81	3.8	474	6.5	62.1	22.2	2.3
Cheesy, KP Snacks*	1 Bag/17g	89	5.0	524	6.2	58.5	29.5	1.0
Pickled Onion, KP Snacks*	1 Bag/13g	67	4.0	512	3.4	56.4	30.3	1.4
Prawn Cocktail, KP Snacks*	1 Bag/17g	89	5.1	523	3.1	60.6	29.9	1.4
SKITTLES								
Mars*	1 Pack/55g	223	2.4	406	0.0	90.6	4.4	0.0
SLICES								
Bacon & Cheese, Pastry, Tesco*	1 Slice/165g	480	32.0	291	7.4	21.7	19.4	1.0
Beef, Minced, Morrisons*	1 Slice/143g	457	29.6	320	8.8	24.6	20.7	1.0
Beef, Minced Steak & Onion, Tesco*	1 Slice/150g	424	27.1	283	8.7	21.3	18.1	1.6
Beef, Minced with Onion, Sainsbury's*	1 Slice/120g	328	19.7	273	6.8	24.5	16.4	1.1
Belgian Chocolate, Weight Watchers*	1 Slice/30g	99	2.0	329	5.9	61.3	6.7	2.3
Cheddar Cheese & Onion, Ginsters*	1 Slice/180g	583	40.9	324	7.1	22.8	22.7	1.0

INFO/WEIGHT	per Measure KCAL	FAT	Nutrition Values per 100g / 100ml KCAL	PROT	CARB	FAT	FIBRE

SLICES

	Measure INFO/WEIGHT	KCAL	FAT	KCAL	PROT	CARB	FAT	FIBRE
Cheese, Potato & Onion, Pastry, Taste!*	1 Slice/155g	501	30.4	323	8.6	28.1	19.6	0.0
Cheese & Ham, Pastry, Sainsbury's*	1 Slice/118g	352	23.2	298	7.8	22.5	19.7	1.8
Cheese & Onion, Pastry, Tesco*	1 Slice/150g	502	37.0	335	8.0	20.1	24.7	1.4
Chicken, Spicy, Deep Fill, Ginsters*	1 Slice/180g	499	30.6	277	9.2	21.8	17.0	1.4
Chicken & Ham, Taste!*	1 Slice/155g	356	15.3	230	10.8	24.2	9.9	0.0
Chicken & Leek, Taste!*	1 Slice/155g	406	19.1	262	10.1	27.6	12.3	0.0
Chicken & Mushroom, Ginsters*	1 Slice/180g	439	26.8	244	8.3	19.1	14.9	1.8
Chicken & Mushroom, Sainsbury's*	1 Slice/164g	427	26.5	259	7.3	21.3	16.1	1.0
Custard, Pastry, Tesco*	1 Slice/108g	275	11.1	255	2.8	37.2	10.3	1.3
Fresh Cream, Tesco*	1 Slice/75g	311	21.0	414	3.5	37.4	27.9	1.0
Ham & Cheese, Pastry, Ginsters*	1 Slice/155g	625	43.7	403	9.8	31.9	28.2	4.2
Meat Feast, Ginsters*	1 Slice/180g	468	32.0	260	8.0	17.2	17.8	2.2
Minced Steak & Onion, Sainsbury's*	1 Slice/165g	475	29.9	288	15.2	16.0	18.1	2.5
Mushroom, Creamy, Quorn*	1 Slice/164g	653	29.5	398	9.8	49.2	18.0	1.6
Pork & Egg, Gala, Tesco*	1 Slice/105g	333	24.1	317	10.3	17.2	23.0	3.4
Prawn & Avocado, Plait, Extra Special, Asda*	1 Serving/198g	331	6.7	167	11.0	23.0	3.4	1.3
Salmon, & Watercress, Honey Roast, Plait, Asda*	1 Plait/166g	421	16.6	254	13.0	28.0	10.0	0.4
Sausage Meat, with Onion Gravy, Lattice, Asda*	1 Serving/278g	595	38.9	214	10.0	12.0	14.0	1.7
Spinach & Ricotta, Sainsbury's*	1 Slice/165g	500	35.3	303	6.5	21.1	21.4	2.9
Steak, Ginsters*	1 Slice/105g	274	14.5	261	9.3	25.0	13.8	1.6
Steak, Peppered, Ginsters*	1 Slice/180g	457	27.0	254	8.4	21.3	15.0	1.6
Steak & Onion, Aberdeen Angus, Tesco*	1 Slice/165g	444	27.7	269	8.7	20.7	16.8	1.3
Westcountry Cheddar & Onion, Ginsters*	1 Slice/180g	486	32.6	270	6.7	20.8	18.1	2.2

SLIMFAST*

Meal Bar, Fruits of the Forest, Slim Fast*	1 Bar/60g	211	6.1	351	23.7	42.1	10.1	7.3
Meal Bar, Yoghurt & Muesli, Slim Fast*	1 Bar/60g	208	6.5	347	23.9	42.2	10.8	7.4
Milk Shake, Banana, Canned, Slim Fast*	1 Can/325ml	214	8.4	66	4.2	10.6	2.6	4.9
Milk Shake, Chocolate, Ready to Drink, Slim Fast*	1 Bottle/325ml	211	5.2	65	4.6	8.0	1.6	1.5
Milk Shake, Peach, Canned, Slim Fast*	1 Can/325ml	214	2.6	66	4.2	10.6	0.8	1.5
Shake, Chocolate, Powder, Dry, Slim Fast*	2 Scoops/38g	136	2.8	363	13.9	59.0	7.5	10.9
Shake, Summer Strawberry, Ready to Drink, Slim Fast*	1 Bottle/325ml	211	6.5	65	4.4	7.4	2.0	1.4
Shake, Vanilla, Powder, Dry, Slim Fast*	2 Scoops/37g	131	2.4	360	13.4	60.9	6.5	11.0
Snacks, Chocolate Caramel Bar, Slim Fast*	1 Bar/26g	99	3.2	382	3.4	69.6	12.4	1.2
Snacks, Sour Cream & Chive Pretzels, Slim Fast*	1 Pack/23g	96	2.0	416	9.5	75.2	8.6	3.4
Soup, Chicken & Vegetable Pasta, Hearty's*	1 Pack/295ml	212	5.6	72	6.6	7.0	1.9	0.7

SMARTIES

Giants, Nestle*	1 Pack/186g	882	35.9	474	4.6	70.4	19.3	0.7
Mini Cones, Nestle*	1 Serving/44g	145	5.8	330	4.5	45.0	13.1	0.0
Mini Eggs, Nestle*	1 Lge Bag/100g	488	20.3	488	3.9	72.5	20.3	1.2
Nestle*	1 Tube/40g	184	6.6	461	4.0	73.6	16.6	0.6
Tree Decoration, Nestle*	1 Chocolate/18g	95	5.4	529	5.6	58.9	30.1	0.8

SMIRNOFF*

Ice, Smirnoff*	1 Bottle/275ml	188	0.0	68	1.8	12.0	0.0	0.0

SMOOTHIE

Apple, Grapes & Blackcurrant, PJ Smoothies*	1 Bottle/250ml	125	0.7	50	0.8	11.1	0.3	0.7
Apple, Kiwi & Lime, SunJuice*	1 Bottle/250ml	132	0.2	53	0.5	13.4	0.1	0.8
Apple, Strawberry, Cherry & Banana, M & S*	1 Bottle/250ml	125	0.7	50	0.5	11.2	0.3	0.6
Apples & Blackcurrants for Kids, Innocent*	1 Carton/180ml	104	0.2	58	0.3	14.1	0.1	0.1
Apricot & Peach, COU, M & S*	1 Bottle/250ml	100	0.9	40	0.9	8.3	0.4	0.4
Banana, M & S*	1 Bottle/500ml	400	2.0	80	1.8	16.8	0.4	1.2
Banana, Shapers, Boots*	1 Bottle/251ml	176	0.8	70	2.8	14.0	0.3	0.8
Banana & Mango, Juice, Calypso*	1 Carton/200ml	106	0.0	53	0.0	12.8	0.0	1.0
Blackberries, Strawberries & Boysenberries, Innocent*	1 Serving/250ml	130	0.0	52	0.6	11.8	0.0	1.3

S

SMOOTHIE	Measure INFO/WEIGHT	per Measure KCAL	FAT	Nutrition Values per 100g / 100ml KCAL	PROT	CARB	FAT	FIBRE
Blackberries & Blueberries, Innocent*	1 Bottle/250ml	120	0.2	48	0.5	12.0	0.1	2.1
Blackcurrants & Gooseberries, for Autumn, Innocent*	1 Bottle/250ml	117	0.2	47	0.5	12.5	0.1	1.0
Blueberry, Blackberry & Strawberry, COU, M & S*	1 Bottle/250ml	150	0.7	60	0.8	13.1	0.3	0.3
Blueberry & Pear, COU, M & S*	1 Bottle/250ml	112	0.7	45	0.3	10.4	0.3	0.3
Cappuccino, with Yoghurt, Island Oasis*	1 Carton/473ml	300	3.5	63	1.7	12.5	0.7	0.4
Cherries & Strawberries, Innocent*	1 Bottle/250ml	122	0.2	49	0.6	12.6	0.1	0.0
Cherry, Grape & Raspberry, Juiceburst*	1 Bottle/250ml	170	0.5	68	0.7	14.9	0.2	1.2
Cranberries, Blueberries, Cherries, Innocent*	1 Serving/250ml	137	0.0	55	0.3	12.8	0.0	1.3
Cranberries, Yumberries & Blackcurrants, Innocent*	1 Bottle/250ml	130	0.2	52	0.5	14.2	0.1	1.5
Cranberries & Raspberries, Innocent*	1 Bottle/250ml	112	0.0	45	0.5	12.0	0.0	2.3
Cranberries & Strawberries, Innocent*	1 Bottle/250ml	102	0.5	41	0.5	9.5	0.2	0.0
Fruit, Cranberry & Raspberry, Juice Republic*	1 Bottle/250ml	182	1.0	73	0.5	16.0	0.4	0.0
Fruit Kick, Orange, Mango & Pineapple, PJ Smoothies*	1 Carton/100ml	54	0.0	54	0.6	12.2	0.0	0.0
Guavas, Mangoes & Goji Berries, Innocent*	1 Bottle/250ml	112	0.2	45	0.6	12.0	0.1	2.1
Kiwi, Apples & Limes, Innocent*	1 Bottle/250ml	125	0.2	50	0.5	11.0	0.1	1.8
Mango, Mini-me, Skinny, Boost*	1 Sm/480ml	178	1.4	37	0.5	7.7	0.3	0.4
Mango & Orange, Smoothie Smile*	1 Bottle/250ml	130	1.0	52	0.4	11.7	0.4	0.0
Mango & Orange, Sweetbird*	1 Serving/330ml	181	0.7	55	0.7	11.9	0.2	0.0
Mango & Passionfruit, Tesco*	1 Glass/250g	125	0.5	50	0.5	11.1	0.2	1.0
Mango & West Indian Cherry, Plus, Tesco*	1 Serving/250ml	133	0.6	53	0.6	12.2	0.2	0.5
Mango Mania, King Parrot Food Company*	1 Drink/450g	248	0.5	55	1.3	12.3	0.1	0.4
Orange, Banana & Pineapple, Innocent*	1 Bottle/250ml	120	1.0	48	0.6	10.8	0.4	0.0
Orange, Mandarin & Guava, PJ Smoothies*	1 Bottle/250ml	122	0.0	49	0.7	10.9	0.0	1.6
Orange, Mango, Banana & Passion Fruit, Asda*	1 Serving/100ml	55	0.2	55	0.8	12.0	0.2	1.1
Orange, Mango & Pumpkin, Love Life, Waitrose*	1 Bottle/250ml	97	0.5	39	0.6	8.8	0.2	1.1
Orange, Strawberry & Guava, Sainsbury's*	1 Serving/300ml	159	0.6	53	0.3	12.0	0.2	0.8
Oranges, Bananas & Pineapples, Innocent*	1 Bottle/250ml	142	0.2	57	0.6	14.1	0.1	0.0
Oranges, Mangoes & Pineapples For Kids, Innocent*	1 Carton/180g	101	0.2	56	0.7	12.7	0.1	0.9
Passionfruit, for Kids, Innocent*	1 Serving/100ml	95	0.0	53	0.6	14.7	0.0	0.9
Peaches, Bananas & Passionfruit, PJ Smoothies*	1 Bottle/250g	127	0.2	51	0.4	12.1	0.1	0.0
Peaches & Passionfruit, for Kids, Innocent*	1 Carton/180ml	95	0.0	53	0.6	14.7	0.0	0.9
Pineapple, Banana & Pear, Asda*	1 Bottle/250ml	147	0.3	59	0.5	13.6	0.1	0.3
Pineapple, Mango & Lime, Way to Five, Sainsbury's*	1 Bottle/250g	120	0.2	48	0.4	11.3	0.1	0.3
Pineapple, Mango & Passion Fruit, Extra Special, Asda*	½ Bottle/250ml	100	0.5	40	0.5	9.0	0.2	1.3
Pineapple, Strawberries & Passion Fruit, PJ Smoothies*	1 Bottle/330ml	152	0.3	46	0.6	10.8	0.1	1.3
Pineapple & Passion Fruit, Sweetbird*	1 Serving/330ml	175	0.3	53	0.8	12.3	0.1	0.0
Pineapples, Bananas & Coconuts, Innocent*	1 Bottle/250ml	172	2.7	69	0.7	13.6	1.1	1.0
Pomegranate, Raspberry & Cranberry, PJ Smoothies*	1 Bottle/250ml	132	0.5	53	1.1	11.6	0.2	0.0
Pomegranates & Raspberries, Innocent*	1 Bottle/250ml	150	0.2	60	0.6	15.4	0.1	2.0
Raspberry, Banana & Peach, Sainsbury's*	1 Bottle/251ml	138	0.3	55	0.8	12.8	0.1	1.5
Raspberry, M & S*	1 Bottle/250ml	137	1.5	55	1.7	12.2	0.6	1.9
Raspberry & Blueberry, Plus, Tesco*	1 Serving/100ml	59	0.3	59	2.6	11.6	0.3	0.5
Raspberry & Boysenberry, Shapers, Boots*	1 Bottle/248ml	109	0.0	44	0.7	10.0	0.0	1.6
Raspberry & Cranberry, Smoothie Plus, Tesco*	1 Bottle/250ml	140	0.4	56	0.6	13.0	0.2	3.0
Strawberries, Blackberries, Raspberries, Kids, Innocent*	1 Carton/180ml	81	0.2	45	0.5	9.9	0.1	1.3
Strawberries & Bananas, PJ Smoothies*	1 Bottle/250ml	117	0.2	47	0.4	11.0	0.1	0.0
Strawberries & Bananas, Pure Fruit, Innocent*	1 Bottle/250ml	132	0.2	53	0.7	13.1	0.1	1.3
Strawberries & Raspberries, Squeezie, Innocent*	1 Squeezie/40g	16	0.0	39	0.3	8.5	0.0	2.1
Strawberry, Dairy, Finest, Tesco*	1 Bottle/250ml	162	0.2	65	2.9	13.2	0.1	0.1
Strawberry, Raspberry, Apple & Banana, PJ Smoothies*	1 Bottle/250ml	132	0.7	53	0.8	11.9	0.3	0.7
Strawberry, Raspberry & Banana, Waitrose*	1 Bottle/250ml	122	0.2	49	0.7	10.8	0.1	0.8
Strawberry, Wild Orchard*	1 Bottle/250ml	120	0.0	48	0.6	11.8	0.0	1.4
Strawberry & Banana, Don Simon, Don Simon*	1 Carton/250ml	132	0.0	53	0.6	12.2	0.0	0.3

INFO/WEIGHT	Measure	per Measure		Nutrition Values per 100g / 100ml				
		KCAL	FAT	KCAL	PROT	CARB	FAT	FIBRE
SMOOTHIE								
Strawberry & Banana, Fruit, Finest, Tesco*	1 Bottle/250ml	135	0.7	54	0.3	12.5	0.3	0.5
Strawberry & Banana, Fruit, Serious Food Company*	1 Bottle/250ml	135	0.0	54	0.5	12.7	0.0	1.3
Strawberry & Banana, Juice, Calypso*	1 Carton/200ml	100	0.0	50	0.0	11.9	0.0	0.0
Strawberry & Cherry, Organic, M & S*	1 Bottle/250ml	137	0.7	55	0.8	12.3	0.3	0.4
Strawberry & Raspberry, Fruity, Sainsbury's*	1 Glass/200ml	106	0.0	53	0.6	11.9	0.0	2.4
Strawberry & Raspberry, Rhapsody, M & S*	1 Glass/200ml	90	0.2	45	0.6	9.4	0.1	0.9
Strawberry & Raspberry, Shapers, Boots*	1 Bottle/250ml	122	0.5	49	0.3	12.0	0.2	0.6
Strawberry & White Chocolate, M & S*	1 Bottle/250ml	100	2.5	40	2.5	5.5	1.0	0.1
Strawberry Fields, King Parrot Food Company*	1 Drink/450g	221	0.9	49	1.4	10.4	0.2	0.6
Strawberry with Yoghurt, Finest, Tesco*	1 Serving/100ml	62	1.2	62	2.1	10.5	1.2	0.6
Summer Fruits, Tesco*	1 Bottle/250ml	140	0.0	56	0.2	13.8	0.0	0.5
Super Berry, M & S*	1 Bottle/250ml	150	1.0	60	0.9	13.0	0.4	1.2
Superfruits, Guavas, Mangoes & Goji Berries, Innocent*	1 Bottle/250g	127	0.5	51	0.6	10.7	0.2	1.9
Vanilla & Honey, Sainsbury's*	1 Bottle/250ml	237	6.0	95	3.2	14.8	2.4	0.3
Vanilla Bean, M & S*	1 Bottle/500ml	450	13.0	90	3.3	13.9	2.6	0.0
Vanilla Bean & Honey, Yoghurt, Serious Food Company*	1 Bottle/250ml	250	7.0	100	3.7	15.2	2.8	0.0
Yoghurt, Vanilla Bean & Honey, Thickie, Innocent*	1 Bottle/250g	242	4.5	97	4.1	16.2	1.8	0.1
SNACK POT								
Chicken & Sweetcorn Noodles, Morrisons*	1 Pot/247g	249	1.5	101	4.1	19.8	0.6	1.6
Chilli Con Carne, Tasty Little Numbers*	1 Pot/200g	200	6.8	100	8.9	8.4	3.4	3.5
Potato & Vegetable, Quick Snack, Made Up, Tru Free*	1 Pack/246g	236	7.4	96	1.0	15.0	3.0	1.0
Rice & Lentil, Quick Snack, Made Up, Tru Free*	1 Pack/270g	291	5.0	108	3.0	20.4	1.8	0.6
Spicy Jerk Chicken, Chosen By You, Asda*	1 Tub/350g	353	3.9	101	7.2	13.8	1.1	3.6
SNACK STOP								
Chicken & Mushroom Flavour Pasta, Crosse & Blackwell*	1 Pot/60g	251	5.3	418	10.3	74.3	8.8	0.0
Creamy Cheese Pasta, Made Up, Crosse & Blackwell*	1 Pot/218g	251	6.3	115	3.0	19.2	2.9	0.0
Creamy Chicken Pasta, Made Up, Crosse & Blackwell*	1 Pot/247g	210	4.0	85	2.7	15.7	1.6	0.0
Macaroni Cheese, Light, Made Up, Crosse & Blackwell*	1 Pot/248g	260	7.4	105	3.2	16.4	3.0	0.9
Roast Onion & Potato, Made Up, Crosse & Blackwell*	1 Pot/210g	210	7.8	100	1.7	14.4	3.7	0.0
SNACK-A-JACKS								
Apple Danish, Jumbo, Quaker Oats*	1 Cake/10g	39	0.2	390	5.0	87.0	2.5	1.0
Barbecue, Jumbo, Quaker Oats*	1 Cake/10g	38	0.2	380	8.0	83.0	2.0	1.7
Barbecue, Snack, Quaker Oats*	1 Bag/30g	123	1.8	410	7.5	81.0	6.0	1.0
Cheese, Jumbo, Quaker Oats*	1 Cake/10g	38	0.2	380	8.5	81.0	2.5	1.7
Cheese, Snack, Quaker Oats*	1 Bag/26g	108	2.1	415	8.5	77.0	8.0	0.9
Cheese & Onion, Snack, Quaker Oats*	1 Bag/30g	120	2.2	400	6.7	77.0	7.5	1.5
Chocolate & Caramel, Delights, Quaker Oats*	1 Cake/15g	62	0.9	415	6.0	83.0	6.0	1.6
Chocolate & Orange, Delights, Quaker Oats*	1 Cake/15g	59	0.7	394	5.5	83.0	4.5	1.0
Mini Bites, Smoked Ham, Quaker Oats*	1 Bag/28g	114	2.1	408	6.5	78.3	7.5	2.0
Mini Bites, Sour Cream & Sweet Chilli, Quaker Oats*	1 Bag/28g	115	2.2	410	6.5	78.0	8.0	2.0
Mini Breadsticks, Cheese & Onion, Quaker Oats*	1 Bag/35g	145	3.1	414	12.9	71.1	8.9	3.7
Prawn Cocktail, Snack-A-Jacks, Quaker Oats*	1 Bag/26g	106	1.9	408	6.9	78.3	7.5	0.9
Roast Chicken, Snack, Quaker Oats*	1 Bag/30g	124	2.4	415	7.0	77.5	8.0	1.0
Salt & Vinegar, Snack-A-Jacks, Quaker Oats*	1 Pack/22g	89	1.6	404	7.0	77.4	7.4	0.8
Sour Cream & Chive, Snack-A-Jacks, Quaker Oats*	1 Bag/22g	92	1.7	418	7.7	78.2	7.7	1.4
Sweet Chilli Flavour, Snack-A-Jacks, Quaker Oats*	1 Packet/26g	107	1.9	412	7.3	78.9	7.5	1.1
SNAILS								
in Garlic Butter, Average	6 Snails/50g	219	20.7	438	9.7	8.0	41.5	1.0
Raw, Average	1 Snail/5g	4	0.1	90	16.1	2.0	1.4	0.0
SNAPPER								
Red, Fried in Blended Oil	*1oz/28g*	*35*	*0.9*	*126*	*24.5*	*0.0*	*3.1*	*0.0*
Red, Weighed with Bone, Raw	*1oz/28g*	*25*	*0.4*	*90*	*19.6*	*0.0*	*1.3*	*0.0*

S

	Measure INFO/WEIGHT	per Measure KCAL	FAT	Nutrition Values per 100g / 100ml KCAL	PROT	CARB	FAT	FIBRE
SNICKERS								
Cruncher, Mars*	1 Bar/40g	209	12.0	523	9.0	57.0	30.0	2.3
Mars*	1 Bar/44g	225	12.5	511	9.4	54.5	28.4	1.2
SORBET								
Blackcurrant, Del Monte*	1oz/28g	30	0.0	106	0.4	27.1	0.1	0.0
Blackcurrant, Iceland*	¼ Pot/100g	100	0.0	100	0.0	25.0	0.0	0.0
Elderflower, Bottle Green*	1 Serving/100g	104	0.0	104	0.1	25.6	0.0	0.0
Exotic Fruit, Sainsbury's*	1 Serving/75g	90	1.5	120	1.2	24.1	2.0	0.0
Jamaican Me Crazy, Ben & Jerry's*	1 Serving/100g	130	0.0	130	0.2	32.0	0.0	0.4
Kiwi & Papaya, World Fruit, Del Monte*	1 Lolly/90ml	61	0.3	68	0.2	16.2	0.3	0.0
Lemon	1 Scoop/60g	79	0.0	131	0.9	34.2	0.0	0.0
Mango, Del Monte*	1 Sorbet/500g	575	0.5	115	0.2	29.6	0.1	0.0
Mango, Organic, M & S*	1 Serving/100g	99	0.1	99	0.3	24.1	0.1	0.9
Mango, Waitrose*	1 Pot/100g	90	0.0	90	0.1	22.1	0.0	0.6
Mango Berry Swirl, Ben & Jerry's*	1 Serving/100g	100	0.0	100	0.2	25.0	0.0	1.5
Mango Lemon, Fruit Ice, BGTY, Sainsbury's*	1 Lolly/72g	84	0.2	116	0.3	28.1	0.3	0.5
Orange, Del Monte*	1 Sorbet/500g	625	0.5	125	0.2	32.1	0.1	0.0
Passion Fruit, Fat Free, M & S*	1 Sorbet/125g	129	0.0	103	0.4	25.0	0.0	0.4
Peach & Vanilla Fruit Swirl, HL, Tesco*	1 Pot/73g	93	0.6	127	1.1	28.9	0.8	0.5
Pineapple, Del Monte*	1 Sorbet/500g	600	0.5	120	0.3	30.6	0.1	0.0
Raspberry, Haagen-Dazs*	½ Cup/105g	120	0.0	114	0.0	28.6	0.0	1.9
Raspberry, Waitrose*	1 Pot/750ml	690	0.7	92	0.5	22.2	0.1	1.1
Raspberry & Blackberry, Fat Free, M & S*	1 Sorbet/125g	140	0.0	112	0.4	27.5	0.0	0.6
Sicilian Lemon, Seriously Fruity, Waitrose*	1/5 Pot/100ml	77	0.1	77	18.8	13.5	0.1	0.2
Strawberry, Fruit Ice, Starburst, Mars*	1 Stick/93ml	99	0.1	106	0.1	26.7	0.1	0.0
Strawberry & Champagne, Sainsbury's*	¼ Pot/89g	95	0.0	107	0.2	25.5	0.0	0.6
Summer Berry, Swirl, Asda*	¼ Pack/89g	97	0.4	109	3.0	26.0	0.4	0.0
SOUFFLE								
Cheese	1oz/28g	71	5.4	253	11.4	9.3	19.2	0.3
Chocolate, Gu*	1 Pot/70g	307	24.9	439	6.3	24.4	35.6	2.9
Chocolate & Toffee, Gu*	1 Pot/95g	353	15.8	372	4.6	46.4	16.6	2.5
Lemon, Finest, Tesco*	1 Pot/80g	270	20.5	338	2.9	24.1	25.6	0.2
Plain	1oz/28g	56	4.1	201	7.6	10.4	14.7	0.3
Raspberry & Amaretto, M & S*	1oz/28g	83	4.7	298	2.8	33.1	16.7	0.1
Ricotta & Spinach, M & S*	1 Serving/120g	186	13.3	155	8.0	6.2	11.1	2.1
Strawberry, M & S*	1 Serving/95g	171	10.1	180	1.6	19.5	10.6	0.9
SOUP								
3 Bean, Chorizo, Low Fat, Solo Slim, Rosemary Conley*	1 Serving/100g	54	0.8	54	4.0	7.6	0.8	5.8
Apple, Carrot, Strawberry, Vie, Knorr*	1 Drink/100g	65	0.6	65	0.8	13.0	0.6	1.5
Aromatic Chicken, Thai Herbs, Deli Inspired, Baxters*	1 Can/415g	349	25.7	84	1.8	5.1	6.2	0.8
Asian Tomato Rice & Ginger, Skinny Soup, Glorious!*	1 Carton/300g	159	5.4	53	1.0	8.2	1.8	0.8
Asparagus, Cream of, Heinz*	1oz/28g	13	1.0	46	1.1	4.5	2.6	0.2
Asparagus, Fresh, M & S*	1 Serving/300g	135	10.8	45	1.1	2.5	3.6	0.9
Asparagus, Hi Taste Low Cal, Cup, Ainsley Harriott*	1 Sachet/22g	36	0.9	164	2.3	29.1	4.1	2.3
Asparagus, in a Cup, BGTY, Sainsbury's*	1 Sachet/18g	72	1.5	400	1.7	77.8	8.3	2.8
Asparagus, M & S*	1 Serving/300g	180	13.5	60	1.1	3.3	4.5	0.7
Asparagus, New Covent Garden Food Co*	½ Carton/300g	132	7.2	44	1.5	4.1	2.4	0.9
Asparagus, Slimline, Cup, Waitrose*	1 Sachet/204ml	51	1.4	25	0.4	4.3	0.7	0.7
Asparagus & Chicken, Waitrose*	1 Can/415g	166	4.6	40	2.1	5.3	1.1	0.7
Asparagus & Creme Fraiche, Morrisons*	½ Pot/300g	186	11.7	62	1.3	5.4	3.9	0.5
Assorted, Meal Replacement, The Biggest Loser*	1 Sachet/55g	210	3.3	382	28.2	50.5	6.0	4.2
Bacon & Lentil, Chosen By You, Asda*	1 Pot/600g	348	7.2	58	3.3	7.7	1.2	1.6
Bean, Italian Style, Tesco*	1 Can/300g	153	3.6	51	2.8	7.3	1.2	1.1
Beef, Mushroom & Red Wine, Farmers Market, Heinz*	1 Can/515g	263	9.3	51	2.4	6.4	1.8	0.7

	Measure INFO/WEIGHT	per Measure		Nutrition Values per 100g / 100ml				
		KCAL	FAT	KCAL	PROT	CARB	FAT	FIBRE
SOUP								
Beef, Spicy, & Tomato, Diet Chef Ltd*	1 Pack/300g	165	5.7	55	2.3	7.3	1.9	1.9
Beef & Mushroom, Big Soup, Heinz*	1 Can/515g	216	2.6	42	2.3	7.0	0.5	0.7
Beef & Tomato, Cup a Soup, Batchelors*	1 Serving/252g	83	1.6	33	0.6	6.3	0.6	0.4
Beef & Tomato, in a Cup, Sainsbury's*	1 Cup/210ml	61	1.1	29	0.6	5.6	0.5	0.2
Beef & Vegetable, Big Soup, Heinz*	1 Can/400g	212	4.0	53	3.5	7.5	1.0	0.9
Beef & Vegetable, Chunky, Canned, Sainsbury's*	1 Can/400g	188	3.2	47	3.2	6.7	0.8	1.3
Beef & Vegetable, Fresh, New Covent Garden Food Co*	½ Carton/300g	177	6.6	59	4.5	5.4	2.2	0.7
Beef & Vegetable, Ten Calorie, Gourmet Cuisine*	1 Sachet/200g	10	0.1	5	0.3	1.0	0.0	0.1
Beef & Vegetable Broth, Chunky, Canned, M & S*	1 Can/415g	166	3.3	40	1.9	6.4	0.8	0.6
Beef Broth, Big Soup, Heinz*	1 Can/400g	184	2.8	46	2.5	7.0	0.7	0.9
Beef Broth, Classic, Heinz*	1 Can/400g	180	2.8	45	2.2	7.2	0.7	0.8
Beetroot, Tomato & Buckwheat, Stay Full, Baxters*	1 Can/400g	264	4.8	66	3.4	8.7	1.2	2.9
Beetroot with Chopped Dill, Duchy Originals*	½ Pot/298g	152	7.4	51	1.1	5.9	2.5	0.9
Big Red Tomato, Heinz*	½ Can/210g	63	0.8	30	0.5	6.4	0.4	0.0
Black Bean, Corn & Chipotle, Fresh, Finest, Tesco*	½ Pot/300g	135	4.0	45	0.9	6.6	1.3	1.3
Bloody Mary, Fresh, Sainsbury's*	½ Carton/300g	65	0.9	22	0.4	4.3	0.3	0.9
Bloody Mary, New Covent Garden Food Co*	1 Serving/300g	69	0.3	23	1.0	3.3	0.1	0.7
Boston Bean & Ham, New Covent Garden Food Co*	½ Carton/300g	171	0.6	57	2.4	7.8	0.2	1.6
Brazilian Beef & Black Bean, Glorious!*	½ Pot/300g	144	6.9	48	2.0	4.8	2.3	0.8
Broccoli, Pea & Mint, Love Life, Waitrose*	1 Pot/400g	200	9.6	50	2.7	4.3	2.4	2.1
Broccoli, Salmon & Watercress, Stay Full, Baxters*	1 Can/400g	244	8.8	61	3.3	5.8	2.2	2.4
Broccoli & Cauliflower, Cup, BFY, Morrisons*	1 Sachet/15g	56	2.1	376	4.9	57.2	14.2	4.9
Broccoli & Cheddar, Heinz*	1 Can/430g	340	24.1	79	2.6	4.4	5.6	0.6
Broccoli & Stilton, Canned, Tesco*	1 Can/400g	240	14.0	60	1.7	5.0	3.5	0.4
Broccoli & Stilton, Classics, Fresh, Tesco*	½ Pot/300g	180	8.4	60	2.9	5.8	2.8	1.1
Broccoli & Stilton, Cup Soup, Ainsley Harriott*	1 Sachet/229ml	87	1.8	38	1.0	7.0	0.8	1.3
Broccoli & Stilton, Farmers Market, Heinz*	1 Can/515g	299	21.1	58	1.3	4.1	4.1	0.4
Broccoli & Stilton, Fresh, Sainsbury's*	½ Pot/300ml	141	9.9	47	2.7	1.8	3.3	1.5
Broccoli & Stilton, New Covent Garden Food Co*	1 Carton/600ml	240	14.4	40	2.2	1.9	2.4	1.1
Butternut Squash, Diet Chef Ltd*	1 Pack/300g	135	5.4	45	0.8	6.5	1.8	1.6
Butternut Squash, Fresh, Waitrose*	½ Pot/300g	153	8.7	51	0.5	5.8	2.9	0.8
Butternut Squash, Sage, New Covent Garden Food Co*	½ Carton/300g	153	6.9	51	0.9	6.6	2.3	0.7
Butternut Squash & Red Pepper, Vegetarian, Baxters*	1 Can/415g	162	4.1	39	0.7	6.9	1.0	0.6
Butternut Squash & Tarragon, Waitrose*	½ Pot/300g	123	6.6	41	0.8	4.5	2.2	1.0
Cantonese Hot & Sour Noodle, Baxters*	1 Serving/215g	133	2.8	62	1.4	11.1	1.3	0.5
Carrot, Butterbean & Coriander Soup, Chunky, Baxters*	1 Can/415g	220	2.5	53	2.1	9.9	0.6	2.2
Carrot, Coriander & Ginger, So Organic, Sainsbury's*	½ Can/197g	75	3.3	38	0.3	5.3	1.7	0.7
Carrot, Onion & Chickpea, Healthy, Baxters*	1 Can/415ml	170	0.8	41	1.9	8.0	0.2	1.2
Carrot, Orange & Coriander, COU, M & S*	1 Pack/415g	145	2.5	35	0.6	6.9	0.6	1.2
Carrot, Orange & Ginger, Go Organic*	1 Jar/495g	119	4.0	24	0.5	3.6	0.8	1.4
Carrot & Butterbean, Diet Chef Ltd*	1 Pack/300g	174	2.1	58	2.7	10.3	0.7	2.8
Carrot & Butterbean, Vegetarian, Baxters*	1 Can/415g	228	7.9	55	1.7	7.7	1.9	1.5
Carrot & Coriander, Average	1 Serving/200g	83	4.3	42	0.6	4.8	2.2	1.0
Carrot & Coriander, Canned, BGTY, Sainsbury's*	½ Can/200g	62	2.0	31	0.8	4.8	1.0	0.9
Carrot & Coriander, Fresh, Organic, Simply Organic*	1 Pot/600g	276	18.0	46	0.5	4.5	3.0	1.3
Carrot & Coriander, Jenny Craig*	1 Packet/300g	69	1.8	23	2.2	2.1	0.6	0.9
Carrot & Coriander, Low Calorie, Average	1 Serving/200g	45	1.3	22	0.6	3.5	0.6	1.1
Carrot & Coriander, Soup-A-Cup, Asda*	1 Serving/26g	102	3.6	392	4.6	62.0	14.0	4.5
Carrot & Coriander, Weight Watchers*	1 Pouch/300g	102	3.9	34	0.4	5.1	1.3	0.6
Carrot & Coriander, with Creme Fraiche, Heinz*	1 Can/515g	232	9.3	45	0.7	6.6	1.8	0.9
Carrot & Coriander Soup, Low Fat, Fresh, Sainsbury's*	1 Tub/600g	114	3.6	19	0.2	3.2	0.6	1.9
Carrot & Ginger, Fresh, Sainsbury's*	1 Pot/600g	150	5.4	25	0.4	3.9	0.9	1.0
Carrot & Ginger, Perfectly Balanced, Waitrose*	½ Pot/300g	66	2.7	22	0.4	3.1	0.9	1.0

S

SOUP

	Measure INFO/WEIGHT	KCAL	FAT	KCAL	PROT	CARB	FAT	FIBRE
Carrot & Lentil, Microwave, Heinz*	1 Can/303g	94	0.3	31	1.5	6.1	0.1	0.8
Carrot & Lentil, Weight Watchers*	1 Can/295g	86	0.3	29	1.3	5.5	0.1	0.7
Carrot & Lentil Soup, Weight Watchers*	1 1/295g	86	0.4	29	1.3	5.7	0.1	0.7
Carrot & Orange	1oz/28g	6	0.1	20	0.4	3.7	0.5	1.0
Cassoulet, Gastropub, M & S*	½ Pot/300g	255	11.4	85	4.7	6.0	3.8	3.1
Cauliflower & Cheese, Tesco*	1oz/28g	13	0.8	47	1.9	3.0	3.0	0.9
Celeriac & Truffle, New Covent Garden Food Co*	1 Serving/300g	225	17.7	75	1.1	4.3	5.9	0.7
Celery, Cream of, Campbell's*	1 Serving/150g	70	5.0	47	0.6	3.2	3.4	0.0
Cheese & Bacon, with Pasta, Meal in a Mug, Tesco*	1 Serving/37g	142	2.8	383	9.1	69.5	7.6	2.8
Chicken, Barley & Veg, Simply Fuller Longer, M & S*	1 Pack/400g	200	6.0	50	4.9	4.5	1.5	1.6
Chicken, Coconut & Lemon Grass, Fresh, Waitrose*	½ Pot/300g	303	24.9	101	2.6	4.1	8.3	0.8
Chicken, Condensed, 99% Fat Free, Campbell's*	1 Can/295g	77	2.1	26	1.0	3.8	0.7	0.1
Chicken, Cream of, Canned	1oz/28g	16	1.1	58	1.7	4.5	3.8	0.0
Chicken, Cup, Calorie Counter, Dry, Co-Op*	1 Sachet/13g	40	1.4	320	6.0	49.0	11.0	7.0
Chicken, Fresh, Sainsbury's*	½ Carton/300g	126	5.7	42	2.2	4.0	1.9	0.3
Chicken, Green Thai, Spiced, M & S*	½ Pot/300g	195	11.4	65	2.0	6.3	3.8	0.6
Chicken, Green Thai, Waitrose*	1 Pot/600g	462	30.0	77	4.4	3.5	5.0	1.6
Chicken, in a Cup, Dry, Symingtons*	1 Serving/22g	93	4.0	424	7.0	57.7	18.4	11.7
Chicken, Jamaican Jerk & Pumpkin, Sainsbury's*	½ Pot/300g	141	5.1	47	2.7	5.1	1.7	0.2
Chicken, Leek & White Wine, Fresh, Finest, Tesco*	1 Pack/300g	216	12.6	72	2.8	5.7	4.2	0.3
Chicken, M & S*	1 Pack/213g	196	15.3	92	1.6	5.5	7.2	0.2
Chicken, Moroccan Inspired, Sainsbury's*	1 Bowl/342g	202	3.1	59	2.6	10.2	0.9	7.5
Chicken, Mushroom, & Potato, Big Soup, Heinz*	½ Can/200g	132	4.6	66	3.4	8.1	2.3	0.4
Chicken, Mushroom & Rice, Chilled, M & S*	½ Pot/300g	225	10.2	75	3.2	7.3	3.4	1.8
Chicken, New Covent Garden Food Co*	1 Carton/600g	510	32.4	85	3.8	5.4	5.4	0.6
Chicken, Noodle, Canned, Asda*	1 Can/400g	148	4.4	37	1.7	5.1	1.1	0.7
Chicken, Potato, & Lentil, Weight Watchers*	1 Can/400g	136	3.6	34	1.2	5.3	0.9	0.3
Chicken, Potato & Bacon, Big Soup, Heinz*	1 Can/515g	294	11.3	57	3.0	6.1	2.2	0.5
Chicken, Potato & Leek, Weight Watchers*	1 Can/295g	97	2.4	33	1.1	5.1	0.8	0.3
Chicken, Red Thai, Waitrose*	1 Pot/6400g	316	14.8	79	6.5	5.1	3.7	0.7
Chicken, Roasted, Canned, Tesco*	1 Can/400g	220	10.8	55	1.0	6.6	2.7	0.3
Chicken, Sweetcorn & Potato, Heinz*	1 Can/400g	204	11.2	51	1.2	5.4	2.8	0.3
Chicken, Ten Calorie, Gourmet Cuisine*	1 Serving/200g	10	0.1	5	0.2	1.1	0.0	0.0
Chicken, Thai, Fresh, Finest, Tesco*	½ Tub/300g	255	16.2	85	4.1	4.2	5.4	1.1
Chicken, Thai, GFY, Asda*	1 Serving/200g	85	3.0	42	1.7	5.5	1.5	0.5
Chicken, Thai Style, Canned, Soupreme*	1 Can/400g	200	10.8	50	2.5	3.8	2.7	1.1
Chicken, Thai Style, Thick & Creamy, in a Mug, Tesco*	1 Sachet/28g	107	4.0	390	3.7	61.3	14.5	5.1
Chicken, Thick & Creamy, M & S*	1oz/28g	31	2.2	110	5.8	3.9	8.0	0.5
Chicken, Weight Watchers*	1 Can/295g	97	2.9	33	1.6	4.4	1.0	0.0
Chicken & Bacon, with Pasta, Meal in a Mug, Tesco*	1 Sachet/37g	142	2.8	384	9.2	69.5	7.6	2.7
Chicken & Broccoli, Soup a Cups, GFY, Asda*	1 Cup/226ml	52	1.4	23	0.5	4.0	0.6	0.4
Chicken & Broccoli, Soup-A-Slim, Asda*	1 Sachet/16g	55	1.4	341	7.0	58.0	9.0	6.0
Chicken & Country Vegetable, Soupfulls, Batchelors*	1 Serving/400g	164	3.6	41	5.1	3.0	0.9	1.3
Chicken & Ham, Big, Heinz*	½ Can/200g	92	2.0	46	2.3	6.9	1.0	0.6
Chicken & Ham, Chunky, Canned, Sainsbury's*	½ Can/200g	80	1.2	40	2.7	6.0	0.6	0.9
Chicken & Herb, Farmers Market, Heinz*	½ Carton/300g	183	6.9	61	2.2	7.8	2.3	0.5
Chicken & King Prawn, Noodle, Fresh, Tesco*	1 Pot/400g	180	1.6	45	4.7	5.5	0.4	0.4
Chicken & Leek, Big Soup, Heinz*	½ Can/258g	162	5.1	63	3.0	8.2	2.0	0.6
Chicken & Leek, Cup, Co-Op*	1 Cup/18g	64	2.5	355	3.0	55.0	14.0	8.0
Chicken & Leek, Cup a Soup, Made Up, Batchelors*	1 Serving/259g	96	4.7	37	0.5	4.7	1.8	0.7
Chicken & Mushroom, BFY, Dry, Morrisons*	1 Serving/14g	47	0.9	337	16.0	54.8	6.1	2.5
Chicken & Mushroom, Canned, Tesco*	½ Can/200g	130	7.6	65	1.4	5.6	3.8	0.1
Chicken & Mushroom, Extra, Slim a Soup, Batchelors*	1 Serving/257g	90	1.5	35	1.4	5.9	0.6	0.3

SOUP

	Measure INFO/WEIGHT	per Measure KCAL	FAT	Nutrition Values per 100g / 100ml KCAL	PROT	CARB	FAT	FIBRE
Chicken & Mushroom, Meal in a Mug, Tesco*	1 Sachet/40g	146	2.7	366	10.8	65.3	6.8	5.1
Chicken & Mushroom, Slim a Soup, Made Up, Batchelors*	1 Sachet/203g	63	2.0	31	0.7	4.7	1.0	0.3
Chicken & Mushroom, Soup-A-Slim, Asda*	1 Sachet/14g	51	1.4	362	10.0	58.0	10.0	4.2
Chicken & Mushroom in a Cup, Sainsbury's*	1 Sachet/223ml	107	4.2	48	0.7	7.1	1.9	0.1
Chicken & Noodle Laksa, Simply Fuller Longer, M & S*	1 Pot/385g	289	7.7	75	7.0	7.1	2.0	0.9
Chicken & Pasta Big, Heinz*	½ Can/200g	68	0.8	34	1.8	5.9	0.4	0.8
Chicken & Red Pepper Noodle, Fresh, Tesco*	1 Serving/400ml	200	1.2	50	3.6	8.5	0.3	0.4
Chicken & Spring Vegetable, M & S*	1 Pot/600g	210	8.4	35	3.0	2.9	1.4	0.8
Chicken & Sweetcorn, Asda*	1 Pot/600g	246	8.4	41	2.2	4.9	1.4	1.6
Chicken & Sweetcorn, Canned, BGTY, Sainsbury's*	½ Can/200g	56	0.8	28	1.5	4.5	0.4	0.2
Chicken & Sweetcorn, Canned, HL, Tesco*	½ Can/200g	70	0.6	35	1.6	6.4	0.3	0.3
Chicken & Sweetcorn, Canned, Tesco*	1 Can/400ml	240	6.0	60	1.6	8.2	1.5	0.7
Chicken & Sweetcorn, Cantonese, Fresh, Sainsbury's*	½ Pot/300ml	135	1.5	45	2.1	7.9	0.5	0.5
Chicken & Sweetcorn, Chosen By You, Asda*	1 Pot/600g	294	9.6	49	4.4	4.1	1.6	0.5
Chicken & Sweetcorn, Cup, Morrisons*	1 Serving/14g	52	2.1	375	8.4	51.2	15.2	0.0
Chicken & Sweetcorn, Cup Soup, Asda*	1 Sachet/200ml	109	3.9	54	0.7	8.5	1.9	0.3
Chicken & Sweetcorn, Fresh, Asda*	1 Pack/500g	260	9.5	52	2.6	6.0	1.9	0.0
Chicken & Sweetcorn, Fresh, Sainsbury's*	½ Pack/300ml	123	3.6	41	2.0	5.5	1.2	1.2
Chicken & Sweetcorn, GFY, Asda*	1 Can/400g	108	2.0	27	1.5	4.2	0.5	0.2
Chicken & Sweetcorn, in a Mug, Tesco*	1 Sachet/28g	122	5.0	434	4.8	63.4	17.9	1.1
Chicken & Sweetcorn, Light Choice, Tesco*	½ Can 200g	84	0.8	42	1.7	7.9	0.4	0.2
Chicken & Sweetcorn, New Covent Garden Food Co*	1 Carton/600g	282	5.4	47	1.0	8.7	0.9	0.5
Chicken & Sweetcorn, Soupreme*	1 Serving/250g	90	0.7	36	2.7	5.6	0.3	1.7
Chicken & Tarragon, Thick & Creamy, Batchelors*	1 Sachet/281g	118	6.5	42	0.8	5.7	2.3	0.3
Chicken & Thyme, Diet Chef Ltd*	1 Pack/300g	147	9.0	49	2.2	3.4	3.0	0.7
Chicken & Vegetable, Big Soup, Heinz*	½ Can/200g	104	2.8	52	3.3	6.7	1.4	0.8
Chicken & Vegetable, Chunky, Canned, Eat Well, M & S*	½ Can/213g	138	4.0	65	4.6	6.9	1.9	1.0
Chicken & Vegetable, Chunky, Canned, Sainsbury's*	½ Can/200g	94	1.6	47	4.0	6.0	0.8	1.6
Chicken & Vegetable, Classic, Heinz*	1 Can/400g	132	1.6	33	1.1	6.2	0.4	0.6
Chicken & Vegetable, Healthy, Baxters*	1 Can/415g	158	2.1	38	1.9	6.6	0.5	1.7
Chicken & Vegetable, Loyd Grossman*	1 Pack/400g	272	15.2	68	0.5	8.0	3.8	0.6
Chicken & Vegetable, M & S*	½ Pot/300g	120	4.2	40	3.0	2.9	1.4	0.8
Chicken & Vegetable, Micro, Tesco*	1 Pot/330g	139	4.9	42	2.1	5.0	1.5	0.5
Chicken & Vegetable, Mighty, Asda*	1 Can/410g	176	5.3	43	2.5	6.8	1.3	0.7
Chicken & Vegetable, Soup to Go, Asda*	1 Pot/330g	145	4.9	44	2.4	5.1	1.5	0.7
Chicken & Vegetable Broth, Canned, BFY, Morrisons*	½ Can/205g	50	0.4	24	1.2	4.5	0.2	0.5
Chicken & Vegetable Casserole, Chunky, Baxters*	1 Can/415g	195	2.9	47	2.4	7.8	0.7	1.1
Chicken & Vegetable Casserole, Taste of Home, Heinz*	1 Pot/430g	331	16.8	77	3.9	6.7	3.9	0.8
Chicken & Vegetable with Pasta, Select, Campbell's*	1 Can/480ml	220	1.0	46	2.9	7.9	0.2	0.8
Chicken & White Wine, Campbell's*	1 Serving/295g	145	9.7	49	1.0	4.0	3.3	0.0
Chicken Broth, Favourites, Baxters*	1 Can/415g	129	1.7	31	1.5	5.4	0.4	0.6
Chicken Curry, Big Soup, Heinz*	1 Can/400g	196	2.8	49	2.8	7.3	0.7	1.0
Chicken Curry, Mild, Indian, Soups of the World, Heinz*	1 Can/515g	381	21.1	74	3.6	5.9	4.1	0.3
Chicken Flavour, Tony Ferguson*	1 Pack/59g	203	1.9	344	25.6	49.8	3.2	5.1
Chicken Leek & Potato Soup, Weight Watchers*	1 Tin/295g	80	1.2	27	0.9	5.0	0.4	0.3
Chicken Miso, Chosen By You, Asda*	1 Pack/350g	266	6.6	76	9.0	5.0	1.9	1.6
Chicken Miso, Noodle, Waitrose*	1 Pot/400g	268	8.8	67	5.9	5.9	2.2	0.9
Chicken Mulligatawny, Asda*	1 Serving/300g	150	2.4	50	3.8	7.0	0.8	0.8
Chicken Mulligatawny, Chunky, Weight Watchers*	1 Pack/340g	163	4.4	48	2.2	6.8	1.3	1.5
Chicken Mulligatawny, Perfectly Balanced, Waitrose*	1 Serving/300g	138	6.0	46	1.7	5.3	2.0	0.4
Chicken Noodle, Batchelors*	1 Pack/284g	71	0.6	25	1.6	4.2	0.2	0.3
Chicken Noodle, Chunky, Campbell's*	½ Can/200g	86	1.2	43	2.8	6.5	0.6	0.0
Chicken Noodle, Classic, Heinz*	1 Can/400g	124	1.2	31	1.2	6.0	0.3	0.2

SOUP

INFO/WEIGHT	Measure	per Measure KCAL	FAT	Nutrition Values per 100g / 100ml KCAL	PROT	CARB	FAT	FIBRE
Chicken Noodle, Clear, Weight Watchers*	1 Can/295g	50	0.6	17	0.8	3.1	0.2	0.2
Chicken Noodle, Cup, GFY, Asda*	1 Sachet/215ml	43	0.2	20	0.6	4.2	0.1	0.1
Chicken Noodle, Cup Soup, Dry, Heinz*	1 Sachet/20g	48	0.5	240	8.0	46.0	2.5	1.5
Chicken Noodle, Cup Soup, Made Up, Heinz*	1 Cup/218ml	48	0.4	22	0.7	4.3	0.2	0.1
Chicken Noodle, Dry, Nissin*	1 Pack/85g	364	14.1	428	9.5	62.0	16.6	3.3
Chicken Noodle, Dry, Symingtons*	½ Pack/15g	48	0.4	318	8.6	65.4	2.4	2.4
Chicken Noodle, Soup in a Cup, Made Up, Sainsbury's*	1 Cup/200ml	44	0.2	22	0.7	4.7	0.1	0.2
Chicken Noodle & Vegetable, Slim a Soup, Batchelors*	1 Serving/203g	55	1.0	27	0.8	4.8	0.5	0.6
Chilli, Meal, Chunky, Canned, Tesco*	½ Can/200g	120	2.4	60	5.0	6.3	1.2	1.6
Chilli Bean, Chosen By You, Asda*	1 Pot/600g	258	1.8	43	2.1	6.8	0.3	2.2
Chilli Bean, M & S*	½ Carton/300g	150	7.5	50	2.5	4.7	2.5	2.7
Chilli Bean, Mexican, Tesco*	1 Carton/600g	270	6.6	45	2.2	6.4	1.1	1.9
Chilli Beef, Lentils & Buckwheat, Deli Inspired, Baxters*	1 Can/415g	237	2.1	57	3.7	9.3	0.5	1.2
Chilli Con Carne, Chunky, Sainsbury's*	½ Can/200g	110	1.8	55	3.6	8.0	0.9	1.5
Chilli Tomato & Pasta, COU, M & S*	1 Serving/300g	150	5.7	50	1.3	7.2	1.9	0.9
Chinese Chicken Noodle, Dry, Knorr*	1 Pack/45g	138	2.0	307	15.1	51.8	4.4	2.9
Chinese Chicken Noodle, Slim a Soup Extra, Batchelors*	1 Sachet/246g	69	0.7	28	1.0	5.3	0.3	0.4
Chorizo & Bean, TTD, Sainsbury's*	1 Pack/298g	161	2.4	54	4.0	7.6	0.8	5.8
Chorizo & Tomato, Vegetables, Canned, Sainsbury's*	½ Can/200g	114	6.0	57	2.6	4.9	3.0	0.3
Chowder, Bacon & Corn, M & S*	½ Pot/300g	195	10.8	65	2.5	6.0	3.6	1.8
Chowder, Clam, New England, Select, Campbell's*	1 Cup/240ml	221	14.4	92	2.5	6.0	6.0	0.8
Chowder, Ham & Sweetcorn, Diet Chef Ltd*	1 Pack/300g	165	3.6	55	1.9	9.2	1.2	0.9
Chowder, Prawn, Manhattan, Fresh, Sainsbury's*	1 Serving/300g	177	6.9	59	1.6	7.9	2.3	0.1
Chowder, Smoked Haddock, Canned, Sainsbury's*	½ Can/200g	128	8.0	64	1.6	5.3	4.0	0.3
Chowder, Sweetcorn & Chicken, Heinz*	1 Serving/200g	148	5.6	74	3.3	9.1	2.8	0.6
Chunky Chilli Beef, Asda*	1 Can/400g	212	4.0	53	4.2	5.7	1.0	2.4
Chunky Vegetable, Diet Chef Ltd*	1 Packet/300g	114	0.9	38	1.4	7.4	0.3	1.3
Ciao Bella, New Covent Garden Food Co*	1 Carton/600g	294	6.6	49	2.9	6.2	1.1	0.9
Cock-A-Leekie, Favourites, Baxters*	1 Can/425g	93	2.1	22	1.2	2.8	0.5	0.4
Country Beef, Celebrity Slim*	1 Pack/55g	211	2.8	384	25.6	56.4	5.1	1.4
Country Garden, Vegetarian, Baxters*	1 Can/415g	116	2.1	28	0.9	4.9	0.5	0.8
Country Vegetable, Chunky, Baxters*	1 Can/415g	199	1.2	48	2.0	8.6	0.3	1.6
Country Vegetable, Fresh, Chilled, Eat Well, M & S*	½ Pot/300g	135	6.0	45	1.0	5.2	2.0	1.4
Country Vegetable, Fresh, Sainsbury's*	½ Pot/300g	123	2.7	41	1.6	6.6	0.9	2.5
Country Vegetable, Knorr*	1 Pack/500ml	160	3.5	32	0.9	5.5	0.7	1.2
Country Vegetable, Weight Watchers*	1 Can/295g	91	0.6	31	1.1	6.1	0.2	1.0
Country Vegetable & Herb, Farmers Market, Heinz*	½ Carton/300g	114	3.6	38	1.2	5.7	1.2	0.9
Country Vegetable Casserole, Taste of Home, Heinz*	1 Pot/430g	206	6.0	48	1.3	7.6	1.4	1.3
Courgette & Parmesan, Fresh, Sainsbury's*	1 Pack/300ml	198	16.8	66	1.5	2.5	5.6	0.4
Cumberland Sausage & Vegetable, Big Soup, Heinz*	1 Can/515g	221	4.1	43	1.9	6.7	0.8	0.8
Dhansak, TTD, Sainsbury's*	½ Pot/300g	180	3.9	60	3.2	9.0	1.3	1.6
Egg, Drop, Average	1 Bowl/500g	470	30.0	94	6.0	4.0	6.0	0.0
English Broccoli & Stilton, Dry, Knorr*	1 Pack/65g	331	24.6	509	11.7	30.3	37.9	1.6
Fabulous Fagioli, Tesco*	1 Pot/400g	284	8.8	71	3.9	9.0	2.2	2.1
Farmhouse Chicken Leek, Dry, Knorr*	1 Pack/54g	248	15.7	459	10.3	39.3	29.0	1.5
Farmhouse Vegetable, Canned, BGTY, Sainsbury's*	½ Can/200ml	52	1.6	26	0.5	4.4	0.8	0.9
Farmhouse Vegetable, Fresh, Avonmore*	½ Carton/250g	137	5.0	55	1.9	7.4	2.0	0.8
Farmhouse Vegetable, Soup-A-Cup, GFY, Asda*	1 Sachet/219ml	59	1.1	27	0.6	4.9	0.5	0.4
Farmhouse Vegetable, Thick, Co-Op*	1 Can/400g	140	1.6	35	1.0	7.0	0.4	0.3
Fire Roasted Tomato & Red Pepper, Asda*	½ Tub/265g	114	6.9	43	0.7	4.1	2.6	1.0
Fish, Bouillabaise, Bistro, M & S*	1 Pack/820g	2665	18.0	325	10.0	4.3	2.2	1.3
Fish, Frozen, Findus*	1 Serving/85g	127	4.7	150	11.0	13.0	5.5	0.0
Florida Spring Vegetable, Dry, Knorr*	1 Pack/36g	104	2.0	290	7.8	52.2	5.6	5.2

S

SOUP

Measure INFO/WEIGHT	per Measure KCAL	per Measure FAT	Nutrition Values per 100g / 100ml KCAL	PROT	CARB	FAT	FIBRE
Forest Mushroom, Heinz*	1oz/28g	12	0.6	43	1.0	4.5	2.3	0.1
Four Mushroom, Loyd Grossman*	1 Pack/420g	202	16.4	48	0.8	2.5	3.9	0.2
Fragrant Thai Carrot, Skinny Soup, Glorious!*	½ Tub/298g	119	5.4	40	0.3	3.5	1.8	1.6
French Onion	1oz/28g	11	0.6	40	0.2	5.7	2.1	1.0
French Onion, Chilled, M & S*	½ Pot/300g	150	4.5	50	2.0	7.2	1.5	1.0
French Onion, Favourites, Baxters*	½ Can/208g	66	1.2	32	0.8	6.0	0.6	0.5
French Onion, GFY, Asda*	½ Pot/253g	91	1.3	36	1.9	6.0	0.5	0.4
French Onion, Heinz*	1 Pack/400g	100	0.4	25	0.5	5.7	0.1	0.4
French Onion, Tinned, M & S*	½ Can/200g	40	0.4	20	0.4	3.9	0.2	0.3
French Onion & Cider, Waitrose*	1 Can/425g	93	0.4	22	0.5	4.8	0.1	0.4
French Onion & Croutons, Dry, Tesco*	1 Serving/30g	106	2.3	353	7.3	63.7	7.7	2.0
Fresh, Leek & Potato, Waitrose*	½ Pot/300g	108	5.1	36	0.7	4.6	1.7	0.9
Fresh, Super Green, M & S*	½ Pot/300g	120	5.7	40	1.5	3.7	1.9	1.7
Fresh Minted Potato with Parsley, Yorkshire Provender*	½ Pot/300g	222	15.0	74	1.3	5.7	5.0	0.7
Garden Pea & Wiltshire Cured Ham, Finest, Tesco*	½ Pot/300g	195	8.1	65	3.4	5.9	2.7	1.6
Garden Vegetable, Dry, Slim Fast*	1 Serving/60g	224	6.2	373	23.8	45.0	10.3	7.0
Garden Vegetable, Heinz*	1 Can/400g	160	3.2	40	0.9	7.2	0.8	0.9
Garden Vegetable Flavour, Celebrity Slim*	1 Pack/55g	211	3.0	384	25.6	56.4	5.4	1.4
Gazpacho, Canned, Average	1 Can/400g	76	0.4	19	2.9	1.8	0.1	0.2
Gazpacho, New Covent Garden Food Co*	1 Carton/600g	276	17.4	46	1.0	3.3	2.9	1.2
Goa Carnival, New Covent Garden Food Co*	½ Carton/300g	144	8.4	48	1.6	4.9	2.8	1.4
Goan Spiced Tomato & Lentil, Skinny Soup, Glorious!*	½ Pot/300g	153	3.3	51	2.1	8.1	1.1	1.2
Goats Cheese & Rocket, Fresh, Sainsbury's*	½ Carton/300g	180	13.2	60	2.0	3.2	4.4	0.3
Golden Vegetable, Asda*	1 Pack/300g	150	6.0	50	1.9	6.0	2.0	0.0
Golden Vegetable, Cup, GFY, Asda*	1 Sachet/217ml	52	1.1	24	0.5	4.4	0.5	0.2
Golden Vegetable, Dry, Knorr*	1 Pack/76g	299	14.4	394	10.4	45.4	19.0	3.3
Golden Vegetable, Slim a Soup, Batchelors*	1 Sachet/207g	58	1.7	28	0.5	4.7	0.8	0.7
Golden Vegetable with Croutons Cup Soup, Co-Op*	1 Sachet/25g	120	6.5	480	4.0	56.0	26.0	2.0
Gumbo, Spicy, Fresh, Sainsbury's*	½ Pot/300g	120	5.4	40	1.5	4.5	1.8	0.9
Haddock, Smoked, Fresh, Finest, Tesco*	1 Pot/550g	302	13.7	55	2.7	5.1	2.5	0.8
Haggis Broth, Favourites, Baxters*	1 Can/415g	187	6.2	45	1.8	6.1	1.5	0.6
Harvest Vegetable, Soupfull, Batchelors*	1 Can/400g	160	0.4	40	1.4	8.4	0.1	1.6
Hearty Vegetable, 99% Fat Free, Prepared, Campbell's*	1 Can/295g	91	1.2	31	0.8	6.1	0.4	0.0
Hearty Vegetable Broth, Weight Watchers*	1 Can/295g	127	0.6	43	2.0	8.2	0.2	1.4
Hey Pesto, New Covent Garden Food Co*	1 Pack/600g	204	9.0	34	1.2	3.5	1.5	0.9
Highlander's Broth, Favourites, Baxters*	1 Can/414g	195	6.2	47	1.8	6.5	1.5	0.6
Hot & Sour, Szechuan, Cup Soup, Ainsley Harriott*	1 Sachet/219ml	57	0.0	26	0.5	5.9	0.0	1.1
Indian Chicken, Glorious!*	½ Pot/300g	201	7.5	67	3.4	7.6	2.5	0.7
Italian, Chunky, New Covent Garden Food Co*	½ Carton/300g	111	4.2	37	1.5	4.7	1.4	0.9
Italian Bean, Fresh, Love Life, Waitrose*	½ Pot/300g	135	7.2	45	2.1	3.7	2.4	2.2
Italian Bean & Pasta, Healthy, Baxters*	1 Can/415g	224	0.8	54	2.2	9.9	0.2	1.7
Italian Meatball & Tomato, Big Soup, Heinz*	1 Can/515g	319	14.9	62	2.5	6.4	2.9	1.8
Italian Meatball & Tomato, Soups of the World, Heinz*	1 Can/515g	319	14.9	62	2.5	6.4	2.9	1.8
Italian Minestrone, Dry, Knorr*	1 Pack/62g	193	2.5	311	11.5	57.1	4.1	7.8
Italian Minestrone, M & S*	1 Can/425g	191	2.1	45	2.2	9.0	0.5	0.8
Italian Style Tomato & Basil, Co-Op*	1 Pack/500g	200	10.0	40	1.0	4.0	2.0	0.6
Italian Tomato & Basil, Go Organic*	1 Jar/495g	183	10.4	37	1.2	3.3	2.1	0.8
Italian Tomato with Basil, Vegetarian, Baxters*	1 Can/415g	199	3.7	48	2.1	7.9	0.9	0.8
Italian Wedding, Deli Inspired, Baxters*	1Can /415g	199	5.4	48	2.1	6.9	1.3	0.9
Jammin Jamaica, New Covent Garden Food Co*	1 Carton/600g	324	15.6	54	1.0	6.0	2.6	1.6
Keralan Spiced Chicken, Waitrose*	½ Pot/300g	222	14.1	74	3.9	4.0	4.7	2.2
King Prawn Noodle, M & S*	1 Pot/600g	180	4.8	30	3.7	2.2	0.8	0.4
Laksa, Chicken & Noodle, Simply Fuller Longer, M & S*	1 Pack/385g	289	7.7	75	7.0	7.1	2.0	0.9

S

	Measure INFO/WEIGHT	per Measure KCAL	FAT	Nutrition Values per 100g / 100ml KCAL	PROT	CARB	FAT	FIBRE
Lamb & Cous Cous, M & S*	½ Can/208g	100	3.7	48	2.1	6.2	1.8	0.9
Lamb & Vegetable, Big Soup, Heinz*	½ Can/200g	120	2.6	60	3.0	9.1	1.3	1.3
Lamb & Vegetable, Mega, Morrisons*	1 Pack/410g	172	4.1	42	1.9	6.3	1.0	0.8
Lamb Casserole, Chunky, Baxters*	1 Can/415g	232	3.3	56	2.4	9.0	0.8	1.6
Lancashire Lamb Hotpot, Taste of Home, Heinz*	1 Pot/430g	299	11.1	70	2.6	8.9	2.6	1.1
Leek, Cream of, Favourites, Baxters*	1 Can/415g	237	17.4	57	1.1	3.8	4.2	0.7
Leek & Chicken, Knorr*	1 Serving/300ml	82	5.2	27	0.6	2.4	1.7	0.1
Leek & Maris Piper Potato, Chilled, M & S*	1 Serving/300g	165	11.4	55	0.6	4.5	3.8	0.9
Leek & Potato, Chunky, Meal, Canned, Tesco*	½ Can/200g	60	2.6	30	1.0	3.5	1.3	1.0
Leek & Potato, Creamy, Fresh, Asda*	1 Serving/300g	106	2.4	35	1.0	5.4	0.8	1.2
Leek & Potato, Cup a Soup, Batchelors*	1 Sachet/28g	121	4.9	432	5.2	63.2	17.6	1.8
Leek & Potato, Cup Soup, GFY, Asda*	1 Sachet/219ml	57	0.9	26	0.4	5.3	0.4	0.2
Leek & Potato, Fresh, Sainsbury's*	½ Pot/300ml	141	7.2	47	1.0	5.3	2.4	0.4
Leek & Potato, Fresh with Cream, Tesco*	½ Tub/300g	180	7.2	60	1.5	8.0	2.4	0.9
Leek & Potato, in a Cup, BGTY, Sainsbury's*	1 Serving/218ml	59	1.5	27	0.3	4.9	0.7	0.2
Leek & Potato, in a Mug, Light Choices, Tesco*	1 Sachet/220g	55	0.9	25	0.5	4.9	0.4	0.6
Leek & Potato, Mix, Asda*	½ Pack/100g	25	0.0	25	0.6	5.7	0.0	1.5
Leek & Potato, New Covent Garden Food Co*	½ Carton/300g	108	4.5	36	0.9	4.2	1.5	1.1
Leek & Potato, Slim a Soup, Batchelors*	1 Serving/204g	57	1.4	28	0.4	5.0	0.7	0.2
Leek & Potato, Smooth, Vie, Knorr*	1 Pack/500ml	155	4.5	31	0.9	4.8	0.9	1.0
Leek & Potato, Solo Slim, Rosemary Conley*	1 Pack/300g	156	6.6	52	0.9	7.2	2.2	1.1
Leek & Potato, Soup in a Cup, Made Up, Waitrose*	1 Sachet/204ml	47	1.0	23	0.3	4.3	0.5	0.5
Leek & Potato, Soup in a Mug, HL, Tesco*	1 Serving/16g	54	0.9	336	4.3	67.1	5.6	7.4
Leek & Potato, Thick & Creamy, Soup in a Mug, Tesco*	1 Serving/25g	94	2.4	378	4.2	68.5	9.7	4.9
Leek & Potato, Weight Watchers*	1 Sachet/215ml	58	1.1	27	0.5	5.1	0.5	0.1
Lemon Rasam, Love Life, Waitrose*	½ Pot/300g	147	4.2	49	3.7	5.3	1.4	1.8
Lentil, & Potato, Spiced, Heinz*	1 Can/295g	118	0.6	40	2.0	7.7	0.2	0.7
Lentil, Average	1 Serving/220g	218	8.4	99	4.4	12.7	3.8	1.1
Lentil, Bacon & Mixed Bean, Low Fat, Aldi*	1 Serving/400g	260	3.6	65	4.7	9.5	0.9	1.6
Lentil, Canned	1 Serving/220g	86	0.4	39	3.1	6.5	0.2	1.2
Lentil, Carrot & Cumin, Canned, BGTY, Sainsbury's*	1 Can/400g	204	3.6	51	2.3	8.4	0.9	0.1
Lentil, Low Fat, Amy's Kitchen*	1 Can/411g	242	7.0	59	3.1	7.7	1.7	3.6
Lentil, Low Fat, Solo Slim, Rosemary Conley*	1 Pack/300g	102	0.9	34	2.0	5.8	0.3	0.3
Lentil, Redemption*	1 Pot/600g	138	1.2	23	1.6	3.2	0.2	0.0
Lentil, Spicy, Organic, Suma*	1 Can/400g	232	4.8	58	2.7	9.0	1.2	1.6
Lentil, Tomato & Vegetable, M & S*	1 Can/415g	170	3.4	41	2.0	6.3	0.8	1.4
Lentil, with Red Lentils, Carrots, Potato & Onion, Asda*	1 Can/400g	192	0.8	48	1.4	10.2	0.2	1.2
Lentil & Bacon, Canned, Tesco*	1 Serving/200g	96	1.4	48	3.2	7.2	0.7	0.5
Lentil & Bacon, Chunky, Fresh, Sainsbury's*	½ Pot/300g	117	2.4	39	2.3	5.7	0.8	2.0
Lentil & Bacon, Favourites, Baxters*	1 Can/425g	234	3.8	55	3.6	8.2	0.9	0.8
Lentil & Bacon, M & S*	1oz/28g	18	0.4	63	4.1	8.6	1.6	0.7
Lentil & Bean, Spicy, Canned, Organic, Asda*	1 Can/400g	212	3.2	53	2.8	8.6	0.8	3.0
Lentil & Chick Pea, Fresh, Organic, Tesco*	1 Serving/300ml	117	2.4	39	1.9	6.1	0.8	0.5
Lentil & Pancetta, Tesco*	½ Can/192g	115	2.5	60	3.1	8.0	1.3	1.6
Lentil & Parsley, Simply Organic*	1 Pot/600g	390	1.8	65	4.4	11.8	0.3	1.4
Lentil & Red Pepper, Sainsbury's*	½ Pot/300g	162	3.6	54	3.5	7.4	1.2	1.6
Lentil & Tomato, New Covent Garden Food Co*	½ Pack/284g	162	3.1	57	3.6	8.1	1.1	0.7
Lentil & Tomato, Spicy, Chunky, Fresh, Tesco*	½ Pot/300g	195	5.4	65	2.6	9.7	1.8	1.3
Lentil & Vegetable, Diet Chef Ltd*	1 Pack/300g	156	0.9	52	2.6	9.6	0.3	2.1
Lentil & Vegetable, Light Choices, Tesco*	1 Can/400g	188	0.8	47	2.5	8.8	0.2	1.1
Lentil & Vegetable with Bacon, Organic, Baxters*	½ Can/211g	93	1.5	44	1.9	7.6	0.7	1.0
Lincolnshire Sausage Hotpot, Taste of Home, Heinz*	1 Pot/430g	301	13.3	70	2.4	7.9	3.1	1.0
Lobster Bisque, Baxters*	1 Can/415g	187	8.7	45	3.0	3.6	2.1	0.2

SOUP

	Measure INFO/WEIGHT	per Measure KCAL	FAT	KCAL	PROT	CARB	FAT	FIBRE
Lobster Bisque, New Covent Garden Food Co*	½ Carton/300g	108	1.8	36	3.2	4.4	0.6	0.4
Lobster Bisque, Waitrose*	½ Carton/300g	201	13.8	67	0.9	5.5	4.6	0.6
Londoner's Pea Souper, New Covent Garden Food Co*	½ Carton/300g	153	6.0	51	4.3	4.1	2.0	1.1
Luxury Game, Baxters*	1 Can/415g	187	2.9	45	3.7	5.9	0.7	0.5
Malaysian Chicken & Sweetcorn, Dry, Knorr*	1 Pack/57g	211	6.5	370	10.6	56.3	11.4	1.8
Mediterranean Fish, Waitrose*	½ Pot/300g	108	2.7	36	3.4	3.5	0.9	0.7
Mediterranean Minestrone, Campbell's*	½ Carton/250ml	95	2.7	38	0.9	6.1	1.1	0.6
Mediterranean Tomato, Campbell's*	1 Can/295g	83	0.0	28	0.6	6.4	0.0	0.0
Mediterranean Tomato, COU, M & S*	1 Pack/415g	104	2.1	25	0.7	4.8	0.5	0.6
Mediterranean Tomato, Dry, Slim Fast*	1 Sachet/62g	213	5.6	343	22.6	39.8	9.0	10.7
Mediterranean Tomato, Fresh, Organic, Sainsbury's*	1 Serving/250ml	77	3.5	31	1.3	3.3	1.4	1.0
Mediterranean Tomato, in a Cup, Waitrose*	1 Sachet/18g	52	1.5	289	8.3	45.6	8.3	10.0
Mediterranean Tomato, Instant, Weight Watchers*	1 Serving/200ml	50	0.2	25	0.7	5.2	0.1	0.1
Mediterranean Tomato, Slim a Soup, Cup, Batchelors*	1 Serving/208g	56	1.2	27	0.5	4.8	0.6	0.4
Mediterranean Tomato, Vegetarian, Baxters*	1 Can/415g	129	0.8	31	0.9	6.3	0.2	0.7
Mediterranean Tomato & Vegetable, Fresh, Tesco*	½ Pot/300g	105	2.1	35	1.0	6.2	0.7	0.7
Mediterranean Vegetable, GFY, Asda*	½ Pot/250g	80	4.2	32	0.5	3.6	1.7	1.6
Mediterranean Vegetable, Homepride*	1 Serving/250ml	82	3.2	33	0.9	4.3	1.3	0.0
Mediterranean Vegetable, Squeeze & Stir, Heinz*	1 Soup/197g	114	8.1	58	1.3	4.1	4.1	0.4
Melon & Carrot, New Covent Garden Food Co*	1 Serving/300g	60	1.2	20	0.6	3.6	0.4	0.6
Mexican Beef Chilli, Mighty, Asda*	1 Can/400g	192	2.8	48	3.3	7.0	0.7	0.9
Mexican Black Bean, Extra Special, Asda*	½ Pot/263g	194	10.8	74	2.3	7.0	4.1	1.7
Mexican Chilli Beef & Bean, Soups of the World, Heinz*	1 Can/515g	360	9.3	70	4.5	9.0	1.8	1.6
Mexican Spicy Bean, Weight Watchers*	1 Can/295g	112	1.5	38	1.2	6.8	0.5	0.9
Minestrone, Average	1 Serving/220g	139	6.6	63	1.8	7.6	3.0	0.9
Minestrone, Calorie Counter, Low Calorie Cup, Co-Op*	1 Sachet/13g	40	0.3	310	7.0	66.0	2.0	3.0
Minestrone, Canned	1oz/28g	9	0.2	32	1.4	5.1	0.8	0.6
Minestrone, Canned, M & S*	½ Can/200g	60	1.0	30	1.2	5.7	0.5	1.5
Minestrone, Chunky, Big Soup, Heinz*	½ Can/200g	74	1.6	37	1.3	6.2	0.8	1.1
Minestrone, Chunky, Canned, Sainsbury's*	½ Can/200g	80	1.2	40	1.5	7.2	0.6	1.2
Minestrone, Chunky, Classic, Fresh, Tesco*	½ Pot/300g	126	2.1	42	1.2	7.8	0.7	1.2
Minestrone, Chunky, COU, M & S*	1 Bowl/400g	300	7.2	75	3.0	11.8	1.8	0.8
Minestrone, Chunky, Fresh, Baxters*	1 Serving/250g	95	1.7	38	1.5	6.5	0.7	1.1
Minestrone, Chunky, Waitrose*	1 Can/415g	195	3.3	47	1.6	8.3	0.8	1.1
Minestrone, Diet Chef Ltd*	1 Pack/300g	123	2.7	41	1.4	6.9	0.9	1.2
Minestrone, for One, Heinz*	1 Can/300g	96	2.1	32	1.4	5.2	0.7	0.7
Minestrone, Fresh, Baxters*	1 Box/568ml	233	5.7	41	1.8	6.2	1.0	0.6
Minestrone, Fresh, Waitrose*	1 Pack/600g	240	8.4	40	1.1	5.8	1.4	0.8
Minestrone, Hearty, 99% Fat Free, Campbell's*	1 Can/295g	77	0.3	26	0.7	5.6	0.1	0.0
Minestrone, Hearty, Chilled, Farmers Market, Heinz*	½ Carton/300g	123	2.7	41	1.4	6.9	0.9	0.5
Minestrone, in a Cup, BGTY, Sainsbury's*	1 Serving/200ml	54	0.2	27	0.8	6.0	0.1	0.6
Minestrone, in a Mug, HL, Tesco*	1 Sachet/21g	72	1.3	342	3.6	67.7	6.3	3.8
Minestrone, in a Mug, Made Up, Morrisons*	1 Sachet/269g	132	1.6	49	1.4	10.4	0.6	0.6
Minestrone, Instant, Under 60 Calories, Tesco*	1 Sachet/19g	58	0.5	307	7.3	63.6	2.6	2.3
Minestrone, Italian, Canned, Sainsbury's*	1 Can/415g	212	7.5	51	2.0	6.6	1.8	1.1
Minestrone, Low Fat, Solo Slim, Rosemary Conley*	100g	41	0.9	41	1.4	6.9	0.9	1.2
Minestrone, Mighty, Dry, Asda*	1 Serving/38g	131	0.5	343	9.0	74.0	1.2	2.4
Minestrone, New Covent Garden Food Co*	½ Carton/300g	111	4.2	37	1.5	4.7	1.4	0.9
Minestrone, Organic, M & S*	1 Pack/208g	83	1.0	40	1.4	8.9	0.5	1.1
Minestrone, Organic, Seeds of Change*	1 Pack/350g	227	11.5	65	1.4	7.4	3.3	0.9
Minestrone, Packet, Dry, Knorr*	1 Pack/61g	178	2.7	292	9.2	53.9	4.4	6.5
Minestrone, Simmer, Dry, Asda*	1 Pack/50g	131	0.5	262	6.0	57.0	1.1	15.0
Minestrone, Simmer & Serve, Dried, Sainsbury's*	1 Pack/600ml	108	0.0	18	0.5	3.9	0.0	0.4

S

SOUP

INFO/WEIGHT	per Measure KCAL	FAT	Nutrition Values per 100g / 100ml KCAL	PROT	CARB	FAT	FIBRE
Minestrone, Soup a Slim, Asda*	1 Serving/17g	53	0.2	311	6.0	69.0	1.2	4.5
Minestrone, Squeeze & Stir, Heinz*	1 Soup/197g	59	1.4	30	0.8	5.0	0.7	0.4
Minestrone, Tuscan, Weight Watchers*	1 Can/295g	121	3.2	41	1.0	6.9	1.1	0.8
Minestrone, with Borlotti Beans, Tuscan Style, Heinz*	½ Can/200g	90	1.5	45	1.4	8.0	0.7	1.1
Minestrone, with Croutons, Cup a Soup, Batchelors*	1 Serving	93	1.3	37	0.7	7.3	0.5	0.3
Minestrone, with Croutons, Dry, Soupreme*	1 Serving/27g	94	1.7	349	7.6	65.3	6.4	4.4
Minestrone, with Croutons, in a Cup, Sainsbury's*	1 Sachet/225ml	72	0.9	32	0.9	6.3	0.4	0.5
Minestrone, with Croutons, in a Mug, Tesco*	1 Sachet/23g	83	1.9	360	9.0	62.6	8.1	2.7
Minestrone, with Croutons, Slim a Soup, Batchelors*	1 Serving/203g	55	1.2	27	0.6	4.8	0.6	0.6
Minestrone, with Meatballs, Simply Fuller Longer, M & S*	1 Pack/400g	260	10.0	65	5.2	5.8	2.5	1.2
Minestrone, with Pasta, Chunky, Co-Op*	1 Pack/400g	140	2.4	35	1.0	6.0	0.6	0.7
Miso, Instant, Blue Dragon*	1 Sachet/18g	25	0.7	139	10.0	14.4	3.9	0.0
Miso, Japanese, Made Up, Yutaka*	1 Serving/250ml	24	0.7	10	0.6	1.1	0.3	0.0
Miso, Organic, Instant, Sanchi*	1 Sachet/10g	27	0.3	270	14.0	47.0	3.0	0.0
Miso, Wakama*	1 Sachet/8g	27	0.6	336	18.7	48.6	7.6	0.0
Miso, with Tofu, Instant, Kikkoman*	1 Sachet/10g	35	1.0	350	30.0	30.0	10.0	0.0
Mixed Bean & Pepper, Organic, M & S*	1 Pack/208g	94	0.6	45	2.3	7.7	0.3	1.8
Mixed Vegetable Flavour, Tony Ferguson*	1 Pack/58g	204	2.1	352	25.7	51.3	3.7	5.4
Moreish Mushroom, New Covent Garden Food Co*	1 Carton/300g	90	3.0	30	1.3	2.9	1.0	1.4
Moroccan Chick Pea, M & S*	1oz/28g	20	0.6	70	3.6	8.8	2.1	2.0
Moroccan Chicken, Finest, Tesco*	½ Pot/300g	180	5.1	60	3.6	6.8	1.7	1.2
Moroccan Chicken, New Covent Garden Food Co*	1 Serving/300g	108	5.7	36	2.1	2.7	1.9	0.4
Moroccan Chicken & Vegetable, Love Life, Waitrose*	½ Pot/300g	192	5.7	64	3.7	7.9	1.9	1.9
Moroccan Lentil, Waitrose*	½ Pot/300g	153	1.5	51	3.5	8.2	0.5	3.4
Moroccan Style Chicken, Chosen By You, Asda*	1 Pot/400g	296	4.8	74	5.0	10.3	1.2	0.8
Mulligatawny	1 Serving/220g	213	15.0	97	1.4	8.2	6.8	0.9
Mulligatawny, Asda*	1 Can/400g	172	4.4	43	2.2	6.0	1.1	0.3
Mulligatawny, Canned, Tesco*	1 Can/400g	188	4.0	47	1.3	8.1	1.0	0.3
Mulligatawny, Classic, Heinz*	1 Can/400g	208	7.2	52	2.0	7.1	1.8	0.6
Mulligatawny, in a Cup, Symingtons*	1 Serving/232ml	95	1.4	41	0.7	8.3	0.6	0.5
Mushroom, 98% Fat Free, Baxters*	1 Can/425g	170	6.8	40	0.9	5.6	1.6	0.3
Mushroom, Canned, HL, Tesco*	1 Can/400g	132	5.6	33	0.5	4.4	1.4	0.2
Mushroom, Chosen By You, Asda*	½ Pot/300g	108	5.1	36	1.0	3.8	1.7	0.9
Mushroom, Cream of, Canned	1 Serving/220g	101	6.6	46	1.1	3.9	3.0	0.1
Mushroom, Cream of, Classics, Heinz*	1 Can/400g	208	11.2	52	1.5	5.2	2.8	0.1
Mushroom, Diet Chef Ltd*	1 Pack/300g	105	5.1	35	1.9	3.2	1.7	0.9
Mushroom, Dry, Symingtons*	1 Serving/23g	80	2.1	348	17.8	48.4	9.2	6.7
Mushroom, Farm Harvest, Green Giant*	1 Pouch/330g	122	5.9	37	0.6	5.2	1.8	1.3
Mushroom, for One, Heinz*	1 Can/290g	148	7.8	51	1.4	5.1	2.7	0.1
Mushroom, Fresh, M & S*	½ Pack/300g	165	11.7	55	1.8	3.5	3.9	0.9
Mushroom, in a Cup, Sainsbury's*	1 Serving/200ml	96	3.8	48	0.5	7.0	1.9	0.2
Mushroom, Low Fat, Fresh, Sainsbury's*	½ Pot/300g	132	8.7	44	0.7	3.7	2.9	0.6
Mushroom, Low Fat, Solo Slim, Rosemary Conley*	100g	35	1.7	35	1.9	3.2	1.7	0.9
Mushroom, Simmer & Serve, Dried, Sainsbury's*	½ Pack/600ml	234	9.6	39	0.6	5.5	1.6	0.3
Mushroom, Weight Watchers*	1 Can/295g	83	2.1	28	1.1	4.5	0.7	0.1
Mushroom, Wild, New Covent Garden Food Co*	1 Carton/600g	222	7.2	37	1.5	4.1	1.2	0.3
Mushroom, with Croutons, Soup in a Mug, Tesco*	1 Pack/26g	113	4.5	435	6.1	63.3	17.5	2.9
Mushroom & Chestnut, Fresh, Finest, Tesco*	1 Serving/250g	130	8.2	52	1.1	4.7	3.3	0.7
Mushroom & Crouton, Cup Soup, Made Up, Heinz*	1 Cup/200ml	80	4.2	40	0.7	4.5	2.1	0.0
Mushroom & Garlic, Slimming Cup a Soup, Tesco*	1 Serving/16g	58	1.6	360	5.8	61.1	10.3	3.2
Mushroom Noodle, Mighty, Dry, Asda*	1 Serving/42g	171	4.6	407	8.0	69.0	11.0	1.9
Mushroom Potage, Baxters*	1 Can/415g	320	21.6	77	1.5	6.1	5.2	0.3
New England Butternut Squash, Skinny Soup, Glorious!*	½ Pot/300g	103	3.6	34	0.6	5.9	1.2	0.7

S

SOUP

	Measure INFO/WEIGHT	per Measure KCAL	FAT	Nutrition Values per 100g / 100ml KCAL	PROT	CARB	FAT	FIBRE
Onion, Ten Calorie, Gourmet Cuisine*	1 Serving/200g	10	0.2	5	0.3	0.8	0.1	0.1
Oxtail, Canned	1 Serving/220g	97	3.7	44	2.4	5.1	1.7	0.1
Oxtail, Condensed, Classics, Diluted, Campbell's*	1 Can/590g	236	8.8	40	1.4	5.3	1.5	0.0
Oxtail, Cup Soup, Co-Op*	1 Sachet/19g	67	1.7	355	7.0	63.0	9.0	1.0
Oxtail, Diet Chef Ltd*	1 Pack/300g	144	3.6	48	1.8	7.5	1.2	0.5
Oxtail, M & S*	1 Serving/415g	207	5.8	50	2.1	6.9	1.4	0.5
Oxtail, New Covent Garden Food Co*	1 Carton/600g	198	3.0	33	2.5	4.5	0.5	0.5
Oxtail, Simmer & Serve, Dried, Sainsbury's*	1 Pack/600ml	180	5.4	30	0.6	4.9	0.9	0.2
Oxtail, Soup in a Cup, Sainsbury's*	1 Serving/223ml	69	1.1	31	1.0	5.7	0.5	0.2
Oxtail, with Croutons, Per Sachet, Morrisons*	1 Sachet/22g	81	2.1	377	5.6	67.0	9.8	5.1
Parsnip, Fresh, Morrisons*	½ Pot/250g	100	3.7	40	0.9	5.8	1.5	1.4
Parsnip, Fresh, VLH Kitchens*	1 Can/400g	180	6.4	45	0.9	5.8	1.6	1.4
Parsnip, Honey & Ginger, COU, M & S*	1 Can/415g	124	2.5	30	0.7	5.3	0.6	0.7
Parsnip, Leek & Ginger, New Covent Garden Food Co*	1 Carton/600g	162	1.8	27	1.2	4.9	0.3	1.3
Parsnip, Spicy, Fresh, Tesco*	1 Serving/300g	123	6.3	41	0.8	4.6	2.1	1.9
Parsnip & Apple, COU, M & S*	1 Can/415g	187	10.4	45	0.7	5.4	2.5	1.2
Parsnip & Butternut Squash, The Best, Morrisons*	1 Can/400g	244	8.4	61	2.4	8.1	2.1	1.6
Parsnip & Chilli, Diet Chef Ltd*	1 Serving /300g	102	4.2	34	0.8	4.6	1.4	1.3
Parsnip & Honey, Diet Chef Ltd*	1 Pack/300g	153	7.5	51	0.9	6.3	2.5	1.8
Parsnip & Honey, Fresh, Sainsbury's*	½ Carton/300g	192	12.6	64	1.1	5.4	4.2	1.5
Parsnip & Orchard Apple, Duchy Originals*	1 Pack/350g	115	3.1	33	0.7	5.4	0.9	1.0
Pasta, Tomato & Basil, Bertolli*	1 Serving/100g	47	1.1	47	1.5	7.9	1.1	1.6
Pea, Artichoke & Parmesan, The Best, Morrisons*	½ Pot/300g	171	7.8	57	2.8	5.6	2.6	1.0
Pea, in a Cup, Symingtons*	1 Sachet/31g	95	2.2	311	7.2	54.1	7.2	6.9
Pea, Organic, Suma*	1 Can /400g	272	8.8	68	2.7	9.4	2.2	0.7
Pea & Ham	1 Serving/220g	154	4.6	70	4.0	9.2	2.1	1.4
Pea & Ham, Creamy, Chunky, Meal, Weight Watchers*	1 Pack/340g	156	3.7	46	2.3	6.8	1.1	2.0
Pea & Ham, Diet Chef Ltd*	1 Portion/300g	138	3.3	46	3.2	5.8	1.1	2.6
Pea & Ham, Eat Well, M & S*	½ Can/207g	93	2.1	45	3.7	5.1	1.0	2.2
Pea & Ham, Extra Thick, in a Cup, Sainsbury's*	1 Sachet/224ml	85	1.8	38	1.1	6.7	0.8	0.4
Pea & Ham, Fresh, Waitrose*	1 Serving/300g	196	10.0	65	2.9	6.2	3.3	1.6
Pea & Ham, Low Fat, Solo Slim, Rosemary Conley*	1 Serving/100g	46	1.1	46	3.2	5.8	1.1	2.6
Pea & Mint, Fresh, M & S*	1 Serving/164g	49	0.2	30	1.8	6.3	0.1	1.5
Pea & Mint, Fresh, Sainsbury's*	½ Pot/300g	102	2.7	34	1.4	5.0	0.9	1.9
Pea & Mint, Fresh, Waitrose*	1 Serving/300g	126	3.9	42	2.8	4.7	1.3	2.9
Pea & Mint, New Covent Garden Food Co*	½ Pack/300g	168	5.7	56	2.5	7.1	1.9	1.7
Peking Shiitake Mushroom Noodle, Baxters*	1 Serving/215g	90	1.7	42	1.3	7.5	0.8	0.2
Pepper & Chorizo, Canned, Sainsbury's*	1 Can/400ml	172	4.0	43	7.0	2.0	1.0	0.0
Peppered Steak Casserole, Taste of Home, Heinz*	1 Pot/430g	216	3.9	50	2.8	7.7	0.9	0.7
Perfect Pea, New Covent Garden Food Co*	1 Carton/300g	93	0.9	31	1.7	4.6	0.3	1.7
Plum Tomato & Basil, New Covent Garden Food Co*	½ Carton/300g	132	6.0	44	1.3	5.2	2.0	1.3
Plum Tomato & Basil Soup, Farmers Market, Heinz*	1 Can/515g	247	13.9	48	0.7	5.3	2.7	0.7
Pork & Orzo, Slow Cooked, Chosen By You, Asda*	1 Pot/1000g	400	9.0	40	2.4	4.8	0.9	1.4
Pork & Stuffing, Taste of Home, Heinz*	1 Pot/410g	241	5.7	59	3.0	8.6	1.4	1.0
Potato, Leek & Bacon, Fresh, Baxters*	½ Pot/300g	249	16.8	83	2.0	6.1	5.6	0.7
Potato, Leek & Chicken, Canned, BGTY, Sainsbury's*	½ Can/200g	62	0.8	31	1.6	5.3	0.4	0.4
Potato, Leek & Thyme, Farmers Market, Heinz*	1 Can/515g	294	15.4	57	0.9	6.7	3.0	0.6
Potato & Leek	1oz/28g	15	0.7	52	1.5	6.2	2.6	0.8
Potato & Leek with Peppers & Chicken, Stockmeyer*	½ Can/200g	118	4.8	59	2.6	6.7	2.4	0.8
Prawn Laksa, Waitrose*	1 Pot/400g	388	25.2	97	2.5	9.7	6.3	0.6
Pumpkin, Creamy, Very Special, Heinz*	1 Sm Can/290g	188	5.5	65	1.3	9.9	1.9	1.1
Pumpkin, New Covent Garden Food Co*	½ Pint/284ml	97	3.1	34	0.4	5.5	1.1	0.6
Pumpkin, Spicy, Fresh, Sainsbury's*	½ Pot/300g	87	3.0	29	0.9	4.2	1.0	1.3

SOUP

	Measure INFO/WEIGHT	per Measure KCAL	FAT	Nutrition Values per 100g / 100ml KCAL	PROT	CARB	FAT	FIBRE
Puy Lentil & Vine Ripened Tomato, Finest, Tesco*	1 Pot/600g	360	7.8	60	2.8	9.2	1.3	1.5
Red Lentil & Chilli, Love Life, Waitrose*	½ Pot/300g	138	4.5	46	1.7	6.4	1.5	1.3
Red Lentil & Ham, Waitrose*	½ Pot/300g	147	3.3	49	3.9	5.8	1.1	2.0
Red Lentil & Tomato, Canned, Tesco*	½ Can/300g	189	3.9	63	4.0	8.9	1.3	1.1
Red Lentil & Vegetable, Favourites, Baxters*	1 Can/415g	199	2.1	48	2.6	8.3	0.5	1.2
Red Pepper, Tomato & Basil, M & S*	1 Can/415g	83	1.2	20	1.3	2.7	0.3	0.8
Red Pepper & Goats Cheese, Diet Chef Ltd*	1 Pack/300g	138	6.6	46	2.2	4.4	2.2	0.9
Red Pepper & Tomato, Canned, Sainsbury's*	1 Can/400g	120	4.4	30	0.9	4.1	1.1	1.6
Red Pepper & Tomato, Canned, Weight Watchers*	1 Can /295g	35	0.2	12	0.4	2.4	0.1	0.4
Red Pepper & Tomato, Vie, Knorr*	1 Pack/500ml	195	6.0	39	0.8	6.4	1.2	1.0
Roast Chicken & Herb Dumplings, Taste of Home, Heinz*	1 Pot/430g	482	27.5	112	3.6	10.1	6.4	0.8
Roast Chicken Flavour, Celebrity Slim*	1 Pack/55g	210	3.1	382	28.5	52.5	5.6	0.9
Roasted Red Pepper, Fresh, Waitrose*	1 Pack/600g	172	9.0	29	0.8	3.0	1.5	1.0
Roasted Red Pepper & Tomato, Weight Watchers*	1 Can/400g	136	0.4	34	0.7	7.7	0.1	0.6
Roasted Vegetable, Chunky, M & S*	1 Can/400g	140	2.4	35	1.3	5.8	0.6	1.1
Root Vegetable, Medley, New Covent Garden Food Co*	1 Pot/600ml	168	4.8	28	0.7	4.9	0.8	1.1
Root Vegetable & Barley, Broth, Special, Heinz*	1 Can/400g	188	6.0	47	0.9	7.4	1.5	1.1
Root Vegetable & Sweet Potato, Farmers Market, Heinz*	1 Can/515g	278	9.8	54	0.9	8.5	1.9	1.1
Royal Game, Favourites, Baxters*	1 Can/415g	149	1.2	36	2.2	6.0	0.3	0.3
San Marzano Tomato & Mascarpone, M & S*	1 Serving/150g	97	6.4	65	1.4	5.7	4.3	2.0
Sausage & Bean, Spicy, Meal, Canned, Tesco*	1 Can/500g	265	7.0	53	2.8	6.4	1.4	1.2
Scotch Broth, British, Sainsbury's*	1 Can/415g	149	2.9	36	1.9	5.4	0.7	0.9
Scotch Broth, Classic, Heinz*	1 Can/400g	168	5.2	42	1.5	6.0	1.3	0.8
Scotch Broth, Favourites, Baxters*	1 Can/415g	199	4.1	48	2.0	7.8	1.0	1.3
Scotch Broth, Fresh, Baxters*	1 Serving/300g	108	2.1	36	1.6	5.9	0.7	0.6
Scotch Broth, M & S*	1 Serving/300g	150	7.2	50	2.1	5.1	2.4	1.1
Scotch Broth, New Covent Garden Food Co*	1 Carton/600g	300	7.2	50	2.4	7.4	1.2	1.2
Scotch Vegetable, with Lamb, Favourites, Baxters*	1 Can/416g	179	2.1	43	2.0	7.6	0.5	1.7
Scottish Vegetable with Lentils & Beef, Heinz*	1 Can/404g	210	2.8	52	3.4	8.2	0.7	1.2
Seafood Chowder, Waitrose*	1 Can/415g	224	11.2	54	2.1	5.3	2.7	0.8
Smoked Bacon & Bean, Diet Chef Ltd*	1 Pack/300g	162	3.3	54	2.8	8.2	1.1	2.1
Smoked Bacon & Three Bean, Chunky, Baxters*	1 Can/415g	241	5.0	58	2.9	8.8	1.2	1.8
Smoked Salmon & Dill, Fresh, Finest, Tesco*	½ Carton/300g	240	16.5	80	2.2	5.3	5.5	0.6
Smokey Bacon, Leek & Potato, Big Soup, Canned, Heinz*	1 Can/515g	278	10.8	54	1.9	6.6	2.1	0.6
Soup, Leek & Potato, Fresh, Sainsbury's*	½ Pot/300g	114	3.6	38	0.7	6.1	1.2	1.3
Spiced Chickpea & Fresh Red Pepper, M & S*	1 Serving/300g	165	6.9	55	2.2	5.8	2.3	2.5
Spiced Lentil & Vegetable, Chosen By You, Asda*	½ Pot/300g	132	2.4	44	2.3	6.5	0.8	1.0
Spicy, Three Bean, Tesco*	½ Carton/300g	165	4.5	55	2.8	7.3	1.5	2.1
Spicy Beef & Tomato, Diet Chef Ltd*	1 Pouch/300g	165	5.7	55	2.3	7.3	1.9	1.9
Spicy Cajun Style Chicken, Chosen By You, Asda*	1 Pot/397g	262	4.8	66	5.2	8.1	1.2	0.8
Spicy Lentil, Chilled, Morrisons*	1 Serving/300ml	271	8.6	90	3.9	12.3	2.9	4.0
Spicy Lentil, COU, M & S*	1 Pack/415g	187	3.7	45	2.6	6.7	0.9	1.2
Spicy Lentil, Cup, Made Up, Ainsley Harriott*	1 Sachet/226ml	86	1.1	38	1.1	7.3	0.5	0.4
Spicy Lentil, in a Mug, Light Choices, Tesco*	1 Sachet/221ml	62	0.0	28	1.1	5.9	0.0	0.0
Spicy Lentil, Seeds of Change*	1 Pack/422g	190	0.8	45	2.5	8.2	0.2	1.9
Spicy Lentil & Vegetable, Chilled, M & S*	½ Serving/600g	300	4.8	50	2.7	8.0	0.8	1.1
Spicy Mixed Bean, Big Soup, Heinz*	1 Serving/200g	78	0.6	39	2.3	6.7	0.3	2.0
Spicy Parsnip, New Covent Garden Food Co*	½ Box/297g	116	3.9	39	0.9	5.8	1.3	1.8
Spicy Parsnip, Vegetarian, Baxters*	1 Can/425g	221	10.6	52	1.2	6.1	2.5	1.5
Spicy Sweetcorn, Fresh, New Covent Garden Food Co*	½ Carton/300g	159	4.8	53	1.4	7.8	1.6	0.7
Spicy Tomato, Cup a Soup, Batchelors*	1 Sachet/23g	74	0.7	322	7.6	65.8	3.2	3.2
Spicy Tomato & Rice with Sweetcorn, Healthy, Baxters*	1 Can414g	211	1.2	51	1.9	10.2	0.3	0.8
Spinach, Creme Fraiche, & Nutmeg, Organic, Waitrose*	½ Pot/300g	243	22.8	81	0.9	2.3	7.6	1.1

	Measure INFO/WEIGHT	per Measure KCAL	FAT	Nutrition Values per 100g / 100ml KCAL	PROT	CARB	FAT	FIBRE
SOUP								
Spinach & Nutmeg, New Covent Garden Food Co*	½ Carton/300g	147	6.6	49	1.9	5.3	2.2	1.0
Spinach & Watercress, New Covent Garden Food Co*	½ Carton/298g	60	1.2	20	1.3	2.8	0.4	0.8
Split Pea & Ham, Asda*	1 Serving/300g	129	0.6	43	3.5	6.9	0.2	0.7
Spring Vegetable, Classic, Heinz*	1 Can/400g	136	1.6	34	0.8	6.8	0.4	0.7
Spring Vegetable, Condensed, Campbell's*	1 Can/295g	62	0.3	21	0.5	4.5	0.1	0.0
Squash, Butternut, & Ginger, Waitrose*	½ Pot/300g	210	17.4	70	0.9	3.5	5.8	1.0
Squash, Butternut, Curried, & Lentil, Seeds of Change*	1 Pack/400g	164	1.2	41	2.3	7.2	0.3	1.9
Steak, Potato & Ale, Chunky, Sainsbury's*	1 Can/400g	152	2.4	38	2.2	5.9	0.6	0.8
Steak & Potato, Big Soup, Heinz*	½ Can/258g	129	2.1	50	3.0	7.7	0.8	0.8
Steak & Potato with Hp Sauce, Taste of Home, Heinz*	1 Serving/410g	286	7.6	70	3.3	9.6	1.8	0.7
Stilton, Celery & Watercress, Morrisons*	1 Serving/250g	272	23.0	109	3.9	3.1	9.2	0.3
Summer Minestrone, with Basil Pesto, M & S*	½ Pot/300g	240	16.2	80	1.9	5.7	5.4	1.2
Summer Vegetable, New Covent Garden Food Co*	1 Carton/600g	336	14.4	56	1.7	6.5	2.4	0.7
Summer Vegetable, with Pasta, Cup a Soup, Batchelors*	1 Serving/33g	16	0.4	50	1.4	8.5	1.1	1.0
Sun Dried Tomato & Basil, Heinz*	1 Serving/275ml	124	5.2	45	0.6	6.5	1.9	0.1
Sun Dried Tomato & Basil, Microwaveable Cup, Heinz*	1 Cup/275ml	118	4.9	43	0.6	6.2	1.8	0.1
Sunny Thai Chicken, Glorious!*	½ Pot/300g	201	6.6	67	3.6	8.3	2.2	1.0
Sunshine Yellow Tomato, New Covent Garden Food Co*	1 Portion/300g	99	2.4	33	0.9	4.9	0.8	1.2
Super Chicken Noodle, Dry, Knorr*	1 Pack/56g	182	2.7	325	14.3	56.0	4.9	1.8
Super Chicken Noodle, in Seconds, Dry, Knorr*	1 Pack/37g	111	1.7	299	17.9	46.1	4.7	0.3
Super Vegetable, M & S*	½ Pot/300g	120	4.2	40	1.0	5.0	1.4	1.2
Sweet Potato & Coconut, Diet Chef Ltd*	1 Pack/300g	147	8.7	49	0.8	4.9	2.9	0.9
Sweetcorn, Cream of, Campbell's*	1 Serving/80g	41	2.2	51	0.6	6.2	2.7	0.5
Sweetcorn & Chicken, Cup, Calorie Counter, Co-Op*	1 Sachet/11g	35	1.2	315	5.0	49.0	11.0	11.0
Sweetcorn & Chilli, COU, M & S*	½ Can/275g	137	6.6	50	0.9	6.1	2.4	0.4
Tangy Tomato, Extra, Slim a Soup, Batchelors*	1 Pack/253g	121	2.0	48	1.2	9.0	0.8	0.4
Tangy Tomato, Slim a Soup, Batchelors*	1 Serving/230ml	81	1.0	35	1.1	6.7	0.4	0.5
Terrific Toulouse Sausage, Tesco*	1 Pot/400g	248	8.8	62	3.7	6.9	2.2	2.0
Thai, Mealpak, All About Weight*	1 Pack/40g	150	4.2	376	35.1	31.0	10.6	8.5
Thai Chicken, Diet Chef Ltd*	1 Pack/300g	114	4.5	38	1.0	5.1	1.5	1.0
Thai Chicken, New Covent Garden Food Co*	½ Carton/300g	174	10.5	58	2.6	4.1	3.5	0.8
Thai Pumpkin Coconut, New Covent Garden Food Co*	1 Carton/568ml	182	7.4	32	1.3	3.5	1.3	1.1
Three Bean, Chunky, M & S*	1 Can/415g	207	5.0	50	2.3	7.5	1.2	1.8
Three Bean & Chorizo, Diet Chef Ltd*	1 Pack/300g	162	2.4	54	4.0	7.6	0.8	5.8
Three Bean & Smoked Bacon, Farmers Market, Heinz*	1 Can/515g	309	9.8	60	2.7	8.1	1.9	1.9
Three Bean & Vegetable, Light Choices, Tesco*	½ Can/200g	110	0.6	55	2.6	9.7	0.3	1.9
Tomato, & Lentil, Mediterranean, Weight Watchers*	1 Can/400g	184	2.4	46	2.3	7.8	0.6	1.0
Tomato, 99% Fat Free, Wattie's*	1 Serving/105g	32	0.4	31	1.0	5.6	0.4	1.1
Tomato, Basil & Chilli, Microwave, Sainsbury's*	1 Pot/345g	100	2.1	29	1.0	5.0	0.6	1.2
Tomato, Canned, HL, Tesco*	½ Can/200g	110	4.0	55	0.7	7.4	2.0	0.5
Tomato, Cannellini & Borlotti Bean, M & S*	½ Pot/300g	195	9.9	65	2.1	6.7	3.3	2.5
Tomato, Cream of, Canned	1oz/28g	15	0.8	52	0.8	5.9	3.0	0.7
Tomato, Cream of, Condensed, Batchelors*	1 Can/295g	454	19.5	154	1.7	21.9	6.6	0.6
Tomato, Cream of, Condensed, Prepared, Heinz*	1oz/28g	15	0.7	55	0.9	7.1	2.6	0.4
Tomato, Cream of, Dry, Knorr*	1 Pack/90g	391	21.2	435	4.3	51.3	23.6	3.3
Tomato, Cream of, in a Cup, Sainsbury's*	1 Sachet/233ml	112	2.1	48	0.7	9.3	0.9	0.1
Tomato, Cream of, Soup & Go, Heinz*	1 Cup/293ml	161	8.5	55	0.9	6.4	2.9	0.4
Tomato, Cream of, with a Hint of Basil, Heinz*	½ Can/200g	114	6.0	57	0.9	6.6	3.0	0.4
Tomato, Cream of, with Red Pepper, Classic, Heinz*	1 Can/400g	232	11.6	58	0.9	7.0	2.9	0.6
Tomato, Cup a Soup, Made Up, Batchelors*	1 Sachet/256g	92	2.3	36	0.3	6.7	0.9	0.3
Tomato, Diet Chef Ltd*	1 Pack/300g	159	5.4	53	1.3	7.7	1.8	1.2
Tomato, Fire Flamed & Red Onion, Fresh, Sainsbury's*	½ Pack/300ml	129	6.6	43	0.8	5.0	2.2	1.0
Tomato, Fresh, Tesco*	1 Serving/100g	44	2.3	44	0.7	5.2	2.3	0.4

S

SOUP

	Measure INFO/WEIGHT	KCAL	FAT	KCAL	PROT	CARB	FAT	FIBRE
Tomato, Hi Taste Low Cal, Cup Soup, Ainsley Harriott*	1 Sachet/22g	70	0.5	318	8.6	65.9	2.3	3.6
Tomato, in a Cup, Symingtons*	1 Sachet/32g	97	1.6	308	3.5	62.0	5.0	3.8
Tomato, Lighter Life*	1 Pack/36g	125	2.6	347	34.7	33.9	7.2	7.5
Tomato, Low Fat, Solo Slim, Rosemary Conley*	100g	56	2.3	56	1.3	7.6	2.3	1.2
Tomato, Mealpak, All About Weight*	1 Pack/37g	152	7.5	416	35.0	22.4	20.6	5.0
Tomato, Mediterranean, in a Mug, Light Choices, Tesco*	1 Sachet/220ml	62	0.4	28	0.6	6.0	0.2	0.6
Tomato, Mediterranean, Rich, Fresh, Baxters*	1 Carton/600g	318	10.2	53	1.8	7.7	1.7	1.1
Tomato, Mixed Bean & Vegetable, Tesco*	1oz/28g	18	0.1	64	2.4	9.8	0.3	1.6
Tomato, Onion & Basil, GFY, Asda*	1 Can/400g	96	2.8	24	1.0	3.4	0.7	1.7
Tomato, Red Lentil & Pepper, Chosen By You, Asda*	½ Pot/300g	177	3.3	59	3.0	8.8	1.1	0.9
Tomato, Red Pepper & Basil, Thick & Creamy, Asda*	1 Sachet/24g	89	2.3	370	5.6	65.7	9.4	5.5
Tomato, Simmer & Serve, Dried, Sainsbury's*	1 Serving/200ml	70	2.2	35	0.3	6.0	1.1	0.4
Tomato, Spicy, & Beef, Diet Chef Ltd*	1 Pack/300ml	144	1.2	48	2.2	6.3	0.4	1.4
Tomato, Squeeze & Stir, Heinz*	1 Soup/197g	114	5.7	58	0.9	6.8	2.9	0.4
Tomato, Sweet Chilli, & Pasta, Classic, Heinz*	½ Can/200g	74	0.2	37	0.8	8.0	0.1	0.3
Tomato, Ten Calorie, Gourmet Cuisine*	1 Sachet/200g	10	0.1	5	0.3	1.0	0.0	0.1
Tomato, Three Bean & Bacon, Sainsbury's*	½ Can/200g	86	2.0	43	3.1	5.4	1.0	3.0
Tomato, Vegetable Garden, Campbell's*	1 Can/310g	240	2.7	77	1.6	16.1	0.9	0.0
Tomato, Vine Ripened, Green Giant*	1 Pouch/330g	129	3.0	39	0.6	7.7	0.9	1.6
Tomato, Weight Watchers*	1 Can/295g	74	1.5	25	0.7	4.5	0.5	0.3
Tomato & Basil, Cup a Soup, Made Up, GFY, Asda*	1 Serving/250ml	50	0.2	20	0.4	4.4	0.1	0.2
Tomato & Basil, Diet Chef Ltd*	1 Pack/300g	159	5.4	53	1.3	7.7	1.8	1.2
Tomato & Basil, Fresh, Finest, Tesco*	½ Pot/300g	219	14.7	73	1.0	6.3	4.9	0.6
Tomato & Basil, Fresh, M & S*	½ Pot/300g	105	3.6	35	0.8	5.2	1.2	1.5
Tomato & Basil, Fresh, So Organic, Sainsbury's*	½ Carton/200g	100	4.0	50	0.5	7.5	2.0	0.2
Tomato & Basil, GFY, Asda*	1 Serving/250ml	100	3.5	40	0.9	6.0	1.4	1.6
Tomato & Basil, Italian, 99% Fat Free, Baxters*	½ Can/208g	119	2.1	57	2.6	9.3	1.0	1.1
Tomato & Basil, Loyd Grossman*	½ Pack/210g	97	4.0	46	0.8	6.4	1.9	0.2
Tomato & Basil, Vie, Knorr*	1 Pack/500ml	145	2.0	29	0.8	5.5	0.4	0.9
Tomato & Brown Lentil, Healthy, Baxters*	1 Can/415g	199	0.8	48	2.6	9.0	0.2	2.7
Tomato & Brown Lentil, Healthy Choice, Heinz*	½ Can/208g	112	0.6	54	3.1	9.6	0.3	1.5
Tomato & Butterbean, Classic, Heinz*	½ Can/200g	92	1.4	46	1.3	8.1	0.7	0.8
Tomato & Butterbean, Vegetarian, Baxters*	1 Can/415g	166	5.0	40	1.2	6.1	1.2	1.0
Tomato & Chorizo, Mediterranean, Tesco*	1 Serving/200g	130	6.8	65	2.0	6.1	3.4	0.3
Tomato & Herb, Campbell's*	1 Carton/500ml	180	6.5	36	1.0	5.0	1.3	0.0
Tomato & Lentil, M & S*	½ Can/211g	95	0.4	45	2.3	8.4	0.2	1.5
Tomato & Orange, Baxters*	1 Can/425g	178	2.1	42	1.0	8.3	0.5	0.4
Tomato & Pesto, Diet Chef Ltd*	1 Pack/300g	171	6.6	57	1.3	7.9	2.2	1.1
Tomato & Puy Lentil, Canned, Tesco*	½ Can/200g	64	0.6	32	0.7	6.5	0.3	0.6
Tomato & Red Pepper, Campbell's*	1 Can/590g	366	19.5	62	0.5	7.7	3.3	0.0
Tomato & Red Pepper, to Go, Asda*	1 Pot/330g	102	4.3	31	0.6	4.3	1.3	0.6
Tomato & Red Pepper with Basil, Farmers Market, Heinz*	½ Carton/300g	117	4.2	39	1.0	5.2	1.4	0.5
Tomato & Roasted Red Pepper, COU, M & S*	1 Serving/415g	145	0.4	35	1.0	7.6	0.1	0.4
Tomato & Spinach, Organic, Waitrose*	1 Serving/300g	126	5.7	42	1.4	4.9	1.9	0.7
Tomato & Three Bean, Canned, BGTY, Sainsbury's*	½ Can/200g	118	1.8	59	3.7	9.1	0.9	1.7
Tomato & Vegetable, Cup a Soup, Batchelors*	1 Serving/218g	107	2.6	49	1.1	8.5	1.2	0.6
Tomato & Vegetable, Organic, Baxters*	1 Can/400g	200	3.2	50	1.6	9.2	0.8	0.8
Tomato & Vegetable, Spicy, Meal in a Mug, Tesco*	1 Sachet/20g	74	2.1	370	5.5	62.3	10.5	4.3
Tomato & Vegetable, with Croutons, Dry, Soupreme*	1 Serving/27g	106	3.8	394	7.2	59.9	13.9	4.8
Tomato Flavoured, Tony Ferguson*	1 Pack/58g	205	2.1	354	26.2	49.2	3.6	5.2
Toulouse Inspired, Sausage & Lentil, Sainsbury's*	1 Pot/400g	249	7.2	62	3.6	6.7	1.8	2.4
Traditional Vegetable, Knorr*	1 Serving/200ml	42	0.2	21	1.0	3.2	0.1	1.0
Turkey Broth, Canned, Baxters*	½ Can/208g	79	1.5	38	1.3	6.5	0.7	0.7

S

Measure INFO/WEIGHT	per Measure KCAL	FAT	Nutrition Values per 100g / 100ml KCAL	PROT	CARB	FAT	FIBRE

SOUP

	Measure INFO/WEIGHT	KCAL	FAT	KCAL	PROT	CARB	FAT	FIBRE
Tuscan Bean, Canned, HL, Tesco*	½ Can/200ml	130	3.6	65	3.5	10.3	1.8	1.3
Tuscan Bean, Chunky, Waitrose*	½ Can/206g	68	0.6	33	3.3	4.2	0.3	3.5
Tuscan Bean, GFY, Asda*	1 Carton/400ml	224	3.6	56	2.9	9.0	0.9	0.8
Tuscan Bean, New Covent Garden Food Co*	½ Carton/300g	84	2.4	28	1.6	3.7	0.8	1.0
Tuscan Bean, Organic, Fresh, Sainsbury's*	1 Pack/400g	171	3.2	43	2.6	6.3	0.8	2.0
Tuscan Bean, Perfectly Balanced, Waitrose*	½ Pot/300g	147	5.4	49	2.0	6.1	1.8	1.8
Tuscan Chicken & Orzo, Glorious!*	½ Pot/300g	135	1.5	45	3.2	7.0	0.5	0.8
Tuscan Style Bean & Sausage, Chunky, M & S*	1 Can/415g	249	9.1	60	2.4	7.7	2.2	1.0
Vegetable, 99% Fat Free, Wattie's*	1 Serving/105g	30	0.2	28	0.8	5.9	0.1	0.8
Vegetable, Average	1 Serving/220g	114	8.8	52	0.9	3.2	4.0	0.9
Vegetable, Bean & Pasta, Organic, Baxters*	1 Can/415g	212	3.3	51	2.2	8.7	0.8	1.4
Vegetable, Canned	1oz/28g	13	0.2	48	1.4	9.9	0.6	1.5
Vegetable, Condensed, Campbell's*	1 Can/295g	103	2.4	35	0.8	6.2	0.8	0.0
Vegetable, Condensed, Classic, Campbell's*	1 Can/295g	221	5.0	75	1.7	13.2	1.7	1.7
Vegetable, Cream of, Cup a Soup, Batchelors*	1 Sachet/33g	134	5.3	406	5.8	59.8	16.0	6.2
Vegetable, Cream of, Cup a Soup, Soupreme*	1 Pack/21g	73	2.2	356	4.9	59.5	10.7	6.3
Vegetable, Cup Soup, Dry, Heinz*	1 Sachet/16g	54	1.1	348	5.8	64.5	7.1	3.2
Vegetable, Cup Soup, Made Up, Heinz*	1 Cup/200g	50	1.0	25	0.4	4.7	0.5	0.2
Vegetable, Extra Thick, Canned, Sainsbury's*	1 Can/400g	184	2.4	46	1.5	8.6	0.6	1.4
Vegetable, for One, Heinz*	1 Can/300g	129	2.1	43	1.1	8.1	0.7	0.9
Vegetable, From Heinz, Canned, Weight Watchers*	1 Can/295g	86	0.9	29	0.9	5.6	0.3	0.8
Vegetable, Golden, in a Mug, Tesco*	1 Sachet/17g	60	1.3	351	8.2	62.0	7.8	3.7
Vegetable, in a Cup, Weight Watchers*	1 Serving/100g	57	1.2	57	1.2	10.4	1.2	0.5
Vegetable, Mediterranean, Canned, Tesco*	½ Can/200g	76	1.8	38	0.6	6.8	0.9	0.5
Vegetable, Mediterranean, Tesco*	½ Pot/300g	105	2.1	35	1.0	6.2	0.7	0.7
Vegetable, Provencal, M & S*	1 Serving/300g	150	7.5	50	1.0	6.0	2.5	1.1
Vegetable, Soup-A-Cups, Asda*	1 Sachet/200ml	59	1.1	29	0.6	5.5	0.5	0.4
Vegetable, Tesco*	½ Carton/200g	78	2.6	39	0.9	5.8	1.3	1.0
Vegetable, Vie, Knorr*	1 Pack/500ml	160	3.5	32	0.9	5.5	0.7	1.2
Vegetable & Chilli, Chunky, Fresh, Sainsbury's*	½ Pot/300g	117	1.8	39	1.6	6.9	0.6	2.6
Vegetable & Rosemary, Fresh, Sainsbury's*	½ Pack/300g	96	3.0	32	0.9	4.9	1.0	1.3
Vegetable Broth, Canned, HL, Tesco*	½ Can/200g	74	0.4	37	1.2	7.4	0.2	1.0
Vegetable Broth, M & S*	1 Pack/213g	85	3.0	40	1.0	6.3	1.4	0.8
Vegetable Chowder, New Covent Garden Food Co*	½ Carton/300g	159	5.1	53	2.9	6.6	1.7	1.1
Vegetable Curry, Chosen By You, Asda*	½ Pot/300g	240	2.1	80	4.5	13.3	0.7	1.1
Vegetable Mulligatawny, Tesco*	½ Pack/300g	210	7.5	70	1.9	9.0	2.5	1.1
Watercress, M & S*	½ Pot/300g	75	5.1	25	1.3	1.5	1.7	0.6
Watercress & Cream, Soup Chef*	1 Jar/780g	413	22.6	53	0.8	5.9	2.9	0.3
Winter Vegetable, Broth, Classic, Heinz*	1 Serving/200g	68	0.3	34	0.8	7.3	0.1	0.8
Winter Vegetable, Chosen By You, Asda*	1 Pot/600g	234	4.2	39	1.6	5.9	0.7	1.1
Winter Vegetable, New Covent Garden Food Co*	½ Pack/300g	117	2.1	39	2.0	5.1	0.7	2.3
Winter Vegetable, Organic, Sainsbury's*	½ Can/200g	100	2.0	50	2.3	7.9	1.0	1.3

SOUP MIX

	Measure INFO/WEIGHT	KCAL	FAT	KCAL	PROT	CARB	FAT	FIBRE
Leek & Potato, Made Up, Sainsbury's*	½ Pack/204g	39	0.4	19	0.6	3.6	0.2	0.5
Minestrone, Made Up, Sainsbury's*	1 Serving/200ml	44	0.0	22	0.3	6.0	0.0	0.3
Pea & Ham, Traditional, King	1 Serving/200ml	66	0.4	33	2.2	5.9	0.2	0.0
Scotch Broth, Made Up, Sainsbury's*	1 Serving/175g	31	0.3	18	0.2	3.8	0.2	0.6
Soup & Broth Mix, Wholefoods, Tesco*	¼ Pack/125g	456	2.4	365	14.7	71.4	1.9	7.3

SOUTHERN COMFORT

	Measure INFO/WEIGHT	KCAL	FAT	KCAL	PROT	CARB	FAT	FIBRE
37.5% Volume	*1 Shot/35ml*	*72*	*0.0*	*207*	*0.0*	*0.0*	*0.0*	*0.0*

SOYA

	Measure INFO/WEIGHT	KCAL	FAT	KCAL	PROT	CARB	FAT	FIBRE
Barbeque Chilli, Vegelicious, Tesco*	1 450g/450g	450	15.7	100	3.1	12.9	3.5	2.7
Bolognese Style, Sainsbury's*	½ Pack/168g	113	1.2	67	3.1	13.9	0.7	2.7

S

	Measure INFO/WEIGHT	per Measure KCAL	FAT	Nutrition Values per 100g / 100ml KCAL	PROT	CARB	FAT	FIBRE
SOYA								
Chunks, Dried, Cooked, Sainsbury's*	1oz/28g	27	0.1	98	14.0	9.8	0.3	1.1
Chunks, Protein, Natural, Nature's Harvest*	1 Serving/50g	172	0.5	345	50.0	38.0	1.0	4.0
Mince, Dry Weight, Sainsbury's*	1 Serving/50g	164	0.4	328	47.2	33.2	0.8	3.6
Mince, Granules	*1oz/28g*	*74*	*1.5*	*263*	*43.2*	*11.0*	*5.4*	*0.0*
SOYA MILK								
Flavoured, Average	1 fl oz/30ml	12	0.5	40	2.8	3.6	1.7	0.0
Light, Sweetened, Dairy Free Alt, with Multivitamins, Alpro*	1 Serving/250ml	77	3.0	31	2.1	2.0	1.2	1.2
No Added Sugar, Unsweetened, Average	*1 Serving/250ml*	*85*	*4.8*	*34*	*3.3*	*0.9*	*1.9*	*0.4*
Omega Vanilla, So Good Beverages*	1 Serving/250ml	130	3.0	52	3.6	7.6	1.2	0.0
Sweetened, Average	*1 Glass/200ml*	*93*	*4.2*	*47*	*3.4*	*3.7*	*2.1*	*0.4*
Sweetened, Calcium Enriched, Average	1 Glass/200ml	91	3.9	46	3.4	3.7	2.0	0.3
Unsweetened, Uht, Organic, Tesco*	1 Serving/150ml	46	2.8	31	3.4	0.1	1.9	0.6
SPAGHETTI								
Brown Rice, Gluten Free, Organic, Dove's Farm*	1 Serving/70g	237	1.0	338	7.9	70.3	1.5	4.1
Chicken, BGTY, Sainsbury's*	1 Serving/300g	281	2.7	94	9.8	11.6	0.9	2.3
Cooked, Average	*1oz/28g*	*33*	*0.2*	*119*	*4.1*	*24.8*	*0.6*	*1.1*
Dry, Average	*1oz/28g*	*98*	*0.4*	*350*	*12.1*	*72.1*	*1.5*	*2.4*
Durum Wheat, Dry, Average	*1oz/28g*	*97*	*0.1*	*347*	*12.3*	*71.7*	*0.3*	*1.4*
Fresh, Cooked, Average	*1 Serving/125g*	*182*	*2.2*	*146*	*6.1*	*26.9*	*1.7*	*1.8*
Fresh, Dry, Average	*1 Serving/100g*	*278*	*3.0*	*278*	*10.8*	*53.0*	*3.0*	*2.2*
in Tomato & Cheese, Sainsbury's*	1 Serving/300g	345	10.2	115	4.4	16.8	3.4	1.4
in Tomato Sauce, Canned	1oz/28g	18	0.1	64	1.9	14.1	0.4	0.7
in Tomato Sauce, Heinz*	½ Can/200g	120	0.6	60	1.7	12.7	0.3	2.4
in Tomato Sauce, HP*	1 Can/410g	247	0.8	60	1.5	13.1	0.2	0.4
In Tomato Sauce, Multigrain, Heinz*	½ Can/200g	120	0.6	60	1.7	12.7	0.3	2.4
in Tomato Sauce, Organic, Sainsbury's*	½ Can/205g	133	0.4	65	1.8	13.9	0.2	1.1
in Tomato Sauce, Whole Wheat, Sainsbury's*	1 Serving/205g	125	1.2	61	2.0	11.9	0.6	1.1
in Tomato Sauce with Parsley, Weight Watchers*	1 Sm Can/200g	96	0.6	48	1.8	9.6	0.3	2.4
TTD, Sainsbury's*	1 Serving/90g	321	1.5	357	12.3	73.1	1.7	2.5
Wheat Free, Tesco*	1 Serving/100g	340	2.0	340	8.0	72.5	2.0	2.5
Whole Wheat, Cooked, Average	*1oz/28g*	*32*	*0.3*	*113*	*4.7*	*23.2*	*0.9*	*3.5*
Whole Wheat, Dry, Average	*1 Serving/100g*	*324*	*2.6*	*324*	*13.5*	*62.2*	*2.6*	*8.0*
with Sausages, in Tomato Sauce, Heinz*	1 Can/400g	352	14.0	88	3.4	10.8	3.5	0.5
with Tomato & Cheese, Tesco*	½ Pack/250g	280	6.5	112	4.0	18.1	2.6	1.1
SPAGHETTI & MEATBALLS								
BGTY, Sainsbury's*	1 Pack/300g	249	2.7	83	5.9	12.7	0.9	3.1
Chicken, in Tomato Sauce, Heinz*	1 Can/400g	332	9.2	83	4.2	11.3	2.3	0.5
COU, M & S*	1 Pack/400g	360	8.0	90	6.0	12.3	2.0	2.6
HL, Tesco*	1 Pack/370g	407	14.4	110	4.7	13.8	3.9	1.6
Italian, Sainsbury's*	1 Pack/450g	495	21.1	110	5.0	11.9	4.7	2.7
Italian Cuisine, Tesco*	1 Pack/400g	500	17.6	125	5.9	14.6	4.4	1.7
Sainsbury's*	1 Pack/400g	497	18.4	124	6.5	14.2	4.6	2.8
Tesco*	1 Serving/475g	641	30.9	135	5.1	14.1	6.5	0.9
SPAGHETTI BOLOGNESE								
Al Forno, Sainsbury's*	1 Pack/400g	460	19.6	115	7.8	10.0	4.9	1.1
Average	1 Serving/450g	580	25.2	129	7.8	12.5	5.6	0.9
BGTY, Sainsbury's*	1 Pack/400g	416	9.2	104	6.3	14.4	2.3	1.1
Canned, Asda*	½ Can/205g	174	5.7	85	4.2	10.7	2.8	0.6
Egg Pasta in Rich Beef Sauce, Waitrose*	1 Pack/400g	404	10.4	101	7.6	11.7	2.6	1.0
GFY, Asda*	1 Pack/400g	352	6.4	88	4.9	13.4	1.6	2.2
Hidden Veg, Heinz*	1 Can/400g	312	6.4	78	3.4	12.6	1.6	0.9
in Tomato & Beef Sauce, Canned, Carlini*	1 Can/410g	324	10.7	79	3.7	10.2	2.6	1.2
Italian, Chilled, Tesco*	1 Pack/400g	520	17.2	130	6.5	15.9	4.3	1.5

S

	Measure INFO/WEIGHT	per Measure		Nutrition Values per 100g / 100ml				
		KCAL	FAT	KCAL	PROT	CARB	FAT	FIBRE
SPAGHETTI BOLOGNESE								
Italiano, Pro-Cuisine, Pro Cuisine*	1 Pack/600g	522	11.4	87	5.7	11.7	1.9	0.0
Lean Cuisine, Findus*	1 Pack/320g	275	7.4	86	4.5	11.5	2.3	1.1
Meat Free, Heinz*	1 Serving/200g	162	3.4	81	3.3	13.1	1.7	0.6
Perfectly Balanced, Waitrose*	1 Pack/400g	380	6.8	95	6.7	13.4	1.7	1.1
Quick Pasta, Dry, Sainsbury's*	1 Serving/63g	231	2.8	367	10.8	71.0	4.4	3.3
Vegetarian, Tesco*	1 Pack/340g	374	13.3	110	5.1	13.7	3.9	1.2
Weight Watchers*	1 Pack/320g	307	7.0	96	5.7	13.1	2.2	0.7
SPAGHETTI CARBONARA								
Chicken, Mushroom & Ham, Asda*	1 Pack/700g	686	14.0	98	10.0	10.0	2.0	1.5
Chicken & Asparagus, Sainsbury's*	1 Pack/450g	657	27.4	146	6.6	16.2	6.1	1.1
COU, M & S*	1 Pack/330g	346	6.6	105	5.7	15.5	2.0	1.8
Italian, Chilled, Sainsbury's*	1 Pack/400g	492	15.6	123	5.5	16.1	3.9	1.4
Italian, Fresh, Chilled, Tesco*	1 Pack/430g	606	26.2	141	7.6	13.9	6.1	1.3
Italian, Tesco*	1 Pack/450g	607	26.5	135	5.4	14.1	5.9	0.6
M & S*	1 Pack/400g	660	36.0	165	6.5	14.2	9.0	0.6
SPAGHETTI HOOPS								
& Sausages, Tesco*	1 Serving/205g	184	6.8	90	3.1	11.9	3.3	0.2
in Tomato Sauce, Heinz*	½ Can/200g	106	0.4	53	1.7	11.1	0.2	0.5
in Tomato Sauce, Multigrain, Snap Pot, Heinz*	1 Pot/190g	112	0.6	59	1.6	12.7	0.3	1.5
in Tomato Sauce, Snap Pot, Heinz*	1 Pot/192g	113	0.6	59	1.6	12.7	0.3	1.5
SPAGHETTI MARINARA								
GFY, Asda*	1 Pack/400g	520	16.8	130	8.0	15.0	4.2	0.9
SPAGHETTI RINGS								
in Tomato Sauce, Canned, Sainsbury's*	1 Serving/213g	136	0.8	64	1.9	13.3	0.4	0.5
SPAGHETTINI								
Wholewheat, Great Stuff, Asda*	1 Serving/100g	99	0.7	99	3.4	19.7	0.7	2.4
SPAM*								
Pork & Ham, Chopped, Spam*	1 Serving/100g	296	24.2	296	14.5	3.2	24.2	0.0
SPELT								
Organic, Easy Grain, Food Doctor*	1 Pack/225g	326	4.0	145	5.2	26.6	1.8	5.9
SPICE BLEND								
Balti, Sharwood's*	1oz/28g	34	2.7	122	1.8	7.1	9.6	1.2
Thai, Sharwood's*	1 Pack 260g	424	30.9	163	1.8	12.0	11.9	1.0
Tikka, Sharwood's*	1 Pack/260g	263	14.0	101	2.7	10.2	5.4	1.7
SPICE MIX								
for Burritos, Old El Paso*	½ Packet/23g	68	0.9	304	13.0	54.0	4.0	0.0
for Fajitas, Old El Paso*	1 Pack/35g	107	2.1	306	9.0	54.0	6.0	0.0
for Mexican Fajitas, Discovery*	½ Pack/15g	34	1.0	230	8.0	35.0	6.5	17.5
From Fajita Dinner Kit, Original Smoky BBQ, Old El Paso*	1 Pack/35g	100	0.6	285	7.9	56.0	1.8	0.0
Tex Mex Chilli Con Carne, Schwartz*	1 Sachet/100g	278	6.6	278	12.9	66.5	6.6	24.5
SPINACH								
Baby, Average	*1 Serving/90g*	*22*	*0.7*	*25*	*2.8*	*1.6*	*0.8*	*2.1*
Boiled Or Steamed, Average	*1 Serving/80g*	*17*	*0.6*	*21*	*2.6*	*0.9*	*0.8*	*2.1*
Canned, Average	*1 Serving/80g*	*18*	*0.4*	*22*	*3.0*	*1.4*	*0.5*	*2.9*
Raw	*1 Bunch/340g*	*75*	*1.2*	*22*	*2.9*	*3.5*	*0.3*	*2.7*
Raw, Average	*1 Serving/80g*	*20*	*0.6*	*25*	*2.8*	*1.6*	*0.8*	*2.1*
SPIRALI								
Dry, Average	*1 Serving/50g*	*176*	*0.8*	*351*	*12.1*	*72.5*	*1.6*	*2.7*
SPIRITS								
37.5% Volume	*1 Shot/35ml*	*72*	*0.0*	*207*	*0.0*	*0.0*	*0.0*	*0.0*
40% Volume	*1 Shot/35ml*	*78*	*0.0*	*222*	*0.0*	*0.0*	*0.0*	*0.0*
SPLENDIPS								
Cheesecake, Philadelphia, Kraft*	1 Pack/85g	200	7.1	235	6.1	34.0	8.3	2.9

S

	Measure INFO/WEIGHT	per Measure KCAL	FAT	Nutrition Values per 100g / 100ml KCAL	PROT	CARB	FAT	FIBRE
SPLENDIPS								
Chives, Philadelphia, Kraft*	1 Pack/85g	159	4.4	187	7.5	27.0	5.2	1.7
Nachos, Philadelphia, Kraft*	1 Pack/85g	150	6.5	177	6.4	20.0	7.6	1.0
Poppadoms & Mango Chutney, Light, Philadelphia, Kraft*	1 Pack/76g	131	3.6	172	5.1	26.5	4.7	1.9
SPLIT PEAS								
Dried, Average	*1oz/28g*	*89*	*0.5*	*319*	*22.1*	*57.4*	*1.7*	*3.1*
Green, Dried, Boiled, Average	*1 Tbsp/35g*	*40*	*0.2*	*115*	*8.3*	*19.8*	*0.6*	*3.9*
Yellow, Morrisons*	1 Serving /120g	338	1.4	282	21.3	62.2	1.2	15.6
Yellow, Wholefoods, Tesco*	1 Serving/15g	52	0.4	345	22.1	58.2	2.4	6.3
SPONGE PUDDING								
Average	1 Portion/170g	578	27.7	340	5.8	45.3	16.3	1.1
Banoffee, Heinz*	¼ Can/78g	239	9.5	307	2.8	46.6	12.2	0.6
Blackcurrant, BGTY, Sainsbury's*	1 Serving/110g	155	1.0	141	2.5	30.7	0.9	3.2
Canned, Average	1 Serving/75g	214	8.5	285	3.1	45.4	11.4	0.8
Chocolate, BGTY, Sainsbury's*	1 Pudding/105g	137	2.5	131	4.4	23.1	2.4	2.7
Chocolate, Cadbury*	1 Pack/370g	1276	73.3	345	4.9	36.7	19.8	0.0
Chocolate, Free From, Sainsbury's*	1 Pudding/110g	388	10.2	353	5.2	62.0	9.3	0.3
Chocolate, Heinz*	¼ Pudding/77g	229	8.9	298	4.6	44.0	11.5	1.2
Chocolate, Less Than 3% Fat, BGTY, Sainsbury's*	1 Pudding/105g	180	2.0	171	4.5	34.0	1.9	0.9
Chocolate, M & S*	¼ Pudding/131g	524	32.2	400	6.1	38.6	24.6	1.8
Chocolate, Waitrose*	1 Pudding/110g	400	22.5	363	3.6	41.4	20.4	1.7
Chocolate, with Cadbury's Caramel Sticky Sauce, Heinz*	1 Serving/200g	762	33.8	381	3.5	52.3	16.9	0.6
Circus, & Custard, Weight Watchers*	1 Serving/140g	239	4.1	171	4.2	32.1	2.9	0.9
Fruit, Co-Op*	1 Can/300g	1110	48.0	370	3.0	53.0	16.0	2.0
Fruited with Brandy Sauce, Sainsbury's*	1 Pudding/125g	261	8.4	209	3.6	33.6	6.7	0.8
Ginger, with Plum Sauce, Waitrose*	1 Pudding/120g	424	17.9	353	3.1	51.7	14.9	0.7
Golden Syrup, Co-Op*	1 Can/300g	945	39.0	315	2.0	47.0	13.0	0.6
Jam & Custard, Co-Op*	1 Pack/244g	598	22.0	245	3.0	37.0	9.0	0.3
Lemon, COU, M & S*	1 Pudding/100g	157	2.3	157	2.0	32.1	2.3	1.9
Lemon, M & S*	1 Pudding/105g	325	16.0	310	4.3	39.4	15.2	2.3
Lemon, Waitrose*	1 Serving/105g	212	2.5	202	3.4	41.7	2.4	1.4
Lemon Curd, Heinz*	¼ Can/78g	236	9.1	302	2.6	46.7	11.7	0.6
Pear & Ginger, COU, M & S*	1 Pudding/100g	175	0.7	175	1.9	39.8	0.7	1.1
Raspberry Jam, Asda*	½ Pudding/147g	481	16.2	327	3.1	54.0	11.0	4.1
Sticky Toffee, COU, M & S*	1 Pack/150g	277	2.5	185	2.5	39.3	1.7	1.8
Sticky Toffee, Microwavable, Heinz*	1 Serving/75g	233	9.0	311	3.3	47.4	12.0	0.7
Strawberry Jam, Heinz*	¼ Can/82g	230	6.2	281	2.6	50.4	7.6	0.6
Sultana, with Toffee Sauce, HL, Tesco*	1 Serving/80g	280	2.2	350	3.2	60.2	2.7	1.0
Syrup, BGTY, Sainsbury's*	1 Pudding/110g	338	4.5	307	2.8	64.6	4.1	0.4
Syrup, Finest, Tesco*	1 Pudding/115g	330	9.0	287	3.1	51.2	7.8	0.6
Syrup, GFY, Asda*	1 Sponge/105g	207	4.3	197	2.0	38.0	4.1	2.6
Syrup, Sainsbury's*	¼ Pudding/110g	408	13.0	371	2.7	63.5	11.8	0.4
Syrup & Custard, Morrisons*	1 Serving/125g	290	8.6	232	3.4	39.1	6.9	0.8
Treacle, Heinz*	1 Serving/160g	445	13.0	278	2.5	48.9	8.1	0.6
Treacle, Waitrose*	1 Pudding/105g	385	13.8	367	2.8	58.9	13.1	0.6
Very Fruity Cherry, M & S*	1 Pot/110g	286	11.3	260	3.5	38.6	10.3	1.8
with Custard	1 Serving/200g	521	24.9	261	4.8	34.1	12.4	0.9
with Dried Fruit	1oz/28g	93	4.0	331	5.4	48.1	14.3	1.2
with Jam or Treacle	1oz/28g	93	4.0	333	5.1	48.7	14.4	1.0
with Lyles Golden Syrup, Heinz*	½ Pudding/95g	368	14.4	386	3.1	53.3	15.1	0.5
SPOTTED DICK								
Average	1 Serving/105g	343	17.5	327	4.2	42.7	16.7	1.0
with Custard	1 Serving/210g	438	15.6	209	3.4	31.5	7.4	1.3

S

	Measure INFO/WEIGHT	per Measure KCAL	FAT	Nutrition Values per 100g / 100ml KCAL	PROT	CARB	FAT	FIBRE
SPRATS								
Fried	*1oz/28g*	*116*	*9.8*	*415*	*24.9*	*0.0*	*35.0*	*0.0*
Raw	*1oz/28g*	*48*	*3.1*	*172*	*18.3*	*0.0*	*11.0*	*0.0*
SPREAD								
British Butterspread, Asda*	1 Serving/10g	70	7.7	699	0.4	0.5	77.3	0.0
Butter Me Up, Tesco*	1 Thin Spread/7g	38	4.1	540	0.8	1.2	59.0	0.0
Butterlicious, Vegetable, Sainsbury's*	1 Thin Spread/7g	44	4.8	628	0.6	1.1	69.0	0.0
Buttersoft, Light, Reduced Fat, Sainsbury's*	1 Thin Spread/7g	38	4.2	544	0.4	0.5	60.0	0.0
Buttery Taste, Benecol*	1 Thin Spread/7g	40	4.4	575	0.0	0.8	63.3	0.0
Clover, Light, Dairy Crest Ltd*	1 Serving/7g	32	3.4	455	0.7	2.9	49.0	0.0
Dairy Free, Organic, Pure Spreads*	1 Thin Spread/7g	37	4.1	533	0.5	0.0	59.0	0.0
Diet, Delight*	1 Thin Spread/7g	16	1.6	228	3.6	1.6	23.0	0.0
Enriched Olive, Tesco*	1 Thin Spread/7g	38	4.1	540	0.2	1.2	59.0	0.0
From Soya, Kallo*	1 Thin Spread/7g	27	2.6	380	7.0	6.0	37.0	0.0
Gold, Lowest Fat, with Omega 3, St Ivel*	1 Thin Spread/7g	13	1.3	192	0.8	4.3	19.0	1.3
Irish, Dairy, Original, Low Low*	1 Thin Spread/7g	24	2.7	346	0.4	0.5	38.0	0.0
Light, Benecol*	1 Thin Spread/7g	23	2.4	333	2.5	0.0	35.0	0.0
Lighter Than Light, Flora*	1 Serving/10g	19	1.8	188	5.0	1.6	18.0	0.0
Low Fat, Average	1 Thin Spread/7g	27	2.8	390	5.8	0.5	40.5	0.0
Olive, Gold, Reduced Fat, Sainsbury's*	1 Thin Spread/7g	38	4.1	536	0.1	1.2	59.0	0.0
Olive, Light, Low Fat, HL, Tesco*	1 Thin Spread/7g	24	2.7	348	1.5	0.0	38.0	0.0
Olive, Reduced Fat, Asda*	1 Thin Spread/7g	38	4.1	536	0.2	1.1	59.0	0.0
Olive, Reduced Fat, M & S*	1 Thin Spread/7g	38	4.1	536	0.2	1.1	59.0	0.0
Olive, Reduced Fat, So Organic, Sainsbury's*	1 Thin Spread/7g	38	4.2	537	0.1	0.4	59.5	0.0
Olive, Waitrose*	1 Thin Spread/7g	37	4.1	534	0.2	0.5	59.0	0.0
Olive Gold, Reduced Fat, Co-Op*	1 Thin Spread/7g	37	4.1	535	0.2	1.0	59.0	0.0
Olive Oil, 55% Reduced Fat, Benecol*	1 Thin Spread/7g	35	3.8	498	0.3	0.5	55.0	0.0
Olive Oil, Bertolli*	1 Thin Spread/7g	38	4.1	536	0.2	1.0	59.0	0.0
Organic, Dairy Free, M & S*	1 Thin Spread/7g	37	4.1	531	0.0	0.0	59.0	0.0
Soft, Economy, Sainsbury's*	1 Thin Spread/7g	31	3.5	450	0.2	0.9	50.0	0.0
Soft, Sainsbury's*	1 Thin Spread/7g	44	4.9	630	0.1	0.1	70.0	0.0
Sunflower, Asda*	1 Thin Spread/7g	44	4.9	635	0.2	1.0	70.0	0.0
Sunflower, Enriched, Tesco*	1 Thin Spread/7g	37	4.1	535	0.1	0.2	59.0	0.0
Sunflower, Light, BGTY, Sainsbury's*	1 Thin Spread/7g	19	2.0	265	0.1	0.8	29.0	0.0
Sunflower, M & S*	1 Thin Spread/7g	44	4.9	630	0.0	0.0	70.0	3.0
Sunflower, Morrisons*	1 Thin Spread/7g	37	4.1	531	0.0	0.2	59.0	0.0
Sunflower, Reduced Fat, Suma*	1 Thin Spread/7g	38	4.2	537	0.0	0.4	59.5	0.0
Sunflower, Sainsbury's*	1 Thin Spread/7g	37	4.1	532	0.1	0.2	59.0	0.0
Sunflower, Waitrose*	1 Thin Spread/7g	44	4.9	631	0.0	0.2	70.0	0.0
Vegetable, Dairy Free, Free From, Sainsbury's*	1 Thin Spread/7g	44	4.9	630	0.0	0.0	70.0	3.0
Vegetable, Soft, Tesco*	1 Thin Spread/7g	46	5.1	661	0.1	1.0	73.0	0.0
Vitalite, St Ivel*	1 Thin Spread/7g	35	3.9	503	0.0	0.0	56.0	0.8
SPRING ROLLS								
Cantonese Selection, Sainsbury's*	1 Serving/35g	68	2.7	193	4.1	26.9	7.7	1.4
Chicken, & Chilli, Cantonese, Sainsbury's*	1 Roll/51g	85	2.8	166	9.7	19.4	5.5	0.6
Chicken, & Chilli, Sainsbury's*	1 Roll/50g	92	4.6	185	9.6	15.6	9.3	2.8
Chicken, Asda*	1 Roll/58g	115	5.2	199	4.6	25.0	9.0	3.4
Chicken, Finest, Tesco*	1 Roll/60g	118	5.0	196	10.1	20.1	8.3	1.0
Chicken, Oriental, Asda*	1 Roll/60g	106	4.2	178	3.7	25.0	7.0	0.4
Chicken, Oriental Snack Selection, Sainsbury's*	1 Roll/15g	38	1.5	256	11.5	30.3	9.9	1.7
Chicken, Tesco*	1 Roll/50g	115	5.6	231	8.1	24.5	11.2	1.5
Chinese Takeaway, Tesco*	1 Roll/50g	100	4.3	201	4.4	26.4	8.6	1.5
Dim Sum, Sainsbury's*	1 Roll/12g	26	1.2	216	4.1	28.2	9.6	2.9
Duck, M & S*	1 Roll/30g	75	3.4	250	9.8	27.7	11.2	1.5

	Measure INFO/WEIGHT	per Measure KCAL	FAT	Nutrition Values per 100g / 100ml KCAL	PROT	CARB	FAT	FIBRE
SPRING ROLLS								
Duck, Mini, Asda*	1 Roll/18g	47	1.9	259	8.7	32.8	10.3	1.9
Duck, Morrisons*	1 Roll/65g	147	6.7	226	6.2	27.2	10.3	1.2
Duck, Party Bites, Sainsbury's*	1 Roll/20g	49	1.8	245	10.1	31.4	8.8	1.0
Duck with Sweet Chilli Sauce, Waitrose*	1 Roll/72g	66	1.4	92	5.1	14.0	1.9	0.9
M & S*	1 Pack/180g	333	15.1	185	3.5	24.2	8.4	2.3
Mini, Sainsbury's*	1 Roll/12g	27	1.2	221	4.2	28.7	9.9	1.6
Prawn, Cantonese, Sainsbury's*	1 Roll/28g	46	1.7	162	6.8	20.3	6.0	2.5
Prawn, Crispy, M & S*	1 Roll/34g	75	3.4	220	10.0	22.2	9.9	1.3
Prawn, Tesco*	1 Roll/33g	70	3.1	211	8.7	22.8	9.4	1.4
Roast Duck, M & S*	1 Roll/31g	85	4.9	275	7.8	26.2	15.7	1.4
Thai, Sainsbury's*	1 Roll/30g	69	3.4	229	2.9	28.8	11.3	3.5
Thai Prawn, Waitrose*	1 Roll/50g	109	4.7	219	8.0	25.4	9.5	2.4
Vegetable, Asda*	1 Roll/62g	126	5.6	203	3.5	27.0	9.0	2.7
Vegetable, Cantonese, Sainsbury's*	1 Roll/36g	84	4.2	233	3.6	28.1	11.7	1.4
Vegetable, Chilled, Tesco*	1 Roll/68g	149	7.6	221	4.0	25.9	11.3	1.6
Vegetable, Chinese, Sainsbury's*	1 Roll/26g	50	2.0	193	4.1	26.9	7.7	1.4
Vegetable, Frozen, Tesco*	1 Roll/60g	123	6.4	205	3.5	23.0	10.6	1.3
Vegetable, M & S*	1 Roll/37g	80	3.6	215	4.3	27.8	9.6	2.0
Vegetable, Mini, Occasions, Sainsbury's*	1 Roll/24g	52	2.3	216	4.1	28.2	9.6	2.9
Vegetable, Mini, Oriental Selection, Waitrose*	1 Roll/18g	35	1.2	192	4.2	28.6	6.8	1.7
Vegetable, Mini, Party Food, M & S*	1 Roll/17g	35	1.6	205	3.5	26.3	9.7	2.0
Vegetable, Mini, Tesco*	1 Roll/18g	36	1.5	205	4.4	26.4	8.6	1.5
Vegetable, Oriental, Sainsbury's*	1 Roll/61g	137	7.2	224	3.8	24.3	11.8	2.9
Vegetable, Tempura, M & S*	1 Pack/140g	280	12.0	200	2.8	27.9	8.6	1.8
Vegetable, Waitrose*	1 Roll/57g	107	5.3	187	3.7	22.1	9.3	3.4
Vegetable & Chicken, Tesco*	1 Roll/60g	110	4.6	183	6.1	22.2	7.7	2.5
SPRITE*								
Sprite*	1 Bottle/500ml	215	0.0	43	0.0	10.5	0.0	0.0
Zero, Sprite*	1 Can/330ml	3	0.0	1	0.0	0.0	0.0	0.0
SPRITZER								
Red Grape, Non-Alcoholic, Extra Special, Asda*	1 Bottle/750ml	330	0.0	44	0.0	11.0	0.0	0.0
Rose & Grape, Non Alcoholic, Extra Special, Asda*	1 Bottle/750ml	90	0.0	12	0.0	3.0	0.0	0.0
with White Zinfandel, Echo Falls*	1 Serving/200ml	216	0.0	108	0.0	0.0	0.0	0.0
SQUARES								
Rice Krispies, Chocolate & Caramel, Kellogg's*	1 Bar/36g	155	5.0	430	4.5	71.0	14.0	2.0
Rice Krispies, Crazy Choc, Kellogg's*	1 Bar/28g	118	3.4	422	3.0	76.0	12.0	1.5
SQUASH								
Apple, Cherry & Raspberry, High Juice, Robinson's*	1 Serving/25ml	49	0.0	196	0.2	47.6	0.1	0.0
Apple, Hi Juice, Tesco*	1 fl oz/30ml	52	0.0	173	0.0	42.5	0.0	0.0
Apple, No Added Sugar, Morrisons*	1 Serving/40ml	8	0.0	21	0.1	4.1	0.0	0.0
Apple & Blackcurrant, No Added Sugar, Tesco*	1 Serving/30ml	4	0.0	15	0.2	2.0	0.0	0.0
Apple & Blackcurrant, Special R, Diluted, Robinson's*	1 fl oz/30ml	2	0.0	8	0.1	1.1	0.1	0.0
Apple & Blackcurrant, Special R, Robinson's*	1 Serving/30ml	2	0.0	8	0.1	1.1	0.0	0.0
Apple & Strawberry High Juice, Sainsbury's*	1 Serving/250ml	82	0.2	33	0.1	8.2	0.1	0.1
Blackcurrant, High Juice, M & S*	1 Glass/250ml	50	0.0	20	0.1	5.2	0.0	0.1
Blackcurrant, No Added Sugar, Tesco*	1 Serving/25ml	3	0.0	14	0.4	1.7	0.0	0.0
Butternut, Courgette & Mange Tout, M & S*	1 Pack/80g	24	0.2	30	2.0	5.8	0.2	2.3
Cherries & Berries, Sugar Free, Diluted, Tesco*	1 Glass/250ml	5	0.0	2	0.0	0.3	0.0	0.0
Cranberry, Light, Classic, Undiluted, Ocean Spray*	1 Serving/50ml	31	0.0	63	0.2	14.1	0.0	0.0
Dandelion & Burdock, Morrisons*	1 Serving/50ml	1	0.0	3	0.0	0.0	0.0	0.0
Forest Fruits, Fruit & Barley, Diluted, Morrisons*	1 fl oz/30ml	4	0.0	12	0.1	1.7	0.0	0.0
Forest Fruits, High Juice, Undiluted, Robinson's*	1 Serving/25ml	51	0.0	206	0.2	50.0	0.1	0.0
Fruit & Barley, No Added Sugar, Robinson's*	1 fl oz/30ml	4	0.0	14	0.3	2.0	0.0	0.0

SQUASH

	Measure INFO/WEIGHT	per Measure KCAL	FAT	Nutrition Values per 100g / 100ml KCAL	PROT	CARB	FAT	FIBRE
Fruit & Barley, Tropical, No Added Sugar, Robinson's*	1 Serving/60ml	7	0.0	12	0.2	1.6	0.0	0.0
Fruit & Barley Orange, Diluted, Robinson's*	1 Serving/50ml	6	0.0	12	0.2	1.7	0.0	0.1
Grape & Passion Fruit, High Juice, Diluted, Sainsbury's*	1 Serving/250ml	100	0.2	40	0.1	9.8	0.1	0.1
Grapefruit, High Juice, No Added Sugar, Sainsbury's*	1 Serving/25ml	1	0.0	6	0.1	1.1	0.0	0.0
Lemon, High Juice, Diluted, Sainsbury's*	1 Glass /250ml	97	0.2	39	0.1	9.1	0.1	0.1
Lemon, High Juice, Tesco*	1 Serving/80ml	141	0.1	176	0.3	43.6	0.1	0.0
Lemon, No Added Sugar, Double Concentrate, Tesco*	1 Serving/25ml	4	0.0	16	0.3	0.7	0.0	0.0
Lemon, No Sugar, Asda*	1 Serving/200ml	5	0.2	2	0.1	0.3	0.1	0.1
Lemon & Lime, Double Strength, No Added Sugar, Asda*	1 Glass/200ml	4	0.0	2	0.0	0.0	0.0	0.0
Mixed Fruit, Diluted, Kia Ora*	1 Serving/250ml	5	0.0	2	0.0	0.3	0.0	0.0
Mixed Fruit, Low Sugar, Sainsbury's*	1 Glass/250ml	5	0.2	2	0.1	0.2	0.1	0.1
Mixed Fruit, Tesco*	1 Serving/75ml	13	0.0	17	0.0	3.5	0.0	0.0
Orange, Fruit & Barley, Chosen By You, Asda*	1 Serving/100ml	2	0.0	2	0.0	0.2	0.0	0.0
Orange, Hi Juice, Tesco*	1 Serving/75ml	140	0.1	187	0.3	45.0	0.1	0.0
Orange, High Juice, Undiluted, Robinson's*	1 Serving/200ml	364	0.2	182	0.3	44.0	0.1	0.0
Orange, No Added Sugar, High Juice, Sainsbury's*	1 Serving/100ml	6	0.1	6	0.1	1.1	0.1	0.1
Orange, No Added Sugar, Undiluted, Pennywise, Crystal*	1 Serving/40ml	3	0.0	8	0.1	1.2	0.0	0.0
Orange, Sainsbury's*	1 Glass/250ml	7	0.2	3	0.1	0.5	0.1	0.1
Orange, Undiluted, Pennywise, Crystal*	1 Serving/40ml	7	0.0	17	0.1	3.5	0.0	0.0
Orange & Mandarin, Fruit Spring, Robinson's*	1 Serving/440ml	26	0.0	6	0.1	0.8	0.0	0.0
Orange & Mango, Low Sugar, Sainsbury's*	1 Serving/250ml	5	0.2	2	0.1	0.2	0.1	0.1
Orange & Mango, No Added Sugar, Robinson's*	1 Serving/25ml	2	0.0	8	0.2	0.9	0.0	0.0
Orange & Mango, Special R, Diluted, Robinson's*	1 Serving/250ml	20	0.0	8	0.2	0.9	0.0	0.0
Orange & Pineapple, No Sugar Added, Robinson's*	1 Serving/25ml	2	0.0	8	0.2	0.7	0.0	0.2
Orange & Pineapple, Original, Undiluted, Robinson's*	1 Serving/250ml	137	0.0	55	1.0	13.0	0.0	0.0
Peach, High Juice, Undiluted, Robinson's*	1 fl oz/30ml	54	0.0	181	0.5	43.0	0.1	0.0
Pink Grapefruit, High Juice, Diluted, Sainsbury's*	1 Serving/250ml	85	0.2	34	0.0	8.1	0.1	0.0
Pink Grapefruit, High Juice, Low Sugar, Tesco*	1 Serving/75ml	12	0.1	16	0.2	3.7	0.1	0.0
Pink Grapefruit, High Juice, Tesco*	1 Serving/75ml	135	0.1	180	0.2	44.6	0.1	0.0
Pink Grapefruit, High Juice, Undiluted, Robinson's*	1 Glass/250ml	455	0.2	182	0.2	43.3	0.1	0.0
Spaghetti, Baked	**1oz/28g**	**6**	**0.1**	**23**	**0.7**	**4.3**	**0.3**	**2.1**
Spaghetti, Including Pips & Rind, Raw	**1oz/28g**	**7**	**0.2**	**26**	**0.6**	**4.6**	**0.6**	**2.3**
Summer Fruit, No Added Sugar, Sainsbury's*	1 Serving/250ml	5	0.2	2	0.1	0.2	0.1	0.1
Summer Fruits, High Juice, Undiluted, Robinson's*	1 fl oz/30ml	61	0.0	203	0.1	49.0	0.1	0.0
Summer Fruits, High Juice, Waitrose*	1 Serving/250ml	102	0.0	41	0.0	10.0	0.0	0.0
Summer Fruits, No Added Sugar, Double Strength, Asda*	1 Serving/50ml	1	0.0	2	0.0	0.2	0.0	0.0
Summer Fruits, No Added Sugar, Made Up, Morrisons*	1 Glass/200ml	3	0.0	1	0.0	0.2	0.0	0.0
Summer Fruits, Robinson's*	1 Measure/25ml	14	0.0	56	0.1	13.0	0.0	0.0
Summer Fruits & Barley, no Added Sugar, Tesco*	1 Serving/50ml	5	0.0	11	0.2	1.7	0.0	0.0
Summerfruits. High Juice, Tesco*	1 Serving/50ml	11	0.0	23	0.2	4.5	0.0	0.0
Tropical, High Juice, Tesco*	1 Glass/75ml	141	0.1	188	0.2	46.6	0.1	0.1
Tropical, No Added Sugar, Diluted, Tesco*	1 Glass/200ml	18	0.0	9	0.2	0.9	0.0	0.0
Tropical Fruits, Sainsbury's*	1 Serving/250ml	95	0.2	38	0.1	9.3	0.1	0.1
Whole Orange, Tesco*	1 Serving/100ml	45	1.0	45	0.2	10.1	1.0	1.0
Winter, Acorn, Baked, Average	**1oz/28g**	**16**	**0.0**	**56**	**1.1**	**12.6**	**0.1**	**3.2**
Winter, Acorn, Raw, Average	**1oz/28g**	**11**	**0.0**	**40**	**0.8**	**9.0**	**0.1**	**2.3**
Winter, All Varieties, Flesh Only, Raw, Average	**1oz/28g**	**10**	**0.0**	**34**	**0.9**	**8.6**	**0.1**	**1.5**
Winter, Butternut, Baked, Average	**1oz/28g**	**9**	**0.0**	**32**	**0.9**	**7.4**	**0.1**	**1.4**
Winter, Butternut, Raw, Unprepared, Average	**1 Serving/80g**	**29**	**0.1**	**36**	**1.1**	**8.3**	**0.1**	**1.6**

SQUID

	Measure INFO/WEIGHT	per Measure KCAL	FAT	Nutrition Values per 100g / 100ml KCAL	PROT	CARB	FAT	FIBRE
Dried, Average	**1oz/28g**	**88**	**1.3**	**313**	**63.3**	**4.8**	**4.6**	**0.0**
in Batter, Fried in Blended Oil, Average	1oz/28g	55	2.8	195	11.5	15.7	10.0	0.5
Raw, Average	**1oz/28g**	**23**	**0.5**	**81**	**15.4**	**1.2**	**1.7**	**0.0**

S

	Measure INFO/WEIGHT	per Measure KCAL	FAT	Nutrition Values per 100g / 100ml KCAL	PROT	CARB	FAT	FIBRE
STAR FRUIT								
*Average, Tesco**	*1oz/28g*	*9*	*0.1*	*32*	*0.5*	*7.3*	*0.3*	*1.3*
STARBAR								
Cadbury*	1 Bar/53g	260	14.8	491	10.7	49.0	27.9	0.0
STARBURST								
Fruit Chews, Tropical, Mars*	1 Tube/45g	168	3.3	373	0.0	76.9	7.3	0.0
Joosters, Mars*	1 Pack/45g	160	0.0	356	0.0	88.8	0.1	0.0
Juicy Gums, Mars*	1 Pack/45g	139	1.8	309	5.9	71.0	4.1	0.0
Mars*	1 Pack/45g	185	3.4	411	0.3	85.3	7.6	0.0
STEAK & KIDNEY PUDDING								
Fray Bentos*	1 Tin/213g	477	26.8	224	7.8	19.8	12.6	0.0
M & S*	1 Pudding/121g	260	13.4	215	9.2	19.4	11.1	3.2
Sainsbury's*	1 Pudding/435g	1135	62.6	261	10.5	22.3	14.4	0.8
Tesco*	1 Serving/190g	437	22.6	230	10.0	20.7	11.9	1.2
Waitrose*	1 Pudding/223g	497	26.1	223	8.9	20.4	11.7	1.2
STEAMED PUDDING								
Apple & Sultana, BGTY, Sainsbury's*	1 Pudding/110g	294	3.2	267	2.9	57.4	2.9	0.8
Apple with Wild Berry Sauce, BGTY, Sainsbury's*	1 Pudding/110g	308	3.7	280	2.6	59.7	3.4	1.4
Chocolate Fudge, Less Than 5% Fat, Aunty's*	1 Pudding/110g	329	5.3	299	3.0	58.2	4.8	1.6
Golden Syrup, Aunty's*	1 Pudding/110g	324	4.5	295	2.9	58.6	4.1	0.7
Lemon, BGTY, Sainsbury's*	1 Pudding/110g	307	3.2	279	3.0	60.2	2.9	0.7
Sticky Toffee, Aunty's*	1 Pudding/110g	331	5.3	301	2.6	58.4	4.8	1.2
Toffee & Date, Aunty's*	1 Pudding/110g	320	5.1	291	2.6	59.1	4.6	1.1
STEW								
Beef, Meal for One, M & S*	1 Pack/440g	350	8.4	80	7.0	8.7	1.9	2.0
Beef & Dumplings	1 Serving/652g	766	32.7	117	7.4	10.7	5.0	0.8
Beef & Dumplings, Birds Eye*	1 Pack/400g	308	8.4	77	4.4	10.0	2.1	0.9
Beef & Dumplings, British Classics, Tesco*	1 Pack/450g	563	29.7	125	7.9	8.6	6.6	0.5
Beef & Dumplings, Frozen, Asda*	1 Pack/400g	392	13.2	98	6.0	11.0	3.3	0.8
Beef & Dumplings, Plumrose*	½ Can/196g	143	3.9	73	6.1	9.0	2.0	0.0
Beef & Dumplings, Ready Meals, Waitrose*	1oz/28g	38	1.6	136	8.0	13.3	5.6	0.8
Beef & Dumplings, Weight Watchers*	1 Pack/327g	262	6.9	80	5.2	10.0	2.1	0.8
Chicken, Morrisons*	1 Pack/400g	492	7.6	123	17.6	8.9	1.9	0.5
Chicken & Dumplings, Birds Eye*	1 Pack/320g	282	8.6	88	7.0	8.9	2.7	0.5
Chicken & Dumplings, Tesco*	1 Serving/450g	567	29.7	126	7.6	9.1	6.6	0.7
Chickpea, Roast Sweet Potato, & Feta, Stewed!*	½ Pot/250g	187	7.2	75	3.3	8.8	2.9	2.7
Irish, Asda*	¼ Can/196g	172	7.8	88	6.0	7.0	4.0	1.0
Irish, Plumrose*	1 Can/392g	318	9.8	81	7.5	7.2	2.5	0.0
Irish, Sainsbury's*	1 Pack/450g	274	9.4	61	5.7	4.8	2.1	0.5
Lentil & Vegetable, Organic, Simply Organic*	1 Pack/400g	284	6.0	71	3.5	11.0	1.5	1.3
Lentil & Winter Vegetable, Organic, Pure & Pronto*	1 Pack/400g	364	9.6	91	3.6	14.0	2.4	4.0
Tuscan Bean, Tasty Veg Pot, Innocent*	1 Pot/400g	320	7.6	80	3.1	12.5	1.9	3.6
STIR FRY								
Baby Leaf, Ready Prepared, M & S*	1 Serving/125g	25	0.1	20	1.7	4.9	0.1	2.5
Baby Leaf, Waitrose*	1 Pack/265g	50	0.3	19	1.7	2.9	0.1	2.0
Baby Vegetable & Pak Choi, Two Step, Tesco*	½ Pack/95g	29	0.8	31	2.1	4.0	0.8	2.3
Bean Sprout, Chinese, Sainsbury's*	1 Pack/300g	144	8.4	48	1.9	5.1	2.8	1.5
Bean Sprout, Ready to Eat, Washed, Sainsbury's*	1 Serving/150g	82	5.8	55	1.5	3.3	3.9	1.8
Bean Sprout & Vegetable, with Red Peppers, Asda*	1 Pack/350g	126	3.9	36	1.8	4.7	1.1	2.3
Bean Sprouts, Asda*	½ Pack/175g	56	0.9	32	2.9	4.0	0.5	1.5
Bean Sprouts & Vegetables, Asda*	½ Pack/173g	107	6.9	62	2.0	4.5	4.0	1.8
Cabbage, Carrot, Broccoli & Onion, Vegetable, Tesco*	1 Serving/100g	31	0.4	31	1.9	4.9	0.4	2.6
Cherry Tomato & Noodle, Waitrose*	1 Pack/400g	304	15.2	76	2.1	8.5	3.8	1.5
Chinese, Eastern Inspirations*	½ Pack/170g	49	0.8	29	2.7	3.5	0.5	1.8

S

STIR FRY

	Measure INFO/WEIGHT	per Measure KCAL	FAT	Nutrition Values per 100g / 100ml KCAL	PROT	CARB	FAT	FIBRE
Chinese, Family, Sainsbury's*	1 Serving/150g	60	3.0	40	2.3	3.3	2.0	3.6
Chinese, with Oriental Sauce, Tesco*	1 Pack/530g	180	2.1	34	2.3	5.4	0.4	1.5
Chinese Bean Sprout, Sainsbury's*	½ Pack/313g	150	8.8	48	1.9	5.1	2.8	1.5
Chinese Exotic Vegetable, Sainsbury's*	1 Pack/350g	133	7.7	38	1.7	2.8	2.2	1.8
Chinese Leaf & Mixed Peppers, Cook Asian, M & S*	1 Pack/260g	65	1.3	25	1.4	3.4	0.5	1.8
Chinese Mushroom, Sainsbury's*	1 Serving/175g	66	4.2	38	1.7	2.4	2.4	1.7
Chinese Noodles, Oriental Express*	1oz/28g	20	0.1	70	2.7	14.7	0.5	1.4
Chinese Prawn, Asda*	1 Serving/375g	345	2.2	92	3.6	18.0	0.6	1.8
Chinese Style, Co-Op*	1 Pack/300g	105	1.2	35	3.0	6.0	0.4	2.0
Chinese Style Prawn, GFY, Asda*	1 Pack/400g	324	6.4	81	3.6	13.0	1.6	1.6
Chinese Style Rice with Vegetables, Tesco*	1 Serving/550g	495	13.7	90	2.2	14.8	2.5	0.3
Chinese Vegetable & Oyster Sauce, Asda*	1 Serving/150g	93	3.7	62	1.9	8.0	2.5	0.0
Chinese Vegetables, Oriental Express*	½ Pack/200g	44	0.4	22	1.4	3.7	0.2	2.2
Chinese Vegetables, Tesco*	1 Serving/175g	93	0.7	53	1.6	10.8	0.4	1.3
Chinese Vegetables, with Chinese Style Sauce, Tesco*	1 Serving/350g	133	3.5	38	1.4	5.6	1.0	1.2
Chinese Vegetables, with Oyster Sauce, Tesco*	1 Pack/350g	98	0.7	28	2.0	4.6	0.2	1.1
Classic Medley, Veg Cuisine*	½ Pack/150g	45	0.6	30	2.5	4.1	0.4	2.1
Edamame Bean & Ginger, Tesco*	1 Pack/290g	145	4.6	50	4.1	4.9	1.6	2.5
Exotic, Tesco*	1 Pack/191g	42	0.4	22	1.3	3.8	0.2	1.5
Family, Tesco*	1 Pack/600g	210	3.0	35	2.3	5.2	0.5	2.1
Green Vegetable, M & S*	1 Pack/220g	165	13.0	75	3.1	2.5	5.9	2.2
Mediterranean Style, Waitrose*	1 Pack/305g	82	1.2	27	1.6	4.6	0.4	2.2
Mixed Pepper, Just Stir Fry, Sainsbury's*	½ Pack/150g	117	8.4	67	1.5	4.6	4.8	1.2
Mixed Pepper, Sainsbury's*	1 Pack/300g	201	14.4	67	1.5	4.6	4.8	1.2
Mixed Pepper, Waitrose*	½ Pack/150g	52	0.6	35	1.9	4.8	0.4	1.9
Mixed Pepper & Sweet Chilli Sauce, Asda*	1 Pack/300g	180	6.0	60	1.6	9.0	2.0	2.6
Mixed Pepper & Vegetable, Asda*	½ Pack/150g	42	1.5	28	1.6	3.2	1.0	2.6
Mixed Vegetable & Peashoot, Tesco*	1 Serving/100g	36	0.5	36	2.1	4.7	0.5	2.0
Mixed Vegetables, Sainsbury's*	½ Pack/140g	70	3.8	50	1.7	4.7	2.7	3.0
Mushroom, Just Stir Fry, Sainsbury's*	1 Pack/350g	171	9.5	49	2.8	3.3	2.7	2.8
Mushroom, Waitrose*	½ Pack/165g	43	0.7	26	2.3	3.3	0.4	1.6
Orient Inspired, M & S*	1 Serving/250g	50	0.7	20	1.6	3.4	0.3	1.6
Oriental, Ready Prepared, M & S*	½ Pack/260g	65	1.6	25	2.3	2.1	0.6	1.9
Oriental Leaf, M & S*	½ Pack/125g	25	0.6	20	1.9	2.5	0.5	2.2
Oriental Style Pak Choi, M & S*	1 Pack/220g	165	12.5	75	2.2	3.5	5.7	2.4
Oriental Vegetable, Frozen, Asda*	1 Serving/150g	115	6.7	77	2.1	7.0	4.5	1.7
Oriental Vegetable, Szechuan, Spicy, Sainsbury's*	1 Pack/350g	224	15.4	64	1.3	4.9	4.4	1.7
Singaporean Noodle, Sainsbury's*	½ Pack/160g	202	11.7	126	3.2	11.9	7.3	2.4
Spicy Thai Style Noodle, Tesco*	1 Pack/500g	335	13.0	67	2.6	8.4	2.6	1.3
Sweet & Sour, Tesco*	1 Pack/350g	161	1.0	46	1.8	9.1	0.3	1.3
Sweet Pepper, M & S*	1 Pack/400g	160	7.2	40	2.3	3.5	1.8	0.6
Tatsoi & Sugar Snap Pea, M & S*	½ Pack/125g	25	0.4	20	2.0	3.0	0.3	1.9
Tender Shoot, Sainsbury's*	½ Pack/126g	113	8.3	90	4.4	2.8	6.6	0.8
Thai Style, M & S*	1 Serving/150g	75	4.5	50	2.3	3.0	3.0	1.2
Vegetable, Cantonese, Sainsbury's*	1 Serving/150g	90	5.2	60	2.8	4.2	3.5	2.7
Vegetable, Chinese Style, Tesco*	1 Pack/360g	79	0.7	22	1.9	3.2	0.2	1.4
Vegetable, Crunchy, Waitrose*	1 Pack/300g	81	0.3	27	1.6	4.8	0.1	2.4
Vegetable, Oriental, Frozen, Freshly, Asda*	1 Serving/100g	25	0.3	25	2.2	3.4	0.3	2.0
Vegetable, Oriental, Just Stir Fry, Sainsbury's*	½ Pack/135g	94	7.2	70	2.2	3.4	5.3	1.3
Vegetable, Premium, Sainsbury's*	½ Pack/150g	90	5.2	60	2.8	4.2	3.5	2.7
Vegetable, Ready Prepared, M & S*	½ Pack/150g	37	0.4	25	2.2	3.5	0.3	2.2
Vegetable, Sweet & Crunchy, Waitrose*	1 Pack/300g	69	0.3	23	1.8	3.6	0.1	1.4
Vegetable, Thai Style, Tesco*	½ Pack/135g	42	0.7	31	2.3	4.2	0.5	2.1

S

	Measure INFO/WEIGHT	per Measure KCAL	FAT	Nutrition Values per 100g / 100ml KCAL	PROT	CARB	FAT	FIBRE
STIR FRY								
Vegetable & Beansprout, Waitrose*	1 Pack/300g	78	0.9	26	1.4	4.5	0.3	2.1
Vegetable & Beansprout, with Peanut Sauce, Tesco*	1 Serving/475g	408	23.7	86	3.9	6.2	5.0	1.9
Vegetable & Mushroom, Asda*	½ Pack/160g	59	2.4	37	2.4	3.4	1.5	3.4
Vegetable Noodles, BGTY, Sainsbury's*	1 Pack/455g	391	9.1	86	3.2	14.0	2.0	1.4
Vegetables, Cantonese Style, Tesco*	1 Serving/125g	40	1.1	32	2.0	4.1	0.9	1.4
Vegetables, Fresh, Asda*	½ Pack/150g	106	7.5	71	1.7	4.9	5.0	1.7
Vegetables, Mixed, with Slices of Pepper, Tesco*	1 Pack/300g	57	0.3	19	1.9	2.6	0.1	1.5
Vegetables, Mixed Pepper, M & S*	½ Pack/150g	52	0.6	35	1.9	4.9	0.4	1.9
Vegetables, Sunshine, Tesco*	½ Pack/150g	42	0.4	28	1.8	4.6	0.3	2.1
Vegetables & Bean Sprout, M & S*	1 Pack/350g	105	1.4	30	1.8	4.6	0.4	2.0
Vegetables with Oyster Sauce, Asda*	1 Serving/150g	93	3.7	62	1.9	8.0	2.5	0.0
Water Chestnut & Bamboo Shoot, Asda*	½ Pack/175g	61	2.4	35	1.4	4.3	1.4	1.7
STOCK								
Beef, As Sold, Stock Pot, Knorr*	1 Serving/5g	5	0.4	89	3.0	3.5	7.0	0.7
Beef, Fresh, Tesco*	1 Serving/300ml	54	0.9	18	2.1	1.6	0.3	0.5
Beef, Made Up, Stock Pot, Knorr*	1 Serving/100ml	5	0.4	5	0.1	0.2	0.4	0.0
Beef, Simply Stock, Knorr*	1 Serving/100ml	6	0.0	6	1.4	0.1	0.0	0.0
Chicken, As Sold, Stock Pot, Knorr*	1 Serving/100ml	5	0.4	95	2.4	4.9	7.3	0.8
Chicken, Asda*	½ Pot/150g	25	1.3	17	1.8	0.7	0.9	0.1
Chicken, Fresh, Sainsbury's*	½ Pot/142ml	23	0.1	16	3.7	0.1	0.1	0.3
Chicken, Fresh, Tesco*	1 Serving/300ml	27	0.3	9	1.6	0.5	0.1	0.5
Chicken, Granules, Knorr*	1 Tsp/5g	10	0.2	232	13.1	36.5	3.7	0.4
Chicken, Home Prepared, Average	*1 fl oz/30ml*	*7*	*0.3*	*24*	*3.8*	*0.7*	*0.9*	*0.3*
Chicken, Prepared, Tesco*	1 Serving/300ml	54	0.3	18	2.4	1.8	0.1	0.5
Chicken, Simply Stock, Knorr*	1 Pack/450ml	27	0.0	6	1.5	0.0	0.0	0.1
Fish, Fresh, Finest, Tesco*	1 Serving/100g	10	0.0	10	0.6	1.8	0.0	0.5
Fish, Home Prepared, Average	*1 Serving/250ml*	*42*	*2.0*	*17*	*2.3*	*0.0*	*0.8*	*0.0*
Vegetable, As Sold, Stock Pot, Knorr*	1 Serving/100ml	6	0.5	117	2.4	5.7	9.4	1.3
Vegetable, Campbell's*	1 Serving/250ml	37	1.7	15	0.3	2.0	0.7	0.0
Vegetable, Concentrated, M & S*	1 Tsp/5g	19	0.9	380	3.3	43.0	19.0	1.2
Vegetable, Granules, Knorr*	2 Tsp/9g	18	0.1	199	8.5	39.9	0.6	0.9
Vegetable, Made Up, Stock Pot, Knorr*	1 Serving/100ml	6	0.5	6	0.1	0.3	0.5	0.1
STOCK CUBES								
Basil, Herb Cubes, Knorr*	1 Cube/10g	47	3.4	472	6.1	35.9	33.8	0.6
Beef, Dry Weight, Bovril*	1 Cube/6g	12	0.2	197	10.8	29.3	4.1	0.0
Beef, Dry Weight, Oxo*	1 Cube/6ml	15	0.3	265	17.3	38.4	4.7	1.5
Beef, Knorr*	1 Cube/10g	31	2.3	310	5.0	19.0	23.0	0.0
Beef, Organic, Kallo*	1 Cube/12g	25	1.0	208	16.7	16.7	8.3	0.0
Beef, Tesco*	1 Cube/7g	17	0.2	260	9.7	48.9	2.8	1.3
Beef Flavour, Made Up, Oxo*	1 Cube/189ml	17	0.4	9	0.6	1.3	0.2	0.1
Chicken	1 Cube/6g	14	0.9	237	15.4	9.9	15.4	0.0
Chicken, Dry, Oxo*	1 Cube/7g	17	0.2	249	10.9	44.0	3.3	0.9
Chicken, Just Bouillon, Kallo*	1 Cube/12g	30	1.3	247	11.8	26.1	10.6	1.0
Chicken, Knorr*	1 Cube/10g	31	2.0	310	4.0	29.0	20.0	0.0
Chicken, Made Up, Sainsbury's*	1 Cube/200ml	16	0.2	8	0.3	1.4	0.1	0.1
Chicken, Prepared, Oxo*	1 Cube/100ml	9	0.1	9	0.4	1.5	0.1	0.1
Chicken, Telma*	1 Cube/15g	25	0.1	167	0.0	0.0	1.0	0.0
Chicken, Tesco*	1 Cube/11g	32	2.5	290	10.5	11.1	22.6	0.7
Fish, Knorr*	1 Cube/10g	32	2.4	321	8.0	18.0	24.0	1.0
Fish, Sainsbury's*	1 Cube/11g	31	2.2	282	19.1	7.3	20.0	0.9
Garlic, Dry Weight, Oxo*	1 Cube/6g	18	0.3	298	13.4	48.5	5.5	3.6
Ham, Knorr*	1 Cube/10g	31	1.9	313	11.8	24.4	18.7	0.0
Indian, Dry Weight, Oxo*	1 Cube/6g	17	0.5	291	11.5	43.9	7.7	6.7

S

	Measure INFO/WEIGHT	per Measure KCAL	FAT	Nutrition Values per 100g / 100ml KCAL	PROT	CARB	FAT	FIBRE
STOCK CUBES								
Italian, Dry Weight, Oxo*	1 Cube/6g	19	0.4	309	11.9	48.9	7.3	4.6
Lamb, Made Up, Knorr*	1 Cube/10g	32	2.5	320	11.0	14.0	25.0	0.0
Parsley & Garlic, Herb Cubes, Knorr*	1 Cube/10g	42	2.7	422	8.6	35.2	27.4	1.8
Vegetable, Average	1 Cube/7g	18	1.2	253	13.5	11.6	17.3	0.0
Vegetable, Knorr*	1 Cube/10g	33	2.4	330	10.0	25.0	24.0	1.0
Vegetable, Made Up, Organic, Kallo*	2 Cubes/100ml	7	0.4	7	0.1	0.5	0.4	0.1
Vegetable, Made up, Oxo*	1 Cube/100ml	9	0.2	9	0.4	1.4	0.2	0.1
Vegetable, Telma*	1 Serving/14g	35	2.4	253	0.0	2.2	17.3	0.0
Vegetable Bouillon, Yeast Free, Made Up, Marigold*	1 Serving/250ml	19	1.6	8	0.0	0.5	0.6	0.0
STORTELLI								
Microwaveable, Dolmio*	1 Serving/220g	299	2.2	136	5.3	26.3	1.0	0.0
STRAWBERRIES								
Dried, Graze*	1 Pack/35g	131	0.2	374	1.0	91.0	0.7	0.0
Fresh, Raw, Average	*1 Berry/12g*	*3*	*0.0*	*28*	*0.8*	*6.0*	*0.1*	*0.9*
in Fruit Juice, Canned, Average	*1/3 Can/127g*	*58*	*0.0*	*45*	*0.4*	*11.0*	*0.0*	*1.0*
in Light Syrup, Canned, Drained, Tesco*	1 Can/149g	100	0.1	67	0.5	16.0	0.1	0.7
STROGANOFF								
Beef, Asda*	1 Serving/120g	276	20.4	230	16.0	3.3	17.0	0.6
Beef, BGTY, Sainsbury's*	1 Pack/400g	416	10.4	104	5.6	14.6	2.6	0.6
Beef, Finest, Tesco*	½ Pack/200g	330	13.4	165	9.4	16.2	6.7	0.7
Beef, HL, Tesco*	1 Pack/400g	400	8.8	100	7.0	13.0	2.2	1.3
Beef, Low Fat with White & Wild Rice, Waitrose*	1 Pack/401g	429	6.4	107	7.9	15.3	1.6	1.0
Beef, Sainsbury's*	1 Can/200g	232	12.0	116	12.5	3.0	6.0	0.2
Beef, Weight Watchers*	1 Pack/330g	297	7.6	90	4.3	13.0	2.3	0.1
Beef, with Rice, Naturally Good Food, Tesco*	1 Pack/400g	425	9.4	106	7.1	13.9	2.3	1.3
Beef, with Rice 'n' Peppers, Tesco*	1 Pack/450g	562	19.8	125	7.5	13.1	4.4	0.4
Beef & Rice, TTD, Sainsbury's*	1 Pack/410g	595	20.9	145	9.6	15.2	5.1	1.7
Chicken, with Rice, BGTY, Sainsbury's*	1 Pack/415g	448	5.4	108	7.0	17.1	1.3	1.1
Chicken & Mushroom, COU, M & S*	1 Serving/400g	400	8.0	100	3.2	16.7	2.0	0.1
Mushroom, Solo Slim, Rosemary Conley*	1 Pack/251g	193	11.3	77	2.7	6.5	4.5	2.7
Mushroom, with Rice, BGTY, Sainsbury's*	1 Serving/450g	418	6.7	93	3.3	16.6	1.5	1.0
Mushroom, with Rice, Vegetarian, HL, Tesco*	1 Pack/450g	526	21.6	117	3.2	15.2	4.8	1.2
STRUDEL								
Apple, Co-Op*	1 Slice/100g	225	12.0	225	3.0	28.0	12.0	3.0
Apple, Sainsbury's*	1/6 Strudel/90g	255	13.9	283	3.2	32.8	15.4	1.9
Apple & Mincemeat, Tesco*	1 Serving/100g	322	16.7	322	3.3	39.6	16.7	2.0
Woodland Fruit, Sainsbury's*	1/6 Strudel/95g	276	14.8	290	3.7	34.0	15.5	2.0
STUFFING								
Apricot & Walnut, Made Up, Celebrations, Paxo*	1 Serving/50g	80	1.7	161	4.3	28.0	3.5	2.8
Olde English Chestnut, Sainsbury's*	1 Serving/110g	216	12.8	196	9.4	13.5	11.6	2.1
Parsley, Thyme & Lemon Stuffing, Paxo*	1 Serving/45g	67	0.9	150	4.3	28.4	2.1	2.4
Parsley & Thyme, Co-Op*	1 Serving/28g	95	0.8	340	10.0	67.0	3.0	6.0
Sage & Onion, for Chicken, Paxo*	1 Serving/50g	61	0.9	123	3.6	23.0	1.8	1.7
Sage & Onion, Made Up, Paxo*	1 Serving/50g	71	0.6	143	3.2	29.9	1.2	1.9
Sage & Onion, with Lemon, Paxo*	1 Serving/50g	61	0.6	122	3.4	24.2	1.2	1.9
Sausagemeat, Sainsbury's*	1 Serving/100g	175	4.2	175	7.0	27.0	4.2	2.3
Sausagemeat & Thyme, Made Up, Celebrations, Paxo*	1 Serving/50g	80	1.7	160	6.3	25.8	3.5	4.0
STUFFING BALLS								
Pork, Sausagemeat, Aunt Bessie's*	1 Ball/26g	55	2.1	212	7.2	27.3	8.2	3.0
Sage & Onion, Aunt Bessie's*	1 Ball/26g	63	2.3	243	6.4	34.4	8.9	3.1
Sage & Onion, Meat-Free, Aunt Bessie's*	1 Ball/28g	54	1.9	193	5.4	28.0	6.7	1.7
STUFFING MIX								
Apple, Mustard & Herb, Paxo*	1 Serving/50g	83	1.0	166	4.2	32.8	2.0	4.0

S

	Measure INFO/WEIGHT	per Measure KCAL	FAT	Nutrition Values per 100g / 100ml KCAL	PROT	CARB	FAT	FIBRE
STUFFING MIX								
Apple & Herb, Special Recipe, Sainsbury's*	1 Serving/41g	68	0.9	165	3.8	32.4	2.2	2.2
Chestnut & Cranberry, Celebration, Paxo*	1 Serving/25g	35	0.5	141	4.0	26.7	2.0	2.4
Date, Walnut & Stilton, Special Recipe, Sainsbury's*	1 Serving/25g	49	2.1	196	5.2	25.0	8.4	2.0
Herb & Onion, Gluten Free, Allergycare*	1 Serving/12g	43	0.3	360	7.9	76.8	2.4	0.0
Parsley, Thyme & Lemon, Sainsbury's*	1 Pack/170g	240	2.2	141	4.2	28.2	1.3	1.3
Sage & Onion, Asda*	1 Serving/27g	29	0.2	107	3.4	22.0	0.6	1.3
Sage & Onion, Made Up, Paxo*	1 Serving/60g	74	1.1	123	3.6	23.0	1.8	1.7
SUET								
Beef, Shredded, Original, Atora*	1 Pack/200g	1592	163.0	796	1.1	14.6	81.5	0.5
Beef, Tesco*	1 Serving/100g	854	91.9	854	0.6	6.2	91.9	0.1
Vegetable, Average	*1oz/28g*	*234*	*24.6*	*836*	*1.2*	*10.1*	*87.9*	*0.0*
SUET PUDDING								
Average	*1oz/28g*	*94*	*5.1*	*335*	*4.4*	*40.5*	*18.3*	*0.9*
SUGAR								
Brown, Soft, Average	*1 Tsp/4g*	*15*	*0.0*	*382*	*0.0*	*96.5*	*0.0*	*0.0*
Caster, Average	*1 Tbsp/12g*	*48*	*0.0*	*399*	*0.0*	*99.8*	*0.0*	*0.0*
Castor, White, Fairtrade, Sainsbury's*	1 Serving/100g	401	0.2	401	0.5	99.9	0.2	0.0
Dark Brown, Muscovado, Average	*1 Tsp/7g*	*27*	*0.0*	*380*	*0.2*	*94.7*	*0.0*	*0.0*
Dark Brown, Soft, Average	*1 Tsp/5g*	*18*	*0.0*	*369*	*0.1*	*92.0*	*0.0*	*0.0*
Demerara, Average	*1 Tsp/5g*	*18*	*0.0*	*367*	*0.2*	*99.1*	*0.0*	*0.0*
for Making Jam, Silver Spoon*	1oz/28g	111	0.0	398	0.0	99.5	0.0	0.0
Fructose, Fruit Sugar, Tate & Lyle*	1 Tsp/4g	16	0.0	400	0.0	100.0	0.0	0.0
Golden, Unrefined, Average	*1 Tsp/4g*	*16*	*0.0*	*399*	*0.0*	*99.8*	*0.0*	*0.0*
Granulated, Organic, Average	*1 Tsp/4g*	*16*	*0.0*	*398*	*0.2*	*99.7*	*0.0*	*0.0*
Icing, Average	*1 Tsp/4g*	*16*	*0.0*	*394*	*0.0*	*102.1*	*0.0*	*0.0*
Icing, Homegrown, Silver Spoon*	1 Serving/100g	400	70.0	400	0.0	99.4	70.0	0.0
Light Or Diet, Average	*1 Tsp/4g*	*16*	*0.0*	*394*	*0.0*	*98.5*	*0.0*	*0.0*
Muscovado, Light, Average	1 Tsp/5g	19	0.0	384	0.0	96.0	0.0	0.0
Vanilla, Fairtrade, Cooks' Ingredients, Waitrose*	1 Serving/100g	399	0.0	399	0.0	99.7	0.0	0.0
Vanilla, Fiddes Payne*	1 Serving/100g	397	0.1	397	0.1	99.2	0.1	0.5
White, Granulated, Average	*1 Tsp/5g*	*20*	*0.0*	*397*	*0.0*	*100.7*	*0.0*	*0.0*
SULTANAS								
Average	*1oz/28g*	*82*	*0.1*	*292*	*2.5*	*69.7*	*0.4*	*2.0*
SUNDAE								
Banoffee, Perfectly Balanced, Waitrose*	1 Pot/115g	143	2.2	124	3.1	23.6	1.9	0.8
Blackcurrant, M & S*	1 Sundae/53g	212	10.2	400	3.0	54.2	19.2	1.9
Chocolate, Mini, Asda*	1 Pot/86g	199	12.9	231	3.1	21.0	15.0	1.7
Chocolate, Sainsbury's*	1 Pot/140g	393	29.8	281	2.5	19.3	21.3	0.6
Chocolate & Cookie, Weight Watchers*	1 Pot/82g	128	2.8	156	2.5	30.3	3.4	2.2
Chocolate & Sticky Toffee, Asda*	1 Sundae/215g	755	51.6	351	2.8	31.0	24.0	0.5
Chocolate & Vanilla, HL, Tesco*	1 Sundae/120g	193	3.1	161	2.8	31.5	2.6	0.6
Chocolate Brownie, Finest, Tesco*	1 Serving/215g	778	56.5	362	2.7	28.7	26.3	2.3
Chocolate Mint, COU, M & S*	1 Pot/90g	108	2.3	120	5.4	17.8	2.6	0.5
Chocolate Nut	1 Serving/70g	195	10.7	278	3.0	34.2	15.3	0.1
Ice Cream	1 Serving/170g	482	15.4	284	5.9	45.3	9.1	0.3
Raspberry, Perfectly Balanced, Waitrose*	1 Pot/175ml	150	1.0	86	1.7	18.9	0.6	0.0
Strawberry, M & S*	1 Sundae/45g	173	8.0	385	3.4	53.3	17.8	1.0
Strawberry & Vanilla, Tesco*	1 Serving/68g	120	3.9	177	2.0	29.5	5.7	0.1
Strawberry & Vanilla, Weight Watchers*	1 Pot/105g	148	2.2	141	1.2	29.1	2.1	0.3
Toffee, Asda*	1 Serving/120g	322	19.2	268	2.1	29.0	16.0	0.0
Toffee & Vanilla, Tesco*	1 Serving/70g	133	4.5	189	2.1	30.7	6.4	0.1
SUNNY DELIGHT*								
Californian Style, No Added Sugar, Sunny Delight*	1 Serving/200ml	20	0.4	10	0.1	1.4	0.2	0.1

S

	Measure INFO/WEIGHT	per Measure		Nutrition Values per 100g / 100ml				
		KCAL	FAT	KCAL	PROT	CARB	FAT	FIBRE
SUNNY DELIGHT*								
Florida Style, Sunny Delight*	1 Serving/200ml	70	0.2	35	0.4	7.4	0.1	0.2
Original, Sunny Delight*	1 Glass/200ml	88	0.4	44	0.1	10.0	0.2	0.0
SUPPLEMENT								
Acai Shake, Fruitein, Nature's Plus*	1 Scoop/34g	110	0.0	324	29.4	44.1	0.0	2.9
Anabolic Nitro Energy Surge, Ultimate Sports Nutrition*	1 Sachet/21g	40	0.0	191	15.6	51.2	0.0	0.5
BCAA Power Punch, Ultimate Sports Nutrition*	2 Tsp/13g	40	0.0	304	0.0	3.0	0.0	0.0
Benefiber, Novartis*	1 Sachet/4g	7	0.0	200	0.1	15.0	0.0	85.0
Cellmass, All Flavours, BSN*	1 Scoop/16g	30	0.0	187	43.7	0.0	0.0	0.0
Chocolate, Forever Lite, Ultra, Powder, Forever Living*	1 Scoop/25g	90	1.0	360	68.0	16.0	4.0	4.0
Chocolate Shake, Micellar Casien, Reflex Nutrition Ltd*	1 Serving/45g	159	0.7	354	80.0	4.0	1.5	0.0
Fibre, Powder, Benefibre*	1 Tsp/3g	6	0.0	200	0.5	15.0	0.0	85.0
Fibre Sure, Protcor & Gamble*	1 Serving/100g	270	0.1	270	16.0	0.0	0.1	81.0
Fruits & Fibres, Ortis*	1 Cube/10g	27	0.2	266	3.9	53.2	1.7	15.6
High Protein Powder, Sanatogen*	2 Tsp/7g	25	0.1	360	81.0	5.8	1.2	0.0
Malt Extract, Holland & Barrett*	1 Tbsp/24g	72	0.0	300	5.3	70.0	0.0	0.0
Myofusion Protein Shake, Gaspari*	1 Scoop/35g	157	3.0	450	71.4	14.3	8.6	2.9
Pro Peptide, Cnp*	1 Scoop/33g	115	1.5	354	69.2	9.2	4.6	0.0
Pro Recover, Cnp*	2 Scoops/80g	297	1.0	371	29.5	60.6	1.3	0.0
Protein, Hot Chocolate, Easy Body*	1 Serving/20g	74	0.2	370	70.7	19.2	1.2	0.0
Protein, Ultra, 80+, Ultimax*	1 Serving/20g	74	0.2	372	80.0	12.5	1.0	1.5
Protein, Vanilla, Precision, EAS*	1 Scoop/26g	91	0.5	357	78.4	4.7	2.0	0.0
Psyllium Husk, Average	1 Tsp/5g	16	0.0	330	0.0	80.0	0.0	80.0
Psyllium Husk, True Dietary Fibre, Ceres Organics*	1 Tsp/5g	9	0.0	190	2.0	4.5	0.0	85.0
Shake, Chocolate, Myoplex, EAS*	1 Serving/76g	279	1.7	367	55.0	31.0	2.2	1.1
Shake, Diet, Chocolate Delight Flavour, Maxitone*	1 Serving/50g	209	6.4	418	33.2	40.0	12.8	4.4
Shake, Strawberry, Max Elle True Diet, My Protein*	1 Scoop/28g	106	2.1	378	63.6	14.7	7.4	3.3
Soya Protein Isolate Powder, Holland & Barrett*	1 Scoop/28g	109	1.3	391	86.6	1.0	4.5	0.0
Sport Gel, Smart Berry Flavour, Science in Sport*	1 Sachet/60ml	86	0.0	144	0.0	36.0	0.0	0.0
Tablet, Berocca*	1 Tablet/5g	5	0.0	109	0.0	5.7	0.1	0.0
Total Nutrition Today, Plain, Natures Sunshine*	1 Scoop/38g	120	0.8	316	2.6	79.0	2.0	32.0
Vextrago, Carbohydrate, Pvl Fit Foods International*	2 Scoops/75g	280	0.5	373	0.7	92.0	0.7	0.0
Whey, Instant, Strawberry Flavour, Reflex Nutrition Ltd*	1 Serving/25g	98	1.4	394	80.0	6.0	5.5	0.2
Whey Protein, Body Fortress*	1 Scoop/25g	98	2.2	392	70.5	7.9	8.9	2.1
Whey Protein, Define*	1 Serving/40g	165	3.8	412	71.5	10.3	9.4	0.5
Whey Protein, Holland & Barrett*	1 Serving/24g	94	1.9	392	73.3	7.1	7.9	0.0
Whey Protein, Super, Precision*	1 Scoop/24g	94	2.0	390	71.5	7.3	8.3	0.0
Whey Protein Isolate, Musashi*	2 Scoop/30g	111	0.2	371	88.7	1.2	0.5	0.0
Xtend, Premium Performance, Scivation*	1 Serving/12g	42	0.0	348	87.0	0.0	0.0	0.0
SUSHI								
Aya Set, Waitrose*	1 Pack/110g	200	4.3	182	5.4	31.7	3.9	1.5
California Roll Box, M & S*	1 Pack/230g	391	12.0	170	7.0	22.0	5.2	1.1
California Set, Waitrose*	1 Pack/120g	223	9.1	186	3.8	25.2	7.6	1.7
Californian, Yakatori, M & S*	1 Serving/200g	340	9.4	170	6.4	25.0	4.7	1.0
Californian Roll, Nigiri & Maki Selection, M & S*	1 Pack/210g	294	4.4	140	4.4	25.9	2.1	2.2
Californian Roll & Nigiri, Selection, M & S*	1 Pack/215g	355	5.8	165	7.1	28.0	2.7	1.1
Chicken, M & S*	1 Pack/186g	260	4.1	140	6.0	24.4	2.2	1.0
Deluxe, Shapers, Boots*	1 Serving/235g	355	3.5	151	5.3	29.0	1.5	2.7
Fish, Large Pack, Tesco*	1 Pack/284g	469	11.1	165	5.5	27.0	3.9	1.5
Fish, Snack, Tesco*	1 Pack/104g	159	2.6	153	4.5	28.0	2.5	1.5
Fish & Veg Selection, Tesco*	1 Pack/150g	247	3.4	165	6.7	29.2	2.3	0.4
Fish Nigiri, Adventurous, Tesco*	1 Pack/200g	270	4.4	135	7.1	21.7	2.2	0.5
Fish Roll, Nigiri & Maki Selection, M & S*	1 Pack/210g	315	4.8	150	6.5	25.8	2.3	1.0
Fish Selection, M & S*	1 Pack/210g	346	6.5	165	7.4	26.3	3.1	1.4

S

	Measure INFO/WEIGHT	per Measure KCAL	FAT	Nutrition Values per 100g / 100ml KCAL	PROT	CARB	FAT	FIBRE
SUSHI								
Fusion, M & S*	1 Pack/186g	260	3.3	140	5.1	23.8	1.8	2.9
GFY, Asda*	1 Pack/220g	352	3.1	160	4.9	32.0	1.4	0.0
Hagi Set, Waitrose*	1 Pack/370g	688	9.6	186	7.1	33.6	2.6	1.1
Hana Set, Waitrose*	1 Serving/175g	324	4.0	185	5.4	35.7	2.3	1.4
Irodori Set, with Fish, Cucumber, & Avocado, Waitrose*	1 Pack/281g	472	12.4	168	5.2	26.7	4.4	1.3
Komachi Set, with Salmon, Whiting & Handroll, Waitrose*	1 Pack/257g	447	13.9	174	5.3	25.8	5.4	1.2
Maki Rolls Box, Sainsbury's*	1 Pack/127g	197	2.2	155	4.5	30.5	1.7	0.8
Maki Selection, Shapers, Boots*	1 Pack/158g	225	2.1	142	3.5	29.0	1.3	1.1
Medium, Vegetarian, Taiko Foods*	1 Pack/267g	403	5.3	151	4.0	36.0	2.0	1.0
Medium Pack, Tesco*	1 Pack/139g	211	3.2	152	6.3	26.6	2.3	2.3
Mini, Boots*	1 Pack/99g	153	1.9	155	5.5	29.0	1.9	0.8
Nigiri, Californian Roll, Maki Roll, Sainsbury's*	1 Pack/195g	283	2.9	145	5.3	27.4	1.5	1.9
Nigiri, M & S*	1 Serving/190g	303	5.9	159	7.3	25.3	3.1	0.6
Nigiri Set, Taiko, Salmon & Tuna, Waitrose*	1 Pack/113g	174	2.3	154	6.3	26.0	2.0	0.6
Oriental Fish Box, M & S*	1 Pack/205g	318	8.4	155	6.1	23.3	4.1	0.9
Prawn & Salmon Selection, M & S*	1 Serving/175g	255	2.9	146	5.5	27.4	1.7	0.6
Prawn Feast, M & S*	1 Pack/219g	350	8.1	160	5.7	25.8	3.7	1.1
Rolls, Shapers, Boots*	1 Pack/168g	259	4.0	154	4.7	28.0	2.4	0.5
Salmon, Nigiri Crayfish, Red Pepper, Sainsbury's*	1 Serving/150g	232	4.5	155	5.5	26.4	3.0	1.0
Salmon & Roll Set, Sainsbury's*	1 Serving/101g	167	2.6	165	4.9	30.4	2.6	0.8
Salmon Feast Box, M & S*	1 Pack/200g	330	5.8	165	5.6	27.0	2.9	1.0
Selection, Shapers, Boots*	1 Pack/162g	245	2.6	151	5.6	29.0	1.6	1.7
Snack Selection, Eat Well, M & S*	1 Pack/96g	134	0.7	140	5.3	28.7	0.7	0.8
to Share, Tesco*	1 Pack/385g	616	6.2	160	5.7	30.6	1.6	0.7
Tokyo Set, M & S*	1 Pack/150g	240	4.6	160	7.3	25.3	3.1	0.6
Tuna, to Snack Selection, Food to Go, M & S*	1 Serving/150g	225	3.9	150	5.2	26.4	2.6	2.3
Vegetarian, Selection, M & S*	1 Pack/171g	248	2.4	145	3.0	28.5	1.4	2.4
Vegetarian, Snack Selection, Tesco*	1 Pack/85g	106	2.8	125	3.7	20.1	3.3	0.6
Vegetarian, with Pickled Vegetables, Waitrose*	1 Pack/135g	244	4.9	181	5.0	27.8	3.6	1.7
SWEDE								
Boiled, Average	*1oz/28g*	*3*	*0.0*	*11*	*0.3*	*2.3*	*0.1*	*0.7*
Raw, Unprepared, Average	*1oz/28g*	*6*	*0.1*	*21*	*0.8*	*4.4*	*0.3*	*1.9*
SWEET & SOUR								
Chicken, & Noodles, BGTY, Sainsbury's*	1 Pack/400g	356	2.4	89	7.5	13.3	0.6	0.7
Chicken, & Noodles, Chinese Takeaway, Tesco*	1 Pack/350g	350	0.7	100	5.7	18.8	0.2	0.2
Chicken, & Rice, Chilled, Tesco*	1 Pack/450g	540	5.8	120	4.9	21.9	1.3	0.9
Chicken, & Rice, Morrisons*	1 Pack/400g	452	10.4	113	3.6	18.8	2.6	0.8
Chicken, Breasts, Tesco*	1 Serving/185g	172	1.8	93	14.6	6.5	1.0	0.1
Chicken, Canned, Tesco*	1 Can/400g	408	6.4	102	9.6	12.4	1.6	1.1
Chicken, Chinese Takeaway, Sainsbury's*	1 Pack/264g	515	16.9	195	13.1	21.3	6.4	1.0
Chicken, Crispy, Fillets, Tesco*	1 Pack/350g	507	19.6	145	7.2	15.3	5.6	0.9
Chicken, Healthy Options, Birds Eye*	1 Meal/348g	390	3.8	112	4.8	20.7	1.1	0.6
Chicken, in Batter, Cantonese, Chilled, Sainsbury's*	1 Pack/350g	560	21.0	160	8.9	22.4	6.0	0.9
Chicken, in Crispy Batter, Morrisons*	1 Pack/350g	511	13.6	146	10.1	17.6	3.9	1.2
Chicken, M & S*	1 Pack/300g	465	10.8	155	6.6	24.4	3.6	0.8
Chicken, Oriental, Tesco*	1 Pack/350g	340	4.0	97	9.3	12.2	1.1	0.8
Chicken, Take It Away, M & S*	1 Pack/200g	200	1.6	100	9.4	13.2	0.8	1.2
Chicken, Waitrose*	1 Serving/400g	372	3.2	93	9.8	11.7	0.8	1.4
Chicken, with Egg Rice, Chilled, HL, Tesco*	1 Pack/450g	499	3.1	111	6.8	19.2	0.7	0.6
Chicken, with Noodles, Feeling Great, Findus*	1 Pack/350g	385	8.7	110	5.0	17.0	2.5	1.5
Chicken, with Rice, Chilled, BGTY, Sainsbury's*	1 Pack/400g	344	3.6	86	6.0	13.5	0.9	1.0
Chicken, with Rice, Oriental Express*	1 Pack/340g	350	2.0	103	4.4	21.3	0.6	0.7
Chicken, with Vegetable Rice, COU, M & S*	1 Pack/400g	400	5.6	100	6.9	14.9	1.4	1.1

	Measure INFO/WEIGHT	per Measure KCAL	FAT	Nutrition Values per 100g / 100ml KCAL	PROT	CARB	FAT	FIBRE
SWEET & SOUR								
Chicken Balls, Chinese Takeaway, Iceland*	1 Pack/255g	311	3.3	122	9.9	17.5	1.3	6.0
Chicken with Egg Fried Rice, GFY, Asda*	1 Pack/400g	500	7.6	125	6.0	20.3	1.9	1.8
Chicken with Rice, Iceland*	1 Pack/450g	513	3.6	114	5.0	21.7	0.8	1.1
Chicken with Rice, Weight Watchers*	1 Pack/330g	310	1.3	94	5.0	17.5	0.4	0.3
Pork	1oz/28g	48	2.5	172	12.7	11.3	8.8	0.6
Pork, Battered, Sainsbury's*	½ Pack/175g	306	8.7	175	7.3	25.1	5.0	0.6
Roasted Vegetables, Cantonese, Sainsbury's*	1 Pack/348g	327	4.2	94	1.1	19.6	1.2	0.9
Vegetables, with Rice, Waitrose*	1 Pack/400g	384	4.4	96	1.9	19.5	1.1	1.1
SWEET POTATO								
Baked, Average	*1 Med/130g*	*149*	*0.5*	*115*	*1.6*	*27.9*	*0.4*	*3.3*
Boiled in Salted Water, Average	*1 Med/130g*	*109*	*0.4*	*84*	*1.1*	*20.5*	*0.3*	*2.3*
Dried	1 Serving/100g	110	3.0	110	1.6	19.7	3.0	3.2
Raw, Unprepared, Average	*1 Med/130g*	*113*	*0.4*	*87*	*1.2*	*21.3*	*0.3*	*2.4*
Steamed, Average	*1 Med/130g*	*109*	*0.4*	*84*	*1.1*	*20.4*	*0.3*	*2.3*
with Rosemary & Garlic, Frozen, McCain*	1 Serving/150g	172	5.5	115	2.1	18.4	3.7	2.8
SWEETBREAD								
Lamb, Fried	*1oz/28g*	*61*	*3.2*	*217*	*28.7*	*0.0*	*11.4*	*0.0*
SWEETCORN								
Baby, Canned, Drained, Average	1 Serving/80g	18	0.3	23	2.9	2.0	0.4	1.5
Baby, Frozen, Average	*1oz/28g*	*7*	*0.1*	*24*	*2.5*	*2.7*	*0.4*	*1.7*
Boiled, Average	*1oz/28g*	*31*	*0.6*	*111*	*4.2*	*19.6*	*2.3*	*2.2*
Canned, in Water, No Sugar & Salt, Average	*½ Can/125g*	*99*	*1.3*	*79*	*2.7*	*14.9*	*1.1*	*1.6*
Canned, with Sugar & Salt, Average	*½ Can/71g*	*79*	*0.8*	*111*	*3.2*	*21.9*	*1.2*	*1.9*
Frozen, Average	*1 Sachet/115g*	*121*	*2.4*	*105*	*3.8*	*17.9*	*2.1*	*1.8*
Supersweet, Field Fresh, Birds Eye*	1 Portion/80g	67	0.6	84	2.6	16.9	0.7	2.4
Tinned, Weight Watchers*	1 Portion/143g	103	1.4	72	2.5	12.0	1.0	2.0
with Peppers, Canned, Average	*1 Serving/50g*	*39*	*0.1*	*79*	*2.6*	*16.4*	*0.3*	*0.6*
SWEETENER								
Aspartamo, Artificial Sugar, Zen*	1 Tbsp/2g	8	0.0	383	1.8	94.0	0.0	0.0
Canderel, Spoonful, Canderel*	1 Tsp/0.5g	2	0.0	384	2.9	93.0	0.0	0.0
Canderel*	1 Tbsp/2g	8	0.0	379	24.7	7.0	0.0	5.3
Granulated, Low Calorie, Splenda*	1 Tsp/0.5g	2	0.0	391	0.0	97.7	0.0	0.0
Granulated, Silver Spoon*	1 Tsp/0.5g	2	0.0	387	1.0	96.8	0.0	0.0
Natural, Pure Via*	1 Sachet/2g	3	0.0	149	0.0	95.7	0.0	0.0
Natural Syrup, Fruit, Sweet Freedom*	1 Tsp/5g	15	0.0	292	0.0	79.0	0.0	0.0
Silver Spoon*	1 Tablet/0.05g	0	0.0	325	10.0	71.0	0.0	0.0
Simply Sweet*	1 Tbsp/2g	7	0.0	375	1.4	92.3	0.0	0.0
Slendasweet, Sainsbury's*	1 Tsp/1g	4	0.0	395	1.8	97.0	0.0	0.1
Spoonfull, Low Calorie, SupaSweet*	1 Tsp/1g	4	0.0	392	3.0	95.0	0.0	0.0
Sweet' N Low*	1 Sachet/1g	3	0.0	368	0.0	92.0	0.0	0.0
Sweetex**	1oz/28g	0	0.0	0	0.0	0.0	0.0	0.0
Tablets, Low Calorie, Canderel*	1 Tablet/0.1g	0	0.0	342	13.0	72.4	0.0	0.0
Tablets, Splenda*	1 Tablet/0.1g	0	0.0	345	10.0	76.2	0.0	1.6
Tablets, Tesco*	1 Tablet/1g	0	0.0	20	2.0	2.0	0.5	0.0
Tagatesse, Granulated, Damhert*	1 Serving/5g	14	2.0	275	0.0	79.8	39.9	20.1
Tagatesse, Tablet, Damhert*	1 Tablet/0.075g	0	0.0	266	2.7	76.3	0.0	0.0
Xylosweet, Xylitol*	1 Serving/4g	10	0.0	240	0.0	100.0	0.0	0.0
SWEETS								
Almonds, Sugared, Dragee*	1 Sweet/4g	17	0.6	472	10.0	68.3	17.9	2.5
Alphabet Candies, Asda*	1 Pack/80g	306	0.0	382	0.5	95.0	0.0	0.0
Banana, Baby Foam, M & S*	1/3 Pack/34g	131	0.0	385	4.1	92.7	0.0	0.0
Big Purple One, Quality Street, Nestle*	1 Sweet/39g	191	9.9	490	4.7	60.5	25.5	0.7
Blackcurrant & Liquorice, M & S*	1 Sweet/8g	32	0.3	400	0.6	89.0	4.3	0.0

INFO/WEIGHT	Measure	per Measure		Nutrition Values per 100g / 100ml				
		KCAL	FAT	KCAL	PROT	CARB	FAT	FIBRE

SWEETS

	INFO/WEIGHT	KCAL	FAT	KCAL	PROT	CARB	FAT	FIBRE
Body Parts, Rowntree's*	1 Pack/42g	146	0.0	348	4.3	82.9	0.0	0.0
Butter Candies, Original, Werther's*	1 Sweet/5g	21	0.4	424	0.1	85.7	8.9	0.1
Campino, Strawberries & Cream, Bendicks*	1oz/28g	117	2.3	418	0.1	86.2	8.1	0.0
Candy Cane, Average	1oz/28g	100	0.0	357	3.6	85.7	0.0	0.0
Candy Floss, Asda*	1 Tub/75g	292	0.0	390	0.0	100.0	0.0	0.0
Cappuccino Cream, Sugar Free, Sula*	1 Sweet/3g	8	0.2	269	0.1	91.2	5.5	0.0
Chewits, Blackcurrant	1 Pack/33g	125	0.9	378	0.3	86.9	2.7	0.0
Chewits, Blackcurrant, Leaf*	1 Chew/3g	12	0.1	385	0.2	87.5	3.0	0.0
Chewits, Cola, Leaf*	1 Chew/3g	12	0.1	385	0.2	87.5	3.0	0.0
Chewits, Fruit Salad, Leaf*	1 Chew/3g	12	0.1	385	0.2	87.5	3.0	0.0
Chewits, Strawberry, Leaf*	1 Chew/3g	12	0.1	385	0.2	87.5	3.0	0.0
Chews, Just Fruit, Fruit-tella*	1 Serving/43g	170	2.8	400	0.9	79.5	6.5	0.0
Chews, Spearmint, Victoria, Aldi*	1 Sweet/10g	40	0.8	405	0.3	83.8	7.6	0.0
Chews, Strawberry Mix, Starburst*	1 Sweet/4g	15	0.3	401	0.0	83.9	7.3	0.0
Chocolate Caramels, Diabetic, Boots*	5 Sweets/40g	109	13.2	272	3.2	33.0	33.0	2.0
Chocolate Caramels, Milk, Tesco*	1 Sweet/3g	15	0.5	444	2.7	72.1	16.1	0.1
Chocolate Eclairs, Cadbury*	1 Sweet/8g	36	1.4	455	4.5	68.9	17.9	0.0
Chocolate Eclairs, Co-Op*	1 Sweet/8g	38	1.6	480	3.0	71.0	20.0	0.6
Chocolate Limes, Pascall*	1 Sweet/8g	27	0.2	333	0.3	77.2	2.5	0.0
Cola Bottles, Fizzy, M & S*	1 Pack/200g	650	0.0	325	6.4	75.0	0.0	0.0
Cough, Herbs, Swiss, Original, Ricola*	1 Packet/37g	148	0.0	400	0.0	98.0	0.0	0.0
Cream Caramel, Sula*	1 Sweet/3g	10	0.0	297	0.4	86.1	0.0	0.0
Crunchies, Fruit, Fruit-tella*	1 Box/23g	90	1.1	390	0.7	86.0	5.0	0.0
Dolly Mix, Bassett's*	1 Bag/45g	171	1.4	380	3.0	85.1	3.1	0.4
Double Lolly, Swizzels Matlow*	1 Lolly/10g	41	0.3	409	0.0	93.2	3.4	0.0
Drops, Lemon & Orange, M & S*	1 Pack42g	97	0.0	230	0.0	61.0	0.0	0.0
Drumstick, Matlow's*	1 Pack/40g	164	2.2	409	0.4	88.3	5.5	0.0
Edinburgh Rock, Gardiners of Scotland*	1 Piece/2g	8	0.0	380	0.1	94.4	0.3	0.8
Fizzy Cola, Weight Watchers*	1 Sweet/2g	5	0.0	249	0.3	98.6	0.6	0.3
Fizzy Lemon Fish, Asda*	1 Sweet/4g	14	0.0	325	5.0	76.0	0.1	0.0
Fizzy Mix, Tesco*	½ Bag/50g	166	0.0	332	5.2	75.2	0.0	0.0
Flipsters, Starburst*	1pack/37g	145	0.0	392	0.0	98.1	0.0	0.0
Flumps, Bassett's*	1 Serving/5g	16	0.0	325	4.0	77.0	0.0	0.0
Flumps, Fluffy Mallow Twists, Fat Free, Bassett's*	1 Twist/13g	30	0.0	230	4.1	77.1	0.0	0.0
Flying Saucers, Asda*	1 Serving/23g	82	0.6	355	0.1	83.0	2.5	0.8
Foamy Mushrooms, Chewy, Asda*	1 Sweet/3g	9	0.0	347	4.2	82.0	0.2	0.0
Fruit, Mentos*	1 Sweet/3g	10	0.0	333	0.0	100.0	0.0	0.0
Fruit Gums & Jellies	1 Tube/33g	107	0.0	324	6.5	79.5	0.0	0.0
Fruit Tingles, Wonka*	1 Sweet/8g	8	0.0	104	0.0	26.0	0.0	0.0
Fruities, Lemon & Lime, Weight Watchers*	1 Sweet/2g	3	0.0	134	0.0	54.0	0.0	33.0
Fruity Babies, Bassett's*	1 Sweet/3g	10	0.0	310	4.6	72.7	0.2	0.0
Fruity Chews, Starburst*	1 Sweet/8g	34	0.6	404	0.0	83.4	7.4	0.0
Fruity Flutterbies, Chewits*	1 Serving/100g	316	0.2	316	3.8	73.9	0.2	0.0
Fruity Frogs, Rowntree's*	1 Serving/40g	128	0.1	321	4.7	74.5	0.2	0.0
Fruity Mallows, Fizzy, Asda*	1 Pack/400g	1252	0.0	313	4.3	74.0	0.0	0.0
Gummy Bears	10 Bears/22g	85	0.0	386	0.0	98.9	0.0	98.9
Gummy Worms	10 Worms/74g	286	0.0	386	0.0	98.9	0.0	98.9
Gummy Zingy Fruits, Bassett's*	1 Sm Bag/40g	135	0.0	337	5.1	79.2	0.0	0.0
Hazardously Sour, Toxic Waste*	1 Sweet/3g	12	0.0	400	0.0	100.0	0.0	0.0
Ice Cream Sundae, Asda*	1 Sweet/2g	8	0.0	343	4.1	81.0	0.2	0.1
Kisses, Hershey*	1 Sweet/5g	28	1.6	561	7.0	59.0	32.0	0.0
Lances, Strawberry & Cream Flavour, Tesco*	1 Bag/75g	276	0.9	368	3.2	86.1	1.2	2.1
Lances, Strawberry Flavour, Fizzy, Tesco*	½ Pack/50g	177	1.3	354	2.8	79.8	2.6	1.8

S

	Measure INFO/WEIGHT	per Measure		Nutrition Values per 100g / 100ml				
		KCAL	FAT	KCAL	PROT	CARB	FAT	FIBRE
SWEETS								
Liquorice and Fruit, Fruit-tella*	1 Sweet/4g	16	0.3	395	0.9	83.0	6.5	0.0
Lovehearts, Giant, Swizzels*	1 Pack/42g	165	0.0	393	0.0	100.0	0.0	0.0
Maynards Sours, Bassett's*	1 Pack/52g	169	0.0	325	6.1	75.0	0.0	0.0
Midget Gems, Maynards*	1 Sweet/1g	3	0.0	340	8.7	76.2	0.0	0.0
Milk Chocolate Eclairs, Sainsbury's*	1 Sweet/8g	33	1.1	442	2.1	75.7	14.5	0.5
Milk Duds, Hershey*	13 Pieces/33g	170	6.0	510	3.0	84.0	18.0	0.0
Parma Violets, Swizzlers*	1 Sml Tube/10g	41	0.0	406	0.9	99.1	0.0	0.0
Percy Pig & Pals, Soft, M & S*	1 Sweet/8g	26	0.0	344	5.8	80.0	0.1	0.0
Randoms, Rowntree's*	1 Pack/50g	164	0.1	328	4.9	75.7	0.3	0.6
Rhubarb & Custard, Sainsbury's*	1 Sweet/8g	28	0.0	351	0.1	87.7	0.0	0.0
Salzige Heringe, Katjes*	1 Serving/50g	172	0.0	345	5.8	80.0	0.1	0.0
Scary Mix, Tesco*	1 Bag/100g	327	0.5	327	9.5	71.1	0.5	0.3
Scary Sours, Rowntree's*	1 Serving/100g	321	0.0	321	3.5	74.7	0.0	0.0
Sherbert Cocktails, Sainsbury's*	1 Sweet/9g	36	0.7	400	0.0	83.1	7.5	0.0
Sherbert Dib Dab, with Strawberry Lolly, Barratt*	1 Pack/23g	88	0.0	383	0.1	95.6	0.1	0.0
Sherbet Lemons, Bassett's*	1 Sweet/7g	25	0.0	375	0.0	93.9	0.0	0.0
Shrimps & Bananas, Sainsbury's*	½ Pack/50g	188	0.0	376	2.5	91.3	0.1	0.5
Snakes, Bassett's*	1 Sweet/9g	30	0.0	320	3.5	76.8	0.1	0.0
Soft Fruits, Trebor*	1 Roll/45g	165	0.0	367	0.0	90.9	0.0	0.0
Sour Squirms, Bassett's*	1 Serving/7g	21	0.0	325	3.1	78.1	0.0	0.0
Strawberry & Cream, Sugar Free, Sula*	1 Sweet/3g	9	0.2	267	0.2	90.5	5.4	0.0
Sugar Free, Sula*	1 Sweet/3g	7	0.0	231	0.0	96.1	0.0	0.0
Sweetshop Favourites, Bassett's*	1 Sweet/5g	17	0.0	340	0.0	84.3	0.0	0.0
Tic Tac, Cool Cherry, Ferrero*	1 Pack/18g	69	0.1	382	0.2	92.2	0.7	0.0
Toffo*	1 Tube/43g	194	9.5	451	2.2	69.8	22.0	0.0
Tootsie Roll, Small Midgees, Tootsie*	1 Sweet/7g	23	0.5	350	2.5	70.0	7.5	0.0
Tooty Frooties, Rowntree's*	1 Bag/28g	111	1.0	397	0.1	91.5	3.5	0.0
Wazzly Wobble Drops, Wonka*	1 Bag/42g	186	6.8	443	3.0	71.6	16.1	0.2
Wiggly Worms, Sainsbury's*	1 Serving/10g	32	0.0	317	5.6	72.7	0.4	0.2
Wine Gummies, Matlow, Swizzels*	1 Pack/16g	52	0.0	324	0.0	58.7	0.0	0.0
Xtra Sour Spiders, Rowntree's*	1 Pack/35g	112	0.0	321	3.5	74.8	0.0	0.0
Yo Yo's, All Flavours, 100% Fruit, We Are Bear*	1 Roll/10g	27	0.0	275	1.9	63.4	0.2	12.0
Yo Yo's, Strawberry 100% Fruit, We Are Bear*	1 Roll/10g	27	0.0	275	1.9	63.4	0.2	12.0
SWORDFISH								
Grilled, Average	*1oz/28g*	*39*	*1.5*	*139*	*22.9*	*0.0*	*5.2*	*0.0*
Raw, Average	*1oz/28g*	*42*	*2.0*	*149*	*21.1*	*0.0*	*7.2*	*0.0*
SYRUP								
Corn, Dark, Average	*1 Tbsp/20g*	*56*	*0.0*	*282*	*0.0*	*76.6*	*0.0*	*0.0*
Golden, Average	*1 Tbsp/20g*	*61*	*0.0*	*304*	*0.4*	*78.2*	*0.0*	*0.0*
Maple, Average	*1 Tbsp/20g*	*52*	*0.0*	*262*	*0.0*	*67.2*	*0.2*	*0.0*

S

	Measure INFO/WEIGHT	per Measure KCAL	FAT	Nutrition Values per 100g / 100ml KCAL	PROT	CARB	FAT	FIBRE
TABOO*								
Average, Taboo*	1 Shot/35ml	80	0.0	230	0.0	33.0	0.0	0.0
TABOULEH								
Average	*1oz/28g*	*33*	*1.3*	*119*	*2.6*	*17.2*	*4.6*	*0.0*
TACO SHELLS								
Corn, Crunchy, Old El Paso*	1 Taco/10g	51	2.6	506	7.0	61.0	26.0	0.0
Old El Paso*	1 Taco/12g	57	2.7	478	7.4	60.8	22.8	0.0
Traditional, Discovery*	1 Taco/11g	55	3.2	489	5.7	53.4	28.1	6.0
TAGINE								
Spicy Chermoula, Tasty Veg Pot, Innocent*	1 Pot/400g	356	9.6	89	3.4	13.8	2.4	5.0
Vegetable, Filo Topped, M & S*	1 Serving/282g	310	6.5	110	3.3	18.7	2.3	3.9
TAGLIATELLE								
Basil, M & S*	1 Serving/100g	365	2.8	365	15.1	69.0	2.8	4.0
Bicolore, Asda*	¼ Pack/125g	202	3.0	162	7.0	28.0	2.4	1.4
Carbonara, Frozen, Tesco*	1 Pack/450g	427	8.5	95	5.2	14.1	1.9	0.9
Carbonara, Naturally Less 5% Fat, Asda*	1 Pack/400g	440	9.6	110	4.2	18.0	2.4	0.8
Carbonara, TTD, Sainsbury's*	1 Pack/405g	644	25.9	159	7.8	17.6	6.4	1.6
Chargrilled Chicken & Tomato, Asda*	1 Pack/400g	392	12.4	98	5.8	11.7	3.1	1.4
Chicken, Italia, M & S*	1 Pack/360g	342	6.5	95	8.1	12.1	1.8	1.2
Chicken & Mushroom, GFY, Asda*	1 Pack/400g	359	7.0	90	7.2	11.2	1.7	0.7
Chicken & Tomato, Italiano, Tesco*	1 Pack/400g	416	8.4	104	6.6	14.8	2.1	0.8
Creamy Mushroom, Chosen By You, Asda*	1 Pak/400g	428	10.8	107	3.7	16.3	2.7	1.4
Dry, Average	*1 Serving/100g*	*356*	*1.8*	*356*	*12.6*	*72.4*	*1.8*	*1.0*
Egg, Dry, Average	*1 Serving/75g*	*271*	*2.5*	*362*	*14.2*	*68.8*	*3.3*	*2.3*
Egg, Fresh, Dry, Average	*1 Serving/125g*	*345*	*3.5*	*276*	*10.6*	*53.0*	*2.8*	*2.1*
Fresh, Dry, Average	*1 Serving/75g*	*211*	*2.0*	*281*	*11.4*	*53.3*	*2.6*	*2.6*
Fresh, Free Range, Morrisons*	¼ Pack/125g	331	2.5	265	11.5	50.2	2.0	3.4
Garlic & Herb, Fresh, Tesco*	1 Serving/125g	361	4.6	289	12.0	51.8	3.7	1.5
Garlic & Herb, Fresh, Waitrose*	1 Serving/125g	327	3.1	262	11.8	48.1	2.5	2.1
Garlic Mushroom, BGTY, Sainsbury's*	1 Pack/400g	416	9.2	104	4.7	16.2	2.3	2.0
Ham & Mushroom, BGTY, Sainsbury's*	1 Pack/450g	486	14.4	108	5.3	14.5	3.2	0.8
Ham & Mushroom, Light Choices, Tesco*	1 Pack/400g	400	8.8	100	6.0	13.8	2.2	1.8
Ham & Mushroom, M & S*	1 Pack/400g	400	18.8	100	4.0	15.1	4.7	0.7
Ham & Roasted Mushroom, Finest, Tesco*	1 Pack/450g	562	23.8	125	7.3	12.0	5.3	2.4
Multigrain, BGTY, Uncooked, Sainsbury's*	1 Serving/190g	294	4.7	155	7.0	26.0	2.5	3.0
Mushroom & Bacon, Sainsbury's*	1 Pack/450g	585	23.4	130	7.1	13.8	5.2	0.5
Mushroom & Ham, GFY, Asda*	1 Pack/399g	323	9.2	81	5.4	9.6	2.3	0.7
Nests, Dry Weight, Napolina*	1oz/28g	93	0.4	332	11.5	68.0	1.5	3.7
Prawn, Primavera, Sainsbury's*	1 Pack/400g	383	6.1	100	6.1	15.3	1.6	1.4
Red Pepper, Organic, Sainsbury's*	½ Bag/125g	182	1.9	146	5.4	27.8	1.5	1.4
Salmon, Perfectly Balanced, Waitrose*	1 Pack/400g	376	10.8	94	5.4	11.7	2.7	0.8
Salmon & King Prawn, HL, Tesco*	1 Pack/400g	480	9.6	120	6.5	17.2	2.4	1.7
Salmon & Prawn, Perfectly Balanced, Waitrose*	1 Pack/401g	341	13.2	85	6.8	7.1	3.3	1.1
Sundried Tomato, Fresh, Morrisons*	1 Pack/250g	747	8.2	299	11.1	56.4	3.3	3.5
Sweet Chilli & Prawn, Tesco*	1 Pack/400g	440	12.4	110	5.5	14.9	3.1	1.3
Tomato & Basil Chicken, Weight Watchers*	1 Pack/330g	322	4.0	98	7.5	14.1	1.2	0.3
Tricolore, Waitrose*	½ Pack/125g	351	3.6	281	12.0	51.6	2.9	1.6
Verdi, Dry, Barilla*	1 Serving/150g	555	5.2	370	14.0	70.5	3.5	0.0
Verdi, Fresh, Average	*1 Serving/125g*	*171*	*1.8*	*137*	*5.5*	*25.5*	*1.5*	*1.8*
TAHINI PASTE								
Average	*1 Tsp/6g*	*36*	*3.5*	*607*	*18.5*	*0.9*	*58.9*	*8.0*
TAMARIND								
Pulp	*1oz/28g*	*76*	*0.1*	*273*	*3.2*	*64.5*	*0.3*	*0.0*
Whole, Raw, Weighed with Pod, Average	*1oz/28g*	*67*	*0.2*	*239*	*2.8*	*62.5*	*0.6*	*5.1*

T

	Measure INFO/WEIGHT	per Measure		Nutrition Values per 100g / 100ml				
		KCAL	FAT	KCAL	PROT	CARB	FAT	FIBRE
TANGERINES								
Fresh, Raw	*1oz/28g*	*10*	*0.0*	*35*	*0.9*	*8.0*	*0.1*	*1.3*
Weighed with Peel & Pips	*1 Med/70g*	*17*	*0.1*	*25*	*0.7*	*5.8*	*0.1*	*0.9*
TANGO*								
Cherry, Britvic*	1 Bottle/500ml	55	0.0	11	0.0	2.4	0.0	0.0
Orange, Britvic*	1 Can/330ml	63	0.0	19	0.1	4.4	0.0	0.0
TAPAS								
Champinones Al Ajillo, Tapas at, Tesco*	½ Pack/85g	123	11.6	145	2.3	2.5	13.6	1.5
Paella Valenciana, Tapas at, Tesco*	½ Pack/75g	105	4.1	140	9.0	12.6	5.5	1.3
Patatas Bravas, Tapas at, Tesco*	½ Pack/125g	169	6.4	135	2.5	18.7	5.1	3.0
Pollo Con Salsa, Tapas at, Tesco*	½ Pack/75g	94	6.5	125	9.4	2.1	8.7	0.7
TAPIOCA								
Creamed, Ambrosia*	½ Can/213g	159	3.4	75	2.6	12.6	1.6	0.2
Raw	*1oz/28g*	*101*	*0.0*	*359*	*0.4*	*95.0*	*0.1*	*0.4*
TARAMASALATA								
Average	1oz/28g	141	14.8	504	3.2	4.1	52.9	0.0
BGTY, Sainsbury's*	1oz/28g	71	5.7	253	4.3	13.5	20.2	0.7
Tesco*	1/8 Tub/25g	115	11.2	460	2.9	10.5	44.8	1.0
TARRAGON								
Dried, Ground	*1 Tsp/2g*	*5*	*0.1*	*295*	*22.8*	*42.8*	*7.2*	*0.0*
Fresh, Average	*1 Tbsp/4g*	*2*	*0.0*	*49*	*3.4*	*6.3*	*1.1*	*0.0*
TART								
Apple & Custard, Asda*	1 Tart/84g	227	11.0	270	3.1	35.0	13.1	0.1
Apple & Fresh Cream, Asda*	½ Tart/50g	133	8.0	267	3.4	33.0	16.0	0.8
Apricot Lattice, Sainsbury's*	1 Slice/125g	321	14.2	257	3.4	35.3	11.4	2.6
Aubergine & Feta, Roast Marinated, Sainsbury's*	1 Serving/105g	227	15.2	216	4.8	16.6	14.5	1.7
Bakewell, Average	1 Tart/50g	228	14.8	456	6.3	43.5	29.7	1.9
Bakewell, Weight Watchers*	1 Tart/43g	156	5.0	363	3.6	65.2	11.7	3.2
Blackcurrant Sundae, Asda*	1 Tart/55g	227	10.4	413	3.5	57.0	19.0	2.3
Cherry Bakewell, Morrisons*	1 Tart/46g	198	9.8	430	4.6	54.9	21.4	1.3
Cherry Tomato & Mascarpone, Asda*	1 Tart/160g	290	18.0	181	4.4	15.6	11.2	1.1
Chocolate, Co-Op*	1 Tart/22g	102	6.8	465	4.0	42.0	31.0	0.7
Coconut, M & S*	1 Tart/53g	220	9.6	415	5.8	57.8	18.1	3.6
Coconut & Cherry, Asda*	1 Serving/50g	215	10.0	430	4.4	58.0	20.0	4.0
Coconut & Raspberry, Waitrose*	1 Tart/48g	204	11.5	426	5.0	45.0	24.0	3.9
Custard, Individual, Average	1 Tart/94g	260	13.6	277	6.3	32.4	14.5	1.2
Date Pecan & Almond, Sticky, Sainsbury's*	1/8 Tart/75g	298	10.3	397	5.0	63.5	13.7	1.7
Egg Custard, Asda*	1 Tart/80g	215	10.4	269	9.0	29.0	13.0	1.2
Egg Custard, Tesco*	1 Tart/82g	214	10.0	261	6.2	31.5	12.2	1.1
Feta Cheese & Spinach, Puff Pastry, Tesco*	1 Tart/108g	306	19.2	283	7.1	23.5	17.8	0.9
Filo Asparagus Tartlette, M & S*	1 Serving/15g	45	3.1	300	4.4	25.2	20.4	2.1
Frangipane, Chocolate & William Pear, Waitrose*	1/6 Pack/80g	219	12.4	274	3.5	29.9	15.5	2.5
Frangipane, Lutowska Cherry Amaretto, Sainsbury's*	1 Serving/66g	264	12.9	400	6.0	50.0	19.5	1.3
Italian Lemon & Almond, Sainsbury's*	1 Slice/49g	182	11.6	371	7.4	31.9	23.7	4.1
Jam, Assorted, VLH Kitchens*	1 Slice/34g	44.2	4.9	130	3.4	56.0	14.4	1.3
Jam, Average	1 Slice/90g	342	13.4	380	3.3	62.0	14.9	1.6
Lemon, M & S*	1/6 Tart/50g	207	14.6	415	5.0	32.7	29.3	0.9
Lemon, Sainsbury's*	1/8 Tart/56g	258	15.8	459	4.4	47.0	28.1	0.6
Lemon & Raspberry, Finest, Tesco*	1 Tart/120g	360	16.8	300	5.2	38.4	14.0	2.9
Lemon Bakewell, Easter, Morrisons*	1 Tart/45g	186	7.1	413	3.1	64.8	15.7	1.8
Lemon Curd, Asda*	1 Tart/30g	121	4.5	402	2.8	64.0	15.0	2.2
Lemon Curd, Lyons*	1 Tart/30g	122	5.1	406	3.7	59.3	17.0	0.0
Mixed Fruit, Waitrose*	1 Tart/146g	318	16.4	218	2.3	27.3	11.2	1.0
Normandy Apple & Calvados, Finest, Tesco*	1/6 Tart/100g	256	7.6	256	3.2	41.4	7.6	1.9

T

	Measure INFO/WEIGHT	per Measure KCAL	FAT	Nutrition Values per 100g / 100ml KCAL	PROT	CARB	FAT	FIBRE
TART								
Raspberry & Blueberry, Tesco*	1 Serving/85g	168	7.5	198	2.7	27.0	8.8	2.8
Red Pepper, Serrano Ham & Goats Cheese, Waitrose*	1 Serving/100g	293	19.2	293	8.7	21.3	19.2	3.2
Roasted Vegetable, Finest, Tesco*	¼ Tart/113g	226	13.2	200	3.1	20.6	11.7	2.3
Strawberries & Cream, Finest, Tesco*	1/6 Tart/74g	210	13.0	280	3.4	27.2	17.3	1.5
Strawberry, Fresh, M & S*	1 Tart/120g	305	18.4	255	3.1	26.4	15.4	2.4
Strawberry, Reduced Sugar, Asda*	1 Tart/37g	141	3.7	380	4.6	67.5	10.1	1.2
Strawberry, Waitrose*	1 Serving/101g	241	12.0	239	3.8	29.2	11.9	1.2
Strawberry & Fresh Cream, Finest, Tesco*	1 Tart/129g	350	19.1	271	3.3	31.1	14.8	1.2
Strawberry Sundae, Asda*	1 Tart/46g	187	8.3	407	3.3	58.0	18.0	1.3
Summer Fruit Crumble, Morrisons*	1 Tart/128g	379	15.1	296	3.6	43.8	11.8	1.3
Toffee Bakewell, Morrisons*	1 Tart/47g	212	8.5	451	3.4	69.5	18.2	1.4
Toffee Bakewell, Sainsbury's*	1 Tart/45g	200	8.7	444	3.4	64.2	19.3	1.1
Toffee Pecan, M & S*	1 Tart/91g	414	24.1	455	6.0	48.5	26.5	2.0
Toffee Pecan, Waitrose*	¼ Tart/133g	564	19.1	423	4.3	69.3	14.3	1.6
Tomato, Mozzarella & Basil Puff, Sainsbury's*	1/3 Tart/120g	318	25.0	265	9.2	10.2	20.8	0.9
Treacle, Average	1 Serving/125g	460	17.6	368	3.7	60.4	14.1	1.1
Treacle Lattice, Mr Kipling*	1/6 Tart/70g	255	8.5	365	4.4	59.8	12.1	1.1
Treacle with Custard	1 Serving/251g	586	23.5	233	3.1	36.1	9.4	0.8
Vegetable & Feta, Deli, M & S*	½ Tart/115g	315	18.4	274	5.0	20.0	16.0	6.0
TARTAR								
Cream of, Leavening Agent	***1 Tsp/3g***	***8***	***0.0***	***258***	***0.0***	***61.5***	***0.0***	***0.0***
TARTE								
Au Citron, Frozen, Tesco*	1/6 Tarte/81g	255	11.8	315	5.4	39.4	14.6	0.7
Au Citron, Frozen, TTD, Sainsbury's*	1/6 Tart/80g	232	13.4	290	4.7	40.7	16.8	7.7
Au Citron, Waitrose*	1 Tarte/100g	325	18.1	325	4.9	35.7	18.1	1.0
Aux Cerises, Finest, Tesco*	1 Serving/98g	219	7.0	225	4.9	35.4	7.2	0.6
Normande, French Style, M & S*	1/6 Tarte/85g	245	16.1	290	3.3	26.8	19.0	0.7
Tatin, Sainsbury's*	1 Serving/120g	244	8.0	203	2.9	32.8	6.7	1.9
TARTLETS								
Caramelised Onion & Gruyere, Sainsbury's*	1 Tartlet/145g	381	27.5	263	5.8	17.3	19.0	1.3
Cheese & Roast Onion, Asda*	1 Tartlet/50g	135	7.5	270	6.0	28.0	15.0	1.9
Cherry Tomato & Aubergine, M & S*	1 Tartlet/160g	320	20.2	200	3.1	17.8	12.6	1.7
Mandarin, Mini, M & S*	1 Tartlet/29g	80	4.7	280	3.4	30.4	16.3	0.6
Mushroom & Watercress, Waitrose*	1 Tartlet/120g	308	24.6	257	8.4	19.1	20.5	2.6
Mushroom Medley, BGTY, Sainsbury's*	1 Serving/80g	134	8.0	167	4.7	14.5	10.0	3.4
Raspberry, Mini, M & S*	1 Tartlet/27g	90	5.4	330	4.3	34.4	19.6	0.5
Red Onion & Goats Cheese, Sainsbury's*	1 Tartlet/113g	335	21.8	297	7.0	23.7	19.3	1.5
Redcurrant & Blackcurrant, Mini, M & S*	1 Tartlet/29g	85	4.9	290	3.9	30.5	16.8	1.1
Roasted Pumpkin & Goats Cheese Filo, Finest, Tesco*	1 Tartlet/160g	320	19.2	200	4.8	18.4	12.0	1.9
Roasted Red Pepper, BGTY, Sainsbury's*	1 Tartlet/80g	143	7.4	179	3.1	21.0	9.2	3.4
Salmon & Watercress, Hot Smoked, Waitrose*	1 Serving/130g	315	19.9	242	8.1	18.0	15.3	3.0
Sausage & Tomato, Sainsbury's*	1 Tartlet/135g	323	21.3	239	4.8	19.5	15.8	1.6
Spinach Ricotta & Sundried Tomato, Filo, Tesco*	1 Tartlet/135g	358	23.1	265	5.2	22.4	17.1	1.9
Tomato & Goats Cheese, Waitrose*	1 Tartlet/130g	295	19.0	227	6.6	17.4	14.6	2.0
TEA								
Assam, Blended, TTD, Sainsbury's*	1 Serving/2g	0	0.0	0	0.0	0.0	0.0	0.0
Damask, Rose, Chinese, Choi Time*	1 Mug/500ml	0	0.3	0	0.0	0.0	0.1	0.0
Decaf, Tetley*	1 Cup/100ml	1	0.0	1	0.0	0.3	0.0	0.0
Earl Grey, Infusion with Water, Average	1 Mug/250ml	2	0.0	1	0.0	0.2	0.0	0.0
Fruit Or Herbal, Made with Water, Twinings*	1 Mug/200ml	8	0.0	4	0.0	1.0	0.0	0.0
Fruits of the Forest, Westminster Tea*	1 Bag/250ml	5	0.0	2	0.0	0.6	0.0	0.0
Ginger, Herbal, Brit & Tang*	1 Tea Bag/1.8g	5	0.0	278	0.0	55.6	0.0	0.0
Green, with Jasmine, Wellbeing Selection, Flavia*	1 Cup/200ml	14	0.2	7	0.5	1.2	0.1	0.0

	Measure INFO/WEIGHT	per Measure		Nutrition Values per 100g / 100ml				
		KCAL	FAT	KCAL	PROT	CARB	FAT	FIBRE
TEA								
Green, with Lemon, Jackson's*	1 Serving/200ml	2	0.0	1	0.0	0.2	0.0	0.0
Green, with Mango, Brewed with Water, Twinings*	1 Cup/200ml	2	0.0	1	0.0	0.2	0.0	0.0
Green Tea Pure, Twinings*	1 Serving/100g	1	0.0	1	0.0	0.2	0.0	0.0
Green with Mint, Whittards of Chelsea*	1 Cup/100ml	1	0.0	1	0.2	0.1	0.0	0.0
Herbal, Wellbeing Blends, Infusions, Twinings*	1 Serving/200ml	4	0.0	2	0.0	0.3	0.0	0.0
Ice, with Lemon, Lipton*	1 Bottle/325ml	91	0.0	28	0.0	6.9	0.0	0.0
Iced, Green, Orange, Lipton*	1 Bottle/500ml	100	0.0	20	0.0	5.0	0.0	0.0
Iced, Lemon, San Benedetto*	1 Bottle/500ml	170	0.0	34	0.1	8.3	0.0	0.0
Iced, No Sugar Peach Flavour, Nestle*	1 Glass/100ml	1	0.0	1	0.0	0.1	0.0	0.0
Iced, Peach, Twinings*	1 Serving/200ml	60	0.2	30	0.1	7.3	0.1	0.0
Iced, Pickwick*	1 Serving/250ml	32	0.0	13	0.0	3.3	0.0	0.0
Lemon, Instant, Original, Lift*	1 Serving/15g	53	0.0	352	0.0	87.0	0.0	0.0
Lemon, Instant, Tesco*	1 Serving/7g	23	0.0	326	1.0	80.5	0.0	0.0
Lemon & Limeflower, Infused, M & S*	1 Bottle/330ml	99	0.0	30	0.0	7.8	0.0	0.0
Light And Delicate, Green with Lemon, Twinings*	1 Cup/100ml	1	0.1	1	0.1	0.2	0.1	0.1
Made with Water	1 Mug/227ml	0	0.0	0	0.1	0.0	0.0	0.0
Made with Water with Semi-Skimmed Milk, Average	1 Cup/200ml	14	0.4	7	0.5	0.7	0.2	0.0
Made with Water with Skimmed Milk, Average	1 Mug/227ml	14	0.5	6	0.5	0.7	0.2	0.0
Made with Water with Whole Milk, Average	1 Cup/200ml	16	0.8	8	0.4	0.5	0.4	0.0
Peach Flavour, Lift*	1 Cup/15g	58	0.0	384	0.3	95.6	0.0	0.0
Red Bush, Made with Water, Tetley*	1 Mug/250ml	2	0.0	1	0.0	0.1	0.0	0.0
TEACAKES								
Average	1 Teacake/60g	178	4.5	296	8.0	52.5	7.5	0.0
Caramel, Highlights, Mallows, Cadbury*	1 Teacake/15g	61	1.9	408	6.2	69.1	12.4	3.6
Coconut Snowballs, Tunnock's*	1 Cake/30g	116	6.5	388	3.9	47.0	21.8	0.0
Currant, Sainsbury's*	1 Teacake/72g	204	2.9	284	8.2	53.7	4.0	2.5
Fruited, M & S*	1 Teacake/60g	156	0.6	260	8.9	53.4	1.0	2.0
Fruity, Warburton's*	1 Teacake/63g	160	2.2	256	8.7	48.0	3.5	2.7
Jam, Castello*	1 Teacake/13g	60	2.4	470	5.3	70.1	18.4	1.3
Mallow, Tesco*	1 Teacake/14g	63	2.7	450	4.1	65.4	19.1	1.0
Marshmallow, Milk Chocolate, Tunnock's*	1 Teacake/24g	106	4.6	440	4.9	61.9	19.2	2.4
Sainsbury's*	1 Teacake/70g	171	2.5	244	8.0	45.0	3.6	2.6
Tesco*	1 Teacake/61g	163	2.1	267	7.8	51.1	3.5	2.4
Toasted, Average	1 Teacake/60g	197	5.0	329	8.9	58.3	8.3	0.0
with Orange Filling, M & S*	1 Teacake/20g	80	2.8	410	4.5	66.6	14.2	0.9
TEMPEH								
Average	*1oz/28g*	*46*	*1.8*	*166*	*20.7*	*6.4*	*6.4*	*4.3*
TEQUILA								
Average	*1 Shot/35ml*	*78*	*0.0*	*224*	*0.0*	*0.0*	*0.0*	*0.0*
TERRINE								
Salmon, Poached, Tesco*	1 Pack/113g	349	30.6	309	15.5	0.8	27.1	0.0
Salmon, Three, M & S*	1 Serving/80g	168	12.2	210	17.6	0.8	15.3	0.9
Salmon, with Prawn & Lobster, M & S*	1 Serving/55g	107	7.4	195	18.2	0.7	13.4	0.7
Salmon & Crayfish, Slice, Finest, Tesco*	1 Serving/110g	148	5.7	135	21.9	0.1	5.2	0.1
Salmon & King Prawn, Waitrose*	1 Serving/75g	97	4.0	130	19.3	1.3	5.3	0.0
Salmon & Lemon, Luxury, Tesco*	1 Serving/50g	98	7.8	196	10.6	3.2	15.7	0.8
THAI BITES								
Mild Thai Flavour, Jacob's*	1 Bag/25g	93	0.8	373	6.9	79.0	3.3	1.0
Roasted Chilli Flavour, Fusions, Jacob's*	1 Bag/30g	109	1.7	363	5.5	72.3	5.8	1.2
Seaweed Flavour, Jacob's*	1 Bag/25g	94	0.8	377	7.1	80.0	3.2	0.5
Sesame & Prawn, Fusions, Jacob's*	1 Bag/25g	91	1.5	366	6.3	71.2	5.9	1.3
Sweet Herb, Jacob's*	1 Bag/25g	93	0.8	372	7.1	78.8	3.2	0.2

T

	Measure INFO/WEIGHT	per Measure KCAL	FAT	Nutrition Values per 100g / 100ml KCAL	PROT	CARB	FAT	FIBRE
THICKENING GRANULES								
McDougalls*	1 Tbsp/10g	46	1.9	463	0.0	73.7	18.7	0.0
THINS								
Cheddar & Black Pepper, Ryvita*	1oz/28g	116	2.5	413	18.1	62.6	9.1	4.0
Multi Seed, Ryvita*	1 Thin/10g	37	0.9	385	16.0	60.0	9.0	9.5
Sweet Chilli, Ryvita*	1 Thin/8g	30	0.1	370	14.3	74.1	1.8	4.9
THYME								
Dried, Ground, Average	*1 Tsp/1g*	*3*	*0.1*	*276*	*9.1*	*45.3*	*7.4*	*0.0*
Fresh, Average	*1 Tsp/1g*	*1*	*0.0*	*95*	*3.0*	*15.1*	*2.5*	*0.0*
TIA MARIA								
Original	*1 Shot/35ml*	*105*	*0.0*	*300*	*0.0*	*0.0*	*0.0*	*0.0*
TIC TAC								
Extra Strong Mint, Ferrero*	2 Tic Tacs/1g	4	0.0	381	0.0	95.2	0.0	0.0
Fresh Mint, Ferrero*	2 Tic Tacs/1g	4	0.0	390	0.0	97.5	0.0	0.0
Lime & Orange, Ferrero*	2 Tic Tacs/1g	4	0.0	386	0.0	95.5	0.0	0.0
Orange, Ferrero*	2 Tic Tacs/1g	4	0.0	385	0.0	95.5	0.0	0.0
Spearmint, Ferrero*	1 Box/16g	62	0.0	390	0.0	97.5	0.0	0.0
TIDGY PUDS								
Aunt Bessie's*	4 Puds/17g	55	2.5	326	9.6	38.4	14.8	2.1
TIDGY TOADS								
Aunt Bessie's*	1 Serving/45g	125	5.9	278	14.7	25.3	13.2	1.1
TIKKA MASALA								
Chicken, & Pilau Rice, GFY, Asda*	1 Pack/450g	495	9.0	110	6.0	17.0	2.0	0.8
Chicken, & Pilau Rice, Takeaway, Asda*	1 Pack/561g	852	27.5	152	7.0	20.0	4.9	1.5
Chicken, & Pilau Rice, Waitrose*	1 Pack/500g	797	34.5	159	8.2	16.1	6.9	0.8
Chicken, & Rice, Light Choices, Tesco*	1 Pack/450g	472	7.2	105	7.9	14.6	1.6	1.3
Chicken, & Rice, M & S*	1 Pack/400g	700	35.2	175	7.4	17.0	8.8	1.0
Chicken, & Vegetable, HL, Tesco*	1 Pack/450g	360	12.1	80	6.8	6.9	2.7	1.8
Chicken, Asda*	1 Pack/340g	388	20.4	114	9.0	6.0	6.0	1.5
Chicken, Birds Eye*	1 Serving/400g	420	7.2	105	5.6	16.6	1.8	0.3
Chicken, Boiled Rice & Nan, Meal for One, GFY, Asda*	1 Pack/605g	823	18.8	136	6.0	21.0	3.1	0.0
Chicken, Breast, GFY, Asda*	1 Pack/380g	486	14.4	128	19.0	4.5	3.8	0.2
Chicken, COU, M & S*	1 Pack/400g	400	6.8	100	7.6	14.1	1.7	1.3
Chicken, Feeling Great, Findus*	1 Pack/350g	420	12.2	120	5.5	17.0	3.5	2.0
Chicken, Hot, Sainsbury's*	1 Pack/400g	604	37.2	151	13.2	3.6	9.3	1.5
Chicken, Hot, Tesco*	1 Pack/400g	588	34.4	147	8.7	8.6	8.6	1.0
Chicken, Indian, Medium, Sainsbury's*	1 Pack/400g	848	61.2	212	13.2	5.3	15.3	0.1
Chicken, Indian, Tesco*	1 Pack/350g	560	32.6	160	11.6	7.2	9.3	0.6
Chicken, Indian Meal for One, BGTY, Sainsbury's*	1 Serving/241g	200	1.9	83	13.9	5.1	0.8	1.0
Chicken, Indian Takeaway, Tesco*	1 Serving/125g	100	3.2	80	8.9	4.9	2.6	2.1
Chicken, Large, Sainsbury's*	1 Pack/650g	1105	68.9	170	11.7	7.0	10.6	0.3
Chicken, Medium Spiced, without Rice, Tesco*	½ Pack/175g	231	13.1	132	10.2	5.9	7.5	0.9
Chicken, Microwave Meal, Good Choice, Iceland*	1 Pack/400g	488	6.0	122	6.6	20.4	1.5	0.6
Chicken, Mild, Diet Chef Ltd*	1 Pack/300g	291	6.6	97	10.4	9.0	2.2	0.6
Chicken, Sharwood's*	1 Pack/375g	562	25.1	150	7.2	15.1	6.7	0.8
Chicken, The Authentic Food Company*	1 Serving/375g	510	31.5	136	10.6	5.5	8.4	0.9
Chicken, Tinned, M & S*	½ Can/213g	309	18.1	145	14.5	2.9	8.5	2.2
Chicken, Waitrose*	½ Pack/200g	298	19.4	149	12.8	2.6	9.7	1.6
Chicken, Weight Watchers*	1 Pack/331g	344	4.6	104	7.0	15.8	1.4	0.2
Chicken, with Fruit & Nut Pilau Rice, Sainsbury's*	1 Pack/500g	885	45.5	177	7.6	16.1	9.1	2.8
Chicken, with Pilau Rice, Perfectly Balanced, Waitrose*	1 Pack/400g	476	10.0	119	8.2	15.8	2.5	1.8
Chicken, with Rice, Sainsbury's*	1 Pack/500g	960	41.0	192	8.3	21.2	8.2	0.1
Cooking Sauce, Under 3% Fat, BGTY, Sainsbury's*	¼ Jar/126g	83	2.3	66	0.8	11.7	1.8	0.6
King Prawn & Rice, Finest, Tesco*	1 Pack/475g	617	30.4	130	6.0	16.6	6.4	1.2

T

	Measure INFO/WEIGHT	per Measure		Nutrition Values per 100g / 100ml				
		KCAL	FAT	KCAL	PROT	CARB	FAT	FIBRE
TIKKA MASALA								
Prawn, COU, M & S*	1 Pack/400g	400	6.4	100	6.9	14.7	1.6	1.9
Prawn, King, Perfectly Balanced, Waitrose*	1 Pack/400g	372	3.6	93	5.2	16.0	0.9	1.7
Spicy, Rice Time, Uncle Ben's*	1 Tub/300g	399	11.7	133	2.3	21.7	3.9	0.9
Vegetable, Asda*	1 Pack/340g	316	20.7	93	2.0	7.4	6.1	1.1
Vegetable, Canned, Waitrose*	1 Can/200g	152	4.4	76	3.6	10.5	2.2	0.0
Vegetable, Indian, Tesco*	1 Pack/225g	234	13.5	104	2.4	10.4	6.0	2.4
Vegetable, Waitrose*	1 Serving/196g	149	4.3	76	3.6	10.5	2.2	3.8
TILAPIA								
Raw, Average	*100g*	*95*	*1.0*	*95*	*20.0*	*0.0*	*1.0*	*0.0*
TIME OUT								
Break Pack, Cadbury*	1 Serving/20g	108	6.3	530	6.2	58.3	30.7	0.0
Chocolate Fingers, Cadbury*	2 Fingers/35g	185	10.7	530	6.2	58.3	30.7	0.0
Orange, Snack Size, Cadbury*	1 Finger/11g	61	3.6	555	5.0	59.4	32.9	0.0
TIRAMISU								
Asda*	1 Pot/100g	252	11.0	252	4.3	34.0	11.0	0.5
BGTY, Sainsbury's*	1 Pot/90g	140	2.4	156	4.5	28.3	2.7	0.3
Choc & Mascarpone, Tiramigu, Gu*	1 Pud/90g	316	23.3	351	3.3	26.1	25.9	1.0
COU, M & S*	1 Tub/95g	138	2.6	145	3.7	26.9	2.7	0.6
Family Size, Tesco*	1 Serving/125g	356	18.1	285	4.3	34.5	14.5	4.3
Italian, Co-Op*	1 Pack/90g	229	9.0	255	5.0	37.0	10.0	0.4
Light Choices, Tesco*	1 Pot/90g	162	3.5	180	7.7	27.6	3.9	2.4
Raspberry, M & S*	1 Serving/84g	197	12.1	235	3.8	22.9	14.4	0.2
Sainsbury's*	1 Serving/100g	263	10.0	263	4.4	40.2	10.0	0.1
Single Size, Tesco*	1 Pot/100g	290	12.9	290	3.8	35.1	12.9	4.5
Waitrose*	1 Pot/90g	221	11.2	246	6.4	27.2	12.4	0.0
TOAD IN THE HOLE								
Average	1 Serving/231g	640	40.2	277	11.9	19.5	17.4	1.1
Vegetarian, Aunt Bessie's*	1 Pack/190g	502	19.4	264	15.6	27.5	10.2	2.7
Vegetarian, Linda McCartney*	1 Pack/190g	359	16.7	189	13.6	13.9	8.8	1.1
Vegetarian, Meat Free, Asda*	1 Serving/173g	407	19.0	235	9.0	25.0	11.0	3.1
Vegetarian, Tryton Foods*	1oz/28g	73	4.0	262	14.8	18.6	14.2	1.6
TOFFEE APPLE								
Average	1 Apple/141g	188	3.0	133	1.2	29.2	2.1	2.3
TOFFEE CRISP								
Biscuit, Nestle*	1 Original/44g	228	12.1	519	3.7	62.8	27.6	1.4
TOFFEES								
Assorted, Bassett's*	1 Toffee/8g	35	1.1	434	3.8	73.1	14.0	0.0
Assorted, Sainsbury's*	1 Sweet/8g	37	1.3	457	2.2	76.5	15.8	0.2
Brazil Nut, Diabetic, Thorntons*	1 Serving/20g	93	7.0	467	3.2	49.0	35.1	0.5
Chewy, Werther's*	1 Toffee/5g	22	0.8	436	3.5	71.3	15.2	0.1
Chocolate Coated, Thorntons*	1 Bag/100g	521	30.7	521	3.5	57.9	30.7	0.3
Dairy, Waitrose*	1 Toffee/14g	64	2.0	458	2.0	80.2	14.3	0.5
Devon Butter, Thorntons*	1 Sweet/9g	40	1.5	444	1.7	72.2	16.7	0.0
English Butter, Co-Op*	1 Toffee/8g	38	1.6	470	2.0	71.0	20.0	0.0
Liquorice, Thorntons*	1 Bag/100g	506	29.4	506	1.9	58.8	29.4	0.0
Milk Chocolate Smothered, Thorntons*	1 Pack/125g	655	38.5	524	4.3	57.5	30.8	1.1
Mixed, Average	1oz/28g	119	5.2	426	2.2	66.7	18.6	0.0
No Added Sugar, Boots*	1 Serving/7g	23	1.0	324	1.3	52.0	14.0	0.0
Original, Hard Candies, Sugar Free, Werther's*	1 Pack/90g	260	7.9	289	0.2	86.8	8.8	0.1
Original, Thorntons*	1 Bag/100g	514	30.1	514	1.8	59.3	30.1	0.0
Squares, No Added Sugar, Russell Stover*	1 Piece/15g	57	3.9	380	6.0	49.3	26.0	1.3
TOFU								
Average	*1 Pack/250g*	*297*	*16.5*	*119*	*13.4*	*1.4*	*6.6*	*0.1*

T

	Measure INFO/WEIGHT	per Measure KCAL	FAT	Nutrition Values per 100g / 100ml KCAL	PROT	CARB	FAT	FIBRE
TOFU								
Beech Smoked, Organic, Cauldron Foods*	½ Pack/110g	124	7.8	113	10.9	1.0	7.1	0.5
Pieces, Marinated, Organic, Cauldron Foods*	1 Pack/160g	363	27.2	227	17.5	1.0	17.0	2.7
Smoked, Organic, Evernat*	1oz/28g	36	1.8	127	16.3	0.8	6.6	0.0
TOMATILLOS								
Raw	*1 Med/34g*	*11*	*0.3*	*32*	*1.0*	*5.8*	*1.0*	*1.9*
TOMATO PASTE								
Average	*1 Tbsp/20g*	*19*	*0.0*	*96*	*4.9*	*19.2*	*0.2*	*1.5*
Sun Dried, Average	*1 Tsp/10g*	*38*	*3.5*	*385*	*3.2*	*13.8*	*35.1*	*0.0*
TOMATO PUREE								
Average	*1oz/28g*	*21*	*0.1*	*76*	*4.5*	*14.1*	*0.2*	*2.3*
Sun Dried, & Olive Oil & Herbs, GIA*	1 Serving/20g	41	4.3	204	2.6	0.5	21.6	0.0
TOMATOES								
Cherry, Average	*1 Serving/80g*	*15*	*0.2*	*19*	*0.9*	*3.3*	*0.3*	*1.0*
Cherry, on the Vine, Average	*1 Serving/80g*	*14*	*0.3*	*18*	*0.7*	*3.1*	*0.3*	*1.0*
Cherry, Raw	*1oz/28g*	*5*	*0.1*	*18*	*0.8*	*3.0*	*0.4*	*1.0*
Chopped, Canned, Branded Average	*1 Serving/130g*	*27*	*0.2*	*21*	*1.1*	*3.8*	*0.1*	*0.8*
Chopped, Canned, Cirio*	½ Can/200g	54	0.4	27	1.1	4.2	0.2	1.1
Chopped, Italian, Average	*½ Can/200g*	*47*	*0.2*	*23*	*1.3*	*4.4*	*0.1*	*0.9*
Chopped, Italian, with Olive Oil & Garlic, Waitrose*	1 Serving/100g	33	1.6	33	1.1	3.6	1.6	0.0
Chopped, Italian, with Olives, Waitrose*	1 Can/400g	184	7.2	46	1.4	6.0	1.8	0.8
Chopped, with Chilli, Sainsbury's*	½ Can/200g	44	1.0	22	1.0	3.5	0.5	0.9
Chopped, with Chilli & Peppers, Asda*	1 Pack/400g	92	1.2	23	1.0	4.0	0.3	0.0
Chopped, with Garlic, Average	*½ Can/200g*	*43*	*0.3*	*21*	*1.2*	*3.8*	*0.1*	*0.8*
Chopped, with Herbs, Average	*½ Can/200g*	*42*	*0.3*	*21*	*1.1*	*3.8*	*0.1*	*0.8*
Chopped, with Olive Oil & Roasted Garlic, Sainsbury's*	1 Pack/390g	187	8.2	48	1.3	5.9	2.1	1.0
Chopped, with Onion & Herbs, Napolina*	1 Can/400g	84	0.4	21	1.0	4.0	0.1	0.4
Chopped, with Onions, Italian, Tesco*	½ Can/200g	46	0.4	23	1.4	4.0	0.2	0.9
Chopped, with Peppers & Onions, Sainsbury's*	½ Can/200g	40	0.2	20	1.2	3.5	0.1	0.9
Creamed, Sainsbury's*	1oz/28g	6	0.0	22	1.5	5.0	0.1	1.6
Fresh, Raw, Average	*1 Med/123g*	*22*	*0.2*	*18*	*0.9*	*3.9*	*0.2*	*1.2*
Fried in Blended Oil	1 Med/85g	77	6.5	91	0.7	5.0	7.7	1.3
Green Tiger, Raw, M & S*	1 Serving/80g	16	0.2	20	0.7	3.1	0.3	1.0
Grilled, Average	1oz/28g	14	0.3	49	2.0	8.9	0.9	2.9
Plum, Baby, Average	*1 Serving/50g*	*9*	*0.2*	*18*	*1.5*	*2.3*	*0.3*	*1.0*
Plum, in Tomato Juice, Average	*1 Can/400g*	*71*	*0.4*	*18*	*0.9*	*3.3*	*0.1*	*0.7*
Plum, in Tomato Juice, Premium, Average	*1 Can/400g*	*93*	*1.2*	*23*	*1.3*	*3.8*	*0.3*	*0.7*
Ripened on the Vine, Average	*1 Med/123g*	*22*	*0.4*	*18*	*0.7*	*3.0*	*0.3*	*0.7*
San Marzano, TTD, Sainsbury's*	½ Can/200g	34	0.2	17	0.9	3.1	0.1	2.9
Stuffed with Rice Based Filling, Average	1oz/28g	59	3.8	212	2.1	22.2	13.4	1.1
Sun Dried, Average	*3 Pieces/20g*	*43*	*3.2*	*213*	*4.7*	*12.9*	*15.9*	*3.3*
Sun Dried, with Herbs & Extra Virgin Olive Oil, Waitrose*	1 Serving/50g	72	5.2	145	3.4	9.1	10.5	7.1
Sun Dried in Oil	100g	301	24.8	301	5.8	13.5	24.8	7.0
TONGUE								
Lunch, Average	*1oz/28g*	*51*	*3.0*	*181*	*20.1*	*1.8*	*10.6*	*0.0*
Slices, Average	*1oz/28g*	*56*	*3.9*	*201*	*18.7*	*0.0*	*14.0*	*0.0*
TONIC WATER								
Average	1 Glass/250ml	82	0.0	33	0.0	8.8	0.0	0.0
Diet, Asda*	1 Glass/200ml	2	0.0	1	0.0	0.0	0.0	0.0
Indian, Diet, Schweppes*	1 Glass/100ml	1	0.0	1	0.0	0.0	0.0	0.0
Indian, Fever-Tree*	1 Bottle/200ml	76	0.0	38	0.0	9.0	0.0	0.0
Indian, Sainsbury's*	1 Can/150ml	46	0.0	31	0.0	7.4	0.0	0.0
Indian, Schweppes*	1 Serving/500ml	110	0.0	22	0.0	5.1	0.0	0.0
Indian, Slimline, Schweppes*	1 Serving/188ml	3	0.0	2	0.4	0.0	0.0	0.0

T

	Measure INFO/WEIGHT	per Measure KCAL	per Measure FAT	Nutrition Values per 100g / 100ml KCAL	PROT	CARB	FAT	FIBRE
TONIC WATER								
Indian, Sugar Free, Essential, Waitrose*	1 Serving/50ml	1	0.0	2	0.0	0.0	0.0	0.0
Indian, with a Hint of Lemon, Low Calorie, Asda*	1 Serving/300ml	3	0.3	1	0.0	0.0	0.1	0.0
Indian with Lime, Low Calorie, Tesco*	1 Glass/250ml	5	0.0	2	0.0	0.0	0.0	0.0
Light, Royal Club*	1 Glass/250ml	2	0.0	1	0.0	0.0	0.0	0.0
Low Calorie, Indian, Co-Op*	1 100ml/100ml	2	0.0	2	0.0	0.0	0.0	0.0
Low Calorie, Tesco*	1 Serving/200ml	4	0.0	2	0.0	0.5	0.0	0.0
M & S*	1 Bottle/500ml	100	0.0	20	0.0	4.8	0.0	0.0
Quinine, Schweppes*	1 Glass/125ml	46	0.0	37	0.0	9.0	0.0	0.0
Soda Stream*	1 Glass/100ml	15	0.0	15	0.0	3.2	0.0	0.0
TONIC WINE								
Original, Sanatogen*	1 Bottle/700ml	889	0.0	127	0.0	124.4	0.0	0.0
TOPIC								
Mars*	1 Bar/47g	234	12.3	498	6.2	59.6	26.2	1.7
TORTE								
Chocolate, Half Fat, Waitrose*	1/6 Torte/70g	135	4.1	193	5.4	29.7	5.8	2.2
Chocolate, Mint, Weight Watchers*	1 Pot/88g	174	4.1	198	4.7	34.3	4.7	5.2
Chocolate, Tesco*	1 Serving/50g	125	5.9	251	3.6	32.3	11.9	1.0
Chocolate & Pecan Brownie, Gu*	1/6 Torte/67g	292	17.7	436	5.3	45.1	26.4	3.1
Chocolate Fondant, Gu*	1/8 Torte/63g	264	18.9	423	5.7	32.0	30.2	1.8
Chocolate Orange & Almond, Gu*	1 Serving/65g	273	19.8	420	5.0	28.2	30.5	2.7
Chocolate Truffle, Waitrose*	1 Serving/116g	359	20.1	309	4.6	30.1	17.3	1.4
Fruit Mix, Apricot, Graze*	1 Pack/45g	137	3.4	305	3.3	59.5	7.6	3.2
Lemon, Tesco*	1 Serving/62g	142	6.1	230	2.3	32.9	9.9	0.5
Lemon & Mango, Waitrose*	1 Serving/80g	142	2.4	177	3.9	33.6	3.0	0.6
Raspberry, BGTY, Sainsbury's*	1 Serving/100g	154	3.9	154	2.6	27.0	3.9	1.2
TORTELLINI								
3 Cheese, Sainsbury's*	1 Serving/50g	195	4.3	391	14.4	63.8	8.7	3.0
Aubergine & Pecorino, Sainsbury's*	½ Pack/150g	354	6.4	236	8.9	40.3	4.3	3.2
Beef & Red Wine, Italian, Asda*	½ Pack/150g	242	4.2	161	9.0	25.0	2.8	0.0
Beef & Red Wine, Italiano, Tesco*	1 Serving/150g	324	4.8	216	11.7	35.3	3.2	3.3
Beef Bolognese, Rich, Italian, Giovanni Rana*	½ Pack/125g	222	9.0	178	7.6	20.6	7.2	4.1
Cheese, Fresh, Sainsbury's*	½ Pack/180g	329	9.0	183	7.6	26.8	5.0	1.7
Cheese, Tomato & Basil, Tesco*	1 Serving/150g	387	8.1	258	13.0	39.5	5.4	3.3
Cheese, Weight Watchers*	1 Can/395g	245	6.3	62	2.3	9.7	1.6	0.4
Cheese & Ham, Italiano, Tesco*	½ Pack/150g	396	12.3	264	12.8	34.8	8.2	3.0
Chicken, Spicy, Big Eat, Heinz*	1 Pot/350g	404	23.1	115	2.9	11.2	6.6	0.4
Four Cheese, Italian, Asda*	1 Serving/150g	295	7.5	197	8.0	30.0	5.0	3.4
Four Cheese, Tesco*	½ Pack/150g	405	11.8	270	12.3	37.3	7.9	3.4
Four Cheese & Tomato, Italian, Asda*	1 Serving/150g	249	5.7	166	8.0	25.0	3.8	0.0
Four Cheese with Tomato & Basil Sauce, Tesco*	1 Pack/400g	500	14.8	125	6.1	16.9	3.7	0.6
Garlic, Basil & Ricotta, Asda*	½ Pack/175g	318	10.5	182	6.0	26.0	6.0	2.6
Garlic & Herb, Fresh, Sainsbury's*	½ Pack/150g	364	11.7	243	11.1	32.2	7.8	1.8
Ham & Cheese, Fresh, Asda*	½ Pack/150g	255	9.0	170	6.0	23.0	6.0	1.7
Ham & Cheese, Tesco*	1 Serving/225g	578	12.6	257	13.5	38.1	5.6	1.8
Italian, Diet Chef Ltd*	1 Pack/300g	234	1.5	78	2.3	16.0	0.5	0.2
Meat, Italian, Tesco*	1 Serving/125g	332	9.5	266	10.6	38.9	7.6	2.3
Mozzarella & Tomato, Fresh, Asda*	1oz/28g	46	1.1	166	8.0	25.0	3.8	0.0
Mushroom, Asda*	1 Serving/125g	217	5.2	174	6.0	28.0	4.2	2.3
Mushroom, BGTY, Sainsbury's*	½ Can/200g	180	6.2	90	2.2	13.2	3.1	0.7
Mushroom, Perfectly Balanced, Waitrose*	1 Pack/250g	572	9.0	229	9.4	39.8	3.6	2.4
Pepperoni, Italian, Asda*	½ Pack/150g	250	6.0	167	6.7	26.0	4.0	0.0
Pesto & Goats Cheese, Fresh, Sainsbury's*	½ Pack/150g	310	12.1	207	8.9	24.6	8.1	2.6
Pork & Beef, BGTY, Sainsbury's*	½ Can/200g	148	3.0	74	3.7	11.2	1.5	0.6

T

	Measure INFO/WEIGHT	per Measure KCAL	FAT	Nutrition Values per 100g / 100ml KCAL	PROT	CARB	FAT	FIBRE
TORTELLINI								
Ricotta & Spinach, Giovanni Rana*	½ Pack/125g	340	13.6	272	10.1	34.6	10.9	10.0
Sausage & Ham, Italiano, Tesco*	1 Pack/300g	816	27.9	272	13.1	34.0	9.3	3.7
Smoked Bacon & Tomato, Asda*	1 Pack/300g	591	15.0	197	9.0	29.0	5.0	0.0
Smoked Ham & Cheese, Ready Meals, Waitrose*	1oz/28g	73	1.7	261	12.9	38.7	6.1	1.3
Spicy Pepperoni, Asda*	½ Pack/150g	252	6.0	168	7.0	26.0	4.0	0.0
Spicy Pepperoni, Fresh, Asda*	½ Pack/150g	249	6.0	166	7.0	26.0	4.0	0.0
Spinach & Ricotta, Italian, Asda*	½ Pack/150g	189	3.6	126	5.0	21.0	2.4	0.6
Spinach & Ricotta, Pasta Reale*	½ Pack/125g	319	5.2	255	11.2	45.5	4.2	2.6
Spinach & Ricotta, Sainsbury's*	1oz/28g	109	2.4	388	15.0	62.5	8.7	2.2
Spinach & Ricotta, Verdi, Asda*	1 Serving/125g	186	5.6	149	6.0	21.0	4.5	2.4
Tomato & Mozzarella, Fresh, Asda*	½ Pack/150g	235	4.2	157	8.0	25.0	2.8	0.0
Tomato & Mozzarella, Fresh, Sainsbury's*	½ Pack/150g	291	12.0	194	7.5	23.0	8.0	3.4
Trio, Fresh, Tesco*	½ Pack/125g	322	8.9	258	12.8	35.8	7.1	2.0
with Tomato, Basil, & Paprika, Easy Cook, Napolina*	1 Pack/120g	481	14.5	401	12.4	60.7	12.1	0.0
TORTELLONI								
Arrabbiata, Sainsbury's*	½ Pack/210g	407	11.8	194	7.1	28.8	5.6	2.6
Basil, Mozzarella & Tomato, Weight Watchers*	½ Pack/125g	278	3.4	222	9.0	40.5	2.7	4.8
Beef & Chianti, TTD, Sainsbury's*	½ Pack/125g	300	8.0	240	11.3	34.3	6.4	1.9
Bell Pepper & Sundried Tomato, Morrisons*	½ Pack/150g	375	6.5	250	12.1	40.7	4.3	2.9
Cheese, Garlic & Herb, Co-Op*	1 Serving/125g	331	7.5	265	10.0	43.0	6.0	0.0
Cheese, Tomato, & Basil, Sainsbury's*	½ Pack/150g	271	9.7	181	8.0	22.7	6.5	1.7
Cheese & Smoked Ham, Tesco*	½ Pack/150g	315	10.6	210	8.9	26.5	7.1	1.7
Cheese & Smoked Ham, Waitrose*	1 Serving/250g	625	17.0	250	11.5	35.8	6.8	1.8
Chicken & Bacon, Italiano, Tesco*	1 Pack/300g	660	21.9	220	7.8	29.8	7.3	2.1
Chicken & Ham, Morrisons*	1 Serving/150g	366	5.8	244	12.3	38.6	3.9	2.4
Chorizo & Tomato, Morrisons*	1 Serving/150g	447	12.9	298	12.8	45.1	8.6	2.6
Five Cheese, Sainsbury's*	1 Serving/125g	285	11.6	228	10.8	25.2	9.3	2.9
Four Cheese, Asda*	½ Pack/150g	312	13.0	208	7.6	24.9	8.7	1.6
Four Cheese, Express, Dolmio*	1 Pack/220g	411	16.7	187	7.6	22.1	7.6	0.0
Four Cheese, Tesco*	1 Serving/200g	390	13.4	195	8.0	25.5	6.7	1.8
Four Cheese, Waitrose*	½ Pack/125g	297	8.4	238	10.3	34.2	6.7	1.6
Fresh, Ham & Cheese, Asda*	½ Pack/150g	315	11.4	210	8.8	26.7	7.6	1.4
Fresh, Morrisons*	1 Serving/150g	430	14.5	287	11.2	41.0	9.7	2.4
Garlic & Herb, Cooked, Pasta Reale*	1 Pack/300g	546	11.7	182	6.7	30.1	3.9	0.9
Goats Cheese & Red Pepper, Morrisons*	1 Pack/150g	450	16.6	300	11.5	38.4	11.1	3.8
Italian Style Sausage & Red Wine, Morrisons*	½ Pack/150g	420	10.8	280	11.1	45.5	7.2	2.7
Meat, Italian, Asda*	½ Pack/150g	265	6.7	177	7.0	27.0	4.5	2.4
Meat & Cheese, Fresh, Sainsbury's*	½ Pack/125g	304	10.5	243	13.5	28.3	8.4	2.6
Mushroom, Perfectly Balanced, Waitrose*	½ Pack/125g	300	4.0	240	10.9	41.8	3.2	2.2
Olive & Ricotta, Sainsbury's*	½ Pack/175g	403	18.4	230	8.8	25.1	10.5	2.3
Pasta, Fresh, Cream Cheese, Garlic & Herb, Morrisons*	1 Serving/150g	400	9.0	267	10.3	46.1	6.0	3.2
Pesto, Italian, Tesco*	1 Pack/300g	885	33.9	295	10.7	36.7	11.3	3.0
Pesto, Light Choices, Tesco*	½ Pack/150g	277	8.7	185	6.5	26.5	5.8	2.0
Ricotta & Basil, Asda*	½ Pack/150g	322	12.9	215	9.2	25.1	8.6	1.6
Ricotta & Tender Spinach, Cooked, Giovanni Rana*	½ Pack/190g	376	12.3	198	7.8	27.0	6.5	3.1
Sausage, Spicy, Italian, Asda*	½ Pack/150g	339	11.7	226	7.4	31.6	7.8	1.5
Sausage & Ham, Italiano, Tesco*	1 Serving/150g	285	10.5	190	8.5	22.5	7.0	1.8
Sicilian Style & Tuna, Morrisons*	½ Pack/150g	397	8.8	265	12.1	43.0	5.9	2.3
Smoked Ham, Bacon & Tomato, Tesco*	½ Packet/150g	450	17.5	300	12.0	35.7	11.7	2.5
Spicy Red Pepper & Tomato, Pasta Reale*	½ Pack/125g	310	5.5	248	10.0	42.0	4.4	3.3
Spinach & Ricotta, Chilled, Italiano, Tesco*	½ Pack/150g	412	12.7	275	10.4	38.1	8.5	3.3
Spinach & Ricotta, Fresh, Waitrose*	½ Pack/125g	327	8.7	262	11.3	38.4	7.0	2.4
Spinach & Ricotta, Sainsbury's*	½ Pack/150g	325	10.8	217	7.8	30.2	7.2	2.4

	Measure INFO/WEIGHT	per Measure		Nutrition Values per 100g / 100ml				
		KCAL	FAT	KCAL	PROT	CARB	FAT	FIBRE
TORTELLONI								
Spinach & Ricotta Cheese, Co-Op*	½ Pack/126g	315	6.3	250	10.0	41.0	5.0	4.0
Tomato & Mozzarella, Sainsbury's*	1 Serving/175g	339	14.0	194	7.5	23.0	8.0	3.4
Walnut & Gorgonzola, Fresh, Sainsbury's*	½ Pack/210g	414	12.2	197	8.4	27.8	5.8	2.4
Wild Mushroom, Italian, Sainsbury's*	½ Pack/150g	309	12.3	206	7.7	25.4	8.2	2.3
Wild Mushroom, Italian, Tesco*	1 Pack/300g	645	24.0	215	6.5	28.5	8.0	2.5
TORTIGLIONI								
Dry, Average	*1 Serving/75g*	*266*	*1.4*	*355*	*12.5*	*72.2*	*1.9*	*2.1*
TORTILLA CHIPS								
Blazing BBQ, Sainsbury's*	1 Serving/50g	237	11.7	474	6.8	58.9	23.5	4.6
Blue, Organic, Sainsbury's*	1 Serving/50g	252	11.7	504	7.7	65.8	23.4	5.6
Chilli, Organic, Evernat*	1oz/28g	137	6.2	490	8.0	65.0	22.0	0.0
Classic Mexican, Phileas Fogg*	1 Serving/35g	162	6.7	464	5.9	67.2	19.1	3.8
Cool, Salted, Sainsbury's*	1 Serving/50g	253	13.6	506	6.5	58.6	27.3	4.3
Cool, Tesco*	1 Serving/40g	190	9.9	474	6.3	56.7	24.7	7.8
Cool Flavour, Sainsbury's*	1 Serving/50g	231	9.3	463	5.7	68.1	18.7	3.7
Easy Cheesy!, Sainsbury's*	1 Serving/50g	249	13.0	498	7.1	58.7	26.1	4.5
Hot Chilli Flavour, Weight Watchers*	1 Bag/18g	83	3.3	461	4.6	67.7	18.2	4.2
Lightly Salted, M & S*	1 Serving/20g	98	4.8	490	7.2	61.5	24.1	4.5
Lightly Salted, Tesco*	1 Serving/50g	247	13.8	495	4.8	56.8	27.6	7.5
Lightly Salted, Waitrose*	1 Serving/40g	187	8.6	468	7.1	61.2	21.6	6.5
Mexicana Cheddar, Kettle Chips*	1 Serving/50g	249	13.3	498	7.9	56.7	26.6	5.1
Nacho Cheese Flavour, M & S*	1 Serving/30g	144	6.7	480	7.5	62.0	22.4	4.2
Nacho Cheese Flavour, Mexican Style, Co-Op*	1 Serving/50g	247	13.5	495	7.0	58.0	27.0	4.0
Nacho Cheese Flavour, Weight Watchers*	1 Pack/18g	83	3.3	459	5.2	66.6	18.2	4.1
Nachos Kit, Asda*	1 Serving/100g	448	24.0	448	7.0	51.0	24.0	0.7
Plain	1 Serving/100g	486	21.1	486	6.8	62.0	21.1	4.2
Salsa, Asda*	1 Serving/25g	122	6.0	488	6.0	62.0	24.0	6.0
Salsa, M & S*	½ Bag/75g	364	18.8	485	5.7	59.1	25.1	6.1
Slightly Salted, Organic, Sainsbury's*	1 Serving/50g	226	6.6	453	10.0	73.3	13.3	13.3
Taco, Tesco*	1 Serving/50g	247	12.7	495	7.4	59.3	25.4	4.4
TORTILLAS								
Ancient Grain, Wrap, Blue Menu*	1 Tortilla/34g	100	2.0	294	8.8	50.0	5.9	5.9
Corn, Gluten Free, Discovery*	1 Tortilla/22g	53	0.5	243	5.4	53.8	2.3	3.8
Corn, Soft, Old El Paso*	1 Tortilla/38g	129	2.6	343	10.0	60.0	7.0	0.0
Flour, 10 Pack, Asda*	1 Tortilla/30g	94	2.1	315	9.0	54.0	7.0	2.5
Flour, American Style, Sainsbury's*	1 Tortilla/35g	108	2.4	313	8.6	53.9	7.0	2.5
Flour, Mexican Style, Morrisons*	1 Tortilla/33g	103	2.3	313	8.6	53.9	7.0	2.5
Flour, Salsa, Old El Paso*	1 Tortilla/41g	132	3.7	323	9.0	52.0	9.0	0.0
Flour, Soft, Chilli & Jalapeno, Discovery*	1 Tortilla/40g	131	5.2	328	7.8	44.8	13.1	2.2
Flour, Soft, Discovery*	1 Tortilla/40g	119	2.8	298	8.0	49.6	7.1	2.4
Flour, Soft, Garlic & Coriander, Discovery*	1 Tortilla/40g	116	2.4	289	8.1	50.6	6.0	1.7
Flour, Tex "N" Mex 12, Sainsbury's*	1 Tortilla/26g	85	2.5	326	8.6	53.9	9.6	2.5
Made with Wheat Flour	1oz/28g	73	0.3	262	7.2	59.7	1.0	2.4
Plain, Morrisons*	1 Serving/35g	92	0.9	263	8.5	51.2	2.7	2.5
Plain, Wraps, Tesco*	1 Tortilla/64g	192	3.8	300	8.4	52.2	5.9	2.7
White, Wraps, M & S*	1 Tortilla/64g	170	2.4	265	7.9	49.0	3.8	1.6
Wholewheat, Asda*	1 Tortilla/35g	88	2.7	252	9.8	35.7	7.8	7.1
Wrap, 8 Pack, Light Choices, Tesco*	1 Tortilla/68g	180	1.9	265	8.5	50.7	2.8	3.4
Wrap, Bueno*	1 Tortilla/63g	171	3.6	272	6.9	48.2	5.7	2.0
Wrap, Flour, Soft, Old El Paso*	1 Tortilla/58g	200	7.2	343	9.3	48.6	12.4	1.7
Wrap, Garlic & Parsley, Sainsbury's*	1 Tortilla/60g	166	3.7	277	7.2	48.0	6.2	1.8
Wrap, Low Carb, Tesco*	1 Tortilla/17g	77	1.5	453	39.4	53.5	8.8	23.5
Wrap, Low Fat, M & S*	1 Serving/180g	225	4.0	125	6.3	20.6	2.2	1.9

T

	Measure INFO/WEIGHT	per Measure		Nutrition Values per 100g / 100ml				
		KCAL	FAT	KCAL	PROT	CARB	FAT	FIBRE
TORTILLAS								
Wrap, Organic, Sainsbury's*	1 Tortilla/56g	167	4.3	298	8.6	48.7	7.7	2.1
Wrap, Organic, Tesco*	1 Tortilla/57g	173	4.4	306	8.1	51.0	7.7	2.0
Wrap, Plain, Mini, Morrisons*	1 Tortilla/34g	91	1.4	267	8.1	48.9	4.0	2.8
Wrap, Tomato & Herb, Tesco*	1 Serving/63g	165	3.5	262	7.9	45.1	5.5	2.1
Wrap, Tomato & Herbs, Sainsbury's*	1 Tortilla/52g	157	3.1	302	7.8	54.1	6.0	2.4
Wrap, Weight Watchers*	1 Wrap/42g	98	0.6	233	7.6	43.6	1.5	7.3
TREACLE								
Black, Average	**1 Tbsp/20g**	**51**	**0.0**	**257**	**1.2**	**67.2**	**0.0**	**0.0**
TRIFLE								
Average	1 Portion/170g	272	10.7	160	3.6	22.3	6.3	0.5
Banana & Mandarin, Co-Op*	¼ Trifle/125g	237	13.7	190	2.0	21.0	11.0	0.1
Black Forest, Asda*	1 Serving/100g	237	9.0	237	3.1	36.0	9.0	0.0
Blackforest, BGTY, Sainsbury's*	1 Pot/125g	171	5.6	137	2.1	21.9	4.5	1.6
Caramel, Galaxy, Mars*	1 Pot/100g	255	13.0	255	4.5	30.0	13.0	1.0
Cherry, Finest, Tesco*	¼ Trifle/163g	340	19.3	209	2.6	22.9	11.9	0.3
Chocolate, Asda*	1 Serving/125g	272	16.3	217	4.1	21.0	13.0	0.5
Chocolate, BGTY, Sainsbury's*	1 Pot/100g	137	2.7	137	4.8	23.4	2.7	1.6
Chocolate, Cadbury*	1 Pot/100g	282	18.5	282	5.2	24.3	18.5	0.0
Chocolate, HL, Tesco*	1 Serving/150g	189	4.0	126	4.0	21.4	2.7	4.6
Chocolate, Light, Cadbury*	1 Pot/90g	166	6.7	185	5.5	23.4	7.5	0.0
Chocolate, Tesco*	1 Serving/125g	312	19.0	250	4.3	24.0	15.2	0.7
Cream Mandarin, GFY, Asda*	1 Serving/113g	151	5.0	134	1.6	27.0	4.4	0.2
Fruit, Sainsbury's*	1 Serving/125g	232	12.5	186	2.3	21.7	10.0	0.3
Fruit Cocktail, COU, M & S*	1 Trifle/140g	175	3.2	125	2.8	23.1	2.3	0.5
Fruit Cocktail, Individual, Shape, Danone*	1 Trifle/115g	136	3.1	118	3.2	19.6	2.7	1.6
Fruit Cocktail, Individual, Tesco*	1 Pot/113g	175	8.8	155	1.7	19.6	7.8	0.6
Fruit Cocktail, Low Fat, Danone*	1 Pot/115g	140	2.1	122	2.2	24.0	1.8	0.4
Fruit Cocktail, Luxury Devonshire, St Ivel*	1 Trifle/125g	211	9.9	169	1.9	22.6	7.9	0.2
Fruit Cocktail, M & S*	1 Serving/165g	272	13.7	165	2.4	19.6	8.3	0.9
Fruit Cocktail, Sainsbury's*	1 Trifle/150g	241	9.0	161	1.8	24.8	6.0	0.4
Mango & Passion Fruit, Danone*	1oz/28g	50	1.4	177	2.6	30.7	4.9	0.4
Peach & Zabaglione, COU, M & S*	1 Glass/130g	149	3.0	115	2.8	20.6	2.3	0.8
Raspberry, Asda*	1 Serving/100g	175	8.0	175	1.8	24.0	8.0	0.1
Raspberry, Co-Op*	1 Trifle/125g	206	10.0	165	2.0	22.0	8.0	0.3
Raspberry, Sainsbury's*	1 Pot/125g	204	9.7	163	1.7	21.5	7.8	0.6
Raspberry, Tesco*	1 Pot/150g	210	9.7	140	1.7	18.5	6.5	1.0
Sainsbury's*	1 Serving/133g	215	10.0	162	2.4	20.1	7.5	0.3
Sherry, BGTY, Sainsbury's*	1 Pot/135g	146	2.3	108	3.0	20.2	1.7	0.5
Strawberry, BGTY, Sainsbury's*	1 Pot/125g	135	2.6	108	2.4	19.9	2.1	0.5
Strawberry, Co-Op*	1 Serving/123g	234	13.5	190	2.0	21.0	11.0	0.2
Strawberry, COU, M & S*	1 Pot/138g	145	2.9	105	2.7	19.2	2.1	1.2
Strawberry, Individual, Shape, Danone*	1 Pot/115g	137	3.1	119	3.3	19.8	2.7	1.6
Strawberry, Individual, Waitrose*	1 Pot/150g	205	8.5	137	1.8	19.7	5.7	1.0
Strawberry, Low Fat, Shape, Danone*	1oz/28g	38	0.9	137	3.8	22.8	3.1	1.8
Strawberry, Low Fat Goodies, Danone*	1 Pot/115g	148	2.1	129	2.2	26.0	1.8	0.3
Strawberry, Luxury Devonshire, St Ivel*	1 Trifle/125g	207	9.9	166	2.0	21.7	7.9	0.2
Strawberry, Sainsbury's*	¼ Tub/150g	261	15.4	174	2.2	18.1	10.3	1.0
Strawberry, St Ivel*	1 Trifle/113g	194	9.8	172	2.4	21.0	8.7	0.2
Strawberry, Tesco*	1 Trifle/605	998	55.7	165	1.5	19.1	9.2	0.8
Summerfruit, BGTY, Sainsbury's*	1 Trifle/125g	151	5.5	121	1.2	19.2	4.4	0.5
TRIFLE MIX								
Strawberry Flavour, Bird's*	1oz/28g	119	2.9	425	2.7	78.0	10.5	1.2

	Measure INFO/WEIGHT	per Measure KCAL	FAT	Nutrition Values per 100g / 100ml KCAL	PROT	CARB	FAT	FIBRE
TRIFLE SPONGES								
Sainsbury's*	1 Sponge/24g	77	0.4	323	5.3	71.9	1.6	1.1
Tesco*	1 Sponge/24g	75	0.6	311	5.3	66.6	2.6	1.1
TRIPE &								
Onions, Stewed	1oz/28g	26	0.8	93	8.3	9.5	2.7	0.7
TROMPRETTI								
Fresh, Waitrose*	1 Serving/125g	339	3.0	271	11.7	50.6	2.4	2.0
Tricolour, Fresh, Tesco*	1 Pack/250g	675	8.5	270	11.2	48.6	3.4	4.0
TROUT								
Brown, Steamed, Average	*1 Serving/120g*	*162*	*5.4*	*135*	*23.5*	*0.0*	*4.5*	*0.0*
Fillets, Scottish, Hot Smoked, TTD, Sainsbury's*	½ Pack/63g	85	3.4	136	20.8	1.0	5.4	0.5
Fillets, Skinless, Chunky, TTD, Sainsbury's*	½ Pack/123g	227	13.0	185	22.4	0.1	10.6	0.6
Grilled, Weighed with Bones & Skin	1 Serving/100g	98	3.9	98	15.7	0.0	3.9	0.0
Rainbow, Fillets, with Thyme & Lemon Butter, Asda*	1 Serving/147g	210	10.3	143	20.0	0.9	7.0	0.5
Rainbow, Grilled, Average	*1 Serving/120g*	*162*	*6.5*	*135*	*21.5*	*0.0*	*5.4*	*0.0*
Rainbow, Raw, Average	*1oz/28g*	*36*	*1.4*	*127*	*20.5*	*0.0*	*5.1*	*0.0*
Rainbow, Smoked, Average	*1 Pack/135g*	*190*	*7.6*	*140*	*21.7*	*0.7*	*5.6*	*0.0*
Raw, Average	*1 Serving/120g*	*159*	*6.5*	*132*	*20.6*	*0.0*	*5.4*	*0.0*
Smoked, Average	*2 Fillets/135g*	*187*	*7.1*	*138*	*22.7*	*0.3*	*5.2*	*0.1*
TUMS								
Extra 750, Sugar Free, Tums*	2 Tablets/2g	5	0.0	250	0.0	50.0	0.0	0.0
Extra 750, Tums*	2 Tablets/2g	10	0.0	500	0.0	100.0	0.0	0.0
Regular, Tums*	1 Tablet/2g	2	0.0	125	0.0	25.0	0.0	0.0
Smoothies, Extra Strength 750, Tums*	2 Tablets/2g	10	0.0	500	0.0	100.0	0.0	0.0
TUNA								
Albacore, in Olive Oil, TTD, Sainsbury's*	1 Serving/80g	162	8.7	203	26.1	0.0	10.9	0.0
Bluefin, Cooked, Dry Heat, Average	*1 Serving/100g*	*184*	*6.3*	*184*	*29.9*	*0.0*	*6.3*	*0.0*
Chunks, in Brine, Average, Drained	*1 Can /130g*	*141*	*0.7*	*108*	*25.9*	*0.0*	*0.5*	*0.0*
Chunks, in Brine, Drained, Value, Morrisons*	1 Can/120g	122	0.6	102	23.1	1.0	0.5	0.0
Chunks, in Brine, Princes*	1oz/28g	29	0.1	105	25.0	0.0	0.5	0.0
Chunks, in Spring Water, Average, Drained	*1 Can /130g*	*140*	*0.8*	*108*	*25.4*	*0.0*	*0.6*	*0.1*
Chunks, in Sunflower Oil, Average, Drained	*1 Can/138g*	*260*	*12.6*	*188*	*26.5*	*0.0*	*9.1*	*0.0*
Chunks, in Sunflower Oil, No Drain, 120g, John West*	1 Can/120g	202	9.1	168	25.0	0.0	7.6	0.0
Chunks, in Sunflower Oil, No Drain, 60g, John West*	1 Can/60g	136	9.5	226	21.0	0.0	15.8	0.0
Chunks, Skipjack, in Brine, Average	*1 Can/138g*	*141*	*0.8*	*102*	*24.3*	*0.0*	*0.6*	*0.0*
Chunks, with a Little Brine, No Drain, 120g, John West*	1 Can/120g	130	1.1	108	25.0	0.0	0.9	0.0
Chunks, with a Little Brine, No Drain, 60g, John West*	1 Can/60g	55	0.5	91	21.0	0.0	0.8	0.0
Coronation, BGTY, Sainsbury's*	1 Can/80g	90	2.1	112	16.5	5.7	2.6	1.0
Coronation Style, Canned, Average	1 Can/80g	122	7.6	152	10.2	6.5	9.5	0.6
Fillets, in Tomato Sauce, Princes*	1 Can/120g	131	3.0	109	19.0	2.5	2.5	0.0
Flakes, in Brine, Average	*1oz/28g*	*29*	*0.2*	*104*	*24.7*	*0.0*	*0.5*	*0.0*
Flakes, with Tomato & Onion, Mermaid Bay*	I Can/85g	93	2.5	110	16.1	4.7	2.9	0.5
French Style, Light Lunch, John West*	1 Pack/240g	204	6.5	85	8.3	6.7	2.7	1.2
in a Light Lemon Mayonnaise, Slimming World, Princes*	1 Can/80g	99	3.8	124	16.8	3.5	4.8	0.0
in a Light Mayonnaise. Slimming World, Princes*	1 Can/80g	96	3.3	120	17.3	3.6	4.1	0.0
in a Red Chilli & Lime Dressing, Princes*	1 Sachet/85g	102	2.8	120	21.5	1.0	3.3	0.0
in a Tikka Dressing, Slimming World, Princes*	1 Can/80g	108	4.6	135	16.8	4.0	5.7	0.0
in Thousand Island Dressing, John West*	1 Can/185g	287	12.9	155	18.0	5.1	7.0	0.2
In Thousand Island Dressing, Weight Watchers*	1 Can/79g	67	1.7	85	8.3	7.8	2.2	0.4
in Water, Average	*1 Serving/120g*	*126*	*1.0*	*105*	*24.0*	*0.1*	*0.8*	*0.0*
Lemon Pepper Flavour, Sensations, Sealord*	1 Can/95g	212	13.8	223	18.5	4.9	14.5	0.0
Light Lunch, Indian Style, John West*	1 Pack/240g	401	23.0	167	7.7	12.3	9.6	0.6
Light Lunch, Mediterranean Style, John West*	1 Pack/240g	218	6.0	91	7.9	9.3	2.5	1.7
Light Lunch, Nicoise Style, John West*	1 Pack/250g	245	5.7	98	10.3	9.0	2.3	2.7

	Measure INFO/WEIGHT	per Measure		Nutrition Values per 100g / 100ml				
		KCAL	FAT	KCAL	PROT	CARB	FAT	FIBRE
TUNA								
Light Lunch, Tomato Salsa Style, John West*	1 Pack/250g	195	3.0	78	7.1	9.7	1.2	1.9
Lime & Black Pepper, John West*	1 Serving/85g	133	7.8	156	15.6	2.8	9.2	0.0
Puertorican Style, Tinned, Natura*	1 Can/185g	157	8.3	85	9.0	1.0	4.5	0.0
Steak, Control Chef, All About Weight*	1 Meal/270g	284	4.3	105	9.8	10.9	1.6	3.9
Steaks, Chargrilled, Italian, Sainsbury's*	1 Serving/125g	199	8.0	159	25.1	0.2	6.4	0.5
Steaks, in Brine, Average	*1 Sm Can/99g*	*106*	*0.5*	*107*	*25.6*	*0.0*	*0.5*	*0.0*
Steaks, in Cajun Marinade, Sainsbury's*	1 Steak/100g	141	2.4	141	29.8	0.0	2.4	0.0
Steaks, in Olive Oil, Average	*1 Serving/111g*	*211*	*10.7*	*190*	*25.8*	*0.0*	*9.6*	*0.0*
Steaks, in Oriental Sauce, Good Choice, Iceland*	1 Pack/260g	333	1.8	128	22.3	8.1	0.7	0.4
Steaks, in Sunflower Oil, Average	*1 Can/150g*	*276*	*12.9*	*184*	*26.7*	*0.0*	*8.6*	*0.0*
Steaks, in Water, Average	*1 Serving/200g*	*215*	*0.8*	*107*	*25.6*	*0.0*	*0.4*	*0.0*
Steaks, John West*	1 Can/130g	140	0.4	108	26.2	0.0	0.3	0.0
Steaks, Lemon & Herb Marinade, Seared, Sainsbury's*	½ Pack/119g	191	8.8	161	23.4	0.1	7.4	0.0
Steaks, Marinated, Sainsbury's*	1 Serving/100g	153	5.3	153	25.1	1.3	5.3	0.5
Steaks, Raw, Average	*1 Serving/140g*	*185*	*2.8*	*132*	*28.5*	*0.1*	*2.0*	*0.2*
Steaks, Skipjack, in Brine, Average	*½ Can/75g*	*73*	*0.4*	*97*	*23.2*	*0.0*	*0.5*	*0.0*
Steaks, Thai Style Butter, Tesco*	1 Serving/110g	191	9.1	174	24.7	0.0	8.3	0.0
Steaks, with a Little Brine, No Drain, John West*	1 Can/130g	140	0.4	108	26.2	0.0	0.3	0.0
Steaks, with a Little Olive Oil, No Drain, John West*	1 Can/130g	209	7.0	161	28.2	0.0	5.4	0.0
Steaks, with Lime & Coriander Dressing, Tesco*	1 Serving/150g	156	0.6	104	21.6	3.6	0.4	0.6
Steaks, with Sweet Red Pepper Glaze, Sainsbury's*	1 Steak/100g	135	0.1	135	28.5	5.0	0.1	0.1
Yellowfin, Cooked, Dry Heat, Average	*1 Serving/100g*	*139*	*1.2*	*139*	*30.0*	*0.0*	*1.2*	*0.0*
TUNA MAYONNAISE								
& Sweetcorn, Canned, BGTY, Sainsbury's*	1 Can/80g	78	1.8	97	15.2	4.0	2.3	0.7
Garlic & Herb, John West*	½ Can/92g	243	20.4	264	12.0	4.0	22.2	0.2
Light, Slimming World*	1 Serving/80g	96	3.3	120	17.3	3.6	4.1	0.0
with Sweetcorn, From Heinz, Weight Watchers*	1 Can/80g	114	6.3	142	11.5	6.2	7.9	0.1
with Sweetcorn, John West*	½ Can/92g	231	19.0	251	12.0	4.5	20.6	0.2
with Sweetcorn & Green Peppers, GFY, Asda*	1 Pack/100g	103	3.0	103	14.0	5.0	3.0	0.8
TURBOT								
Grilled	*1oz/28g*	*34*	*1.0*	*122*	*22.7*	*0.0*	*3.5*	*0.0*
Raw	*1oz/28g*	*27*	*0.8*	*95*	*17.7*	*0.0*	*2.7*	*0.0*
TURKEY								
Breast, Butter Basted, Average	*1 Serving/75g*	*110*	*3.6*	*146*	*23.7*	*1.9*	*4.9*	*0.4*
Breast, Canned, Average	*1 Can/200g*	*194*	*4.7*	*97*	*18.3*	*0.7*	*2.3*	*0.0*
Breast, Diced, Healthy Range, Average	*1oz/28g*	*30*	*0.4*	*107*	*23.8*	*0.0*	*1.3*	*0.0*
Breast, Honey Roast, Sliced, Average	*1 Serving/50g*	*57*	*0.7*	*114*	*24.0*	*1.6*	*1.3*	*0.2*
Breast, Joint, Raw, Average	*1 Serving/125g*	*134*	*2.6*	*107*	*21.3*	*0.7*	*2.1*	*0.6*
Breast, Raw, Average	*1oz/28g*	*33*	*0.6*	*117*	*24.1*	*0.5*	*2.0*	*0.1*
Breast, Roasted, Average	*1oz/28g*	*37*	*0.9*	*131*	*24.6*	*0.7*	*3.3*	*0.1*
Breast, Roll, Cooked, Average	*1 Slice/10g*	*9*	*0.1*	*92*	*17.6*	*3.5*	*0.8*	*0.0*
Breast, Slices, Cooked, Average	*1 Slice/20g*	*23*	*0.3*	*114*	*24.0*	*1.2*	*1.4*	*0.3*
Breast, Smoked, Sliced, Average	*1 Slice/20g*	*23*	*0.4*	*113*	*23.4*	*0.7*	*1.9*	*0.0*
Breast, Steaks, in Crumbs, Average	1 Steak/76g	217	14.1	286	13.7	16.4	18.5	0.2
Breast, Steaks, Raw, Average	*1oz/28g*	*30*	*0.3*	*107*	*24.3*	*0.0*	*1.1*	*0.0*
Breast, Steaks, Thai, Bernard Matthews*	1 Serving/175g	280	4.7	160	29.4	4.6	2.7	0.0
Breast, Strips, Chinese Style, Sainsbury's*	¼ Pack/163g	318	7.3	196	26.4	12.5	4.5	0.5
Breast, Strips, for Stir Fry, Average	*1 Serving/175g*	*205*	*2.7*	*117*	*25.6*	*0.1*	*1.6*	*0.0*
Breast, Stuffed, Just Roast, Sainsbury's*	1 Serving/100g	155	6.6	155	21.1	2.9	6.6	0.6
Dark Meat, Raw, Average	*1oz/28g*	*29*	*0.7*	*104*	*20.4*	*0.0*	*2.5*	*0.0*
Dark Meat, Roasted, Average	*1oz/28g*	*50*	*1.8*	*177*	*29.4*	*0.0*	*6.6*	*0.0*
Drummers, Golden, Bernard Matthews*	1 Drummer/57g	147	10.3	258	13.1	11.0	18.0	1.1
Drummers, Golden, Grilled, Bernard Matthews*	1 Drummer/50g	147	10.6	294	15.6	10.0	21.2	1.0

T

	Measure INFO/WEIGHT	per Measure KCAL	FAT	Nutrition Values per 100g / 100ml KCAL	PROT	CARB	FAT	FIBRE
TURKEY								
Drumsticks, Tesco*	1 Serving/200g	272	12.6	136	19.9	0.0	6.3	0.0
Escalope, Average	*1 Piece/138g*	*341*	*19.3*	*247*	*13.5*	*16.7*	*14.0*	*0.6*
Escalope, Creamy Pepper Topped, Tesco*	1 Piece/165g	337	17.7	204	11.5	15.3	10.7	1.7
Escalope, Lemon & Pepper, Average	1 Piece/143g	371	22.6	259	12.6	16.7	15.8	0.4
Escalope, Spicy Mango, Bernard Matthews*	1 Piece/136g	354	17.4	260	11.6	24.6	12.8	0.0
Escalope, Tomato & Herb, Bernard Matthews*	1 Piece/143g	336	19.2	236	10.5	18.0	13.5	0.0
Fillets, Chinese Marinated, Bernard Matthews*	1 Pack/200g	304	6.6	152	23.4	7.2	3.3	0.0
Goujons, Cooked, Bernard Matthews*	4 Goujons/128g	355	23.3	277	11.8	16.6	18.2	1.1
Light Meat, Raw, Average	*1oz/28g*	*29*	*0.2*	*105*	*24.4*	*0.0*	*0.8*	*0.0*
Light Meat, Roasted	*1 Cup/140g*	*220*	*4.5*	*157*	*29.9*	*0.0*	*3.2*	*0.0*
Medallions, Tomato Salsa, Morrisons*	½ Pack/125g	184	3.1	147	30.4	0.8	2.5	0.9
Mince, Average	*1oz/28g*	*45*	*2.0*	*161*	*23.9*	*0.0*	*7.2*	*0.0*
Mince, Lean, Healthy Range, Average	*1oz/28g*	*33*	*1.1*	*118*	*20.3*	*0.0*	*4.1*	*0.0*
Rashers, Average	*1 Rasher/26g*	*26*	*0.4*	*101*	*19.1*	*2.3*	*1.6*	*0.0*
Rashers, Smoked, Average	*1 Serving/75g*	*76*	*1.3*	*101*	*19.8*	*1.5*	*1.8*	*0.0*
Roast, Meat & Skin, Average	*1oz/28g*	*48*	*1.8*	*171*	*28.0*	*0.0*	*6.5*	*0.0*
Roast, Meat Only, Average	*1 Serving/100g*	*157*	*3.2*	*157*	*29.9*	*0.0*	*3.2*	*0.0*
Roast, Sugar Marinade, Slices, M & S*	½ Pack/120g	156	1.9	130	29.0	0.2	1.6	0.5
Roast, Wafer Thin, Tesco*	1 Slice/8g	8	0.2	105	20.0	1.5	2.0	0.0
Roll, Dinosaur, Cooked, Bernard Matthews*	1 Slice/10g	17	1.0	170	13.6	6.0	10.2	1.1
Steaks, Breaded, Bernard Matthews*	1 Steak/110g	319	20.0	290	11.0	20.5	18.2	1.5
Sticks, Honey Roast, Mini, Tesco*	1 Serving/90g	101	1.7	112	20.0	3.6	1.9	0.0
Strips, Stir-Fried, Average	1oz/28g	46	1.3	164	31.0	0.0	4.5	0.0
Thigh, Diced, Average	*1oz/28g*	*33*	*1.2*	*117*	*19.6*	*0.0*	*4.3*	*0.0*
Wafer Thin, Cooked, Average	1 Slice/10g	12	0.4	122	19.0	3.2	3.7	0.0
Wafer Thin, Honey Roast, Average	1 Slice/10g	11	0.2	109	19.2	4.2	1.7	0.2
Wafer Thin, Smoked, Average	1 Slice/10g	12	0.4	119	18.1	3.6	3.7	0.0
Whole, Raw, Average	*½ Joint/254g*	*389*	*16.8*	*153*	*22.5*	*0.8*	*6.6*	*0.0*
TURKEY DINNER								
Roast, Asda*	1 Pack/400g	344	6.4	86	7.0	11.0	1.6	2.0
Roast, Iceland*	1 Meal/400g	374	7.2	93	8.4	10.9	1.8	1.3
Roast, Meal for One, M & S*	1 Pack/370g	462	16.3	125	9.1	12.4	4.4	2.7
Roast, Sainsbury's*	1 Pack/450g	354	9.0	79	6.8	8.4	2.0	1.9
Traditional, Birds Eye*	1 Pack/340g	292	7.8	86	6.1	10.3	2.3	1.7
TURKEY HAM								
Average	*1 Serving/75g*	*81*	*2.9*	*108*	*15.6*	*2.8*	*3.9*	*0.0*
TURKISH DELIGHT								
Assorted Flavours, Julian Graves*	1 Square/30g	110	0.0	366	0.5	91.1	0.1	0.0
Co-Op*	1 Bar/53g	207	4.2	390	2.0	78.0	8.0	0.1
Dark Chocolate Covered, Thorntons*	1 Chocolate/10g	39	1.1	390	2.7	69.0	11.0	2.0
Fry's*	1 Bar/51g	186	3.7	365	2.0	73.3	7.2	0.0
Milk Chocolate, M & S*	1 Pack/55g	220	4.7	400	1.6	79.0	8.5	0.0
Sultans*	1 Serving/16g	58	0.0	360	0.0	90.0	0.0	0.0
with Mixed Nuts, Hazer Baba*	1 Piece/12g	47	0.2	389	1.6	88.5	1.7	0.0
with Rose, Hazer Baba*	1 Square/18g	70	0.3	389	1.6	88.6	1.7	0.0
TURMERIC								
Powder	*1 Tsp/3g*	*11*	*0.3*	*354*	*7.8*	*58.2*	*9.9*	*0.0*
TURNIP								
Boiled, Average	*1oz/28g*	*3*	*0.1*	*12*	*0.6*	*2.0*	*0.2*	*1.9*
Mash, Direct Foods*	½ Pack/190g	49	3.4	26	0.6	2.0	1.8	1.9
Raw, Unprepared, Average	*1oz/28g*	*6*	*0.1*	*23*	*0.9*	*4.7*	*0.3*	*2.4*
TURNOVER								
Apple, Bramley, Tesco*	1 Turnover/88g	304	22.8	346	2.7	25.4	25.9	0.9

T

	Measure INFO/WEIGHT	per Measure KCAL	FAT	Nutrition Values per 100g / 100ml KCAL	PROT	CARB	FAT	FIBRE
TURNOVER								
Apple, Co-Op*	1 Turnover/77g	308	20.8	400	4.0	35.0	27.0	1.0
Apple, Dutch, Sainsbury's*	1 Serving/33g	130	5.5	393	3.6	56.9	16.8	1.4
Apple, Fresh Cream, Sainsbury's*	1 Turnover/84g	292	20.9	347	4.1	26.9	24.8	2.5
Apple, Tesco*	1 Turnover/88g	294	19.7	334	3.2	29.8	22.4	0.9
Mincemeat, Fresh Cream, Tesco*	1 Turnover/83g	334	22.2	405	3.1	37.5	26.9	1.1
Raspberry, Fresh Cream, Asda*	1 Turnover/100g	411	23.0	411	6.0	45.0	23.0	2.1
Raspberry, Tesco*	1 Turnover/84g	290	20.2	345	4.0	27.2	24.1	2.1
TWIGLETS								
Curry, Jacob's*	1 Bag/30g	134	6.4	448	8.0	55.7	21.5	6.0
Original, Jacob's*	1 Bag/30g	115	3.5	383	12.7	57.0	11.6	11.8
Tangy, Jacob's*	1 Bag/30g	136	6.6	454	8.1	55.9	22.0	5.4
TWIRL								
Cadbury*	1 Finger/22g	118	6.8	535	7.6	56.0	30.9	0.8
Treat Size, Cadbury*	1 Bar/21g	115	6.6	535	7.6	56.0	30.9	0.8
TWIRLS								
Prawn Cocktail, Bobby's*	1 Pack/26g	116	4.8	445	3.4	65.9	18.6	0.0
Salt & Vinegar, Co-Op*	1 Bag/40g	170	8.0	425	5.0	57.5	20.0	5.0
Salt & Vinegar, Sainsbury's*	½ Bag/40g	167	5.6	418	3.0	70.1	14.0	3.0
Salt & Vinegar, Tesco*	1 Bag/80g	349	14.0	436	3.9	65.8	17.5	2.4
TWISTS								
Black Olive & Basil, Finest, Tesco*	¼ Pack/31g	151	7.9	483	11.3	53.1	25.1	3.9
Gruyere & Poppy Seed, TTD, Sainsbury's*	1 Serving/8g	41	2.3	509	13.7	50.5	28.0	2.6
Parmesan, All Butter, TTD, Sainsbury's*	1 Serving/8g	38	2.0	487	13.8	51.0	25.3	2.8
Strawberry, Sainsbury's*	1 Serving/10g	37	0.3	375	1.7	82.7	3.0	0.1
Tomato & Herb, Shapers, Boots*	1 Pack/20g	94	4.2	468	3.7	66.0	21.0	3.9
TWIX								
Fun Size, Mars*	1 Bar/21g	103	5.0	492	4.7	65.5	23.7	1.5
Standard, Mars*	1 Pack/58g	284	13.7	490	4.7	65.5	23.7	1.5
Top, Mars*	1 Bar/28g	143	7.8	511	5.2	60.2	27.7	0.0
Twixels, Mars*	1 Finger/6g	31	1.6	513	5.0	64.0	26.1	0.0
Xtra, Mars*	1 Pack/85g	416	20.1	490	4.7	65.5	23.7	1.5
TZATZIKI								
Average	1 Serving/50g	33	2.4	66	3.7	2.0	4.9	0.2

T

	Measure INFO/WEIGHT	per Measure KCAL	FAT	Nutrition Values per 100g / 100ml KCAL	PROT	CARB	FAT	FIBRE
VANILLA								
Bean, Average	*1 Pod/2g*	*6*	*0.0*	*288*	*0.0*	*13.0*	*0.0*	*0.0*
Flavouring, Supercook*	1 Tsp/4g	2	0.0	50	6.2	0.0	0.0	0.0
VANILLA EXTRACT								
Average	*1 Tbsp/13g*	*37*	*0.0*	*288*	*0.1*	*12.6*	*0.1*	*0.0*
VEAL								
Chop, Loin, Raw, Weighed with Bone, Average	1 Chop/195g	495	27.8	254	29.5	0.0	14.3	0.0
Escalope, Fried, Average	1oz/28g	55	1.9	196	33.7	0.0	6.8	0.0
Escalopes, Breaded, M & S*	1 Piece/130g	292	13.9	225	13.6	18.7	10.7	0.4
Mince, Raw, Average	*1oz/28g*	*40*	*2.0*	*144*	*20.3*	*0.0*	*7.0*	*0.0*
Shoulder, Lean & Fat, Roasted, Average	*1oz/28g*	*52*	*2.3*	*183*	*25.5*	*0.0*	*8.2*	*0.0*
Shoulder, Lean Only, Roasted, Average	*1oz/28g*	*46*	*1.6*	*164*	*26.1*	*0.0*	*5.8*	*0.0*
Sirloin, Lean & Fat, Roasted, Average	*1oz/28g*	*57*	*3.0*	*202*	*25.1*	*0.0*	*10.4*	*0.0*
Sirloin, Lean Only, Roasted, Average	*1oz/28g*	*48*	*1.8*	*168*	*26.3*	*0.0*	*6.2*	*0.0*
VEGEMITE								
Australian, Kraft*	1 Tsp/5g	9	0.0	173	23.5	19.7	0.0	0.0
VEGETABLE CHIPS								
Beetroot, Carrot & Parsnips, Hand Fried, Tyrrells*	½ Pack/25g	103	7.0	413	3.9	36.0	28.1	11.5
Cassava, Average	1oz/28g	99	0.1	353	1.8	91.4	0.4	4.0
Mixed Root, Tyrrells*	1oz/28g	133	8.3	476	5.7	35.4	29.8	12.8
Parsnip, Golden, Kettle Chips*	½ Pack/50g	257	18.8	515	4.6	39.5	37.6	8.4
Sweet Potato, Kettle Chips*	½ Pack/50g	241	16.4	483	2.4	44.4	32.8	9.3
VEGETABLE FAT								
Pure, Trex*	1 Tbsp/12g	108	12.0	900	0.0	0.0	100.0	0.0
VEGETABLE FINGERS								
Crispy, Birds Eye*	2 Fingers/60g	107	4.8	179	3.2	23.5	8.0	2.3
Crispy Crunchy, Dalepak*	1 Finger/28g	62	3.1	223	4.2	26.7	11.0	15.0
Sweetcorn, Tesco*	1 Finger/28g	66	3.5	236	7.7	23.0	12.6	3.0
VEGETABLE MEDLEY								
Asparagus Tips, Perfectly Balanced, Waitrose*	1 Serving/225g	121	7.6	54	1.3	4.6	3.4	1.4
Basil & Oregano Butter, Waitrose*	1 Serving/113g	59	3.8	52	1.7	3.7	3.4	1.9
Buttered, Sainsbury's*	½ Pack/175g	122	6.8	70	1.7	7.0	3.9	1.8
Carrot, Courgette, Fine Bean & Baby Corn, Tesco*	1 Serving/100g	36	2.4	36	1.1	2.4	2.4	3.0
Crunchy, M & S*	1 Pack/250g	75	2.0	30	3.1	2.8	0.8	2.5
Frozen, M & S*	1 Pack/500g	175	4.0	35	3.4	3.9	0.8	3.1
Green, HL, Tesco*	1 Serving/125g	59	2.2	47	3.7	4.1	1.8	4.1
Green, M & S*	1 Serving/250g	62	1.2	25	3.0	1.8	0.5	1.8
Green, Sainsbury's*	1 Pack/220g	178	14.3	81	3.0	2.5	6.5	2.9
HL, Tesco*	1 Serving/100g	23	1.2	23	0.8	2.3	1.2	1.3
Roast, Four Seasons*	1 Pack/375g	202	12.0	54	2.8	3.5	3.2	2.7
Roasted, Waitrose*	½ Pack/200g	282	15.6	141	1.2	16.4	7.8	3.7
with Herby Butter, M & S*	1 Pack/300g	225	15.0	75	1.5	6.2	5.0	2.6
VEGETABLE SELECTION								
Chefs, M & S*	1 Pack/250g	87	1.2	35	2.6	4.5	0.5	2.9
Five, Sainsbury's*	½ Pack/125g	42	1.0	34	2.6	4.3	0.8	3.1
Fresh, Finest, Tesco*	1 Pack/250g	182	14.5	73	1.9	3.2	5.8	2.2
Garden, Tesco*	1 Pack/275g	124	9.1	45	1.2	2.7	3.3	1.2
Lightly Buttered & Seasoned, M & S*	1 Pack/300g	195	10.8	65	1.6	6.3	3.6	2.8
Oriental with Soy Dressing, Sainsbury's*	1 Serving/100g	44	0.8	44	2.0	5.5	0.8	3.3
Ready to Cook, Morrisons*	1 Serving/150g	51	0.9	34	2.4	4.8	0.6	2.3
Roast, COU, M & S*	1 Serving/250g	95	2.0	38	1.2	6.1	0.8	0.6
Winter, M & S*	1 Bag/400g	80	0.0	20	2.2	3.2	0.0	3.1
with Chilli & Garlic Dressing, Finest, Tesco*	1 Serving/250g	257	12.2	103	2.0	12.8	4.9	1.0
with Herb Butter, Waitrose*	1 Pack/300g	270	16.8	90	1.9	8.1	5.6	2.1

V

VEGETABLES

	Measure INFO/WEIGHT	per Measure KCAL	FAT	Nutrition Values per 100g / 100ml KCAL	PROT	CARB	FAT	FIBRE
Asparagus & Tenderstem Broccoli, Finest, Tesco*	½ Pack/95g	28	0.4	29	3.7	2.7	0.4	2.7
Baby, Frozen, Asda*	1 Serving/100g	25	0.3	25	1.9	3.7	0.3	1.9
Baby Mix, Freshly Frozen, Iceland*	1 Serving/100g	26	0.3	26	1.8	3.9	0.3	1.9
Bean & Vegetable Layer, M & S*	1 Pack/285g	271	13.7	95	3.6	7.2	4.8	3.7
Broccoli & Cauliflower, Layered, M & S*	½ Pack/135g	94	4.6	70	1.5	7.6	3.4	1.2
Butternut Squash, Broccoli & Spinach, M & S*	½ Pack/138g	55	0.7	40	2.7	4.5	0.5	2.3
Carrot, Broccoli & Cauliflower, Organic, Sainsbury's*	1 Serving/250g	62	1.5	25	1.9	3.0	0.6	2.2
Carrot & Sprouts, Microwaved, Fresh Tastes, Asda*	1 Pack/300g	150	0.9	50	1.9	8.7	0.3	2.3
Carrots, Peas & Sweetcorn, Steam, Tesco*	½ Pack/150g	150	4.2	100	3.4	15.0	2.8	3.2
Casserole, Cooks' Ingredients, Waitrose*	¼ Pack/125g	37	0.4	30	1.0	5.9	0.3	4.0
Casserole, Mixed, Co-Op*	1 Serving/100g	40	0.3	40	1.2	7.5	0.3	2.1
Chargrilled with Tomato Sauce, GFY, Asda*	1 Serving/260g	164	7.3	63	1.4	8.0	2.8	0.0
Chinese Glazed, Tesco*	1 Pack/200g	110	4.4	55	1.3	7.7	2.2	1.2
Chinese Inspired, Crisp, M & S*	1 Pack/250g	62	0.7	25	1.7	4.6	0.3	1.9
Classic Layered, M & S*	1 Pack/320g	224	12.5	70	1.2	7.3	3.9	1.2
Crisp & Crunchy, Stir Fry, M & S*	½ Pack/115g	29	0.2	25	1.9	3.9	0.2	1.7
Crispy, Ready to Cook, Sainsbury's*	1 Serving/100g	24	0.3	24	1.8	3.6	0.3	2.2
Farmhouse Mix, Frozen, Asda*	1 Serving/100g	25	0.8	25	2.5	2.2	0.8	0.0
Favourite Five Selection, M & S*	½ Pack/125g	25	0.7	20	1.8	2.4	0.6	2.9
for Roasting, M & S*	½ Pack/224g	190	12.5	85	1.2	7.7	5.6	2.4
Garden, Washed, Tesco*	1 Bag/250g	65	1.7	26	3.0	1.9	0.7	2.0
Green, Minted, Love Life, Waitrose*	1 Pack/265g	154	6.9	58	3.0	4.1	2.6	3.2
Green Medley, Microwaved, Chosen By You, Asda*	1 Pack/220g	132	3.3	60	3.8	6.8	1.5	2.2
Grilled, Frozen, Sainsbury's*	1 Serving/80g	42	2.9	52	1.2	3.8	3.6	1.5
Italiano Marinated, Roasted, Tesco*	½ Tub/100g	121	8.6	121	1.7	9.2	8.6	0.8
Julienne, Tesco*	1 Serving/100g	30	0.3	30	1.1	5.7	0.3	1.9
Kale, Spinach, Pak Choi & Jagallo Nero, Asda*	¼ Bag/45g	13	0.5	29	2.4	1.0	1.1	2.8
Layered, GFY, Asda*	½ Pack/150g	81	4.2	54	1.2	6.0	2.8	2.0
Layered, Tesco*	1 Serving/280g	202	14.6	72	1.6	4.8	5.2	1.6
Layered, with Butter, Waitrose*	1 Pack/280g	207	16.2	74	1.7	3.6	5.8	2.4
Mediterranean, Ready to Roast, Sainsbury's*	½ Pack/182g	111	4.2	61	1.8	6.8	2.3	2.8
Mediterranean, Ready to Roast, Waitrose*	1 Serving/200g	128	8.0	64	1.3	5.6	4.0	1.6
Mediterranean, Sainsbury's*	1 Pack/400g	180	9.6	45	1.2	4.5	2.4	3.1
Mediterranean Roasted, Sainsbury's*	1 Serving/150g	118	5.4	79	2.2	9.5	3.6	3.4
Mediterranean Style, Asda*	½ Pack/205g	113	3.7	55	1.7	7.9	1.8	1.3
Mediterranean Style, COOK!, M & S*	½ Pack/200g	60	1.8	30	1.2	5.5	0.9	1.0
Mediterranean Style, Finest, Tesco*	½ Pack/150g	155	12.2	103	1.5	5.5	8.1	3.0
Mediterranean Style, M & S*	½ Pack/214g	75	1.9	35	1.2	5.5	0.9	1.0
Mexican Chilli Bean, Lovely Vegetables, M & S*	1 Pack/300g	270	6.9	90	2.9	11.6	2.3	4.6
Mixed, Frozen, Chosen By You, Asda*	1 Serving/80g	47	0.8	59	2.6	8.5	1.0	0.0
Mixed, Frozen, Sainsbury's*	1 Serving/100g	50	0.7	50	2.9	7.9	0.7	3.5
Mixed, Hacendado*	1 Jar/320g	147	1.0	46	2.0	0.2	0.3	0.0
Moroccan, COU, M & S*	1 Pack/300g	165	4.5	55	2.4	8.2	1.5	1.7
Oriental, Waitrose*	1 Pack/300g	108	0.6	36	0.8	7.8	0.2	1.4
Oriental Inspired, M & S*	1 Pack/260g	78	1.3	30	1.9	4.6	0.5	2.7
Oriental Stir Fry, Frozen, Sainsbury's*	½ Pack/225g	142	8.8	63	1.5	5.4	3.9	1.5
Ribbon, Pan Fry, Waitrose*	½ Pack/134g	47	0.5	35	1.3	5.4	0.4	2.4
Roast, M & S*	1 Pack/420g	273	17.6	65	1.4	4.9	4.2	0.4
Roasted, Italian, M & S*	1 Serving/95g	218	19.9	230	1.8	7.1	21.0	1.7
Roasted, Mediterranean, Tesco*	½ Pack/173g	95	3.1	55	1.3	7.6	1.8	2.0
Roasted, Selection, COU, M & S*	1 Pack/250g	87	2.0	35	1.2	6.1	0.8	0.6
Roasted Root, Extra Special, Asda*	½ Pack/205g	160	3.1	78	1.1	15.0	1.5	6.0
Roasted Winter, HL, Tesco*	½ Pack/200g	160	5.0	80	1.9	12.7	2.5	3.6

	Measure INFO/WEIGHT	per Measure KCAL	per Measure FAT	Nutrition Values per 100g / 100ml KCAL	PROT	CARB	FAT	FIBRE
VEGETABLES								
Roasting, Tesco*	1 Serving/350g	152	1.9	43	1.2	8.0	0.5	3.0
Root, Honey Roast, BGTY, Sainsbury's*	½ Pack/150g	174	2.2	116	2.5	23.1	1.5	5.5
Root, Honey Roast, Sainsbury's*	1 Pack/400g	748	34.8	187	0.0	25.8	8.7	5.2
Root, Ready to Roast, Sainsbury's*	½ Pack/200g	188	8.6	94	1.3	13.0	4.3	2.2
Seasonal, Pack, Sainsbury's*	1 Serving/261g	60	0.8	23	0.7	4.6	0.3	2.0
Soup Mix, Prepared, Tesco*	1/3 Pack/163g	51	1.0	31	1.1	5.3	0.6	2.8
Special Mix, Sainsbury's*	1 Serving/80g	54	1.4	68	3.4	9.7	1.7	3.2
Steam & Serve, Morrisons*	1 Serving/120g	66	1.3	55	2.4	8.8	1.1	2.6
Stir Fry, Frozen, Sainsbury's*	1 Serving/80g	19	0.2	24	1.3	3.9	0.3	2.0
Stir Fry, Tesco*	1 Serving/150g	37	0.1	25	0.9	5.0	0.1	1.4
Summer, Layered with Butter, Asda*	¼ Pack/80g	50	1.7	62	2.6	8.2	2.1	0.0
Summer, Rainbow, Roasting, Fresh Tastes, Asda*	½ Pack/175g	84	4.7	48	1.4	3.5	2.7	0.0
Summer, Roasting, Tesco*	½ Pack/175g	105	6.6	60	1.0	5.1	3.8	1.6
Sun Dried Tomato, Selection, Finest, Tesco*	1 Pack/340g	303	17.3	89	1.8	8.9	5.1	1.1
Sweet & Crunchy, Tesco*	1 Serving/50g	21	0.3	43	2.3	7.0	0.6	2.4
Szechuan Style, Ready Prepared, Waitrose*	1 Pack/300g	132	3.9	44	2.3	5.7	1.3	1.9
Tender, Green, Medley, Sainsbury's*	½ Pack/88g	35	0.5	40	3.6	5.1	0.6	3.3
Tender, Green, Selection, Waitrose*	½ Pack/140g	66	1.1	47	3.9	3.8	0.8	3.8
Tindora, Ivy Goud, Kovakkai, Dadoo's Market*	1 Serving/100g	27	0.1	27	0.0	5.2	0.1	0.0
Trivoglio, Peas, Potatoes & Carrots, Bonduelle*	½ Tin/200g	114	1.0	57	3.3	7.5	0.5	4.8
Vietnamese, Wok, Findus*	1 Serving/100g	25	0.5	25	1.5	4.5	0.5	0.0
Winter, Fresh, Asda*	1 Bag/250g	75	2.5	30	3.0	2.2	1.0	2.3
Winter, Ready to Roast, Fresh, Sainsbury's*	1 Pack/272g	226	7.6	83	1.2	13.2	2.8	0.0
Winter, Sainsbury's*	1 Serving/125g	37	1.0	30	2.0	3.6	0.8	2.2
Winter Crunchy, M & S*	½ Pack/125g	31	1.0	25	2.0	3.1	0.8	2.7
Winter Soup Mix, Sainsbury's*	1 Portion/149g	61	0.3	41	1.1	7.9	0.2	1.7
Wok, Chinese, Stir Fry, Classic, Findus*	1 Pack/500g	150	2.5	30	1.0	5.0	0.5	3.5
Wok, Sambal Oelek, Findus*	1 Serving/200g	170	0.8	85	3.0	17.0	0.4	0.0
Wok, Thai, Findus*	½ Pack/250g	87	0.7	35	1.5	7.0	0.3	0.0
Wok Mix, Stir Fry, Frozen, Essential, Waitrose*	1 Serving/200g	60	0.4	30	1.2	4.0	0.2	3.4
VEGETARIAN								
Chicken Style Pieces, Sainsbury's*	1 Pack/375g	754	26.2	201	25.5	9.0	7.0	0.6
Fingers, Fish Style, Breaded, The Redwood Co*	1 Finger/36g	94	5.2	262	16.5	16.0	14.5	0.0
Pepperoni Style, Cheatin', The Redwood Co*	1 Slice/10g	28	1.8	282	25.3	5.2	17.7	0.2
Roast, Chicken Style, Vegeroast, Realeat*	4 Slices/114g	211	10.2	186	23.0	3.2	9.0	1.5
Roast, Linda McCartney*	¼ Roast/114g	222	10.2	196	19.4	9.4	9.0	1.5
Slices, Sage & Onion, Vegi Deli, The Redwood Co*	1 Slice/10g	23	1.4	233	21.4	5.0	14.1	0.5
Slices, Vegetable, Tesco*	1 Slice/165g	452	30.5	274	5.6	21.4	18.5	3.3
VEGETARIAN MINCE								
Chicken Style Pieces, Realeat*	¼ Pack/88g	119	1.4	136	29.0	1.5	1.6	4.4
Easy Cook, Linda McCartney*	1oz/28g	35	0.1	126	21.4	9.3	0.4	1.7
Frozen, Meatfree, Improved Recipe, Sainsbury's*	1Pack/454g	799	31.8	176	18.3	10.7	7.0	6.7
Meat Free, Boiled, Chosen By You, Asda*	1 Serving/75g	83	2.5	111	13.7	6.7	3.3	4.4
Meat Free, Tesco*	1 Serving/76g	113	3.8	150	19.0	7.0	5.0	6.0
Vegemince, Realeat*	1 Serving/125g	217	12.5	174	18.0	3.0	10.0	3.0
VENISON								
Grill Steak, Average	*1 Steak/150g*	*178*	*3.7*	*119*	*19.0*	*5.0*	*2.5*	*0.9*
Minced, Cooked, Average	*1 Serving/100g*	*187*	*8.2*	*187*	*26.4*	*0.0*	*8.2*	*0.0*
Minced, Raw, Average	*1 Serving/100g*	*157*	*7.1*	*157*	*21.8*	*0.0*	*7.1*	*0.0*
Raw, Haunch, Meat Only, Average	1 Serving/100g	103	1.6	103	22.2	0.0	1.6	0.0
Roasted, Average	*1oz/28g*	*46*	*0.7*	*165*	*35.6*	*0.0*	*2.5*	*0.0*
Steak, Raw, Average	*1oz/28g*	*30*	*0.5*	*108*	*22.8*	*0.0*	*1.9*	*0.0*

V

	Measure INFO/WEIGHT	per Measure KCAL	FAT	Nutrition Values per 100g / 100ml KCAL	PROT	CARB	FAT	FIBRE
VERMICELLI								
Dry	*1oz/28g*	*99*	*0.1*	*355*	*8.7*	*78.3*	*0.4*	*0.0*
Egg, Cooked, Average	*1 Serving/185g*	*239*	*2.6*	*129*	*5.0*	*24.0*	*1.4*	*1.0*
VERMOUTH								
Dry	*1 Shot/50ml*	*54*	*0.0*	*109*	*0.1*	*3.0*	*0.0*	*0.0*
Sweet	*1 Shot/50ml*	*75*	*0.0*	*151*	*0.0*	*15.9*	*0.0*	*0.0*
VIMTO*								
Cordial, No Added Sugar, Diluted, Vimto Soft Drinks*	1 Glass/250ml	6	0.2	2	0.1	0.4	0.1	0.0
Cordial, Original, Diluted, Vimto Soft Drinks*	1 Glass/200ml	60	0.0	30	0.0	7.4	0.0	0.0
VINAIGRETTE								
Balsamic, Hellmann's*	1 Tbsp/15ml	12	0.4	82	0.1	9.6	2.7	0.6
Balsamic, Newman's Own*	1 Serving/20g	67	7.0	333	0.5	3.9	35.0	0.0
Balsamic Vinegar & Pistachio, Finest, Tesco*	1 Tbsp/15ml	55	5.9	370	0.2	2.8	39.2	0.0
Blush Wine, Briannas*	2 Tbsp/30ml	100	6.0	333	0.0	40.0	20.0	0.0
Fat Free, Hellmann's*	1 Serving/15ml	7	0.0	49	0.1	10.9	0.0	0.3
Frank Cooper*	1 Pot/28g	46	3.2	163	1.0	14.1	11.4	0.3
French, Real, Briannas*	2 Tbsp/30ml	150	17.0	500	0.0	0.0	56.7	0.0
French Style, Finest, Tesco*	1 Tbsp/15ml	93	9.8	620	0.6	6.3	65.3	0.2
Luxury French, Hellmann's*	1 Tsp/5ml	15	1.3	305	0.8	16.0	26.1	0.4
Olive Oil & Lemon, Amoy*	½ Sachet/15ml	37	3.6	250	0.3	3.0	24.0	0.0
Perfectly Balanced, Waitrose*	1 Tsp/5ml	4	0.0	89	0.4	20.9	0.4	0.5
Portuguese, Nando's*	1 Tbsp/15g	61	6.6	409	1.0	2.0	44.0	0.3
Waistline, 99% Fat Free, Crosse & Blackwell*	1 Tbsp/15ml	1	0.0	9	1.0	0.7	0.2	0.2
VINE LEAVES								
Preserved in Brine	*1oz/28g*	*4*	*0.0*	*15*	*3.6*	*0.2*	*0.0*	*0.0*
Stuffed, Mediterranean Deli, M & S*	1 Leaf/37g	39	1.5	105	2.6	14.2	4.1	1.2
Stuffed with Rice	1oz/28g	73	5.0	262	2.8	23.8	18.0	0.0
Stuffed with Rice & Mixed Herbs, Sainsbury's*	1 Leaf/37g	44	1.8	120	2.6	16.3	4.9	1.2
VINEGAR								
Apple Balsamic, Aspall*	1 Serving/100g	123	0.1	123	0.5	26.1	0.1	0.0
Balsamic, Average	*1 Tsp/5ml*	*4*	*0.0*	*88*	*0.5*	*17.0*	*0.0*	*0.0*
Cider	*1 Tbsp/15ml*	*2*	*0.0*	*14*	*0.0*	*5.9*	*0.0*	*0.0*
Cyder, Aspall*	1 fl oz/30ml	5	0.0	18	0.0	0.1	0.0	0.0
Malt, Average	*1 Tbsp/15g*	*1*	*0.0*	*4*	*0.4*	*0.6*	*0.0*	*0.0*
Red Wine, Average	1 Tbsp/15ml	3	0.0	19	0.0	0.3	0.0	0.0
Rice, Mizkan*	1 Tbsp/15ml	4	0.0	26	0.2	2.6	0.0	0.0
Rice, White, Amoy*	1 Tsp/5ml	0	0.0	4	0.0	1.0	0.0	0.0
VODKA								
37.5% Volume	*1 Shot/35ml*	*72*	*0.0*	*207*	*0.0*	*0.0*	*0.0*	*0.0*
40% Volume	*1 Shot/35ml*	*78*	*0.0*	*222*	*0.0*	*0.0*	*0.0*	*0.0*
VODKA &								
Tonic, Ready Mixed, M & S*	1 Can/250ml	202	0.0	81	0.0	6.3	0.0	0.0
VOL AU VENTS								
Broccoli, M & S*	1oz/28g	105	7.4	375	6.8	28.5	26.4	1.0
Chicken & Mushroom, M & S*	1oz/28g	98	6.8	350	7.7	25.2	24.3	2.1
Garlic Mushroom, Mini, Asda*	1 Serving/17g	59	4.6	347	5.0	21.0	27.0	0.0
Ham & Cheese, M & S*	1oz/28g	106	7.5	380	8.8	25.7	26.7	1.8
Mushroom, Sainsbury's*	1 Serving/14g	49	3.1	350	6.9	30.8	22.1	1.4
Mushroom & Roast Garlic, M & S*	1 Serving/19g	65	4.6	345	6.2	25.2	24.3	1.9
Prawn, M & S*	1oz/28g	101	6.9	360	8.0	26.2	24.7	1.9
Seafood, Party, Youngs*	1 Serving/17g	60	4.2	354	8.3	26.0	24.8	1.0
Tomato, M & S*	1oz/28g	87	5.7	310	4.5	26.7	20.4	1.7

V

	Measure INFO/WEIGHT	per Measure KCAL	per Measure FAT	Nutrition Values per 100g / 100ml KCAL	PROT	CARB	FAT	FIBRE
WAFERS								
Apricot & Peach, Highlights, Cadbury*	1 Wafer/19g	80	2.7	430	5.2	70.6	14.3	1.4
Cafe Curls, Rolled, Askeys*	1 Wafer/5g	21	0.4	422	5.8	80.3	8.6	0.0
Caramel, Dark Chocolate, Tunnock's*	1 Wafer/26g	128	6.6	492	5.2	60.7	25.4	0.0
Caramel, M & S*	1oz/28g	136	6.6	486	5.4	63.1	23.5	0.5
Caramel, Milk Chocolate, M & S*	1oz/28g	133	6.4	475	5.9	61.9	22.8	3.1
Caramel, Tunnock's*	1 Wafer/26g	116	4.5	448	3.6	69.2	17.4	2.5
Caramel Log, Tunnock's*	1 Wafer/32g	152	7.7	474	4.2	64.3	24.0	0.0
Cheese Footballs, Jacob's*	1 Serving/25g	137	9.1	549	10.5	44.5	36.6	1.7
Chocolate, Cadbury*	1oz/28g	147	8.3	526	7.0	61.2	29.8	0.0
Cream, Tunnock's*	1 Wafer/20g	103	5.6	513	6.6	63.2	28.0	0.0
Desiree, Assortment of, Hans Freitag*	4 Biscuits/29g	161	9.6	555	3.6	59.5	33.2	2.1
Filled, Average	1oz/28g	150	8.4	535	4.7	66.0	29.9	0.0
Florida Orange, Tunnock's*	1 Wafer/20g	104	5.8	519	5.1	64.0	29.0	0.0
for Ice Cream, Askeys*	1 Wafer/1.5g	6	0.0	388	11.4	79.0	2.9	0.0
Hazelnut, Elledi*	1 Wafer/8g	38	1.9	493	6.3	62.4	24.3	0.0
Lemon, Sugar Free, Wawel*	3 Biscuits/35g	170	11.0	486	11.4	51.4	31.4	1.4
Milk Chocolate, Sainsbury's*	1 Wafer/10g	51	2.7	506	6.2	60.5	26.7	1.4
Orange, Highlights, Cadbury*	1 Wafer/19g	80	2.7	430	5.2	70.6	14.3	1.4
WAFFLES								
Belgian, TTD, Sainsbury's*	1 Waffle/25g	122	7.3	490	6.0	50.6	29.3	1.2
Caramel, Asda*	1 Waffle/8g	37	1.8	459	3.3	62.0	22.0	1.1
Milk Chocolate, Tregroes*	1 Waffle/49g	220	20.5	450	4.5	57.0	42.0	0.5
Sweet, American Style, Sainsbury's*	1 Waffle/35g	160	8.9	457	7.2	50.6	25.3	1.1
Toasting, McVitie's*	1 Waffle/25g	118	6.3	474	6.0	52.6	25.5	0.6
Toffee, Tregroes, Aldi*	1 Waffle/35g	160	6.2	463	3.5	71.7	18.0	2.2
WAGON WHEEL								
Chocolate, Burton's*	1 Biscuit/39g	165	5.7	424	5.3	67.4	14.6	1.9
Jammie, Burton's*	1 Biscuit/40g	168	5.6	420	5.1	67.7	14.1	1.9
WALNUT WHIP								
Nestle*	1 Whip/35g	173	8.8	494	5.3	61.3	25.2	0.7
The, Classics, M & S*	1 Whip/26g	127	7.1	490	7.2	54.9	27.4	1.1
Vanilla, Nestle*	1 Whip/34g	165	8.4	486	5.7	60.5	24.6	0.0
WALNUTS								
Average	**6 Halves/20g**	**138**	**13.7**	**691**	**15.6**	**3.2**	**68.5**	**3.5**
Cocoa Cream, Dusted, Julian Graves*	1 Bag/200g	1124	70.6	562	8.2	52.9	35.3	2.0
Halves, Average	**1 Serving/25g**	**167**	**16.2**	**669**	**17.4**	**6.3**	**65.0**	**4.7**
WASABI								
Paste, Ready Mixed, Japanese, Yutaka*	1 Tsp/5g	14	0.3	286	2.7	53.0	7.0	0.0
WATER								
Berry Blast, Revive, Volvic*	1 Bottle/500ml	9	0.0	2	0.3	0.4	0.0	0.0
Blackcurrant Flavour, Still, Danone*	1 Serving/120ml	25	0.0	21	0.0	5.0	0.0	0.0
Cranberry & Raspberry Flavoured, Morrisons*	1 Serving/200ml	3	0.0	2	0.2	0.1	0.0	0.0
Cranberry & Raspberry Still, MacB*	1 Bottle/500ml	4	0.0	1	0.1	0.0	0.0	0.0
Elderflower & Pear, Detox, V Water*	1 Bottle/500ml	40	0.0	8	0.0	1.9	0.0	0.0
Ginger & Mango, Kick, V Water*	1 Bottle/500ml	40	0.0	8	0.0	1.9	0.0	0.0
Grapefruit, Slightly Sparkling, Tesco*	1 Serving/200ml	4	0.0	2	0.0	0.2	0.0	0.0
Green Tea, De-Stress, V Water*	1 Bottle/500ml	40	0.0	8	0.0	1.9	0.0	0.0
Lemon, Vittel*	1 Bottle/500ml	5	0.0	1	0.0	0.0	0.0	0.0
Lemon & Lime, Sparkling, M & S*	1 Bottle/500ml	15	0.0	3	0.0	0.4	0.0	0.0
Lemon & Lime, Still, M & S*	1 Bottle/500ml	5	0.0	1	0.0	0.2	0.0	0.0
Lemon & Lime, Sugar Free, Touch of Fruit, Volvic*	1 Bottle/150ml	2	0.0	1	0.0	0.0	0.0	0.0
Lemon & Lime Flavour Sparkling Spring, Co-Op*	1 Serving/200ml	2	0.0	1	0.0	0.0	0.0	0.0
Lemon & Lime Flavoured, Strathmore*	1 Bottle/500g	85	0.0	17	0.0	4.0	0.0	0.0

W

	Measure INFO/WEIGHT	per Measure KCAL	FAT	Nutrition Values per 100g / 100ml KCAL	PROT	CARB	FAT	FIBRE
WATER								
Mandarin & Cranberry, Still, M & S*	1 Bottle/500ml	100	0.0	20	0.0	5.0	0.0	0.0
Mineral, Energy, Vittel*	1 fl oz/30ml	7	0.0	23	0.0	5.5	0.0	0.0
Mineral Or Tap	**1 Glass/200ml**	**0**	**0.0**	**0**	**0.0**	**0.0**	**0.0**	**0.0**
Orange & Passion Fruit, Vital V, V Water*	1 Bottle/500ml	45	0.0	9	0.0	2.1	0.0	0.0
Peach, Slightly Sparkling, Tesco*	1 Serving/200ml	4	0.0	2	0.0	0.2	0.0	0.0
Peach & Lemon, Still, M & S*	1 Bottle/500ml	100	0.0	20	0.0	5.0	0.0	0.0
Peach & Orange Flavoured, Morrisons*	1 Serving/200ml	3	0.0	2	0.2	0.1	0.0	0.0
Peach & Raspberry, Still, M & S*	1 Bottle/500ml	10	0.0	2	0.0	0.0	0.0	0.0
Pomegranate & Blueberry, Glow, V Water*	1 Bottle/500ml	40	0.0	8	0.0	2.0	0.0	0.0
Raspberry & Apple, Still, Shapers, Boots*	1 Serving/250ml	10	0.0	4	0.0	0.8	0.0	0.0
Skinny, Bo-Synergy*	1 Bottle/500ml	9	0.0	2	0.0	0.3	0.0	0.0
Sparkling, Blueberry & Pomegranate, M & S*	1 Glass/250ml	5	0.0	2	0.0	0.4	0.0	0.0
Sparkling, Fruit, Aqua Libra*	1 Glass/200ml	54	0.0	27	0.0	5.1	0.0	0.0
Sparkling, San Pellegrino*	1 Glass/200ml	0	0.0	0	0.0	0.0	0.0	0.0
Spring, Apple & Blackcurrant, Hadrian*	1 Bottle/365ml	3	0.0	1	0.1	0.1	0.0	0.0
Spring, Apple & Mango, Sparkling, Asda*	1 Glass/200ml	2	0.0	1	0.0	0.2	0.0	0.0
Spring, Apple & Raspberry, Shapers, Boots*	1 Bottle/500ml	10	0.0	2	0.0	0.2	0.0	0.0
Spring, Cranberry & Raspberry, Drench*	1 Bottle/440ml	145	0.4	33	0.1	7.7	0.1	0.0
Spring, Elderflower & Pear, Sainsbury's*	1 Glass/250g	5	0.2	2	0.1	0.2	0.1	0.1
Spring, Lemon & Lime, Slightly Sparkling, Tesco*	1 Serving/200ml	4	0.2	2	0.1	0.2	0.1	0.1
Spring, Lemon & Lime Flavour, Sparkling, Superdrug*	1 Bottle/500ml	8	0.5	2	0.1	0.1	0.1	0.1
Spring, Lemon & Lime Flavoured, Sparkling, Sainsbury's*	1 Glass/250ml	4	0.2	2	0.1	0.1	0.1	0.1
Spring, Orange & Passionfruit, Drench*	1 Serving/250ml	95	0.5	38	0.1	9.0	0.2	0.0
Spring, Raspberry & Cranberry, Shapers, Boots*	1 Bottle/500ml	10	0.0	2	0.0	0.5	0.0	0.0
Spring, Strawberry & Aloe Vera, Botanical, M & S*	1 Bottle/500ml	5	0.0	1	0.0	0.2	0.0	0.0
Spring, Strawberry & Kiwi, Still, Shapers, Boots*	1 Glass/250ml	2	0.0	1	0.0	0.1	0.0	0.9
Spring, Strawberry & Vanilla, Sainsbury's*	1 Glass/250ml	5	0.2	2	0.1	0.2	0.1	0.1
Spring, White Grape & Blackberry, Tesco*	1 Glass/200ml	4	0.0	2	0.0	0.5	0.0	0.0
Spring, with a Hint of Orange, Slightly Sparkling, Tesco*	1 Serving/250ml	5	0.0	2	0.0	0.2	0.0	0.0
Spring, with Cranberry, Tesco*	1 Glass/250ml	2	0.0	1	0.0	0.2	0.0	0.0
Spring, with Grapefruit, Tesco*	1 Serving/200ml	4	0.0	2	0.0	0.2	0.0	0.0
Still, Raspberry & Mango, Shapers, Boots*	1 Bottle/500g	5	0.0	1	0.0	0.0	0.0	0.0
Strawberry, Original, Touch of Fruit, Volvic*	1 Bottle/500ml	99	0.0	20	0.0	4.8	0.0	0.0
Strawberry, Sugar Free, Touch of Fruit, Volvic*	1 Bottle/500ml	7	0.0	1	0.0	0.1	0.0	0.0
Strawberry & Guava, Still, M & S*	1 Glass/250ml	5	0.0	2	0.0	0.1	0.0	0.0
Touch of Fruit, Blackcurrant, Volvic*	1 250ml/250ml	42	0.0	17	0.0	4.0	0.0	0.0
Vitamin, Xxx, Triple Berry, Glaceau*	1 Bottle/500ml	95	0.0	19	0.0	4.6	0.0	0.0
WaterVit, Refresh & Revive, Shapers, Boots*	1 Bottle/500ml	10	0.0	2	0.0	0.2	0.0	0.0
WATER CHESTNUTS								
Raw, Average	**1oz/28g**	**10**	**0.0**	**34**	**1.0**	**7.8**	**0.0**	**0.1**
Whole, in Water, Drained, Sainsbury's*	1 Can/140g	25	0.1	18	0.8	3.4	0.1	0.4
with Bamboo Shoots, Sainsbury's*	1 Serving/50g	29	0.1	58	2.0	12.0	0.2	1.1
WATERCRESS								
Baby, Steve's Leaves*	1 Bag/40g	10	0.2	25	2.6	2.5	0.5	2.1
Raw, Trimmed, Average	**1 Sprig/3g**	**1**	**0.0**	**22**	**3.0**	**0.4**	**1.0**	**1.5**
WATERMELON								
Flesh Only, Average	**1 Serving/250g**	**75**	**0.7**	**30**	**0.4**	**7.0**	**0.3**	**0.4**
Raw	**1 Wedge/286g**	**92**	**1.2**	**32**	**0.6**	**7.2**	**0.4**	**0.5**
WHEAT								
Whole Grain, Split, Average	**1 Serving/60g**	**205**	**1.0**	**342**	**11.3**	**75.9**	**1.7**	**12.2**
WHEAT BRAN								
Average	**1 Tbsp/7g**	**14**	**0.4**	**206**	**14.1**	**26.8**	**5.5**	**36.4**
Coarse, Holland & Barrett*	1 Tbsp/4g	8	0.2	206	14.1	26.8	5.5	36.4

W

	Measure INFO/WEIGHT	per Measure KCAL	FAT	Nutrition Values per 100g / 100ml KCAL	PROT	CARB	FAT	FIBRE
WHEAT BRAN								
Natural, Jordans*	1 Tbsp/7g	13	0.4	188	16.3	17.4	5.9	44.5
WHEAT CRUNCHIES								
Golden Wonder*	1 Pack/35g	172	8.7	491	11.1	55.9	24.8	0.0
Salt & Vinegar, Golden Wonder*	1 Bag/34g	165	8.5	484	10.5	54.5	24.9	2.8
Worcester Sauce, Golden Wonder*	1 Bag/35g	172	8.9	492	9.3	56.4	25.5	3.9
WHEAT GERM								
Average	*1oz/28g*	*100*	*2.6*	*357*	*26.7*	*44.7*	*9.2*	*15.6*
Natural, Jordans*	2 Tbsp/16g	54	1.5	340	28.0	36.0	9.3	13.1
WHELKS								
Boiled, Weighed without Shell	*1oz/28g*	*25*	*0.3*	*89*	*19.5*	*0.0*	*1.2*	*0.0*
WHISKEY								
37.5% Volume	*1 Shot/35ml*	*72*	*0.0*	*207*	*0.0*	*0.0*	*0.0*	*0.0*
40% Volume	*1 Shot/35ml*	*78*	*0.0*	*222*	*0.0*	*0.0*	*0.0*	*0.0*
Bells & Ginger Ale, Premixed, Canned, Diageo*	1 Can/250ml	170	0.0	68	0.0	76.0	0.0	0.0
Jack Daniel's*	1 Shot/35ml	78	0.0	222	0.0	0.0	0.0	0.0
Teacher's*	1 Shot/35ml	78	0.0	222	0.0	0.0	0.0	0.0
WHISKY								
Scotch, 37.5% Volume	*1 Shot/35ml*	*72*	*0.0*	*207*	*0.0*	*0.0*	*0.0*	*0.0*
Scotch, 40% Volume	*1 Shot/35ml*	*78*	*0.0*	*222*	*0.0*	*0.0*	*0.0*	*0.0*
WHITE PUDDING								
Average	*1oz/28g*	*126*	*8.9*	*450*	*7.0*	*36.3*	*31.8*	*0.0*
WHITEBAIT								
in Flour, Fried	*1oz/28g*	*147*	*13.3*	*525*	*19.5*	*5.3*	*47.5*	*0.2*
WHITECURRANTS								
Raw, Average	*1oz/28g*	*7*	*0.0*	*26*	*1.3*	*5.6*	*0.0*	*3.4*
WHITING								
in Crumbs, Fried in Blended Oil	1 Serving/180g	344	18.5	191	18.1	7.0	10.3	0.2
Raw	*1oz/28g*	*23*	*0.2*	*81*	*18.7*	*0.0*	*0.7*	*0.0*
Steamed	*1 Serving/85g*	*78*	*0.8*	*92*	*20.9*	*0.0*	*0.9*	*0.0*
WIENER SCHNITZEL								
Average	1oz/28g	62	2.8	223	20.9	13.1	10.0	0.4
WINE								
Elderberry & Lemon, Ame*	1 Glass/125ml	46	0.0	37	0.0	6.4	0.0	0.0
Fruit, Average	*1 Glass/125ml*	*115*	*0.0*	*92*	*0.0*	*5.5*	*0.0*	*0.0*
Madeira, Henriques & Henriques*	1 Glass/100ml	130	0.0	130	0.0	0.0	0.0	0.0
Mulled, Homemade, Average	*1 Glass/125ml*	*245*	*0.0*	*196*	*0.1*	*25.2*	*0.0*	*0.0*
Original, Lambrini*	1 Glass/125ml	88	0.0	70	0.0	0.0	0.0	0.0
Red, Amarone, Average	1 Glass/125ml	120	0.0	96	0.1	3.0	0.0	0.0
Red, Average	*1 Glass/125ml*	*85*	*0.0*	*68*	*0.1*	*2.5*	*0.0*	*0.0*
Red, Burgundy, 12.9% Abv, Average	1 Glass/125ml	110	0.0	88	0.1	3.7	0.0	0.0
Red, Cabernet Sauvignon, 13.1% Abv, Average	1 Glass/125ml	105	0.0	84	0.1	2.6	0.0	0.0
Red, Cabernet Sauvignon, Non Alcoholic, Ariel*	1 Glass/240ml	50	0.0	21	0.0	4.8	0.0	0.0
Red, Claret, 12.8% Abv, Average	1 Glass/125ml	105	0.0	84	0.1	3.0	0.0	0.0
Red, Gamay, 12.3% Abv, Average	1 Glass/125ml	99	0.0	79	0.1	2.4	0.0	0.0
Red, Low Calorie, Asda*	1 Glass/125ml	49	0.0	39	0.0	0.1	0.0	0.0
Red, Merlot, 13.3% Abv, Average	1 Glass/125ml	105	0.0	84	0.1	2.5	0.0	0.0
Red, Non Alcoholic, Ame*	1 Glass/125ml	42	0.0	34	0.0	5.7	0.0	0.0
Red, Petit Sirah, 13.5% Abv, Average	1 Glass/125ml	107	0.0	86	0.1	2.7	0.0	0.0
Red, Pinot Noir, 13% Abv, Average	1 Glass/125ml	104	0.0	83	0.1	2.3	0.0	0.0
Red, Sangiovese, 13.6% Abv, Average	1 Glass/125ml	109	0.0	87	0.1	2.6	0.0	0.0
Red, Smooth, Weight Watchers*	1 Glass/125ml	75	0.1	60	0.1	1.4	0.1	0.1
Red, Syrah, 13.1% Abv, Average	1 Glass/125ml	105	0.0	84	0.1	2.6	0.0	0.0
Red, Zinfandel, 13.9% Abv, Average	1 Glass/125ml	111	0.0	89	0.1	2.9	0.0	0.0

W

	Measure INFO/WEIGHT	per Measure KCAL	FAT	Nutrition Values per 100g / 100ml KCAL	PROT	CARB	FAT	FIBRE
WINE								
Rose, Medium, Average	**1 Glass/125ml**	**89**	**0.0**	**71**	**0.1**	**2.5**	**0.0**	**0.0**
Rose, Refreshing, Weight Watchers*	1 Glass/125ml	80	0.0	64	0.0	1.6	0.0	0.0
Rose, The Pink Chill, Co-Op*	1 Glass/125ml	85	0.0	68	0.0	0.0	0.0	0.0
Rose, Weight Watchers*	1 Bottle/187ml	112	0.2	60	0.1	1.8	0.1	0.1
Rose, White Grenache, Blossom Hill*	1 Glass/125ml	105	0.0	84	0.0	3.2	0.0	0.0
Rose, White Zinfandel, Ernest & Julio Gallo*	1 Glass/125ml	89	0.0	71	0.0	0.0	0.0	0.0
Sangria, Average	1 Glass/125ml	95	0.0	76	0.1	9.9	0.0	0.1
Spritzer, White, Echo Falls*	1 Glass/125ml	78	0.0	39	0.0	0.0	0.0	0.0
White, Californian, Chardonnay, Light Choices, Tesco*	1 Bottle/181ml	96	0.0	53	0.0	1.8	0.0	0.0
White, Chardonnay, Low Alcohol, McGuigan*	1 Glass/125ml	75	0.1	60	0.1	2.2	0.1	0.0
White, Chardonnay, Southern Australia, Kissing Tree*	1 Bottle/185ml	85	0.0	46	0.0	0.0	0.0	0.0
White, Chenin Blanc, 12% Abv, Average	1 Glass/125ml	101	0.0	81	0.1	3.3	0.0	0.0
White, Dry, Average	**1 Glass/125ml**	**87**	**0.0**	**70**	**0.1**	**0.6**	**0.0**	**0.0**
White, Fume Blanc, 13.1% Abv, Average	1 Glass/125ml	104	0.0	83	0.1	2.3	0.0	0.0
White, Gewurztraminer, 12.6% Abv, Average	1 Glass/125ml	102	0.0	82	0.1	2.6	0.0	0.0
White, Late Harvest, 10.6% Abv, Average	1 Glass/125ml	141	0.0	113	0.1	13.4	0.0	0.0
White, Medium, Average	**1 Glass/125ml**	**92**	**0.0**	**74**	**0.1**	**3.0**	**0.0**	**0.0**
White, Muller-Thurgau, 11.3% Abv, Average	1 Glass/125ml	96	0.0	77	0.1	3.5	0.0	0.0
White, Muscat, 11% Abv, Average	1 Glass/125ml	104	0.0	83	0.1	5.2	0.0	0.0
White, Non Alcoholic, Ame*	1 Glass/125ml	47	0.0	38	0.0	9.5	0.0	0.0
White, Pinot Blanc, 13.3% Abv, Average	1 Glass/125ml	102	0.0	82	0.1	0.0	0.0	0.0
White, Pinot Grigio, 13.4% Abv, Average	1 Glass/125ml	105	0.0	84	0.1	2.1	0.0	0.0
White, Riesling, 11.9% Abv, Average	1 Glass/125ml	101	0.0	81	0.1	3.7	0.0	0.0
White, Sauvignon Blanc, 13.1% Abv, Average	1 Glass/125ml	102	0.0	82	0.1	2.0	0.0	0.0
White, Semillon, 12.5% Abv, Average	1 Glass/125ml	104	0.0	83	0.1	3.1	0.0	0.0
White, Sparkling, Average	**1 Glass/125ml**	**92**	**0.0**	**74**	**0.3**	**5.1**	**0.0**	**0.0**
White, Sweet, Average	**1 Glass/120ml**	**113**	**0.0**	**94**	**0.2**	**5.9**	**0.0**	**0.0**
WINE GUMS								
Average	1 Sweet/6g	19	0.0	315	5.0	73.4	0.2	0.1
Light, Maynards*	1 Pack/42g	90	0.1	215	4.6	48.0	0.2	27.9
Sour, Bassett's*	¼ Bag/50g	159	0.0	319	3.7	78.0	0.0	0.0
WINKLES								
Boiled	**1oz/28g**	**20**	**0.3**	**72**	**15.4**	**0.0**	**1.2**	**0.0**
WISPA								
Bite, with Biscuit in Caramel, Cadbury*	1 Bar/47g	240	13.4	510	6.4	56.9	28.6	0.0
Cadbury*	1 Bar/40g	210	12.9	525	6.7	53.0	32.2	0.7
Gold, Cadbury*	1 Bar/52g	265	15.1	510	5.3	56.0	29.0	0.7
Mint, Cadbury*	1 Bar/50g	275	16.8	550	7.0	54.7	33.6	0.0
WONTON								
Prawn, Dim Sum Selection, Sainsbury's*	1 Wonton/10g	26	1.2	259	11.3	26.8	11.8	1.3
Prawn, Oriental Selection, Waitrose*	1 Wonton/18g	45	2.0	252	9.1	29.2	11.0	1.1
Prawn, Oriental Snack Selection, Sainsbury's*	1 Wonton/20g	53	2.7	265	10.6	25.6	13.4	2.0
WOTSITS								
BBQ, Walkers*	1 Bag/21g	108	6.3	515	4.5	57.0	30.0	1.3
Flamin' Hot, Walkers*	1 Bag/19g	99	5.7	520	5.0	57.0	30.0	1.2
Prawn Cocktail, Walkers*	1 Bag/19g	101	5.9	530	5.5	57.0	31.0	1.1
Really Cheesy, Big Eat, Walkers*	1 Bag/36g	196	11.9	545	5.5	56.0	33.0	1.1
Really Cheesy, Walkers*	1 Bag/19g	104	6.3	545	5.5	56.0	33.0	1.1
WRAP								
All Day Breakfast, M & S*	1 Pack/196g	529	31.4	270	10.8	21.2	16.0	1.4
American Deli, Shapers, Boots*	1 Pack/172g	249	4.5	145	9.5	21.0	2.6	2.0
BBQ Beef, Ginsters*	1 Pack/210g	404	12.2	192	6.7	28.4	5.8	1.8
Beef & Duck, Mouli with Salad, Eat Well, M & S*	1 Pack/88g	48	0.4	55	4.6	7.8	0.4	1.3

W

WRAP

INFO/WEIGHT	Measure	per Measure		Nutrition Values per 100g / 100ml				
		KCAL	FAT	KCAL	PROT	CARB	FAT	FIBRE
Beef Fajita, Boots*	1 Pack/200g	352	8.4	176	9.5	25.5	4.2	3.1
Beef in Black Bean, M & S*	1 Pack/150g	337	17.1	225	10.2	20.5	11.4	1.6
Bombay Potato, Whistlestop*	1 Wrap/180g	343	15.0	191	4.2	24.7	8.3	0.3
Brie & Cranberry, M & S*	1 Pack/225g	550	27.8	245	6.1	27.3	12.4	1.7
Butternut Squash, COU, M & S*	1 Pack/182g	245	4.7	135	4.3	22.2	2.6	2.9
Cajun, GFY, Asda*	1 Pack/176g	231	2.1	131	9.0	21.0	1.2	0.9
Cajun Chicken, Sandwich King*	1 Pack/138g	386	19.9	279	12.3	25.0	14.4	0.0
Cajun Chicken, Tesco*	1 Pack/184g	415	16.6	225	9.8	25.1	9.0	1.9
Chargrilled Chicken, Perfectly Balanced, Waitrose*	1 Pack/230g	361	6.7	157	10.3	22.7	2.9	2.9
Cheese & Bean, Tesco*	1 Pack/105g	235	9.4	224	7.0	28.6	9.0	1.0
Chicken, Barbecue, GFY, Asda*	1 Pack/176g	294	4.4	167	9.6	26.4	2.5	1.8
Chicken, Barbecue, Shapers, Boots*	1 Pack/181g	283	4.9	156	10.0	23.0	2.7	3.3
Chicken, Cheddar & Peppers, Cajun, Sainsbury's*	1 Pack/242g	535	26.6	221	10.4	19.8	11.0	2.1
Chicken, Chilli, GFY, Asda*	1 Pack/194g	277	4.3	143	9.1	21.6	2.2	2.3
Chicken, M & S*	1 Pack/247g	530	24.9	215	8.2	23.4	10.1	1.6
Chicken, Mediterranean Style, Waitrose*	1 Pack/183g	296	11.0	162	8.3	18.6	6.0	2.3
Chicken, Mexican Style, Co-Op*	1 Pack/163g	367	14.7	225	11.0	26.0	9.0	3.0
Chicken, Moroccan, BGTY, Sainsbury's*	1 Pack/207g	315	3.1	152	9.4	25.3	1.5	0.0
Chicken, Nacho, No Mayo, Asda*	1 Pack/183g	392	13.9	214	12.0	24.3	7.6	3.1
Chicken, Salsa, Light Choices, Tesco*	1 Pack/219g	340	5.9	155	9.7	22.6	2.7	1.9
Chicken, Southern Fried, Fresh for You, Tesco*	1 Pack/206g	485	24.4	235	8.6	22.7	11.8	2.0
Chicken, Southern Style, Ginsters*	1 Wrap/210g	491	22.0	234	6.4	28.3	10.5	1.8
Chicken, Tasties*	1 Pack/149g	324	10.6	218	11.7	26.5	7.1	0.0
Chicken, Thai, Spiced, Salad, Eat Well, M & S*	1 Pack/122g	91	1.5	75	5.2	9.5	1.2	1.5
Chicken & Bacon, Simple Solutions, Tesco*	1 Pack/300g	474	23.4	158	20.7	1.2	7.8	0.5
Chicken & Bacon Caesar, COU, M & S*	1 Pack/170g	260	4.2	153	10.6	22.0	2.5	2.1
Chicken & Bacon Caesar Salad, Asda*	1 Pack/160g	565	35.2	353	18.0	20.8	22.0	0.9
Chicken & Cous Cous, BGTY, Sainsbury's*	1 Pack/230g	359	9.0	156	8.8	21.5	3.9	0.0
Chicken & Cous Cous, Moroccan Style, GFY, Asda*	1 Pack/164g	307	2.0	187	12.0	32.0	1.2	1.8
Chicken & Sweetfire Pepper, Light Choices, Tesco*	1 Wrap/175g	350	7.9	200	10.2	28.5	4.5	1.4
Chicken Caesar, HL, Tesco*	1 Pack/200g	296	4.0	148	10.2	22.3	2.0	2.2
Chicken Caesar, Tesco*	1 Pack /215g	516	24.3	240	11.6	23.0	11.3	1.2
Chicken Caesar, Weight Watchers*	1 Pack/173g	298	4.7	172	11.2	24.5	2.7	1.3
Chicken Fajita, Asda*	1 Pack/180g	369	16.9	205	9.4	20.6	9.4	0.4
Chicken Fajita, Daily Bread*	1 Pack/191g	392	10.5	205	9.4	29.4	5.5	0.0
Chicken Fajita, Finest, Tesco*	1 Pack/213g	422	15.6	198	9.0	24.0	7.3	1.9
Chicken Fajita, Shapers, Boots*	1 Pack/216g	291	5.2	135	14.0	15.0	2.4	3.1
Chicken Fajita, Tesco*	1 Pack/220g	407	11.7	185	10.6	23.2	5.3	1.8
Chicken Fajita, VLH Kitchens*	1 Wrap/170g	311	8.8	183	10.6	25.0	5.2	0.0
Chicken Fillet with Cheese & Bacon, Asda*	1 Pack/164g	366	21.3	223	25.0	1.4	13.0	0.0
Chicken Jalfrezi, Boots*	1 Pack/215g	456	15.7	212	8.6	28.0	7.3	1.7
Chicken Korma, Patak's*	1 Pack/150g	294	14.2	196	7.6	20.0	9.5	0.0
Chicken Louisiana, Benedicts*	1 Pack/250g	410	5.5	164	13.4	24.2	2.2	0.0
Chicken Nacho, HL, Tesco*	1 Pack/223g	390	10.0	175	12.3	21.2	4.5	2.6
Chicken Salad, Roast, Sainsbury's*	1 Pack/214g	443	19.9	207	10.0	20.9	9.3	2.5
Chicken Sweet & Sour, Ginsters*	1 Pack/150g	378	5.8	252	13.4	40.8	3.9	2.4
Chicken Thai Style, Boots*	1 Pack/156g	290	10.0	186	11.0	21.0	6.4	2.2
Chicken Tikka, Average	1 Wrap/183g	277	7.3	151	9.7	18.5	4.0	1.1
Chicken Tikka Masala, Patak's*	1 Pack/150g	252	9.9	168	7.8	19.3	6.6	0.0
Chilli Bean & Cheese, Meat Free, Asda*	1 Wrap/151g	263	7.1	174	7.9	25.1	4.7	4.9
Chilli Beef, Co-Op*	1 Pack/163g	310	9.8	190	10.0	26.0	6.0	2.0
Chilli Beef, COU, M & S*	1 Pack/179g	268	2.9	150	10.1	23.4	1.6	2.6
Chilli Chicken, BGTY, Sainsbury's*	1 Pack/180g	313	4.3	174	10.2	28.0	2.4	0.0

W

WRAP

Chinese Chicken, Asda*	1 Pack/200g	404	12.0	202	9.0	28.0	6.0	0.0
Chinese Chicken, M & S*	1 Pack/155g	239	1.5	154	14.0	22.3	1.0	2.0
Coronation Chicken, Waitrose*	1 Pack/164g	283	8.3	173	10.1	21.3	5.1	2.2
Crayfish, Lemon Dressing & Rocket, COU, M & S*	1 Pack/183g	274	4.9	150	9.5	22.5	2.7	1.2
Crayfish & Rocket, HL, Tesco*	1 Pack/164g	270	5.1	165	7.5	25.9	3.1	1.9
Dhansak Prawn, M & S*	1 Pack/208g	385	15.0	185	7.1	23.3	7.2	2.4
Duck, Food to Go, M & S*	1 Pack/257g	475	13.9	185	8.5	25.5	5.4	1.0
Duck, Hoi Sin, Delicious, Boots*	1 Pack/160g	295	4.3	184	11.0	28.0	2.7	2.0
Duck, Hoisin, M & S*	1 Pack/225g	405	8.3	180	8.4	27.7	3.7	1.5
Duck, Hoisin, No Mayo, Tesco*	1 Pack/184g	340	8.5	185	9.4	26.1	4.6	1.8
Egg Mayonnaise, Tomato & Cress, Sainsbury's*	1 Pack/255g	592	38.2	232	7.3	17.7	15.0	0.0
Fajita, Steak, Delicatessen, Waitrose*	1 Pack/232g	489	21.1	211	10.5	22.7	9.1	2.7
Feta Cheese, GFY, Asda*	1 Pack/165g	256	7.1	155	7.0	22.0	4.3	2.1
Feta Cheese Flat Bread, COU, M & S*	1 Pack/180g	225	4.0	125	6.3	20.6	2.2	1.9
Fiery Cheese, Ginsters*	1 Pack/210g	424	17.6	202	6.8	24.8	8.4	1.8
Fiery Mexican Cheese, Ginsters*	1 Pack/150g	291	10.9	194	7.4	25.0	7.3	1.8
Goats Cheese, & Grilled Pepper, Asda*	1 Serving/75g	194	11.2	259	5.0	26.0	15.0	2.1
Greek Feta, Tortilla, Shapers, Boots*	1 Pack/169g	271	4.6	160	6.7	27.0	2.7	1.6
Greek Feta Salad, Shapers, Boots*	1 Pack/158g	241	5.7	153	6.4	24.0	3.6	1.2
Greek Salad, COU, M & S*	1 Pack/180g	288	4.9	160	6.0	27.2	2.7	2.3
Greek Salad, M & S*	1 Pack/179g	250	4.5	140	8.1	21.5	2.5	1.0
Greek Salad, Sainsbury's*	1 Pack/167g	242	6.2	145	6.7	21.2	3.7	1.8
Green Thai Prawn, BGTY, Sainsbury's*	1 Pack/200g	237	3.0	118	7.0	19.2	1.5	1.5
Ham, Cheese & Pickle Tortilla, Weight Watchers*	1 Pack/170g	296	4.8	174	10.9	26.4	2.8	1.2
Houmous, Royal London Hospital*	1 Pack/200g	318	13.4	159	6.3	20.0	6.7	0.0
Houmous, Taste!*	1 Pack/170g	291	8.3	171	5.4	26.4	4.9	0.0
Houmous & Chargrilled Vegetables, Shapers, Boots*	1 Pack/186g	301	5.0	162	5.8	29.0	2.7	3.2
Italian Chicken, Sainsbury's*	½ Pack/211g	395	23.2	187	15.7	6.2	11.0	0.9
King Prawn, Shapers, Boots*	1 Pack/154g	227	2.2	147	9.2	24.0	1.4	2.1
Mexican Bean, BGTY, Sainsbury's*	1 Pack/216g	341	5.3	158	9.2	24.9	2.5	1.5
Mexican Bean, GFY, Asda*	1 Pack/173g	303	5.9	175	5.0	31.0	3.4	2.3
Mexican Bean & Potato in Spinach Tortilla, Daily Bread*	1 Pack/196g	329	10.6	168	4.9	25.0	5.4	0.0
Mexican Chicken, M & S*	1 Serving/218g	447	22.5	205	8.6	19.7	10.3	1.3
Mexican Three Bean, M & S*	1 Pack/188g	405	19.2	215	6.9	24.3	10.2	2.2
Mexican Tortilla, Ainsley Harriott*	1 Pack/230g	421	17.2	183	7.1	22.4	7.5	0.0
Mild Chicken Curry, Patak's*	1 Pack/150g	238	9.0	159	8.1	21.3	6.0	2.8
Minted Lamb, Darwins Deli*	1 Pack/250g	287	6.3	115	3.2	19.9	2.5	0.0
Monterey Jack & Ham, Tesco*	1 Pack/200g	522	28.2	261	7.9	25.9	14.1	0.2
Nacho Chicken, COU, M & S*	1 Pack/175g	280	4.2	160	10.2	24.4	2.4	2.0
Peking Duck, Average	1 Serving/183g	356	10.5	194	9.2	26.5	5.7	1.1
Pork Caribbean Spicy, Ginsters*	1 Pack/150g	396	13.6	264	11.3	34.1	9.1	2.3
Red Thai Chicken, BGTY, Sainsbury's*	1 Pack/194g	384	7.6	198	11.3	29.3	3.9	1.0
Red Thai Chicken, Shapers, Boots*	1 Pack/172g	234	3.6	136	9.5	20.0	2.1	2.4
Red Thai Chicken Panini, W38	1 Wrap/186g	402	13.6	216	13.3	28.6	7.3	1.4
Roasted Vegetable & Feta, BGTY, Sainsbury's*	1 Serving/200g	318	8.0	159	5.8	25.0	4.0	0.0
Selection, Chicken, BBQ Steak, Hoisin Duck, M & S*	1 Pack/334g	685	23.7	205	10.9	24.3	7.1	1.7
Sicilian Lemon & Roasted Vegetable, COU, M & S*	1 Pack/178g	240	3.7	135	4.9	23.8	2.1	1.9
Smoked Salmon, Finest, Tesco*	1 Pack/58g	113	8.4	194	15.5	0.6	14.4	0.3
Smoked Salmon & Prawn, Finest, Tesco*	1 Serving/59g	84	5.3	143	14.3	1.0	9.1	0.0
Soft Cheese & Spinach, to Go*	1 Serving/250g	278	6.7	111	4.5	17.4	2.7	0.0
Southern Fried Chicken, Tesco*	1 Pack/214g	395	14.7	185	9.9	20.8	6.9	2.1
Sushi Salmon & Cucumber, Waitrose*	1 Pack/180g	299	6.5	166	6.3	27.2	3.6	1.6
Sweet Chilli & King Prawn, COU, M & S*	1 Pack/155g	225	2.6	145	8.0	24.2	1.7	2.1

W

	Measure INFO/WEIGHT	per Measure KCAL	FAT	Nutrition Values per 100g / 100ml KCAL	PROT	CARB	FAT	FIBRE
WRAP								
Sweet Chilli Chicken, Shapers, Boots*	1 Pack/195g	302	3.7	155	10.0	24.0	1.9	3.0
Sweet Chilli Chicken, Waitrose*	1 Pack/200g	390	14.7	195	10.2	22.0	7.3	2.4
Sweet Chilli King Prawn, M & S*	1 Pack/155g	225	3.1	145	8.0	24.2	2.0	2.1
Sweet Chilli Noodle, Sainsbury's*	1 Pack/210g	399	10.1	190	10.6	26.1	4.8	2.1
Tandoori Chicken, GFY, Asda*	1 Pack/167g	281	4.5	168	10.0	26.0	2.7	1.7
Thai Prawn, COU, M & S*	1 Pack/181g	235	2.9	130	8.3	20.4	1.6	1.9
Tuna, Sweetcorn & Red Pepper, BGTY, Sainsbury's*	1 Pack/178g	306	8.2	172	11.5	21.2	4.6	2.1
Tuna Nicoise, BGTY, Sainsbury's*	1 Pack/181g	273	7.1	151	11.0	18.0	3.9	0.0
Tuna Salsa, Healthy Eating, Wild Bean Cafe*	1 Pack/159g	245	2.7	154	11.3	23.5	1.7	1.5
Turkey, Bacon & Cranberry, COU, M & S*	1 Pack/144g	230	2.2	160	9.6	27.1	1.5	2.3
Yellow Thai Prawn, COU, M & S*	1 Pack/171g	266	5.0	155	7.6	23.4	2.9	1.7

	Measure INFO/WEIGHT	per Measure KCAL	FAT	Nutrition Values per 100g / 100ml KCAL	PROT	CARB	FAT	FIBRE
YAM								
Baked	**1oz/28g**	**43**	**0.1**	**153**	**2.1**	**37.5**	**0.4**	**1.7**
Boiled, Average	**1oz/28g**	**37**	**0.1**	**133**	**1.7**	**33.0**	**0.3**	**1.4**
Raw	**1oz/28g**	**32**	**0.1**	**114**	**1.5**	**28.2**	**0.3**	**1.3**
YEAST								
Dried, Average	**1 Tbsp/6g**	**10**	**0.1**	**169**	**35.6**	**3.5**	**1.5**	**0.0**
Extract	**1 Tsp/9g**	**16**	**0.0**	**180**	**40.7**	**3.5**	**0.4**	**0.0**
YOGHURT								
Activia, Danone*	1 Pot/132g	125	4.2	94	3.5	12.8	3.2	2.0
Activia, Pouring, Natural, Danone*	1 Carton/950g	484	16.1	51	4.1	4.9	1.7	0.0
Activia, Snackpot, Peach, Fat Free, Bio, Danone*	1 Pot/165g	99	0.2	60	4.6	10.2	0.1	1.0
Activia, Snackpot, Raspberry, Fat Free, Bio, Danone*	1 Pot/165g	81	0.2	48	4.6	6.9	0.1	2.5
Activia, Snackpot, Vanilla, Fat Free, Bio, Danone*	1 Pot/165g	87	0.2	53	5.0	8.1	0.1	0.9
Activia Snackpot, Mango, Fat Free, Bio, Danone*	1 Pot/165g	86	0.2	52	4.8	8.1	0.1	0.2
Apple, Light, Muller*	1 Pot/175g	94	0.2	54	4.4	9.0	0.1	0.0
Apple & Blackberry, Bio, Sainsbury's*	1 Pot/125g	134	3.4	107	4.1	16.6	2.7	0.2
Apple & Blackberry, Organic, Yeo Valley*	1 Pot/125g	121	4.1	97	4.3	12.5	3.3	0.1
Apple & Cinnamon, COU, M & S*	1 Pot/150g	67	0.1	45	4.2	6.1	0.1	0.2
Apple & Cinnamon, Dessert, Low Fat, Sainsbury's*	1 Pot/125g	115	2.1	92	4.5	14.7	1.7	0.1
Apple & Cinnamon, Jubileum, Tine*	1 Pot/125g	166	6.5	133	3.2	18.5	5.2	0.0
Apple & Cinnamon Farmhouse, Twekkelo*	1 Bowl/125g	142	4.1	114	4.1	17.0	3.3	0.4
Apple & Custard, Low Fat, Sainsbury's*	1 Pot/125g	116	1.9	93	4.3	15.5	1.5	0.2
Apple & Pear, Low Fat, Sainsbury's*	1 Pot/125g	115	1.9	92	4.3	15.2	1.5	0.2
Apple & Prune, Fat Free, Yeo Valley*	1 Pot/125g	97	0.1	78	5.1	14.1	0.1	0.2
Apple & Spice Bio, Virtually Fat Free, Shape, Danone*	1 Pot/120g	67	0.1	56	5.6	7.3	0.1	0.2
Apple Pie, Simply Desserts, Muller*	1 Pot/175g	278	8.0	159	4.6	24.7	4.6	0.7
Apricot, Bio, Low Fat, Benecol*	1 Pot/125g	98	0.8	78	3.9	14.3	0.6	0.0
Apricot, Bio Activia, Danone*	1 Pot/125g	121	4.0	97	3.7	13.3	3.2	1.7
Apricot, Fat Free, Activ8, Ski, Nestle*	1 Pot/120g	88	0.8	73	4.5	13.6	0.7	0.2
Apricot, Fat Free, Bio Live, Rachel's Organic*	1 Pot/142g	81	0.1	57	3.5	10.5	0.1	0.0
Apricot, Fruity, Mullerlight, Muller*	1 Pot/175g	87	0.2	50	4.2	7.5	0.1	0.1
Apricot, Low Fat, Organic, Average	1 Serving/100g	84	1.0	84	5.8	13.3	1.0	0.6
Apricot, Low Fat, Tesco*	1 Pot/125g	112	2.2	90	4.3	14.1	1.8	0.0
Apricot, Pro Activ, Flora*	1 Pot/125ml	70	0.6	56	4.0	7.9	0.5	1.8
Apricot & Mango, 25% Extra Fruit, Low Fat, Asda*	1 Pot/125g	120	1.4	96	4.6	17.0	1.1	0.0
Apricot & Mango, Best There Is, Yoplait*	1 Pot/125g	130	2.0	104	4.7	17.4	1.6	0.0
Apricot & Mango, Thick & Creamy, Sainsbury's*	1 Pot/150g	178	5.4	119	4.3	17.3	3.6	0.2
Apricot & Mango, Tropical Fruit, Activ8, Ski, Nestle*	1 Pot/120g	112	2.0	93	4.3	15.1	1.7	0.2
Apricot & Nectarine, Sunshine Selection, Sainsbury's*	1 Pot/125g	115	1.9	92	4.4	15.3	1.5	0.1
Apricot & Passion Fruit, Fat Free, Yeo Valley*	1 Pot/125g	94	0.1	75	5.3	13.2	0.1	0.1
Banana, Childrens, Co-Op*	1 Pot/125g	124	3.2	99	3.7	15.1	2.6	0.2
Banana, Custard Style, Asda*	1 Pot/150g	223	9.0	149	3.7	20.0	6.0	0.2
Banana, Low Fat, Average	1 Serving/100g	98	1.4	98	4.6	16.7	1.4	0.1
Banana & Custard, Smooth, Mullerlight, Muller*	1 Pot/175g	94	0.2	54	4.1	8.6	0.1	0.6
Banana & Mango, Oatie Breakfast, Moma Foods*	1 Pot/235g	314	4.7	134	4.2	26.0	2.0	1.7
Banana & Orange, Low Fat, 25% Extra Fruit, Asda*	1 Pot/125g	125	1.4	100	4.6	18.0	1.1	0.0
Banana Smooth, M & S*	1 Pot/150g	165	2.5	110	4.8	19.3	1.7	0.2
Banoffee, Dessert, Low Fat, Sainsbury's*	1 Pot/125g	122	2.1	98	4.5	16.1	1.7	0.2
Banoffee, Low Fat, Asda*	1 Pot/125g	126	1.5	101	4.6	18.2	1.2	1.0
Bio, Low Fat, Spelga*	1 Pot/125g	125	2.1	100	3.9	17.0	1.7	0.0
Bio Fruits with Cherries, 0% Fat, Danone*	1 Pot/125g	65	0.1	52	3.6	9.1	0.1	0.0
Black Cherry, Average	1 Serving/100g	96	2.2	96	3.4	16.5	2.2	0.1
Black Cherry, Greek Style, Corner, Muller*	1 Pot/150g	172	4.5	115	5.0	16.2	3.0	0.1
Black Cherry, Live Bio, Perfectly Balanced, Waitrose*	1 Pot/125g	115	0.1	92	4.6	18.3	0.1	0.1

Y

YOGHURT

INFO/WEIGHT	per Measure KCAL	per Measure FAT	Nutrition Values per 100g / 100ml KCAL	PROT	CARB	FAT	FIBRE
Black Cherry, Low Fat, Average	1 Serving/100g	69	0.6	69	3.8	12.2	0.6	0.3
Black Cherry, Swiss, Finest, Tesco*	1 Pot/150g	195	8.8	130	3.5	15.7	5.9	0.5
Black Cherry, Thick & Creamy, Waitrose*	1 Pot/125g	139	3.1	111	3.7	18.3	2.5	0.4
Black Cherry, Very Cherry, Activ8, Ski, Nestle*	1 Pot/120g	116	2.0	97	4.3	16.1	1.7	0.2
Black Cherry, VLH Kitchens*	1 Pot/150g	188	5.6	125	3.7	19.6	3.7	1.0
Blackberry, Alpro*	1 Pot/125g	99	2.6	79	3.7	9.2	2.1	1.2
Blackberry, Boysenberry & William Pear, M & S*	1 Pot/150g	187	9.7	125	4.0	13.6	6.5	2.4
Blackberry, Farmhouse, BGTY, Sainsbury's*	1 Pot/150g	106	0.6	71	3.4	13.5	0.4	1.6
Blackberry, Fat Free, BGTY, Sainsbury's*	1 Pot/150g	100	0.1	67	3.4	13.6	0.1	1.6
Blackberry, Fat Free, Danone, Shape*	1 Pot/120g	74	0.2	62	6.7	8.4	0.2	2.4
Blackberry, Very Berry, Activ8, Ski, Nestle*	1 Pot/120g	114	2.0	95	4.4	15.5	1.7	0.7
Blackberry & Apple, BGTY, Sainsbury's*	1 Pot/122g	61	0.2	50	4.7	7.2	0.2	0.3
Blackberry & Apple, HL, Tesco*	1 Pot/176g	86	0.2	49	2.1	10.0	0.1	1.5
Blackberry & Bramley Apple, Loseley*	1 Jar/150g	186	6.3	124	4.8	16.7	4.2	0.0
Blackberry & Raspberry, Fruit Corner, Muller*	1 Pot/175g	184	6.8	105	3.8	13.1	3.9	0.9
Blackberry & Raspberry Flip, Morrisons*	1 Pot/175g	206	8.0	118	3.4	15.8	4.6	0.5
Blackcurrant, BGTY, Sainsbury's*	1 Pot/200g	100	0.4	50	4.8	7.3	0.2	0.1
Blackcurrant, Extra Special, Asda*	1 Pot/100g	163	9.0	163	2.6	18.0	9.0	0.0
Blackcurrant, Fat Free, BGTY, Sainsbury's*	1 Pot/125g	64	0.1	51	4.6	8.0	0.1	1.6
Blackcurrant, Fruity, Mullerlight, Muller*	1 Pot/175g	89	0.2	51	4.1	7.9	0.1	0.8
Blackcurrant, Longley Farm*	1 Pot/150g	168	5.5	112	4.9	14.7	3.7	0.0
Blackcurrant, Low Fat, Chosen By You, Asda*	1 Pot/125g	104	1.6	83	3.6	14.2	1.3	0.0
Blackcurrant, Low Fat, Sainsbury's*	1 Pot/125g	116	1.7	93	4.2	15.9	1.4	0.6
Blackcurrant, Munch Bunch, Nestle*	1 Pot/100g	107	3.1	107	4.4	15.3	3.1	0.5
Blackcurrant, Probiotic, Organic, Yeo Valley*	1 Pot/150g	151	5.8	101	4.1	12.4	3.9	0.2
Blackcurrant, Thick & Creamy, Sainsbury's*	1 Pot/150g	171	5.4	114	4.3	15.9	3.6	0.4
Blackcurrant, Virtually Fat Free, Morrisons*	1 Pot/200g	114	0.4	57	5.4	8.4	0.2	0.2
Blackcurrant & Raspberry, Layers, Mullerlight, Muller*	1 Pot/175g	94	0.2	54	3.1	9.7	0.1	0.7
Blackcurrant with Liquorice, Tesco*	1 Pot/150g	138	1.6	92	4.6	15.8	1.1	0.4
Blueberry, Bio, Co-Op*	1 Pot/125g	141	3.5	113	4.5	16.5	2.8	0.4
Blueberry, Extremely Fruity, Low Fat, Probiotic, M & S*	1 Pot/150g	142	2.1	95	4.7	14.7	1.4	1.5
Blueberry, Fat Free, Activia, Danone*	1 Pot/125g	64	0.1	51	4.7	7.8	0.1	2.4
Blueberry, Flip, Morrisons*	1 Pot/175g	201	8.0	115	3.1	15.1	4.6	0.5
Blueberry, Fruit Bottom, Stonyfield*	1 Pot/170g	120	2.0	71	3.5	12.3	1.2	0.6
Blueberry, Fruit Corner, Muller*	1 Pot/175g	182	6.8	104	3.8	12.8	3.9	0.4
Blueberry, Loganberry, Layered, Bio, Sainsbury's*	1 Pot/125g	134	3.4	107	4.0	16.6	2.7	0.2
Blueberry, Oatie Breakfast, Moma Foods*	1 Pot/235g	318	6.0	135	4.5	24.6	2.5	1.9
Blueberry, Probiotic, Natural Balance, Asda*	1 Pot/125g	102	2.9	82	2.1	13.1	2.3	2.6
Blueberry, Wholemilk, Organic, Sainsbury's*	1 Pot/150g	123	5.2	82	3.5	9.2	3.5	0.1
Blueberry & Elderberry, with Wholegrains, Bio, Optifit*	1 Pot/250g	150	3.5	60	4.9	7.0	1.4	1.6
Boysenberry, Low Fat, Yoplait*	1 Pot/100g	49	0.1	49	5.3	6.7	0.1	0.0
Bramble & Apple, Virtually Fat Free, Longley Farm*	1 Pot/150g	118	0.1	79	5.5	13.9	0.1	0.0
Breakfast Crunch, Strawberry, Corner, Muller*	1 Pack/135g	163	3.5	121	5.5	0.0	2.6	0.0
Caramel, Organic, Onken*	1 Serving/50g	55	1.6	111	4.6	15.6	3.3	0.0
Cereals, Fibre, Bio Activia, Danone*	1 Pot/120g	119	4.1	99	3.7	13.5	3.4	3.0
Champagne Rhubarb & Vanilla, M & S*	1 Pot/150g	195	8.7	130	3.8	15.7	5.8	0.8
Cherry, 0% Fat, Yoplait*	1 Pot/125g	70	0.1	56	3.8	9.8	0.1	0.0
Cherry, 0.1% Fat, Shape, Danone*	1 Pot/120g	56	0.1	47	4.6	6.8	0.1	2.1
Cherry, Bio, Low Fat, Benecol*	1 Pot/150g	121	0.9	81	3.8	15.2	0.6	0.0
Cherry, Fat Free, Activia, Danone*	1 Pot/125g	71	0.1	57	4.7	9.4	0.1	0.9
Cherry, Fat Free, M & S*	1 Pot/200g	170	0.2	85	4.3	16.7	0.1	0.5
Cherry, Fruit, Biopot, Onken*	1 Serving/100g	107	2.7	107	3.7	16.7	2.7	0.2
Cherry, Fruity, Mullerlight, Muller*	1 Pot/175g	86	0.2	49	4.3	7.0	0.1	0.2

YOGHURT

	Measure INFO/WEIGHT	per Measure KCAL	FAT	Nutrition Values per 100g / 100ml KCAL	PROT	CARB	FAT	FIBRE
Cherry, Greek Style, Shape, Danone*	1 Pot/125g	143	3.4	114	6.0	16.4	2.7	0.0
Cherry, Light, Fat Free, Muller*	1 Pot/190g	89	0.2	47	4.1	6.7	0.1	0.2
Cherry, Low Fat, Asda*	1 Pot/125g	120	1.4	96	4.6	17.0	1.1	0.0
Cherry, Low Fat, Chosen By You, Asda*	1 Pot/125g	90	1.6	72	3.6	11.4	1.3	0.3
Cherry, Noir De Basle, 0.06% Fat, TTD, Sainsbury's*	1 Pot/150g	195	8.7	130	3.7	15.7	5.8	0.3
Cherry, Pots, Probiotic, Yeo Valley*	1 Pot /119g	124	4.4	104	4.9	12.8	3.7	0.1
Cherry & Vanilla Flavour, Light, Brooklea*	1 Pot/200g	138	0.2	69	5.5	11.4	0.1	0.6
Cherry Bakewell Tart Flavour, M & S*	1 Pot/150g	315	13.2	210	3.0	17.0	8.8	1.0
Cherry Bakewell Tart Flavour, Muller*	1 Pot/175g	119	0.3	68	4.8	11.8	0.2	0.2
Cherry Bio, Co-Op*	1 Pot/125g	144	3.5	115	4.5	17.0	2.8	0.1
Cherry Flip, BFY, Morrisons*	1 Pot/175g	93	0.5	53	3.9	8.7	0.3	0.4
Choc Chip Granola, Naturally Creamy, Nom Dairy UK*	1 Pot/150g	196	8.5	131	4.2	15.8	5.7	0.4
Chocolate, GFY, Asda*	1 Pot/200g	110	1.0	55	4.7	8.0	0.5	0.1
Chocolate, Seriously Smooth, Waitrose*	1 Pot/125g	157	3.0	126	6.0	20.1	2.4	0.1
Chocolate, Village Dairy*	1 Pot/125g	181	3.7	145	6.3	23.5	3.0	0.0
Chocolate, Vitaline*	1 Pot/125g	102	0.6	82	3.5	15.8	0.5	0.0
Chocolate Raisins, Naturally Creamy, Nom Dairy UK*	1 Pot/155g	245	9.5	158	3.4	22.4	6.1	0.2
Citrus Fruit, Tesco*	1 Serving/117g	53	0.1	45	4.2	6.5	0.1	0.1
Coconut, Biopot, Onken*	1 Pot/450g	562	23.4	125	3.9	15.6	5.2	0.9
Country Rhubarb, Naturally Light, Nom Dairy UK*	1 Pot/180g	131	0.2	73	4.3	13.8	0.1	0.4
Cranberry, Bio Activia, Danone*	1 Pot/125g	115	4.0	92	3.6	12.3	3.2	1.7
Creamy Cranberry & Raspberry, Shapers, Boots*	1 Pot/150g	85	1.6	57	4.0	7.0	1.1	1.1
Dessert with Honey, Perfectly Balanced, Waitrose*	1 Pot/125ml	127	1.5	102	3.5	19.4	1.2	0.1
Devon Toffee, Low Fat, Sainsbury's*	1 Pot/126g	137	1.9	109	4.3	19.6	1.5	0.0
Devonshire Fudge, 0.06% Fat, TTD, Sainsbury's*	1 Pot/150g	219	9.0	146	3.5	19.5	6.0	0.0
Drink, Actimel, Peach & Mango, Danone*	1 Bottle/100g	27	0.1	27	2.7	3.1	0.1	0.4
Exotic, Alpro*	1 Pot/125g	97	2.4	78	3.6	11.1	1.9	0.9
Exotic Fruits, Soya, Savia, Danone*	1 Pot/125g	104	2.1	83	2.9	12.6	1.7	0.5
Exotic Fruits French Set Wholemilk, Asda*	1 Pot/125g	125	4.0	100	3.6	14.1	3.2	0.0
Farmhouse, Forest Fruits, Twekkelo, De Zuivelhoeve*	1 Pot/500g	555	16.5	111	4.2	16.0	3.3	0.5
Fat Free, Probiotic Peach & Nectarine, Waitrose*	1 Pot/150g	108	0.0	72	4.4	13.3	0.0	0.2
Fig, Bio, Activia, Danone*	1 Pot/125g	121	4.0	97	3.7	13.3	3.2	1.6
Forest Fruits, 0.1% Fat, Shape, Danone*	1 Pot/120g	55	0.1	46	4.6	6.7	0.1	2.1
Forest Fruits, Bio, Activia, Fat Free, Danone*	1 Pot/125g	66	0.1	53	4.5	8.5	0.1	1.1
Forest Fruits, Layered Greek Style, Shapers, Boots*	1 Pot/150g	85	2.1	57	3.2	7.9	1.4	2.2
Forest Fruits, M & S*	1 Pot/150g	148	2.4	99	4.7	16.8	1.6	0.5
French Set, Low Fat, Iceland*	1 Pot/125g	100	1.5	80	3.6	13.6	1.2	0.0
French Set, Waitrose*	1 Pot/125g	120	3.9	96	3.5	13.4	3.1	0.0
French Style, Whole Milk, Smooth Set, Tesco*	1 Pot/125g	122	3.7	98	3.6	14.1	3.0	0.0
Frozen, Cherry Garcia, Low Fat, Ben & Jerry's*	1 Serving/100g	143	2.4	143	3.0	26.0	2.4	1.0
Frozen, Choc Fudge Brownie, Low Fat, Ben & Jerry's*	1 Serving/100g	180	3.0	180	4.0	34.0	3.0	1.5
Frozen, Chocolate, Snog*	1 Serving/100g	109	1.6	109	4.5	19.9	1.6	1.7
Frozen, Frae*	1 Small/83ml	56	0.0	67	2.4	12.0	0.0	0.0
Frozen, Strawb Cheesecake, Low Fat, Ben & Jerry's*	1 Serving/100g	170	3.0	170	4.0	31.0	3.0	1.0
Fruit, Brooklea*	1 Pot/120g	97	0.1	81	2.7	15.0	0.1	0.0
Fruit, Low Fat	1 Pot/120g	108	0.8	90	4.1	17.9	0.7	0.0
Fruit, Luscious, Low Fat, Bio-Live, Rachel's Organic*	1 Pot/125g	115	2.0	92	4.0	15.3	1.6	0.0
Fruit, Whole Milk	1 Pot/150g	157	4.2	105	5.1	15.7	2.8	0.0
Fruit Bio, Low Fat, Sainsbury's*	1 Pot/150g	156	1.6	104	4.6	18.9	1.1	0.3
Fruits of the Forest, Nestle*	1 Pot/125g	122	2.0	98	3.4	16.7	1.6	0.0
Fruits of the Forest, Smooth Set, Co-Op*	1 Pot/125g	95	1.1	76	3.7	12.5	0.9	0.0
Fruity Favourites, Organic, Yeo Valley*	1 Pot/125g	126	4.9	101	4.1	12.4	3.9	0.2
Fudge, Devonshire Style, Finest, Tesco*	1 Pot/150g	281	13.8	187	3.7	22.4	9.2	0.0

Y

YOGHURT

INFO/WEIGHT	Measure	per Measure KCAL	FAT	Nutrition Values per 100g / 100ml KCAL	PROT	CARB	FAT	FIBRE
Fudge, Thick & Creamy, Co-Op*	1 Pot/150g	196	7.5	131	3.8	17.6	5.0	0.0
Fudge, Thick & Creamy, M & S*	1 Pot/150g	195	7.5	130	4.4	17.3	5.0	0.7
Fudge, Thick & Creamy, Waitrose*	1 Pot/150g	196	4.5	131	4.4	21.5	3.0	0.0
Garden Fruit, Wholemilk, Bio Live, Rachel's Organic*	1 Pot/125g	109	4.2	87	3.5	10.5	3.4	0.0
Get Up & Go, Get Fresh At Home*	1 Pack/100g	113	0.5	113	8.0	19.0	0.5	1.9
Goats Whole Milk	**1 Carton/150g**	**94**	**5.7**	**63**	**3.5**	**3.9**	**3.8**	**0.0**
Gooseberry, Custard Style, Co-Op*	1 Pot/150g	216	7.9	144	3.7	19.3	5.3	0.3
Gooseberry, Custard Style, Shapers, Boots*	1 Pot/151g	106	1.1	70	3.9	12.0	0.7	0.2
Gooseberry, Low Fat, Average	1 Serving/100g	90	1.4	90	4.5	14.5	1.4	0.2
Gooseberry, Low Fat, Chosen By You, Asda*	1 Pot/125g	102	1.7	82	3.6	13.7	1.4	0.0
Gooseberry, Luxury Farmhouse, Stapleton*	1 Yogurt/150g	132	3.7	88	3.3	13.7	2.5	0.7
Gooseberry, Virtually Fat Free, Longley Farm*	1 Pot/150g	121	0.1	81	4.2	15.7	0.1	0.0
Greek, 0% Fat, Strained, Authentic, Total, Fage*	¼ Pot/125g	65	0.0	52	9.0	4.0	0.0	0.0
Greek, 2% Fat, Strained, Authentic, Total, Fage*	1 Pot/150g	100	3.0	67	8.4	3.8	2.0	0.0
Greek, Low Fat, Easiyo*	1 Pot/150g	99	1.9	66	5.6	8.4	1.3	0.0
Greek, Strained, Authentic, Original, Total, Fage*	1 Pot/200g	260	20.0	130	6.8	3.2	10.0	0.0
Greek, with Honey, Strained, Authentic, Total, Fage*	1 Pot/150g	255	12.0	170	5.4	19.0	8.0	0.0
Greek, with Strawberry, 2% Fat, Total, Fage*	1 Pot/150g	139	2.4	93	6.7	12.9	1.6	0.0
Greek Style, & Granola, Sainsbury's*	1 Pot/140g	262	7.6	187	5.8	29.0	5.4	0.6
Greek Style, & Nectarines, Food to Go, M & S*	1 Pack/200g	100	4.2	50	2.9	6.3	2.1	1.0
Greek Style, Fat Free, Natural, Chosen By You, Asda*	1 Tub/200g	114	0.4	57	7.9	5.8	0.2	0.1
Greek Style, Honey, Selection Pack, Organic, Tesco*	1 Pot/100g	156	8.7	156	4.1	15.3	8.7	0.0
Greek Style, Honey Topped, Tesco*	1 Pot/140g	203	12.0	145	3.6	13.4	8.6	0.0
Greek Style, Layered, Honey, Shapers, Boots*	1 Pot/150g	136	3.0	91	4.2	14.0	2.0	0.0
Greek Style, Low Fat, M & S*	1 Serving/100g	75	2.7	75	6.1	6.9	2.7	0.5
Greek Style, Luxury, Loseley*	1 Pot/175g	226	17.8	129	4.8	4.5	10.2	0.0
Greek Style, Natural, Fat Free, Tesco*	½ Pot/100g	55	0.2	55	7.5	4.8	0.2	0.4
Greek Style, Summer Berry Compote & Granola, M & S*	1 Pot/205g	336	16.4	164	5.6	17.3	8.0	0.1
Greek Style, with Golden Honey, Activia, Danone*	1 Pack/126g	122	3.5	97	5.0	13.0	2.8	0.1
Greek Style with Black Cherry Compote, M & S*	1 Pot/241g	205	3.4	85	3.4	15.0	1.4	0.5
Greek Style with Honey, Asda*	1 Pot/150g	225	13.0	150	4.0	13.9	8.7	0.0
Greek Style with Strawberries, Asda*	1 Pot/125g	159	8.2	127	3.2	13.6	6.6	0.2
Greek Style with Strawberry, Morrisons*	1 Pot/125g	162	8.2	130	3.3	14.4	6.6	0.0
Greek Style with Toffee & Hazelnuts, Asda*	1 Pot/125g	230	10.7	184	3.7	23.1	8.6	0.1
Greek Style with Tropical Fruits, Asda*	1 Pot/125g	164	8.2	131	3.3	14.5	6.6	0.3
Guava & Orange, Fat Free, Organic, Yeo Valley*	1 Pot/125g	92	0.1	74	5.3	13.0	0.1	0.2
Guava & Passion Fruit, Virtually Fat Free, Tesco*	1 Pot/125g	56	0.7	45	4.2	6.7	0.2	1.2
Hazelnut, Longley Farm*	1 Pot/150g	201	8.5	134	5.5	16.0	5.7	0.0
Hazelnut, Low Fat, Average	1 Serving/100g	106	2.3	106	4.5	16.9	2.3	0.1
Hazelnut, Sainsbury's*	1 Serving/150g	183	3.4	122	5.0	20.3	2.3	0.2
Hazelnut, Yoplait*	1 Pot/125g	166	5.0	133	4.6	19.6	4.0	0.0
Hazelnut Crunchy, Jordans*	1 Pot/150g	231	6.0	154	5.2	22.2	4.0	1.1
Honey, Greek Style, Co-Op*	1 Pot/150g	228	12.7	152	4.0	13.8	8.5	0.0
Honey, Greek Style, Organic, Sainsbury's*	1 Pot/100g	156	8.7	156	4.1	15.3	8.7	0.1
Honey, Low Fat, Asda*	1 Pot/125g	130	1.4	104	4.6	19.0	1.1	0.0
Honey & Ginger, Tesco*	1 Pot/150g	150	1.6	100	4.6	18.0	1.1	0.0
Honey & Ginger, Waitrose*	1 Pot/150g	226	11.4	151	3.7	17.0	7.6	0.1
Honey & Muesli, Breakfast Break, Tesco*	1 Pot/170g	207	4.6	122	3.9	20.5	2.7	0.6
Honey & Multigrain, Breakfast Selection, Sainsbury's*	1 Pot/125g	126	1.9	101	4.4	17.4	1.5	0.2
Honey Granola, Creamy, Nom Dairy UK*	1 Pot/150g	186	7.5	124	4.3	15.6	5.0	0.5
Honeyed Apricot, Greek Style, Corner, Muller*	1 Pot/150g	168	4.5	112	5.0	15.5	3.0	0.1
Italian Lemon, Amore Luxury, Muller*	1 Pot/150g	219	11.7	146	2.8	16.2	7.8	0.1
Jaffa Orange, Low Fat, Co-Op*	1 Pot/150g	126	1.3	84	3.9	15.0	0.9	0.4

YOGHURT

	Measure INFO/WEIGHT	per Measure KCAL	per Measure FAT	Nutrition Values per 100g / 100ml KCAL	PROT	CARB	FAT	FIBRE
Jubileum Kiwi, Tine*	1 Pot/135g	148	6.6	110	3.2	13.5	4.9	0.0
Jubileum Raspberry, Tine*	1 Pot/135g	163	6.5	121	3.2	16.1	4.8	0.0
Kiwi, Activia, Danone*	1 Pot/125g	119	4.1	95	3.6	12.7	3.3	0.3
Kiwi, Cereal, Fibre, Bio Activia, Danone*	1 Pot/120g	124	4.0	103	3.8	14.5	3.3	3.0
Kiwi & Gooseberry, Naturally Creamy, Nom Dairy UK*	1 Pot/175g	189	6.6	108	3.1	15.3	3.8	0.1
Lemon, COU, M & S*	1 Pot/200g	90	0.2	45	4.2	6.6	0.1	0.4
Lemon, Greek Style, GFY, Asda*	1 Pot/150g	124	4.3	83	4.1	10.0	2.9	0.1
Lemon, Greek Style, Shape, Danone*	1 Pot/125g	140	3.4	112	5.9	15.9	2.7	0.0
Lemon, Longley Farm*	1 Pot/150g	159	5.5	106	5.0	13.4	3.7	0.0
Lemon, Low Fat, Average	1 Serving/100g	95	0.9	95	4.6	17.3	0.9	0.1
Lemon, Smooth Set French, Low Fat, Sainsbury's*	1 Pot/125g	100	1.5	80	3.5	13.6	1.2	0.0
Lemon, Summer, Biopot, Onken*	1 Pot/150g	154	3.9	103	3.9	15.9	2.6	0.1
Lemon, Thick & Fruity, Citrus Fruits, Weight Watchers*	1 Pot/120g	49	0.1	41	4.0	5.8	0.1	0.1
Lemon & Lime, BGTY, Sainsbury's*	1 Pot/125g	66	0.1	53	4.6	8.3	0.1	1.1
Lemon & Lime, Fat Free, Shape, Danone*	1 Pot/120g	61	0.1	51	4.5	7.3	0.1	0.1
Lemon Cheesecake, Average	1 Serving/100g	55	0.2	55	4.3	8.8	0.2	0.2
Lemon Curd, Indulgent, Dessert, Waitrose*	1 Pot/150g	277	13.8	185	4.1	21.5	9.2	0.0
Lemon Lime Mousse, Shapers, Boots*	1 Pot/90g	89	3.8	99	4.2	11.0	4.2	0.1
Lemon Meringue, Sveltesse, Nestle*	1 Pot/125g	60	0.1	48	4.1	7.7	0.1	0.0
Light, Fat Free, Apricot, Muller*	1 Pot/190g	93	0.2	49	4.1	7.3	0.1	0.1
Light, Summer Fruits, Limited Edition, Muller*	1 Pot/175g	87	0.2	50	4.1	7.6	0.1	0.4
Light, Vanilla with Dark Chocolate Flakes, Brooklea*	1 Pot/165g	96	1.6	58	4.9	7.0	1.0	0.5
Loganberry, 0.06% Fat, TTD, Sainsbury's*	1 Pot/150g	186	8.7	124	3.7	14.2	5.8	0.8
Loganberry, Low Fat, Sainsbury's*	1 Pot/125g	111	1.9	89	4.2	14.5	1.5	0.1
Loganberry, Sainsbury's*	1 Pot/150g	193	9.3	129	3.9	14.2	6.2	0.6
Low Calorie	1 Pot/120g	49	0.2	41	4.3	6.0	0.2	0.0
Low Fat, Bio, Strawberry, Dale Farm*	1 Pot/125g	125	2.1	100	3.9	17.0	1.7	0.2
Low Fat, Totally Strawberry, Chosen By You, Asda*	1 Pot/125g	104	1.2	83	4.1	14.2	1.0	0.4
Luxury Strawberry & Clotted Cream, Stapleton Farm*	1 Pot/150g	147	5.7	98	3.2	13.2	3.8	0.6
Madagascan Vanilla, 0.06% Fat, TTD, Sainsbury's*	1 Pot/150g	210	9.0	140	3.7	17.8	6.0	0.0
Madagascan Vanilla, Indulgent, Dessert, Waitrose*	1 Pot/150g	240	11.4	160	3.7	19.2	7.6	0.0
Madagascan Vanilla, West Country, TTD, Sainsbury's*	¼ Pot/113g	145	6.3	128	3.9	15.5	5.6	0.0
Mandarin, Fat Free, Mullerlight, Muller*	1 Pot/190g	103	0.2	54	4.2	8.5	0.1	0.0
Mandarin, Longley Farm*	1 Pot/150g	141	5.7	94	4.9	13.3	3.8	0.0
Mandarin, Low Fat, Asda*	1 Pot/125g	101	1.5	81	4.6	13.0	1.2	0.0
Mango, Bio Activia, Danone*	1 Pot/125g	121	4.0	97	3.7	13.4	3.2	1.6
Mango, Fat Free, Shape Danone*	1 Pot/120g	74	0.1	62	6.6	8.6	0.1	2.2
Mango, Light, HL, Tesco*	1 Serving/125g	56	0.3	45	4.1	6.6	0.2	0.9
Mango, Light, Muller*	1 Pot/175g	96	0.2	55	4.3	9.2	0.1	0.0
Mango, Swiss, Emmi*	1 Serving/175g	184	4.4	105	3.5	17.0	2.5	0.3
Mango, Thick & Fruity, Tropical Fruit, Weight Watchers*	1 Pot/120g	49	0.1	41	3.9	6.0	0.1	1.1
Mango, Virtually Fat Free, Tesco*	1 Pot/125g	56	0.2	45	4.1	6.6	0.2	0.9
Mango, Zer0% Fat, No Added Sugar, Shape, Danone*	1 Pot/120g	72	0.1	60	6.0	8.8	0.1	0.9
Mango & Apple, Fat Free, Onken*	1 Serving/150g	79	0.3	53	4.9	6.6	0.2	0.2
Mango & Guava, Sunshine Selection, Sainsbury's*	1 Pot/125g	145	2.4	116	5.4	19.3	1.9	0.3
Mango & Passion Fruit, Creamy, Nom Dairy UK*	1 Pot/175g	189	6.6	108	3.1	15.4	3.8	0.3
Mango & Passion Fruit, Layered, Nom Dairy UK*	1 Pot/125g	114	3.0	91	3.2	14.2	2.4	0.3
Mango & Passionfruit, Fruit Corner, Muller*	1 Yoghurt/165g	177	6.4	107	3.8	13.5	3.9	0.3
Mango & Pineapple, BGTY, Sainsbury's*	1 Pot/124g	63	0.2	51	4.6	7.6	0.2	0.2
Mango 0% Fat, Shape Delights*	1 Pot/120g	80	0.1	67	5.5	10.9	0.1	0.9
Maple & Cinnamon Granola, Low Fat, Natural, Asda*	1 Pot/140g	196	4.6	140	6.1	21.5	3.3	0.8
Mississippi Mud Pie, Crunchable, Brooklea*	1 Pot/140g	237	6.3	169	4.0	28.0	4.5	0.3
Mixed Berries, Jogood, Imlek*	1 Pot/200g	172	4.4	86	2.9	13.4	2.2	0.0

YOGHURT

INFO/WEIGHT	Measure		Nutrition Values per 100g / 100ml				
	KCAL	FAT	KCAL	PROT	CARB	FAT	FIBRE
Mixed Seeds, Probiotic, Yoplait* — 1 Pot/125g	139	5.6	111	4.5	13.2	4.5	3.1
Morello Cherry, Amore Luxury, Muller* — 1 Pot/150g	216	11.7	144	2.8	16.3	7.8	0.1
Morello Cherry, HL, Tesco* — 1 Pot/125g	56	0.2	45	4.1	6.6	0.2	0.9
Muesli Nut, Low Fat — 1 Pot/120g	134	2.6	112	5.0	19.2	2.2	0.0
Multifruits, Yop Petit Déjeuner, Yoplait* — 1 Bottle/180g	155	2.2	86	2.7	16.0	1.2	0.0
Natural, Bio Life, Easiyo* — 1 Pot/150g	95	2.7	63	5.0	6.7	1.8	0.0
Natural, Greek Style, Average — 1 Serving/100g	138	10.6	138	4.7	6.1	10.6	0.0
Natural, Greek Style, Low Fat, Average — 1 Serving/100g	77	2.7	77	6.1	7.3	2.7	0.2
Natural, Greek Style, with Honey Sauce, Sainsbury's* — 1 Pot/140g	206	11.1	147	3.3	15.7	7.9	0.0
Natural, Low Fat, Average — **1 Pot/125g**	**75**	**1.6**	**60**	**5.4**	**7.0**	**1.3**	**0.0**
Natural, Low Fat, Organic, Average — 1 Serving/100g	87	1.2	87	5.7	7.7	1.2	0.0
Natural, Low Fat, Stirred, Sainsbury's* — 1 Serving/124g	83	1.9	67	5.5	7.8	1.5	0.0
Natural, Luxury, Bio Live, Jersey Dairy* — 1 Pot/150g	225	12.0	150	4.6	8.2	8.0	0.0
Natural, Organic, Evernat* — 1 Serving/100g	104	4.0	104	3.9	12.9	4.0	0.0
Natural, Organic, Yeo Valley* — 1 Pot/150g	120	5.5	80	4.7	6.9	3.7	0.0
Natural, Probiotic, 2% Fat, Sainsbury's* — ¼ Pot/125g	76	1.9	61	4.9	7.0	1.5	0.0
Natural, Probiotic, Crunchy Sultana Granola, M & S* — 1 Pack/180g	306	9.9	170	6.6	23.6	5.5	0.7
Natural, Probiotic, Fat Free, Organic, Yeo Valley* — 1 Pot/150g	87	0.1	58	5.9	8.4	0.1	0.0
Natural, Probiotic, Organic, Yeo Valley* — 1 Pot/150g	123	6.3	82	4.5	6.6	4.2	0.0
Natural, Set, Asda* — 1 Pot/450g	256	4.5	57	5.1	6.8	1.0	0.0
Natural, Set, Low Fat, Waitrose* — 1 Pot/150g	99	1.8	66	5.7	8.1	1.2	0.0
Natural, Sojasun* — 1 Serving/100g	51	2.7	51	4.6	2.0	2.7	0.0
Natural, Whole Milk, Set, Biopot, Onken* — 1 Pot/150g	108	5.5	72	3.9	5.7	3.7	0.0
Natural, Wholemilk, Live Bio, Organic, Waitrose* — 1 Serving/100g	88	4.4	88	5.1	7.1	4.4	0.0
Natural, with Cow's Milk, Greek Style, Sainsbury's* — ½ Pot/100g	143	10.9	143	4.5	6.6	10.9	0.0
Natural Probiotic, 0.1% Fat, BGTY, Sainsbury's* — 1 Serving/125g	69	0.1	55	5.6	8.0	0.1	0.0
Natural with Honey, Greek Style, Sainsbury's* — 1 Sm Pot/150g	243	14.1	162	4.0	15.4	9.4	0.0
Nectarine & Orange, Best There Is, Yoplait* — 1 Pot/122g	131	2.0	107	4.7	18.0	1.6	0.0
Nectarine & Orange, Channel Island, M & S* — 1 Pot/150g	157	4.9	105	4.5	14.7	3.3	0.3
Nectarine & Orange, Fat Free, Average — 1 Serving/100g	46	0.1	46	4.4	6.7	0.1	0.0
Nectarine & Orange, Fat Free, BFY, Morrisons* — 1 Serving/200g	128	0.6	64	5.9	9.5	0.3	0.1
Nectarine & Orange, M & S* — 1 Pot/150g	147	2.4	98	4.9	16.0	1.6	0.3
Nectarine & Passion Fruit, 0.1% Fat, Shape, Danone* — 1 Pot/120g	55	0.1	46	4.6	6.7	0.1	2.1
Nectarine & Passion Fruit, BGTY, Sainsbury's* — 1 Pot/151g	122	0.6	81	3.2	16.3	0.4	0.6
Nectarine & Passion Fruit, Low Fat, Stapleton Farm* — 1 Pot/150g	120	0.7	80	3.2	16.3	0.5	0.6
Orange, BGTY, Sainsbury's* — 1 Pot/125g	62	0.1	50	4.5	7.7	0.1	1.1
Orange, Greek Style, Boots* — 1 Pot/140g	207	12.0	148	3.7	14.0	8.6	0.2
Orange, Greek Style, Shape, Danone* — 1 Pot/125g	140	3.4	112	6.0	16.0	2.7	0.1
Orange, Low Fat, Tesco* — 1 Pot/125g	114	2.2	91	4.3	14.5	1.8	0.0
Orange, Sprinkled with Dark Chocolate, Light, Muller* — 1 Pot/165g	84	0.8	51	4.0	7.1	0.5	0.1
Orange & Lemon, BGTY, Sainsbury's* — 1 Pot/125g	62	0.2	50	4.7	7.3	0.2	0.2
Orange & Mango, Thick & Fruity, Probiotic, COU, M & S* — 1 Pot/145g	65	0.1	45	4.2	6.5	0.1	0.5
Orange & Pineapple, Tropical Fruit, Activ8, Ski, Nestle* — 1 Pot/120g	112	2.0	93	4.4	15.1	1.7	0.2
Orange Blossom Honey, Finest, Tesco* — 1 Pot/150g	237	10.6	158	3.5	20.1	7.1	0.0
Passion Fruit with Elderflower Extract, Tesco* — 1 Pot/150g	147	1.6	98	4.7	17.3	1.1	0.2
Peach, BGTY, Sainsbury's* — 1 Pot/125g	61	0.2	49	4.7	7.2	0.2	0.2
Peach, Bio, Activia, Fat Free, Danone* — 1 Sm Pot/125g	71	0.1	57	4.7	9.3	0.1	1.0
Peach, Custard Style, Low Fat, Sainsbury's* — 1 Pot/125g	110	1.9	88	4.4	14.2	1.5	0.1
Peach, Economy, Sainsbury's* — 1 Pot/125g	92	0.5	74	2.8	14.7	0.4	0.0
Peach, Fat Free, Activ8, Ski, Nestle* — 1 Yogurt/120g	89	0.1	74	4.5	13.7	0.1	0.7
Peach, Fat Free, Probiotic, Chosen By You, Asda* — 1 Yoghurt/125g	88	0.1	70	3.9	12.1	0.1	2.6
Peach, Forbidden Fruits, Rachel's Organic* — 1 Pot/125g	156	7.6	125	3.4	14.0	6.1	0.0
Peach, Low Fat, Average — 1 Serving/100g	86	1.1	86	4.5	14.6	1.1	0.1

YOGHURT

	Measure INFO/WEIGHT	per Measure KCAL	FAT	Nutrition Values per 100g / 100ml KCAL	PROT	CARB	FAT	FIBRE
Peach, Low Fat, Probiotic, Tesco*	1 Pot/125g	106	1.7	85	3.9	14.3	1.4	0.3
Peach, Luscious, Low Fat, Rachel's Organic*	1 Pot/125g	112	2.0	90	4.0	14.9	1.6	0.2
Peach, Smooth Style, Mullerlight, Muller*	1 Pot/125g	59	0.1	47	4.1	6.9	0.1	0.2
Peach & Apricot, 0.1% Fat, Shape, Danone*	1 Pot/120g	55	0.1	46	4.6	6.7	0.1	2.1
Peach & Apricot, Fruit Corner, Muller*	1 Pot/175g	189	6.8	108	3.8	13.6	3.9	0.5
Peach & Apricot, HL, Tesco*	1 Pot/92g	42	0.1	46	4.0	7.4	0.1	1.0
Peach & Apricot, Light, HL, Tesco*	1 Pot/200g	82	0.2	41	3.9	6.2	0.1	1.0
Peach & Lemon Balm, Biowild, Onken*	1 Pot/175g	157	2.6	90	4.3	14.9	1.5	0.1
Peach & Mango, 0.1% Actimel, Danone*	1 Serving/100g	29	0.1	29	2.7	3.6	0.1	0.1
Peach & Mango, Dairy Free, Organic, Yofu, Provamel*	1 Pot/125g	100	2.7	80	3.9	10.4	2.2	0.8
Peach & Mango, Juicy, Shapers, Boots*	1 Pot/150g	88	1.6	59	4.0	8.3	1.1	0.5
Peach & Mango, Thick & Creamy, Waitrose*	1 Pot/125g	136	3.1	109	3.7	17.8	2.5	0.3
Peach & Mango, Truly Fruity, Brooklea, Aldi*	1 Pot/200g	162	2.8	81	4.6	12.4	1.4	0.0
Peach & Maracuya, Mullerlight, Muller*	1 Pot/200g	102	0.2	51	4.5	8.1	0.1	0.0
Peach & Papaya, Fat Free, Yeo Valley*	1 Pot/125g	94	0.1	75	5.3	13.1	0.1	0.1
Peach & Papaya, Waitrose*	1 Pot/150g	129	0.1	86	4.2	17.1	0.1	0.2
Peach & Passion Fruit, Average	1 Serving/100g	66	0.7	66	4.5	10.6	0.7	0.4
Peach & Passion Fruit, Fat Free, Shape, Danone*	1 Pot/120g	74	0.1	62	6.6	8.6	0.1	2.3
Peach & Passion Fruit, Fruit Layered, Bio, GFY, Asda*	1 Pot/126g	77	0.1	61	4.0	11.0	0.1	0.5
Peach & Passion Fruit, Layers, Mullerlight, Muller*	1 Pot/175g	94	0.2	54	3.1	9.7	0.1	0.2
Peach & Passion Fruit, Lite Biopot, Onken*	1/5 Pot/100g	45	0.2	45	4.6	6.0	0.2	0.2
Peach & Passionfruit, BGTY, Sainsbury's*	1 Pot/125g	69	0.1	55	4.9	8.6	0.1	0.1
Peach & Pear, Seriously Fruity, Low Fat, Waitrose*	1 Pot/125g	110	1.2	88	4.5	15.3	1.0	0.3
Peach & Vanilla, Thick & Creamy, Co-Op*	1 Pot/150g	180	6.9	120	3.6	16.0	4.6	0.1
Peach & Vanilla Flip, Morrisons*	1 Pot/175g	212	8.0	121	3.4	16.5	4.6	0.6
Peach Melba, Low Fat, Average	1 Serving/100g	75	0.7	75	2.6	14.5	0.7	0.0
Peach Melba, Sveltesse, Nestle*	1 Pot/126g	70	0.1	56	4.7	9.1	0.1	0.2
Peaches, Farmhouse, BGTY, Sainsbury's*	1 Pot/150g	133	0.6	89	3.2	17.8	0.4	0.3
Peach-Nectarine, Bio Activia, Fat Free, Danone*	1 Pot/125g	70	0.1	56	4.5	9.3	0.1	1.0
Pear, Jubileum, Tine*	1 Carton/125g	167	6.5	134	3.2	18.6	5.2	0.0
Pear & Butterscotch, Finest, Tesco*	1 Pot/150g	412	21.0	275	5.0	32.3	14.0	0.5
Pear & Vanilla, Thick & Creamy, Weight Watchers*	1 Pot/120g	54	0.6	45	4.2	5.8	0.5	0.2
Phish Food, Frozen, Lower Fat, Ben & Jerry's*	½ Pot/211g	464	10.5	220	4.0	40.0	5.0	1.5
Pineapple, Average	1 Serving/100g	73	1.1	73	4.4	11.3	1.1	0.5
Pineapple, Bio Activia, Fat Free, Danone*	1 Pot/125g	62	0.1	50	4.7	7.5	0.1	1.7
Pineapple, Channel Island, M & S*	1 Pot/150g	165	4.9	110	4.3	15.9	3.3	0.3
Pineapple, Extremely Fruity, M & S*	1 Pot/200g	200	2.8	100	4.3	17.6	1.4	0.2
Pineapple, Low Fat, Average	1 Serving/100g	89	1.2	89	4.6	14.7	1.2	0.0
Pineapple, Low Fat, Bio, Asda*	1 Pot/150g	144	1.6	96	4.6	17.0	1.1	0.1
Pineapple, Thick & Creamy, Waitrose*	1 Pot/125g	136	3.1	109	3.6	17.9	2.5	0.2
Pineapple, Virtually Fat Free, Tesco*	1 Pot/125g	55	0.2	44	4.1	6.5	0.2	0.9
Pineapple, Vitality, Low Fat, with Omega 3, Muller*	1 Pot/150g	138	2.8	92	4.2	13.8	1.9	0.7
Pineapple & Grapefruit, BGTY, Sainsbury's*	1 Pot/125g	67	0.1	54	4.4	8.8	0.1	0.1
Pineapple & Passion Fruit, Soya, Light, Alpro*	1 Pot/120g	62	1.3	52	2.1	7.3	1.1	0.8
Pineapple & Peach, Fruity, Mullerlight, Muller*	1 Pot/175g	89	0.2	51	4.2	7.7	0.1	0.2
Pink Grapefruit, Low Fat, Sainsbury's*	1 Pot/125g	116	1.7	93	4.2	15.9	1.4	0.1
Pink Grapefruit, Thick & Fruity, Weight Watchers*	1 Pot/120g	49	0.1	41	3.9	6.2	0.1	1.0
Plain, Low Fat, Average	*1 Serving/100g*	*63*	*1.5*	*63*	*5.2*	*7.0*	*1.5*	*0.0*
Plain, Whole Milk, Average	*1oz/28g*	*22*	*0.8*	*79*	*5.7*	*7.8*	*3.0*	*0.0*
Plum, BGTY, Sainsbury's*	1 Pot/125g	69	0.1	55	4.8	8.8	0.1	0.1
Plum, Low Fat, Sainsbury's*	1 Pot/125g	117	2.1	94	4.5	15.2	1.7	0.1
Plum, Probiotic, Summer Selection, Yeo Valley*	1 Pot/125g	126	4.9	101	4.1	12.4	3.9	0.1
Plum, Soya, Dairy Free, Organic, with Fibre, Provamel*	1 Serving/125g	90	2.5	72	3.7	7.5	2.0	4.0

Y

YOGHURT

INFO/WEIGHT	Measure	per Measure KCAL	FAT	Nutrition Values per 100g / 100ml KCAL	PROT	CARB	FAT	FIBRE
Pouring, Strawberry, Activia, Danone*	1 Serving/100g	59	1.6	59	3.9	7.3	1.6	0.1
Probiotic, Aldi*	1 Serving/200g	178	2.8	89	4.1	14.2	1.4	0.0
Probiotic, Low Fat, Organic, Glenisk Organic Dairy Co*	1 Serving/150g	91	2.8	61	4.5	6.4	1.9	0.0
Prune, Bifidus, Activo, Mercadona*	1 Pot/125g	70	0.1	56	4.5	6.8	0.1	3.0
Prune, Bio Activia, Danone*	1 Pot/125g	110	3.5	88	3.5	12.2	2.8	0.2
Prune, Breakfast Selection, Sainsbury's*	1 Pot/125g	119	1.7	95	4.2	16.3	1.4	0.2
Prune, Probiotic, Tesco*	1 Serving/170g	145	2.4	85	3.9	14.3	1.4	1.0
Prune, Vitality, Low Fat, with Omega 3, Muller*	1 Pot/150g	144	2.8	96	4.7	15.0	1.9	1.1
Raspberry, Bio, Activia, Danone*	1 Pot/125g	112	3.5	90	3.5	12.8	2.8	2.0
Raspberry, Bio, Activia, Fat Free, Danone*	1 Pot/125g	59	0.1	47	4.6	6.9	0.1	2.5
Raspberry, Bio, Low Fat, Benecol*	1 Pot/125g	99	0.8	79	3.8	14.5	0.6	0.0
Raspberry, Bio, Pur Natur*	1 Pot/150g	150	4.6	100	1.4	14.5	3.1	0.0
Raspberry, Economy, Sainsbury's*	1 Pot/125g	85	1.2	68	3.0	11.9	1.0	0.0
Raspberry, Extremely Fruity, M & S*	1 Pot/200g	190	3.0	95	5.0	15.6	1.5	0.5
Raspberry, Fat Free, Average	1 Serving/100g	64	0.1	64	4.9	11.0	0.1	1.7
Raspberry, Fat Free, Probiotic, Organic, Yeo Valley*	1 Pot/125g	97	0.1	78	5.2	14.0	0.1	0.4
Raspberry, Forbidden Fruit, Rachel's Organic*	1 Pot/125g	155	7.6	124	3.4	13.8	6.1	0.1
Raspberry, French Set, Waitrose*	1 Pot/125g	120	3.9	96	3.5	13.4	3.1	2.0
Raspberry, Incredibly Fruity, Fat Free, Tesco*	1 Pot/150g	112	0.1	75	4.8	13.1	0.1	1.0
Raspberry, Lactose Free, Lactofree, Arla*	1 Pot/125g	130	3.4	104	3.3	16.5	2.7	0.7
Raspberry, Light, HL, Tesco*	1 Pot/200g	88	0.2	44	3.9	7.0	0.1	1.7
Raspberry, Low Fat, Average	1 Serving/100g	83	1.1	83	4.1	14.1	1.1	0.8
Raspberry, Low Fat, Bio, Sainsbury's*	1 Pot/150g	145	1.6	97	4.7	17.0	1.1	0.7
Raspberry, Low Fat, Bio Live, Rachel's Organic*	1 Pot/125g	109	2.0	87	4.0	14.2	1.6	0.1
Raspberry, Low Fat, Organic, Sainsbury's*	1 Serving/125g	106	1.2	85	5.1	14.0	1.0	0.2
Raspberry, Low Fat, Probiotic, Tesco*	1 Pot/170g	144	2.4	85	3.9	14.3	1.4	0.3
Raspberry, Low Fat, Stapleton*	1 Serving/150g	105	0.7	70	3.3	13.6	0.5	2.0
Raspberry, Meadow Fresh*	1 Sm Pot/125g	130	1.2	104	4.5	18.9	1.0	0.0
Raspberry, Naturally Light, Nom Dairy UK*	1 Pot/180g	133	0.2	74	4.3	13.9	0.1	0.2
Raspberry, Organic, Yeo Valley*	1 Pot/150g	151	5.8	101	4.2	12.3	3.9	0.4
Raspberry, Probiotic, Live, Yeo Valley*	1 Pot/125g	106	1.2	85	5.1	14.0	1.0	0.4
Raspberry, Probiotic, Low Fat, Organic, M & S*	1 Pot/170g	127	2.4	75	4.4	11.5	1.4	0.4
Raspberry, Scottish, The Best, Morrisons*	1 Pot/150g	208	10.3	139	3.6	15.6	6.9	1.3
Raspberry, Smooth, Activ8, Ski, Nestle*	1 Pot/120g	113	2.0	94	4.6	14.8	1.7	0.7
Raspberry, Smooth, Mullerlight, Muller*	1 Pot/125g	64	0.1	51	4.2	7.8	0.1	0.6
Raspberry, Summer, Biopot, Onken*	1/5 Pot/90g	91	2.4	101	3.8	15.0	2.7	0.6
Raspberry, Thick & Creamy, Sainsbury's*	1 Pot/150g	178	5.5	119	4.4	17.2	3.7	0.2
Raspberry, Thick & Fruity, Probiotic, COU, M & S*	1 Pot/170g	76	0.2	45	4.2	6.9	0.1	0.6
Raspberry, Virtually Fat Free, Tesco*	1 Pot/125g	51	0.2	41	4.1	5.8	0.2	1.1
Raspberry, Vitality, Low Fat, with Omega 3, Muller*	1 Pot/125g	115	2.5	92	4.3	13.4	2.0	1.3
Raspberry, with Fruit Layer, Bio Activia, Danone*	1 Pot/125g	107	3.5	86	3.5	11.6	2.8	2.0
Raspberry & Blackberry, Rich & Creamy, Spelga*	1 Serving/150g	187	7.0	125	3.7	17.2	4.7	0.1
Raspberry & Blackberry, Thick & Creamy, Co-Op*	1 Pot/150g	187	6.9	125	3.6	17.3	4.6	0.1
Raspberry & Cranberry, BGTY, Sainsbury's*	1 Pot/125g	65	0.1	52	4.4	8.4	0.1	0.5
Raspberry & Cranberry, Fat Free, Mullerlight, Muller*	1 Pot/175g	89	0.2	51	4.2	7.8	0.1	0.5
Raspberry & Cranberry, Light, HL, Tesco*	1 Pot/125g	55	0.2	44	4.2	6.3	0.2	1.1
Raspberry & Elderberry, Organic, Onken*	1 Serving/50g	53	1.5	106	3.8	15.0	3.1	0.0
Raspberry & Orange, Fat Free, Organic, Yeo Valley*	1 Serving/100g	77	0.1	77	5.1	13.7	0.1	0.1
Raspberry & Redcurrant, Low Fat, Morrisons*	1 Pot/125g	117	2.0	94	4.4	15.4	1.6	0.7
Raspberry & Redcurrant, Low Fat, Sainsbury's*	1 Pot/125g	109	1.7	87	4.2	14.5	1.4	0.5
Raspberry or Strawberry, Smooth, No Bits, Ski, Nestle*	1 Pot/120g	118	3.2	98	3.9	13.6	2.7	0.0
Raspberry Smooth, Favourites, Nom Dairy UK*	1 Pot/125g	111	3.0	89	3.2	13.7	2.4	0.3
Rhubarb, Bio Activia, Danone*	1 Pot/125g	112	4.0	90	3.5	11.8	3.2	2.2

YOGHURT

INFO/WEIGHT	Measure	per Measure		Nutrition Values per 100g / 100ml				
		KCAL	FAT	KCAL	PROT	CARB	FAT	FIBRE
Rhubarb, Custard Style, Co-Op*	1 Pot/150g	202	7.9	135	3.7	17.2	5.3	0.3
Rhubarb, Extremely Fruity, Low Fat, Probiotic, M & S*	1 Pot/170g	153	1.7	90	4.4	15.5	1.0	0.7
Rhubarb, Fruity, Mullerlight, Muller*	1 Pot/175g	91	0.2	52	4.2	7.9	0.1	0.0
Rhubarb, Greek Style, Corner, Muller*	1 Pot/150g	169	4.5	113	5.0	15.8	3.0	0.1
Rhubarb, Longley Farm*	1 Pot/150g	165	5.5	110	4.9	14.3	3.7	0.0
Rhubarb, Low Fat, Average	1 Serving/100g	83	1.2	83	4.6	13.3	1.2	0.2
Rhubarb, Luscious, Low Fat, Bio Live, Rachel's Organic*	1 Pot/125g	104	2.0	83	4.0	13.1	1.6	0.1
Rhubarb, M & S*	1 Pot/150g	148	2.1	99	4.4	17.4	1.4	0.3
Rhubarb, Spiced, Thick & Creamy, COU, M & S*	1 Pot/170g	68	0.2	40	4.3	5.8	0.1	0.5
Rhubarb & Champagne, Truly Irresistible, Co-Op*	1 Pot/150g	195	8.2	130	3.5	16.6	5.5	0.2
Rhubarb & Orange, Tesco*	1 Pot/150g	145	1.6	97	4.6	17.1	1.1	0.5
Rhubarb & Vanilla, Summer, Biopot, Onken*	1/5 Pot/90g	94	2.4	104	3.7	16.0	2.7	0.3
Rhubarb Crumble, Crunch Corner, Muller*	1 Pot/150g	238	8.4	159	3.6	23.5	5.6	0.5
Sheep's Milk, Total, Fage*	1 Pot/200g	180	12.0	90	4.8	4.3	6.0	0.0
Simply, Bio Lite, Ideal World*	1 Serving/100g	57	1.5	57	4.6	6.8	1.5	0.0
Simply, Lemon, Ideal World*	1 Serving/100g	108	3.9	108	4.6	19.4	3.9	0.0
Smooth Toffee, Mullerlight, Muller*	1 Pot/190g	97	0.2	51	4.0	7.9	0.1	0.0
Smooth Toffee & Apple, Low Fat, Co-Op*	1 Pot/125g	150	1.2	120	6.0	22.0	1.0	0.1
Smoothie, Apple, Strawb & Peach, Sveltesse, Nestle*	1 Pot/125g	61	0.1	49	4.8	7.3	0.1	0.1
Smoothie, Strawb, Rasp, & Mint, Sveltesse, Nestle*	1 Pot/125g	62	0.1	50	4.8	7.4	0.1	0.2
Soya, Peach, Dairy Free, Organic, Yofu, Provamel*	1 Serving/125g	100	2.7	80	3.9	10.3	2.2	0.8
Soya, Plain, Average	*1oz/28g*	*20*	*1.2*	*72*	*5.0*	*3.9*	*4.2*	*0.0*
Soya, Raspberry, Alpro*	1 Pot/125g	99	2.4	79	3.7	10.4	1.9	1.2
Spanish Orange, Amore Luxury, Muller*	1 Pot/150g	226	11.7	151	2.9	17.2	7.8	0.1
Spiced Apple, 6% Fat, TTD, Sainsbury's*	1 Pot/15g	16	0.6	107	2.7	15.6	3.8	0.5
Spiced Orange, Dessert, Low Fat, Sainsbury's*	1 Pot/125g	121	2.1	97	4.5	16.0	1.7	0.1
Strawberries & Cream, 0.06% Fat, TTD, Sainsbury's*	1 Pot/150g	183	8.2	122	3.5	14.7	5.5	0.4
Strawberries & Cream, Finest, Tesco*	1 Pot/150g	205	10.3	137	3.4	15.4	6.9	0.5
Strawberry, & Muesli, Breakfast, Tesco*	1 Pot/170g	192	4.8	113	4.1	17.9	2.8	0.5
Strawberry, & Whole Grain, Bio Break, Tesco*	1 Pot/175g	175	1.9	100	4.7	17.8	1.1	0.2
Strawberry, Amore for Me, Muller*	1 Pot/150g	216	10.9	144	2.6	17.0	7.3	0.2
Strawberry, Balanced Lifestyle, Aldi*	1 Pot/150g	72	0.4	48	4.1	7.1	0.3	0.5
Strawberry, BGTY, Sainsbury's*	1 Pot/125g	64	0.1	51	4.8	7.7	0.1	1.2
Strawberry, Bio, Granola, Corner, Muller*	1 Pot/135g	161	3.5	119	5.5	17.8	2.6	0.8
Strawberry, Bio Activia, Danone*	1 Pot/125g	117	4.0	94	3.5	12.8	3.2	2.0
Strawberry, Cereals, Fibre, Bio Activia, Danone*	1 Pot/120g	113	3.8	94	3.7	12.7	3.2	3.0
Strawberry, Childrens, Co-Op*	1 Pot/125g	121	3.4	97	3.5	14.9	2.7	0.2
Strawberry, Custard Style, Shapers, Boots*	1 Pot/150g	117	1.0	78	3.9	14.0	0.7	0.5
Strawberry, Duo, Co-Op*	1 Pot/175g	219	8.7	125	3.0	17.0	5.0	0.7
Strawberry, Everyday Low Fat, Co-Op*	1 Pot/125g	87	0.9	70	3.0	13.0	0.7	0.0
Strawberry, Farmhouse, BGTY, Sainsbury's*	1 Pot/150g	106	0.6	71	3.2	13.7	0.4	0.5
Strawberry, Fat Free, Average	1 Serving/100g	66	0.1	66	4.9	11.1	0.1	0.6
Strawberry, Fruit Corner, Snack Size, Muller*	1 Pot/95g	108	3.8	114	3.9	15.6	4.0	0.4
Strawberry, Fruit 'n' Creamy, Ubley*	1 Pot/151g	167	4.4	111	4.3	16.9	2.9	0.3
Strawberry, Fruity, Mullerlight, Muller*	1 Pot/175g	102	0.2	51	4.1	7.9	0.1	0.0
Strawberry, Granose*	1 Pot/120g	108	1.9	90	4.5	15.5	1.6	0.0
Strawberry, Great Stuff, Asda*	1 Pot/60g	58	1.5	97	4.7	14.0	2.5	0.5
Strawberry, Healthy Balance, Corner, Muller*	1 Pot/135g	161	3.5	119	5.4	17.9	2.6	0.8
Strawberry, Light, Brooklea*	1 Pot/200g	154	0.2	77	6.1	12.9	0.1	0.4
Strawberry, Light, HL, Tesco*	1 Pot/200g	80	0.2	40	3.5	6.4	0.1	0.8
Strawberry, Light & Refreshing, Campina*	1 Pot/125g	110	1.4	88	2.5	16.9	1.1	0.0
Strawberry, Light Choices, Tesco*	1 Pot/200g	86	0.2	43	4.1	6.3	0.1	0.6
Strawberry, Little Town Dairy*	1 Pot/125g	82	2.0	66	2.9	9.9	1.6	0.0

YOGHURT

	INFO/WEIGHT	KCAL	FAT	KCAL	PROT	CARB	FAT	FIBRE
Strawberry, Live, Turners Dairies*	1 Pot/125g	86	0.4	69	4.9	11.9	0.3	0.0
Strawberry, Low Fat, Average	1 Serving/100g	81	1.0	81	4.5	13.6	1.0	0.2
Strawberry, Low Fat, Probiotic, Organic, M & S*	1 Pot/170g	136	2.4	80	4.8	11.6	1.4	0.4
Strawberry, Luscious, Shapers, Boots*	1 Pot/150g	82	1.6	55	4.0	7.3	1.1	0.6
Strawberry, Luxury, Bio Live, Jersey Dairy*	1 Pot/150g	159	8.5	106	3.8	10.2	5.7	0.5
Strawberry, Naturally Creamy, Nom Dairy UK*	1 Pot/175g	185	6.6	106	3.1	15.0	3.8	0.3
Strawberry, Naturally Light, Nom Dairy UK*	1 Pot/180g	137	0.2	76	4.5	13.4	0.1	0.3
Strawberry, Organic, Yeo Valley*	1 Pot/150g	144	4.9	96	4.3	12.4	3.3	0.1
Strawberry, Perfectly Balanced, Waitrose*	1 Pot/150g	136	0.2	91	4.6	17.8	0.1	0.1
Strawberry, Petit Filou, Yoplait*	1 Pot/60g	62	1.7	104	6.6	12.6	2.9	0.2
Strawberry, Probiotic, Natural Balance, Asda*	1 Pot/125g	109	3.0	87	3.1	13.3	2.4	2.4
Strawberry, Probiotic, Organic, Yeo Valley*	1 Pot/125g	125	5.0	100	4.4	11.7	4.0	0.1
Strawberry, Redcurrant, Bio Layered, Sainsbury's*	1 Serving/125g	134	3.4	107	4.1	16.5	2.7	0.2
Strawberry, Smooth, Activ8, Ski, Nestle*	1 Pot/120g	113	2.0	94	4.6	14.8	1.7	0.7
Strawberry, Smooth Set French, Low Fat, Sainsbury's*	1 Pot/125g	112	4.0	90	3.7	11.8	3.2	0.0
Strawberry, Soya, Dairy Free, Organic, Yofu, Provamel*	1 Pot/125g	101	2.7	81	3.9	10.6	2.2	0.8
Strawberry, Soyage, GranoVita*	1 Pot/145g	112	0.6	77	1.8	16.5	0.4	0.0
Strawberry, Sveltesse, Nestle*	1 Serving/125g	61	0.1	49	4.8	7.1	0.1	0.2
Strawberry, Swiss, Emmi*	1 Pot/175g	177	4.4	101	3.5	16.0	2.5	0.3
Strawberry, Thick & Creamy, Co-Op*	1 Pot/150g	181	6.9	121	3.6	16.4	4.6	0.1
Strawberry, Thick & Creamy, Waitrose*	1 Pot/125g	135	3.1	108	3.7	17.6	2.5	0.4
Strawberry, Thick & Fruity, Probiotic, COU, M & S*	1 Pot/170g	76	0.2	45	4.1	7.3	0.1	0.4
Strawberry, Very Berry, Activ8, Ski, Nestle*	1 Pot/120g	110	2.0	92	4.3	15.0	1.7	0.3
Strawberry, Virtually Fat Free, Average	1 Serving/100g	65	0.2	65	4.7	11.3	0.2	0.2
Strawberry, Vitality, Low Fat, with Omega 3, Muller*	1 Pot/150g	139	2.8	93	4.3	14.0	1.9	0.8
Strawberry, Wholemilk, Organic, Sainsbury's*	1 Pot/150g	123	5.2	82	3.5	9.2	3.5	0.1
Strawberry, Yoplait*	1 Pot/125g	61	0.2	49	4.2	7.6	0.2	0.9
Strawberry & Banana, Oatie Breakfast, Moma Foods*	1 Pot/235g	320	5.6	136	4.3	25.4	2.4	1.7
Strawberry & Cornish Clotted Cream, M & S*	1 Pot/150g	217	11.5	145	3.2	15.4	7.7	0.5
Strawberry & French Vanilla, Amore Luxury, Muller*	1 Pot/150g	225	11.7	150	2.9	17.0	7.8	0.1
Strawberry & Raspberry, HL, Tesco*	1 Pot/125g	57	0.1	46	4.2	7.0	0.1	0.0
Strawberry & Raspberry, Layered, Bio, GFY, Asda*	1 Pot/72g	43	0.1	60	3.8	11.0	0.1	0.4
Strawberry & Raspberry, Low Fat, Asda*	1 Pot/150g	142	1.5	95	4.6	17.4	1.0	0.2
Strawberry & Raspberry, Low Fat, Sainsbury's*	1 Pot/125g	109	1.7	87	4.2	14.3	1.4	0.2
Strawberry & Raspberry, Probiotic, Organic, Yeo Valley*	1 Pot/125g	125	4.9	100	4.2	12.0	3.9	0.1
Strawberry & Redcurrant, Farmhouse, Ann Forshaw's*	1 Pot/150g	193	7.3	129	3.8	17.4	4.9	0.2
Strawberry & Rhubarb, Channel Island, M & S*	1 Pot/150g	157	4.5	105	3.9	15.4	3.0	0.0
Strawberry & Rhubarb, Low Fat, Sainsbury's*	1 Pot/125g	107	1.7	86	4.2	14.1	1.4	0.2
Strawberry & Rhubarb, Onken*	1 Serving/100g	85	0.1	85	4.6	16.2	0.1	0.4
Strawberry Crumble, Crunch Corner, Muller*	1 Pot/150g	234	8.4	156	3.6	22.9	5.6	0.5
Strawberry Lactose Free, Lactofree, Arla*	1 Pot/125g	126	3.2	101	3.5	15.9	2.6	0.4
Strawberry Mousse, Shapers, Boots*	1 Pot/91g	88	3.7	97	4.1	11.0	4.1	0.1
Strawberry Orange Balls. Crunch Corner, Muller*	1 Pot/150g	222	8.1	148	4.0	20.8	5.4	0.2
Strawberry Rice - Low Fat, Muller*	1 Pot/190g	203	4.4	107	3.2	18.4	2.3	0.4
Strawberry Shortcake, Crunch Corner, Muller*	1 Pot/150g	232	8.7	155	3.9	21.0	5.8	0.1
Strawberry Smooth, Nom Dairy UK*	1 Yoghurt/125g	112	3.0	90	3.2	13.8	2.4	0.3
Summer Berries, Fat Free, Mullerlight, Muller*	1 Pot /175g	87	0.2	50	4.1	7.6	0.1	0.4
Summer Berries, Wholegrain, Biopot, Onken*	1 Portion/100g	110	2.9	110	4.1	16.9	2.9	0.7
Summer Fruits, Cool Country*	1 Serving/150g	136	2.2	91	3.0	16.3	1.5	0.0
Summer Fruits, Greek Style, Corner, Muller*	1 Pot/150g	165	4.5	110	5.1	15.0	3.0	0.5
Summer Fruits, Light, Spelga*	1 Pot/175g	79	0.3	45	4.4	7.1	0.2	0.0
Summer Selection, Fat Free, Organic, Yeo Valley*	1 Pot/125g	89	0.1	71	5.2	12.3	0.1	0.2
Summer Selection, Thick & Fruity, COU, M & S*	1 Pot/145g	75	0.2	52	4.2	7.8	0.1	0.5

YOGHURT

	Measure INFO/WEIGHT	per Measure KCAL	FAT	Nutrition Values per 100g / 100ml KCAL	PROT	CARB	FAT	FIBRE
Summerfruits, Fat Free, Bio Live, Rachel's Organic*	1 Pot/125g	120	2.2	96	4.7	15.3	1.8	0.0
Summerfruits Bio, Boots*	1 Pot/150g	139	4.0	93	4.1	13.0	2.7	0.4
Sweet Treat, Low Fat, Tesco*	1 Pot/125g	131	2.9	105	3.1	18.0	2.3	0.3
Thick & Fruity Black Cherry, COU, M & S*	1 Pot/145g	72	0.1	50	4.2	7.8	0.1	0.5
Timperley Rhubarb, Seriously Fruity, Waitrose*	1 Pot/150g	127	1.5	85	4.6	14.4	1.0	0.0
Timperley Rhubarb, TTD, Sainsbury's*	1 Pot/150g	168	7.3	112	3.4	13.6	4.9	0.4
Toffee, Benecol*	1 Pot/125g	124	0.9	99	3.8	19.3	0.7	0.0
Toffee, COU, M & S*	1 Pot/145g	65	0.3	45	4.2	7.7	0.2	0.0
Toffee, Economy, Sainsbury's*	1 Pot/126g	91	1.3	72	3.0	12.8	1.0	0.0
Toffee, Light, HL, Tesco*	1 Pot/200g	80	0.2	40	3.9	5.9	0.1	1.0
Toffee, Live Bio, Perfectly Balanced, Waitrose*	1 Pot/150g	156	0.4	104	4.2	21.1	0.3	0.0
Toffee, Low Fat, Co-Op*	1 Pot/150g	124	1.3	83	3.8	15.0	0.9	0.2
Toffee, Low Fat, M & S*	1 Pot/150g	180	2.5	120	4.9	21.6	1.7	0.0
Toffee, Seriously Smooth, Low Fat, Waitrose*	1 Pot/150g	156	3.1	104	4.7	16.5	2.1	0.1
Toffee, Smooth, Mullerlight, Fat Free, Muller*	1 Pot/190g	95	0.2	50	4.0	7.7	0.1	0.0
Toffee, Smooth & Creamy, Fat Free, Weight Watchers*	1 Pot/120g	48	0.1	40	3.9	5.9	0.1	0.8
Toffee, Virtually Fat Free, Boots*	1 Pot/125g	69	0.1	55	5.1	8.3	0.1	0.0
Toffee & Vanilla, Fat Free, Multipack, Weight Watchers*	1 Vanilla/120g	47	0.1	40	3.9	5.9	0.1	0.8
Toffee Flavour, Bio, Virtually Fat Free, Morrisons*	1 Serving/150g	82	0.3	55	5.3	8.1	0.2	0.0
Toffee Fudge, Low Fat, Sainsbury's*	1 Pot/125g	146	2.5	117	4.3	20.4	2.0	0.0
Toffee with Chocolate Hoops, Crunch Corner, Muller*	1 Pot/150g	229	8.2	153	4.0	21.1	5.5	0.2
Total 0% Greek with Blueberries, Total, Fage*	1 Serving/150g	123	0.0	82	8.3	12.3	0.0	0.0
Totally Vanilla, Low Fat, Asda*	1 Pot/150g	133	1.6	89	4.7	15.1	1.1	0.0
Treacle Toffee, Dessert, Low Fat, Sainsbury's*	1 Pot/125g	149	2.4	119	4.3	21.2	1.9	0.0
Tropical, Luscious, Low Fat, Rachel's Organic*	1 Pot/125g	115	2.0	92	4.0	15.3	1.6	0.0
Tropical Crunch, Healthy Balance, Fruit Corner, Muller*	1 Pot/150g	169	3.1	113	4.7	18.2	2.1	0.5
Tropical Fruit, Bio, Granola, Corner, Muller*	1 Pot/135g	161	3.2	119	5.4	18.2	2.4	0.6
Tropical Fruit, Greek Style, Asda*	1 Pot/125g	170	8.7	136	3.3	15.0	7.0	0.0
Tropical Fruit, Greek Style, Shapers, Boots*	1 Pot/150g	100	2.2	67	3.6	9.8	1.5	0.8
Tropical Fruit, HL, Tesco*	1 Serving/125g	56	0.2	45	4.1	6.6	0.2	0.9
Valencia Orange, Layered, Bio, GFY, Asda*	1 Pot/125g	80	0.1	64	3.7	12.0	0.1	0.0
Valencia Orange, Seriously Fruity, Low Fat, Waitrose*	1 Pot/150g	147	1.5	98	4.3	18.0	1.0	0.3
Vanilla, Average	1 Serving/120g	100	5.4	83	4.5	12.4	4.5	0.8
Vanilla, Benecol*	1 Serving/125g	99	0.8	79	3.7	14.6	0.6	0.0
Vanilla, BGTY, Sainsbury's*	1 Pot/200g	98	0.2	49	4.5	7.5	0.1	0.0
Vanilla, Bio, BFY, Morrisons*	1 Pot/150g	82	0.4	55	5.7	8.4	0.3	0.0
Vanilla, Breakfast, Tesco*	1 Pot/150g	108	0.7	72	2.9	13.9	0.5	0.0
Vanilla, Brooklea*	1 Pot/180g	135	0.4	75	4.8	13.4	0.2	0.0
Vanilla, Chocolate, & Black Cherry, Mullerlight, Muller*	1 Pot/175g	103	0.7	59	3.1	10.3	0.4	0.3
Vanilla, Creamy, Smarties, Nestle*	1 Pot/120g	200	7.4	167	4.1	23.7	6.2	0.0
Vanilla, Delite, Yoplait*	1 Serving/125g	66	0.1	53	4.6	7.4	0.1	2.2
Vanilla, Fat Free, Onken*	1 Serving/150g	73	0.1	49	4.7	7.3	0.1	0.1
Vanilla, Lifestyle, Co-Op*	1 Pot/180g	81	0.2	45	5.0	6.0	0.1	0.1
Vanilla, Live, Bio, Bio Green Dairy*	1 Bottle/250ml	262	7.2	105	2.5	17.7	2.9	0.0
Vanilla, Live Bio, Low Fat, Perfectly Balanced, Waitrose*	1 Pot/150g	114	0.1	76	4.1	14.7	0.1	0.0
Vanilla, Low Fat, Bio, Sainsbury's*	1 Pot/150g	147	1.6	98	4.8	17.2	1.1	0.0
Vanilla, Low Fat, Probiotic, Organic, M & S*	1 Serving/100g	85	1.8	85	6.2	10.9	1.8	0.0
Vanilla, Low Fat, Tesco*	1 Pot/125g	125	2.1	100	4.9	16.3	1.7	0.0
Vanilla, Onken*	1 Serving/100g	100	2.7	100	3.1	15.9	2.7	0.0
Vanilla, Organic, Low Fat, Sainsbury's*	1 Pot/125g	114	1.2	91	5.3	15.3	1.0	0.0
Vanilla, Organic, Probiotic, Fat Free, Yeo Valley*	1 Pot/500g	400	0.5	80	5.4	14.2	0.1	0.0
Vanilla, Smooth, Light, Fat Free, Muller*	1 Pot/175g	87	0.2	50	4.3	7.2	0.1	0.0
Vanilla, Smooth & Creamy, Fat Free, Weight Watchers*	1 Pot/120g	50	0.1	42	3.9	6.5	0.1	0.1

Y

	Measure INFO/WEIGHT	per Measure KCAL	FAT	Nutrition Values per 100g / 100ml KCAL	PROT	CARB	FAT	FIBRE

YOGHURT

	Measure INFO/WEIGHT	per Measure KCAL	FAT	KCAL	PROT	CARB	FAT	FIBRE
Vanilla, Soya, Dairy Free, Organic, Yofu, Provamel*	1 Pot/125g	114	2.7	91	3.8	13.3	2.2	0.7
Vanilla, Thick & Creamy, Channel Island, M & S*	1 Pot/150g	187	6.6	125	4.5	17.5	4.4	1.0
Vanilla, Thick & Creamy, Probiotic, COU, M & S*	1 Pot/170g	76	0.2	45	4.2	6.9	0.1	0.6
Vanilla, Virtually Fat Free, Shapers, Boots*	1 Pot/125g	84	0.6	67	3.6	12.0	0.5	0.0
Vanilla, Virtually Fat Free, Yeo Valley*	1 Pot/150g	121	0.1	81	5.1	15.0	0.1	0.0
Vanilla & Chocolate, Muller*	1 Pot/165g	86	0.8	52	4.0	7.2	0.5	0.1
Vanilla Choco Balls, Crunch Corner, Muller*	1 Pot/150g	223	8.2	149	4.1	20.2	5.5	0.2
Vanilla Flavour, Healthy Living, Light, Tesco*	1 Pot/200g	90	0.2	45	4.1	7.0	0.1	0.0
Vanilla Flavour, Organic, Low Fat, Tesco*	1 Pot/125g	114	1.2	91	5.3	15.3	1.0	0.0
Vanilla Toffee, Low Fat, Sainsbury's*	1 Pot/125g	145	2.2	116	4.3	20.6	1.8	0.0
Very....Lemon Curd, Morrisons*	1 Pot/150g	262	13.6	175	4.1	19.2	9.1	0.0
Walnut & Greek Honey, Amore Luxury, Muller*	1 Pot/150g	241	13.0	161	3.0	17.6	8.7	0.1
White & Milk Chocolate Puffed Rice, Nom Dairy UK*	1 Pot/150g	226	8.8	151	3.8	20.7	5.9	0.1
White Peach, Seriously Fruity, Waitrose*	1 Pot/150g	151	2.5	101	4.8	16.5	1.7	0.2
Wholegrain, Lite, Fig, Date & Grape, Biopot, Onken*	¼ Pot/120g	102	0.2	85	4.8	16.0	0.2	1.0
Wholegrain, Lite, Summer Berries, Biopot, Onken*	¼ Pot/120g	100	0.2	83	4.6	15.8	0.2	1.4
Wholegrain, Peach, Biopot, Onken*	1 Serving/100g	114	2.8	114	4.0	17.8	2.8	0.5
Wholegrain, Strawberry, Biopot, Onken*	1 Serving/100g	111	2.9	111	4.1	17.2	2.9	0.5
Wholemilk, Maple Syrup, Bio Live, Rachel's Organic*	1 Pot/142g	139	5.0	98	3.5	13.0	3.5	0.0
Wholemilk, Organic, M & S*	1 Pot/454ml	409	16.3	90	6.1	7.4	3.6	0.0
Wicked Wholemilk Vanilla, Bio Live, Rachel's Organic*	1 Pot/125g	125	4.4	100	5.2	12.1	3.5	0.0
Wild Berry, Oatie Breakfast, Moma Foods*	1 Pot/235g	301	5.6	128	4.4	23.1	2.4	2.2
Wild Blackberry, Seriously Fruity, Waitrose*	1 Pot/125g	120	1.3	96	4.4	17.2	1.0	0.4
Wild Blueberry, Finest, Tesco*	1 Pot/150g	211	10.2	141	3.4	16.6	6.8	0.5
Wild Blueberry, Light, Fat Free, Muller*	1 Pot/175g	82	0.2	47	4.1	6.9	0.1	0.7
Winter Medley, COU, M & S*	1 Pot/150g	67	0.1	45	4.2	6.2	0.1	0.1
with Coconut, Greek Style, Organic, Bio-live, Rachel's*	1 Pot/120g	187	13.3	156	3.6	10.4	11.1	0.2
with Large Fruit Chunks, Bio, Waitrose*	1 Serving/170g	170	4.1	100	3.7	15.8	2.4	0.4
with Reduce Sugar Rhubarb Jam, Bonne Maman*	1 Pot/125g	141	4.8	113	2.4	16.8	3.8	0.4
with Reduced Sugar, Apricot Jam, Bonne Maman*	1 Pot/125g	141	4.1	113	2.4	16.8	3.3	0.4
with Reduced Sugar, Strawberry Jam, Bonne Maman*	1 Pot/125g	141	4.1	113	2.4	16.8	3.3	0.4
Yellow Fruit, Yoplait*	1 Pot/125g	139	3.6	111	3.3	18.0	2.9	0.0
Yoo Fruity Thing, Cherry, Split Pot, Yoo, Nom Dairy UK*	1 Pot/175g	192	6.5	110	3.3	14.9	3.7	0.0
Yoo Light Thing, Fat Free, Cherry, Yoo, Nom Dairy UK*	1 Pot/180g	135	0.4	75	4.4	13.3	0.2	0.3
Yoo Light Thing, Fat Free, Raspberry, Nom Dairy UK*	1 Pot/180g	135	0.2	75	4.5	13.4	0.1	0.3
Yoo Light Thing, Fat Free, Toffee, Yoo, Nom Dairy UK*	1 Pot/150g	127	0.3	85	4.6	15.4	0.2	0.1
Yoo Light Thing, Fat Free, Vanilla, Yoo, Nom Dairy UK*	1 Pot/180g	135	0.2	75	4.8	13.6	0.1	0.1
Yoo Light Thing, Rhubarb, Yoo, Nom Dairy UK*	1 Pot/180g	135	0.2	75	4.8	13.6	0.1	0.1
Yoo Light Thing, Strawberry, Yoo, Nom Dairy UK*	1 Pot/180g	135	0.2	75	4.5	13.4	0.1	0.3
Yoo Tasty Thing, Prune, Layered, Yoo, Nom Dairy UK*	1 Pot/125g	106	3.0	85	3.7	11.8	2.4	0.0
Zesty Lemon, Intensely Creamy, Activia, Danone*	1 Pot/120g	119	3.6	99	4.8	13.3	3.0	0.1

YOGHURT BREAK

	Measure INFO/WEIGHT	per Measure KCAL	FAT	KCAL	PROT	CARB	FAT	FIBRE
Blueberry, Go Ahead, McVitie's*	1 Slice/18g	72	1.8	401	5.5	72.1	10.0	2.2
Plain, Go Ahead, McVitie's*	1 Bar/18g	72	2.1	394	6.5	66.0	11.5	3.3
Strawberry, Go Ahead, McVitie's*	1 Slice/18g	72	2.0	397	5.9	68.0	11.1	2.1
Tropical, Go Ahead, McVitie's*	1 Slice/18g	77	2.0	430	5.9	76.3	11.0	2.3

YOGHURT DRINK

	Measure INFO/WEIGHT	per Measure KCAL	FAT	KCAL	PROT	CARB	FAT	FIBRE
Actimel, Mixed Fruit, Danone*	1 Bottle/100ml	88	1.5	88	2.7	16.0	1.5	0.0
Actimel, Multi Fruit, Danone*	1 Bottle/100g	85	1.5	85	2.7	14.4	1.5	0.1
Actimel, Orange, Danone*	1 Bottle/100g	74	1.5	74	2.9	11.5	1.5	0.0
Actimel, Original, 0.1% Fat, Danone*	1 Bottle/100g	28	0.1	28	2.8	3.3	0.1	1.9
Actimel, Original, Danone*	1 Bottle/100g	80	1.6	80	2.8	12.8	1.6	0.0
Actimel, Pineapple, 0.1% Fat, Danone*	1 Bottle/100g	33	0.0	33	2.7	5.5	0.0	1.8

Y

YOGHURT DRINK	Measure INFO/WEIGHT	per Measure KCAL	FAT	Nutrition Values per 100g / 100ml KCAL	PROT	CARB	FAT	FIBRE
Actimel, Strawberry, Danone*	1 Bottle/100g	74	1.5	74	2.9	11.5	1.5	0.0
Average	1 fl oz/30ml	19	0.0	62	3.1	13.1	0.0	0.0
Ayran, Gazi*	1 Can/330ml	34	1.9	10	0.5	0.8	0.6	0.0
Banana & Honey, Ski Up & Go, Nestle*	1 Bottle/250g	215	2.2	86	0.0	16.0	0.9	0.0
Blueberry, Low Fat, Prebiotic and Probiotic, Muller*	1 Pot/100g	66	1.4	66	2.6	10.3	1.4	2.2
Blueberry & Blackcurrant, Orchard Maid*	1 Carton/250ml	147	0.1	59	1.6	13.6	0.0	0.0
Cholesterol Lowering, Asda*	1 Bottle/100g	76	1.4	76	2.9	13.0	1.4	1.0
Danacol, Original, Danone*	1 Bottle/100ml	64	1.0	64	3.2	10.0	1.0	0.0
Danacol, Strawberry, Danone*	1 Bottle/100g	68	1.2	68	3.2	11.2	1.2	0.0
Fristi*	1 Carton/330g	191	0.3	58	2.6	13.6	0.1	0.0
Light, Benecol*	1 Bottle/68g	40	1.4	60	2.8	7.3	2.1	0.1
Light, Yakult*	1 Bottle/65ml	27	0.0	42	1.4	10.2	0.0	1.8
Mango, Probiotic, Mundella Foods*	1 Glass/250g	191	2.5	76	2.4	12.3	1.0	1.4
Mixed Berry, Up & Go, Ski, Nestle*	1 Bottle/250g	217	2.2	87	3.1	16.0	0.9	0.2
Multifruit, Natural Defences, Tesco*	1 Bottle/100g	70	1.1	70	3.2	11.8	1.1	0.7
Omega 3 Plus, Raspberry, Pro Biotic, Flora*	1 Bottle/100g	58	1.6	58	2.6	8.5	1.6	0.0
Orange, Banana & Passion Fruit, One a Day, Muller*	1 Bottle/310ml	208	0.3	67	2.1	14.1	0.1	0.0
Original, Benecol*	1 Serving/70g	62	1.6	88	2.6	14.2	2.3	0.0
Peach & Apricot, Benecol*	1 Bottle/68g	38	1.5	56	2.8	6.2	2.2	0.0
Peach & Mango, Fristi*	1 Carton/330g	191	0.3	58	2.6	13.6	0.1	0.0
Pomegranate & Raspberry Pro Active, Mini Drink, Flora*	1 Serving/100g	45	1.5	45	2.6	4.7	1.5	1.1
Pro Activ, Orange, Cholesterol, Flora*	1 Bottle/100g	45	1.5	45	3.2	5.6	1.5	1.1
Pro Activ, Original, Cholesterol, Flora*	1 Bottle/100g	45	1.5	45	2.6	4.8	1.5	1.1
Pro Activ, Strawberry, Cholesterol, Flora*	1 Bottle/100g	45	1.5	45	2.6	4.7	1.5	0.0
Raspberry & Passion Fruit, Everybody, Yoplait*	1 Bottle/90g	60	0.8	67	2.6	12.2	0.9	0.0
Strawberry, Benecol*	1 Bottle/68g	38	1.5	56	2.9	6.2	2.2	0.0
Strawberry, Fristi*	1 Carton/250g	165	0.2	66	2.6	13.6	0.1	0.0
Strawberry, Low Fat, Pre & Probiotic, Muller*	1 Pot/100g	67	1.4	67	2.5	10.7	1.4	2.4
Strawberry, Probiotic, Mundella Foods*	1 Glass/250g	191	2.5	76	2.4	12.3	1.0	1.4
Strawberry, Yop, Yoplait*	1 Bottle/330g	261	4.3	79	2.8	14.0	1.3	0.0
Sveltesse, 0%, Nestle*	1 Pot/125g	61	0.1	49	4.8	7.3	0.1	0.1
Vanilla, Activate, Probiotic, Little Town Dairy*	1 Bottle/265g	167	3.7	63	2.7	10.0	1.4	0.2
Vanilla, Probiotic, Mundella Foods*	1 Glass/250g	191	2.5	76	2.4	12.3	1.0	1.4
Yakult*	1 Pot/65ml	51	0.1	78	1.4	17.8	0.1	0.0
YORK FRUITS								
Terry's*	1 Sweet/9g	30	0.0	328	0.0	81.4	0.0	1.0
YORKIE								
Honeycomb, Nestle*	1 Bar/65g	331	16.8	509	5.7	63.6	25.8	0.0
King Size, Nestle*	1 Bar/83g	445	26.1	537	6.1	57.3	31.5	0.0
Original, Nestle*	1 Bar/65g	365	21.4	537	6.1	57.3	31.5	0.7
Raisin & Biscuit, Nestle*	1 Bar/67g	331	17.4	497	5.5	59.7	26.2	0.9
YORKSHIRE PUDDING								
& Beef Dripping, M & S*	4 Pudding/100g	410	30.4	410	9.4	25.2	30.4	3.2
Average	1 Pudding/30g	62	3.0	208	6.6	24.7	9.9	0.9
Batters, in Foils, Ready to Bake, Frozen, Aunt Bessie's*	1 Pudding/17g	47	1.8	276	9.1	32.6	10.8	1.4
Chicken & Vegetable, COU, M & S*	1 Pudding/150g	195	3.3	130	12.2	14.3	2.2	1.3
Filled, with Beef, Morrisons*	1 Serving/350g	514	21.0	147	7.4	15.7	6.0	0.5
Filled, with Sausage, Sainsbury's*	1 Pack/300g	576	31.2	192	6.9	17.5	10.4	0.9
Filled with Beef, Tesco*	1 Pudding/300g	408	15.6	136	6.1	16.2	5.2	1.1
Filled with Chicken, GFY, Asda*	1 Pack/381g	438	9.9	115	9.0	14.0	2.6	1.5
Filled with Chicken, Tesco*	1 Pack/300g	366	8.7	122	6.5	17.4	2.9	1.3
Filled with Chicken & Vegetable, GFY, Asda*	1 Pack/380g	376	9.9	99	6.0	13.0	2.6	1.1
Frozen, Ovenbaked, Iceland*	1 Pudding/12g	36	1.0	290	9.7	45.1	7.9	4.1

Y

INFO/WEIGHT	per Measure KCAL	per Measure FAT	Nutrition Values per 100g / 100ml KCAL	PROT	CARB	FAT	FIBRE

YORKSHIRE PUDDING

Item	Measure	KCAL	FAT	KCAL	PROT	CARB	FAT	FIBRE
Fully Prepared, M & S*	1 Pudding/22g	63	2.9	285	9.4	31.6	13.2	1.2
Giant, Aunt Bessie's*	1 Pudding/110g	290	9.9	264	8.5	37.4	9.0	2.0
Giant, VLH Kitchens*	1 Pud/110g	284	11.0	259	8.5	33.6	10.0	2.3
Large, Aunt Bessie's*	1 Pudding/40g	111	4.6	277	8.5	35.3	11.4	1.5
Large, The Real Yorkshire Pudding Co*	1 Pudding/34g	103	4.1	304	11.5	37.3	12.1	2.5
Minced Beef Filled, Waitrose*	1 Serving/350g	525	24.8	150	7.5	14.1	7.1	1.0
Mini, Co-Op*	1 Serving/16g	50	2.0	312	6.2	43.7	12.5	2.5
Premium, Bisto*	1 Pudding/30g	74	3.3	248	7.3	30.3	10.9	2.1
Roast Chicken Filled, COU, M & S*	1 Pudding/150g	210	4.0	140	12.6	15.7	2.7	0.9
Sage & Onion, Tesco*	1 Pudding/19g	53	2.3	280	8.0	35.0	12.0	2.6
Sausage Filled, Frozen, Tesco*	1 Pack/340g	510	19.7	150	6.6	17.8	5.8	1.8
Steak Filled, COU, M & S*	1 Serving/150g	187	3.7	125	11.0	14.7	2.5	0.8
Traditional, Giant, Asda*	1 Pudding/110g	310	11.0	282	10.0	38.0	10.0	2.3

YULE LOG

Item	Measure	KCAL	FAT	KCAL	PROT	CARB	FAT	FIBRE
Chocolate, Sainsbury's*	1/8 Log/49g	186	9.5	382	5.1	46.5	19.6	0.7
Christmas Range, Tesco*	1 Serving/30g	131	6.4	442	4.9	56.8	21.7	2.8
Mini, M & S*	1 Cake/36g	165	8.4	460	5.7	56.9	23.3	1.1

	Measure INFO/WEIGHT	per Measure KCAL	FAT	Nutrition Values per 100g / 100ml KCAL	PROT	CARB	FAT	FIBRE

BAGEL FACTORY
BAGEL

	Measure INFO/WEIGHT	KCAL	FAT	KCAL	PROT	CARB	FAT	FIBRE
Bacon, Bagel Factory*	1 Bagel/100g	613	25.9	613	32.2	62.1	25.9	3.8
Salmon & Cream Cheese, Bagel Factory*	1 Bagel/300g	515	18.3	172	9.9	19.1	6.1	0.7
with Marmite, Wholemeal, Bagel Factory*	1 Bagel/85g	312	1.6	367	24.4	63.4	1.9	11.6

BURGER KING
APPLE

Fries, Burger King*	1 Serving/60g	28	0.1	47	0.1	12.0	0.1	2.0

BITES

Chicken, Kids, Burger King*	1 Serving/56g	158	7.3	282	16.0	25.0	13.0	2.0

BURGERS

Angus, Double, Burger King*	1 Burger/323g	795	45.2	246	16.0	14.0	14.0	1.0
Angus, Mini, Burger King*	1 Burger/97g	272	10.7	280	14.0	31.0	11.0	1.0
Angus, Mini with Cheese, Burger King*	1 Burger/110g	321	15.4	292	15.0	27.0	14.0	1.0
Angus, Smoked Bacon & Cheddar, Burger King*	1 Burger/270g	678	37.8	251	14.0	17.0	14.0	1.0
Angus, Steakhouse, Burger King*	1 Burger/239g	554	28.7	232	12.0	18.0	12.0	1.0
Bean, Veggie, Kids, Burger King*	1 Burger/116g	278	7.0	240	6.0	42.0	6.0	3.0
Big King, Burger King*	1 Burger/190g	503	26.6	265	15.0	17.0	14.0	1.0
Big King, XL, Burger King*	1 Burger/338g	902	54.1	267	16.0	14.0	16.0	1.0
BK, Veggie Bean Burger, Burger King*	1 Burger/280g	588	19.6	210	6.0	30.0	7.0	3.0
Cheeseburger, Bacon Double, Burger King*	1 Burger/160g	478	25.6	299	19.0	19.0	16.0	1.0
Cheeseburger, Burger King*	1 Burger/123g	320	13.5	260	13.0	25.0	11.0	1.0
Cheeseburger, Double, Burger King*	1 Burger/173g	465	22.5	269	17.0	18.0	13.0	1.0
Cheeseburger, Kids, Burger King*	1 Burger/113g	318	13.6	281	14.0	27.0	12.0	1.0
Chicken, Chargrilled, Mini, Burger King*	1 Burger/109g	214	3.3	196	15.0	28.0	3.0	1.0
Chicken, Piri Piri, Sandwich, Burger King*	1 Sandwich/196g	335	5.9	171	13.0	21.0	3.0	1.0
Chicken Royale, Burger King*	1 Burger/210g	607	31.5	289	11.0	25.0	15.0	1.0
Chicken Royale, Sweet Chilli, Burger King*	1 Burger/210g	542	23.1	258	11.0	28.0	11.0	1.0
Chicken Royale, with Cheese, Burger King*	1 Burger/263g	695	39.0	264	10.6	20.9	14.8	0.4
Hamburger, Burger King*	1 Burger/110g	275	8.8	250	13.0	28.0	8.0	1.0
Hamburger, Kids, Burger King*	1 Burger/100g	272	9.0	272	14.0	31.0	9.0	1.0
Ocean Catch, Burger King*	1 Burger/188g	494	26.3	263	9.0	23.0	14.0	1.0
Whopper, Burger King*	1 Burger/274g	633	35.6	231	11.0	18.0	13.0	1.0
Whopper, Double, Burger King*	1 Burger/355g	877	53.2	247	14.0	14.0	15.0	1.0
Whopper, Double, with Cheese, Burger King*	1 Burger/380g	961	60.8	253	14.0	13.0	16.0	1.0
Whopper, Junior, Burger King*	1 Burger/148g	343	16.3	232	9.0	21.0	11.0	1.0
Whopper, with Cheese, Burger King*	1 Burger/299g	721	41.9	241	11.0	16.0	14.0	1.0
Whopper, with Cheese, Junior, Burger King*	1 Burger/161g	388	19.3	241	10.0	19.0	12.0	1.0

BUTTY

Bacon, with Heinz Ketchup, Burger King*	1 Butty/77g	221	6.0	287	13.0	41.6	7.8	2.6
Bacon, with HP Sauce, Burger King*	1 Butty/77g	222	6.0	288	13.0	41.6	7.8	2.0
Bacon & Egg, with Heinz Ketchup, Burger King*	1 Butty/140g	362	17.0	259	12.9	25.0	12.1	11.4
Bacon & Egg, with HP Sauce, Burger King*	1 Butty/140g	363	17.0	259	12.9	25.0	12.1	1.4
Big Breakfast, with Heinz Ketchup, Burger King*	1 Butty/297g	849	50.5	286	14.0	18.0	17.0	1.0
Egg & Cheese, with Heinz Ketchup, Burger King*	1 Butty/126g	300	17.6	238	10.3	27.0	14.0	1.6
Sausage, with Heinz Ketchup, Burger King*	1 Butty/119g	312	13.0	262	13.4	26.9	10.9	1.7
Sausage, with HP Sauce, Burger King*	1 Butty/119g	313	13.0	263	13.4	26.9	10.9	1.7
Sausage & Egg, with HP Sauce, Burger King*	1 Butty/182g	454	24.0	249	13.2	19.2	13.2	1.1

CHICKEN

Bites, Burger King*	14 Bites/112g	317	15.0	283	16.1	25.0	13.4	0.9

COFFEE

Black, Large, Burger King*	1 Serving/284ml	6	0.0	2	0.0	0.0	0.0	0.0
Black, Regular, Burger King*	1 Regular/200ml	4	0.0	2	0.0	0.0	0.0	0.0
Cappuccino, Large, Burger King*	1 Large/59g	81	2.9	137	10.0	15.0	5.0	0.0

INFO/WEIGHT	Measure	per Measure		Nutrition Values per 100g / 100ml				
		KCAL	FAT	KCAL	PROT	CARB	FAT	FIBRE
BURGER KING								
COFFEE								
Cappuccino, Regular, Burger King*	1 Regular/46g	64	1.8	139	9.0	15.0	4.0	0.0
Latte, Large, Burger King*	1 Regular/45g	60	1.8	133	11.0	13.0	4.0	0.0
Latte, Regular, Burger King*	1 Large/62g	82	3.1	132	10.0	15.0	5.0	0.0
COLA								
Coca Cola, Burger King*	1 Regular/400g	168	0.0	42	0.0	11.0	0.0	0.0
Coke, Diet, Burger King*	1 Regular/400g	4	0.0	1	0.0	0.0	0.0	0.0
DIP POT								
Barbeque Sauce, Heinz, Burger King*	1 Pot/40g	48	0.0	120	0.1	28.0	0.1	0.1
Sweet Chilli, Heinz, Burger King*	1 Pot/40g	96	0.0	240	0.0	60.0	0.0	0.0
DRESSING								
French, Burger King*	1 Sachet/40g	7	0.0	17	0.0	2.5	0.0	0.0
Honey & Mustard, Burger King*	1 Sachet/40g	32	1.0	80	2.5	15.0	2.5	0.0
FANTA								
Orange, Burger King*	1 Reg/400g	156	0.4	39	0.1	10.0	0.1	0.0
Orange, Small, Burger King*	1 Sm/300g	117	0.3	39	0.1	10.0	0.1	0.0
FRIES								
Large, Burger King*	1 Large/141g	381	18.3	270	3.0	38.0	13.0	4.0
Regular, Burger King*	1 Regular/111g	300	15.5	270	3.0	39.0	14.0	4.0
Small, Burger King*	1 Small/74g	200	10.4	270	3.0	38.0	14.0	4.0
Super, Burger King*	1 Super/174g	470	22.6	270	3.0	39.0	13.0	4.0
HASH BROWNS								
Large, Burger King*	1 Large/130g	403	27.3	310	3.0	27.0	21.0	4.0
Regular, Burger King*	1 Regular/102g	316	22.4	310	3.0	27.0	22.0	4.0
KETCHUP								
Heinz, Sachet, Burger King*	1 Sachet/10g	10	0.0	100	0.1	20.0	0.1	0.1
MAYONNAISE								
Heinz, Sachet, Burger King*	1 Sachet/12g	80	9.0	667	0.0	0.0	75.0	0.0
MILK								
Semi Skimmed, Kids, Burger King*	1 Carton/258g	117	3.9	47	3.5	4.6	1.5	0.0
MILK SHAKE								
Chocolate, Large, Burger King*	1 Large/519g	612	10.4	118	3.0	22.0	2.0	0.0
Chocolate, Regular, Burger King*	1 Regular/401g	449	8.0	112	3.0	20.0	2.0	0.1
Chocolate, Small, Burger King*	1 Small/276g	301	8.3	109	3.0	19.0	3.0	0.1
Strawberry, Large, Burger King*	1 Large/519g	581	10.4	112	3.0	20.0	2.0	0.0
Strawberry, Regular, Burger King*	1 Regular/401g	433	8.0	108	3.0	19.0	2.0	0.0
Strawberry, Small, Burger King*	1 Small/276g	293	8.3	106	3.0	18.0	3.0	0.0
ONION RINGS								
Large, Burger King*	1 Large/190g	697	36.0	367	6.3	43.2	18.9	4.7
Regular, Burger King*	1 Regular/126g	462	24.0	367	6.3	42.9	19.0	4.8
Super, Burger King*	1 Super/253g	929	48.0	367	6.3	43.1	19.0	4.7
SALAD								
Chicken, Flame Grilled, Burger King*	1 Salad/240g	127	2.4	53	8.0	3.0	1.0	1.0
Garden, Burger King*	1 Serving/165g	33	1.6	20	1.0	4.0	1.0	1.0
SPRITE								
Burger King*	1 Regular/400g	148	0.0	37	0.0	9.0	0.0	0.0
TEA								
Regular, White, No Sugar, Burger King*	1 Regular/200ml	22	4.0	11	1.0	1.0	2.0	0.0
WRAP								
Sweet Chilli, Chicken, Burger King*	1 Wrap/160g	296	6.4	185	14.0	22.0	4.0	1.0
CAFFE NERO								
BARS								
Fruit & Seed Bar, Caffe Nero*	1 Bar/65g	197	5.8	303	7.5	48.2	8.9	8.7

	Measure INFO/WEIGHT	per Measure KCAL	FAT	Nutrition Values per 100g / 100ml KCAL	PROT	CARB	FAT	FIBRE

CAFFE NERO

BARS
Organic Granola, Caffe Nero*	1 Bar/64g	275	13.4	429	6.5	53.7	20.9	4.6

BISCOTTI
Organic Almond, Caffe Nero*	1 Serving/40g	155	6.1	388	9.2	53.1	15.3	2.8
Organic Chocolate, Caffe Nero*	1 Serving/37g	136	4.3	369	7.0	59.1	11.6	2.7

BROWNIE
Organic Gluten Free Double Chocolate, Caffe Nero*	1 Serving/75g	318	15.5	425	4.3	55.4	20.7	2.0

CAKE
Belgian Chocolate Brownie, Caffe Nero*	1 Serving/75g	314	14.7	419	4.6	54.6	19.6	2.9
Chocolate Crunch, Caffe Nero*	1 Serving/65g	308	16.5	473	6.2	54.3	25.3	4.2
Chocolate Fudge, Caffe Nero*	1 Serving/126g	517	26.4	410	4.9	50.6	20.9	1.1
Organic Carrot & Raisin, Wheat Free, Caffe Nero*	1 Serving/70g	295	17.7	421	4.1	44.8	25.3	3.4
Organic Carrot & Raisin, Wrapped, Caffe Nero*	1 Serving/70g	290	17.5	414	4.5	43.4	25.0	3.9
Organic Lemon Drizzle, Caffe Nero*	1 Serving/70g	248	11.1	354	4.2	48.5	15.9	0.8
Panettone, Mini Chocolate, Caffe Nero*	1 Serving/100g	404	18.8	404	9.5	49.0	18.8	1.2
Panettone, Mini Classic, Caffe Nero*	1 Serving/100g	366	14.6	366	7.8	51.1	14.6	1.2

CHEESECAKE
Sicilian Lemon, Caffe Nero*	1 Serving/107g	400	26.0	374	5.0	33.0	24.3	1.4
White & Dark Chocolate Truffle, Caffe Nero*	1 Serving/131g	538	36.6	410	5.8	33.7	27.9	0.9

CHOCOLATE
Coated Coffee Beans, Caffe Nero*	1 Serving/25g	117	6.5	469	8.5	50.0	26.2	11.9
Coin, Caffe Nero*	1 Serving/25g	129	6.9	516	6.3	59.7	27.8	2.1
Milk Bar, Caffe Nero*	1 Serving/40g	223	13.6	558	8.0	55.0	34.0	1.0
Milk Bar with Hazelnuts, Caffe Nero*	1 Serving/40g	229	15.2	572	8.0	49.5	38.0	1.8

COFFEE
Cappuccino, Regular, Semi Skimmed Milk, Caffe Nero*	1 Serving/80g	37	1.4	46	3.5	4.7	1.7	0.0
Cappuccino, Regular, Skimmed Milk, Caffe Nero*	1 Serving/79g	27	0.1	34	3.5	4.8	0.1	0.0
Cappuccino, Regular, Soya Milk, Caffe Nero*	1 Serving/80g	36	1.8	45	3.7	2.5	2.2	0.6
Caramelatte, Semi Skimmed Milk, Caffe Nero*	1 Serving/422g	485	25.3	115	2.3	12.3	6.0	0.0
Latte, Regular, Semi Skimmed Milk, Caffe Nero*	1 Serving/150g	69	2.5	46	3.5	4.7	1.7	0.0
Latte, Regular, Skimmed Milk, Caffe Nero*	1 Serving/150g	51	0.4	34	3.5	4.8	0.3	0.0
Latte, Regular, Soya Milk, Caffe Nero*	1 Serving/151g	68	3.3	45	3.7	2.5	2.2	0.6
Mocha, No Cream, Regular, Skimmed Milk, Caffe Nero*	1 Serving/179g	156	1.3	87	3.8	16.6	0.7	0.8

COOKIES
Milk Chocolate Chunk, Caffe Nero*	1 Serving/72g	338	17.9	470	5.8	55.8	24.9	1.7
Organic Chocolate Chip, Caffe Nero*	1 Serving/60g	263	12.1	438	4.5	56.6	20.1	1.5
Organic Oat & Raisin Cookie, Caffe Nero*	1 Serving/60g	282	14.0	470	4.4	60.5	23.4	2.6
Triple Chocolate, Caffe Nero*	1 Serving/72g	333	17.5	463	5.6	55.6	24.3	3.3

CRISPS
Mature Cheddar & Spring Onion, Caffe Nero*	1 Serving/40g	192	11.4	481	6.1	54.0	28.6	4.4
Sea Salt, Caffe Nero*	1 Serving/40g	197	10.8	493	7.0	54.0	27.1	4.5
Sea Salt & Balsamic Vinegar, Caffe Nero*	1 Serving/40g	192	11.0	482	7.0	54.1	27.5	4.0

CROISSANTS
Almond, Caffe Nero*	1 Serving/83g	350	19.8	422	10.0	41.7	23.9	2.6
Apricot, Caffe Nero*	1 Serving/100g	273	11.3	273	5.4	37.3	11.3	1.2
Butter, Caffe Nero*	1 Serving/52g	216	12.1	417	8.5	43.0	23.4	1.7
Cheese Twist, Caffe Nero*	1 Serving/76g	316	18.4	416	13.4	36.1	24.2	2.6
Chocolate Twist, Caffe Nero*	1 Serving/85g	314	13.3	369	6.8	42.2	15.6	2.9
Pain au Chocolat, Caffe Nero*	1 Serving/62g	269	15.0	435	8.3	46.0	24.2	1.8
Pain au Raisin, Caffe Nero*	1 Serving/90g	279	10.5	310	5.8	44.6	11.7	1.9

CUPCAKE
Chocolate, Caffe Nero*	1 Serving/68g	311	19.1	457	3.1	48.7	28.1	0.5
Lemon, Caffe Nero*	1 Serving/72g	340	19.6	472	2.9	54.0	27.2	0.3

	Measure INFO/WEIGHT	per Measure KCAL	FAT	KCAL	PROT	CARB	FAT	FIBRE
CAFFE NERO								
CUPCAKE								
Raspberry, Caffe Nero*	1 Serving/67g	295	15.1	440	3.4	55.7	22.5	0.5
DESSERTS								
Tiramisu, Caffe Nero*	1 Serving/95g	311	20.6	327	3.9	28.4	21.7	1.0
FRAPPE								
Double Chocolate, Caffe Nero*	1 Serving/455g	355	4.6	78	3.0	14.9	1.0	0.3
Frappe Latte, Caffe Nero*	1 Serving/431g	267	3.9	62	2.8	11.1	0.9	0.0
Frappe Latte, Skimmed Milk, Caffe Nero*	1 Serving/429g	240	0.9	56	2.8	11.1	0.2	0.0
Frappe Latte, Soya Milk, Caffe Nero*	1 Serving/388g	101	5.0	26	2.2	1.5	1.3	0.4
Mocha Frappe Latte, Caffe Nero*	1 Serving/455g	355	4.6	78	3.0	14.9	1.0	0.3
Mocha Frappe Latte, Skimmed Milk, Caffe Nero*	1 Serving/456g	328	1.4	72	3.0	15.0	0.3	0.3
FRUIT SALAD								
Fruit Salad, Caffe Nero*	1 Serving/171g	70	0.2	41	0.5	9.8	0.1	1.3
JUICE								
Apple & Mango Juice, Caffe Nero*	1 Serving/250g	125	0.0	50	0.2	12.3	0.0	0.1
Fresh Orange, 100% Squeezed Juice, Caffe Nero*	1 Serving/250g	95	0.0	38	0.5	8.8	0.0	0.1
Fruit Booster, Mango & Passionfruit, Caffe Nero*	1 Serving/597g	191	0.6	32	0.4	7.8	0.1	0.6
Fruit Booster, Orange, Lemon & Lime, Caffe Nero*	1 Serving/591g	207	0.6	35	0.5	7.6	0.1	0.9
Fruit Booster, Strawberry & Raspberry, Caffe Nero*	1 Serving/589g	206	1.8	35	0.4	7.5	0.3	1.6
Organic Apple Juice Carton, Caffe Nero*	1 Serving/200g	94	0.0	47	0.5	11.2	0.0	0.0
Pressed Apple, 100% Premium Juice, Caffe Nero*	1 Serving/250g	120	0.0	48	0.1	11.8	0.0	0.0
LEMONADE								
Sicilian Still, Caffe Nero*	1 Serving/250g	115	0.0	46	0.0	11.2	0.0	0.0
MILKSHAKE								
Banana Frappe, Caffe Nero*	1 Serving/420g	315	4.6	75	3.0	13.5	1.1	0.0
Mint Frappe, Semi Skimmed Milk, Caffe Nero*	1 Serving/419g	310	4.6	74	3.0	13.3	1.1	0.0
Strawberry Frappe, Caffe Nero*	1 Serving/416g	316	4.6	76	3.0	13.6	1.1	0.0
Vanilla Frappe, Caffe Nero*	1 Serving/420g	315	4.6	75	3.0	13.6	1.1	0.0
MINTS								
Mints, Caffe Nero*	1 Serving/14g	35	0.1	249	0.6	97.0	0.8	0.0
MUFFINS								
Raspberry & White Chocolate, Caffe Nero*	1 Serving/120g	454	23.5	378	4.9	45.2	19.6	0.9
Reduced Fat Cranberry & Orange, Caffe Nero*	1 Serving/120g	322	9.8	269	4.5	44.3	8.2	3.1
Spiced Apple & Pecan, Caffe Nero*	1 Serving/120g	474	26.5	395	4.7	43.5	22.1	1.5
Triple Belgian Chocolate, Caffe Nero*	1 Serving/120g	495	26.2	413	5.6	47.2	21.9	2.0
PANINI								
All Day Breakfast Panini, Caffe Nero*	1 Serving/223g	409	17.7	183	8.7	19.2	7.9	1.6
Breakfast Panini, Bacon & Tomato Sauce, Caffe Nero*	1 Serving/105g	263	9.7	251	11.1	30.6	9.3	1.4
Chicken, Bacon & Arrabbiata Sauce, Caffe Nero*	1 Serving/214g	346	8.5	162	11.2	20.2	4.0	1.3
Chicken Milanese Panini, Caffe Nero*	1 Serving/249g	428	13.9	172	8.5	21.9	5.6	1.2
Ham & Mozzarella Panini, Caffe Nero*	1 Serving/204g	421	16.1	206	13.0	20.7	7.9	1.1
Meatball & Mozzarella Napoletana Panini, Caffe Nero*	1 Serving/218g	483	21.8	222	10.8	22.2	10.0	1.2
Mushroom with Gorgonzola Cheese Panini, Caffe Nero*	1 Serving/181g	377	17.4	208	7.0	23.4	9.6	1.5
Napoli Salami & Mozzarella Panini, Caffe Nero*	1 Serving/193g	404	17.8	209	10.1	21.5	9.2	1.2
Pesto Chicken Panini, Caffe Nero*	1 Serving/210g	385	13.3	183	11.8	19.7	6.3	1.1
Tostati, Ham, Mozzarella & Emmental, Caffe Nero*	1 Serving/77g	172	7.1	223	15.6	19.4	9.2	0.8
Tostati, Three Cheese & Roasted Tomato, Caffe Nero*	1 Serving/71g	170	8.4	240	11.8	21.5	11.8	1.1
Tuna Melt Panini, Caffe Nero*	1 Serving/201g	389	13.4	194	11.6	21.2	6.7	1.1
Vine Tomato, Mozzarella & Basil Panini, Caffe Nero*	1 Serving/212g	398	17.4	188	8.3	20.3	8.2	1.3
PASTA								
Red Pepper Penne, Caffe Nero*	1 Serving/303g	197	3.0	65	2.8	11.4	1.0	1.3
SALADS								
Chicken with Caesar Dressing, Caffe Nero*	1 Serving/170g	156	9.8	92	6.2	3.2	5.8	0.9

	Measure INFQ/WEIGHT	per Measure		Nutrition Values per 100g / 100ml				
		KCAL	FAT	KCAL	PROT	CARB	FAT	FIBRE
CAFFE NERO								
SANDWICH								
Chicken Salad, Caffe Nero*	1 Serving/174g	368	16.9	211	10.1	20.9	9.7	1.7
Free Range Egg Mayonnaise, Caffe Nero*	1 Serving/159g	325	12.5	205	9.8	23.5	7.9	1.9
Ham & Cheddar, Caffe Nero*	1 Serving/179g	418	17.8	233	15.2	20.8	9.9	1.4
Mature Cheddar & Pickle, Caffe Nero*	1 Serving/186g	458	23.3	246	9.8	22.9	12.5	1.6
Tuna Salad, Caffe Nero*	1 Serving/147g	268	5.3	182	11.7	25.8	3.6	1.8
SCONES								
Luxury Fruit, Caffe Nero*	1 Serving/100g	337	10.9	337	6.6	53.3	10.9	2.1
SOUP								
Organic Sundried Tomato & Basil, Caffe Nero*	1 Serving/300g	144	6.9	48	2.2	4.7	2.3	0.5
TART								
Apple & Blackcurrant, Caffe Nero*	1 Serving/101g	279	12.9	276	2.9	37.4	12.8	2.2
Portuguese Custard, Caffe Nero*	1 Serving/69g	184	6.5	266	3.9	41.5	9.4	2.4
TEA								
Chai Latte, Semi Skimmed Milk, Caffe Nero*	1 Serving/406g	284	10.5	70	3.8	8.3	2.6	0.0
Chai Latte, Skimmed Milk, Caffe Nero*	1 Serving/405g	239	5.3	59	3.8	8.4	1.3	0.0
WRAP								
Chicken Caesar Wrap, Caffe Nero*	1 Serving/165g	434	22.8	263	12.8	21.9	13.8	0.8
Falafel Wrap, Caffe Nero*	1 Serving/157g	424	21.8	270	8.7	29.4	13.9	1.8
COSTA								
BISCUITS								
Gingerbread George, Costa*	1 Biscuit/55g	234	5.7	425	5.9	77.8	10.4	0.0
Stem Ginger, Costa*	1 Pack/60g	286	13.0	476	4.8	65.6	21.6	0.0
BREAKFAST								
All Day Roll, Costa*	1 Pack/230g	663	33.6	288	11.7	27.5	14.6	0.0
Bacon Roll, Costa*	1 Pack/130g	367	11.0	282	15.6	35.8	8.5	1.7
Egg & Mushroom Roll, Costa*	1 Pack/155g	354	12.3	228	8.4	30.9	7.9	1.8
BROWNIES								
Brownies	1 Serving/72g	342	22.1	475	5.4	44.3	30.7	0.0
Chocolate, Gluten Free, Costa*	1 Serving/80g	400	25.4	500	7.3	46.2	31.8	0.0
CAKE								
Carrot, Costa*	1 Slice/138g	514	23.4	374	5.1	48.6	17.0	0.0
Chocolate, Costa*	1 Slice/150g	575	23.6	383	4.8	76.7	15.7	0.0
Lemon, Costa*	1 Slice/144g	576	25.4	399	3.6	56.0	17.6	0.0
Victoria Sandwich, Costa*	1 Slice/136g	546	25.6	401	3.5	54.0	18.8	0.0
COFFEE								
Americano, Massimo, No Added Milk, Costa*	1 Massimo/600ml	12	0.4	2	0.1	0.3	0.1	0.0
Americano, Medio, No Added Milk, Costa*	1 Medio/480ml	8	0.3	2	0.1	0.2	0.1	0.0
Americano, Primo, No Added Milk, Costa*	1 Primo/360ml	6	0.2	2	0.1	0.2	0.1	0.0
Babyccino, Full Fat, Solo, Costa*	1 Solo/30ml	101	4.3	337	14.0	38.3	14.3	0.0
Babyccino, Skimmed, Solo, Costa*	1 Solo/30ml	65	0.1	217	14.3	39.7	0.3	0.0
Babyccino, Soya, Solo, Costa*	1 Solo/30ml	70	2.2	233	13.0	28.7	7.3	0.0
Caffe Latte, Full Fat, Massimo, Costa*	1 Massimo/600ml	260	14.4	43	2.2	3.2	2.4	0.0
Caffe Latte, Full Fat, Medio, Costa*	1 Medio/480ml	202	11.2	42	2.2	3.2	2.3	0.0
Caffe Latte, Full Fat, Primo, Costa*	1 Primo/360ml	151	8.5	42	2.2	3.1	2.4	0.0
Caffe Latte, Skimmed, Massimo, Costa*	1 Massimo/600ml	149	0.7	25	2.4	3.6	0.1	0.0
Caffe Latte, Skimmed, Medio, Costa*	1 Medio/480ml	114	0.5	24	2.3	3.5	0.1	0.0
Caffe Latte, Skimmed, Primo, Costa*	1 Primo/360ml	86	0.3	24	2.4	3.5	0.1	0.0
Caffe Latte, Soya, Massimo, Costa*	1 Massimo/600ml	165	7.7	27	2.1	1.8	1.3	0.0
Caffe Latte, Soya, Medio, Costa*	1 Medio/480ml	124	5.8	26	2.0	1.7	1.2	0.0
Caffe Latte, Soya, Primo, Costa*	1 Primo/360ml	93	4.4	26	2.0	1.6	1.2	0.0
Cappuccino, Full Fat, Massimo, Costa*	1 Massimo/600ml	123	6.7	22	1.1	1.6	1.2	0.0
Cappuccino, Full Fat, Medio, Costa*	1 Medio/480ml	160	8.8	33	1.7	2.5	1.8	0.0

COSTA
COFFEE

INFO/WEIGHT	Measure	per Measure KCAL	FAT	Nutrition Values per 100g / 100ml KCAL	PROT	CARB	FAT	FIBRE
Cappuccino, Full Fat, Primo, Costa*	1 Primo/360ml	94	5.1	26	1.4	2.0	1.4	0.0
Cappuccino, Skimmed, Massimo, Costa*	1 Massimo/600ml	113	0.7	19	1.8	2.7	0.1	0.0
Cappuccino, Skimmed, Medio, Costa*	1 Medio/480ml	91	0.7	19	2.4	3.7	0.1	0.0
Cappuccino, Skimmed, Primo, Costa*	1 Primo/360ml	56	0.3	16	1.5	2.3	0.1	0.0
Cappuccino, Soya, Massimo, Costa*	1 Massimo/600ml	126	5.8	21	1.6	1.4	1.0	0.0
Cappuccino, Soya, Medio, Costa*	1 Medio/480ml	100	4.6	21	1.6	1.4	1.0	0.0
Cappuccino, Soya, Primo, Costa*	1 Primo/360ml	62	2.8	17	1.3	1.2	0.8	0.0
Espresso, Ristretto, Doppio, Costa*	1 Doppio/60ml	6	0.2	10	0.7	1.3	0.3	0.0
Espresso, Ristretto, Solo, Costa*	1 Solo/30ml	3	0.1	10	0.7	1.3	0.3	0.0
Flat White made with Full Fat Milk, Primo, Costa*	1 Primo/360ml	135	7.6	37	1.9	2.8	2.1	0.0
Flat White Made with Skimmed Milk, Primo, Costa*	1 Primo/360ml	77	0.3	21	2.1	3.1	0.1	0.0
Flat White Made with Soya Milk, Primo, Costa*	1 Primo/360ml	85	4.0	24	1.9	1.5	1.1	0.0
Iced, Latte, Full Fat Milk, Medio, Costa*	1 Medio/454ml	114	6.6	25	1.3	1.8	1.4	0.0
Iced, Latte, Full Fat Milk, Primo, Costa*	1 Primo/340ml	79	4.5	23	1.2	1.7	1.3	0.0
Iced, Latte, Skimmed Milk, Medio, Costa*	1 Medio/454ml	62	0.6	14	1.3	1.9	0.1	0.0
Iced, Latte, Skimmed Milk, Primo, Costa*	1 Primo/340ml	43	0.5	13	1.3	1.8	0.1	0.0
Iced, Latte, Soya Milk, Medio, Costa*	1 Medio/454ml	75	3.3	17	1.3	1.1	0.7	0.0
Iced, Latte, Soya Milk, Primo, Costa*	1 Primo/340ml	52	2.3	15	1.2	1.1	0.7	0.0
Light, Massimo, Costa*	1 Massimo/600ml	98	0.5	16	1.6	2.4	0.1	0.0
Light, Medio, Costa*	1 Medio/480ml	88	0.4	18	1.8	2.7	0.1	0.0
Light, Primo, Costa*	1 Primo/360ml	65	0.3	18	1.8	2.7	0.1	0.0
Mocha, Full Fat, Massimo, Costa*	1 Massimo/600ml	373	15.7	62	2.5	7.0	2.6	0.0
Mocha, Full Fat, Medio, Costa*	1 Medio/480ml	316	12.6	66	2.5	7.8	2.6	0.0
Mocha, Full Fat, Primo, Costa*	1 Primo/360ml	206	6.3	57	1.7	5.0	1.7	0.0
Mocha, Skimmed, Massimo, Costa*	1 Massimo/600ml	264	3.3	44	2.5	7.1	0.5	0.0
Mocha, Skimmed, Medio, Costa*	1 Medio/480ml	242	3.1	50	2.7	8.2	0.6	0.0
Mocha, Skimmed, Primo, Costa*	1 Primo/360ml	153	1.9	42	2.4	6.9	0.5	0.0
Mocha, Soya, Massimo, Costa*	1 Massimo/600ml	285	9.5	47	2.4	5.6	1.6	0.0
Mocha, Soya, Medio, Costa*	1 Medio/480ml	258	8.3	54	2.5	6.6	1.7	0.0
Mocha, Soya, Primo, Costa*	1 Primo/360ml	164	4.1	46	1.6	4.1	1.1	0.0
Mocha Flake, Full Fat, Massimo, Costa*	1 Massimo/600ml	548	29.7	91	2.7	8.8	4.9	0.0
Mocha Flake, Full Fat, Medio, Costa*	1 Medio/480ml	492	26.6	102	2.8	10.0	5.5	0.0
Mocha Flake, Full Fat, Primo, Costa*	1 Primo/360ml	356	20.0	99	2.6	9.4	5.6	0.0
Mocha Flake, Skimmed, Massimo, Costa*	1 Massimo/600ml	440	17.3	73	2.8	8.9	2.9	0.0
Mocha Flake, Skimmed, Medio, Costa*	1 Medio/480ml	418	17.1	87	3.0	10.4	3.6	0.0
Mocha Flake, Skimmed, Primo, Costa*	1 Primo/360ml	303	13.5	84	2.7	9.6	3.7	0.0
Mocha Flake, Soya, Massimo, Costa*	1 Massimo/600ml	461	23.6	77	2.6	7.4	3.9	0.0
Mocha Flake, Soya, Medio, Costa*	1 Medio/480ml	433	22.3	90	2.8	8.8	4.6	0.0
Mocha Flake, Soya, Primo, Costa*	1 Primo/360ml	314	17.0	87	2.6	8.2	4.7	0.0

COFFEE COOLERS

INFO/WEIGHT	Measure	per Measure KCAL	FAT	Nutrition Values per 100g / 100ml KCAL	PROT	CARB	FAT	FIBRE
Mocha with Full Fat Milk, Massimo, Costa*	1 Massimo/600ml	615	5.3	102	0.9	22.7	0.9	0.0
Mocha with Full Fat Milk, Medio, Costa*	1 Medio/480ml	489	4.5	102	1.0	22.4	0.9	0.0
Mocha with Full Fat Milk, Primo, Costa*	1 Primo/360ml	369	4.0	102	1.1	22.0	1.1	0.0
Mocha with Skimmed Milk, Massimo, Costa*	1 Massimo/600ml	579	1.1	96	1.0	22.8	0.2	0.0
Mocha with Skimmed Milk, Medio, Costa*	1 Medio/480ml	458	0.8	95	1.0	22.5	0.2	0.0
Mocha with Skimmed Milk, Primo, Costa*	1 Primo/360ml	340	0.6	94	1.2	22.1	0.2	0.0
Mocha with Soya Milk, Massimo, Costa*	1 Massimo/600ml	583	3.1	97	0.9	22.2	0.5	0.0
Mocha with Soya Milk, Medio, Costa*	1 Medio/480ml	462	2.6	96	0.9	21.9	0.5	0.0
Mocha with Soya Milk, Primo, Costa*	1 Primo/360ml	344	2.3	96	1.1	21.4	0.6	0.0
with Full Fat Milk, Massimo, Costa*	1 Massimo/600ml	457	4.7	76	0.8	16.6	0.8	0.0
with Full Fat Milk, Medio, Costa*	1 Medio/480ml	371	4.1	77	0.8	16.6	0.8	0.0
with Full Fat Milk, Primo, Costa*	1 Primo/360ml	290	37.1	81	1.0	16.9	10.3	0.0

COSTA

INFO/WEIGHT	Measure INFO/WEIGHT	per Measure KCAL	FAT	KCAL	PROT	CARB	FAT	FIBRE
COFFEE COOLERS								
with Skimmed Milk, Massimo, Costa*	1 Massimo/600ml	421	0.5	70	0.8	16.6	0.1	0.0
with Skimmed Milk, Medio, Costa*	1 Medio/480ml	340	0.4	71	0.8	16.7	0.1	0.0
with Skimmed Milk, Primo, Costa*	1 Primo/360ml	262	0.3	73	1.0	17.0	0.1	0.0
with Soya Milk, Massimo, Costa*	1 Massimo/600ml	426	2.5	71	0.7	16.1	0.4	0.0
with Soya Milk, Medio, Costa*	1 Medio/480ml	344	2.2	72	0.7	16.1	0.5	0.0
with Soya Milk, Primo, Costa*	1 Primo/360ml	266	2.0	74	0.9	16.3	0.6	0.0
COOKIES								
Choc Chunk, Double, Costa*	1 Pack/60g	296	15.2	493	5.2	61.1	25.3	3.7
Fruit & Oat, Costa*	1 Pack/60g	283	12.7	472	5.1	65.2	21.2	2.0
CROISSANT								
Almond, Costa*	1 Croissant/88g	336	16.9	382	9.3	43.0	19.2	0.0
Butter, Costa*	1 Croissant/64g	276	16.7	431	8.3	40.6	26.1	0.0
Ham & Cheese, Costa*	1 Croissant/100g	337	19.3	337	12.1	28.8	19.3	0.0
Tomato & Emmental, Costa*	1 Croissant/98g	342	21.0	349	9.0	30.0	21.4	0.0
CUPCAKES								
Banoffee, Costa *	1 Cupcake/112g	431	17.7	385	3.7	56.7	15.8	0.0
Lemon, Costa*	1 Cupcake/97g	512	32.5	528	2.8	53.2	33.5	0.0
Rocky Road, Costa*	1 Cupcake/101g	427	17.7	421	5.1	58.9	17.5	0.0
FLAPJACK								
Fruity, Costa*	1 Serving/85g	353	12.1	415	4.9	67.0	14.2	12.5
Nutty, Costa*	1 Serving/85g	391	20.0	460	7.4	54.8	23.5	5.0
FLATBREAD								
Cajun Chicken, Costa*	1 Pack/168g	310	5.1	184	12.7	26.6	3.0	0.0
Cheddar & Caramelised Onion Chutney, Costa*	1 Pack/118g	340	13.3	288	11.9	34.8	11.3	0.0
Chicken, Green Thai, Costa*	1 Pack/173g	325	6.4	188	12.2	26.6	3.7	0.0
Emmenthal & Mushroom, Costa*	1 Pack/158g	391	16.1	248	13.1	25.9	10.2	0.0
FLAVOURING FOR COFFEE								
Caramel, Massimo, Costa*	1 Massimo/600ml	66	0.0	11	0.0	2.7	0.0	0.0
Caramel, Medio, Costa*	1 Medio/480ml	49	0.0	10	0.0	2.5	0.0	0.0
Caramel, Primo, Costa*	1 Primo/360ml	33	0.0	9	0.0	2.2	0.0	0.0
Cinnamon, Massimo, Costa*	1 Massimo/600ml	66	0.0	11	0.0	2.7	0.0	0.0
Cinnamon, Medio, Costa*	1 Medio/480ml	49	0.0	10	0.0	2.5	0.0	0.0
Cinnamon, Primo, Costa*	1 Primo/360ml	33	0.0	9	0.0	2.2	0.0	0.0
Gingerbread, Massimo, Costa*	1 Massimo/600ml	68	0.0	11	0.0	2.8	0.0	0.0
Gingerbread, Medio, Costa*	1 Medio/480ml	51	0.0	11	0.0	2.6	0.0	0.0
Gingerbread, Primo, Costa*	1 Primo/360ml	34	0.0	9	0.0	2.3	0.0	0.0
Roasted Hazelnut, Massimo, Costa*	1 Massimo/600ml	63	0.0	10	0.0	2.6	0.0	0.0
Roasted Hazelnut, Medio, Costa*	1 Medio/480ml	48	0.0	10	0.0	2.4	0.0	0.0
Roasted Hazelnut, Primo, Costa*	1 Primo/360ml	32	0.0	9	0.0	2.2	0.0	0.0
Vanilla, Massimo, Costa*	1 Massimo/600ml	68	0.0	11	0.0	2.8	0.0	0.0
Vanilla, Medio, Costa*	1 Medio/480ml	51	0.0	11	0.0	2.6	0.0	0.0
Vanilla, Primo, Costa*	1 Primo/360ml	34	0.0	9	0.0	2.3	0.0	0.0
FRESCATO								
Coffee, Full Fat Milk, Medio Coffee Only, Costa*	1 Medio/454ml	423	7.9	93	1.5	17.9	1.7	0.0
Coffee, Full Fat Milk, Primo, Coffee Only, Costa*	1 Primo/340ml	302	5.6	89	1.4	17.1	1.6	0.0
Coffee, Skimmed Milk, Medio Coffee Only, Costa*	1 Medio/454ml	359	0.5	79	1.6	18.0	0.1	0.0
Coffee, Skimmed Milk, Primo Coffee Only, Costa*	1 Primo/340ml	256	0.5	75	1.5	17.2	0.1	0.0
Coffee, Soya Milk, Medio Coffee Only, Costa*	1 Medio/454ml	375	3.9	83	1.5	17.1	0.9	0.0
Coffee, Soya Milk, Primo, Coffee Only, Costa*	1 Primo/340ml	267	2.8	79	1.4	16.3	0.8	0.0
Coffee Caramel, Full Fat Milk, Medio, Costa*	1 Medio/454ml	488	7.9	107	1.5	21.5	1.7	0.0
Coffee Caramel, Skimmed Milk, Primo, Costa*	1 Primo/340ml	289	0.5	85	1.5	19.6	0.1	0.0
Coffee Caramel, Soya Milk, Primo, Costa*	1 Primo/340ml	300	2.8	88	1.4	18.6	0.8	0.0

	Measure INFO/WEIGHT	per Measure		Nutrition Values per 100g / 100ml				
		KCAL	FAT	KCAL	PROT	CARB	FAT	FIBRE
COSTA								
FRESCATO								
Coffee Mocha, Full Fat Milk, Medio, Costa*	1 Medio/454ml	540	8.3	119	1.6	24.0	1.8	0.0
Coffee Mocha, Skimmed Milk, Medio, Costa*	1 Medio/454ml	477	1.2	105	1.7	24.1	0.3	0.0
Coffee Mocha, Skimmed Milk, Primo, Costa*	1 Primo/340ml	335	0.8	99	1.6	22.6	0.2	0.0
Coffee Vanilla, Full Fat Milk, Medio, Costa*	1 Medio/454ml	491	7.9	108	1.5	21.6	1.7	0.0
Coffee Vanilla, Full Fat Milk, Primo, Costa*	1 Primo/340ml	336	5.6	99	1.4	19.6	1.6	0.0
Coffee Vanilla, Skimmed Milk, Medio, Costa*	1 Medio/454ml	427	0.7	94	1.6	21.7	0.1	0.0
Coffee Vanilla, Skimmed Milk, Primo, Costa*	1 Primo/340ml	290	0.5	85	1.5	19.7	0.1	0.0
FRUIT COOLERS								
Mango & Passionfruit, Massimo, Costa*	1 Massimo/600ml	290	0.6	48	0.1	11.6	0.1	0.0
Mango & Passionfruit, Medio, Costa*	1 Medio/480ml	232	0.5	48	0.1	11.6	0.1	0.0
Mango & Passionfruit, Primo, Costa*	1 Primo/360ml	173	0.3	48	0.1	11.6	0.1	0.0
Peach, Massimo, Costa*	1 Massimo/600ml	406	0.3	68	0.2	16.3	0.0	0.0
Peach, Medio, Costa*	1 Medio/480ml	325	0.2	68	0.2	16.3	0.0	0.0
Peach, Primo, Costa*	1 Primo/360ml	243	0.2	67	0.2	16.3	0.1	0.0
Red Berry, Massimo, Costa*	1 Massimo/600ml	409	0.6	68	0.2	16.3	0.1	0.0
Red Berry, Medio, Costa*	1 Medio/480ml	327	0.5	68	0.2	16.3	0.1	0.0
Red Berry, Primo, Costa*	1 Primo/360ml	245	0.3	68	0.2	16.3	0.1	0.0
Sicilian Lemonade, Medio, Costa*	1 Medio/454ml	264	0.2	59	0.0	14.0	0.0	0.0
Sicilian Lemonade, Primo, Costa*	1 Primo/340ml	197	0.2	58	0.1	14.0	0.1	0.0
HOT CHOCOLATE								
with Frothed Milk, Full Fat, Massimo, Costa*	1 Massimo/600ml	433	19.4	72	3.0	7.6	3.2	0.0
with Frothed Milk, Full Fat, Medio, Costa*	1 Medio/480ml	360	15.2	75	2.9	8.4	3.2	0.0
with Frothed Milk, Full Fat, Primo, Costa*	1 Primo/360ml	238	6.6	66	2.6	7.2	1.8	0.0
with Frothed Milk, Skimmed, Massimo, Costa*	1 Massimo/600ml	296	3.0	49	3.1	7.9	0.5	0.0
with Frothed Milk, Skimmed, Medio, Costa*	1 Medio/480ml	262	2.9	55	3.1	8.8	0.6	0.0
with Frothed Milk, Skimmed, Primo, Costa*	1 Primo/360ml	167	1.8	46	2.8	7.5	0.5	0.0
with Frothed Milk, Soya, Massimo, Costa*	1 Massimo/600ml	319	11.3	53	2.8	5.8	1.9	0.0
with Frothed Milk, Soya, Medio, Costa*	1 Medio/480ml	280	9.4	58	2.9	6.8	2.0	0.0
with Frothed Milk, Soya, Primo, Costa*	1 Primo/360ml	181	6.3	50	2.6	5.7	1.7	0.0
with Marshmallows & Cream, Soya, Massimo, Costa*	1 Massimo/600ml	468	21.0	78	3.0	8.2	3.5	0.0
with Marshmallows & Cream, Soya, Medio, Costa*	1 Medio/480ml	429	19.2	89	3.1	9.8	4.0	0.0
with Marshmallows & Cream, Soya, Primo, Costa*	1 Primo/360ml	305	13.6	85	2.8	9.5	3.8	0.0
ICE DESSERTS								
Double Choc Flake, Full Fat Milk, Medio, Costa*	1 Medio/454ml	786	29.9	173	2.1	26.4	6.6	0.0
Simply Vanilla, Full Fat Milk, Medio, Costa*	1 Medio/454ml	421	7.8	93	1.4	17.9	1.7	0.0
Simply Vanilla, Full Fat Milk, Primo, Costa*	1 Primo/340ml	301	5.6	89	1.4	17.1	1.6	0.0
Simply Vanilla, Skimmed Milk, Primo, Costa*	1 Primo/340ml	255	0.5	75	1.5	17.1	0.1	0.0
Simply Vanilla, Soya Milk, Medio, Costa*	1 Medio/454ml	373	3.8	82	1.4	17.0	0.8	0.0
Simply Vanilla, Soya Milk, Primo, Costa*	1 Primo/340ml	267	2.7	79	1.4	16.2	0.8	0.0
Strawberry Shortcake, Full Fat Milk, Primo, Costa*	1 Primo/340ml	569	23.9	167	1.8	24.3	7.0	0.0
Strawberry Shortcake, Skimmed Milk, Medio, Costa*	1 Medio/454ml	694	19.0	153	1.9	27.2	4.2	0.0
LOAF								
Breakfast, Banana & Pecan, Costa*	1 Loaf/108g	422	22.3	391	5.1	44.0	20.7	0.0
MOCHA								
Iced, Full Fat Milk, Medio, Costa*	1 Medio/454ml	209	0.0	46	1.2	7.7	0.0	0.0
Iced, Full Fat Milk, Primo, Costa*	1 Primo/340ml	142	3.7	42	1.1	6.9	1.1	0.0
Iced, Skimmed Milk, Medio, Costa*	1 Medio/454ml	170	1.1	37	1.2	7.7	0.2	0.0
Iced, Skimmed Milk, Primo, Costa*	1 Primo/340ml	115	0.8	34	1.1	7.0	0.2	0.0
Iced, Soya Milk, Primo, Costa*	1 Primo/340ml	122	2.1	36	1.1	6.4	0.6	0.0
MUFFIN								
Banana & Pecan Breakfast Loaf, Costa*	1 Muffin/113g	442	23.4	391	5.1	44.0	20.7	0.0
Blueberry, Costa*	1 Muffin/132g	475	20.9	360	4.0	50.4	15.8	0.0

	Measure			Nutrition Values per 100g / 100ml				
	INFO/WEIGHT	KCAL	FAT	KCAL	PROT	CARB	FAT	FIBRE

COSTA

MUFFIN

Chocolate, Mini, Costa*	1 Muffin/19g	73	3.9	383	4.3	44.5	20.5	0.0
Lemon & Orange, Low Fat, Costa*	1 Muffin/135g	319	3.1	236	4.6	49.4	2.3	1.1
Lemon & Poppyseed, Costa*	1 Muffin/131g	532	28.0	406	4.3	49.0	21.4	0.0
Lemon & White Chocolate, Costa*	1 Muffin/129g	472	20.4	366	5.4	52.3	15.8	0.0
Original Breakfast Loaf, Costa*	1 Muffin/128g	443	18.6	346	5.0	48.9	14.5	0.0
Raspberry & White Chocolate, Costa*	1 Muffin/135g	511	26.0	376	4.8	46.4	19.1	0.0
Raspberry & White Chocolate, Mini, Costa*	1 Muffin/19g	72	3.7	379	4.1	45.9	19.4	0.0
Triple Chocolate, Costa*	1 Muffin/130g	530	27.8	408	5.3	48.6	21.4	0.0

PAIN AU RAISIN

Costa*	1 Pastry/119g	356	13.7	299	5.1	43.7	11.5	0.0

PANETTINO

Chocolate, Costa*	1 Cake/100g	423	19.8	423	9.7	50.8	19.8	0.0
Classic, Costa*	1 Cake/100g	365	12.7	365	7.6	54.3	12.7	0.0

PANINI

Brie & Tomato Chutney, Costa*	1 Panini/177g	453	16.5	256	9.8	33.3	9.3	2.8
Chicken & Pesto, Costa*	1 Panini/210g	419	21.4	200	22.5	57.9	10.2	0.0
Goats Cheese & Caramelised Onion Chutney, Costa*	1 Panini/172g	431	5.3	251	4.9	19.5	3.1	0.0
Goats Cheese & Pepper, Costa*	1 Panini/197g	424	11.0	215	9.9	30.3	5.6	0.0
Ham & Cheese, Costa*	1 Panini/175g	461	21.2	263	12.5	26.2	12.1	0.0
Mozzarella, Tomato & Basil, Costa*	1 Panini/190g	400	11.0	211	8.3	29.8	5.8	0.0
Ragu Meatball, Costa*	1 Panini/190g	477	15.8	251	11.7	31.2	8.3	0.0
Steak & Cheese, Costa*	1 Panini/228g	492	16.4	216	11.3	25.7	7.2	0.0
Tuna Melt, Costa*	1 Panini/190g	462	14.3	243	14.4	29.5	7.5	0.0

PASTRY

Cinnamon Swirl, Costa*	1 Pastry/92g	341	22.8	369	4.0	31.9	24.7	0.0

SALAD

Chargrilled Vegetable & Cous Cous, Costa*	1 Pack/291g	352	7.6	121	3.0	21.5	2.6	0.0
Chicken & Pasta, Costa*	1 Pack/270g	427	11.1	158	8.4	21.9	4.1	0.0
Chicken & Pesto Pasta, Costa*	1 Pack/271g	420	11.4	155	7.8	21.3	4.2	1.7
Cous Cous, Moroccan Styles, Costa*	1 Pack/290g	392	7.3	135	3.6	24.6	2.5	2.2
Tuna, Costa*	1 Serving/181g	274	4.0	151	10.3	22.6	2.2	0.0

SANDWICH

Bacon & Tomato Sauce, Tostato, Costa*	1 Tostato/132g	316	6.6	239	8.5	40.2	5.0	0.0
BLT, Costa*	1 Pack/169g	397	15.7	235	11.0	26.8	9.3	0.0
Brie, Apple & Grape, Costa*	1 Pack/225g	535	24.5	238	8.3	28.7	10.9	0.0
Chicken, Coronation, Costa*	1 Pack/258g	600	26.1	232	12.5	23.0	10.1	2.5
Chicken, Roast, Costa*	1 Pack/177g	325	7.1	184	13.0	23.8	4.0	0.0
Club, All Day Breakfast, Costa*	1 Pack/243g	592	20.9	244	11.0	30.6	8.6	0.0
Club, Chicken & Bacon, Costa*	1 Pack/213g	484	13.2	227	13.6	29.3	6.2	0.0
Egg, Free Range, Costa*	1 Pack/172g	377	14.6	219	9.7	25.9	8.5	0.0
Egg Mayonnaise & Tomato, Free Range, Costa*	1 Pack/174g	389	24.1	223	8.6	18.3	13.8	0.0
Ham Hock & Mustard Pickle, Roll, Costa*	1 Pack/163g	286	5.2	176	10.6	26.1	3.2	0.0
Houmous, Costa*	1 Pack/165g	263	4.7	160	6.4	25.9	2.8	0.0
Ploughmans, Cheese, Roll, Costa*	1 Pack/175g	431	21.3	247	9.4	25.0	12.2	0.0
Prawn, Tiger, with Lime & Chilli Dressing, Costa*	1 Pack/185g	367	19.0	198	8.2	21.2	10.2	0.0
Salmon, & Salad, Poached, Oatmeal, Costa*	1 Pack/151g	224	4.2	148	7.7	22.9	2.8	0.0
Sausage, Chorizo, & Vine Ripened Tomato, Costa*	1 Pack/181g	315	3.8	174	15.5	26.1	2.1	0.0
Tuna, & Salad, Costa*	1 Pack/177g	289	4.1	163	11.9	25.7	2.3	0.0

SCONE

Fruit, Costa*	1 Scone/110g	370	11.8	336	5.6	55.1	10.7	

SHORTBREAD

Mini, Bag, Costa*	1 Bag/65g	316	15.7	486	4.1	63.0	24.1	0.0

	Measure INFO/WEIGHT	per Measure KCAL	per Measure FAT	Nutrition Values per 100g / 100ml KCAL	PROT	CARB	FAT	FIBRE

COSTA

SHORTCAKE

	Measure INFO/WEIGHT	KCAL	FAT	KCAL	PROT	CARB	FAT	FIBRE
Raspberry, Costa*	1 Shortcake/45g	215	10.7	477	2.4	63.5	23.7	0.0
SLICES								
Cheese, Twist, Pastry, Costa*	1 Pastry/103g	346	20.4	336	11.1	29.5	19.8	0.0
Pecan, Pastry, Costa*	1 Pastry/105g	465	29.9	443	5.6	42.1	28.5	3.0
SOUP								
Fish, Bouillabaisse, Costa*	1 Serving/400g	180	5.6	45	5.8	2.2	1.4	0.0
TEA								
Iced, Lemon, Costa*	1 Bottle/275ml	91	0.0	33	0.0	8.0	0.0	0.0
Iced, Original, Massimo, Costa*	1 Massimo/600ml	179	0.0	30	0.0	9.1	0.0	0.0
Iced, Original, Medio, Costa*	1 Medio/480ml	135	0.0	28	0.0	6.9	0.0	0.0
Iced, Original, Primo, Costa*	1 Primo/360ml	88	0.0	24	0.0	6.0	0.0	0.0
Iced, Peach, Massimo, Costa*	1 Massimo/600ml	121	0.0	20	0.0	4.8	0.0	0.0
Iced, Peach, Medio, Costa*	1 Medio/480ml	91	0.0	19	0.0	4.5	0.0	0.0
Iced, Peach, Primo, Costa*	1 Primo/360ml	60	0.0	17	0.0	4.0	0.0	0.0
Iced, Raspberry, Massimo, Costa*	1 Massimo/600ml	133	0.0	22	0.0	5.4	0.0	0.0
Iced, Raspberry, Medio, Costa*	1 Medio/480ml	100	0.0	21	0.0	5.1	0.0	0.0
Iced, Raspberry, Primo, Costa*	1 Primo/360ml	67	0.0	19	0.0	4.5	0.0	0.0
TRAYBAKE								
Chocolate Tiffin Triangle, Costa*	1 Serving/85g	433	25.7	509	4.9	54.6	30.2	0.0
Fruit, Seed, Nut & Honey Bar, Costa*	1 Serving/75g	317	15.2	423	7.5	52.5	20.3	0.0
Granola Bar, Costa*	1 Bar/75g	317	15.2	423	7.5	52.5	20.3	0.0
Raspberry & Almond, Costa*	1 Serving/100g	451	28.2	451	8.5	40.8	28.2	1.0
Shortbread, Caramel, Costa*	1 Serving/77g	426	26.5	553	4.7	55.9	34.4	0.0
WRAP								
Chicken Caesar, Costa*	1 Wrap/194g	420	15.6	216	11.8	24.1	8.0	1.4
Chicken Fajita, Costa*	1 Wrap/186g	416	12.9	223	12.1	28.0	6.9	0.0
Spicy Three Bean, Costa*	1 Wrap/235g	456	14.3	194	7.1	27.7	6.1	0.0
YOGHURT								
Honey & Granola, Costa*	1 Pot/190g	303	6.1	159	5.3	27.3	3.2	0.0
Strawberry & Granola, Costa*	1 Pot/190g	253	7.4	133	5.4	19.0	3.9	0.0

COSTA

SALAD

	Measure INFO/WEIGHT	KCAL	FAT	KCAL	PROT	CARB	FAT	FIBRE
Sunblush Tomato & Feta Pasta, Costa *	1 Pack/267g	360	13.6	135	4.4	17.1	5.1	2.2

CRUSSH JUICE BARS

BREAKFAST CEREAL

	Measure INFO/WEIGHT	KCAL	FAT	KCAL	PROT	CARB	FAT	FIBRE
Acai Strawberry Bowl, Large, Crussh Juice Bars*	1 Serving/400g	476	11.2	119	2.0	19.7	2.8	3.1
Blueberry Bircher Muesli, Crussh Juice Bars*	1 Serving/190g	199	4.0	105	4.4	17.2	2.1	1.4
Breakfast Berry Muesli Pot, Crussh Juice Bars*	1 Serving/225g	294	13.7	131	5.1	13.9	6.1	1.3
Cinnamon Porridge, Large, Crussh Juice Bars*	1 Serving/400g	380	8.4	95	3.1	15.7	2.1	1.8
Cinnamon Porridge, Medium, Crussh Juice Bars*	1 Serving/331g	314	6.9	95	3.1	15.7	2.1	1.8
Strawberries & Blueberries, Crussh Juice Bars*	1 Serving/171g	60	0.2	35	0.8	8.0	0.1	1.8
Strawberry Bircher, Crussh Juice Bars*	1 Serving/190g	211	4.7	111	4.6	17.5	2.5	1.4
Summer Porridge, Large, Crussh Juice Bars*	1 Serving/460g	602	18.8	131	4.8	18.8	4.1	1.4
Summer Porridge, Medium, Crussh Juice Bars*	1 Serving/330g	432	13.5	131	4.8	18.8	4.1	1.4
Traditional Organic Porridge, Large, Crussh Juice Bars*	1 Serving/400g	380	8.4	95	3.1	15.7	2.1	1.8
FRESHLY PRESSED JUICES								
Apple Juice, Large, Crussh Juice Bars*	1 Serving/451g	185	0.5	41	0.1	9.8	0.1	0.0
Apple Juice, Medium, Crussh Juice Bars*	1 Serving/339g	139	0.3	41	0.1	9.8	0.1	0.0
Carrot Juice, Large, Crussh Juice Bars*	1 Serving/448g	112	0.4	25	0.5	5.4	0.1	0.8
Carrot Juice, Medium, Crussh Juice Bars*	1 Serving/340g	85	0.3	25	0.5	5.4	0.1	0.8
Clean & Lean, Large, Crussh Juice Bars*	1 Serving/449g	211	0.4	47	0.4	11.1	0.1	2.4
Clean & Lean, Medium, Crussh Juice Bars*	1 Serving/338g	159	0.3	47	0.4	11.1	0.1	2.4

	Measure INFO/WEIGHT	per Measure KCAL	FAT	KCAL	PROT	CARB	FAT	FIBRE
CRUSSH JUICE BARS								
FRESHLY PRESSED JUICES								
Energiser, Large, Crussh Juice Bars*	1 Serving/450g	180	0.9	40	0.5	9.0	0.2	2.9
Energiser, Medium, Crussh Juice Bars*	1 Serving/340g	136	0.7	40	0.5	9.0	0.2	2.9
Green Goddess, Large, Crussh Juice Bars*	1 Serving/449g	175	1.3	39	0.8	8.4	0.3	2.6
Green Goddess, Medium, Crussh Juice Bars*	1 Serving/338g	132	1.0	39	0.8	8.4	0.3	2.6
Love Juice, Large, Crussh Juice Bars*	1 Serving/449g	193	0.4	43	0.6	9.9	0.1	0.5
Love Juice, Medium, Crussh Juice Bars*	1 Serving/340g	146	0.3	43	0.6	9.9	0.1	0.5
Orange Juice, Large, Crussh Juice Bars*	1 Serving/448g	148	0.0	33	0.6	7.7	0.0	0.1
Orange Juice, Medium, Crussh Juice Bars*	1 Serving/339g	112	0.0	33	0.6	7.7	0.0	0.1
Purifier, Large, Crussh Juice Bars*	1 Serving/463g	162	0.9	35	0.6	7.6	0.2	2.8
Purifier, Medium, Crussh Juice Bars*	1 Serving/340g	119	0.7	35	0.6	7.6	0.2	2.8
Super Juice, Large, Crussh Juice Bars*	1 Serving/450g	144	1.3	32	0.8	6.5	0.3	2.7
Super Juice, Medium, Crussh Juice Bars*	1 Serving/338g	108	1.0	32	0.8	6.5	0.3	2.7
Tropical Crussh, Large, Crussh Juice Bars*	1 Serving/451g	203	0.9	45	0.4	10.5	0.2	2.1
Tropical Crussh, Medium, Crussh Juice Bars*	1 Serving/340g	153	0.7	45	0.4	10.5	0.2	2.1
Zinger, Large, Crussh Juice Bars*	1 Serving/463g	162	0.9	35	0.6	7.6	0.2	1.9
Zinger, Medium, Crussh Juice Bars*	1 Serving/340g	119	0.7	35	0.6	7.6	0.2	1.9
FRUIT								
Seasonal Fruit, Crussh Juice Bars*	1 Serving/150g	61	0.3	41	0.5	10.0	0.2	1.1
HEALTHPOTS								
Black Lentil Feta & Mint Healthpot, Crussh Juice Bars*	1 Serving/150g	384	19.9	256	12.2	21.7	13.3	5.7
Classic Potato Dressing, Crussh Juice Bars*	1 Serving/25g	21	1.0	83	4.7	6.8	4.1	0.2
Classic Potato Side Salad, Crussh Juice Bars*	1 Serving/150g	166	8.1	111	2.8	12.9	5.4	1.2
Crussh Detox Healthpot, Crussh Juice Bars*	1 Serving/163g	104	4.5	64	3.7	6.0	2.8	1.6
Goats Cheese & Sweet Potato, Crussh Juice Bars*	1 Serving/160g	203	9.8	127	7.1	11.6	6.1	1.9
Great Greens, Crussh Juice Bars*	1 Serving/150g	91	3.7	61	6.2	3.4	2.5	4.1
Sesame Sauce, Crussh Juice Bars*	1 Serving/25g	73	6.8	292	5.8	5.9	27.3	2.7
Superfoods Healthpot, Crussh Juice Bars*	1 Serving/160g	440	24.2	275	10.7	23.9	15.1	4.3
Tuna Lean Bean Healthpot, Crussh Juice Bars*	1 Serving/160g	214	9.7	134	8.0	11.6	6.1	2.0
SALADS								
New Potato Tuna Nicoise Salad, Crussh Juice Bars*	1 Serving/250g	135	5.2	54	6.7	4.5	2.1	1.2
NY:LON Cobb Salad, Crussh Juice Bars*	1 Serving/215g	230	15.5	107	8.9	1.5	7.2	7.2
O-Me-Good Dressing, Crussh Juice Bars*	1 Serving/50g	55	3.8	111	3.2	7.3	7.6	0.7
Super Greens, Crussh Juice Bars*	1 Serving/230g	78	3.0	34	2.9	2.5	1.3	2.6
Zesty Dressing Tuna Nicoise, Crussh Juice Bars*	1 Serving/40g	118	12.9	295	0.4	1.0	32.3	0.0
SANDWICH								
5 a Day Wheat Free, Crussh Juice Bars*	1 Pack/200g	326	14.6	163	4.2	22.2	7.3	1.2
Classic Chicken Club Sandwich, Crussh Juice Bars*	1 Pack/235g	411	15.3	175	11.8	17.5	6.5	1.3
Smokey Ham Swiss, Crussh Juice Bars*	1 Pack/244g	490	19.3	201	12.1	20.2	7.9	3.0
Tu Cumber Mayo, Crussh Juice Bars*	1 Pack/180g	373	16.9	207	11.6	17.3	9.4	2.7
SMOOTHIES								
Bananarama, Large, Crussh Juice Bars*	1 Serving/450g	243	2.7	54	3.7	8.6	0.6	0.4
Bananarama, Medium, Crussh Juice Bars*	1 Serving/339g	183	2.0	54	3.7	8.6	0.6	0.4
Blueberry Hill, Large, Crussh Juice Bars*	1 Serving/449g	211	1.8	47	1.8	9.1	0.4	1.6
Blueberry Hill, Medium, Crussh Juice Bars*	1 Serving/338g	159	1.4	47	1.8	9.1	0.4	1.6
Crusshberry Blast, Large, Crussh Juice Bars*	1 Serving/449g	211	1.8	47	1.8	9.0	0.4	1.6
Crusshberry Blast, Medium, Crussh Juice Bars*	1 Serving/338g	159	1.4	47	1.8	9.0	0.4	1.6
Mango Madness, Large, Crussh Juice Bars*	1 Serving/449g	238	1.8	53	1.8	10.6	0.4	0.8
Mango Madness, Medium, Crussh Juice Bars*	1 Serving/340g	180	1.4	53	1.8	10.6	0.4	0.8
Peach Passion, Large, Crussh Juice Bars*	1 Serving/449g	211	1.3	47	2.0	9.0	0.3	0.6
Peach Passion, Medium, Crussh Juice Bars*	1 Serving/338g	159	1.0	47	2.0	9.0	0.3	0.6
Pineapple Pleasure, Large, Crussh Juice Bars*	1 Serving/450g	234	1.8	52	1.7	10.5	0.4	0.6
Pineapple Pleasure, Medium, Crussh Juice Bars*	1 Serving/338g	176	1.4	52	1.7	10.5	0.4	0.6

	Measure INFO/WEIGHT	per Measure KCAL	FAT	Nutrition Values per 100g / 100ml KCAL	PROT	CARB	FAT	FIBRE

CRUSSH JUICE BARS

SMOOTHIES

	Measure INFO/WEIGHT	KCAL	FAT	KCAL	PROT	CARB	FAT	FIBRE
Strawberry Cool, Large, Crussh Juice Bars*	1 Serving/450g	207	1.3	46	1.9	8.9	0.3	0.9
Strawberry Cool, Medium, Crussh Juice Bars*	1 Serving/339g	156	1.0	46	1.9	8.9	0.3	0.9

SNACKS & DESSERTS

Carrot Cake, Crussh Juice Bars*	1 Serving/167g	533	30.7	319	5.0	33.3	18.4	4.1
Chocolate Cake, Crussh Juice Bars*	1 Serving/115g	469	22.3	408	4.2	54.7	19.4	0.0
Crussh Brownie, Crussh Juice Bars*	1 Serving/75g	315	17.8	420	5.4	47.6	23.8	1.3
Natural Wasabi Peas, Crussh Juice Bars*	1 Serving/71g	294	6.3	412	15.7	66.6	8.8	10.8
Organic Double Chocolate Cookie, Crussh Juice Bars*	1 Serving/50g	210	8.8	421	5.0	60.8	17.6	2.7
Organic Oat & Raisin Cookie, Crussh Juice Bars*	1 Serving/50g	203	9.1	406	4.8	55.8	18.2	2.7
Organic Popcorn, Honey, Crussh Juice Bars*	1 Serving/30g	135	5.2	449	4.1	75.6	17.3	6.4
Organic Popcorn, Sea Salt, Crussh Juice Bars*	1 Serving/30g	118	4.7	394	11.0	64.9	15.8	13.0

SOUP

Bean & Vegetable Garden, Large, Crussh Juice Bars*	1 Serving/440g	295	2.2	67	3.2	10.6	0.5	3.9
Bean & Vegetable Garden, Medium, Crussh Juice Bars*	1 Serving/330g	221	1.6	67	3.2	10.6	0.5	3.9
Beef & Vegetable Pot, Large, Crussh Juice Bars*	1 Serving/440g	198	2.2	45	2.9	7.1	0.5	1.2
Beef & Vegetable Pot, Medium, Crussh Juice Bars*	1 Serving/330g	148	1.6	45	2.9	7.1	0.5	1.2
Beef Chilli, Large, Crussh Juice Bars*	1 Serving/440g	321	14.1	73	5.4	5.6	3.2	1.6
Beef Chilli, Medium, Crussh Juice Bars*	1 Serving/329g	240	10.5	73	5.4	5.6	3.2	1.6
Butternut & Spinach Coconut Curry, Crussh Juice Bars*	1 Serving/501g	551	13.0	110	2.6	19.0	2.6	1.7
Chicken Chilli Stew, Large, Crussh Juice Bars*	1 Serving/441g	216	1.8	49	6.1	5.3	0.4	1.5
Chicken Chilli Stew, Medium, Crussh Juice Bars*	1 Serving/329g	161	1.3	49	6.1	5.3	0.4	1.5
Chickpea Spinach & Dhal, Large, Crussh Juice Bars*	1 Serving/440g	246	7.5	56	3.5	6.6	1.7	1.4
Fit Meatballs Sicilian Style, Crussh Juice Bars*	1 Serving/500g	635	18.5	127	45.6	17.5	3.7	1.3
Ginger Chicken Miso, Crussh Juice Bars*	1 Serving/600g	204	6.6	34	2.8	3.3	1.1	0.7
Green Thai Chicken & Veg Curry, Crussh Juice Bars*	1 Serving/499g	544	11.0	109	3.7	3.5	2.2	1.6
Hungarian Goulash, Large, Crussh Juice Bars*	1 Serving/439g	202	3.1	46	3.8	6.3	0.7	0.9
Hungarian Goulash, Medium, Crussh Juice Bars*	1 Serving/330g	152	2.3	46	3.8	6.3	0.7	0.9
Italian Minestrone, Large, Crussh Juice Bars*	1 Serving/440g	172	1.3	39	2.1	6.8	0.3	2.0
Italian Minestrone, Mediumium, Crussh Juice Bars*	1 Serving/330g	129	1.0	39	2.1	6.8	0.3	2.0
Leek & Potato, Large, Crussh Juice Bars*	1 Serving/440g	176	6.6	40	0.9	5.5	1.5	0.7
Leek & Potato, Mediumium, Crussh Juice Bars*	1 Serving/330g	132	4.9	40	0.9	5.5	1.5	0.7
Lentil & Herbs, Large, Crussh Juice Bars*	1 Serving/440g	229	1.8	52	3.8	8.3	0.4	1.4
Lentil & Herbs, Mediumium, Crussh Juice Bars*	1 Serving/330g	172	1.3	52	3.8	8.3	0.4	1.4
Louisiana Chicken Gumbo, Large, Crussh Juice Bars*	1 Serving/411g	189	9.9	46	3.2	2.9	2.4	1.2
Louisiana Chicken Gumbo, Medium, Crussh Juice Bars*	1 Serving/309g	142	7.4	46	3.2	2.9	2.4	1.2
Organic Armenian Dhal, Large, Crussh Juice Bars*	1 Serving/440g	349	6.6	79	4.6	11.8	1.5	1.4
Organic Armenian Dhal, Medium, Crussh Juice Bars*	1 Serving/330g	262	5.0	79	4.6	11.8	1.5	1.4
Organic Farmhouse Chicken, Large, Crussh Juice Bars*	1 Serving/400g	232	10.4	58	3.4	5.2	2.6	3.0
Organic Leek & Potato, Large, Crussh Juice Bars*	1 Serving/440g	242	12.3	55	1.2	6.5	2.8	1.0
Organic Leek & Potato, Medium, Crussh Juice Bars*	1 Serving/329g	181	9.2	55	1.2	6.5	2.8	1.0
Organic Pea, Mint & Lemon, Large, Crussh Juice Bars*	1 Serving/440g	164	2.6	37	1.9	4.6	0.6	2.7
Organic Spanish Vegetable, Large, Crussh Juice Bars*	1 Serving/440g	176	0.9	40	1.8	5.7	0.2	1.9
Organic Thai Tomato, Large, Crussh Juice Bars*	1 Serving/400g	324	24.8	81	0.9	5.4	6.2	1.6
Organic Thai Tomato, Medium, Crussh Juice Bars*	1 Serving/330g	267	20.5	81	0.9	5.4	6.2	1.6
Organic Tomato & Lentil, Large, Crussh Juice Bars*	1 Serving/440g	231	4.0	52	2.9	8.3	0.9	11.4
Organic Tomato & Lentil, Medium, Crussh Juice Bars*	1 Serving/330g	173	3.0	52	2.9	8.3	0.9	11.4
Organic Wild Mushroom, Large, Crussh Juice Bars*	1 Serving/439g	224	12.7	51	1.1	5.3	2.9	0.5
Organic Wild Mushroom, Medium, Crussh Juice Bars*	1 Serving/329g	168	9.6	51	1.1	5.3	2.9	0.5
Pea & Homemade Pesto, Large, Crussh Juice Bars*	1 Serving/440g	238	13.6	54	2.4	4.0	3.1	1.7
Pea & Homemade Pesto Medium, Crussh Juice Bars*	1 Serving/330g	178	10.2	54	2.4	4.0	3.1	1.7
Thai Jungle Curry Chicken, Large, Crussh Juice Bars*	1 Serving/441g	539	27.4	122	7.9	8.6	6.2	4.3
Thai Jungle Curry Chicken, Medium, Crussh Juice Bars*	1 Serving/330g	403	20.5	122	7.9	8.6	6.2	4.3

	Measure INFO/WEIGHT	per Measure KCAL	FAT	Nutrition Values per 100g / 100ml KCAL	PROT	CARB	FAT	FIBRE
CRUSSH JUICE BARS								
SOUP								
Thai Red Lentil, Large, Crussh Juice Bars*	1 Serving/440g	220	13.6	50	1.8	3.8	3.1	0.6
Thai Red Lentil, Medium, Crussh Juice Bars*	1 Serving/330g	165	10.2	50	1.8	3.8	3.1	0.6
Vegetable Chilli, Large, Crussh Juice Bars*	1 Serving/440g	211	7.0	48	2.3	6.3	1.6	2.2
Vegetable Chilli, Medium, Crussh Juice Bars*	1 Serving/329g	158	5.3	48	2.3	6.3	1.6	2.2
SUPER SMOOTHIES								
Brainstorm, Large, Crussh Juice Bars*	1 Serving/449g	220	1.8	49	1.7	9.8	0.4	1.1
Brainstorm, Medium, Crussh Juice Bars*	1 Serving/339g	166	1.4	49	1.7	9.8	0.4	1.1
Brazilian, Large, Crussh Juice Bars*	1 Serving/450g	297	2.7	66	1.8	10.1	0.6	0.9
Brazilian, Medium, Crussh Juice Bars*	1 Serving/339g	224	2.0	66	1.8	10.1	0.6	0.9
Breakfast Smoothie, Large, Crussh Juice Bars*	1 Serving/450g	459	6.3	102	4.6	17.8	1.4	1.3
Breakfast Smoothie, Medium, Crussh Juice Bars*	1 Serving/339g	346	4.7	102	4.6	17.8	1.4	1.3
Detox Cactus, Large, Crussh Juice Bars*	1 Serving/400g	268	0.8	67	1.8	14.2	0.2	0.7
Detox Cactus, Medium, Crussh Juice Bars*	1 Serving/330g	221	0.7	67	1.8	14.2	0.2	0.7
Energy Explosion, Large, Crussh Juice Bars*	1 Serving/450g	243	1.8	54	1.7	10.8	0.4	0.9
Energy Explosion, Medium, Crussh Juice Bars*	1 Serving/339g	183	1.4	54	1.7	10.8	0.4	0.9
Fat Burner, Large, Crussh Juice Bars*	1 Serving/450g	207	1.8	46	1.7	9.0	0.4	1.4
Fat Burner, Medium, Crussh Juice Bars*	1 Serving/339g	156	1.4	46	1.7	9.0	0.4	1.4
Good Morning, Large, Crussh Juice Bars*	1 Serving/449g	220	0.9	49	1.9	9.5	0.2	1.2
Good Morning, Medium, Crussh Juice Bars*	1 Serving/339g	166	0.7	49	1.9	9.5	0.2	1.2
Peach Performance, Large, Crussh Juice Bars*	1 Serving/456g	310	6.4	68	12.0	13.8	1.4	0.7
Peach Performance, Medium, Crussh Juice Bars*	1 Serving/346g	235	4.8	68	12.0	13.8	1.4	0.7
Protein Power, Large, Crussh Juice Bars*	1 Serving/450g	306	5.4	68	9.9	14.0	1.2	0.8
Protein Power, Medium, Crussh Juice Bars*	1 Serving/346g	235	4.1	68	9.9	14.0	1.2	0.8
Sporty Spicy, Large, Crussh Juice Bars*	1 Serving/400g	280	1.2	70	1.8	14.8	0.3	0.6
Sporty Spicy, Medium, Crussh Juice Bars*	1 Serving/329g	230	1.0	70	1.8	14.8	0.3	0.6
You're Cherry Fit, Large, Crussh Juice Bars*	1 Serving/400g	296	0.8	74	1.9	11.6	0.2	0.6
You're Cherry Fit, Medium, Crussh Juice Bars*	1 Serving/329g	243	0.7	74	1.9	11.6	0.2	0.6
SUSHI								
Chicken Salad Sushi Wrap, Crussh Juice Bars*	1 Wrap/275g	360	3.6	131	5.7	24.1	1.3	1.2
Salmon Sushi Salad Box, Crussh Juice Bars*	1 Box/280g	344	5.6	123	4.3	21.9	2.0	0.0
Spicy Tuna Sushi Wrap, Crussh Juice Bars*	1 Wrap/280g	397	7.5	142	5.4	24.4	2.7	1.4
Veggie Sushi Salad Box, Crussh Juice Bars*	1 Box/325g	559	16.9	172	5.8	26.3	5.2	1.6
TOASTIES								
Jalapeno & Spinach Melt, Crussh Juice Bars*	1 Toastie/150g	403	16.0	269	13.9	29.3	10.7	0.3
Pesto Chicken & Cheddar Toastie, Crussh Juice Bars*	1 Toastie/190g	541	26.8	285	17.8	21.7	14.1	0.0
Skinny Ham & Edam, Crussh Juice Bars*	1 Toastie/130g	329	8.7	253	15.4	32.9	6.7	0.0
Tasty Cheddar Cheese, Crussh Juice Bars*	1 Toastie/105g	310	10.0	295	14.5	37.9	9.5	0.0
Tuna Swiss Melt, Crussh Juice Bars*	1 Toastie/170g	379	11.6	223	16.3	24.0	6.8	0.1
WRAP								
Citrus, Herb & Yoghurt Chicken, Crussh Juice Bars*	1 Wrap/260g	426	15.9	164	20.3	18.0	6.1	0.8
King Prawn Cocktail Wrap, Crussh Juice Bars*	1 Wrap/240g	389	13.0	162	7.3	21.0	5.4	1.9
Simply Caesar Wrap, Crussh Juice Bars*	1 Wrap/190g	538	16.7	283	10.3	40.4	8.8	1.5
Sweet Potato Falafel Salad Wrap, Crussh Juice Bars*	1 Wrap/245g	448	20.8	183	6.0	20.7	8.5	4.0
Tuna Salad Wrap, Crussh Juice Bars*	1 Wrap/210g	365	10.3	174	12.0	20.4	4.9	0.4
Vietnamese Beef Salad Wrap, Crussh Juice Bars*	1 Wrap/230g	375	10.8	163	9.1	18.7	4.7	1.4
CUISINE DE FRANCE								
BREAD								
Baguette, Demi, Cuisine De France*	1 Baguette/140g	360	2.0	257	6.7	56.0	1.4	1.7
Baguette, la Premier, Cuisine De France*	1 Baguette/70g	180	0.7	257	7.6	54.3	1.0	1.8
Baguette, Parisien, Cuisine De France*	1 Baguette/70g	171	0.6	245	8.5	51.0	0.8	1.9
Baps, Brown, Soft, Cuisine De France*	1 Bap/99g	236	0.9	238	11.5	46.0	0.9	7.3
Ciabattina, Cuisine De France*	1 Roll/120g	299	1.9	249	8.3	50.3	1.6	1.5

	Measure INFO/WEIGHT	per Measure KCAL	FAT	Nutrition Values per 100g / 100ml KCAL	PROT	CARB	FAT	FIBRE
CUISINE DE FRANCE								
BREAD								
French, Cuisine De France*	½ Stick/200g	490	1.6	245	8.5	51.0	0.8	1.9
MUFFIN								
Cappuccion, Iced, Luxury, Iced, Cuisine De France*	1 Muffin/105g	457	22.6	435	5.6	54.8	21.5	0.0
Carrot Cake, Cuisine De France*	1 Muffin/105g	373	12.6	355	4.7	56.9	12.0	0.0
DOMINO'S PIZZA								
BREAD								
Garlic, Pizza, Domino's Pizza*	1 Slice/50g	137	4.7	271	16.4	30.3	9.4	2.8
BROWNIES								
Chocolate, Squares, Domino's Pizza*	1 Brownie/22g	104	5.7	474	5.9	54.2	25.9	1.8
CHICKEN								
Kickers, Domino's Pizza*	7 Kickers/168g	366	14.6	218	18.0	17.0	8.7	0.9
Strippers, Domino's Pizza*	7 Strippers/189g	442	23.4	234	17.0	13.5	12.4	1.1
COLESLAW								
Domino's Pizza*	1 Tub/200g	328	29.6	164	1.3	6.6	14.8	1.7
COOKIES								
Domino's Pizza*	1 Cookie/40g	175	7.2	438	5.6	66.6	18.0	3.1
DIP								
BBQ, Domino's Pizza*	1 Pot/28g	46	0.1	163	0.0	39.5	0.5	0.0
Chocolate Sauce, Domino's Pizza*	1 Pot/28g	88	0.1	313	0.5	76.6	0.4	0.8
Garlic & Herb, Domino's Pizza*	1 Pot/28g	194	21.1	693	1.1	1.9	75.4	0.1
Honey & Mustard, Domino's Pizza*	1 Pot/28g	129	13.0	459	1.8	7.5	46.5	0.2
Mango, Domino's Pizza*	1 Pot/28g	52	0.3	185	0.2	42.5	1.1	0.6
Sweet Chilli, Domino's Pizza*	1 Pot/28g	61	0.3	217	4.0	51.0	0.9	0.6
Toffee, Domino's Pizza*	1 Pot/28g	94	0.9	335	1.5	75.1	3.2	0.1
PIZZA								
American Hot, Dominator, Large, Domino's Pizza*	1 Slice/109g	306	12.0	279	13.2	31.7	11.0	1.9
American Hot, Regular Crust, Large, Domino's Pizza*	1 Slice/87g	217	7.6	250	13.6	29.0	8.8	2.2
American Hot, Regular Crust, Medium, Domino's Pizza*	1 Slice/79g	194	7.0	245	13.3	28.0	8.9	2.2
American Hot, Regular Crust, Personal, Domino's Pizza*	1 Pizza/244g	644	20.3	264	14.7	32.6	8.3	2.2
American Hot, Regular Crust, Small, Domino's Pizza*	1 Slice/712g	181	6.6	253	14.0	28.5	9.2	2.2
American Hot, Thin Crust, Large, Domino's Pizza*	1 Slice/67g	202	9.7	303	14.7	28.4	14.5	2.2
American Hot, Thin Crust, Medium, Domino's Pizza*	1 Slice/62g	191	9.3	308	15.0	28.4	15.0	2.5
Americano, Dominator, Large, Domino's Pizza*	1 Slice/114g	334	11.4	293	14.1	37.0	10.0	1.8
Americano, Regular Crust, Large, Domino's Pizza*	1 Slice/91g	268	8.5	295	15.7	37.2	9.3	1.9
Americano, Regular Crust, Medium, Domino's Pizza*	1 Slice/84g	248	7.8	295	15.7	37.2	9.3	1.9
Americano, Regular Crust, Personal, Domino's Pizza*	1 Pizza/257g	738	19.8	287	19.4	35.0	7.7	2.5
Americano, Regular Crust, Small, Domino's Pizza*	1 Slice/76g	224	7.1	295	15.7	37.2	9.3	1.9
Americano, Thin Crust, Large, Domino's Pizza*	1 Slice/71g	257	10.6	362	17.4	39.3	15.0	2.1
Americano, Thin Crust, Medium, Domino's Pizza*	1 Slice/67g	243	10.0	362	17.4	39.3	15.0	2.1
Cheese & Tomato, Dominator, Lge, Domino's Pizza*	1 Slice/92g	265	8.7	288	13.0	37.6	9.5	2.3
Cheese & Tomato, Regular Crust, Lge, Domino's Pizza*	1 Slice/69g	183	5.4	265	14.0	34.7	7.8	2.4
Cheese & Tomato, Regular Crust, Sm, Domino's Pizza*	1 Slice/56g	148	4.4	264	14.1	34.5	7.8	2.5
Cheese & Tomato, Stuffed Crust, Lge, Domino's Pizza*	1 Slice/75g	216	7.3	288	14.4	34.6	9.8	2.3
Cheese & Tomato, Stuffed Crust, Med, Domino's Pizza*	1 Slice/69g	199	6.8	288	14.4	34.6	9.8	2.3
Cheese & Tomato, Thin Crust, Large, Domino's Pizza*	1 Slice/49g	162	7.4	330	15.6	32.9	15.2	3.1
Cheese & Tomato, Thin Crust, Med, Domino's Pizza*	1 Slice/46g	160	7.1	347	15.7	36.2	15.5	2.9
Chicken Feast, Dominator, Large, Domino's Pizza*	1 Slice/112g	289	9.2	258	13.9	32.3	8.2	2.0
Chicken Feast, Reg Crust, Personal, Domino's Pizza*	1 Pizza/248g	613	15.1	247	15.7	32.3	6.1	2.1
Chicken Feast, Regular Crust, Large, Domino's Pizza*	1 Slice/89g	201	5.6	226	14.6	27.8	6.3	2.1
Chicken Feast, Regular Crust, Medium, Domino's Pizza*	1 Slice/81g	183	5.1	226	14.6	27.8	6.3	2.1
Chicken Feast, Regular Crust, Small, Domino's Pizza*	1 Slice/72g	163	4.6	226	14.6	27.8	6.3	2.1
Chicken Feast, Thin Crust, Large, Domino's Pizza*	1 Slice/69g	195	8.0	283	16.5	28.1	11.6	2.4

	Measure INFO/WEIGHT	per Measure KCAL	per Measure FAT	Nutrition Values per 100g / 100ml KCAL	PROT	CARB	FAT	FIBRE
DOMINO'S PIZZA								
PIZZA								
Chicken Feast, Thin Crust, Medium, Domino's Pizza*	1 Slice/64g	181	7.4	283	16.5	28.1	11.6	2.4
Domino's Meateor, Dominator, Large, Domino's Pizza*	1 Slice/114g	357	14.5	313	13.3	36.6	12.7	1.8
Domino's Meateor, Regular Crust, Lge, Domino's Pizza*	1 Slice/88g	280	11.2	319	14.5	36.7	12.7	1.8
Domino's Meateor, Regular Crust, Sm, Domino's Pizza*	1 Slice/74g	236	9.4	319	14.5	36.7	12.7	1.8
Domino's Meateor, Thin Crust, Large, Domino's Pizza*	1 Slice/68g	239	12.0	352	15.3	32.8	17.7	1.7
Domino's Meateor, Thin Crust, Med, Domino's Pizza*	1 Slice/64g	250	12.3	392	16.0	38.6	19.3	2.0
Extravaganza, Dominator, Large, Domino's Pizza*	1 Slice/127g	338	14.1	266	13.3	28.2	11.1	1.9
Extravaganza, Regular Crust, Large, Domino's Pizza*	1 Slice/104g	252	10.7	242	13.7	23.4	10.3	1.9
Extravaganza, Regular Crust, Medium, Domino's Pizza*	1 Slice/95g	230	9.8	242	13.7	23.4	10.3	1.9
Extravaganza, Regular Crust, Personal, Domino's Pizza*	1 Pizza/298g	781	31.0	262	15.2	26.7	10.4	1.9
Extravaganza, Thin Crust, Large, Domino's Pizza*	1 Slice/84g	235	12.8	280	15.0	20.7	15.2	2.2
Extravaganza, Thin Crust, Medium, Domino's Pizza*	1 Slice/78g	227	12.1	291	15.1	22.6	15.5	2.1
Farmhouse, Double Decadence, Med, Domino's Pizza*	1 Slice/100g	277	13.4	277	12.7	26.5	13.4	2.3
Farmhouse, Regular Crust, Large, Domino's Pizza*	1 Slice/88g	195	6.0	222	13.4	26.8	6.8	2.1
Farmhouse, Regular Crust, Medium, Domino's Pizza*	1 Slice/81g	180	5.5	222	13.4	26.8	6.8	2.1
Farmhouse, Regular Crust, Personal, Domino's Pizza*	1 Pizza/248g	605	16.1	244	14.8	31.5	6.5	2.1
Farmhouse, Regular Crust, Small, Domino's Pizza*	1 Slice/73g	162	5.0	222	13.4	26.8	6.8	2.1
Farmhouse, Thin Crust, Large, Domino's Pizza*	1 Slice/68g	180	8.1	265	14.8	24.6	11.9	2.5
Farmhouse, Thin Crust, Medium, Domino's Pizza*	1 Slice/63g	175	7.7	277	15.1	26.9	12.2	2.4
Firenze, Thin Crust, Fresh, Large, Domino's Pizza*	1 Slice/54g	179	8.2	332	15.5	32.0	15.3	2.5
Firenze, Thin Crust, Fresh, Medium, Domino's Pizza*	1 Slice/48g	159	7.3	332	15.5	32.0	15.3	2.5
Firenze, Thin Crust, Fresh, Small, Domino's Pizza*	1 Slice/43g	143	6.6	332	15.5	32.0	15.3	2.5
Florentine, Thin Crust, Fresh, Large, Domino's Pizza*	1 Slice/48g	152	6.6	317	13.4	33.8	13.7	2.2
Florentine, Thin Crust, Fresh, Medium, Domino's Pizza*	1 Slice/42g	133	5.7	317	13.4	33.8	13.7	2.2
Florentine, Thin Crust, Fresh, Small, Domino's Pizza*	1 Slice/37g	117	5.1	317	13.4	33.8	13.7	2.2
Full House, Dominator, Large, Domino's Pizza*	1 Slice/119g	312	11.5	262	12.6	31.0	9.7	2.0
Full House, Double Decadence, Med, Domino's Pizza*	1 Slice/107g	306	15.7	286	12.4	25.9	14.7	2.2
Full House, Regular Crust, Large, Domino's Pizza*	1 Slice/96g	231	8.5	241	13.2	27.0	8.9	2.1
Full House, Regular Crust, Medium, Domino's Pizza*	1 Slice/88g	208	7.8	236	13.0	26.0	8.9	2.0
Full House, Regular Crust, Small, Domino's Pizza*	1 Slice/80g	194	7.4	242	13.5	26.3	9.2	2.1
Full House, Thin Crust, Large, Domino's Pizza*	1 Slice/76g	210	10.6	276	14.0	23.7	13.9	2.4
Full House, Thin Crust, Medium, Domino's Pizza*	1 Slice/71g	206	10.2	290	14.3	25.9	14.3	2.3
Ham & Pineapple, Dominator, Large, Domino's Pizza*	1 Slice/106g	281	9.3	265	13.2	33.3	8.8	2.0
Ham & Pineapple, Regular Crust, Lge, Domino's Pizza*	1 Slice/84g	194	5.9	231	13.7	28.5	7.0	2.0
Ham & Pineapple, Regular Crust, Med, Domino's Pizza*	1 Slice/77g	178	5.4	231	13.7	28.5	7.0	2.0
Ham & Pineapple, Regular Crust, Sm, Domino's Pizza*	1 Slice/70g	162	4.9	231	13.7	28.5	7.0	2.0
Ham & Pineapple, Thin Crust, Large, Domino's Pizza*	1 Slice/64g	181	8.1	283	15.4	26.8	12.7	2.5
Ham & Pineapple, Thin Crust, Medium, Domino's Pizza*	1 Slice/60g	175	7.6	292	15.4	29.0	12.7	2.3
Hawaiian, Dominator, Large, Domino's Pizza*	1 Slice/117g	296	9.9	252	12.7	31.6	8.4	2.0
Hawaiian, Double Decadence, Med, Domino's Pizza*	1 Slice/106g	289	13.9	274	12.5	26.6	13.2	2.2
Hawaiian, Regular Crust, Large, Domino's Pizza*	1 Slice/94g	213	6.3	226	13.4	27.9	6.7	2.0
Hawaiian, Regular Crust, Medium, Domino's Pizza*	1 Slice/86g	189	5.7	219	13.1	26.8	6.6	2.0
Hawaiian, Regular Crust, Personal, Domino's Pizza*	1 Pizza/265g	636	16.7	240	14.4	31.3	6.3	2.0
Hawaiian, Regular Crust, Small, Domino's Pizza*	1 Slice/78g	176	5.3	224	13.7	27.2	6.7	2.1
Hawaiian, Thin Crust, Large, Domino's Pizza*	1 Slice/74g	194	8.6	260	14.4	24.6	11.6	2.4
Hawaiian, Thin Crust, Medium, Domino's Pizza*	1 Slice/69g	189	8.2	273	14.6	26.9	11.9	2.3
Hot & Spicy, Dominator, Large, Domino's Pizza*	1 Slice/107g	284	9.9	264	12.2	33.0	9.2	2.2
Hot & Spicy, Double Decadence, Med, Domino's Pizza*	1 Slice/96g	276	13.7	288	11.8	28.0	14.3	2.4
Hot & Spicy, Regular Crust, Large, Domino's Pizza*	1 Slice/84g	201	6.5	238	12.7	29.5	7.7	2.3
Hot & Spicy, Regular Crust, Medium, Domino's Pizza*	1 Slice/77g	178	5.8	232	12.3	28.7	7.6	2.3
Hot & Spicy, Regular Crust, Personal, Domino's Pizza*	1 Pizza/237g	602	17.1	254	13.9	33.3	7.2	2.3
Hot & Spicy, Regular Crust, Small, Domino's Pizza*	1 Slice/69g	163	5.3	237	12.8	29.3	7.7	2.3

	Measure INFO/WEIGHT	per Measure KCAL	FAT	Nutrition Values per 100g / 100ml KCAL	PROT	CARB	FAT	FIBRE

DOMINO'S PIZZA

PIZZA

	Measure INFO/WEIGHT	KCAL	FAT	KCAL	PROT	CARB	FAT	FIBRE
Hot & Spicy, Thin Crust, Large, Domino's Pizza*	1 Slice/65g	181	8.6	280	9.3	26.5	13.3	2.7
Hot & Spicy, Thin Crust, Medium, Domino's Pizza*	1 Slice/59g	175	8.1	294	13.7	29.2	13.6	2.6
Meat Lovers, Dominator, Large, Domino's Pizza*	1 Slice/111g	320	12.5	288	15.1	31.4	11.3	1.9
Meat Lovers, Regular Crust, Large, Domino's Pizza*	1 Slice/89g	235	9.3	264	16.1	26.5	10.4	1.9
Meat Lovers, Regular Crust, Medium, Domino's Pizza*	1 Slice/81g	214	8.4	264	16.1	26.5	10.4	1.9
Meat Lovers, Regular Crust, Personal, Domino's Pizza*	1 Pizza/244g	683	22.9	280	16.8	31.8	9.4	2.0
Meat Lovers, Regular Crust, Small, Domino's Pizza*	1 Slice/74g	195	7.7	264	16.1	26.5	10.4	1.9
Meat Lovers, Thin Crust, Large, Domino's Pizza*	1 Slice/69g	219	11.4	318	18.3	24.2	16.5	2.3
Meat Lovers, Thin Crust, Medium, Domino's Pizza*	1 Slice/64g	211	10.7	330	18.5	26.5	16.7	2.2
Meatilicious, Stuffed Crust, Large, Domino's Pizza*	1 Slice/82g	235	9.4	286	16.1	28.5	11.5	1.9
Meatilicious, Stuffed Crust, Medium, Domino's Pizza*	1 Slice/76g	217	8.7	286	16.1	28.5	11.5	1.9
Mighty Meaty, Dominator, Large, Domino's Pizza*	1 Slice/118g	326	13.1	276	14.0	30.0	11.1	1.9
Mighty Meaty, Regular Crust, Large, Domino's Pizza*	1 Slice/95g	243	9.7	256	15.0	26.1	10.2	2.0
Mighty Meaty, Regular Crust, Medium, Domino's Pizza*	1 Slice/87g	218	9.0	251	14.7	25.0	10.3	1.9
Mighty Meaty, Regular Crust, Personal, Domino's Pizza*	1 Pizza/265g	715	26.2	270	15.5	29.7	9.9	2.0
Mighty Meaty, Regular Crust, Small, Domino's Pizza*	1 Slice/80g	206	8.5	257	15.3	25.2	10.6	2.0
Mighty Meaty, Stuffed Crust, Large, Domino's Pizza*	1 Slice/100g	274	11.6	274	15.2	26.5	11.6	1.9
Mighty Meaty, Stuffed Crust, Medium, Domino's Pizza*	1 Slice/94g	258	10.9	274	15.2	26.5	11.6	1.9
Mighty Meaty, Thin Crust, Large, Domino's Pizza*	1 Slice/75g	222	11.8	296	16.2	22.6	15.7	2.3
Mighty Meaty, Thin Crust, Medium, Domino's Pizza*	1 Slice/70g	216	11.2	309	16.5	24.6	16.0	2.1
Pepperoni Passion, Dominator, Large, Domino's Pizza*	1 Slice/115g	351	14.9	305	16.1	30.4	13.0	1.8
Pepperoni Passion, Regular Crust, Lge, Domino's Pizza*	1 Slice/92g	269	11.5	292	17.6	26.5	12.5	1.8
Pepperoni Passion, Stuffed Crust, Lge, Domino's Pizza*	1 Slice/97g	299	13.4	308	17.7	26.8	13.8	1.8
Pepperoni Passion, Thin Crust, Large, Domino's Pizza*	1 Slice/72g	248	13.5	344	19.6	22.9	18.8	2.1
Pepperoni Passion, Thin Crust, Med, Domino's Pizza*	1 Slice/68g	242	13.0	356	19.8	25.1	19.1	2.0
Rustica, Thin Crust, Fresh, Large, Domino's Pizza*	1 Slice/57g	164	6.0	288	15.2	32.0	10.5	2.5
Rustica, Thin Crust, Fresh, Medium, Domino's Pizza*	1 Slice/50g	144	5.2	288	15.2	32.0	10.5	2.5
Rustica, Thin Crust, Fresh, Small, Domino's Pizza*	1 Slice/45g	130	4.7	288	15.2	32.0	10.5	2.5
Tandoori Hot, Dominator, Large, Domino's Pizza*	1 Slice/112g	280	9.0	250	12.7	31.8	8.0	2.1
Tandoori Hot, Regular Crust, Large, Domino's Pizza*	1 Slice/89g	199	5.6	223	13.4	28.1	6.3	2.2
Tandoori Hot, Regular Crust, Medium, Domino's Pizza*	1 Slice/81g	176	5.0	217	13.0	27.2	6.2	2.2
Tandoori Hot, Regular Crust, Personal, Domino's Pizza*	1 Pizza/248g	595	14.9	240	14.5	31.9	6.0	2.2
Tandoori Hot, Regular Crust, Small, Domino's Pizza*	1 Slice/73g	162	4.6	222	13.5	27.9	6.3	2.3
Tandoori Hot, Thin Crust, Large, Domino's Pizza*	1 Slice/69g	178	7.7	257	14.3	24.9	11.1	2.6
Tandoori Hot, Thin Crust, Medium, Domino's Pizza*	1 Slice/64g	173	7.3	270	14.5	27.4	11.4	2.5
Texas BBQ, Dominator, Large, Domino's Pizza*	1 Slice/110g	311	10.1	283	12.9	37.3	9.2	1.8
Texas BBQ, Double Decadence, Med, Domino's Pizza*	1 Slice/98g	319	13.6	326	13.5	36.6	13.9	1.8
Texas BBQ, Regular Crust, Large, Domino's Pizza*	1 Slice/87g	240	7.0	276	14.4	36.6	8.0	1.8
Texas BBQ, Regular Crust, Medium, Domino's Pizza*	1 Slice/79g	218	6.3	276	14.4	36.6	8.0	1.8
Texas BBQ, Regular Crust, Personal, Domino's Pizza*	1 Pizza/244g	659	16.1	270	18.4	34.4	6.6	2.4
Texas BBQ, Regular Crust, Small, Domino's Pizza*	1 Slice/71g	196	5.7	276	14.4	36.6	8.0	1.8
Texas BBQ, Thin Crust, Large, Domino's Pizza*	1 Slice/67g	194	7.8	289	15.3	30.8	11.6	1.7
Texas BBQ, Thin Crust, Medium, Domino's Pizza*	1 Slice/62g	203	8.1	328	16.0	36.8	13.0	2.0
The Sizzler, Dominator, Large, Domino's Pizza*	1 Slice/117g	344	13.4	293	13.7	34.1	11.4	2.1
The Sizzler, Medium, Regular Crust, Domino's Pizza*	1 Slice/75g	172	5.2	230	12.9	29.1	6.9	2.3
The Sizzler, Regular Crust, Large, Domino's Pizza*	1 Slice/95g	270	10.6	285	14.7	31.5	11.2	2.2
The Sizzler, Regular Crust, Medium, Domino's Pizza*	1 Slice/87g	247	9.7	285	14.7	31.5	11.2	2.2
The Sizzler, Regular Crust, Personal, Domino's Pizza*	1 Pizza/261g	707	22.7	271	15.6	32.6	8.7	2.4
The Sizzler, Regular Crust, Small, Domino's Pizza*	1 Slice/78g	223	8.8	285	14.7	31.5	11.2	2.2
The Sizzler, Thin Crust, Large, Domino's Pizza*	1 Slice/74g	227	10.8	303	14.7	28.4	14.5	2.2
The Sizzler, Thin Crust, Medium, Domino's Pizza*	1 Slice/70g	242	11.9	347	16.1	32.1	17.1	2.4
Veg Supreme, Stuffed Crust, Lge, Domino's Pizza*	1 Slice/93g	223	7.3	240	11.9	29.3	7.9	2.2

	Measure INFO/WEIGHT	per Measure KCAL	per Measure FAT	Nutrition Values per 100g / 100ml KCAL	PROT	CARB	FAT	FIBRE
DOMINO'S PIZZA								
PIZZA								
Veg Supreme, Thin Crust, Large, Domino's Pizza*	1 Slice/68g	171	7.5	252	11.8	26.1	11.1	2.7
Veg Supreme, Thin Crust, Medium, Domino's Pizza*	1 Slice/63g	168	7.2	266	12.0	28.7	11.5	2.6
Veg-A-Roma, Regular Crust, Large, Domino's Pizza*	1 Slice/86g	240	8.9	279	12.3	34.3	10.4	2.4
Veg-A-Roma, Regular Crust, Medium, Domino's Pizza*	1 Slice/78g	218	8.1	279	12.3	34.3	10.4	2.4
Veg-A-Roma, Regular Crust, Personal, Domino's Pizza*	1 Pizza/242g	641	19.4	265	13.7	34.7	8.0	2.5
Veg-A-Roma, Regular Crust, Small, Domino's Pizza*	1 Slice/70g	195	7.3	279	12.3	34.3	10.4	2.4
Veg-A-Roma, Thin Crust, Large, Domino's Pizza*	1 Slice/66g	180	7.8	273	12.5	29.2	11.8	2.8
Veg-A-Roma, Thin Crust, Medium, Domino's Pizza*	1 Slice/61g	167	7.2	273	12.5	29.2	11.8	2.8
Vegetarian Supreme, Dominator, Lge, Domino's Pizza*	1 Slice/111g	274	8.9	247	11.2	32.6	8.0	2.2
Vegetarian Supreme, Reg Crust, Sm, Domino's Pizza*	1 Slice/72g	156	4.5	217	11.5	28.9	6.2	2.3
Vegi-Volcano, Dominator, Large, Domino's Pizza*	1 Slice/113g	288	10.2	253	12.1	31.1	9.0	2.1
Vegi-Volcano, Regular Crust, Large, Domino's Pizza*	1 Slice/91g	202	6.7	222	12.2	26.5	7.4	2.2
Vegi-Volcano, Regular Crust, Medium, Domino's Pizza*	1 Slice/83g	184	6.1	222	12.2	26.5	7.4	2.2
Vegi-Volcano, Regular Crust, Personal, Domino's Pizza*	1 Pizza/254g	617	18.0	243	13.7	31.0	7.1	2.2
Vegi-Volcano, Regular Crust, Small, Domino's Pizza*	1 Slice/75g	166	5.5	222	12.2	26.5	7.4	2.2
Vegi-Volcano, Thin Crust, Large, Domino's Pizza*	1 Slice/72g	189	9.0	262	13.3	23.9	12.5	2.6
Vegi-Volcano, Thin Crust, Medium, Domino's Pizza*	1 Slice/66g	181	8.4	275	13.5	26.5	12.8	2.5
POTATO								
Wedges, Domino's Pizza*	1 Serving/190g	298	12.3	157	2.5	21.9	6.5	2.2
POTATO SKINS								
Cheese & Bacon, Loaded 3, Domino's Pizza*	1 Skin/56g	99	4.9	176	5.3	19.0	8.8	3.9
Cheese & Onion, Loaded 3, Domino's Pizza*	1 Skin/56g	96	3.8	172	3.8	23.8	6.8	4.1
SAUCE								
Hot, Domino's Pizza*	1 Pot/28g	7	0.3	25	0.8	1.8	1.1	1.1
WAFFLES								
Domino's Pizza*	1 Serving/104g	491	25.4	472	5.0	58.2	24.4	1.2
EAT								
BREAD								
Bag of Croutons, EAT*	1 Serving/15g	69	2.8	463	11.1	63.1	18.5	2.8
Chunk of Freshly Baked Brown Bread, EAT*	1 Serving/67g	141	1.3	211	7.4	44.0	1.9	2.7
Chunk of Freshly Baked White Bread, EAT*	1 Serving/67g	162	2.9	242	7.3	46.4	4.3	1.9
Wheat Free Seeded Rye Bread, EAT*	1 Serving/144g	331	6.0	230	6.7	48.0	4.2	6.7
BREAKFAST								
Almond Croissant, EAT*	1 Serving/83g	350	19.8	422	10.0	41.7	23.9	2.9
Apple, Almond & Cinnamon Bircher Muesli, EAT*	1 Serving/210g	361	12.2	172	6.1	23.3	5.8	2.3
Bacon Butty Hot Toasted Muffin, EAT*	1 Serving/90g	291	10.9	324	17.1	36.1	12.1	0.8
Banana, Honey & Grapenuts, EAT*	1 Serving/228g	349	6.4	153	6.3	25.4	2.8	1.5
Belgian Chocolate Muffin, EAT*	1 Serving/124g	511	26.4	412	5.0	48.9	21.3	2.1
Cheese Twist, EAT*	1 Serving/74g	313	19.0	421	14.0	33.7	25.6	2.2
Chocolate Croissant, EAT*	1 Serving/81g	361	21.3	445	6.9	45.4	26.2	3.0
Cinnamon Swirl, EAT*	1 Serving/77g	360	24.5	470	5.1	40.4	32.0	4.4
Croissant, EAT*	1 Serving/71g	305	17.1	427	9.4	43.4	23.9	2.7
Egg, Mushroom & Cheddar Hot Toasted Muffin, EAT*	1 Serving/125g	240	6.9	192	9.1	26.2	5.5	1.0
Egg & Bacon Half Baguette, EAT*	1 Serving/112g	311	12.2	278	13.5	30.5	10.9	1.8
Egg & Tomato Half Baguette New Improved, EAT*	1 Serving/140g	304	12.2	217	9.0	24.8	8.7	1.7
Eggs Benedict Hot Toasted Muffin, EAT*	1 Serving/120g	265	8.9	220	10.2	27.6	7.4	0.8
Full English Breakfast Muffin, EAT*	1 Serving/295g	687	24.5	233	10.7	28.4	8.3	0.7
Ham & Jarlsberg Croissant, EAT*	1 Serving/128g	339	21.1	265	15.6	20.8	16.5	0.0
Ham & Jarlsberg Half Baguette, EAT*	1 Serving/123g	297	13.3	242	14.5	21.8	10.8	1.5
Large Bacon Butty Hot Toasted Muffin, EAT*	1 Serving/190g	589	18.4	310	15.4	39.7	9.7	0.9
Large Salmon & Cream Cheese Bagel, EAT*	1 Serving/186g	399	12.7	214	13.3	26.0	6.8	1.2
Low Fat Blueberry Muffin, EAT*	1 Serving/124g	324	3.8	261	5.5	51.6	3.1	2.2

	Measure INFO/WEIGHT	per Measure KCAL	per Measure FAT	Nutrition Values per 100g / 100ml KCAL	PROT	CARB	FAT	FIBRE

EAT
BREAKFAST

	Measure INFO/WEIGHT	KCAL	FAT	KCAL	PROT	CARB	FAT	FIBRE
Maple Pecan Plait, EAT*	1 Serving/83g	377	26.0	454	4.7	38.4	31.3	5.2
Pain au Chocolate, EAT*	1 Serving/78g	329	18.4	422	9.8	42.6	23.6	3.6
Plain Porridge Big, EAT*	1 Serving/280g	227	3.4	81	4.4	13.3	1.2	1.2
Plain Porridge Small, EAT*	1 Serving/180g	146	2.2	81	4.4	13.3	1.2	1.2
Porridge with Apple & Blackberry Compote Big, EAT*	1 Serving/331g	291	3.6	88	3.9	16.0	1.1	1.5
Porridge with Apple & Blackberry Compote Small, EAT*	1 Serving/231g	210	2.3	91	3.6	17.2	1.0	1.7
Porridge with Banana & Maple Syrup Big, EAT*	1 Serving/315g	287	3.5	91	4.0	16.4	1.1	1.2
Porridge with Banana & Maple Syrup Small, EAT*	1 Serving/215g	206	2.4	96	3.8	17.8	1.1	1.2
Porridge with Banana Big, EAT*	1 Serving/301g	247	3.3	82	4.2	13.9	1.1	1.3
Porridge with Banana Small, EAT*	1 Serving/200g	166	2.2	83	4.1	14.2	1.1	1.3
Porridge with Maple Syrup Big, EAT*	1 Serving/296g	266	3.5	90	4.2	16.0	1.2	1.1
Porridge with Maple Syrup Small, EAT*	1 Serving/195g	185	2.1	95	4.1	17.3	1.1	1.1
Smoked Salmon & Egg Hot Toasted Muffin, EAT*	1 Serving/126g	325	10.0	258	11.8	37.1	7.9	1.5
Sunshine Muffin, EAT*	1 Serving/124g	498	25.1	402	5.7	47.2	20.3	3.8
Swiss Bircher Muesli, EAT*	1 Serving/205g	246	3.1	120	4.7	21.7	1.5	2.0
Toasted Fruited Brioche without butter, EAT*	1 Serving/120g	414	13.4	345	7.3	50.2	11.2	2.2
Tomato & Jarlsberg Croissant, EAT*	1 Serving/123g	291	19.1	236	9.0	22.6	15.5	0.4
Yoghurt, Granola & Mixed Red Berries, EAT*	1 Serving/180g	306	8.8	170	5.8	26.1	4.9	2.4
Yoghurt & Mango Passionfruit, EAT*	1 Serving/124g	145	3.6	117	5.6	17.1	2.9	0.2
Yoghurt & Mixed Red Berries, EAT*	1 Serving/124g	131	3.6	106	5.6	14.1	2.9	0.3

COFFEE

	Measure INFO/WEIGHT	KCAL	FAT	KCAL	PROT	CARB	FAT	FIBRE
Cappuccino, Skimmed Milk, EAT*	1 Tall/12oz	118	4.0	33	2.4	3.4	1.1	0.0
Cappuccino, Soya Milk, EAT*	1 Tall/12oz	131	4.9	37	3.2	3.5	1.4	0.9
Cappuccino, Whole Milk, EAT*	1 Tall/12oz	168	9.1	47	2.4	3.4	2.6	0.0
Espresso, Macchiato, Skimmed Milk, EAT*	1 Espresso/4oz	8	0.3	7	0.5	0.6	0.3	0.0
Espresso, Macchiato, Soya Milk, EAT*	1 Espresso/4oz	9	0.4	8	0.6	0.7	0.3	0.2
Espresso, Macchiato, Whole Milk, EAT*	1 Espresso/4oz	11	0.6	9	0.5	0.6	0.5	0.0
Latte, Chai, Skimmed Milk, EAT*	1 Tall/12oz	305	1.0	86	3.2	17.7	0.3	0.0
Latte, Chai, Soya Milk, EAT*	1 Tall/12oz	279	5.3	79	2.4	13.9	1.5	0.5
Latte, Chai, Whole Milk, EAT*	1 Tall/12oz	408	12.9	115	3.1	17.5	3.6	0.0
Latte, Chiller, Skimmed Milk, EAT*	1 Tall/12oz	241	3.3	68	3.1	11.9	0.9	0.0
Latte, Chiller, Whole Milk, EAT*	1 Tall/12oz	412	14.8	116	1.8	17.7	4.2	0.2
Latte, Iced, Skimmed Milk, EAT*	1 Tall/12oz	95	3.2	27	1.9	2.7	0.9	0.0
Latte, Iced, Soya Milk, EAT*	1 Tall/12oz	105	3.9	30	2.5	2.8	1.1	0.7
Latte, Iced, Whole Milk, EAT*	1 Tall 12oz	135	7.3	38	1.9	2.7	2.0	0.0
Latte, Matcha, Skimmed Milk, EAT*	1 Tall/12oz	204	1.0	57	3.0	10.6	0.3	0.3
Latte, Matcha, Soya Milk, EAT*	1 Tall/12oz	201	5.8	57	3.0	7.4	1.6	0.3
Latte, Matcha, Whole Milk, EAT*	1 Tall/12oz	297	11.8	84	3.0	10.4	3.3	0.3
Latte, Skimmed Milk, EAT*	1 Tall/12oz	142	4.8	42	3.0	4.2	1.4	0.0
Latte, Soya Milk, EAT*	1 Tall/12oz	157	5.9	46	4.0	4.3	1.7	1.1
Latte, Whole Milk, EAT*	1 Tall/12oz	202	10.9	59	3.0	4.2	3.2	0.0
Matcha, Chiller, Whole Milk, EAT*	1 Tall/12oz	418	14.9	118	1.9	18.2	4.2	0.3
Mocha, Chiller, Skimmed Milk, EAT*	1 Tall/12oz	243	3.4	68	2.5	12.6	0.9	0.0
Mocha, Chiller, Whole Milk, EAT*	1 Tall/12oz	283	7.5	80	2.5	12.6	2.1	0.0
Mocha, Skimmed Milk, EAT*	1 Tall/12oz	157	5.0	44	3.0	4.8	1.4	0.0
Mocha, Soya Milk, EAT*	1 Tall/12oz	173	6.1	49	4.0	5.0	1.7	1.2
Mocha, Whole Milk, EAT*	1 Tall/12oz	219	11.4	62	3.0	4.8	3.2	0.0
White, Flat, Skimmed Milk, EAT*	1 Tall/12oz	198	0.7	58	5.8	8.5	0.2	0.0
White, Flat, Soya Milk, EAT*	1 Tall/12oz	205	12.6	60	6.3	0.2	3.7	1.0
White, Flat, Whole Milk, EAT*	1 Tall/12oz	389	20.5	114	5.8	8.2	6.0	0.0

DESSERTS

	Measure INFO/WEIGHT	KCAL	FAT	KCAL	PROT	CARB	FAT	FIBRE
Bag of Cherries, EAT*	1 Serving/125g	55	0.1	44	0.8	9.0	0.1	1.8

EAT

DESSERTS

Food	Measure INFO/WEIGHT	per Measure KCAL	per Measure FAT	KCAL	PROT	CARB	FAT	FIBRE
Banana Toffee & Pecan Cake, EAT*	1 Serving/79g	247	10.8	313	3.3	45.1	13.7	0.9
Banoffee Pie, EAT*	1 Serving/112g	395	24.1	353	3.7	36.0	21.5	1.4
Belgian Chocolate Brownie, EAT*	1 Serving/54g	227	11.3	420	4.5	50.5	20.9	3.2
Big Fruit Salad, EAT*	1 Serving/279g	120	0.3	43	0.6	10.9	0.1	1.8
Caramel Tiffen, EAT*	1 Serving/73g	351	18.9	481	3.6	60.0	25.9	0.7
Carrot Cake, EAT*	1 Serving/100g	319	20.0	319	2.8	33.1	20.0	1.6
Chilli & Herb Olives, EAT*	1 Serving/75g	99	10.1	132	0.8	1.8	13.5	3.5
Chocolate Cake, EAT*	1 Serving/63g	236	13.0	374	4.1	43.8	20.6	1.5
Chocolate Cookie, EAT*	1 Serving/90g	401	16.8	446	6.6	61.4	18.7	2.7
Chunky Chocolate Fudge, EAT*	1 Serving/116g	452	25.7	389	3.2	44.5	22.1	1.5
Coconut & Raspberry Slice, EAT*	1 Serving/75g	306	17.5	408	5.9	44.1	23.4	4.5
Fresh Fruit Salad, EAT*	1 Serving/160g	77	0.2	48	0.6	11.3	0.1	0.5
Frozen Yoghurt Brownie Sundae, EAT*	1 Serving/176g	308	6.0	175	3.6	34.1	3.4	2.0
Frozen Yoghurt Plain, EAT*	1 Serving/140g	169	0.3	121	3.5	29.0	0.2	2.0
Frozen Yoghurt with Fresh Berries, EAT*	1 Serving/200g	190	0.4	95	2.7	22.0	0.2	2.5
Grape Bag, EAT*	1 Serving/133g	80	0.1	60	0.4	15.4	0.1	1.0
Haagen Das Belgian Chocolate, EAT*	1 Serving/100g	227	18.4	227	3.9	23.8	18.4	1.7
Haagen Das Cookies & Cream, EAT*	1 Serving/100g	225	14.4	225	3.7	20.0	14.4	0.7
Haagen Das Strawberries & Cream, EAT*	1 Serving/100g	221	14.1	221	3.5	20.0	14.1	0.3
Haagen Das Vanilla, EAT*	1 Serving/100g	225	15.2	225	3.8	18.1	15.2	0.0
Honey & Chilli Nuts, EAT*	1 Serving/100g	496	31.7	496	15.9	44.4	31.7	5.6
Honey Toasted Nut & Fruit, EAT*	1 Serving/50g	227	12.8	453	11.5	44.5	25.5	5.6
Lemon Cheesecake, EAT*	1 Serving/114g	446	34.7	391	2.9	25.7	30.4	0.4
Lemon Drizzle Cake, EAT*	1 Serving/70g	232	10.8	332	3.5	44.8	15.5	0.8
Muesli Cookie, EAT*	1 Serving/90g	376	13.4	418	5.7	63.5	14.9	3.6
Nougat, EAT*	1 Serving/30g	126	2.7	420	3.7	80.5	9.1	0.5
Oat & Fruit Slice, EAT*	1 Serving/70g	284	12.5	405	5.1	56.0	17.8	4.8
Rainbow Fruit Salad, EAT*	1 Serving/141g	86	0.6	61	0.8	12.5	0.4	2.6
Summer Berries, EAT*	1 Serving/130g	48	0.3	37	0.8	6.8	0.2	3.1
Summer Berry & Elderflower Jelly, EAT*	1 Serving/130g	100	0.3	77	2.2	17.7	0.2	1.2
Toffee Waffles, EAT*	1 Serving/69g	320	12.4	463	3.5	71.7	18.0	2.2
Victoria Sponge Cake, EAT*	1 Serving/72g	166	7.9	230	2.5	30.5	10.9	0.6
Wasabi Peas, EAT*	1 Serving/38g	158	4.6	416	20.0	57.0	12.0	7.0

JUICE DRINK

Food	Measure INFO/WEIGHT	per Measure KCAL	per Measure FAT	KCAL	PROT	CARB	FAT	FIBRE
Mango & Lime, Blast, EAT*	1 Tall/12oz	253	0.3	71	0.3	17.7	0.1	0.1
Peach & Mint, Blast, EAT*	1 Tall/12oz	216	0.2	61	0.2	15.1	0.1	0.0
Wild Berry, Blast, EAT*	1 Tall/12oz	330	0.2	93	0.2	23.5	0.1	0.5

PIES

Food	Measure INFO/WEIGHT	per Measure KCAL	per Measure FAT	KCAL	PROT	CARB	FAT	FIBRE
Beef & Stilton, Pie Only, EAT*	1 Pie/270g	629	31.6	233	10.2	21.1	11.7	1.6
Beef & Stilton with Mash & Gravy, EAT*	1 Meal/560g	885	40.3	158	5.9	15.9	7.2	1.9
Cheese & Onion, Pie Only, EAT*	1 Pie/270g	724	43.5	268	8.6	21.3	16.1	2.2
Cheese & Onion with Mash & Gravy, EAT*	1 Meal/560g	980	52.6	175	5.1	16.0	9.4	2.2
Chicken & Mushroom Pie Only, EAT*	1 Pie/270g	597	29.4	221	9.3	20.5	10.9	1.8
Chicken & Mushroom with Mash & Gravy, EAT*	1 Meal/560g	851	38.6	152	5.4	15.6	6.9	2.0
Goats Cheese & Sweet Potato, Mash & Gravy, EAT*	1 Meal/560g	946	45.9	169	4.1	18.4	8.2	2.0
Goats Cheese & Sweet Potato, Pie Only, EAT*	1 Pie/270g	694	36.7	257	6.6	26.2	13.6	1.9
Steak & Ale, Pie Only, EAT*	1 Pie/270g	643	30.8	238	9.1	24.4	11.4	0.1
Steak & Ale with Mash & Gravy, EAT*	1 Meal/560g	896	39.8	160	5.3	17.5	7.1	1.1

SALADS

Food	Measure INFO/WEIGHT	per Measure KCAL	per Measure FAT	KCAL	PROT	CARB	FAT	FIBRE
Mezze Salad with Dressing, EAT*	1 Serving/306g	425	26.6	139	3.6	12.0	8.7	2.7
Mezze Salad without Dressing, EAT*	1 Serving/286g	349	20.3	122	3.8	11.0	7.1	2.9
Prawn Cocktail Side Salad, EAT*	1 Serving/163g	346	29.5	212	9.6	2.4	18.1	0.7

EAT

	Measure INFO/WEIGHT	per Measure KCAL	FAT	Nutrition Values per 100g / 100ml KCAL	PROT	CARB	FAT	FIBRE

SALADS

	Measure INFO/WEIGHT	KCAL	FAT	KCAL	PROT	CARB	FAT	FIBRE
Rainbow Superfood with Dressing, EAT*	1 Serving/310g	437	22.9	141	5.5	12.2	7.4	2.6
Rainbow Superfood without Dressing, EAT*	1 Serving/285g	339	14.5	119	5.9	11.3	5.1	2.7
Spicy Chicken Noodles less than 5% Fat, EAT*	1 Serving/288g	412	11.8	143	9.2	16.9	4.1	0.7
Spicy Crayfish Noodles New Improved, EAT*	1 Serving/299g	433	14.3	145	6.8	19.0	4.8	0.6
Spicy Thai Beef with Dressing, EAT*	1 Serving/167g	174	6.0	104	10.0	8.0	3.6	1.4
Spicy Thai Beef without Dressing, EAT*	1 Serving/142g	129	4.8	91	11.3	3.1	3.4	1.5
Summer Ham & Potato with Dressing, EAT*	1 Serving/331g	480	36.7	145	6.0	4.9	11.1	0.8
Summer Ham & Potato without Dressing, EAT*	1 Serving/303g	370	26.4	122	6.4	4.3	8.7	0.9
Tandoori Chicken, Mango & Rice, no Dressing, EAT*	1 Serving/186g	227	3.9	122	8.7	16.5	2.1	1.7
Tandoori Chicken, Mango & Rice with Dressing, EAT*	1 Serving/206g	251	5.6	122	8.3	15.6	2.7	1.6

SANDWICH

	Measure INFO/WEIGHT	KCAL	FAT	KCAL	PROT	CARB	FAT	FIBRE
Bacon, Lettuce & Tomato, EAT*	1 Pack/204g	479	25.1	235	11.1	19.9	12.3	1.7
Chicken, Avocado & Basil, EAT*	1 Pack/233g	452	24.0	194	10.3	17.9	10.3	2.7
Chicken & Bacon, EAT*	1 Pack/229g	483	23.1	211	12.2	17.7	10.1	1.6
Club, EAT*	1 Pack/296g	624	28.7	211	12.9	17.7	9.7	1.3
Crayfish, Lemon & Rocket, EAT*	1 Pack/198g	348	13.6	176	9.4	19.9	6.9	1.4
Free Range Egg Mayo & Tomato Bloomer, EAT*	1 Pack/262g	627	38.8	239	7.3	19.1	14.8	1.5
Free Range Egg Mayonnaise & Cress, EAT*	1 Pack/183g	410	20.9	224	8.7	21.6	11.4	1.8
Ham, Tomato & Mustard, EAT*	1 Pack/203g	394	17.5	194	9.8	19.3	8.6	1.6
Houmous, Avocado & Harissa, EAT*	1 Pack/228g	397	20.5	174	5.0	21.5	9.0	3.9
New York Pastrami, EAT*	1 Pack/224g	358	11.4	160	9.9	18.6	5.1	1.3
Simple Chicken Salad less than 5% Fat, EAT*	1 Pack/203g	339	8.7	167	12.1	19.2	4.3	1.7
Skipjack Tuna & Cucumber less than 5% Fat, EAT*	1 Pack/187g	305	7.1	163	10.8	21.3	3.8	1.7
Smoked Chicken, Tomato & Pesto Bloomer, EAT*	1 Pack/262g	517	21.3	197	11.2	19.0	8.1	1.4
Smoked Scottish Salmon & Soft Cheese, EAT*	1 Pack/173g	362	12.8	209	13.8	22.2	7.4	1.6
Turkey & Cranberry less than 5% Fat, EAT*	1 Pack/218g	369	8.7	169	11.1	22.4	4.0	1.5
Very Small Chicken & Bacon, EAT*	1 Pack/114g	241	11.5	211	12.2	17.7	10.1	1.6
Very Small Crayfish, Lemon & Rocket, EAT*	1 Pack/99g	174	6.8	176	9.4	19.9	6.9	1.4
Very Small Turkey & Cranberry less than 5% Fat, EAT*	1 Pack/109g	184	4.4	169	11.1	22.4	4.0	1.5

SOUP

	Measure INFO/WEIGHT	KCAL	FAT	KCAL	PROT	CARB	FAT	FIBRE
Cauliflower Cheese, EAT*	1 Serving/400ml	288	18.4	72	2.5	5.1	4.6	1.0
Chicken, Leek & Bacon Risotto with garnish, EAT*	1 Serving/370ml	359	18.9	97	4.7	8.1	5.1	0.5
Chicken, Leek & Bacon Risotto without garnish, EAT*	1 Serving/400ml	344	23.2	86	5.2	3.0	5.8	0.4
Chicken Laksa with garnish, EAT*	1 Serving/310ml	276	15.2	89	4.9	5.0	4.9	0.2
Chicken Laksa without garnish, EAT*	1 Serving/625ml	569	31.3	91	5.0	5.1	5.0	0.1
Chicken Pho, EAT*	1 Serving/786ml	291	4.7	37	3.7	3.6	0.6	0.3
Chicken Pot Pie with garnish, EAT*	1 Serving/415ml	432	22.4	104	4.8	9.0	5.4	1.0
Chicken Pot Pie with Garnish, EAT*	1 Serving/500ml	280	21.5	56	4.6	8.0	4.3	1.0
Chicken Pot Pie without garnish, EAT*	1 Serving/625ml	450	18.7	72	4.6	6.8	3.0	1.0
Chorizo & Chickpea, EAT*	1 Serving/402ml	358	16.5	89	5.0	8.1	4.1	1.6
Chunky Minestrone with Pesto with garnish, EAT*	1 Serving/319ml	201	9.3	63	1.9	6.9	2.9	1.5
Chunky Minestrone with Pesto without garnish, EAT*	1 Serving/300ml	123	1.2	41	1.8	7.3	0.4	1.5
Creamy Chicken, EAT*	1 Serving/300ml	237	14.4	79	4.2	4.5	4.8	0.6
Fire Roasted Red Pepper & Goats Cheese, EAT*	1 Serving/400ml	196	10.8	49	1.9	4.0	2.7	0.9
French Onion with garnish, EAT*	1 Serving/316ml	136	3.8	43	1.6	6.2	1.2	0.5
French Onion without garnish, EAT*	1 Serving/400ml	112	1.2	28	0.7	5.4	0.3	0.5
Garden Vegetable, EAT*	1 Serving/300ml	165	8.7	55	0.9	6.1	2.9	1.2
Gazpacho, EAT*	1 Serving/279ml	78	1.4	28	1.0	4.5	0.5	1.0
Ham, Pea & Mint with garnish, EAT*	1 Serving/321ml	202	4.5	63	4.8	7.5	1.4	1.1
Ham, Pea & Mint without garnish, EAT*	1 Serving/626ml	388	8.8	62	4.7	7.4	1.4	0.6
Hoisin Duck Gyoza Dumpling, EAT*	1 Serving/847ml	432	7.6	51	2.3	8.4	0.9	0.5
Hungarian Goulash with garnish, EAT*	1 Serving/403ml	314	8.5	78	7.7	7.2	2.1	0.8

	Measure INFO/WEIGHT	per Measure		Nutrition Values per 100g / 100ml				
		KCAL	FAT	KCAL	PROT	CARB	FAT	FIBRE
EAT								
SOUP								
Hungarian Goulash without garnish, EAT*	1 Serving/400ml	312	8.4	78	7.7	7.2	2.1	0.8
Mexican Chicken Chilli with garnish, EAT*	1 Serving/300ml	264	7.5	88	6.1	10.2	2.5	1.4
Mexican Chicken Chilli without garnish, EAT*	1 Serving/300ml	282	8.1	94	6.5	10.8	2.7	1.4
Prawn Tom Yum, EAT*	1 Serving/814ml	285	9.0	35	1.8	4.1	1.1	0.5
Slow Roasted Tomato, EAT*	1 Serving/625ml	494	37.5	79	1.3	5.0	6.0	1.2
Smokey Bacon & Lentil, EAT*	1 Serving/625ml	519	8.1	83	5.9	11.4	1.3	1.2
Spicy Moroccan Vegetable, EAT*	1 Serving/400ml	184	2.8	46	1.7	7.8	0.7	1.9
Spicy Tomato & Basil, EAT*	1 Serving/400ml	104	1.2	26	0.9	4.6	0.3	0.9
Steak & Ale Pot Pie with garnish, EAT*	1 Serving/415ml	415	13.3	100	8.3	9.2	3.2	1.2
Steak & Ale Pot Pie without garnish, EAT*	1 Serving/625ml	550	13.7	88	8.4	8.3	2.2	1.2
Summer Chicken & Garden Veg with Garnish, EAT*	1 Serving/644ml	264	3.2	41	4.5	4.5	0.5	0.7
Sweet Potato & Chilli, EAT*	1 Serving/300ml	261	13.2	87	1.3	9.6	4.4	1.7
Thai Butternut Squash, EAT*	1 Serving/300ml	168	6.6	56	1.0	6.9	2.2	1.5
Thai Green Chicken Curry with garnish, EAT*	1 Serving/340ml	306	15.0	90	4.3	6.9	4.4	0.6
Thai Green Chicken Curry without garnish, EAT*	1 Serving/300ml	246	14.1	82	4.5	3.8	4.7	0.5
Vegetarian Gyoza Dumpling, EAT*	1 Serving/798ml	431	11.2	54	2.3	7.6	1.4	0.6
Wild Forest Mushroom, EAT*	1 Serving/300ml	150	8.7	50	2.0	3.7	2.9	0.8
SUSHI								
EAT Fish without Soy Sauce, EAT*	1 Serving/289g	474	9.8	164	6.4	26.0	3.4	2.2
EAT Vegetarian without Soy Sauce, EAT*	1 Serving/165g	253	2.3	153	2.5	31.7	1.4	1.6
TEA								
Chai Latte, Soya, EAT*	1 Cup/355ml	208	6.4	59	4.2	7.1	1.8	0.0
GREGGS								
BAGUETTES								
Chicken & Sweetcorn, Greggs*	1 Baguette/235g	480	11.0	204	10.2	29.8	4.7	0.0
Chicken Club, Greggs*	1 Baguette/265g	570	16.0	215	11.7	28.9	6.0	0.0
Chicken Pesto, Greggs*	1 Baguette/214g	520	16.0	243	11.7	32.5	7.5	0.0
Chicken Tikka, Greggs*	1 Baguette/250g	490	10.5	196	10.2	29.0	4.2	0.0
Ham & Cheese, Greggs*	1 Baguette/219g	560	17.0	256	13.7	32.4	7.8	0.0
Prawn Mayonnaise, Greggs*	1 Baguette/235g	500	15.0	213	8.7	4.5	6.4	0.0
Tuna Crunch, Greggs*	1 Baguette/230g	500	11.5	217	11.1	31.1	5.0	0.0
BLOOMERS								
Chicken, Bacon & Sweetcorn, Malted Brown, Greggs*	1 Bloomer/235g	520	18.0	221	11.3	26.8	7.7	0.0
Chicken, Bacon & Sweetcorn On White, Greggs*	1 Bloomer/235g	520	18.5	221	11.1	27.0	7.9	0.0
Chicken Mango On Malted Brown, Greggs*	1 Bloomer/217g	510	18.5	235	11.3	28.3	8.5	0.0
Chicken Mango On White, Greggs*	1 Bloomer/217g	510	19.5	235	11.3	26.7	9.0	0.0
Ham, Cheese & Pickle On Malted Brown, Greggs*	1 Bloomer/228g	540	19.0	237	11.2	28.9	8.3	0.0
Ham, Cheese & Pickle On White, Greggs*	1 Bloomer/228g	510	18.0	224	11.2	27.4	7.9	0.0
Sweet Chilli Chicken On White, Greggs*	1 Bloomer/242g	430	2.5	178	11.2	30.6	1.0	0.0
Tuna Crunch On Malted Brown, Greggs*	1 Bloomer/217g	440	13.0	203	11.3	25.8	6.0	0.0
Tuna Crunch On White, Greggs*	1 Bloomer/217g	430	13.5	198	10.8	24.6	6.2	0.0
BREAKFAST ROLLS								
Breakfast Bacon & Sausage Roll, Greggs*	1 Roll/174g	510	26.0	293	12.9	27.0	14.9	0.0
Breakfast Bacon Roll, Greggs*	1 Roll/152g	460	23.5	303	14.6	26.0	15.5	0.0
Breakfast Sausage Roll, Greggs*	1 Roll/174g	490	24.5	282	10.9	28.2	14.1	0.0
CAKE								
Christmas Slice, Greggs*	1 Slice/86g	360	11.5	419	5.8	67.4	13.4	0.0
Iced, Sweet Mince Pie, Greggs*	1 Pie/63g	230	6.5	365	2.4	62.7	10.3	0.0
Sweet Mince Pie, Greggs*	1 Pie/70g	290	11.0	414	4.3	61.4	15.7	0.0
COLD DRINKS								
Capri-Sun, Greggs*	1 Serving/330ml	143	0.0	43	0.0	10.5	0.0	0.0
Coca-Cola, Greggs*	1 Serving/500ml	210	0.0	42	0.0	10.6	0.0	0.0

GREGGS

	Measure INFO/WEIGHT	per Measure KCAL	FAT	Nutrition Values per 100g / 100ml KCAL	PROT	CARB	FAT	FIBRE
COLD DRINKS								
Coca-Cola, Greggs*	1 Serving/330ml	139	0.0	42	0.0	10.6	0.0	0.0
Coke Zero, Greggs*	1 Serving/500ml	3	0.0	1	0.0	0.0	0.0	0.0
Cranberry/Raspberry Water, Greggs*	1 Serving/500ml	5	0.0	1	0.0	0.0	0.0	0.0
Diet Coca-Cola, Greggs*	1 Serving/330ml	2	0.0	1	0.0	0.0	0.0	0.0
Diet Coca-Cola, Greggs*	1 Serving/500ml	3	0.0	1	0.0	0.0	0.0	0.0
Diet Irn-Bru, Greggs*	1 Serving/330ml	2	0.0	1	0.0	0.0	0.0	0.0
Diet Irn-Bru, Greggs*	1 Serving/500ml	4	0.0	1	0.0	0.0	0.0	0.0
Dr Pepper, Greggs*	1 Serving/500ml	210	0.0	42	0.0	2.1	0.0	0.0
Fairtrade Apple Juice, Greggs*	1 Serving/500ml	220	0.0	44	0.0	11.0	0.0	0.0
Fairtrade Orange Juice, Greggs*	1 Serving/500ml	220	0.0	44	0.1	10.2	0.0	0.0
Fanta Orange, Greggs*	1 Serving/500ml	150	0.0	30	0.0	7.1	0.0	0.0
Irn-Bru, Greggs*	1 Serving/330ml	145	0.0	44	0.0	10.5	0.0	0.0
Irn-Bru, Greggs*	1 Serving/500ml	215	0.0	43	0.0	10.5	0.0	0.0
Lucozade Energy Orange, Greggs*	1 Serving/500ml	350	0.0	70	0.0	17.2	0.0	0.0
Lucozade Sport, Greggs*	1 Serving/500ml	140	0.0	28	0.0	6.4	0.0	0.0
Oasis Citrus Punch, Greggs*	1 Serving/500ml	90	0.0	18	0.0	4.1	0.0	0.0
Oasis Summer Fruits, Greggs*	1 Serving/500ml	90	0.0	18	0.0	4.2	0.0	0.0
Ribena, Greggs*	1 Serving/288ml	124	0.0	43	0.0	10.5	0.0	0.0
Ribena, Greggs*	1 Serving/500ml	215	0.0	43	0.0	10.5	0.0	0.0
Smoothie Mango & Orange, Greggs*	1 Serving/250ml	145	0.0	58	0.6	13.2	0.0	0.0
Smoothie Raspberry & Banana, Greggs*	1 Serving/250ml	135	0.0	54	0.6	12.2	0.0	0.0
Sprite, Greggs*	1 Serving/500ml	220	0.0	44	0.0	10.6	0.0	0.0
FRESHLY BAKED SAVOURIES								
Cheese & Onion Pasty, Greggs*	1 Pasty/125g	380	23.0	304	6.8	27.6	18.4	0.0
Cheese & Tomato Pizza, Greggs*	1 Pizza/111g	330	13.0	297	10.8	37.8	11.7	0.0
Chicken Bake, Greggs*	1 Bake/138g	450	29.0	326	8.3	25.4	21.0	0.0
Cornish Pasty, Greggs*	1 Pasty/190g	510	31.5	268	6.3	23.4	16.6	0.0
Pepperoni Pizza, Greggs*	1 Pizza/120g	340	12.0	283	11.7	37.5	10.0	0.0
Sausage, Bean & Cheese Melt, Greggs*	1 Bake/140g	460	28.0	329	7.5	28.6	20.0	0.0
Sausage Roll, Greggs*	1 Roll/92g	320	20.0	348	8.7	29.9	21.7	0.0
Steak Bake, Greggs*	1 Bake/139g	420	22.5	302	10.4	27.7	16.2	0.0
HOT BAGUETTES								
Chargrill Chicken Club, Greggs*	1 Baguette/167g	450	16.0	269	14.1	31.7	9.6	0.0
Chicken Fajita, Greggs*	1 Baguette/185g	440	12.0	238	12.7	32.4	6.5	0.0
Ham & Cheese, Greggs*	1 Baguette/156g	566	15.5	363	14.1	28.2	9.9	0.0
Meatball Melt, Greggs*	1 Baguette/200g	440	16.0	220	12.0	24.0	8.0	0.0
Mozzarella & Tomato, Greggs*	1 Baguette/154g	420	14.5	273	12.3	34.7	9.4	0.0
Tuna Crunch Melt, Greggs*	1 Baguette/187g	440	13.0	235	13.4	29.9	6.9	0.0
HOT DRINKS								
Espresso Double Shot, Greggs*	1 Serving/60ml	10	0.1	17	0.0	3.3	0.2	0.0
Regular Black Coffee, Greggs*	1 Serving/455ml	18	0.0	4	0.0	0.8	0.0	0.0
Regular Cappuccino No Chocolate Topping, Greggs*	1 Serving/455ml	180	5.0	40	1.7	5.6	1.1	0.0
Regular Hot Chocolate, Greggs*	1 Serving/455ml	390	10.0	86	2.3	11.3	2.2	0.0
Regular Latte, Greggs*	1 Serving/455ml	190	5.2	42	0.9	6.1	1.1	0.0
Regular White Coffee, Greggs*	1 Serving/455ml	87	2.3	19	0.4	3.3	0.5	0.0
Regular White Tea, Greggs*	1 Serving/455ml	32	1.4	7	0.4	0.5	0.3	0.0
Small Black Coffee, Greggs*	1 Serving/340ml	17	0.0	5	0.0	0.8	0.0	0.0
Small Cappuccino No Chocolate Topping, Greggs*	1 Serving/340ml	130	3.6	38	1.3	5.9	1.1	0.0
Small Hot Chocolate, Greggs*	1 Serving/340ml	280	7.7	82	2.4	11.3	2.3	0.0
Small Latte, Greggs*	1 Serving/340ml	130	3.7	38	0.5	6.6	1.1	0.0
Small White Coffee, Greggs*	1 Serving/340ml	68	2.0	20	0.3	3.5	0.6	0.0
Small White Tea, Greggs*	1 Serving/340ml	30	1.2	9	0.0	1.3	0.3	0.0

	Measure INFO/WEIGHT	per Measure KCAL	FAT	Nutrition Values per 100g / 100ml KCAL	PROT	CARB	FAT	FIBRE

GREGGS

OVAL BITES

	Measure INFO/WEIGHT	KCAL	FAT	KCAL	PROT	CARB	FAT	FIBRE
Chargrill Chicken, Greggs*	1 Pack/207g	430	17.5	208	11.6	21.7	8.4	0.0
Cheese Ploughman's, Greggs*	1 Pack/197g	450	20.5	228	9.9	24.4	10.4	0.0
Ham Salad, Greggs*	1 Pack/173g	320	9.5	185	9.0	25.1	5.5	0.0
Mexican Chicken, Greggs*	1 Pack/175g	420	15.5	240	13.1	26.3	8.9	0.0

SANDWICHES

Cheese & Tomato On Malted Brown, Greggs*	1 Pack/168g	450	18.0	268	10.4	32.1	10.7	0.0
Cheese Savoury On Seeded White, Greggs*	1 Pack/174g	510	24.0	293	11.2	27.0	13.8	0.0
Chicken Salad On Malted Brown, Greggs*	1 Pack/220g	480	17.5	218	10.9	25.2	7.9	0.0
Christmas Dinner, Greggs*	1 Pack/205g	365	18.5	178	12.2	35.4	9.0	0.0
Egg Mayonnaise On Seeded White, Greggs*	1 Pack/174g	420	17.5	241	11.2	26.7	10.1	0.0
Festive Oval Bite, Greggs*	1 Pack/160g	410	18.0	256	13.4	23.7	11.2	0.0
Tuna Mayonnaise On Malted Brown, Greggs*	1 Pack/203g	440	13.5	217	12.3	26.6	6.6	0.0

SOUP

Heinz Tomato Soup, Greggs*	1 Serving/296ml	200	7.4	68	0.9	10.5	2.5	0.0

SUB ROLL

Chicken Mayonnaise On Plain White, Greggs*	1 Roll/186g	430	15.0	231	14.5	24.5	8.1	0.0
Egg Mayonnaise & Bacon On Plain White, Greggs*	1 Roll/181g	430	16.5	238	12.1	26.2	9.1	0.0
Ham Salad On Plain White, Greggs*	1 Roll/220g	440	16.5	200	10.2	22.9	7.5	0.0
Tuna Mayonnaise On Seeded White, Greggs*	1 Roll/222g	430	14.0	194	11.5	22.7	6.3	0.0

WRAPS

Chargrill Chicken Salad, Greggs*	1 Pack/192g	360	14.5	187	9.9	19.8	7.5	0.0
Chicken Caesar, Greggs*	1 Pack/189g	410	20.0	217	11.9	18.8	10.6	0.0

ITSU

HOT DISHES

Chicken Potsu, Itsu*	1 Serving/100g	397	0.7	397	1.5	5.8	0.7	0.5
Chicken Rice Bowl, Medium, Itsu*	1 Bowl/100g	499	3.0	499	2.0	12.5	3.0	0.2
Chicken Rice Bowl, Original, Itsu*	1 Bowl/100g	623	3.5	623	2.1	12.1	3.5	0.2
Detox 7 Vegetables, Itsu*	1 Serving/100g	184	0.7	184	1.2	3.5	0.7	0.8
Prawn Rice Bowl, Medium, Itsu*	1 Bowl/100g	414	3.2	414	4.3	12.6	3.2	0.2
Prawn Rice Bowl, Original, Itsu*	1 Bowl/100g	517	3.8	517	3.6	12.2	3.8	0.3
Vegetable Dumpling Potsu, Itsu*	1 Serving/100g	80	0.7	80	2.1	2.1	0.7	0.0
Vegetable Rice Bowl, Medium, Itsu*	1 Bowl/100g	385	3.7	385	2.5	15.2	3.7	0.3
Vegetable Rice Bowl, Original, Itsu*	1 Bowl/100g	481	4.0	481	2.4	14.4	4.0	0.3

MAKI BOXES & SUSHI SANDWICHES

California Crab Sandwich, Itsu*	1 Pack/166g	393	17.6	237	6.1	6.0	10.6	1.0
Duck Hoi Sin, Itsu*	1 Box/198g	455	9.4	230	3.9	6.9	4.7	0.3
Salmon Supreme Sandwich, Itsu*	1 Pack/114g	202	13.3	177	6.6	6.2	11.7	1.2
Special Salmon Salad, Itsu*	1 Box/422g	1443	13.8	342	6.3	6.8	3.3	0.6
Spicy Salmon & Avocado, Itsu*	1 Box/172g	458	19.9	266	5.5	6.2	11.6	1.2
Tuna Sushi Sandwich, Itsu*	1 Pack/116g	179	7.9	154	6.3	7.2	6.8	0.9
Veggie Club, Itsu*	1 Pack/161g	258	9.4	160	1.5	8.8	5.8	1.2

RICE CAKES

Chocolate, Dark, Itsu*	1 Pack/50g	255	25.2	510	16.8	196.8	50.4	23.4
Chocolate, Milk, Itsu*	1 Pack/50g	249	11.4	498	6.0	65.4	22.8	3.0
Yoghurt, Itsu*	1 Pack/50g	240	9.6	480	9.0	66.0	19.2	3.0

SALAD BOXES

Hip & Healthy, Itsu*	1 Box/371g	853	9.4	230	1.7	8.6	2.5	0.9
Low Carb Salmon & Tuna Tartar, Itsu*	1 Box/137g	173	5.3	126	8.2	3.6	3.9	0.8

SNACKS

Peanut Rice Crackers, Itsu*	1 Pack/70g	239	16.1	342	17.0	55.0	23.0	0.0
Yoghurt Fruit & Goji Berries, Itsu*	1 Pack/70g	211	12.6	302	2.0	66.0	18.0	0.0

	Measure INFO/WEIGHT	per Measure KCAL	FAT	Nutrition Values per 100g / 100ml KCAL	PROT	CARB	FAT	FIBRE
ITSU								
SUSHI								
Best Of Itsu, Itsu*	1 Serving/422g	2156	34.5	511	6.3	5.7	8.2	0.8
Health & Happiness, Itsu*	1 Serving/626g	3211	30.7	513	5.3	3.6	4.9	1.5
Omega 3 Salmon Supreme, Itsu*	1 Serving/100g	396	25.4	396	29.5	81.1	25.4	0.0
Salmon & Salmon, Itsu*	1 Serving/200g	518	13.4	259	7.0	6.5	6.7	0.7
Salmon Sashimi & Salad, Itsu*	1 Serving/555g	1970	19.4	355	6.8	2.3	3.5	1.5
Salmon Sushi, Itsu*	1 Serving/100g	167	4.4	167	8.2	7.6	4.4	0.1
Sashimi, Itsu*	1 Serving/587g	2395	13.6	408	8.1	1.2	2.3	1.4
Slim Salmon, Itsu*	1 Serving/100g	375	7.7	375	7.4	7.0	7.7	0.7
Super Salmon 3 Ways, Itsu*	1 Serving/591g	2719	29.4	460	5.2	3.5	5.0	1.6
Tuna & Salmon Junior, Itsu*	1 Serving/132g	211	3.8	160	10.9	14.0	2.9	0.0
Tuna & Salmon Sushi, Itsu*	1 Serving/253g	567	5.2	224	7.6	7.2	2.1	0.2
J D WETHERSPOON								
BAGUETTE								
BLT, Malted Grain, J D Wetherspoon*	1 Baguette/399g	823	45.5	206	8.3	17.8	11.4	1.3
Chicken, BBQ & Bacon, J D Wetherspoon*	1 Baguette/342g	1271	49.0	371	20.6	37.4	14.4	2.9
Chicken, Southn Fried, Creole Mayo, J D Wetherspoon*	1 Baguette/250g	817	35.7	327	12.6	37.7	14.3	2.0
Club, Malted Grain, J D Wetherspoon*	1 Baguette/388g	768	36.8	198	9.8	18.5	9.5	1.4
Crayfish, Malted Grain, J D Wetherspoon*	1 Baguette/314g	594	25.5	189	6.1	23.2	8.1	1.7
Hot Sausage & Tomato Chutney, J D Wetherspoon*	1 Baguette/250g	839	33.4	336	14.1	40.7	13.4	3.8
Mature Cheddar & Pickle, on Malted, J D Wetherspoon*	1 Baguette/361g	696	30.0	193	7.9	21.9	8.3	1.6
Ploughmans, Lloyds, J D Wetherspoon*	1 Baguette/346g	778	34.3	225	8.6	25.5	9.9	2.2
Tuna Mayonnaise, Malted Grain, J D Wetherspoon*	1 Baguette/401g	710	31.3	177	8.9	18.1	7.8	1.3
Wiltshire Ham, J D Wetherspoon*	1 Baguette/346g	536	13.1	155	9.9	20.4	3.8	1.5
BALTI								
Chicken, Rice, Naan, & Pdoms, J D Wetherspoon*	1 Meal/650g	927	27.0	143	6.0	21.0	4.2	1.3
BEEF DINNER								
Roast, with Yorkshire Pudding & Veg, J D Wetherspoon*	1 Portion/836g	1305	63.0	156	6.1	17.7	7.5	2.3
BHAJI								
Onion, J D Wetherspoon*	1 Bhaji/30g	43	2.2	143	5.3	18.7	7.3	5.7
BIRYANI								
Chicken, without Naan, J D Wetherspoon*	1 Meal/614g	700	24.6	114	4.7	14.8	4.0	1.3
Chicken with Naan, Club Dinner, J D Wetherspoon*	1 Meal/706g	897	27.0	127	5.1	18.1	3.8	1.3
BREAD								
Garlic, Ciabatta, J D Wetherspoon*	1 Serving/142g	406	17.9	286	8.0	1.0	12.6	1.5
Naan, J D Wetherspoon*	1 Naan/90g	197	2.5	219	7.6	41.0	2.8	1.4
BREAKFAST								
Baguette, Quorn Sausage, J D Wetherspoon*	1 Baguette/285g	622	18.3	218	10.5	29.4	6.4	3.4
Blueberry Muffin, J D Wetherspoon*	1 Muffin/124g	467	25.8	374	4.7	43.2	20.7	0.4
Bran, Fruit & Nut Muffin, J D Wetherspoon*	1 Serving/145g	571	31.7	394	7.2	43.0	21.9	1.1
Children's, J D Wetherspoon*	1 Serving/341g	613	37.1	180	10.4	10.8	10.9	2.3
Chocolate Muffin, J D Wetherspoon*	1 Muffin/125g	490	28.4	392	5.0	43.6	22.7	4.8
Farmhouse, with Toast, J D Wetherspoon*	1 Serving/796g	1647	101.8	207	9.4	14.0	12.8	1.9
Morning Roll, with Bacon, J D Wetherspoon*	1 Roll/183g	546	34.6	298	11.1	21.7	18.9	1.1
Morning Roll, with Fried Egg, J D Wetherspoon*	1 Roll/143g	400	21.3	280	9.7	27.8	14.9	1.4
Morning Roll, with Quorn Sausage, J D Wetherspoon*	1 Roll/143g	367	16.1	257	10.1	29.5	11.3	2.6
Morning Roll, with Sausage, J D Wetherspoon*	1 Roll/158g	517	28.0	327	13.8	30.1	17.7	2.3
Sandwich, Sausage, Bacon & Egg, J D Wetherspoon*	1 Sandwich/357g	840	56.0	235	12.6	11.3	15.6	1.5
Scrambled Egg, on Toast, J D Wetherspoon*	1 Serving/265g	503	24.9	190	8.4	17.4	9.4	1.1
Toast & Preserves, J D Wetherspoon*	1 Serving/148g	420	15.2	284	5.7	41.8	10.3	3.2
Traditional, J D Wetherspoon*	1 Breakfast/523g	904	60.1	173	8.4	9.4	11.5	1.8
Vegetarian, J D Wetherspoon*	1 Breakfast/562g	804	47.2	143	6.7	10.2	8.4	2.1

J D WETHERSPOON

	Measure INFO/WEIGHT	per Measure KCAL	FAT	Nutrition Values per 100g / 100ml KCAL	PROT	CARB	FAT	FIBRE
BROWNIES								
Chocolate, Fudge with Ice Cream, J D Wetherspoon*	1 Portion/108g	334	18.0	309	4.5	35.6	16.2	1.5
BURGERS								
Beef, Dbl, Bacon, Cheese, & Chips, J D Wetherspoon*	1 Serving/729g	1891	119.3	259	18.1	9.4	16.4	0.4
Beef, Double, & Chips, J D Wetherspoon*	1 Serving/598g	1382	81.6	231	16.8	11.4	13.6	0.5
Beef, Double, Cheese, & Chips, J D Wetherspoon*	1 Serving/654g	1565	91.4	239	17.2	10.7	14.0	0.5
Beef, with Bacon, Cheese & Chips, J D Wetherspoon*	1 Serving/531g	1295	78.9	244	15.2	12.6	14.8	0.5
Beef, with Cheese, & Chips, J D Wetherspoon*	1 Serving/456g	966	53.8	212	13.7	13.8	11.8	0.5
Beef, with Chips, J D Wetherspoon*	1 Serving/428g	881	46.4	206	12.8	15.7	10.8	0.6
Chicken, Fillet, with Chips, J D Wetherspoon*	1 Serving/465g	727	17.1	156	10.9	16.7	3.7	0.8
Lamb, Double, Minted, with Chips, J D Wetherspoon*	1 Serving/598g	1077	47.2	180	14.6	14.1	7.9	0.9
Lamb, Minted, with Chips, J D Wetherspoon*	1 Serving/428g	712	27.8	166	11.3	17.2	6.5	0.9
Vegetable, with Chips, J D Wetherspoon*	1 Meal/488g	839	25.9	172	4.7	27.2	5.3	2.0
BUTTY								
Bacon, Brown Bloomer, J D Wetherspoon*	1 Serving/309g	869	39.6	281	23.3	18.3	12.8	1.2
Bacon & Egg, Brown Bloomer, J D Wetherspoon*	1 Serving/269g	702	31.1	261	18.2	21.0	11.6	1.4
Bacon & Egg, White Bloomer, J D Wetherspoon*	1 Serving/269g	689	32.7	256	16.7	20.9	12.2	1.2
Chip, Brown Bloomer, J D Wetherspoon*	1 Serving/204g	478	14.7	234	7.6	35.7	7.2	1.9
Chip, White Bloomer, J D Wetherspoon*	1 Serving/204g	465	16.3	228	5.6	35.6	8.0	1.6
Chip & Cheese, Brown Bloomer, J D Wetherspoon*	1 Serving/232g	593	24.4	256	9.7	31.4	10.5	1.6
Chip & Cheese, White Bloomer, J D Wetherspoon*	1 Serving/232g	580	26.0	250	7.9	31.3	11.2	1.4
Sausage & Egg, Brown Bloomer, J D Wetherspoon*	1 Serving/331g	885	49.0	267	16.8	20.8	14.8	1.3
Sausage & Egg, White Bloomer, J D Wetherspoon*	1 Serving/331g	872	50.6	263	11.4	20.7	15.3	1.1
CAKE								
Chocolate Fudge, & Ice Cream, J D Wetherspoon*	1 Serving/239g	822	47.3	344	4.0	37.6	19.8	0.4
CAULIFLOWER CHEESE								
J D Wetherspoon*	1 Portion/220g	275	15.2	125	4.1	3.6	6.9	0.8
CHEESECAKE								
Chocolate Chip, J D Wetherspoon*	1 Serving/100g	270	11.5	270	4.9	36.8	11.5	0.5
White Chocolate & Raspberry, J D Wetherspoon*	1 Serving/175g	656	36.9	375	5.6	40.8	21.1	0.9
CHICKEN								
Wings, Buffalo, J D Wetherspoon*	1 Portion/328g	636	42.9	194	15.2	4.0	13.1	0.5
Wings, Buffalo, Wild West Sharer, J D Wetherspoon*	1 Portion/1402g	2833	143.0	202	12.2	15.5	10.2	1.3
CHICKEN ALFREDO								
Pasta, with Dressed Side Salad, J D Wetherspoon*	1 Meal/576g	950	52.4	165	8.7	12.0	9.1	0.3
Pasta, with Garlic Bread, J D Wetherspoon*	1 Meal/501g	1007	47.6	201	10.8	13.0	9.5	0.3
Pasta, without Garlic Bread, J D Wetherspoon*	1 Meal/430g	804	38.7	187	11.3	15.0	9.0	0.1
CHICKEN DINNER								
Roast, Yorkshire Pudding & Veg, J D Wetherspoon*	1 Meal/993g	1529	64.0	154	10.8	14.6	6.4	2.1
CHICKEN FORESTIERRE								
J D Wetherspoon*	1 Serving/684g	626	26.0	91	7.7	8.7	3.8	1.0
CHICKEN PHAAL								
Meal, J D Wetherspoon*	1 Serving/720g	1234	46.0	171	7.5	21.0	6.4	1.6
CHICKEN ROAST								
Chips, Peas, Tomato & Mushrooms, J D Wetherspoon*	1 Meal/742g	904	38.6	122	13.0	5.6	5.2	1.2
with BBQ Sauce, J D Wetherspoon*	1 Meal/742g	948	37.5	128	11.3	9.2	5.0	0.6
with Chips & BBQ Sauce, J D Wetherspoon*	1 Meal/768g	1183	53.0	154	11.5	12.2	6.9	0.9
with Chips & Salad, J D Wetherspoon*	1 Meal/695g	983	52.1	141	13.1	5.9	7.5	0.6
with Dressed Salad & BBQ Sauce, J D Wetherspoon*	1 Meal/666g	913	46.0	137	12.2	6.0	6.9	0.9
with Jacket Potato, Salad, & Salsa, J D Wetherspoon*	1 Meal/785g	1193	57.3	152	12.2	10.2	7.3	1.3
with Piri Piri Sauce, J D Wetherspoon*	1 Serving/994g	994	47.1	100	8.4	5.8	4.7	0.8
CHICKEN VINDALOO								
J D Wetherspoon*	1 Meal/500g	704	18.9	141	6.4	21.0	3.8	1.3

J D WETHERSPOON

	Measure INFO/WEIGHT	per Measure		Nutrition Values per 100g / 100ml				
		KCAL	FAT	KCAL	PROT	CARB	FAT	FIBRE
CHILLI								
5 Bean, Yellow Rice & Tortilla Chips, J D Wetherspoon*	1 Portion/390g	511	9.0	131	3.6	24.0	2.3	1.7
Con Carne, Rice, & Tortilla Chips, J D Wetherspoon*	1 Serving/585g	744	20.0	127	6.5	17.8	3.4	1.6
CHIPS								
Bowl, J D Wetherspoon*	1 Serving/300g	750	30.4	250	3.5	36.5	10.1	2.9
with Cheese, J D Wetherspoon*	1 Serving/501g	1002	51.6	200	5.2	21.9	10.3	1.8
with Roast Gravy, J D Wetherspoon*	1 Serving/400g	392	12.4	98	2.5	17.6	3.1	0.0
CHUTNEY								
Mango, J D Wetherspoon*	1 Serving/25g	47	0.2	188	0.4	44.8	0.8	0.4
CIABATTA								
BBQ Chicken & Bacon Melt, J D Wetherspoon*	1 Ciabatta/333g	716	33.6	215	11.3	20.4	10.1	1.8
BLT, J D Wetherspoon*	1 Ciabatta/390g	789	47.3	202	8.2	15.4	12.1	1.5
Club, J D Wetherspoon*	1 Ciabatta/378g	734	38.6	194	9.7	16.1	10.2	1.6
Crayfish, J D Wetherspoon*	1 Ciabatta/305g	561	27.4	184	5.8	20.3	9.0	1.9
Mature Cheddar Cheese & Pickle, J D Wetherspoon*	1 Ciabatta/350g	662	31.5	189	7.8	19.4	9.0	1.7
Tuna Mayonnaise, J D Wetherspoon*	1 Ciabatta/391g	676	32.8	173	8.8	15.8	8.4	1.5
Wiltshire Ham, J D Wetherspoon*	1 Ciabatta/335g	503	14.8	150	9.8	17.7	4.4	1.7
CRUMBLE								
Apple, Pear, & Rasp Ice Cream, J D Wetherspoon*	1 Serving/300g	579	24.0	193	2.6	27.0	8.1	2.1
Apple, Pear, & Raspberry & Custard, J D Wetherspoon*	1 Serving/372g	648	24.0	174	2.5	26.3	6.4	0.0
CURRY								
Beef, Rendang, with Naan, J D Wetherspoon*	1 Meal/706g	1144	41.0	162	6.8	20.1	5.8	1.1
Beef, Rendang, without Naan, J D Wetherspoon*	1 Meal/615g	947	38.0	154	6.7	17.0	6.2	1.0
Goan, Vegetable, without Naan, J D Wetherspoon*	1 Meal/748g	1017	41.9	136	3.1	18.3	5.6	1.3
Kashmiri, Lamb, with Naan, J D Wetherspoon*	1 Meal/704g	1021	33.1	145	7.2	19.5	4.7	1.2
Kashmiri, Lamb, without Naan, J D Wetherspoon*	1 Meal/615g	824	30.7	134	7.1	16.3	5.0	1.1
Kerala, Fish, with Naan, J D Wetherspoon*	1 Meal/706g	1066	36.0	151	7.0	20.0	5.1	1.0
Kerala, Fish, without Naan, J D Wetherspoon*	1 Meal/616g	869	33.3	141	6.9	16.9	5.4	0.9
Mushroom Dopiaza, No Naan, J D Wetherspoon*	1 Meal/617g	580	14.0	94	2.6	16.7	2.3	1.4
Mushroom Dopiaza, with Naan, J D Wetherspoon*	1 Meal/719g	899	24.5	125	3.5	21.5	3.4	1.5
Royal Thali, with Naan, J D Wetherspoon*	1 Meal/948g	1336	48.3	141	7.1	16.8	5.1	1.3
Thai, Green Chicken, without Naan, J D Wetherspoon*	1 Meal/617g	1037	46.9	168	7.5	17.6	7.6	0.5
Vegetable, Goan, with Naan Bread, J D Wetherspoon*	1 Meal/707g	1032	36.8	146	3.6	21.2	5.2	1.3
Vegetarian, Thali, with Naan, J D Wetherspoon*	1 Meal/950g	1320	42.7	139	5.3	20.3	4.5	2.4
DHANSAK								
Lamb, Meal, J D Wetherspoon*	1 Meal/720g	983	26.1	137	7.2	19.6	3.6	0.8
FISH & CHIPS								
Haddock, J D Wetherspoon*	1 Meal/496g	806	40.7	162	7.2	14.4	8.2	2.4
Plaice, Breaded, & Peas, J D Wetherspoon*	1 Serving/460g	550	15.6	120	6.8	15.0	3.4	1.7
Traditional, J D Wetherspoon*	1 Serving/495g	804	40.6	162	7.2	14.4	8.2	2.4
FISH CAKES								
Salmon & Lime, with Tartare Sauce, J D Wetherspoon*	1 Serving/355g	569	31.3	160	5.8	14.5	8.8	1.0
GAMMON								
Egg, Jacket Pot, Tom & Mroom, J D Wetherspoon*	1 Meal/660g	963	39.0	146	10.8	13.5	5.9	1.3
Egg, Jacket Potato & Dressed Salad, J D Wetherspoon*	1 Meal/707g	1040	45.0	147	10.1	13.1	6.4	1.3
Pineapple, Chips & Dressed, J D Wetherspoon*	1 Meal/654g	830	41.8	127	9.3	9.3	6.4	0.3
Pineapple, Jacket, Peas & Mrooms, J D Wetherspoon*	1 Meal/763g	931	34.0	122	8.7	12.8	4.4	1.3
Pineapple, Jacket Spud & Salad, J D Wetherspoon*	1 Meal/697g	767	36.0	110	8.8	8.3	5.1	0.4
Steak, 8oz, Eggs, Chips & Pineapple, J D Wetherspoon*	1 Meal/609g	1036	51.8	170	13.4	10.2	8.5	0.8
Steak, Egg, Chips & Side Salad, J D Wetherspoon*	1 Meal/593g	801	41.5	135	10.2	9.0	7.0	0.3
GAMMON &								
Chips, Peas, Tomato, & Egg, J D Wetherspoon*	1 Meal/564g	844	41.2	150	15.0	6.7	7.3	1.3
Chips, Peas, Tomato, & Pineapple, J D Wetherspoon*	1 Meal/575g	799	36.2	139	13.6	7.8	6.3	1.4

J D WETHERSPOON

	Measure INFO/WEIGHT	per Measure KCAL	FAT	Nutrition Values per 100g / 100ml KCAL	PROT	CARB	FAT	FIBRE
HAGGIS								
with Neeps & Tatties, J D Wetherspoon*	1 Meal/682g	982	52.5	144	4.6	15.0	7.7	1.9
HAM								
& Eggs, J D Wetherspoon*	1 Serving/396g	253	12.7	64	4.9	3.5	3.2	0.0
ICE CREAM								
Bombe, Mint Chocolate, J D Wetherspoon*	1 Portion/135g	300	13.4	222	2.6	30.6	9.9	0.8
Chocolate, Bomb, J D Wetherspoon*	1 Portion/100g	259	13.4	259	5.9	34.3	13.4	5.4
Neopolitan, Movenpick, J D Wetherspoon*	1 Bowl/100g	181	9.6	181	3.0	20.0	9.6	0.0
JALFREZI								
Chicken, Meal, with Naan Bread, J D Wetherspoon*	1 Meal/705g	916	19.7	130	6.8	19.9	2.8	1.3
Chicken, without Naan Bread, J D Wetherspoon*	1 Meal/614g	719	17.2	117	6.7	16.9	2.8	1.3
KORMA								
Chicken, Meal, without Naan, J D Wetherspoon*	1 Meal/617g	944	38.2	153	6.4	17.0	6.2	0.8
Chicken, with Naan, J D Wetherspoon*	1 Meal/704g	1141	40.8	162	6.6	20.1	5.8	0.9
LAMB								
Braised, Mashed Potato & Veg, J D Wetherspoon*	1 Meal/844g	1114	67.0	132	8.9	6.8	7.9	1.0
LASAGNE								
Al Forno with Dressed Side Salad, J D Wetherspoon*	1 Meal/658g	823	40.8	125	5.5	11.4	6.2	0.8
MASALA								
Chicken, Hot, with Naan, J D Wetherspoon*	1 Meal/707g	1033	31.1	146	6.9	20.1	4.4	1.2
Chicken, Hot, without Naan, J D Wetherspoon*	1 Meal/614g	835	28.2	136	6.8	17.1	4.6	1.1
Prawn, Sri Lankan, with Naan, J D Wetherspoon*	1 Meal/708g	1027	36.0	145	5.7	19.7	5.1	0.8
Prawn, Sri Lankan, without Naan, J D Wetherspoon*	1 Meal/617g	827	33.0	134	5.4	16.6	5.4	1.0
Vegetable, Tandoori, Meal, J D Wetherspoon*	1 Serving/720g	1020	36.0	142	3.4	20.7	5.0	2.3
MEATBALLS								
with Linguine Pasta, J D Wetherspoon*	1 Serving/511g	614	24.0	120	6.3	13.1	4.7	1.9
MELT								
BBQ Chicken, & Chips, & Salad, J D Wetherspoon*	1 Serving/643g	849	42.4	132	10.4	8.2	6.6	0.4
MIXED GRILL								
with Chips, & Dressed Side Salad, J D Wetherspoon*	1 Serving/784g	1324	87.0	169	12.0	5.6	11.1	0.3
MOUSSAKA								
Vegetarian, J D Wetherspoon*	1 Serving/555g	582	38.8	105	2.7	7.6	7.0	2.7
NACHOS								
J D Wetherspoon*	1 Serving/366g	1139	67.3	311	7.0	29.2	18.4	3.2
with Chilli Con Carne, J D Wetherspoon*	1 Meal/570g	1505	88.9	264	8.6	22.2	15.6	1.8
with Fajita Chicken, J D Wetherspoon*	1 Serving/486g	1225	70.5	252	5.7	24.7	14.5	2.9
with Five Bean Chilli, J D Wetherspoon*	1 Serving/571g	1399	81.1	245	7.3	21.8	14.2	2.7
NOODLES								
Thai, with Chicken, J D Wetherspoon*	1 Serving/100g	516	20.8	516	20.8	39.0	20.8	4.4
PANINI								
BBQ Chicken & Bacon, Melt, J D Wetherspoon*	1 Panini/337g	650	27.6	193	9.9	19.9	8.2	1.7
Cheese, Tomato, & Bacon, J D Wetherspoon*	1 Panini/261g	630	29.0	241	14.3	21.6	11.1	0.8
Cheese & Tuna, J D Wetherspoon*	1 Panini/221g	551	22.3	249	15.5	24.9	10.1	0.7
Club, J D Wetherspoon*	1 Panini/378g	734	38.6	194	9.7	16.1	10.2	1.6
Fajita Chicken, J D Wetherspoon*	1 Panini/235g	359	6.1	153	4.4	28.8	2.6	1.7
Mature, Cheddar Cheese & Tomato, J D Wetherspoon*	1 Panini/330g	750	27.1	227	10.4	18.0	8.2	1.7
Pepperoni & Mozzarella, J D Wetherspoon*	1 Panini/205g	617	33.4	301	11.6	27.5	16.3	1.0
Tomato, Mozzarella & Green Pesto, J D Wetherspoon*	1 Panini/245g	502	22.9	205	7.3	23.0	9.3	1.4
Wiltshire Ham & Mature Cheese, J D Wetherspoon*	1 Panini/354g	868	50.0	245	12.7	16.7	14.1	1.5
PASTA								
5 Cheese & Bacon, Garlic Ciabatta, J D Wetherspoon*	1 Meal/469g	563	23.0	120	3.6	9.7	5.0	1.5
5 Cheese & Bacon, with Side Salad, J D Wetherspoon*	1 Meal/544g	506	29.0	93	2.3	9.1	5.3	1.3
Spirale, Vegetable, Sundried Tomato, J D Wetherspoon*	1 Meal/500g	600	2.0	120	3.6	15.2	0.5	0.7

	Measure INFO/WEIGHT	per Measure KCAL	FAT	Nutrition Values per 100g / 100ml KCAL	PROT	CARB	FAT	FIBRE

J D WETHERSPOON

PASTA BAKE

	Measure	KCAL	FAT	KCAL	PROT	CARB	FAT	FIBRE
Mediterranean, J D Wetherspoon*	1 Serving/450g	577	22.1	128	4.3	16.4	4.9	0.9

PEAS

& Ham, with Poppy Seed Bloomer, J D Wetherspoon*	1 Portion/456g	474	17.8	104	4.4	12.5	3.9	2.0

PIE

Aberdeen Angus, Chips, & Veg, J D Wetherspoon*	1 Serving/780g	1356	86.6	174	5.5	15.7	11.1	0.9
Beef & Ale, Chips, Veg & Gravy, J D Wetherspoon*	1 Meal/850g	1258	68.0	148	4.0	14.9	8.0	1.0
Cottage, with Chips & Peas, J D Wetherspoon*	1 Meal/682g	846	33.4	124	3.7	15.6	4.9	1.9
Fish, Carrot & Broccoli, Herb Butter, J D Wetherspoon*	1 Serving/550g	612	37.9	111	4.6	9.7	6.9	2.4
Scotch, J D Wetherspoon*	1 Serving/145g	302	15.4	208	13.1	7.8	10.6	0.9
Scotch, with Chips & Beans, J D Wetherspoon*	1 Serving/435g	603	22.2	139	6.8	14.9	5.1	1.5

PLATTER

Italian Style, J D Wetherspoon*	1 Platter/1020g	1985	75.5	195	10.4	22.9	7.4	0.6
Mexican, Chilli, Sour Cream, J D Wetherspoon*	1 Platter/1062g	2560	141.2	241	7.5	22.6	13.3	2.8
Mexican, with Five Bean Chilli, J D Wetherspoon*	1 Platter/1002g	2358	123.2	235	6.2	25.6	12.3	3.6
Western, J D Wetherspoon*	1 Platter/1454g	2973	168.7	204	16.9	9.1	11.6	0.4

POPPADOMS

& Dips, J D Wetherspoon*	1 Serving/134g	425	10.9	317	4.6	28.4	8.1	2.5
J D Wetherspoon*	1 Poppadom/12g	35	0.2	281	6.7	45.0	1.9	10.0

PORK DINNER

Roast, with Yorkshires & Vegetables, J D Wetherspoon*	1 Meal/1022g	1543	63.0	151	10.4	14.6	6.2	2.1

POTATO BOMBAY

J D Wetherspoon*	1 Serving/300g	285	14.7	95	1.8	10.8	4.9	2.5

POTATO SKINS

Cheese & Bacon, Loaded, J D Wetherspoon*	1 Serving/439g	949	58.4	216	8.9	15.2	13.3	1.5
Cheese & Red Onion, Loaded, J D Wetherspoon*	1 Serving/414g	835	51.3	202	6.0	16.5	12.4	1.6
Chilli Con Carne, Loaded, J D Wetherspoon*	1 Serving/503g	735	35.7	146	5.0	15.7	7.1	1.9

POTATO WEDGES

Spicy, J D Wetherspoon*	1 Serving/270g	434	15.7	161	2.2	27.7	5.8	1.8
Spicy, with Sour Cream, J D Wetherspoon*	1 Serving/330g	558	27.4	169	2.3	23.4	8.3	1.5

POTATOES

Baked, Crayfish, with M Rose Sauce, J D Wetherspoon*	1 Meal/524g	796	41.0	152	3.5	18.2	7.8	1.7
Baked, Jacket, Coleslaw, J D Wetherspoon*	1 Meal/596g	918	48.9	154	2.3	17.1	8.2	1.8
Jacket, Baked Beans, & Salad, J D Wetherspoon*	1 Meal/575g	725	25.0	126	3.3	19.6	4.3	2.4
Jacket, Chilli, Sour Cream & Salad, J D Wetherspoon*	1 Meal/615g	775	30.0	126	4.4	17.0	4.9	1.9
Jacket, Mature, Cheddar Cheese, J D Wetherspoon*	1 Meal/496g	858	45.0	173	5.6	18.7	9.0	1.8
Jacket, with 5 Bean Chilli, & Salad, J D Wetherspoon*	1 Meal/597g	705	26.0	118	3.0	17.9	4.3	2.4
Jacket, with Tuna Mayo, & Salad, J D Wetherspoon*	1 Meal/645g	845	40.0	131	5.4	14.6	6.1	1.3
Mashed, Creamy, J D Wetherspoon*	1 Portion/279g	349	21.2	125	1.5	15.0	7.6	1.1
Roast, J D Wetherspoon*	1 Portion/200g	290	9.4	145	2.5	23.0	4.7	2.3

RIBS

Double, J D Wetherspoon*	1 Serving/350g	767	40.9	219	16.7	11.9	11.7	0.4
Double, with Chips, J D Wetherspoon*	1 Serving/500g	949	46.5	190	12.5	14.9	9.3	0.3
Double, with Jacket Potato, J D Wetherspoon*	1 Serving/590g	1159	50.7	196	11.4	19.2	8.6	1.3

RICE

Basmati, Yellow, J D Wetherspoon*	1 Portion/200g	286	1.2	143	3.4	31.1	0.6	0.2
J D Wetherspoon*	1 Serving/200g	274	0.4	137	2.9	30.9	0.2	0.2

ROGAN JOSH

Lamb, Meal, without Naan, J D Wetherspoon*	1 Meal/617g	820	27.7	133	7.1	17.0	4.5	1.0
Lamb, with Naan, J D Wetherspoon*	1 Meal/706g	1017	30.4	144	7.2	20.1	4.3	1.1

SALAD

Caesar, Chicken, J D Wetherspoon*	1 Meal/230g	507	36.4	220	14.3	5.1	15.8	0.8
Caesar, J D Wetherspoon*	1 Meal/211g	448	38.0	212	6.8	5.8	18.0	1.1

J D WETHERSPOON

	Measure INFO/WEIGHT	per Measure KCAL	FAT	Nutrition Values per 100g / 100ml KCAL	PROT	CARB	FAT	FIBRE
SALAD								
Chicken, BBQ, Croutons & Dressing, J D Wetherspoon*	1 Portion/350g	315	8.4	90	9.4	7.5	2.4	0.8
Chicken & Bacon, Warm, J D Wetherspoon*	1 Meal/426g	600	41.3	141	9.8	3.8	9.7	0.6
Crayfish, J D Wetherspoon*	1 Meal/317g	247	18.0	78	4.4	2.7	5.7	0.6
Side, No Dressing, J D Wetherspoon*	1 Salad/195g	125	4.5	64	2.0	8.9	2.3	1.1
Side, with Dressing, J D Wetherspoon*	1 Salad/215g	263	19.6	122	2.2	8.1	9.1	1.0
Side, with Dressing & Croutons, J D Wetherspoon*	1 Portion/140g	221	18.3	158	2.1	8.6	13.1	1.1
Side, with Dressing & No Croutons, J D Wetherspoon*	1 Portion/129g	145	14.0	112	1.0	3.2	10.8	0.9
Side, without Croutons, J D Wetherspoon*	1 Portion/111g	157	10.8	141	9.8	3.8	9.7	0.6
Thai Noodle, J D Wetherspoon*	1 Portion/394g	433	21.3	110	2.7	12.7	5.4	1.4
Thai Noodle, with Chicken, J D Wetherspoon*	1 Meal/554g	637	27.7	115	9.2	9.6	5.0	1.4
Tiger Prawn, Dressing, & Chilli Jam, J D Wetherspoon*	1 Portion/340g	500	33.0	147	4.7	10.1	9.7	0.9
Tuna, with Eggs, Olives, & Croutons, J D Wetherspoon*	1 Portion/395g	679	51.7	172	10.3	3.2	13.1	0.7
SALMON								
Fillet, Watercress, Chips & Salad, J D Wetherspoon*	1 Meal/585g	912	56.0	156	6.7	10.7	9.6	1.1
Fillet, Watercress, Jacket & Salad, J D Wetherspoon*	1 Meal/655g	995	51.0	152	6.8	14.5	7.8	1.4
SAMOSAS								
Lamb, J D Wetherspoon*	1 Samosa/90g	160	3.8	178	7.9	29.9	4.2	3.9
Vegetable, J D Wetherspoon*	1 Samosa/50g	92	3.1	184	5.4	28.4	6.2	2.2
SANDWICH								
Beef, Hot, Brown Bloomer, J D Wetherspoon*	1 Sandwich/299g	618	27.2	207	11.4	19.9	9.1	1.3
Beef, Hot, Poppy Seed Bloomer, J D Wetherspoon*	1 Sandwich/299g	605	28.7	202	10.0	19.8	9.6	1.1
BLT, Brown Bloomer, J D Wetherspoon*	1 Sandwich/404g	885	39.6	219	18.0	14.6	9.8	1.2
BLT, White Bloomer, J D Wetherspoon*	1 Sandwich/404g	872	32.7	216	17.0	14.6	8.1	1.0
Cheddar, & Pickle, Brown Bloomer, J D Wetherspoon*	1 Sandwich/260g	665	31.9	256	11.0	25.4	12.3	1.9
Cheddar, & Pickle, White Bloomer, J D Wetherspoon*	1 Sandwich/260g	638	32.8	245	9.2	0.0	12.6	1.5
Chicken, Cheese, Bacon, Mayo, J D Wetherspoon*	1 Sandwich/312g	710	39.6	228	13.5	18.8	12.7	1.2
Chicken, Half Fat Mayo, Brown, Hot, J D Wetherspoon*	1 Sandwich/289g	628	28.3	217	11.8	20.7	9.8	1.7
Chicken, Half Fat Mayo, White, Hot, J D Wetherspoon*	1 Sandwich/289g	615	29.8	213	11.3	20.6	10.3	1.5
Egg Mayonnaise, Brown Bloomer, J D Wetherspoon*	1 Sandwich/295g	704	39.5	239	10.1	19.7	13.4	1.3
Egg Mayonnaise, White Bloomer, J D Wetherspoon*	1 Sandwich/295g	692	41.0	235	8.7	19.6	13.9	1.1
Ham, & Tomato, Brown Bloomer, J D Wetherspoon*	1 Sandwich/239g	514	17.2	215	11.4	24.4	7.2	1.8
Ham, & Tomato, White Bloomer, J D Wetherspoon*	1 Sandwich/239g	501	18.6	210	9.7	24.4	7.8	1.5
Prawn Mayonnaise, Brown Bloomer, J D Wetherspoon*	1 Sandwich/244g	579	26.6	237	11.0	23.8	10.9	1.6
Prawn Mayonnaise, White Bloomer, J D Wetherspoon*	1 Sandwich/244g	567	28.3	232	9.3	23.7	11.6	1.4
Salmon, Lemon Mayo, Bloomer, J D Wetherspoon*	1 Sandwich/229g	637	33.7	278	11.4	25.4	14.7	1.7
Salmon, Lemon Mayo, Bloomer, J D Wetherspoon*	1 Sandwich/229g	625	35.0	273	9.6	25.2	15.4	1.4
Tuna Mayo, Half Fat Mayo, White, J D Wetherspoon*	1 Sandwich/389g	828	47.1	213	11.2	15.6	12.1	1.0
SAUSAGE & MASH								
with Red Wine Gravy, J D Wetherspoon*	1 Portion/677g	887	50.8	131	6.0	10.2	7.5	1.8
SAUSAGES WITH								
Bacon & Egg, J D Wetherspoon*	1 Serving/582g	1040	57.6	179	11.7	11.3	9.9	1.0
Chips & Beans, J D Wetherspoon*	1 Meal/554g	897	42.6	162	7.3	16.4	7.7	2.3
SCAMPI								
Chips, Peas, Tartare Sauce, J D Wetherspoon*	1 Serving/561g	987	43.7	176	5.2	19.9	7.8	2.3
SORBET								
Mango & Passionfruit, J D Wetherspoon*	1 Serving/135g	115	0.1	85	0.2	20.0	0.1	0.2
SOUP								
Leek & Potato, & Malted Baguette, J D Wetherspoon*	1 Bowl/490g	490	9.0	100	3.2	17.9	1.8	1.7
Leek & Potato, No Bread & Butter, J D Wetherspoon*	1 Bowl/420	105	0.8	25	0.9	5.1	0.2	1.0
Mushroom, No Bread, J D Wetherspoon*	1 Serving/305g	252	16.5	83	2.8	5.5	5.4	0.4
Mushroom, with Brown Bloomer, J D Wetherspoon*	1 Serving/429g	561	23.7	131	3.4	16.0	5.5	1.2
Mushroom, with White Bloomer, J D Wetherspoon*	1 Serving/429g	549	25.2	128	3.4	15.9	5.9	1.1

	Measure INFO/WEIGHT	per Measure KCAL	FAT	Nutrition Values per 100g / 100ml KCAL	PROT	CARB	FAT	FIBRE

J D WETHERSPOON

SOUP

	Measure	KCAL	FAT	KCAL	PROT	CARB	FAT	FIBRE
Tomato, No Bread, J D Wetherspoon*	1 Serving/305g	198	14.0	65	0.9	3.9	4.6	0.6
Tomato, with Brown Bloomer, J D Wetherspoon*	1 Serving/429g	576	25.8	134	3.7	15.7	6.0	1.3
Tomato, with White Bloomer, J D Wetherspoon*	1 Serving/429g	563	27.3	131	2.8	15.6	6.4	1.2
Tomato & Basil, Organic, & Baguette, J D Wetherspoon*	1 Bowl/491g	584	23.0	119	2.9	15.8	4.7	1.2
Tomato & Basil, Organic, J D Wetherspoon*	1 Serving/491g	584	23.1	119	2.9	15.8	4.7	1.2
Tomato & Basil, Organic, No Bread, J D Wetherspoon*	1 Bowl/350g	199	15.0	57	0.7	3.0	4.3	0.6
Tomato & Basil, Organic, with Bread, J D Wetherspoon*	1 Bowl/450g	396	9.0	88	1.0	6.0	1.9	1.1

SPONGE PUDDING

Treacle, with Hot Custard, J D Wetherspoon*	1 Serving/515g	1267	71.1	246	2.3	41.8	13.8	0.2

SQUASH

Butternut, Roast Dinner, J D Wetherspoon*	1 Meal/847g	1211	55.9	143	4.9	17.5	6.6	2.9

STEAK

Ribeye, 8oz, Chips & Side Salad, J D Wetherspoon*	1 Meal/562g	1006	71.9	179	8.0	8.9	12.8	0.3
Ribeye, Chips, Peas & Mushroom, J D Wetherspoon*	1 Portion/531g	945	64.0	178	9.3	9.3	12.0	0.3
Ribeye, Jacket, Peas & Mushroom, J D Wetherspoon*	1 Meal/674g	1253	154.0	186	7.8	11.5	22.8	1.9
Ribeye, Jacket & Dressed Salad, J D Wetherspoon*	1 Meal/620g	850	43.0	137	8.2	10.1	7.0	1.1
Ribeye, Prawn Skew, Chips, & Salad, J D Wetherspoon*	1 Meal/714g	1093	56.0	153	11.0	7.7	7.9	0.3
Ribeye, Prawn Skew, Chips, Peas, J D Wetherspoon*	1 Meal/768g	1083	51.0	141	11.0	7.0	6.6	0.9
Ribeye, Prawn Skew, Jacket, Peas, J D Wetherspoon*	1 Meal/779g	1169	60.0	150	10.8	6.9	7.7	0.9
Ribeye, Prawn Skew, Jacket, Salad, J D Wetherspoon*	1 Meal/727g	1178	57.0	162	10.8	7.7	7.9	0.3
Rump, 16oz, Chips, Peas, Tomato, J D Wetherspoon*	1 Meal/759g	1268	71.0	167	14.9	6.5	9.3	0.2
Rump, 16oz, Chips & Salad, J D Wetherspoon*	1 Meal/787g	1283	72.0	163	14.3	6.3	9.1	0.2
Rump, 16oz, Jacket, Peas, Tomato, J D Wetherspoon*	1 Meal/839g	1451	70.0	173	14.1	11.0	8.3	1.1
Rump, 16oz, Jacket & Salad, J D Wetherspoon*	1 Meal/867g	1466	71.0	169	13.6	10.7	8.2	1.0
T-Bone, 12oz, Chips, & Salad, J D Wetherspoon*	1 Meal/673g	1313	98.0	195	9.4	7.4	14.5	0.2
T-Bone, 12oz, Jacket, Peas, Tomato, J D Wetherspoon*	1 Meal/722g	1481	95.0	205	9.5	12.7	13.2	1.2
T-Bone, 12oz, Jacket & Salad, J D Wetherspoon*	1 Meal/756g	1496	97.0	198	9.1	12.3	12.8	1.2

STEAK &

Breaded Scampi, Chips, & Peas, J D Wetherspoon*	1 Meal/816g	1369	72.6	168	10.1	11.3	8.9	1.2

STEAK WITH

Chips, & Dressed Side Salad, Rump, J D Wetherspoon*	1 Meal/634g	922	60.2	145	9.5	6.3	9.5	0.3
Chips, & Dressed Side Salad, Sirloin, J D Wetherspoon*	1 Meal/577g	979	73.3	170	7.6	6.9	12.7	0.3
Jacket, Salad, & Salsa, Rump, J D Wetherspoon*	1 Meal/724g	1132	64.4	156	9.0	10.9	8.9	1.1
Jacket, Salad, & Salsa, Sirloin, J D Wetherspoon*	1 Meal/667g	1189	77.4	178	7.3	11.8	11.6	1.2

STEW

Irish, J D Wetherspoon*	1 Portion/600g	516	23.4	86	7.3	5.6	3.9	0.9

STUFFING BALLS

Sage & Onion, J D Wetherspoon*	1 Portion/70g	137	1.1	196	6.6	32.3	1.6	3.6

TART

Apple, with Ice Cream, J D Wetherspoon*	1 Portion/235g	464	20.0	197	1.6	29.8	8.5	0.4

TIKKA

Mixed Grill, Starter, J D Wetherspoon*	1 Portion/374g	460	23.9	123	13.4	3.2	6.4	0.9

TIKKA MASALA

Chicken, Rice & No Naan Bread, J D Wetherspoon*	1 Meal/614g	872	33.2	142	6.9	16.9	5.4	1.2

WAFFLES

Belgian, Ice Cream & Maple Syrup, J D Wetherspoon*	1 Serving/395g	934	33.6	236	13.8	28.4	8.5	0.8

WRAP

Caesar Wetherwrap, J D Wetherspoon*	1 Wrap/159g	478	32.6	301	7.0	23.1	20.5	1.5
Caesar Wetherwrap, Tortillas & Salsa, J D Wetherspoon*	1 Serving/244g	624	38.8	256	5.7	23.4	15.9	1.6
Caesar Wrap & Potato Wedges, J D Wetherspoon*	1 Serving/289g	687	40.2	238	5.0	25.2	13.9	1.6
Chicken, Cheese, & Potato Wedges, J D Wetherspoon*	1 Serving/401g	762	34.1	190	8.0	22.2	8.5	1.5
Chicken, Cheese, Tortilla Chips, J D Wetherspoon*	1 Serving/356g	699	32.4	196	8.8	20.6	9.1	1.5

J D WETHERSPOON

	Measure INFO/WEIGHT	per Measure KCAL	FAT	Nutrition Values per 100g / 100ml KCAL	PROT	CARB	FAT	FIBRE
WRAP								
Chicken, Guacamole, Tortillas, Salsa, J D Wetherspoon*	1 Serving/273g	474	16.9	174	8.2	21.9	6.2	2.0
Chicken, Guacamole, Wedges, J D Wetherspoon*	1 Serving/318g	537	18.4	169	7.2	23.7	5.8	2.0
Chicken, Southern & Creole Mayo, J D Wetherspoon*	1 Wrap/320g	553	30.0	173	7.1	16.3	9.4	1.4
Chicken, with Chicken Breast, J D Wetherspoon*	1 Wrap/292g	450	21.6	154	9.4	14.5	7.4	1.5
Chicken, with Potato Wedges, J D Wetherspoon*	1 Serving/373g	647	24.2	173	6.7	23.9	6.5	1.7
Chicken, with Tortilla Chips & Salsa, J D Wetherspoon*	1 Serving/328g	584	23.0	178	7.5	22.3	7.0	1.6
Chicken & Cheese, J D Wetherspoon*	1 Wrap/271g	553	26.3	204	10.7	19.6	9.7	1.4
Club, J D Wetherspoon*	1 Wrap/286g	711	40.0	249	12.1	19.2	14.1	1.0
Club Wrap, Tortilla Chips, Salsa, J D Wetherspoon*	1 Serving/336g	759	42.0	226	12.2	17.1	12.5	1.1
Club Wrap, with Potato Wedges, J D Wetherspoon*	1 Serving/381g	822	43.1	216	10.9	19.2	11.3	1.2
Fajita Chicken, J D Wetherspoon*	1 Wrap/228g	345	14.1	151	3.8	21.2	6.2	1.9
Fajita Chicken, Tortilla Chips, Salsa, J D Wetherspoon*	1 Serving/313g	491	20.3	157	3.5	21.9	6.5	1.9
Fajita Chicken, with Potato Wedges, J D Wetherspoon*	1 Serving/358g	554	21.8	155	3.2	23.5	6.1	1.9
Poached Salmon, Tortilla Chips, J D Wetherspoon*	1 Serving/203g	573	32.9	282	9.9	25.8	16.2	1.6
Poached Salmon, with Wedges, J D Wetherspoon*	1 Serving/298g	656	34.3	220	7.1	24.2	11.5	1.5
Poached Salmon & Prawn Salad, J D Wetherspoon*	1 Wrap/355g	512	34.1	144	9.8	4.5	9.6	0.5
YORKSHIRE PUDDING								
J D Wetherspoon*	2 Puddings/56g	132	4.6	236	8.2	32.9	8.2	1.1
KFC								
BEANS								
BBQ, Large, KFC*	1 Serving/188g	158	1.4	84	5.3	15.1	0.7	0.0
BBQ, Regular, KFC*	1 Serving/130g	200	1.5	154	6.1	30.0	1.1	6.9
BURGERS								
Fillet, KFC*	1 Burger/245g	479	19.8	196	11.1	19.5	8.1	0.0
Fillet, Mini, KFC*	1 Burger/114g	275	11.2	241	14.8	23.9	9.8	0.0
Fillet Tower Burger, KFC*	1 Burger/163g	617	21.0	378	24.3	41.4	12.9	0.0
Mini Fillet, Kids, KFC*	1 Burger/114g	253	6.4	222	15.8	27.0	5.6	0.0
Tower, KFC*	1 Burger/210g	628	20.8	299	15.9	30.0	9.9	0.0
Tower, Zinger, KFC*	1 Burger/264g	655	32.7	248	11.2	24.3	12.4	0.0
Zinger, Fillet, KFC*	1 Burger/185g	445	19.6	241	13.9	22.4	10.6	1.4
Zinger, KFC*	1 Burger/219g	481	20.8	220	12.2	22.0	9.5	0.0
CHEESECAKE								
Boysenberry, Chateau, KFC*	1 Serving/85g	196	9.3	230	4.0	30.0	11.0	0.0
Cookies & Cream, KFC*	1 Serving/80g	261	17.1	326	4.3	29.1	21.4	0.0
CHICKEN								
Breast, Original Recipe, KFC*	1 Breast/137g	285	13.3	207	24.9	5.6	9.7	0.0
Drumsticks, Original Recipe, KFC*	1 Drumstick/95g	161	9.5	170	11.9	9.1	10.0	0.0
Fillet, Mini, Not In a Bun, KFC*	1 Fillet/50g	116	4.0	232	26.6	14.0	8.0	0.0
Popcorn, Kids, KFC*	1 Portion/66g	144	8.4	219	14.1	13.2	12.7	0.0
Popcorn, Large, KFC*	1 Serving/188g	494	29.8	262	17.5	13.5	15.8	0.0
Ribs, Original Recipe, KFC*	1 Rib/126g	238	13.4	188	19.8	4.1	10.6	0.0
Strips, Crispy, KFC*	1 Strip/46g	112	5.4	243	15.4	20.4	11.7	0.0
Thighs, Original Recipe, KFC*	1 Thigh/134g	218	14.2	162	12.6	4.4	10.6	0.0
Wings, Hot, KFC*	1 Wing/58g	102	7.0	175	9.4	7.5	12.1	0.0
Wings, Original Recipe, KFC*	1 Wing/48g	126	3.8	262	25.0	8.3	8.0	0.0
COLESLAW								
Large, KFC*	1 Serving/200g	268	22.4	134	0.8	9.5	11.2	0.0
Regular, KFC*	1 Serving/100g	134	11.2	134	0.8	9.5	11.2	0.0
CORN								
Cobs, Cobette, KFC*	1 Serving/70g	141	8.5	201	4.3	20.1	12.1	0.0
DRESSING								
Caesar, KFC*	1 Sachet/35g	103	10.9	295	19.2	2.7	31.1	0.0

	Measure INFO/WEIGHT	per Measure KCAL	FAT	Nutrition Values per 100g / 100ml KCAL	PROT	CARB	FAT	FIBRE

KFC
DRESSING

	Measure INFO/WEIGHT	KCAL	FAT	KCAL	PROT	CARB	FAT	FIBRE
French, KFC*	1 Sachet/45g	30	1.3	66	0.2	2.9	2.9	0.0
Vinaigrette, Low Fat, KFC*	1 Sachet/35g	21	0.8	59	0.5	8.9	2.2	0.0
Yoghurt, Coriander & Chilli, KFC*	1 Sachet/45g	166	16.2	369	2.2	9.3	36.0	0.0

FRIES
Large, KFC*	1 Serving/162g	375	19.3	231	3.1	32.4	11.9	0.0
Regular, KFC*	1 Serving/111g	257	13.2	232	3.1	32.4	11.9	0.0

GRAVY
Large, KFC*	1 Serving/204g	144	8.0	71	2.3	7.3	3.9	0.0
Regular, KFC*	1 Serving/102g	72	4.0	71	2.3	7.3	3.9	0.0

ICE CREAM
Avalanche, KFC*	1 Pot/28g	114	5.1	407	10.4	51.4	18.2	0.0
Soft, KFC*	1 Serving/110g	171	7.0	155	3.7	20.6	6.4	0.0

PIE
Apple Slice, Colonel's Pies, KFC*	1 Slice/113g	310	13.9	274	1.7	38.9	12.3	0.0
Strawberry Creme, Slice, KFC*	1 Slice/78g	279	15.0	358	5.4	41.0	19.2	2.5

SALAD
Chicken, Original Recipe, No Dressing, KFC*	1 Salad/292g	270	9.5	92	9.0	7.0	3.3	0.0
Chicken, Zinger, No Dressing, KFC*	1 Salad/285g	307	14.8	108	7.8	8.0	5.2	0.0
Potato, KFC*	1 Portion/160g	229	13.9	143	2.5	14.3	8.7	1.8

WRAP
Twister, Salsa, Toasted, KFC*	1 Wrap/222g	516	24.9	232	8.7	24.6	11.2	0.0
Twister, Toasted, KFC*	1 Wrap/217g	509	24.8	235	8.9	24.6	11.5	0.0
Wrapstar, KFC*	1 Wrapstar/239g	642	36.6	269	11.4	25.9	15.3	0.0

KRISPY KREME
DOUGHNUTS

Blueberry, Powdered, Filled, Krispy Kreme*	1 Doughnut/86g	307	17.2	357	7.0	36.0	20.0	5.0
Butterscotch Fudge, Krispy Kreme*	1 Doughnut/93g	372	16.7	400	6.0	53.0	18.0	0.0
Chocolate, Glazed, Krispy Kreme*	1 Doughnut/80g	309	13.6	387	4.0	55.0	17.0	3.0
Chocolate Dreamcake, Krispy Kreme*	1 Doughnut/92g	358	19.3	389	6.0	43.0	21.0	0.0
Chocolate Iced, Creme Filled, Krispy Kreme*	1 Doughnut/87g	339	17.4	390	6.0	47.0	20.0	4.0
Chocolate Iced, Custard Filled, Krispy Kreme*	1 Doughnut/87g	307	14.8	353	6.0	43.0	17.0	2.0
Chocolate Iced, Glazed, Krispy Kreme*	1 Doughnut/66g	270	13.2	410	5.0	51.0	20.0	3.0
Chocolate Iced, with Creme Filling, Krispy Kreme*	1 Doughnut/87g	350	20.9	402	3.0	42.0	24.0	1.0
Chocolate Iced, with Sprinkles, Krispy Kreme*	1 Doughnut/71g	293	13.5	413	5.0	56.0	19.0	3.0
Cinnamon Apple, Filled, Krispy Kreme*	1 Doughnut/81g	269	14.6	332	7.0	37.0	18.0	5.0
Cookies & Kreme, Krispy Kreme*	1 Doughnut/93g	379	16.7	408	4.0	57.0	18.0	0.0
Cruller, Glazed, Krispy Kreme*	1 Doughnut/54g	254	15.6	471	4.0	49.0	29.0	3.0
Glazed, with a Creme Filling, Krispy Kreme*	1 Doughnut/86g	309	15.5	359	5.0	44.0	18.0	4.0
Lemon Filled, Glazed, Krispy Kreme*	1 Doughnut/66g	218	10.5	331	5.0	41.0	16.0	4.0
Lemon Meringue Pie, Krispy Kreme*	1 Doughnut/83g	290	14.9	350	6.0	40.0	18.0	0.0
Maple Iced, Krispy Kreme*	1 Doughnut/66g	279	15.2	422	5.0	49.0	23.0	3.0
Original, Glazed, Krispy Kreme*	1 Doughnut/52g	217	13.0	417	6.0	43.0	25.0	4.0
Raspberry, Glazed, Krispy Kreme*	1 Doughnut/86g	307	13.8	357	6.0	47.0	16.0	4.0
Sour Cream, Krispy Kreme*	1 Doughnut/80g	340	18.4	425	4.0	53.0	23.0	1.0
Strawberries & Kreme, Krispy Kreme*	1 Doughnut/90g	323	15.3	359	5.0	45.0	17.0	0.0
Strawberry Filled, Powdered, Krispy Kreme*	1 Doughnut/74g	248	13.3	335	7.0	36.0	18.0	5.0
Vanilla, Krispy Kreme*	1 Doughnut/80g	315	13.7	391	4.0	57.0	17.0	2.0

LEON RESTAURANTS
BITS IN BETWEEN

Better Brownie, Leon Restaurants*	1 Serving/86g	402	28.4	467	7.6	38.0	33.0	0.0
Cranberry & Pecan Flapjack, Leon Restaurants*	1 Serving/83g	359	21.2	432	4.8	49.8	25.5	0.0
Dark Chocolate Tart, Leon Restaurants*	1 Serving/118g	593	46.3	503	3.6	35.8	39.2	0.0

LEON RESTAURANTS

	Measure INFO/WEIGHT	per Measure KCAL	FAT	Nutrition Values per 100g / 100ml KCAL	PROT	CARB	FAT	FIBRE
BITS IN BETWEEN								
Double Chocolate Muffin, Leon Restaurants*	1 Serving/100g	403	21.1	403	6.7	48.8	21.1	0.0
Lemon Ginger Crunch, Leon Restaurants*	1 Serving/83g	418	31.5	504	8.2	33.0	37.9	0.0
Life By Chocolate Mousse, Leon Restaurants*	1 Serving/50g	152	12.2	304	5.6	26.2	24.4	0.0
Organic Oat & Raisin Cookie, Leon Restaurants*	1 Serving/50g	203	9.1	406	4.8	55.8	18.2	0.0
Pecan, Bran & Maple Muffin, Leon Restaurants*	1 Serving/100g	399	22.3	399	5.8	46.5	22.3	0.0
Pecan Pie, Leon Restaurants*	1 Serving/125g	605	45.5	484	7.4	33.8	36.4	0.0
Sweet Sevilla Torta Biscuit, Leon Restaurants*	1 Serving/26g	124	6.6	477	7.3	54.2	25.4	0.0
White Chocolate & Cranberry Muffin, Leon Restaurants*	1 Serving/100g	372	19.7	372	5.6	46.0	19.7	0.0
BREAKFAST								
New York Breakfasts, Bacon & Egg, Leon Restaurants*	1 Serving/137g	279	12.8	204	10.8	20.7	9.3	0.0
New York Breakfasts, Classic, Leon Restaurants*	1 Serving/130g	229	8.7	176	8.5	22.2	6.7	0.0
New York Breakfasts, Egg & Tomato, Leon Restaurants*	1 Serving/137g	243	10.5	177	8.0	20.6	7.7	0.0
BREAKFAST CEREAL								
Organic Porridge, Banana, Leon Restaurants*	1 Serving/85g	81	0.3	95	1.2	23.2	0.3	0.0
Organic Porridge, Compote, Leon Restaurants*	1 Serving/40g	42	0.0	105	0.7	27.2	0.0	0.0
Organic Porridge, Granola, Leon Restaurants*	1 Serving/25g	127	7.6	508	10.8	49.6	30.4	0.0
Organic Porridge, Honey, Leon Restaurants*	1 Serving/40g	115	0.0	287	0.5	76.5	0.0	0.0
Organic Porridge, Plain, Leon Restaurants*	1 Serving/270g	305	9.5	113	4.2	16.1	3.5	0.0
Organic Porridge, Seeds, Leon Restaurants*	1 Serving/20g	112	9.6	560	20.0	11.5	48.0	0.0
DINNER								
Bar Snacks, Chilli Roasted Nuts, Leon Restaurants*	1 Serving/80g	489	49.7	611	19.0	6.4	62.1	0.0
Bar Snacks, Olives, Leon Restaurants*	1 Serving/105g	108	11.6	103	0.9	0.0	11.0	0.0
Grazing Dishes, Aioli Chicken, Leon Restaurants*	1 Serving/165g	276	12.6	167	21.5	2.8	7.6	0.0
Grazing Dishes, Brown Rice, Leon Restaurants*	1 Serving/165g	312	7.8	189	4.3	32.4	4.7	0.0
Grazing Dishes, Chilli Chicken, Leon Restaurants*	1 Serving/165g	239	8.3	145	21.3	3.1	5.0	0.0
Grazing Dishes, Fresh Slaw, Leon Restaurants*	1 Serving/115g	156	13.0	136	3.0	5.6	11.3	0.0
Grazing Dishes, Greek Flatbread, Leon Restaurants*	1 Serving/94g	218	4.7	232	5.6	43.8	5.0	0.0
Grazing Dishes, Grilled Halloumi, Leon Restaurants*	1 Serving/140g	538	45.1	384	22.9	0.6	32.2	0.0
Grazing Dishes, Hot Grilled Chorizo, Leon Restaurants*	1 Serving/189g	227	10.6	120	15.8	1.6	5.6	0.0
Grazing Dishes, Leon Gobi, Leon Restaurants*	1 Serving/230g	223	15.4	97	2.6	7.7	6.7	0.0
Grazing Dishes, Leon Mash, Leon Restaurants*	1 Serving/215g	384	14.6	179	5.3	25.8	6.8	0.0
Grazing Dishes, Sunshine Salad, Leon Restaurants*	1 Serving/127g	145	9.6	114	6.2	6.5	7.6	0.0
DRINKS								
Blackcurrant Quencher, Leon Restaurants*	1 Serving/300ml	120	0.0	40	0.1	9.8	0.0	0.0
Carrot & Orange Juice, Leon Restaurants*	1 Serving/300ml	81	0.3	27	0.5	5.9	0.1	0.0
Cloudy Apple with Lime & Mint, Leon Restaurants*	1 Serving/300ml	120	0.0	40	0.1	9.5	0.0	0.0
Fresh Leon, Made Lemonade, Leon Restaurants*	1 Serving/300ml	93	0.0	31	0.1	7.8	0.0	0.0
Fresh Orange Juice, Leon Restaurants*	1 Serving/300ml	99	0.0	33	0.6	7.7	0.0	0.0
Lemon, Ginger & Mint Quencher, Leon Restaurants*	1 Serving/300ml	54	0.0	18	0.1	4.1	0.0	0.0
Leon Kids Menu, Small Lemonade, Leon Restaurants*	1 Serving/250ml	78	0.0	31	0.1	8.2	0.0	0.0
Power Smoothie, Leon Restaurants*	1 Serving/300ml	312	14.4	104	4.0	11.3	4.8	0.0
Strawberry Power Smoothie, Leon Restaurants*	1 Serving/300ml	348	14.4	116	4.1	14.1	4.8	0.0
LUNCH								
Hot Boxes, Chilli Chicken, Leon Restaurants*	1 Serving/494g	815	42.3	165	8.1	13.8	8.6	0.0
Hot Boxes, Grilled Chicken with Aiol, Leon Restaurants*	1 Serving/464g	799	41.8	172	8.5	14.2	9.0	0.0
Hot Boxes, Leon Chicken Curry, Leon Restaurants*	1 Serving/505g	799	42.0	158	7.6	14.5	8.3	0.0
Hot Boxes, Meatball Lunchbox, Leon Restaurants*	1 Serving/335g	506	16.7	151	7.7	20.2	5.0	0.0
Hot Boxes, Moroccan Meatballs, Leon Restaurants*	1 Serving/475g	785	44.5	165	5.9	15.4	9.4	0.0
Hot Boxes, Pork Jambabalya, Leon Restaurants*	1 Serving/533g	590	23.2	111	4.7	14.2	4.3	0.0
Hot Boxes, The Leon Gobi, Leon Restaurants*	1 Serving/524g	709	37.6	135	2.9	14.8	7.2	0.0
Hot Wraps, Chicken & Chorizo Wrap, Leon Restaurants*	1 Serving/286g	420	17.1	147	13.4	17.5	6.0	0.0
Hot Wraps, Chilli Chicken Wrap, Leon Restaurants*	1 Serving/318g	440	8.7	138	11.4	16.0	2.7	0.0

	Measure INFO/WEIGHT	per Measure KCAL	FAT	Nutrition Values per 100g / 100ml KCAL	PROT	CARB	FAT	FIBRE

LEON RESTAURANTS

LUNCH

Hot Wraps, Fish Finger Wrap, Leon Restaurants*	1 Serving/292g	627	27.9	215	8.0	25.9	9.5	0.0
Hot Wraps, Grilled Chicken Wrap, Leon Restaurants*	1 Serving/280g	429	11.1	153	12.9	17.5	4.0	0.0
Hot Wraps, Sweet Potato Falafel, Leon Restaurants*	1 Serving/298g	542	11.9	182	5.3	33.5	4.0	0.0
Leon Kids Menu, Fish Finger, Leon Restaurants*	1 Serving/277g	461	13.1	166	5.3	27.1	4.7	0.0
Leon Kids Menu, Grilled Chicken, Leon Restaurants*	1 Serving/290g	479	13.8	165	10.2	20.4	4.8	0.0
Leon Kids Menu, Meatballs, Leon Restaurants*	1 Serving/283g	432	12.3	153	7.6	20.7	4.3	0.0
Meaty Soups, Magreb Chicken, Leon Restaurants*	1 Serving/375ml	272	10.5	73	5.6	6.8	2.8	0.0
Meaty Soups, Pea, Bacon & Basil, Leon Restaurants*	1 Serving/370ml	199	7.0	54	4.0	5.5	1.9	0.0
Salads, Grilled Chicken Salad, Leon Restaurants*	1 Serving/400g	619	34.3	155	13.5	6.2	8.6	0.0
Salads, Original Superfood Salad, Leon Restaurants*	1 Serving/359g	493	39.9	137	5.1	4.4	11.1	0.0
Sauces, Aioli, Leon Restaurants*	1 Serving/30g	126	12.5	420	4.0	1.3	41.7	0.0
Sauces, Hot Chilli, Leon Restaurants*	1 Serving/30g	14	0.5	47	1.3	7.7	1.7	0.0
Sauces, Ketchup, Leon Restaurants*	1 Serving/30g	3	0.5	9	1.3	9.3	1.7	0.0
Sauces, Vinaigrette, Leon Restaurants*	1 Serving/30g	183	20.1	610	0.7	0.3	67.0	0.0
Sides, Brown Rice, Leon Restaurants*	1 Serving/165g	312	7.8	189	4.3	32.4	4.7	0.0
Sides, Green Sunshine Salad, Leon Restaurants*	1 Serving/147g	294	24.9	200	6.3	5.6	16.9	0.0
Sides, Grilled Chicken Nuggets, Leon Restaurants*	1 Serving/100g	247	13.7	247	29.0	2.0	13.7	0.0
Sides, Hummus & Flatbread, Leon Restaurants*	1 Serving/210g	544	22.1	259	7.8	35.6	10.5	0.0
Sides, Hummus without Flatbread, Leon Restaurants*	1 Serving/130g	283	20.4	218	6.6	12.5	15.7	0.0
Sides, Khobez, Leon Restaurants*	1 Serving/80g	243	0.9	304	8.9	68.7	1.1	0.0
Sides, Moroccan Meatballs, Leon Restaurants*	1 Serving/140g	198	11.5	141	12.4	5.0	8.2	0.0
Sides, Slaw, Leon Restaurants*	1 Serving/115g	156	13.0	136	3.0	5.6	11.3	0.0
Sides, Sweet Potato Falafel, Leon Restaurants*	1 Serving/101g	207	10.2	205	6.2	24.1	10.1	0.0
Veggie Soups, Bean & Cheddar, Leon Restaurants*	1 Serving/365ml	275	16.4	75	3.1	6.1	4.5	0.0
Veggie Soups, French Pea & Mint, Leon Restaurants*	1 Serving/370ml	249	14.2	67	2.5	6.0	3.8	0.0
Veggie Soups, Harira, Leon Restaurants*	1 Serving/375ml	211	5.1	56	3.1	8.2	1.4	0.0
Veggie Soups, Roy's Tomato Soup, Leon Restaurants*	1 Serving/360ml	108	3.6	30	1.1	4.3	1.0	0.0

PUDDINGS

Puds, Banana Split, Leon Restaurants*	1 Serving/525g	1196	84.8	228	2.8	18.8	16.1	0.0
Puds, Better Brownie, Leon Restaurants*	1 Serving/178g	658	45.9	370	5.8	30.5	25.8	0.0
Puds, Dark Chocolate Tart, Leon Restaurants*	1 Serving/226g	823	46.9	364	5.0	40.6	20.7	0.0
Puds, Lemon & Ginger Crunch, Leon Restaurants*	1 Serving/160g	562	39.8	351	5.4	28.1	24.9	0.0
Puds, Pecan Pie, Leon Restaurants*	1 Serving/125g	605	45.5	484	7.4	33.8	36.4	0.0

WRAP

Fish Finger, Hot, Leon Restaurants*	1 Wrap/292g	627	27.9	215	8.0	25.9	9.5	0.0

YOGHURT

Yoghurt & Fruit, Blueberry Boost, Leon Restaurants*	1 Serving/230g	328	18.8	143	5.6	11.6	8.2	0.0
Yoghurt & Fruit, Strawberry & Mango, Leon Restaurants*	1 Serving/225g	241	16.5	107	5.2	5.0	7.3	0.0
Yoghurt & Fruit, Sunshine Salad, Leon Restaurants*	1 Serving/168g	76	0.3	45	0.8	10.4	0.2	0.0

MCDONALD'S

BAGEL

Plain, Toasted, McDonald's*	1 Bagel/85g	210	0.8	248	9.0	50.0	1.0	3.0
Toasted, with Strawberry Jam, McDonald's*	1 Bagel/105g	260	1.0	248	8.0	52.0	1.0	3.0
with Bacon, Egg & Cheese, McDonald's*	1 Bagel/173g	455	22.5	263	13.0	26.0	13.0	2.0
with Butter & Jam, McDonald's*	1 Bagel/122g	399	10.2	326	5.9	58.8	8.3	2.2
with Flora & Jam, McDonald's*	1 Bagel/120g	369	6.9	305	6.0	59.4	5.7	2.2
with Philadelphia, McDonald's*	1 Bagel/125g	317	5.9	254	7.7	47.5	4.7	2.1
with Sausage, Egg & Cheese, McDonald's*	1 Bagel/203g	540	28.4	266	14.0	22.0	14.0	2.0
with Sausage & Egg, McDonald's*	1 Bagel/207g	551	26.5	266	13.3	23.3	12.8	1.6

BREAKFAST

Big Breakfast, McDonald's*	1 Breakfast/264g	595	37.0	225	11.0	15.0	14.0	1.0
Big Breakfast Bun, McDonald's*	1 Bun/242g	571	32.2	236	13.0	15.1	13.3	0.9

MCDONALD'S

	Measure INFO/WEIGHT	per Measure KCAL	FAT	Nutrition Values per 100g / 100ml KCAL	PROT	CARB	FAT	FIBRE
BREAKFAST CEREAL								
Porridge, Oatso Simple, & Jam, McDonald's*	1 Serving/232g	246	5.3	106	4.0	17.0	2.3	0.9
Porridge, Oatso Simple, & Sugar, McDonald's*	1 Serving/215g	205	5.4	95	4.3	13.7	2.5	0.9
Porridge, Oatso Simple, Plain, McDonald's*	1 Serving/212g	195	4.2	92	5.0	13.0	2.0	1.0
BROWNIE								
Belgian Bliss, McDonald's*	1 Serving/85g	390	22.1	459	6.0	51.0	26.0	2.0
BURGERS								
1955 Burger, McDonald's*	1 Burger/281g	655	33.7	233	14.0	18.0	12.0	2.0
Bacon, Chicken & Onion, McDonald's*	1 Burger/255g	660	33.1	259	14.0	22.0	13.0	2.0
Big Mac, McDonald's*	1 Burger/214g	491	25.7	229	13.0	19.0	12.0	2.0
Big Mac, No Sauce, No Cheese, McDonald's*	1 Burger/181g	400	16.0	221	12.1	23.8	8.8	1.1
Big Tasty, McDonald's*	1 Burger/346g	835	52.0	241	13.0	14.0	15.0	1.0
Big Tasty, with Bacon, McDonald's*	1 Burger/359g	890	57.4	248	14.0	14.0	16.0	1.0
Bigger Big Mac, McDonald's*	1 Burger/324g	714	34.0	220	12.9	18.5	10.5	1.6
Cheeseburger, Bacon, McDonald's*	1 Burger/127g	336	15.3	264	16.0	24.0	12.0	2.0
Cheeseburger, Double, McDonald's*	1 Burger/169g	440	23.7	260	17.0	19.0	14.0	1.0
Cheeseburger, McDonald's*	1 Burger/119g	300	12.0	253	14.3	26.2	10.1	2.5
Chicken Legend, with Bacon, Cool Mayo, McDonald's*	1 Burger/227g	590	22.7	260	15.0	27.0	10.0	2.0
Festive, Deluxe, McDonald's*	1 Burger/296g	805	44.4	272	16.0	19.0	15.0	1.0
Filet-O-Fish, McDonald's*	1 Burger/150g	350	18.1	232	10.0	24.0	12.0	1.0
Filet-O-Fish, No Tartar Sauce, McDonald's*	1 Burger/124g	290	9.0	234	12.1	30.6	7.3	0.8
Hamburger, McDonald's*	1 Burger/104g	250	8.3	240	13.0	29.0	8.0	2.0
Mayo Chicken, McDonald's*	1 Burger/122g	310	13.4	254	10.0	30.0	11.0	2.0
McChicken Sandwich, McDonald's*	1 Sandwich/171g	385	17.2	224	9.0	26.0	10.0	2.0
Quarter Pounder, Bacon with Cheese, McDonald's*	1 Burger/230g	592	33.2	259	16.5	15.4	14.5	1.3
Quarter Pounder, Deluxe, McDonald's*	1 Burger/253g	521	26.8	206	11.4	16.1	10.6	1.7
Quarter Pounder, Double, with Cheese, McDonald's*	1 Burger/275g	710	40.3	259	19.5	12.2	14.7	1.1
Quarter Pounder, McDonald's*	1 Burger/178g	424	19.0	238	14.5	20.9	10.7	2.1
Quarter Pounder, with Cheese, McDonald's*	1 Burger/194g	490	25.3	252	16.0	19.0	13.0	2.0
Summer Chorizo, McDonald's*	1 Burger/238g	650	35.7	273	17.0	17.0	15.0	1.0
The M, McDonald's*	1 Serving/240g	580	28.8	242	16.0	18.0	12.0	1.0
The M with Bacon, McDonald's*	1 Serving/249g	620	32.4	249	17.0	18.0	13.0	1.0
BURGERS VEGETARIAN								
Vegetable, Deluxe, McDonald's*	1 Burger/181g	411	16.3	227	6.0	30.0	9.0	6.0
BUTTER								
Country Life, McDonald's*	1 Pack/11g	85	9.0	752	0.0	0.0	80.0	0.0
CAKE								
Birthday, McDonald's*	1 Portion/158g	640	22.6	405	2.7	65.4	14.3	1.0
CARROTS								
Sticks, McDonald's*	1 Bag/80g	30	0.0	38	0.0	8.0	0.0	2.0
CHEESE								
Soft, Philadelphia, Light, McDonald's*	1 Serving/35g	55	3.9	157	9.0	3.0	11.0	0.0
CHICKEN								
McNuggets, 4 Pieces, McDonald's*	4 Pieces/70g	170	9.1	243	13.0	19.0	13.0	1.0
McNuggets, 6 Pieces, McDonald's*	6 Pieces/105g	250	13.7	238	13.0	19.0	13.0	1.0
McNuggets, 9 Pieces, McDonald's*	9 Pieces/157g	375	20.4	239	13.0	19.0	13.0	1.0
Selects, 3 Pieces, McDonald's*	3 Pieces/130g	365	19.6	280	16.0	20.0	15.0	1.0
Selects, 5 Pieces, McDonald's*	5 Pieces/219g	612	32.8	280	16.0	20.0	15.0	1.0
COFFEE								
Black, Large, McDonald's*	1 Large/428ml	0	0.0	0	0.0	0.0	0.0	0.0
Black, Regular, McDonald's*	1 Regular/312ml	0	0.0	0	0.0	0.0	0.0	0.0
Cappuccino, Large, McDonald's*	1 Large/307ml	120	3.1	39	3.0	4.0	1.0	0.0
Cappuccino, Regular, McDonald's*	1 Regular/231ml	90	2.3	39	3.0	4.0	1.0	0.0

MCDONALD'S

	Measure INFO/WEIGHT	per Measure KCAL	FAT	Nutrition Values per 100g / 100ml KCAL	PROT	CARB	FAT	FIBRE
COFFEE								
Espresso, Single Shot, McDonald's*	1 Shot/30ml	0	0.0	0	0.0	0.0	0.0	0.0
Latte, Large, McDonald's*	1 Large/451ml	185	4.5	41	3.0	4.0	1.0	0.0
Latte, Regular, McDonald's*	1 Regular/337ml	135	3.4	40	3.0	4.0	1.0	0.0
White, Large, McDonald's*	1 Large/428ml	30	0.0	7	0.0	1.0	0.0	0.0
White, Regular, McDonald's*	1 Regular/313ml	25	0.0	8	1.0	1.0	0.0	0.0
COLA								
Coca-Cola, Diet, McDonald's*	1 Medium/405ml	4	0.0	1	0.0	0.0	0.0	0.0
Coca-Cola, McDonald's*	1 Medium/405ml	170	0.0	42	0.0	10.0	0.0	0.0
Coke, Zero, McDonald's*	1 Small/200ml	2	0.0	1	0.0	0.0	0.0	0.0
CREAMER								
Uht, McDonald's*	1 Cup/14ml	17	1.4	123	4.2	4.2	10.0	0.0
CROUTONS								
McDonald's*	1 Sachet/14g	60	2.0	426	11.8	63.4	14.0	2.7
DIP								
BBQ, McDonald's*	1 Pot/50g	83	0.0	166	0.0	37.0	0.0	0.0
Caramelised Onion, McDonald's*	1 Pot/31g	45	1.9	144	3.0	19.0	6.0	3.0
Sour Cream & Chive, McDonald's*	1 Pot/50g	150	16.0	300	2.0	2.0	32.0	4.0
Sweet Chilli, McDonald's*	1 Pot/31g	80	0.9	256	0.0	58.0	3.0	0.0
DOUGHNUTS								
Chocolate Donut, McDonald's*	1 Donut/79g	345	16.2	437	5.7	43.8	20.5	1.0
Chocolate Donut, McMini, McDonald's*	1 Donut/17g	64	3.0	375	6.8	46.9	17.8	1.6
Cinnamon Donut, McDonald's*	1 Donut/72g	302	18.1	419	5.1	43.1	25.1	3.8
Sugared Donut, McDonald's*	1 Donut/49g	205	14.7	418	6.0	35.0	30.0	4.0
DRESSING								
Balsamic, Low Fat, McDonald's*	1 Sachet/33g	20	1.0	60	0.0	9.0	3.0	0.0
Caesar, Low Fat, McDonald's*	1 Sachet/80g	55	1.6	68	2.0	10.0	2.0	0.0
French, Low Fat, McDonald's*	1 Serving/22g	13	0.6	58	0.5	7.1	2.6	1.0
FANTA								
Orange, McDonald's*	1 Super/750ml	315	0.0	42	0.0	10.0	0.0	0.0
FISH FINGERS								
McDonald's*	3 Fingers/84g	195	9.2	232	15.0	19.0	11.0	1.0
FRIES								
French, Large, McDonald's*	1 Large/160g	460	22.4	288	3.0	38.0	14.0	4.0
French, Medium, McDonald's*	1 Medium/114g	330	16.0	289	3.0	37.0	14.0	4.0
French, Small, McDonald's*	1 Small/80g	230	11.2	288	2.0	38.0	14.0	4.0
FRUIT								
Bag, McDonald's*	1 Bag/80g	40	0.8	50	0.0	12.0	1.0	2.0
FRUIT SHOOT								
Robinsons, McDonald's*	1 Bottle200ml	10	0.0	5	0.0	1.0	0.0	0.0
HASH BROWNS								
McDonald's*	1 Hash Brown/53g	140	9.0	264	2.0	26.0	17.0	2.0
HOT CHOCOLATE								
McDonald's*	1 Serving/330ml	164	3.6	50	0.7	8.8	1.1	0.0
HOT DOG								
& Ketchup, McDonald's*	1 Serving/116g	296	14.6	255	9.6	25.8	12.6	1.3
ICE CREAM								
Smartie, McDonald's*	1 Pot/120g	260	9.5	216	3.4	33.3	7.9	1.0
ICE CREAM CONE								
McDonald's*	1 Cone/90g	141	4.5	156	4.5	24.4	5.0	0.0
with Flake, McDonald's*	1 Cone/107g	204	7.7	191	4.8	27.0	7.2	0.0
JAM								
Strawberry, McDonald's*	1 Pack/20g	50	0.0	250	0.0	60.0	0.0	0.0

MCDONALD'S

JUICE								
Tropicana, McDonald's*	1 Bottle/250ml	107	0.0	43	1.0	9.0	0.0	0.4
KETCHUP								
Tomato, McDonald's*	1 Portion/23g	25	0.0	109	0.0	26.0	0.0	0.0
LEMONADE								
Sprite, Z, McDonald's*	1 Large/500ml	5	0.0	1	0.0	0.0	0.0	0.0
MARGARINE								
Flora, Original, McDonald's*	1 Portion/10g	55	6.0	550	0.0	0.0	60.0	0.0
MCFLURRY								
After Eight, McDonald's*	1 McFlurry/204g	381	11.0	187	2.8	31.4	5.4	0.5
Cadbury, Shortcake, Limited Edition, McDonald's*	1 McFlurry/206g	385	14.4	187	3.0	28.0	7.0	1.0
Chocolate, Cornetto, McDonald's*	1 McFlurry/207g	400	16.6	193	3.0	29.0	8.0	1.0
Cornetto, Mint Choc, McDonald's*	1 McFlurry/207g	400	16.6	193	3.0	29.0	8.0	1.0
Creme Egg, Cadbury's, McDonald's*	1 McFlurry/203g	381	12.9	188	2.9	29.8	6.3	0.5
Crunchie, McDonald's*	1 McFlurry/185g	330	11.1	178	3.0	28.0	6.0	1.0
Dairy Milk, McDonald's*	1 McFlurry/184g	340	12.9	184	3.0	28.0	7.0	1.0
Dairy Milk, with Caramel, McDonald's*	1 McFlurry/206g	385	13.0	187	2.9	29.1	6.3	0.0
Flake, Chocolate, McDonald's*	1 McFlurry/206g	400	14.4	194	3.0	29.0	7.0	0.0
Flake, Raspberry, McDonald's*	1 McFlurry/205g	370	12.3	180	3.0	27.0	6.0	0.0
Jammie Dodger, McDonald's*	1 McFlurry/128g	256	8.2	200	3.9	33.6	6.4	0.3
Raspberry, McDonald's*	1 McFlurry/206g	370	12.3	180	3.0	27.0	6.0	0.0
Rolo, McDonald's*	1 McFlurry/205g	390	13.3	190	4.0	29.2	6.5	0.1
Smarties, McDonald's*	1 McFlurry/185g	330	11.1	178	3.0	28.0	6.0	1.0
Strawberry, Cornetto, McDonald's*	1 McFlurry/207g	375	12.4	181	3.0	29.0	6.0	0.0
Terry's Chocolate Orange, McDonald's*	1 McFlurry/203g	405	16.3	199	3.0	28.0	8.0	0.0
Toffee Swirl, Oreo Cookie, McDonald's*	1 McFlurry/206g	400	12.4	194	3.0	31.0	6.0	1.0
Yorkie, McDonald's*	1 McFlurry/204g	379	14.9	186	3.4	27.0	7.3	0.8
MCMUFFIN								
Bacon & Egg, Double, McDonald's*	1 McMuffin/161g	395	21.0	244	15.0	16.0	13.0	1.0
Bacon & Egg, McDonald's*	1 McMuffin/143g	340	17.2	237	14.0	18.0	12.0	1.0
Sausage & Egg, Double, McDonald's*	1 McMuffin/222g	560	35.6	252	16.0	12.0	16.0	1.0
Sausage & Egg, McDonald's*	1 McMuffin/174g	420	24.3	242	14.0	16.0	14.0	1.0
Scrambled Egg, McDonald's*	1 McMuffin/147g	294	14.1	200	10.9	17.5	9.6	1.3
MELT								
Toasted Ham & Cheese, McDonald's*	1 Melt/100g	239	8.0	239	11.2	30.6	8.0	1.8
MILK								
Fresh, Portion, McDonald's*	1 Portion/14ml	10	0.0	69	0.0	7.0	0.0	0.0
Organic, McDonald's*	1 Bottle/250ml	117	5.0	47	4.0	5.0	2.0	0.0
MILKSHAKE								
Banana, Large, McDonald's*	1 Large/432ml	545	13.0	126	3.0	21.0	3.0	0.0
Banana, Medium, McDonald's*	1 Medium/338ml	425	10.1	126	3.0	21.0	3.0	0.0
Banana, Small, McDonald's*	1 Small/178ml	226	5.3	127	3.0	21.0	3.0	0.0
Cadbury Dairy Milk, Caramel Flavour, Sm, McDonald's*	1 Medium/177ml	220	5.3	124	3.0	20.0	3.0	1.0
Cadburys Dairy Milk, Caramel, Large, McDonald's*	1 Large/417ml	505	16.7	121	3.0	19.0	4.0	1.0
Cadburys Dairy Milk, Caramel, Medium, McDonald's*	1 Medium/394ml	480	15.8	122	3.0	19.0	4.0	1.0
Chocolate, Large, McDonald's*	1 Large/431ml	530	12.9	123	3.0	20.0	3.0	0.0
Chocolate, Medium, McDonald's*	1 Medium/337ml	425	10.1	126	3.0	21.0	3.0	0.0
Chocolate, Small, McDonald's*	1 Small/177ml	225	5.3	127	3.0	21.0	3.0	0.0
Strawberry, Large, McDonald's*	1 Large/432ml	540	13.0	125	3.0	21.0	3.0	0.0
Strawberry, Medium, McDonald's*	1 Medium/336ml	420	10.1	125	3.0	21.0	3.0	0.0
Strawberry, Small, McDonald's*	1 Small/177ml	220	5.3	124	3.0	21.0	3.0	0.0
Vanilla, Large, McDonald's*	1 Large/431ml	535	12.9	124	3.0	21.0	3.0	0.0
Vanilla, Medium, McDonald's*	1 Medium/336ml	420	10.1	125	3.0	21.0	3.0	0.0

MCDONALD'S

	Measure INFO/WEIGHT	per Measure		Nutrition Values per 100g / 100ml				
		KCAL	FAT	KCAL	PROT	CARB	FAT	FIBRE
MILKSHAKE								
Vanilla, Small, McDonald's*	1 Small/177ml	220	5.3	124	3.0	21.0	3.0	0.0
MOZZARELLA								
Dippers, McDonald's*	3 Dippers/85g	265	13.6	312	13.0	27.0	16.0	1.0
MUFFIN								
Blueberry, Low Fat, McDonald's*	1 Muffin/126g	300	3.8	238	5.0	50.0	3.0	2.0
Double Chocolate, McDonald's*	1 Muffin/123g	515	28.3	419	6.0	46.0	23.0	2.0
ONION RINGS								
McDonald's*	1 Serving/99g	245	11.9	247	4.0	31.0	12.0	3.0
PANCAKE								
& Sausage, with Syrup, McDonald's*	1 Portion/223g	615	20.1	275	8.0	42.0	9.0	2.0
& Syrup, McDonald's*	1 Pack/175g	515	14.0	294	4.0	52.0	8.0	2.0
PIE								
Apple, McDonald's*	1 Pie/80g	231	12.8	289	2.0	35.0	16.0	0.0
POTATO WEDGES								
McDonald's*	1 Portion/177g	349	17.7	197	3.3	23.3	10.0	2.8
QUORN*								
Burger, Premiere, McDonald's*	1 Burger/210g	311	6.1	148	9.1	24.2	2.9	2.7
ROLL								
Bacon, McBacon, McDonald's*	1 Roll/122g	349	14.0	286	13.5	30.5	11.5	1.7
Bacon, with Brown Sauce, McDonald's*	1 Roll/126g	350	8.8	278	15.0	37.0	7.0	2.0
Bacon, with Tomato Ketchup, McDonald's*	1 Roll/126g	345	8.8	273	15.0	36.0	7.0	2.0
SALAD								
Chicken, No Bacon, Grilled, McDonald's*	1 Salad/255g	115	2.6	45	7.0	2.0	1.0	1.0
Chicken, with Bacon, Grilled, McDonald's*	1 Salad/266g	164	5.3	62	9.0	2.0	2.0	1.0
Crispy Chicken, No Bacon, McDonald's*	1 Salad/281g	270	11.2	96	8.0	6.0	4.0	1.0
Crispy Chicken, with Bacon, McDonald's*	1 Serving/292g	326	14.6	111	10.0	7.0	5.0	1.0
Garden, Side, No Dressing, McDonald's*	1 Salad/91g	10	0.0	11	1.0	2.0	0.0	1.0
Garden, Side, with Balsamic Dressing, McDonald's*	1 Salad/128g	91	3.8	71	1.0	11.0	3.0	1.0
Garden, Side & Low Fat Caesar Dressing, McDonald's*	1 Salad/63g	40	1.3	63	2.0	8.0	2.0	2.0
SANDWICH								
Deli, Chicken, Salad, McDonald's*	1 Sandwich/216g	350	8.6	162	7.0	24.0	4.0	2.0
Deli, Chicken, Sweet Chilli, McDonald's*	1 Sandwich/250g	570	22.5	228	12.0	28.0	9.0	2.0
Deli, Chicken & Bacon, McDonald's*	1 Sandwich/192g	405	13.4	211	10.0	27.0	7.0	2.0
Deli, Spicy Veggie, McDonald's*	1 Sandwich/216g	555	21.6	257	6.0	36.0	10.0	4.0
SAUCE								
Barbeque, McDonald's*	1 Portion/50g	85	1.0	170	0.0	38.0	2.0	0.0
Curry, Sweet, McDonald's*	1 Portion/29g	50	0.9	171	0.0	38.0	3.0	3.0
Mustard, Mild, McDonald's*	1 Portion/30g	64	3.6	212	1.0	24.8	12.1	0.0
Sweet & Sour, McDonald's*	1 Portion/29g	50	0.0	172	0.0	38.0	0.0	0.0
SUNDAE								
Hot Caramel, McDonald's*	1 Sundae/189g	357	8.3	189	3.8	33.9	4.4	0.0
Hot Fudge, McDonald's*	1 Sundae/187g	352	10.7	188	4.5	30.0	5.7	0.0
No Topping, McDonald's*	1 Sundae/149g	219	7.6	147	4.2	21.6	5.1	0.0
Strawberry, McDonald's*	1 Sundae/214g	360	8.6	168	2.0	33.0	4.0	0.0
Toffee, McDonald's*	1 Sundae/182g	350	9.1	192	3.0	34.0	5.0	1.0
SYRUP								
Pancake, McDonald's*	1 Pot/55g	190	0.0	345	0.0	84.0	0.0	0.0
TEA								
with Milk, McDonald's*	1 Serving/333ml	10	3.3	3	0.0	1.0	1.0	0.0
WRAP								
Breakfast with Brown Sauce, McDonald's*	1 Wrap/235g	595	30.6	253	11.0	23.0	13.0	2.0
Breakfast with Tomato Ketchup, McDonald's*	1 Wrap/235g	595	30.6	253	11.0	23.0	13.0	2.0

MCDONALD'S

	Measure INFO/WEIGHT	per Measure KCAL	FAT	Nutrition Values per 100g / 100ml KCAL	PROT	CARB	FAT	FIBRE
WRAP								
Chicken, Cajun, McDonald's*	1 Wrap/222g	585	33.4	263	9.0	22.0	15.0	2.0
Chicken, Cheese & Bacon Snack, McDonald's*	1 Wrap/100g	360	18.0	360	14.0	33.0	18.0	2.0
Chicken, Grilled, Salad, McDonald's*	1 Wrap/221g	335	11.0	152	7.2	19.9	5.0	1.8
Chicken, Snack, McDonald's*	1 Wrap/112g	266	11.2	237	10.0	29.0	10.0	2.0
Chicken Fajita, McDonald's*	1 Wrap/259g	647	31.1	250	8.9	26.7	12.0	1.2
Garlic & Herb, Snack, McDonald's*	1 Wrap/121g	335	18.2	276	12.0	25.0	15.0	2.0
Oriental, Snack, McDonald's*	1 Wrap/127g	265	10.1	209	10.0	25.0	8.0	2.0
Sweet Chilli, Crispy Chicken, McDonald's*	1 Wrap/206g	465	18.5	226	10.0	27.0	9.0	2.0

NANDO'S

	Measure INFO/WEIGHT	per Measure KCAL	FAT	Nutrition Values per 100g / 100ml KCAL	PROT	CARB	FAT	FIBRE
BREAD								
Garlic, Nando's*	1 Portion/101g	330	15.5	327	8.5	38.8	15.3	1.7
BURGERS								
Bean, Nando's*	1 Burger/235g	468	13.4	199	9.5	26.5	5.7	2.4
Chicken Breast Fillet, Nando's*	1 Burger/108g	381	5.7	353	38.6	37.8	5.3	1.9
Double Chicken Breast, Nando's*	1 Burger/351g	545	8.0	155	22.2	11.6	2.3	0.6
Veggie, Nando's*	1 Burger/246g	387	6.5	157	8.2	23.2	2.6	3.1
CHICKEN								
¼, Leg, Peri Peri, Nando's*	1 Portion/95g	218	13.2	229	25.9	0.1	13.9	0.0
¼ Breast, Peri Peri, Nando's*	¼ Breast/90g	135	2.4	150	28.1	3.4	2.7	0.0
½ Peri Peri, Nando's*	½ Chicken/185g	353	15.6	191	27.0	1.7	8.4	0.0
Breast, Fillet Strips, Nando's*	1 Serving/108g	152	2.2	141	30.6	0.2	2.0	0.0
Butterfly, Peri Peri, Flame Grilled, Nando's*	1 Portion/193g	315	9.1	163	30.1	0.1	4.7	0.5
Whole, Nando's*	1 Chicken/370g	705	31.3	191	27.0	1.7	8.5	0.0
Wings, 10, Nando's*	10 Wings/246g	593	34.7	241	28.4	0.1	14.1	0.2
Wings, 3, Nando's*	3 Wings/71g	189	11.3	267	30.8	0.1	16.0	0.6
Wings, 5, Nando's*	5 Wings/123g	296	17.3	241	28.4	0.1	14.1	0.0
CHIPS								
Large, Nando's*	1 Serving/480g	1071	43.7	223	2.9	33.6	9.1	2.5
Per Peri, Regular, Nando's*	1 Portion/161g	359	14.6	223	2.9	33.5	9.1	2.5
Peri Peri, Large, Nando's*	1 Large/482g	1074	43.7	223	2.9	33.6	9.1	2.5
Regular, Nando's*	1 Regular/160g	357	14.6	223	2.9	33.6	9.1	2.5
COLESLAW								
Large, Nando's*	1 Large/100g	531	45.9	177	0.8	6.3	15.3	1.1
Regular, Nando's*	1 Serving/150g	265	23.0	177	0.8	6.3	15.3	1.1
CORN								
On the Cob, Large, Nando's*	1 Large/69g	99	1.9	144	5.6	26.7	2.7	4.6
DESSERT								
Bolo De Coco, Portuguese Coconut Tart, Nando's*	1 Serving/70g	277	16.0	396	11.9	35.6	22.9	6.6
Carrot Cake, Nando's*	1 Serving/191g	726	30.6	380	4.0	32.0	16.0	1.0
Choc-a-Lot Cake, Nando's*	1 Serving/157g	534	31.4	340	5.0	40.0	20.0	2.0
Chocolate Cheesecake, Nando's*	1 Serving/134g	496	34.8	370	6.0	29.0	26.0	1.0
Mango & Passion Fruit Cheesecake, Nando's*	1 Serving/131g	419	26.2	320	50.4	29.0	20.0	0.0
Nata, Custard Tart, Nando's*	1 Serving/75g	210	8.1	280	5.5	40.3	10.8	2.0
White Choc Raspberry Swirl, Cheesecake, Nando's*	1 Serving/137g	493	34.3	360	5.0	28.0	25.0	1.0
HOUMOUS WITH								
Peri Peri Drizzle & Pitta, Nando's*	1 Serving/295g	876	32.1	297	9.5	40.9	10.9	6.2
ICE CREAM								
Chocolate, Nando's*	1 Serving/90g	194	8.8	216	4.4	27.6	9.8	0.6
Rum & Raisin Flavour, Nando's*	1 Serving/95g	210	8.4	221	2.9	32.6	8.8	0.5
Strawberry, Nando's*	1 Serving/105g	223	11.5	212	3.1	25.3	10.9	0.5
Vanilla Chilli & Toffee Flavour Sauce, Nando's*	1 Serving/100g	219	10.4	219	3.2	28.1	10.4	0.5

	Measure INFO/WEIGHT	per Measure KCAL	FAT	Nutrition Values per 100g / 100ml KCAL	PROT	CARB	FAT	FIBRE
NANDO'S								
ICED LOLLY								
Chilly Billy, Apple & Blackcurrant, Nando's*	1 Lolly/115g	49	0.1	43	0.2	10.1	0.1	0.0
MASH								
Creamy, Large, Nando's*	1 Large/100g	544	31.6	136	1.7	13.0	7.9	2.5
Creamy, Regular, Nando's*	1 Regular/200g	272	15.8	136	1.7	13.0	7.9	2.5
Sweet Potato, Fino Side, Nando's*	1 Serving/200g	236	4.2	118	2.2	22.7	2.1	2.7
OLIVES								
Spicy, Mixed, Nando's*	1 Bowl/100g	106	10.4	106	0.9	0.6	10.4	3.0
PEAS								
Macho, Large, Nando's*	1 Serving/280g	316	20.7	113	4.7	7.0	7.4	4.2
Macho, Regular, Nando's*	1 Serving/140g	158	10.4	113	4.7	7.0	7.4	4.2
PITTA								
Bean, Nando's*	1 Pitta/235g	477	12.9	203	8.5	28.8	5.5	2.4
Chicken Breast, Nando's*	1 Pitta/223g	386	5.1	173	17.7	20.4	2.3	0.9
Veggie, Nando's*	1 Pitta/235g	384	5.9	163	7.6	26.3	2.5	3.2
RATATOUILLE								
Fino Side, Nando's*	1 Serving/180g	185	13.0	103	1.2	6.3	7.2	4.1
RICE								
Spicy, Large, Nando's*	1 Large/100g	398	10.7	153	3.1	25.9	4.1	3.0
Spicy, Regular, Nando's*	1 Regular/130g	199	5.3	153	3.1	25.9	4.1	3.0
ROLL								
Portuguese with Chicken Livers, Nando's*	1 Serving/251g	641	29.8	255	21.2	16.0	11.9	0.9
Prego Steak, Nando's*	1 Roll/230g	435	11.4	189	18.3	17.7	5.0	0.9
SALAD								
Caesar, No Chicken, Nando's*	1 Serving/220g	265	21.3	120	3.4	4.9	9.7	1.2
Couscous with Chicken, Nando's*	1 Salad/270g	371	24.8	137	2.9	10.2	9.2	1.9
Mediterranean, Nando's*	1 Salad/240g	230	17.4	96	3.8	3.0	7.2	1.8
Mixed Leaf, Fino Side, Nando's*	1 Portion/115g	17	0.4	15	0.7	0.3	0.3	1.1
Mixed Leaf, Nando's*	1 Portion/115g	17	0.4	15	0.7	0.3	0.3	1.1
SORBET								
Mango, Nando's*	1 Serving/135g	186	0.3	138	0.3	33.4	0.2	0.7
WRAP								
Beanie, Nando's*	1 Wrap/320g	698	29.2	218	7.2	25.3	9.1	2.1
Chicken, Breast, Fillet, Nando's*	1 Wrap/308g	608	21.4	197	13.7	19.1	6.9	1.0
Double Chicken, Breast, Fillet, Nando's*	1 Wrap/426g	774	23.7	182	18.4	13.8	5.6	0.7
Portobello Mushroom & Halloumi Cheese, Nando's*	1 Wrap/303g	618	33.1	204	5.5	19.7	10.9	1.3
Veggie, Nando's*	1 Wrap/320g	605	22.2	189	6.5	23.4	6.9	2.7
YOGHURT								
Banana, Frozen, Nando's*	1 Serving/100g	87	0.1	87	3.3	18.2	0.1	0.1
Chocolate, Frozen, Nando's*	1 Serving/100g	107	0.3	107	4.0	22.3	0.3	0.8
Strawberry, Frozen, Nando's*	1 Serving/100g	87	0.1	87	3.3	18.2	0.1	0.1
Vanilla, Frozen, Nando's*	1 Serving/100g	87	0.1	87	3.3	18.2	0.1	0.1
PIZZA HUT								
BACON BITS								
Pizza Hut*	1 Serving/12g	60	3.6	496	8.3	48.7	29.8	0.0
BEANS								
Chocolate Coated, Ice Cream Factory, Pizza Hut*	1 Serving/30g	142	5.4	475	5.5	72.2	18.1	0.0
BEETROOT								
Pizza Hut*	1 Portion/25g	14	0.0	55	0.9	12.0	0.1	0.0
BREAD								
Ciabatta, Garlic, Pizza Hut*	2 Pieces/253g	820	32.1	324	9.1	43.4	12.7	0.0
Garlic, Dipsters, Pizza Hut*	1 Piece/90g	308	14.2	342	6.8	43.1	15.8	0.0
Garlic, Pizza Hut*	1 Slice/30g	95	4.6	318	6.8	38.1	15.4	0.0

PIZZA HUT

	Measure INFO/WEIGHT	per Measure KCAL	per Measure FAT	Nutrition Values per 100g / 100ml KCAL	PROT	CARB	FAT	FIBRE
BREAD								
Garlic, with Cheese, Pizza Hut*	4 Pieces/187g	568	34.0	304	15.9	19.0	18.2	0.0
BREADSTICKS								
Garlic, Pizza Hut*	1 Stick/50g	173	6.7	347	9.8	46.9	13.4	1.0
BRUSCHETTA								
Light Lunch, Pizza Hut*	3 Pieces/211g	369	16.0	175	4.1	22.4	7.6	0.0
CAKE								
Chocolate Fudge, Dessert, Pizza Hut*	1 Piece/178g	684	31.9	384	4.2	51.4	17.9	0.0
Chocolate Fudge, Pizza Hut*	1 Piece/179g	686	32.0	384	4.2	51.4	17.9	0.0
CARBONARA								
Ham, Buffet, Pizza Hut*	1 Portion/200g	180	4.6	90	3.4	14.4	2.3	0.0
CHEESE								
4 & Vegetable, Buffet, Pizza Hut*	1 Portion/200g	210	8.6	105	4.0	12.6	4.3	0.0
Hard, Grated, Pizza Hut*	1 Serving/30g	121	9.0	404	33.0	0.1	30.0	0.0
Hard, Grated, Pizza Hut*	1 Serving/30g	121	9.0	404	33.0	0.1	30.0	0.0
Parmesan Reggiano, Grated at table, Pizza Hut*	1 Serving/5g	20	1.4	400	34.0	0.0	28.0	0.0
Three Cheese Melt, Starter, Pizza Hut*	3 Pieces/209g	546	38.1	261	11.1	12.3	18.2	0.0
CHEESECAKE								
Chocolate, Pizza Hut*	1 Serving/63g	228	11.1	360	5.6	44.9	17.5	0.0
Clotted Cream, Pizza Hut*	1 Serving/63g	205	10.4	323	4.6	39.3	16.4	0.0
Lemon & Ginger, Pizza Hut*	1 Serving/63g	205	9.7	323	4.2	42.4	15.2	0.0
New York Style, Baked, Pizza Hut*	1 Slice/113g	442	16.2	391	6.6	62.3	14.3	0.0
Vanilla, Madagascan, Dessert, Pizza Hut*	1 Serving/133g	397	18.1	298	4.8	39.2	13.6	0.0
CHICKEN								
Cheesy Jalapeno Poppers, Pizza Hut*	6 Pieces/150g	408	19.9	272	5.2	32.8	13.3	0.0
Dippin, Pizza Hut*	1 Serving/155g	332	14.4	214	15.7	17.1	9.3	0.0
Goujons, Pizza Hut*	5 Pieces/169g	311	13.5	184	17.0	11.0	8.0	1.5
Strips, Breaded, Five Strips, Pizza Hut*	5 Pieces/175g	283	13.2	162	15.9	8.9	7.5	0.0
Strips, Hot 'n' Kicking, Pizza Hut*	7 Pieces/140g	276	12.6	197	17.0	12.0	9.0	0.0
Wings, BBQ, Delivery Only, Pizza Hut*	6 Pieces/156g	303	14.4	194	23.2	4.6	9.2	0.0
Wings, BBQ, Pizza Hut*	6 Pieces/171g	306	14.5	179	21.3	4.4	8.5	0.0
Wings, BBQ, Saucy, Pizza Hut*	6 Wings/159g	355	21.8	223	21.4	3.6	13.7	0.0
Wings, Buffalo, Saucy, Pizza Hut*	6 Wings/181g	380	22.2	209	21.0	3.7	12.2	0.0
Wings, Spicy, Crunch, Delivery Only, Pizza Hut*	1 Portion/218g	510	30.5	234	17.0	10.0	14.0	0.0
Wings, Texan BBQ Chicken, Pizza Hut*	6 Pieces/159g	355	21.8	223	21.4	3.6	13.7	0.0
Wings, with Sour Cream & Chive Dip, Pizza Hut*	1 Pack/178g	680	56.1	382	22.8	1.9	31.5	1.3
CHICKEN STRIPS								
Breaded, with Wedges, 2, Kids, Pizza Hut*	1 Serving/231g	386	11.6	167	6.7	23.9	5.0	0.0
Breaded, with Wedges, 3, Kids, Pizza Hut*	1 Serving/265g	451	14.3	170	8.1	22.2	5.4	0.0
Breaded, Wrap Factory, 2, Kids, Pizza Hut*	1 Serving/247g	434	12.1	176	8.3	24.8	4.9	0.0
Breaded, Wrap Factory, 3, Kids, Pizza Hut*	1 Serving/325g	617	17.9	190	9.2	25.9	5.5	0.0
COLESLAW								
Pizza Hut*	1 Pot/38g	54	4.6	143	0.9	7.1	12.3	0.0
Pots, Delivery Only, Pizza Hut*	1 Pot/28g	38	3.1	134	0.8	7.4	11.2	0.0
COOKIE								
Dough, Ice Cream Factory, Delivery Only, Pizza Hut*	1 Portion/145g	650	30.0	448	5.9	59.4	20.7	0.0
CREAM								
Single, Dessert, Pizza Hut*	1 Serving/40g	75	7.2	188	2.6	3.9	18.0	0.0
UHT, Portion, Pizza Hut*	1 Portion/12g	23	2.2	188	2.7	3.9	18.0	0.0
CROUTONS								
Pizza Flavoured, Pizza Hut*	1 Serving/12g	23	3.1	196	10.1	55.2	26.1	0.0
Salad, Large, Pizza Hut*	1 Portion/20g	94	4.2	470	11.0	59.1	21.1	0.0

PIZZA HUT	Measure INFO/WEIGHT	per Measure KCAL	FAT	Nutrition Values per 100g / 100ml KCAL	PROT	CARB	FAT	FIBRE
DESSERT								
Cherries in Sauce, Pizza Hut*	1 Serving/20g	28	0.0	142	0.5	34.9	0.1	0.0
Chocolate Obsession, Pizza Hut*	1 Serving/100g	157	6.8	157	2.0	22.1	6.8	0.0
Cookie Dough, Pizza Hut*	1 Serving/345g	1063	47.6	308	4.0	41.9	13.8	0.0
Cookie Dough, Pizza Hut*	1 Serving/145g	650	30.0	448	5.9	59.4	20.7	0.0
Toffee Apple Meltdown, Pizza Hut*	1 Serving/120g	325	11.0	271	3.3	43.7	9.2	0.0
Vanilla Ice Cream Pots, Pizza Hut*	1 Serving/55g	110	6.4	200	2.8	19.9	11.6	0.0
DIP								
BBQ Sauce Portion In Restaurant, Pizza Hut*	1 Pot/28g	34	0.0	121	1.4	29.3	0.1	0.0
BBQ Tabasco, Pizza Hut*	1 Pot/25g	36	0.1	142	1.2	33.6	0.2	0.0
Garlic & Herb, Delivery Only, Pizza Hut*	1 Pot/28g	93	9.2	331	1.4	7.6	32.6	0.0
Garlic & Herb, Pizza Hut*	1 Pot/28g	93	9.2	331	1.4	7.6	32.6	0.0
Mayonnaise, Light, Restaurant Only, Pizza Hut*	1 Dippot/50g	163	16.5	326	0.6	6.0	33.0	0.0
Sour Cream & Chive, Restaurant Only, Pizza Hut*	1 Pot/28g	83	8.7	296	0.7	3.6	31.1	0.0
Sweet Chilli Sauce, Pizza Hut*	1 Pot/28g	48	0.2	172	0.3	32.9	0.8	0.0
Sweet Chilli Sauce, Restaurant Only, Pizza Hut*	1 Pot/28g	48	0.2	171	0.4	32.9	0.7	0.0
Tomato Ketchup, Restaurant Only, Pizza Hut*	1 Pot/28g	39	0.0	139	1.4	34.3	0.0	0.0
DOUGH BALLS								
Cheese & Jalapeno, Delivery Only, Pizza Hut*	1 Portion/198g	70	16.2	250	9.7	33.8	8.2	0.0
DRESSING								
1000 Island, Pizza Hut*	1 Serving/38g	107	9.7	280	0.7	11.5	25.5	0.0
Blue Cheese, Pizza Hut*	1 Serving/35g	91	8.0	258	1.7	11.5	22.7	0.0
Caesar, Pizza Hut*	1 Serving/40g	27	1.1	68	1.5	8.9	2.8	0.0
Ranch, Pizza Hut*	1 Serving/32g	163	18.0	510	1.2	1.5	56.4	0.0
Vinaigrette, Low Fat, Pizza Hut*	1 Serving/30ml	23	0.1	77	0.3	17.2	0.5	0.0
FISH								
Goujons 5 Strips, Pizza Hut*	5 Strips/210g	416	20.9	198	9.9	17.1	9.9	0.0
FRIES								
Seasoned, Savoury, Express Only, Pizza Hut*	1 Portion/145g	247	11.1	171	2.3	23.0	7.7	0.0
FUDGE BROWNIE								
Pizza Hut*	1 Serving/105g	418	16.4	398	4.3	60.1	15.6	0.0
ICE CREAM								
Coco Mango, Pizza Hut*	1 Serving/100g	88	1.8	88	0.6	17.3	1.8	0.0
Cookie Craving, Pizza Hut*	1 Serving/100g	149	6.9	149	1.6	20.1	6.9	0.0
Dairy, Dessert, Pizza Hut*	1 Serving/142g	272	12.6	192	4.6	23.3	8.9	0.2
Mix, Ice Cream Factory, Pizza Hut*	1 Serving/100g	147	6.2	147	4.0	18.8	6.2	0.0
Mix, Pizza Hut*	1 Serving/100g	147	6.2	147	4.0	18.8	6.2	0.0
Traditional, Dessert, Pizza Hut*	1 Serving/130g	251	13.5	193	2.6	22.4	10.4	0.0
Traditional, Kids, Pizza Hut*	1 Serving/89g	171	9.2	193	2.6	22.4	10.4	0.0
Traditional, Pizza Hut*	1 Serving/132g	254	13.7	193	2.6	22.4	10.4	0.0
Vanilla, Pots, Ice Cream Factory, Deliv Only, Pizza Hut*	1 Pot/55g	110	6.4	200	2.8	19.9	11.6	0.0
KETCHUP								
Heinz, Pizza Hut*	1 Serving/12g	14	0.0	119	0.5	28.4	0.1	0.0
Tomato, Sachet, Heinz, Express Only, Pizza Hut*	1 Sachet/12g	14	0.0	119	0.0	28.4	0.1	0.0
MACARONI CHEESE								
Pizza Hut*	1 Serving/41g	57	2.4	140	4.9	16.6	6.0	0.0
MARSHMALLOWS								
Mini, Ice Cream Factory, Pizza Hut*	1 Serving/30g	96	0.0	320	5.4	74.3	0.0	0.0
MAYONNAISE								
Heinz, Pizza Hut*	1 Serving/12g	88	9.7	731	1.3	1.8	81.2	0.0
Sachet, Heinz, Express Only, Pizza Hut*	1 Sachet/12g	88	9.7	731	1.3	1.8	81.2	0.0
Sachet, Pizza Hut*	1 Sachet/12g	88	9.8	731	1.3	1.8	81.2	0.0

	Measure INFO/WEIGHT	per Measure		Nutrition Values per 100g / 100ml				
		KCAL	FAT	KCAL	PROT	CARB	FAT	FIBRE
PIZZA HUT								
MEATBALLS								
in Pomodoro Sauce, Light Lunch, Pizza Hut*	1 Portion/253g	342	18.2	135	6.6	11.0	7.2	0.0
MILK								
Half Fat, Portions, Millac Maid, Pizza Hut*	1 Portion/14g	6	0.2	45	6.0	5.1	1.6	0.0
MILKSHAKE								
Strawberry Cheesecake, Pizza Hut*	1 Serving/236g	371	14.1	157	3.4	22.3	5.9	0.0
The Chocoholic, Pizza Hut*	1 Serving/248g	442	20.4	178	3.6	22.8	8.2	0.0
Toffee Banoffee Shake, Pizza Hut*	1 Serving/404g	763	22.6	189	2.4	32.3	5.6	0.0
MUFFIN								
Cheesecake, Sicilian Lemon, Pizza Hut*	1 Portion/130g	508	24.2	391	5.1	50.9	18.6	0.0
Fruity, Pizza Hut*	1 Serving/115g	366	13.7	318	4.1	48.4	11.9	0.0
Mixed Berry, Pizza Hut*	1 Muffin/108g	402	22.6	372	4.4	41.6	20.9	0.0
Sicilian Lemon Cheesecake, Pizza Hut*	1 Serving/130g	508	24.2	391	5.1	50.9	18.6	0.0
Strawberry & White Chocolate, Pizza Hut*	1 Muffin/108g	402	22.6	372	4.4	41.6	20.9	0.0
MUSHROOMS								
Blue Cheese, Pizza Hut*	1 Serving/256g	514	40.7	201	7.2	7.5	15.9	0.0
Breaded, Pizza Hut*	1 Serving/180g	410	14.4	228	4.5	26.1	8.0	0.0
Garlic, 2, Pizza Hut*	1 Serving/230g	570	43.4	248	7.9	7.0	18.9	0.0
Garlic, Crispy Coated, Pizza Hut*	1 Serving/135g	240	10.1	178	4.1	23.4	7.5	0.0
Garlic, with BBQ Dip, Pizza Hut*	1 Serving/112g	263	11.2	234	6.2	30.5	10.0	3.4
Garlic, with Sour Cream & Chive Dip, Pizza Hut*	1 Serving/112g	426	34.6	380	6.4	20.0	30.8	3.4
NACHOS								
Chilli, Pizza Hut*	1 Serving/190g	550	33.1	289	8.8	27.2	17.4	0.0
Sharing Starters, Pizza Hut*	1 Serving/356g	1087	76.3	305	7.9	24.6	21.4	0.0
Side, Delivery Only, Pizza Hut*	1 Serving/222g	669	40.3	301	7.7	30.2	18.1	0.0
OLIVES								
Mixed, Pizza Hut*	1 Serving/70g	140	9.0	200	1.5	19.6	12.8	0.0
ONION								
Chilli, Rings, Delivery Only, Pizza Hut*	1 Ring/12g	26	1.2	212	3.2	28.2	9.6	0.0
ONION RINGS								
Chilli, Pizza Hut*	8 Rings/100g	212	9.6	212	3.2	28.2	9.6	0.0
ONIONS								
White, Pizza Hut*	1 Serving/24g	10	0.0	42	1.0	10.0	0.0	0.0
PANCAKE								
Fruity, Kids, Pizza Hut*	1 Serving/155g	227	3.3	146	1.9	30.6	2.1	0.0
PASTA								
3 Cheese & Vegetable, Pizza Hut*	1 Serving/300g	315	12.9	105	4.0	12.6	4.3	0.0
4 Cheese, Sharing, Delivery Only, Pizza Hut*	1 Pack/1200g	1860	102.0	155	6.1	13.5	8.5	0.0
4 Cheese, Sharing, Pizza Hut*	1 Serving/1200g	1860	102.0	155	6.1	13.5	8.5	0.0
Alfredo, Chicken, Sharing, Delivery Only, Pizza Hut*	1 Pack/1200g	1680	40.8	140	8.1	19.1	3.4	0.0
Alfredo, Light Lunch, Pizza Hut*	1 Portion/226g	294	5.0	130	4.1	23.3	2.2	0.0
Alfredo, Pizza Hut*	1 Serving/400g	520	8.8	130	4.1	23.3	2.2	0.0
Alfredo, Pizza Hut*	1 Portion/400g	520	8.8	130	4.1	23.3	2.2	0.0
Arrabiata, Light Lunch, Pizza Hut*	1 Portion/226g	221	6.6	98	2.9	15.0	2.9	0.0
Arrabiata, Pizza Hut*	1 Portion/450g	441	13.0	98	2.9	15.0	2.9	0.0
Arrabiata, Pizza Hut*	1 Serving/450g	441	13.0	98	2.9	15.0	2.9	0.0
Bolognese, Sharing, Delivery Only, Pizza Hut*	1 Pack/1200g	1500	64.8	125	7.2	11.9	5.4	0.0
Bolognese, Sharing, Pizza Hut*	1 Serving/1200g	1500	64.8	125	7.2	11.9	5.4	0.0
Cannelloni, Spinach & Ricotta, Pizza Hut*	1 Serving/404g	565	27.4	140	6.2	13.1	6.8	0.0
Cannelloni, Spinach & Ricotta, Pizza Hut*	1 Portion/404g	566	27.5	140	6.2	13.1	6.8	0.0
Chicken Alfredo, Sharing, Pizza Hut*	1 Serving/1200g	1680	40.8	140	8.1	19.1	3.4	0.0
Ham & Mushroom, Pizza Hut*	1 Serving/450g	473	10.4	105	4.2	17.0	2.3	0.0
Lasagne, Traditional, Pizza Hut*	1 Serving/460g	589	26.7	128	5.9	13.0	5.8	0.0

	INFO/WEIGHT	KCAL	FAT	KCAL	PROT	CARB	FAT	FIBRE
PIZZA HUT								
PASTA								
Lasagne, Traditional, Pizza Hut*	1 Portion/460g	589	26.7	128	5.9	13.0	5.8	0.0
Macaroni Cheese, Kids, Pizza Hut*	1 Portion/250g	332	16.2	133	4.0	14.8	6.5	0.0
Mezzaluna, Tomato & Mozzarella, Pizza Hut*	1 Portion/350g	339	10.1	97	3.1	14.7	2.9	0.0
Salmone Penne Al Forno, Pizza Hut*	1 Serving/496g	832	49.1	168	7.5	10.6	9.9	0.0
Spaghetti Bolognese, New Kids, Pizza Hut*	1 Portion/235g	211	3.5	90	7.6	11.4	1.5	0.0
Tagliatelle, Alla Carbonara, Pizza Hut*	1 Serving/400g	548	32.4	137	5.6	10.4	8.1	0.0
Tagliatelle, Meatball, Italian Recipe, Pizza Hut*	1 Portion/240g	324	10.6	135	6.9	16.6	4.4	0.0
Tomato & Pepperoni, Pizza Hut*	1 Serving/300g	312	8.1	104	3.6	16.3	2.7	0.0
PASTA BAKE								
Salmon, Light Lunch, Pizza Hut*	1 Portion/200g	344	20.0	172	7.5	13.0	10.0	0.0
Salmon, Pizza Hut*	1 Portion/400g	692	42.8	173	7.9	11.3	10.7	0.0
PASTA SALAD								
Sweetcorn & Pepper, Pizza Hut*	1 Serving/47g	75	2.5	159	4.6	23.1	5.3	0.0
Tomato & Basil, Pizza Hut*	1 Serving/50g	50	0.7	100	3.7	17.8	1.5	0.0
PENNE								
Mediterranean Vegetable, Pizza Hut*	1 Portion/448g	592	19.7	132	3.7	18.3	4.4	0.0
PEPPERS								
Red & Green Wedges, Pizza Hut*	1 Serving/40g	6	0.1	15	0.8	2.6	0.3	0.0
Romano, Stuffed, Pizza Hut*	1 Serving/208g	250	13.3	120	2.7	13.3	6.4	0.0
PIE								
Banoffee, Dessert, Pizza Hut*	1 Serving/125g	428	25.3	340	2.5	37.3	20.1	0.0
Banoffee, Pizza Hut*	1 Serving/100g	350	21.5	350	4.2	34.9	21.5	0.0
PIZZA								
BBQ Deluxe, Cheesy Bites, Pizza Hut*	1 Slice/143g	358	11.6	251	11.7	34.4	8.1	0.0
BBQ Deluxe, Individual Italian, Pizza Hut*	1 Serving/78g	185	6.1	238	10.9	34.3	7.9	0.0
BBQ Deluxe, Individual Pan, Pizza Hut*	1 Serving/79g	200	7.9	253	12.7	28.0	10.0	0.0
BBQ Deluxe, Italian, Individual, Pizza Hut*	1 Slice/78g	185	6.1	238	10.9	34.3	7.9	0.0
BBQ Deluxe, Italian, Large, Pizza Hut*	1 Slice/95g	239	8.0	252	14.3	29.7	8.4	0.0
BBQ Deluxe, Italian, Medium, Pizza Hut*	1 Slice/105g	253	8.0	241	12.0	31.1	7.6	0.0
BBQ Deluxe, Pan, Individual, Pizza Hut*	1 Slice/79g	200	7.9	253	12.7	28.0	10.0	0.0
BBQ Deluxe, Pan, Large, Pizza Hut*	1 Slice/122g	306	12.1	251	11.8	28.6	9.9	0.0
BBQ Deluxe, Pan, Medium, Pizza Hut*	1 Slice/107g	276	11.3	257	11.7	28.8	10.5	0.0
BBQ Deluxe, Stuffed Crust, Pizza Hut*	1 Slice/155g	337	10.4	217	11.6	31.9	6.7	0.0
Cajun Chicken, Hot One, Italian, Medium, Pizza Hut*	1 Slice/100g	250	9.3	250	12.5	29.1	9.3	0.0
Cajun Chicken, Hot One, Pan, Large, Pizza Hut*	1 Slice/125g	321	14.7	257	12.9	24.7	11.8	0.0
Cajun Chicken, Hot One, Pan, Medium, Pizza Hut*	1 Slice/105g	273	12.3	259	12.7	25.6	11.7	0.0
Cajun Chicken, Hot One, Stuffed Crust, Pizza Hut*	1 Slice/135g	331	10.8	245	13.3	30.0	8.0	0.0
Cheese Feast, Italian, Medium, Pizza Hut*	1 Slice/96g	260	11.3	272	12.3	29.1	11.8	0.0
Cheese Feast, Pan, Medium, Pizza Hut*	1 Slice/106g	299	15.0	283	14.6	24.2	14.2	0.0
Cheese Feast, Stuffed Crust, Pizza Hut*	1 Slice/132g	361	13.8	273	14.3	30.5	10.4	0.0
Chicken, Hi Light, Medium, Pizza Hut*	1 Slice/83g	189	5.5	230	13.2	29.2	6.7	0.0
Chicken Feast, Italian, Medium, Pizza Hut*	1 Slice/100g	249	8.6	248	14.1	28.6	8.6	0.0
Chicken Feast, Pan, Medium, Pizza Hut*	1 Slice/109g	283	12.0	259	15.5	24.6	11.0	0.0
Chicken Feast, Stuffed Crust, Pizza Hut*	1 Slice/133g	337	12.6	254	14.8	27.3	9.5	0.0
Chicken Supreme, Cheesy Bites, Delivery, Pizza Hut*	1 Serving/113g	247	7.7	218	11.8	29.5	6.8	0.0
Chicken Supreme, Cheesy Bites, Pizza Hut*	1 Slice/148g	322	10.0	218	11.8	29.5	6.8	0.0
Chicken Supreme, Cheesy Bites, Pizza Hut*	1 Serving/142g	309	9.6	218	11.8	29.5	6.8	0.0
Chicken Supreme, Individual Italian, Pizza Hut*	1 Serving/74g	169	4.4	229	10.7	35.4	5.9	0.0
Chicken Supreme, Individual Pan, Pizza Hut*	1 Serving/80g	186	8.0	231	11.6	26.9	9.9	0.0
Chicken Supreme, Italian, Individual, Pizza Hut*	1 Slice/74g	169	4.4	229	10.7	35.4	5.9	0.0
Chicken Supreme, Italian, Large, Delivery, Pizza Hut*	1 Serving/74g	158	4.9	213	11.1	30.7	6.6	0.0
Chicken Supreme, Italian, Large, Pizza Hut*	1 Slice/111g	217	6.4	196	9.8	29.3	5.8	0.0

PIZZA HUT

PIZZA

	Measure INFO/WEIGHT	per Measure KCAL	FAT	Nutrition Values per 100g / 100ml KCAL	PROT	CARB	FAT	FIBRE
Chicken Supreme, Italian, Medium, Delivery, Pizza Hut*	1 Serving/65g	133	4.3	203	10.9	28.3	6.5	0.0
Chicken Supreme, Italian, Medium, Pizza Hut*	1 Slice/102g	220	6.3	215	10.3	31.9	6.2	0.0
Chicken Supreme, Pan, Individual, Pizza Hut*	1 Slice/81g	186	8.0	231	11.6	26.9	9.9	0.0
Chicken Supreme, Pan, Large, Delivery, Pizza Hut*	1 Serving/99g	216	9.3	219	10.9	26.1	9.4	0.0
Chicken Supreme, Pan, Large, Pizza Hut*	1 Slice/124g	271	11.6	219	10.9	26.1	9.4	0.0
Chicken Supreme, Pan, Medium, Delivery, Pizza Hut*	1 Serving/86g	189	7.4	219	11.2	26.6	8.6	0.0
Chicken Supreme, Pan, Medium, Pizza Hut*	1 Slice/115g	251	9.9	219	11.2	26.6	8.6	0.0
Chicken Supreme, Stuffed Crust, Delivery, Pizza Hut*	1 Serving/122g	293	8.8	240	11.6	34.8	7.2	0.0
Chicken Supreme, Stuffed Crust, Pizza Hut*	1 Slice/153g	367	11.0	240	11.6	34.8	7.2	0.0
Country Feast, Italian, Medium, Pizza Hut*	1 Slice/109g	252	9.6	232	9.7	28.6	8.8	0.0
Country Feast, Pan, Medium, Pizza Hut*	1 Slice/115g	279	12.1	243	11.4	25.8	10.5	0.0
Country Feast, Stuffed Crust, Pizza Hut*	1 Slice/144g	326	10.8	227	11.5	28.4	7.5	0.0
Express, Chicken Supreme, Pizza Hut*	1 Serving/65g	143	5.8	221	10.1	28.1	9.0	0.0
Express, Hawaiian, Pizza Hut*	1 Serving/60g	147	6.4	245	10.5	29.9	10.6	0.0
Express, Supreme, Pizza Hut*	1 Serving/69g	165	7.6	242	10.7	27.8	11.2	0.0
Farmhouse, Cheesy Bites, Delivery, Pizza Hut*	1 Serving/106g	266	10.1	250	13.2	30.7	9.5	0.0
Farmhouse, Cheesy Bites, Pizza Hut*	1 Slice/133g	332	12.6	250	13.2	30.7	9.5	0.0
Farmhouse, Italian, Individual, Pizza Hut*	1 Slice/74g	188	6.0	253	11.8	33.1	8.1	0.0
Farmhouse, Italian, Large, Delivery, Pizza Hut*	1 Serving/63g	141	4.8	225	11.5	32.1	7.7	0.0
Farmhouse, Italian, Large, Pizza Hut*	1 Slice/92g	206	6.7	224	10.2	34.0	7.3	0.0
Farmhouse, Italian, Medium, Delivery, Pizza Hut*	1 Serving/56g	126	4.0	226	10.7	33.0	7.1	0.0
Farmhouse, Italian, Medium, Pizza Hut*	1 Slice/84g	192	5.4	229	10.2	35.7	6.4	0.0
Farmhouse, Pan, Individual, Pizza Hut*	1 Slice/70g	179	7.4	256	11.3	31.6	10.6	0.0
Farmhouse, Pan, Large, Delivery, Pizza Hut*	1 Serving/85g	206	8.9	242	11.4	29.7	10.4	0.0
Farmhouse, Pan, Large, Pizza Hut*	1 Slice/106g	257	11.0	242	11.4	29.7	10.4	0.0
Farmhouse, Pan, Medium, Delivery, Pizza Hut*	1 Serving/75g	182	7.8	242	11.3	28.6	10.4	0.0
Farmhouse, Pan, Medium, Pizza Hut*	1 Slice/100g	242	10.4	242	11.3	28.6	10.4	0.0
Farmhouse, Stuffed Crust, Delivery, Pizza Hut*	1 Serving/106g	235	8.0	222	11.8	30.0	7.6	0.0
Farmhouse, Stuffed Crust, Pizza Hut*	1 Slice/132g	387	10.0	293	11.8	30.0	7.6	0.0
Ham, Hi Light, Medium, Pizza Hut*	1 Slice/82g	184	5.5	225	12.1	29.1	6.7	0.0
Happy Hour, Chicken & Mushroom, Pizza Hut*	1 Serving/80g	165	5.4	207	9.6	27.6	6.8	0.0
Happy Hour, Ham & Sweetcorn, Pizza Hut*	1 Serving/86g	174	5.6	202	9.4	27.0	6.5	0.0
Happy Hour, Margherita, Pizza Hut*	1 Serving/78g	183	6.9	234	10.5	28.6	8.8	0.0
Happy Hour, Pepper & Tomato, Pizza Hut*	1 Serving/86g	163	5.4	189	8.0	26.1	6.3	0.0
Happy Hour, Pepperoni & Onion, Pizza Hut*	1 Serving/80g	179	6.9	224	9.4	28.2	8.6	0.0
Hawaiian, Cheesy Bites, Delivery, Pizza Hut*	1 Serving/109g	253	8.5	232	11.6	31.2	7.8	0.0
Hawaiian, Cheesy Bites, Pizza Hut*	1 Slice/136g	316	10.6	232	11.6	31.2	7.8	0.0
Hawaiian, Italian, Individual, Pizza Hut*	1 Serving/71g	164	4.2	229	9.8	37.9	5.8	0.0
Hawaiian, Italian, Large, Delivery, Pizza Hut*	1 Serving/68g	148	5.0	217	10.6	31.1	7.3	0.0
Hawaiian, Italian, Large, Pizza Hut*	1 Slice/99g	221	7.0	223	10.0	33.2	7.1	0.0
Hawaiian, Italian, Medium, Delivery, Pizza Hut*	1 Serving/60g	131	3.9	219	10.0	33.8	6.5	0.0
Hawaiian, Italian, Medium, Pizza Hut*	1 Slice/92g	201	5.6	219	9.8	33.3	6.1	0.0
Hawaiian, Pan, Individual, Pizza Hut*	1 Serving/73g	175	6.5	240	10.9	32.2	8.9	0.0
Hawaiian, Pan, Large, Delivery, Pizza Hut*	1 Serving/89g	234	10.2	262	10.6	32.6	11.4	0.0
Hawaiian, Pan, Large, Pizza Hut*	1 Slice/112g	293	12.7	262	10.6	32.6	11.4	0.0
Hawaiian, Pan, Medium, Pizza Hut*	1 Slice/109g	245	9.7	224	10.1	28.5	8.9	0.0
Hawaiian, Pan, Medium, Delivery, Pizza Hut*	1 Serving/82g	184	7.3	224	10.1	28.5	8.9	0.0
Hawaiian, Stuffed Crust, Delivery, Pizza Hut*	1 Serving/113g	245	8.2	217	11.0	30.7	7.3	0.0
Hawaiian, Stuffed Crust, Pizza Hut*	1 Slice/141g	306	10.3	217	11.0	30.7	7.3	0.0
Hot 'n' Spicy, Cheesy Bites, Pizza Hut*	1 Slice/127g	331	12.6	261	12.6	33.7	9.9	0.0
Hot 'n' Spicy, Italian, Individual, Pizza Hut*	1 Slice/66g	180	6.9	272	11.0	36.5	10.4	0.0
Hot 'n' Spicy, Italian, Large, Pizza Hut*	1 Slice/93g	236	9.4	254	11.2	32.7	10.1	0.0

PIZZA HUT

PIZZA

INFO/WEIGHT	Measure	per Measure KCAL	per Measure FAT	Nutrition Values per 100g / 100ml KCAL	PROT	CARB	FAT	FIBRE
Hot 'n' Spicy, Italian, Medium, Pizza Hut*	1 Slice/86g	222	8.4	259	11.0	34.5	9.8	0.0
Hot 'n' Spicy, Large Pan, Pizza Hut*	1 Serving/105g	266	11.4	254	12.0	30.2	10.9	0.0
Hot 'n' Spicy, Pan, Individual, Pizza Hut*	1 Slice/71g	183	7.9	259	10.9	30.4	11.2	0.0
Hot 'n' Spicy, Pan, Large, Pizza Hut*	1 Slice/105g	266	11.4	254	12.0	30.2	10.9	0.0
Hot 'n' Spicy, Pan, Medium, Pizza Hut*	1 Slice/93g	237	10.6	254	11.5	29.2	11.4	0.0
Hot 'n' Spicy, Stuffed Crust, Pizza Hut*	1 Slice/139g	329	11.0	236	11.8	33.1	7.9	0.0
Margherita, Cheesy Bites, Delivery, Pizza Hut*	1 Serving/103g	270	10.4	263	12.8	33.1	10.1	0.0
Margherita, Cheesy Bites, Pizza Hut*	1 Serving/128g	337	12.9	263	12.8	33.1	10.1	0.0
Margherita, Fingers, Kids, Pizza Hut*	1 Serving/95g	258	12.1	273	11.0	28.4	12.8	0.0
Margherita, Italian, Individual, Pizza Hut*	1 Slice/67g	177	5.4	264	11.9	39.2	8.0	0.0
Margherita, Italian, Large, Delivery, Pizza Hut*	1 Serving/61g	154	5.8	251	12.2	31.8	9.5	0.0
Margherita, Italian, Large, Pizza Hut*	1 Slice/91g	229	8.6	252	10.4	34.2	9.5	0.0
Margherita, Italian, Medium, Delivery, Pizza Hut*	1 Serving/54g	138	5.0	257	10.6	35.6	9.4	0.0
Margherita, Italian, Medium, Pizza Hut*	1 Slice/80g	205	7.0	256	11.0	35.7	8.8	0.0
Margherita, Pan, Individual, Pizza Hut*	1 Slice/70g	189	8.1	268	11.6	32.4	11.5	0.0
Margherita, Pan, Large, Delivery, Pizza Hut*	1 Serving/84g	219	10.0	261	11.6	29.8	11.9	0.0
Margherita, Pan, Large, Pizza Hut*	1 Slice/104g	273	12.4	261	11.6	29.8	11.9	0.0
Margherita, Pan, Medium, Delivery, Pizza Hut*	1 Serving/72g	192	8.6	265	11.6	30.6	11.8	0.0
Margherita, Pan, Medium, Pizza Hut*	1 Slice/97g	248	11.4	256	11.6	30.6	11.8	0.0
Margherita, Stuffed Crust, Delivery, Pizza Hut*	1 Serving/102g	255	9.0	248	14.0	31.6	8.8	0.0
Margherita, Stuffed Crust, Pizza Hut*	1 Slice/140g	349	12.4	248	14.0	31.6	8.8	0.0
Margherita, Thick, Kids, Pizza Hut*	1 Serving/202g	506	17.9	251	9.0	33.0	8.9	0.0
Meat Feast, Cheesy Bites, Delivery, Pizza Hut*	1 Serving/114g	310	13.0	272	13.9	30.3	11.4	0.0
Meat Feast, Cheesy Bites, Pizza Hut*	1 Slice/142g	387	16.2	272	13.9	30.3	11.4	0.0
Meat Feast, Italian, Individual, Pizza Hut*	1 Slice/81g	220	8.8	270	13.9	32.3	10.8	0.0
Meat Feast, Italian, Large, Delivery, Pizza Hut*	1 Serving/74g	187	8.0	251	12.5	29.6	10.7	0.0
Meat Feast, Italian, Large, Pizza Hut*	1 Slice/111g	279	12.7	251	12.9	27.3	11.4	0.0
Meat Feast, Italian, Medium, Delivery, Pizza Hut*	1 Serving/66g	169	7.4	257	12.0	29.8	11.2	0.0
Meat Feast, Italian, Medium, Pizza Hut*	1 Slice/100g	257	11.0	258	13.0	30.0	11.0	0.0
Meat Feast, Pan, Individual, Pizza Hut*	1 Slice/84g	220	9.9	262	13.3	27.6	11.8	0.0
Meat Feast, Pan, Large, Delivery, Pizza Hut*	1 Serving/99g	275	13.1	277	12.6	29.1	13.2	0.0
Meat Feast, Pan, Large, Pizza Hut*	1 Slice/124g	344	16.4	277	12.6	29.1	13.2	0.0
Meat Feast, Pan, Medium, Delivery, Pizza Hut*	1 Serving/84g	221	10.5	262	12.2	28.0	12.4	0.0
Meat Feast, Pan, Medium, Pizza Hut*	1 Slice/112g	294	13.9	262	12.2	28.0	12.4	0.0
Meat Feast, Stuffed Crust, Delivery, Pizza Hut*	1 Serving/122g	301	12.7	247	13.5	28.0	10.4	0.0
Meat Feast, Stuffed Crust, Pizza Hut*	1 Slice/152g	376	15.8	247	13.5	28.0	10.4	0.0
Meaty, The Edge, Medium, Pizza Hut*	1 Slice/36g	110	5.7	308	17.0	20.4	16.1	0.0
Meaty BBQ, Cheesy Bites, Delivery, Pizza Hut*	1 Serving/115g	282	10.8	245	11.3	31.1	9.4	0.0
Meaty BBQ, Italian, Medium, Delivery, Pizza Hut*	1 Serving/70g	154	5.0	220	10.9	30.0	7.2	0.0
Meaty BBQ, Pan, Medium, Delivery, Pizza Hut*	1 Serving/92g	215	8.7	234	11.1	25.9	9.5	0.0
Meaty BBQ, Pan, Large, Delivery, Pizza Hut*	1 Serving/111g	313	9.2	282	10.7	26.4	8.3	0.0
Meaty BBQ, Stuffed Crust, Delivery, Pizza Hut*	1 Serving/122g	259	9.0	213	12.0	28.3	7.4	0.0
Mediterranean Meat Deluxe, Italian, Individ, Pizza Hut*	1 Slice/72g	206	8.8	288	12.6	34.7	12.3	0.0
Mediterranean Meat Deluxe, Italian, Medium, Pizza Hut*	1 Slice/91g	245	9.4	270	12.8	33.5	10.4	0.0
Mediterranean Meat Deluxe, Pan, Individual, Pizza Hut*	1 Slice/75g	212	10.4	284	13.5	29.5	13.9	0.0
Mediterranean Meat Deluxe, Pan, Medium, Pizza Hut*	1 Slice/98g	245	11.2	249	11.7	28.1	11.4	0.0
Mountain Fantastico, Italian, Individual, Pizza Hut*	1 Slice/75g	183	6.3	245	9.3	36.4	8.5	0.0
Pepperoni Feast, Cheesy Bites, Delivery, Pizza Hut*	1 Serving/108g	306	13.4	284	15.8	29.6	12.4	0.0
Pepperoni Feast, Cheesy Bites, Pizza Hut*	1 Slice/135g	382	16.7	284	15.8	29.6	12.4	0.0
Pepperoni Feast, Italian, Individual, Pizza Hut*	1 Slice/73g	205	8.4	282	11.4	36.3	11.6	0.0
Pepperoni Feast, Italian, Large, Delivery, Pizza Hut*	1 Serving/68g	195	9.5	286	12.0	30.8	14.0	0.0
Pepperoni Feast, Italian, Large, Pizza Hut*	1 Slice/103g	286	13.3	278	12.2	30.9	12.9	0.0

	Measure INFO/WEIGHT	per Measure KCAL	FAT	KCAL	PROT	CARB	FAT	FIBRE
PIZZA HUT								
PIZZA								
Pepperoni Feast, Italian, Medium, Delivery, Pizza Hut*	1 Serving/63g	171	7.5	270	12.4	30.6	11.9	0.0
Pepperoni Feast, Italian, Medium, Pizza Hut*	1 Slice/93g	254	9.8	273	12.3	35.0	10.5	0.0
Pepperoni Feast, Pan, Individual, Pizza Hut*	1 Slice/79g	227	10.8	286	12.3	30.3	13.6	0.0
Pepperoni Feast, Pan, Large, Delivery, Pizza Hut*	1 Serving/92g	278	16.2	302	12.0	26.4	17.6	0.0
Pepperoni Feast, Pan, Large, Pizza Hut*	1 Slice/115g	347	20.2	302	12.0	26.4	17.6	0.0
Pepperoni Feast, Pan, Medium, Delivery, Pizza Hut*	1 Serving/80g	223	11.9	279	12.6	26.2	14.9	0.0
Pepperoni Feast, Pan, Medium, Pizza Hut*	1 Slice/106g	297	15.9	279	12.6	26.2	14.9	0.0
Pepperoni Feast, Stuffed Crust, Delivery, Pizza Hut*	1 Serving/115g	300	13.0	261	13.1	30.4	11.3	0.0
Pepperoni Feast, Stuffed Crust, Pizza Hut*	1 Slice/143g	375	16.2	261	13.1	30.4	11.3	0.0
Seafood Fantastico, Italian, Individual, Pizza Hut*	1 Slice/81g	173	4.6	213	15.3	25.1	5.7	0.0
Seafood Fantastico, Italian, Large, Pizza Hut*	1 Slice/106g	228	6.6	215	15.1	24.6	6.2	0.0
Seafood Lovers, Italian, Individual, Pizza Hut*	1 Slice/66g	170	5.4	258	9.8	38.4	8.2	0.0
Seafood Lovers, Italian, Large, Pizza Hut*	1 Slice/90g	215	6.8	239	10.2	35.3	7.6	0.0
Seafood Lovers, Italian, Medium, Pizza Hut*	1 Slice/82g	202	6.6	245	10.1	35.3	8.0	0.0
Seafood Lovers, Pan, Individual, Pizza Hut*	1 Slice/69g	160	6.0	232	10.7	31.3	8.7	0.0
Seafood Lovers, Pan, Large, Pizza Hut*	1 Serving/106g	260	12.0	245	10.4	28.2	11.3	0.0
Seafood Lovers, Pan, Medium, Pizza Hut*	1 Slice/98g	233	10.4	237	9.7	28.3	10.6	0.0
Seafood Lovers, Stuffed Crust, Pizza Hut*	1 Slice/131g	314	10.9	239	12.3	31.8	8.3	0.0
Spicy, Hot One, Pan, Medium, Pizza Hut*	1 Slice/115g	274	13.0	239	11.2	23.1	11.3	0.0
Stuffed Crust, Cheesy Bites, Delivery, Pizza Hut*	1 Serving/129g	312	12.7	241	11.9	29.0	9.8	0.0
Stuffed Crust, Italian, Large, Delivery, Pizza Hut*	1 Serving/85g	198	8.6	234	11.7	26.9	10.2	0.0
Stuffed Crust, Italian, Medium, Delivery, Pizza Hut*	1 Serving/76g	170	7.8	225	11.0	25.3	10.3	0.0
Stuffed Crust, Pan, Large, Delivery, Pizza Hut*	1 Serving/120g	289	14.5	241	10.9	25.0	12.1	0.0
Stuffed Crust, Pan, Medium, Delivery, Pizza Hut*	1 Serving/100g	234	12.0	234	11.6	22.9	12.0	0.0
Stuffed Crust, Stuffed Crust, Delivery, Pizza Hut*	1 Serving/136g	305	12.6	225	11.5	27.2	9.3	0.0
Super Supreme, Cheesy Bites, Pizza Hut*	1 Slice/162g	393	16.2	242	12.4	26.9	10.0	0.0
Super Supreme, Italian, Individual, Pizza Hut*	1 Slice/97g	260	11.0	267	13.9	27.3	11.3	0.0
Super Supreme, Italian, Large, Pizza Hut*	1 Slice/128g	281	13.2	219	10.6	24.4	10.3	0.0
Super Supreme, Italian, Medium, Pizza Hut*	1 Slice/119g	267	11.5	225	11.1	26.3	9.7	0.0
Super Supreme, Pan, Individual, Pizza Hut*	1 Slice/96g	228	10.9	237	11.9	24.8	11.3	0.0
Super Supreme, Pan, Large, Pizza Hut*	1 Slice/148g	346	17.7	234	11.4	22.5	12.0	0.0
Super Supreme, Pan, Medium, Pizza Hut*	1 Slice/127g	323	18.5	255	11.4	22.8	14.6	0.0
Super Supreme, Stuffed Crust, Pizza Hut*	1 Serving/165g	366	16.5	222	11.9	25.2	10.0	0.0
Super Supreme, Stuffed Crust, Pizza Hut*	1 Slice/165g	397	14.3	241	11.7	29.0	8.7	0.0
Supreme, Cheesy Bites, Delivery, Pizza Hut*	1 Serving/118g	296	11.6	251	12.6	29.9	9.8	0.0
Supreme, Cheesy Bites, Pizza Hut*	1 Serving/147g	369	14.4	251	12.6	29.9	9.8	0.0
Supreme, Italian, Individual, Pizza Hut*	1 Slice/81g	204	7.5	251	10.9	33.5	9.2	0.0
Supreme, Italian, Large, Delivery, Pizza Hut*	1 Serving/74g	178	7.6	240	11.4	28.7	10.3	0.0
Supreme, Italian, Large, Pizza Hut*	1 Slice/113g	264	11.0	233	9.7	29.6	9.7	0.0
Supreme, Italian, Medium, Delivery, Pizza Hut*	1 Serving/69g	155	6.3	224	10.0	28.8	9.1	0.0
Supreme, Italian, Medium, Pizza Hut*	1 Slice/110g	286	11.7	261	12.2	28.9	10.7	0.0
Supreme, Pan, Individual, Pizza Hut*	1 Slice/84g	209	9.6	248	11.0	28.0	11.4	0.0
Supreme, Pan, Large, Delivery, Pizza Hut*	1 Serving/106g	242	12.3	228	10.4	24.0	11.6	0.0
Supreme, Pan, Large, Pizza Hut*	1 Serving/132g	302	15.4	228	10.4	24.0	11.6	0.0
Supreme, Pan, Medium, Delivery, Pizza Hut*	1 Serving/90g	232	11.7	259	10.5	27.0	13.1	0.0
Supreme, Pan, Medium, Pizza Hut*	1 Serving/120g	310	15.7	259	10.5	27.0	13.1	0.0
Supreme, Stuffed Crust, Pizza Hut*	1 Slice/160g	371	13.8	232	11.9	29.7	8.6	0.0
The Sizzler, Cajun Chicken, Italian, Large, Pizza Hut*	1 Serving/83g	177	6.1	213	11.2	28.1	7.4	0.0
The Sizzler, Cajun Chicken, Italian, Medium, Pizza Hut*	1 Serving/67g	147	4.8	220	11.8	30.2	7.2	0.0
The Sizzler, Cajun Chicken, Pan, Large, Pizza Hut*	1 Serving/90g	215	7.9	238	10.8	27.2	8.8	0.0
The Sizzler, Cajun Chicken, Pan, Medium, Pizza Hut*	1 Serving/75g	166	7.0	221	10.3	27.3	9.3	0.0
The Sizzler, Cajun Chicken, Stuffed Crust, Pizza Hut*	1 Serving/114g	270	9.8	236	11.7	31.7	8.6	0.0

	Measure INFO/WEIGHT	per Measure KCAL	per Measure FAT	Nutrition Values per 100g / 100ml KCAL	PROT	CARB	FAT	FIBRE

PIZZA HUT
PIZZA

	Measure INFO/WEIGHT	KCAL	FAT	KCAL	PROT	CARB	FAT	FIBRE
The Sizzler, Spicy Beef, Italian, Large, Pizza Hut*	1 Serving/80g	179	5.9	223	9.6	33.1	7.4	0.0
The Sizzler, Spicy Beef, Italian, Medium, Pizza Hut*	1 Serving/68g	163	6.1	240	10.9	31.6	9.0	0.0
The Sizzler, Spicy Beef, Pan, Large, Pizza Hut*	1 Serving/96g	240	11.0	250	10.5	29.1	11.5	0.0
The Sizzler, Spicy Beef, Pan, Medium, Pizza Hut*	1 Serving/76g	173	7.7	228	10.3	32.0	10.1	0.0
The Sizzler, Spicy Mushroom, Italian, Large, Pizza Hut*	1 Serving/79g	165	5.5	209	9.3	31.2	7.0	0.0
The Sizzler, Spicy Mushroom, Italian, Med, Pizza Hut*	1 Serving/65g	146	5.4	223	10.5	30.1	8.2	0.0
The Sizzler, Spicy Mushroom, Stuffed Crust, Pizza Hut*	1 Serving/116g	244	7.9	210	9.7	31.7	6.8	0.0
The Works, The Edge, Medium, Pizza Hut*	1 Slice/64g	150	6.7	235	12.7	19.5	10.4	0.0
Tortilla, Thin, Kids, Pizza Hut*	1 Serving/108g	264	14.4	245	9.1	20.9	13.4	0.0
Tuscani, Caprina, Pizza Hut*	1 Pizza/474g	990	45.5	209	9.0	20.6	9.6	0.0
Tuscani, Chicken & Mushroom, Pizza Hut*	1 Pizza/491g	1032	55.0	210	10.5	16.9	11.2	0.0
Tuscani, Mediterranean Meats, Pizza Hut*	1 Pizza/379g	1065	56.8	281	13.6	21.8	15.0	0.0
Tuscani, Rocket & Proscuitto, Pizza Hut*	1 Pizza/434g	829	36.9	191	9.2	19.2	8.5	0.0
Tuscani, Verde, Pizza Hut*	1 Serving/460g	878	42.3	191	8.0	18.6	9.2	0.0
Vegetable Supreme, Cheesy Bites, Delivery, Pizza Hut*	1 Serving/116g	250	8.0	215	10.0	30.7	6.9	0.0
Vegetable Supreme, Cheesy Bites, Pizza Hut*	1 Slice/145g	312	10.0	215	10.0	30.7	6.9	0.0
Vegetable Supreme, Italian, Individual, Pizza Hut*	1 Slice/77g	160	4.7	207	8.7	32.4	6.1	0.0
Vegetable Supreme, Italian, Large, Delivery, Pizza Hut*	1 Serving/74g	143	4.8	193	8.4	27.9	6.5	0.0
Vegetable Supreme, Italian, Large, Pizza Hut*	1 Slice/111g	222	6.3	200	7.4	32.5	5.7	0.0
Vegetable Supreme, Italian, Medium, Delivery, Pizza Hut*	1 Serving/66g	129	3.9	196	7.8	30.6	5.9	0.0
Vegetable Supreme, Italian, Medium, Pizza Hut*	1 Slice/99g	196	6.0	198	8.3	30.7	6.1	0.0
Vegetable Supreme, Pan, Individual, Pizza Hut*	1 Slice/84g	180	7.6	214	8.6	27.7	9.0	0.0
Vegetable Supreme, Pan, Large, Delivery, Pizza Hut*	1 Serving/101g	206	9.3	204	8.1	25.7	9.2	0.0
Vegetable Supreme, Pan, Large, Pizza Hut*	1 Slice/126g	258	11.6	204	8.1	25.7	9.2	0.0
Vegetable Supreme, Pan, Medium, Delivery, Pizza Hut*	1 Serving/82g	197	8.4	241	9.9	30.0	10.3	0.0
Vegetable Supreme, Pan, Medium, Pizza Hut*	1 Slice/109g	263	11.2	241	9.9	30.0	10.3	0.0
Vegetable Supreme, Stuffed Crust, Delivery, Pizza Hut*	1 Serving/125g	246	8.6	197	9.3	27.8	6.9	0.0
Vegetable Supreme, Stuffed Crust, Pizza Hut*	1 Slice/156g	307	10.8	197	9.3	27.8	6.9	0.0
Vegetarian, Hi Light, Medium, Pizza Hut*	1 Slice/77g	170	5.1	221	10.3	30.0	6.6	0.0
Vegetarian Hot One, Cheesy Bites, Pizza Hut*	1 Slice/142g	302	10.1	212	9.8	30.3	7.1	0.0
Vegetarian Hot One, Italian, Individual, Pizza Hut*	1 Slice/78g	164	4.5	211	8.1	34.6	5.8	0.0
Vegetarian Hot One, Italian, Large, Pizza Hut*	1 Slice/114g	165	6.7	145	7.5	19.1	5.9	0.0
Vegetarian Hot One, Italian, Medium, Pizza Hut*	1 Slice/98g	188	5.4	192	9.3	29.5	5.5	0.0
Vegetarian Hot One, Pan, Individual, Pizza Hut*	1 Slice/82g	174	6.0	211	8.8	29.6	7.3	0.0
Vegetarian Hot One, Pan, Large, Pizza Hut*	1 Slice/126g	290	12.1	231	9.4	29.7	9.6	0.0
Vegetarian Hot One, Pan, Medium, Pizza Hut*	1 Slice/115g	234	9.9	204	8.4	26.6	8.6	0.0
Vegetarian Hot One, Stuffed Crust, Pizza Hut*	1 Slice/161g	334	11.1	208	10.1	30.2	6.9	0.0
Veggie, The Edge, Medium, Pizza Hut*	1 Slice/60g	136	5.4	227	11.2	22.2	9.0	0.0

PLATTER

		KCAL	FAT	KCAL	PROT	CARB	FAT	FIBRE
Favourites, Pizza Hut*	1 Platter/732g	1385	82.4	189	8.7	13.5	11.3	0.0

POTATO SKINS

		KCAL	FAT	KCAL	PROT	CARB	FAT	FIBRE
Cheese & Bacon 6 Skins, Pizza Hut*	6 Skins/246g	408	17.8	166	6.4	20.1	7.2	0.0
Jacket, Loaded, with Cheese, Pizza Hut*	1 Portion/267g	571	34.2	214	13.6	11.2	12.8	0.0
Jacket, Pizza Hut*	1 Portion/ 223g	571	37.2	255	3.4	23.0	16.6	2.1
Jacket, with Sour Cream & Chive Dip, Pizza Hut*	1 Portion/224g	311	24.1	139	1.4	9.3	10.8	0.8

POTATO WEDGES

		KCAL	FAT	KCAL	PROT	CARB	FAT	FIBRE
without Dip, Pizza Hut*	1 Serving/390g	569	23.8	146	2.5	20.3	6.1	0.0

POTATOES

		KCAL	FAT	KCAL	PROT	CARB	FAT	FIBRE
Savoury Seasoned Fries, Pizza Hut*	1 Serving/144g	238	11.5	165	2.4	20.8	8.0	0.0

PROFITEROLES

		KCAL	FAT	KCAL	PROT	CARB	FAT	FIBRE
Dessert, Pizza Hut*	1 Serving/100g	381	31.3	381	4.6	20.1	31.3	0.0

PIZZA HUT

	Measure INFO/WEIGHT	per Measure KCAL	FAT	Nutrition Values per 100g / 100ml KCAL	PROT	CARB	FAT	FIBRE
PUDDING								
Sticky Toffee, Pizza Hut*	1 Serving/105g	400	18.2	380	5.5	50.6	17.3	0.0
RAISINS								
Chocolate, Ice Cream Factory, Pizza Hut*	1 Serving/30g	121	4.3	405	5.4	63.3	14.2	0.0
SALAD								
4 Leaf Mix, Pizza Hut*	1 Serving/100g	14	0.5	14	0.8	1.7	0.5	0.0
Caesar, Chicken, Small, Light Lunch, Pizza Hut*	1 Portion/172g	263	12.7	153	14.1	7.4	7.4	0.0
Caesar, Classic, Pizza Hut*	1 Portion/194g	367	23.1	189	7.2	13.0	11.9	0.0
Caesar, Classic, Small, Light Lunch, Pizza Hut*	1 Portion/97g	183	11.5	189	7.2	13.0	11.9	0.0
Caesar, Pizza Hut*	1 Salad/195g	344	20.2	177	6.0	14.8	10.4	0.0
Caesar, Prawn, Small, Light Lunch, Pizza Hut*	1 Portion/172g	229	12.0	133	9.6	7.6	7.0	0.0
SALAD								
Chicken & Bacon, Pizza Hut*	1 Serving/323g	514	32.0	159	10.3	6.9	9.9	0.0
Chicken Caesar, Pizza Hut*	1 Portion/175g	297	14.9	170	11.5	11.7	8.5	0.0
Chicken Caesar, Pizza Hut*	1 Serving/344g	527	25.5	153	14.1	7.4	7.4	0.0
Chicken Caesar, Small, Happy Hour, Pizza Hut*	1 Serving/172g	263	12.7	153	14.1	7.4	7.4	0.0
Chicken Caesar, with Bacon, Pizza Hut*	1 Serving/374g	588	29.6	157	14.4	6.8	7.9	0.0
Classic Caesar, Pizza Hut*	1 Serving/194g	366	23.1	189	7.2	13.0	11.9	0.0
Classic Caesar, Small, Happy Hour, Pizza Hut*	1 Serving/97g	183	11.5	189	7.2	13.0	11.9	0.0
Dressed, Pasta, Tomato, Med, Pizza Hut*	1 Serving/100g	112	1.5	112	3.5	21.2	1.5	0.0
Dressed, Tabbouleh, Pizza Hut*	1 Serving/100g	189	8.1	189	4.2	24.9	8.1	0.0
Fresh, Apple & Grape, Mix, Pizza Hut*	1 Portion/80g	39	0.8	49	0.4	12.0	1.0	0.0
Fresh, Carrot, Grated, Pizza Hut*	1 Serving/17g	5	0.1	30	0.7	6.0	0.5	0.0
Fresh, Cucumber, Slices, Pizza Hut*	1 Serving/80g	8	0.1	10	0.7	1.5	0.1	0.0
Fresh, Onion, Red, Slices, Pizza Hut*	1 Portion/80g	29	0.2	36	1.2	7.9	0.2	0.0
Fresh, Seasonal, Pizza Hut*	1 Serving/80g	12	0.5	15	0.7	1.8	0.6	0.0
Fresh, Tomatoes, Cherry, Pizza Hut*	1 Serving/80g	15	0.3	19	0.8	3.0	0.4	0.0
Goats Cheese, Pizza Hut*	1 Portion/340g	524	40.1	154	7.5	4.4	11.8	0.0
Grated Hard Cheese, Pizza Hut*	1 Serving/50g	202	15.0	404	33.0	0.0	30.0	0.0
Leaf Mix, Pizza Hut*	1 Serving/41g	7	0.5	17	2.9	6.3	1.1	0.0
Mozzarella & Tomato, Light Lunch, Pizza Hut*	1 Serving/188g	387	30.6	206	12.3	2.4	16.3	0.0
Mozzarella & Tomato, Pizza Hut*	1 Salad/160g	234	19.0	146	7.7	2.1	11.9	0.0
Olive & Feta, Pizza Hut*	1 Portion/406g	345	26.0	85	3.8	3.6	6.4	0.0
Potato, Whole, Pizza Hut*	1 Serving/100g	154	10.1	154	1.6	13.5	10.1	0.0
Prawn Caesar, Small, Happy Hour, Pizza Hut*	1 Serving/172g	229	12.1	133	9.6	7.6	7.0	0.0
Prawn, Caesar, Pizza Hut*	1 Portion/345g	459	24.1	133	9.6	7.6	7.0	0.0
Seasonal, Pizza Hut*	1 Serving/80g	12	0.5	15	0.7	1.8	0.6	0.0
Tuna, Pizza Hut*	1 Portion/461g	378	8.8	82	10.4	5.9	1.9	2.0
Warm Chicken, Pizza Hut*	1 Salad/342g	403	17.4	118	11.0	6.8	5.1	0.0
SALAD BAR								
Adults Pasta, Pizza Hut*	1 Serving/100g	250	10.9	250	5.7	16.8	10.9	0.0
Apple & Grape Mix, Fresh, Pizza Hut*	1 Serving/80g	39	0.1	49	0.4	12.0	0.1	0.0
Baby Potatoes, Pizza Hut*	1 Serving/80g	63	1.4	79	1.2	14.6	1.8	0.0
Beetroot & Carrot, with Balsamic Vinaigrette, Pizza Hut*	1 Serving/80g	24	0.2	30	1.1	5.7	0.3	0.0
Carrot Batons, Fresh, Pizza Hut*	1 Serving/80g	28	0.2	35	0.6	7.9	0.3	0.0
Cherry Tomatoes, Fresh, Pizza Hut*	1 Serving/80g	15	0.3	19	0.8	3.0	0.4	0.0
Coleslaw, Pizza Hut*	1 Serving/80g	149	14.6	186	1.1	4.5	18.2	0.0
Cos Lettuce, Fresh, Pizza Hut*	1 Serving/80g	10	0.2	13	0.7	1.9	0.3	0.0
Cous Cous, Pizza Hut*	1 Serving/100g	219	9.0	219	5.0	30.0	9.0	0.0
Cucumber, Fresh, Pizza Hut*	1 Serving/80g	8	0.1	10	0.7	1.5	0.1	0.0
Gemelli Pasta, Pizza Hut*	1 Serving/100g	155	4.4	155	4.3	26.0	4.4	0.0
Kids Pasta, Pizza Hut*	1 Serving/100g	180	9.4	180	6.9	16.5	9.4	0.0
Melon Pieces, Fresh, Pizza Hut*	1 Serving/80g	27	0.0	34	0.8	8.2	0.0	0.0

	Measure INFO/WEIGHT	per Measure		Nutrition Values per 100g / 100ml				
		KCAL	FAT	KCAL	PROT	CARB	FAT	FIBRE

PIZZA HUT

SALAD BAR
Mixed Peppers, Fresh, Pizza Hut*	1 Serving/80g	12	0.2	15	0.8	2.6	0.3	0.0
Potato Salad, Pizza Hut*	1 Serving/80g	123	9.5	154	1.7	10.0	11.9	0.0
Red Onion, Fresh, Pizza Hut*	1 Serving/80g	29	0.2	36	1.2	7.9	0.2	0.0
Seasonal Salad, Fresh, Pizza Hut*	1 Serving/80g	12	0.5	15	0.7	1.8	0.6	0.0
Sweetcorn, Fresh, Pizza Hut*	1 Serving/80g	63	0.6	79	1.8	16.8	0.8	0.0
Tomato Pasta, Pizza Hut*	1 Serving/80g	149	7.4	186	3.7	21.8	9.3	0.0
Tomato Slices, Fresh, Pizza Hut*	1 Serving/80g	14	0.2	17	0.7	3.1	0.3	0.0

SAUCE
Caramel, Ice Cream Factory, Pizza Hut*	1 Serving/25g	77	1.0	307	0.7	67.2	3.9	0.0
Chocolate, Ice Cream Factory, Pizza Hut*	1 Serving/25g	74	0.6	298	2.0	66.8	2.5	0.0
Strawberry, Ice Cream Factory, Pizza Hut*	1 Serving/25g	70	0.0	280	0.0	69.5	0.0	0.0

SMOOTHIE
BananaBerry Split, Pizza Hut*	1 Serving/171g	258	0.4	151	1.5	33.6	0.2	0.0
Truly Tropical, Pizza Hut*	1 Serving/239g	234	0.3	98	0.6	24.0	0.1	0.0
Very Berry, Pizza Hut*	1 Serving/220g	189	0.3	86	0.6	20.4	0.1	0.0

SPAGHETTI BOLOGNESE
Pizza Hut*	1 Portion/475g	745	31.3	157	6.2	17.8	6.6	0.0

SUNDAE
Double Chocolate, Pizza Hut*	1 Sundae/145g	307	16.2	212	3.1	27.0	11.2	0.0

SWEETCORN
Pizza Hut*	1 Serving/30g	24	0.2	79	1.8	16.8	0.8	0.0

TIRAMISU
Delivery, Pizza Hut*	1 Serving/75g	223	10.3	297	3.9	39.5	13.7	0.0
Pizza Hut*	1 Serving/83g	248	11.4	297	3.9	39.5	13.7	0.0

TOMATO
Spicy & Red Pepper, Buffet, Pizza Hut*	1 Portion/200g	170	1.8	85	3.1	16.7	0.9	0.0

TOPPINGS
Caramel Sauce, Pizza Hut*	1 Serving/100g	307	3.9	307	0.7	67.2	3.9	0.0
Chocolate Raisins, Pizza Hut*	1 Serving/100g	405	14.2	405	5.4	63.3	14.2	0.0
Chocolate Sauce, Pizza Hut*	1 Serving/100g	298	2.5	298	2.0	66.8	2.5	0.0
Coated Chocolate Beans, Pizza Hut*	1 Serving/100g	475	18.1	475	5.5	72.2	18.1	0.0
Lemon Sauce, Pizza Hut*	1 Serving/100g	280	0.0	280	0.1	69.0	0.0	0.0
Mini Marshmallows, Pizza Hut*	1 Serving/100g	320	0.0	320	5.4	74.3	0.0	0.0
Strawberry Sauce, Pizza Hut*	1 Serving/100g	280	0.0	280	0.0	69.5	0.0	0.0

TUSCANI PLATTER
Pizza Hut*	1 Serving/461g	1223	89.5	265	8.8	13.2	19.4	0.0

PRET A MANGER

BAGUETTE
Chicken Caesar & Bacon on Artisan, Pret a Manger*	1 Pack/230g	619	29.4	269	14.2	24.0	12.8	1.8
Italian Prosciutto Artisan Baguette, Pret a Manger*	1 Pack/268g	570	26.3	213	9.1	21.9	9.8	1.9
Sweet Chilli Chicken & Coriander, Pret a Manger*	1 Pack/210g	390	11.4	186	10.2	23.8	5.4	1.5

BARS
Choc Bar, Pret a Manger*	1 Bar/76g	380	21.7	500	4.7	54.3	28.5	3.5
Chocolate Brownie Bar, Pret a Manger*	1 Bar/65g	289	17.0	445	4.6	47.7	26.1	1.4
Love Bar, Pret a Manger*	1 Bar/72g	324	18.3	450	6.0	49.2	25.4	3.5
Pret Bar, Pret a Manger*	1 Bar/65g	265	15.6	408	6.8	41.4	24.0	6.1

BISCUIT
Fruit & Oat Biscuits, Pret a Manger*	1 Pack/40g	187	9.8	467	8.2	50.0	24.5	6.2

BREAD
Artisan Soup Bread, Pret a Manger*	1 Serving/80g	175	0.6	219	7.2	45.6	0.7	2.0

BREAKFAST CEREAL
Bircher Muesli Bowl, Pret a Manger*	1 Bowl/206g	304	9.7	148	6.3	20.2	4.7	1.4

PRET A MANGER

INFO/WEIGHT	Measure	per Measure		Nutrition Values per 100g / 100ml				
		KCAL	FAT	KCAL	PROT	CARB	FAT	FIBRE
BREAKFAST CEREAL								
Honey & Granola Pret Pot, Pret a Manger*	1 Pot/133g	263	7.8	198	7.3	28.8	5.9	1.3
Hot & Cold Granola, Pret a Manger*	1 Serving/226g	579	19.9	256	6.4	38.4	8.8	3.5
Porridge, Pret a Manger*	1 Serving/300g	242	8.4	81	3.0	9.6	2.8	1.7
Porridge with Compote, Pret a Manger*	1 Serving/324g	267	8.4	82	2.8	10.8	2.6	1.7
Porridge with Honey, Pret a Manger*	1 Serving/321g	307	8.4	96	2.8	14.0	2.6	1.6
CAKE								
Apple Cake Slice, Pret a Manger*	1 Slice/100g	303	14.7	303	3.8	38.8	14.7	1.9
Banana Cake Slice, Pret a Manger*	1 Slice/103g	345	18.3	335	4.6	39.0	17.8	1.9
Carrot Cake Slice, Pret a Manger*	1 Slice/112g	402	22.3	359	4.0	41.0	19.9	2.3
Chocolate Cake Slice, Pret a Manger*	1 Slice/88g	354	20.9	402	5.3	41.7	23.7	1.4
Lemon Cake Slice, Pret a Manger*	1 Slice/100g	330	15.1	330	4.2	44.0	15.1	0.9
CHEESECAKE								
Lemon Cheesecake Pot, Pret a Manger*	1 Pot/120g	390	25.9	325	2.7	29.3	21.6	1.4
COFFEE								
Americano, Pret a Manger*	1 Serving/360ml	35	1.3	10	0.7	0.9	0.4	0.0
Cappuccino, Pret a Manger*	1 Serving/280ml	280	9.7	100	7.0	10.1	3.5	0.0
Espresso, Pret a Manger*	1 Serving/137ml	0	0.0	0	0.0	0.0	0.0	0.0
Filter Coffee, Pret a Manger*	1 Serving/360ml	35	1.3	10	0.7	0.9	0.4	0.0
Flat White, Pret a Manger*	1 Serving/250ml	75	2.7	30	2.2	2.9	1.1	0.0
Latte, Pret a Manger*	1 Serving/330ml	112	4.1	34	2.4	3.3	1.2	0.0
Mocha, Pret a Manger*	1 Serving/330ml	177	4.4	54	2.5	7.9	1.3	0.0
COOKIES								
Chocolate Chunk Cookie, Pret a Manger*	1 Cookie/90g	319	12.2	354	4.8	52.6	13.6	3.7
White Chocolate & Orange Cookie, Pret a Manger*	1 Cookie/90g	369	13.3	410	4.9	62.3	14.8	2.6
CRISPS								
Croxton Manor & Red Onion Crisps, Pret a Manger*	1 Pack/40g	181	9.9	452	6.5	50.5	24.7	7.0
Double Cheddar & Onion Topcorn, Pret a Manger*	1 Pack/25g	123	6.5	492	8.0	55.6	26.0	9.6
Maldon Sea Salt Crisps, Pret a Manger*	1 Pack/40g	184	10.4	460	5.5	51.2	26.0	7.5
Parsnip, Beetroot & Carrot Crisps, Pret a Manger*	1 Pack/25g	120	8.6	480	4.4	38.4	34.4	15.2
Sea Salt & Organic Cider Vinegar, Pret a Manger*	1 Pack/40g	178	9.7	445	5.2	52.0	24.2	7.0
Spicy Piri Chilli Crisps, Pret a Manger*	1 Pack/40g	190	10.1	475	5.2	56.7	25.2	5.2
Sweet Potato & Chipotle Chilli Crisps, Pret a Manger*	1 Pack/25g	123	8.2	492	5.2	44.8	32.8	9.6
CROISSANT								
Almond Croissant, Pret a Manger*	1 Croissant/100g	365	21.1	365	8.8	34.9	21.1	1.1
Chocolate Croissant, Pret a Manger*	1 Croissant/95g	406	24.3	427	7.9	45.2	25.6	3.6
Egg & Bacon Croissant, Pret a Manger*	1 Croissant/167g	483	20.1	289	11.3	20.6	12.0	1.8
French Butter Croissant, Pret a Manger*	1 Croissant/80g	304	15.9	380	8.5	41.7	19.9	2.6
Ham, Bacon & Cheese Croissant, Pret a Manger*	1 Croissant/110g	352	22.5	320	13.2	20.6	20.4	1.5
Mozzarella & Tomato Croissant, Pret a Manger*	1 Croissant/110g	373	24.6	339	13.4	20.2	22.4	1.3
Pain au Raisin, Pret a Manger*	1 Croissant/110g	311	13.5	283	5.1	37.4	12.3	1.6
DRIED FRUIT								
Dried Mango, Pret a Manger*	1 Serving/60g	200	0.2	333	1.5	84.5	0.3	3.7
FRUIT								
Five Berry Bowl, Pret a Manger*	1 Bowl/219g	368	15.1	168	5.2	20.3	6.9	1.4
Five Berry Pot, Pret a Manger*	1 Pot/148g	147	4.7	99	6.0	11.6	3.2	0.2
Kid's Fruit Pot, Pret a Manger*	1 Pot/140g	43	0.1	31	0.5	7.4	0.1	1.0
Mango & Lime, Pret a Manger*	1 Serving/135g	70	0.3	52	0.7	12.0	0.2	2.3
Pret's Fruit Salad, Pret a Manger*	1 Serving/250g	115	0.3	46	0.7	11.0	0.1	1.6
Seedless Grapes, Pret a Manger*	1 Serving/150g	96	0.2	64	0.4	15.4	0.1	1.0
Superfruit Bowl, Pret a Manger*	1 Serving/155g	71	0.2	46	0.8	11.0	0.1	2.0
Tropical Fruit Sticks, Pret a Manger*	1 Serving/200g	78	0.4	39	0.6	8.9	0.2	1.4

PRET A MANGER

Measure INFO/WEIGHT	per Measure KCAL	FAT	Nutrition Values per 100g / 100ml KCAL	PROT	CARB	FAT	FIBRE

GINGER BEER

	Measure INFO/WEIGHT	KCAL	FAT	KCAL	PROT	CARB	FAT	FIBRE
Pure Pret Ginger Beer, Pret a Manger*	1 Serving/330ml	152	0.0	46	0.0	11.4	0.0	0.0
GINGERBREAD								
Godfrey, Pret's Gingerbread Man, Pret a Manger*	1 Serving/54g	198	7.5	367	4.8	55.7	13.9	1.8
HOT CHOCOLATE								
Hot Chocolate, Pret a Manger*	1 Serving/305ml	268	5.9	88	3.5	14.1	1.9	0.0
JELLY								
Jelly, Elderflower & Raspberry, Pret a Manger*	1 Serving/135g	96	0.0	71	0.3	17.5	0.0	0.4
JUICE								
Apple Juice, Pret a Manger*	1 Serving/250ml	120	0.3	48	0.1	11.8	0.1	0.0
Carrot Juice, Pret a Manger*	1 Serving/250ml	60	0.3	24	0.5	5.7	0.1	0.0
Large Orange Juice, Pret a Manger*	1 Serving/520ml	229	0.0	44	0.6	11.0	0.0	0.1
Orange Juice, Pret a Manger*	1 Serving/260ml	114	0.0	44	0.6	11.0	0.0	0.1
JUICE DRINK								
Pure Pret Apple, Pret a Manger*	1 Serving/330ml	159	0.0	48	0.0	11.6	0.0	0.0
Pure Pret Grape & Elderflower, Pret a Manger*	1 Serving/330ml	146	0.0	44	0.0	10.6	0.0	0.0
Pure Pret Orange, Pret a Manger*	1 Serving/330ml	200	0.0	61	0.1	3.1	0.0	0.0
MOUSSE								
Chocolate Mousse, Pret a Manger*	1 Serving/100g	375	29.2	375	3.4	24.6	29.2	1.2
MUFFIN								
Double Berry Muffin, Pret a Manger*	1 Muffin/140g	537	26.8	384	5.5	46.0	19.1	2.1
High Fibre Muffin, Pret a Manger*	1 Muffin/130g	455	23.4	350	7.2	36.0	18.0	7.4
POPCORN								
Rock Salt, Skinny, Topcorn, Pret a Manger*	1 Pack/23g	115	6.1	500	8.3	53.5	26.5	10.4
Savoury, Skinny, Topcorn, Pret a Manger*	1 Pack/23g	96	3.0	417	9.6	65.3	12.9	12.0
Sweet 'n' Salt, Skinny, Topcorn, Pret a Manger*	1 Pack/25g	123	6.1	492	7.1	60.0	24.6	9.5
PRETZELS								
Pretzel, Pret a Manger*	1 Serving/120g	371	7.8	309	10.9	51.6	6.5	2.5
SALAD								
Chef's Italian Chicken Salad, Pret a Manger*	1 Serving/303g	323	23.5	107	6.7	2.6	7.8	1.9
Chicken & Pasta Salad, Pret a Manger*	1 Serving/267g	507	21.9	190	7.4	21.0	8.2	1.3
Crayfish & Thai Noodle Salad, Pret a Manger*	1 Serving/239g	174	5.2	73	4.7	8.4	2.2	1.5
Edamame Bowl, Pret a Manger*	1 Serving/125g	125	5.6	100	8.4	6.5	4.5	0.0
No Bread Crayfish & Avocado, Pret a Manger*	1 Serving/206g	182	15.0	88	4.7	1.5	7.3	2.2
Pole & Line Caught Tuna Nicoise Salad, Pret a Manger*	1 Serving/281g	138	3.8	49	6.7	2.7	1.3	1.0
Smoke Roast Salmon Salad, Pret a Manger*	1 Serving/323g	455	30.5	141	5.8	8.4	9.4	1.5
Superfood Salad, Pret a Manger*	1 Serving/327g	345	15.9	105	4.5	11.1	4.9	1.9
Wiltshire Cured Ham & Potato Salad, Pret a Manger*	1 Serving/294g	272	14.2	93	6.4	6.0	4.8	1.1
SANDWICH								
Beech Smoked BLT, Pret a Manger*	1 Pack/248g	493	28.8	199	8.5	15.4	11.6	1.6
Chicken, Ham & Swiss Cheese Club, Pret a Manger*	1 Pack/318g	492	20.0	155	11.5	12.9	6.3	1.3
Chicken & Pesto Bloomer, Pret a Manger*	1 Pack/273g	477	17.1	175	10.2	18.0	6.3	1.9
Chicken Avocado, Pret a Manger*	1 Pack/244g	463	24.8	190	8.6	16.0	10.2	2.8
Classic Ham & Eggs Bloomer, Pret a Manger*	1 Pack/225g	598	25.7	266	14.1	21.3	11.4	2.0
Classic Super Club, Pret a Manger*	1 Pack/274g	551	30.3	201	10.8	14.6	11.1	1.5
Coronation Chicken & Fruit Chutney, Pret a Manger*	1 Pack/290g	529	27.3	182	7.9	16.5	9.4	1.7
Cracking Egg Salad, Pret a Manger*	1 Pack/262g	439	23.6	168	6.6	15.1	9.0	1.5
Crunchy Humous Bloomer, Pret a Manger*	1 Pack/224g	511	17.5	228	10.1	30.1	7.8	7.0
Emmental Cheese Salad, Pret a Manger*	1 Pack/239g	494	28.2	207	8.3	16.9	11.8	1.8
Falafel & Humous, Moroccan, Pret a Manger*	1 Pack/285g	525	17.6	184	5.8	22.9	6.2	3.3
Free Range Egg Mayo, Pret a Manger*	1 Pack/185g	426	23.4	231	9.1	19.9	12.7	1.6
Kid's Cheese Sandwich, Pret a Manger*	1 Pack/127g	399	20.2	314	13.9	28.9	15.9	2.2
Kid's Ham Sandwich, Pret a Manger*	1 Pack/127g	289	8.2	228	13.4	28.9	6.5	2.2

PRET A MANGER

	Measure INFO/WEIGHT	per Measure KCAL	FAT	Nutrition Values per 100g / 100ml KCAL	PROT	CARB	FAT	FIBRE
SANDWICH								
Kid's Tuna Mayo, Pret a Manger*	1 Pack/150g	372	17.3	248	10.9	24.9	11.5	1.9
Mature Cheddar & Pret Pickle, Pret a Manger*	1 Pack/266g	486	25.2	183	7.1	17.5	9.5	1.6
Pret's All Day Breakfast, Pret a Manger*	1 Pack/329g	654	37.7	199	9.9	14.1	11.5	1.4
Red Pepper Tapenade & Soft Cheese, Pret a Manger*	1 Pack/225g	394	18.3	175	6.0	19.5	8.1	2.7
Scottish Smoked Salmon, Pret a Manger*	1 Pack/158g	348	11.5	220	16.5	21.8	7.3	1.7
Sweet Chilli Crayfish & Mango Bloomer, Pret a Manger*	1 Pack/215g	401	12.2	187	9.3	24.6	5.7	2.3
The New York Bloomer, Pret a Manger*	1 Pack/223g	525	23.9	235	11.9	25.2	10.7	2.5
Wensleydale & Chutney Bloomer, Pret a Manger*	1 Pack/276g	564	26.1	204	8.9	20.9	9.5	2.2
Wild Crayfish & Rocket, Pret a Manger*	1 Pack/195g	370	17.1	190	8.3	19.4	8.8	1.6
SMOOTHIE								
Mango Smoothie, Pret a Manger*	1 Serving/250ml	143	0.5	57	0.6	13.7	0.2	3.0
Strawberry Smoothie, Pret a Manger*	1 Serving/250ml	128	0.8	51	0.9	11.2	0.3	0.0
Vitamin Volcano Smoothie, Pret a Manger*	1 Serving/250ml	135	0.8	54	4.6	12.4	0.3	2.3
SOUP								
Carrot & Coriander Soup, Pret a Manger*	1 Serving/370g	181	10.7	49	0.9	4.5	2.9	0.7
Chicken & Mushroom Soup, Pret a Manger*	1 Serving/370g	269	14.4	73	6.6	2.7	3.9	0.5
Chilli Beef & Rice Soup, Pret a Manger*	1 Serving/370g	270	9.2	73	5.4	7.3	2.5	2.8
Garden Pea & Mint Soup, Pret a Manger*	1 Serving/370g	215	8.9	58	2.4	5.9	2.4	1.8
Italian Meatball Soup, Pret a Manger*	1 Serving/370g	263	15.5	71	2.4	5.8	4.2	1.0
Leek & Potato Soup, Pret a Manger*	1 Serving/370g	189	9.3	51	1.2	5.5	2.5	0.9
Lentil & Smoked Bacon Soup, Pret a Manger*	1 Serving/370g	274	11.5	74	5.9	6.3	3.1	1.2
Malaysian Chicken Curry Soup, Pret a Manger*	1 Serving/370g	270	14.8	73	2.7	5.5	4.0	2.0
Moroccan Chicken Soup, Pret a Manger*	1 Serving/370g	304	9.9	82	4.5	8.8	2.7	2.4
Mushroom Risotto Soup, Pret a Manger*	1 Serving/347g	215	9.9	62	1.6	7.5	2.8	1.3
Pret's Classic Tomato Soup, Pret a Manger*	1 Serving/370g	259	17.8	70	1.6	4.7	4.8	0.7
Sag Aloo Soup, Pret a Manger*	1 Serving/375g	245	11.5	65	1.6	7.9	3.1	0.2
Spanish Chorizo & Butterbean Soup, Pret a Manger*	1 Serving/370g	233	8.9	63	3.8	6.1	2.4	1.1
SUSHI								
California Rolls, Pret a Manger*	1 Pack/206g	354	9.3	172	5.1	27.5	4.5	1.4
Deluxe Bento Box, Pret a Manger*	1 Box/267g	369	10.9	138	5.9	19.3	4.1	1.1
Maki & Nigiri, Pret a Manger*	1 Serving/200g	314	8.4	157	5.4	23.4	4.2	1.0
Salmon & Prawn Sushi, Pret a Manger*	1 Serving/232g	382	9.3	165	6.2	25.8	4.0	1.3
TART								
Pret's Bakewell Tart, Pret a Manger*	1 Serving/68g	315	17.7	463	7.2	50.0	26.0	2.2
TEA								
Pure Pret Still, Peach Iced Tea, Pret a Manger*	1 Serving/500ml	78	0.0	16	0.0	3.8	0.0	0.0
Red Berries Tea, Pret a Manger*	1 Serving/60ml	0	0.0	0	0.0	0.0	0.0	0.0
Tropical Green Tea, Pret a Manger*	1 Serving/60ml	0	0.0	0	0.0	0.0	0.0	0.0
TOASTIE								
Ham, Cheese & Mustard Toastie, Pret a Manger*	1 Toastie/215g	601	29.0	280	17.8	21.8	13.5	2.1
Italian Mozzarella & Pesto Toastie, Pret a Manger*	1 Toastie/233g	498	23.2	214	10.3	20.6	10.0	2.1
New York Deli Toastie, Pret a Manger*	1 Toastie/233g	586	28.0	251	15.2	21.3	12.0	2.4
Tuna Melt Toastie, Pret a Manger*	1 Toastie/218g	561	25.3	257	16.8	21.3	11.6	2.4
WRAP								
Avocado & Herb Salad Wrap, Pret a Manger*	1 Wrap/252g	461	30.2	183	4.8	14.1	12.0	2.7
Chunky Humous Salad Wrap, Pret a Manger*	1 Wrap/207g	340	18.3	164	5.1	16.1	8.8	1.3
Falafel & Halloumi, Hot, Pret a Manger*	1 Wrap/275g	567	22.6	206	6.5	21.6	8.2	1.2
Hoisin Duck Wrap, Pret a Manger*	1 Wrap/211g	433	20.1	205	9.5	20.7	9.5	1.4
Italian Pizza Hot Wrap, Pret a Manger*	1 Wrap/200g	391	17.2	195	8.7	20.8	8.6	2.4
Jalapeno Chicken Hot Wrap, Pret a Manger*	1 Wrap/243g	431	16.4	177	11.8	17.2	6.7	1.5
Swedish Meatball Hot Wrap, Pret a Manger*	1 Wrap/219g	566	26.0	259	13.3	24.9	11.9	2.2
Sweet Chilli Crayfish Salad Wrap, Pret a Manger*	1 Wrap/223g	282	10.1	126	5.9	15.5	4.5	1.3

	Measure INFO/WEIGHT	per Measure KCAL	per Measure FAT	Nutrition Values per 100g / 100ml KCAL	PROT	CARB	FAT	FIBRE

PRET A MANGER

YOGHURT

	Measure INFO/WEIGHT	KCAL	FAT	KCAL	PROT	CARB	FAT	FIBRE
Pure Pret Yoga Bunny, Pret a Manger*	1 Serving/330g	132	0.0	40	0.0	9.7	0.0	0.0
Yoga Bunny Bowl, Pret a Manger*	1 Serving/233g	210	5.0	90	5.2	10.9	2.1	1.0
Yoghurt Nuts, Pret a Manger*	1 Pack/75g	430	33.2	573	6.9	29.7	44.3	6.9

YOGHURT DRINK

Blueberry Probiotic Yoghurt Drink, Pret a Manger*	1 Serving/250ml	185	4.3	74	2.3	12.4	1.7	0.0
Vanilla Probiotic Yoghurt Drink, Pret a Manger*	1 Serving/250ml	200	4.5	80	2.5	13.2	1.8	0.0

STARBUCKS

BAGEL

Cheese, & Jalapeno, Starbucks*	1 Bagel/115g	292	3.6	254	10.8	45.8	3.1	1.5
Cheesy, Starbucks*	1 Bagel/90g	253	6.6	281	11.9	41.7	7.3	2.2
Cinnamon & Raisin, Starbucks*	1 Bagel/83g	190	1.2	229	44.8	9.4	1.4	1.3
Fruity, Starbucks*	1 Bagel/90g	338	16.1	376	9.7	44.5	17.9	3.4
Smoked Salmon & Dill Soft Cheese, Starbucks*	1 Bagel/145g	323	7.5	223	12.3	30.8	5.2	1.9

BARS

Almond, Cranberry & Yoghurt, Starbucks*	1 Bar/50g	220	12.7	440	6.6	46.0	25.5	10.2
Chocolate, Milk, Starbucks*	1 Bar/45g	252	16.5	559	8.4	48.8	36.7	0.0
Granola, Starbucks*	1 Bar/80g	348	19.7	435	7.3	46.4	24.6	4.4
Mango, Pistachio & Cashew, Fruit & Nut, Starbucks*	1 Bar/50g	200	10.5	401	7.7	45.0	21.1	16.9
Mini, Dark Chocolate, Starbucks*	1 Bar/43g	236	17.0	548	6.1	46.6	39.5	4.2
Mini, Salted Pecan, Starbucks*	1 Bar/50g	247	13.0	495	3.6	60.8	26.0	2.0
Rocky Road, Starbucks*	1 Bar/65g	366	26.7	563	4.2	46.6	41.1	2.2

BISCOTTI

Almond, Starbucks*	1 Biscuit/27g	120	4.8	446	10.4	61.6	17.6	11.4

BISCUITS

Ginger Snaps, Organic, Starbucks*	3 Biscuits/60g	267	9.2	445	4.8	71.9	15.4	1.5
Golden Crunch, Starbucks*	1 Biscuit/30g	144	6.6	481	5.1	65.4	22.1	2.0
Oat & Fruit, Starbucks*	1 Biscuit/60g	258	10.5	430	4.2	64.0	17.5	2.2

BREAD

Fruit, Luxury, Starbucks*	1 Serving/145g	486	12.0	335	7.0	58.0	8.3	2.3

BREAKFAST CEREAL

Porridge, Dried Fruit, Made with Full Fat Milk, Starbucks*	1 Serving/244g	344	9.5	141	4.3	23.1	3.9	1.6
Porridge, Dried Fruit, Made with Soy Milk, Starbucks*	1 Serving/244g	307	6.3	126	4.3	21.6	2.6	2.0

BROWNIES

Chocolate, Belgian, Fairtrade, Gluten Free, Starbucks*	1 Slice/65g	334	20.6	514	4.1	51.9	31.7	2.6

BUTTIE

Bacon, Starbucks*	1 Buttie/118g	376	13.6	319	19.6	33.6	11.5	1.2
Sausage, Starbucks*	1 Buttie/176g	479	22.2	272	12.3	27.0	12.6	0.9

CAKE

Almond Pops, Starbucks*	1 Serving/41g	211	13.0	515	7.2	49.2	31.7	2.2
Banana & Date, Skinny, Starbucks*	1 Slice/120g	300	3.5	250	3.9	52.1	2.9	2.5
Banana Date & Raisin, Wholemeal, Low Fat, Starbucks*	1 Slice/70g	169	2.0	242	5.0	49.1	2.9	3.4
Butterfly, Starbucks*	1 Slice/80g	361	18.2	451	3.4	58.2	22.7	0.5
Carrot, Skinny, Starbucks*	1 Slice/75g	192	2.5	256	4.0	54.1	3.3	2.1
Carrot, Starbucks*	1 Slice/125g	561	35.4	449	5.5	43.5	28.3	2.5
Carrot & Valencia Orange, Low Fat, Starbucks*	1 Slice/80g	200	2.4	250	3.3	53.0	3.0	3.0
Carrot Loaf, Starbucks*	1 Slice/100g	352	19.9	352	4.7	38.4	19.9	2.3
Chocolate, Fairtrade, Starbucks*	1 Serving/70g	330	19.8	471	10.9	40.7	28.3	4.6
Chocolate Decadence, Starbucks*	1 Slice/170g	717	41.0	422	4.4	46.9	24.1	1.4
Chocolate Hazelnut, Loaf, Starbucks*	1 Slice/120g	467	29.4	389	4.0	38.4	24.5	3.2
Chocolate Orange, Starbucks*	1 Slice/70g	276	14.8	395	5.7	45.4	21.2	1.9
Chocolate Velvet, Starbucks*	1 Slice/130g	534	25.1	411	4.8	53.0	19.3	3.1
Chocolate Whoopies, Starbucks*	1 Cake/35g	152	8.3	433	5.8	48.9	23.7	0.5

	Measure INFO/WEIGHT	per Measure KCAL	FAT	Nutrition Values per 100g / 100ml KCAL	PROT	CARB	FAT	FIBRE
STARBUCKS								
CAKE								
Coconut & Raspberry, Starbucks*	1 Cake/62g	267	14.6	430	4.0	49.9	23.6	1.6
Fruit, Starbucks*	1 Slice/80g	236	7.0	295	3.6	50.1	8.7	2.8
Ginger, Square, Starbucks*	1 Square/45g	202	12.7	450	4.3	45.0	28.2	0.9
Iced Fancies, Starbucks*	1 Cake/81g	307	10.5	379	2.3	63.7	13.0	0.6
Loaf, Lemon, Starbucks*	1 Cake/120g	445	27.1	371	4.6	37.5	22.6	1.0
Loaf, Raspberry & Coconut, Starbucks*	1 Cake/120g	524	33.7	437	4.3	41.8	28.1	2.1
Marshmallow, Chocolate, Twizzle, Starbucks*	1 Cake/35g	143	2.9	410	4.2	78.6	8.3	2.2
Mini, Raspberry & White Chocolate, Starbucks*	1 Cake/64g	302	15.9	472	3.9	57.1	24.9	1.9
Orange, Wheat & Gluten Free, Starbucks*	1 Serving/55g	138	7.3	251	7.4	25.8	13.2	3.3
Passion, Starbucks*	1 Slice/145g	528	31.9	364	4.3	37.2	22.0	1.8
Pops Sparkle, Starbucks*	1 Serving/40g	192	9.7	479	3.3	60.6	24.3	2.2
Red Velvet, Whoopies, Starbucks*	1 Cake/36g	161	8.7	448	5.4	52.0	24.1	0.8
Rocky Road Pops, Starbucks*	1 Cake Pop/44g	225	13.6	512	7.5	49.8	31.0	2.0
Victoria Sponge, Classic, Starbucks*	1 Slice/127g	490	25.1	385	3.2	48.4	19.7	0.8
Victoria Sponge, Mini, Starbucks*	1 Cake/65g	243	12.2	375	3.7	47.5	18.8	0.9
Yoghurt & Berry Loaf, Low Fat, Starbucks*	1 Slice/94g	254	4.8	270	5.3	50.8	5.1	1.7
CHEESECAKE								
Blueberry Swirl, Starbucks*	1 Slice/125g	482	31.6	386	5.5	33.6	25.3	0.8
Chocolate, Starbucks*	1 Serving/185g	723	49.6	391	6.9	30.5	26.8	0.8
COFFEE								
Brewed, Grande, Starbucks*	1 Grande/473ml	5	0.1	1	0.1	0.0	0.0	0.0
Brewed, Short, Starbucks*	1 Short/236ml	3	0.2	1	0.1	0.0	0.1	0.0
Brewed, Tall, Starbucks*	1 Tall/254ml	4	0.1	2	0.2	0.0	0.0	0.0
Brewed, Venti, Starbucks*	1 Venti/591ml	6	0.0	1	0.1	0.0	0.0	0.0
Caffe Americano, Grande, Starbucks*	1 Grande/473ml	17	0.0	4	0.2	0.6	0.0	0.0
Caffe Americano, Short, Starbucks*	1 Short/236ml	6	0.0	3	0.2	0.4	0.0	0.0
Caffe Americano, Tall, Starbucks*	1 Tall/335ml	11	0.0	3	0.1	0.3	0.0	0.0
Caffe Americano, Venti, Starbucks*	1 Venti/591ml	23	0.0	4	0.2	0.7	0.0	0.0
Caffe Latte, Grande, Semi Skimmed Milk, Starbucks*	1 Grande/473ml	188	7.0	40	2.6	4.0	1.5	0.0
Caffe Latte, Grande, Skimmed Milk, Starbucks*	1 Grande/473ml	131	0.3	28	2.7	4.0	0.1	0.0
Caffe Latte, Grande, Soy, Starbucks*	1 Grande/473ml	148	5.3	31	2.2	2.7	1.1	0.3
Caffe Latte, Grande, Whole Milk, Starbucks*	1 Grande/473ml	223	11.5	47	2.6	3.8	2.4	0.0
Caffe Latte, Short, Semi Skimmed Milk, Starbucks*	1 Short/236ml	95	3.5	40	2.7	3.8	1.5	0.0
Caffe Latte, Short, Skimmed Milk, Starbucks*	1 Short/236ml	67	0.1	28	2.7	4.2	0.0	0.0
Caffe Latte, Short, Soy, Starbucks*	1 Short/236ml	75	2.7	32	2.2	3.0	1.1	0.3
Caffe Latte, Short, Whole Milk, Starbucks*	1 Short/236ml	113	5.8	48	2.6	3.8	2.5	0.0
Caffe Latte, Tall, Semi Skimmed Milk, Starbucks*	1 Tall/335ml	148	5.6	44	2.9	4.2	1.7	0.0
Caffe Latte, Tall, Skimmed Milk, Starbucks*	1 Tall/335ml	102	0.2	30	3.0	4.5	0.1	0.0
Caffe Latte, Tall, Soy, Starbucks*	1 Tall/335ml	116	4.3	35	2.4	3.0	1.3	0.3
Caffe Latte, Tall, Whole Milk, Starbucks*	1 Tall/335ml	176	9.2	53	2.8	4.2	2.7	0.0
Caffe Latte, Venti, Semi Skimmed Milk, Starbucks*	1 Venti/591ml	242	9.1	41	2.7	4.1	1.5	0.0
Caffe Latte, Venti, Skimmed Milk, Starbucks*	1 Venti/591ml	210	0.4	36	2.8	4.2	0.1	0.0
Caffe Latte, Venti, Soy, Starbucks*	1 Venti/591ml	190	7.0	32	2.3	2.7	1.2	0.3
Caffe Latte, Venti, Whole Milk, Starbucks*	1 Venti/591ml	289	15.0	49	2.6	3.9	2.5	0.0
Caffe Misto, Cafe Au Lait, Grande, Soy, Starbucks*	1 Grande/473ml	82	3.2	17	1.2	1.3	0.7	0.2
Caffe Misto, Cafe Au Lait, Short, Whole Milk, Starbucks*	1 Short/236ml	65	3.5	28	1.5	2.1	1.5	0.0
Caffe Misto, Cafe Au Lait, Tall, Soy, Starbucks*	1 Tall/335ml	63	2.4	19	1.3	1.5	0.7	0.0
Caffe Misto, Cafe Au Lait, Tall, Whole Milk, Starbucks*	1 Tall/335ml	97	5.2	29	1.6	2.1	1.5	0.0
Caffe Misto, Cafe Au Lait, Venti, Soy, Starbucks*	1 Venti/591ml	104	4.0	18	1.3	1.3	0.7	0.2
Caffe Misto, Cafe Au Lait, Venti, Whole Milk, Starbucks*	1 Venti/591ml	160	8.6	27	1.5	2.0	1.5	0.0
Caffe Misto, Skimmed Milk, Starbucks*	1 Tall/354ml	64	0.0	18	1.8	2.5	0.0	0.0
Caffe Misto, Whole Milk, Starbucks*	1 Grande/442ml	134	7.0	30	1.6	2.3	1.6	0.0

STARBUCKS
COFFEE

INFO/WEIGHT	KCAL	FAT	KCAL	PROT	CARB	FAT	FIBRE
Caffe Mocha, Skimmed Milk, Starbucks*	1 Tall/354ml	175	1.3	49	0.3	9.3	0.4	0.4
Caffe Mocha, Skimmed Milk, with Whip, Starbucks*	1 Grande/473ml	324	11.6	68	3.0	9.3	2.4	0.4
Caffe Mocha, Whole Milk, Starbucks*	1 Tall/354ml	233	9.3	66	2.8	8.8	2.6	0.4
Caffe Mocha, Whole Milk, with Whip, Starbucks*	1 Tall/354ml	313	17.3	88	2.8	9.0	4.9	0.4
Caffe Mocha, with Whip, Short, Soy, Starbucks*	1 Short/236ml	167	8.5	71	2.5	8.5	3.6	0.6
Caffe Mocha, with Whip, Short, Whole Milk, Starbucks*	1 Short/236ml	198	11.0	84	2.8	9.3	4.7	0.4
Caffe Mocha, with Whip, Tall, Skimmed Milk, Starbucks*	1 Tall/335ml	228	8.0	68	3.2	10.1	2.4	0.4
Caffe Mocha, with Whip, Tall, Soy, Starbucks*	1 Tall/254ml	239	11.4	94	3.6	11.4	4.5	0.9
Caffe Mocha, with Whip, Tall, Whole Milk, Starbucks*	1 Tall/335ml	290	15.5	87	3.0	9.8	4.6	0.4
Caffe Mocha, with Whip, Venti, Soy, Starbucks*	1 Venti/591ml	366	15.7	62	2.5	8.1	2.7	0.6
Caffe Mocha, with Whip, Venti, Whole Milk, Starbucks*	1 Venti/591ml	448	22.5	76	2.8	9.0	3.8	0.4
Caffe Mocha & Whip, Grande, Whole Milk, Starbucks*	1 Grande/473ml	364	18.7	77	2.7	8.9	3.9	0.4
Caffe Mocha & Whip, Short, Skimmed Milk, Starbucks*	1 Short/236ml	160	6.4	68	2.9	9.3	2.7	0.4
Caffe Mocha & Whip, Tall, Semi Skimmed, Starbucks*	1 Short/254ml	266	12.5	105	4.1	13.0	4.9	0.5
Caffe Mocha & Whip, Venti, Skimmed Milk, Starbucks*	1 Venti/591ml	347	10.2	59	2.9	9.3	1.7	0.4
Cappuccino, Grande, Semi Skimmed Milk, Starbucks*	1 Grande/473ml	115	4.1	24	1.6	2.5	0.9	0.0
Cappuccino, Grande, Soy, Starbucks*	1 Grande/473ml	92	3.2	19	1.3	1.7	0.7	0.2
Cappuccino, Grande, Whole Milk, Starbucks*	1 Grande/473ml	136	6.8	29	1.6	2.3	1.4	0.0
Cappuccino, Short, Semi Skimmed Milk, Starbucks*	1 Short/236ml	78	2.8	33	2.2	3.4	1.2	0.0
Cappuccino, Short, Skimmed Milk, Starbucks*	1 Short/236ml	55	0.1	23	2.2	3.4	0.0	0.0
Cappuccino, Short, Soy, Starbucks*	1 Short/236ml	62	2.2	26	1.8	2.5	0.9	0.2
Cappuccino, Short, Whole Milk, Starbucks*	1 Short/236ml	92	4.7	39	2.1	3.4	2.0	0.0
Cappuccino, Tall, Semi Skimmed Milk, Starbucks*	1 Tall/335ml	91	3.4	27	1.8	2.7	1.0	0.0
Cappuccino, Tall, Skimmed Milk, Starbucks*	1 Tall/335ml	64	0.1	19	1.8	2.7	0.0	0.0
Cappuccino, Tall, Soy, Starbucks*	1 Tall/335ml	72	2.6	21	1.5	1.8	0.8	0.2
Cappuccino, Tall, Whole Milk, Starbucks*	1 Tall/335ml	108	5.6	32	1.8	2.7	1.7	0.0
Cappuccino, Venti, Semi Skimmed Milk, Starbucks*	1 Venti/591ml	155	5.7	26	1.7	2.5	1.0	0.0
Cappuccino, Venti, Skimmed Milk, Starbucks*	1 Venti/591ml	109	0.2	18	1.8	2.7	0.0	0.0
Cappuccino, Venti, Soy, Starbucks*	1 Venti/591ml	123	4.4	21	1.5	1.9	0.7	0.2
Cappuccino, Venti, Whole Milk, Starbucks*	1 Venti/591ml	184	9.3	31	1.7	2.5	1.6	0.0
Caramel Macchiato, Grande, Skimmed Milk, Starbucks*	1 Grande/473ml	193	1.1	41	2.3	7.4	0.2	0.0
Caramel Macchiato, Grande, Soy, Starbucks*	1 Grande/473ml	207	5.3	44	1.9	6.1	1.1	0.2
Caramel Macchiato, Grande, Whole Milk, Starbucks*	1 Grande/473ml	269	10.5	57	2.2	7.2	2.2	0.0
Caramel Macchiato, Short, Skimmed Milk, Starbucks*	1 Short/236ml	97	0.9	41	2.4	7.2	0.4	0.0
Caramel Macchiato, Short, Soy, Starbucks*	1 Short/236ml	104	3.0	44	1.9	5.9	1.3	0.2
Caramel Macchiato, Short, Whole Milk, Starbucks*	1 Short/236ml	137	5.7	58	2.2	6.8	2.4	0.0
Caramel Macchiato, Skimmed Milk, Starbucks*	1 Tall/354ml	173	0.8	49	3.1	8.5	0.2	0.0
Caramel Macchiato, Tall, Skimmed Milk, Starbucks*	1 Tall/335ml	142	0.9	42	2.4	7.5	0.3	0.0
Caramel Macchiato, Tall, Soy, Starbucks*	1 Tall/335ml	153	4.2	46	2.0	6.3	1.2	0.3
Caramel Macchiato, Tall, Whole Milk, Starbucks*	1 Tall/335ml	201	8.2	60	2.3	7.2	2.4	0.0
Caramel Macchiato, Venti, Skimmed Milk, Starbucks*	1 Venti/591ml	239	1.2	40	2.3	7.4	0.2	0.0
Caramel Macchiato, Venti, Soy, Starbucks*	1 Venti/591ml	256	6.5	43	1.9	6.3	1.1	0.2
Caramel Macchiato, Venti, Whole Milk, Starbucks*	1 Venti/591ml	337	13.1	57	2.2	7.1	2.2	0.0
Caramel Macchiato, Whole Milk, Starbucks*	1 Tall/354ml	244	10.4	69	2.8	7.9	2.9	0.0
Espresso, Doppio, Starbucks*	1 Doppio/60ml	11	0.0	18	1.2	3.3	0.0	0.0
Espresso, Solo, Starbucks*	1 Solo/30ml	6	0.0	20	1.3	3.3	0.0	0.0
Espresso Con Panna, Doppio, Starbucks*	1 Doppio/60ml	36	2.5	60	1.5	5.0	4.2	0.0
Espresso Con Panna, Solo, Starbucks*	1 Solo/30ml	31	2.5	103	1.7	6.7	8.3	0.0
Espresso Macchiato, Doppio, Skimmed Milk, Starbucks*	1 Doppio/60ml	13	0.0	22	1.7	3.3	0.0	0.0
Espresso Macchiato, Doppio, Soy, Starbucks*	1 Doppio/60ml	13	0.1	22	1.5	3.3	0.2	0.0
Espresso Macchiato, Doppio, Whole Milk, Starbucks*	1 Doppio/60ml	15	0.2	25	1.5	3.3	0.3	0.0
Espresso Macchiato, Solo, S/Skimmed Milk, Starbucks*	1 Solo/30ml	8	0.1	27	1.7	3.3	0.3	0.0

STARBUCKS

COFFEE

	Measure INFO/WEIGHT	per Measure KCAL	FAT	Nutrition Values per 100g / 100ml KCAL	PROT	CARB	FAT	FIBRE
Espresso Macchiato, Solo, Skimmed Milk, Starbucks*	1 Solo/30ml	7	0.0	23	1.7	3.3	0.0	0.0
Espresso Macchiato, Solo, Soy, Starbucks*	1 Solo/30ml	7	0.1	23	1.7	3.3	0.3	0.0
Espresso Macchiato, Solo, Whole Milk, Starbucks*	1 Solo/30ml	8	0.2	27	1.7	3.3	0.7	0.0
Hazelnut Mocha, with Whip, Grande, Soy, Starbucks*	1 Grande/473ml	369	13.3	78	2.3	12.0	2.8	0.6
Hazelnut Mocha, with Whip, Venti, Soy, Starbucks*	1 Venti/591ml	448	15.2	76	2.4	11.8	2.6	0.6
Iced, Caffe Americano, Grande, Starbucks*	1 Grande/473ml	17	0.0	4	0.2	0.6	0.0	0.0
Iced, Caffe Americano, Tall, Starbucks*	1 Tall/335ml	11	0.0	3	0.2	0.6	0.0	0.0
Iced, Caffe Americano, Venti, Starbucks*	1 Venti/591ml	23	0.0	4	0.2	0.7	0.0	0.0
Iced, Caffe Latte, Grande, S/Skimmed Milk, Starbucks*	1 Grande/473ml	126	4.5	27	1.8	2.7	0.9	0.0
Iced, Caffe Latte, Grande, Skimmed Milk, Starbucks*	1 Grande/473ml	90	0.2	19	1.8	2.7	0.0	0.0
Iced, Caffe Latte, Grande, Soy, Starbucks*	1 Grande/473ml	104	3.6	22	1.5	1.9	0.8	0.2
Iced, Caffe Latte, Grande, Whole Milk, Starbucks*	1 Grande/473ml	149	7.5	31	1.7	2.5	1.6	0.0
Iced, Caffe Latte, Tall, Semi Skimmed Milk, Starbucks*	1 Tall/335ml	97	3.6	29	1.9	3.0	1.1	0.0
Iced, Caffe Latte, Tall, Skimmed Milk, Starbucks*	1 Tall/335ml	68	0.2	20	1.9	3.0	0.1	0.0
Iced, Caffe Latte, Tall, Soy, Starbucks*	1 Tall/335ml	80	2.9	24	1.7	2.1	0.9	0.2
Iced, Caffe Latte, Tall, Whole Milk, Starbucks*	1 Tall/335ml	115	5.9	34	1.8	2.7	1.8	0.0
Iced, Caffe Latte, Venti, Semi Skimmed Milk, Starbucks*	1 Venti/591ml	142	5.1	24	1.6	2.4	0.9	0.0
Iced, Caffe Latte, Venti, Skimmed Milk, Starbucks*	1 Venti/591ml	100	0.2	17	1.6	2.5	0.0	0.0
Iced, Caffe Latte, Venti, Soy, Starbucks*	1 Venti/591ml	118	4.2	20	1.4	1.9	0.7	0.2
Iced, Caffe Latte, Venti, Whole Milk, Starbucks*	1 Venti/591ml	168	8.5	28	1.5	2.4	1.4	0.0
Iced, Caffe Mocha, with Whip, Venti, Soy, Starbucks*	1 Venti/591ml	322	16.0	54	1.6	7.1	2.7	0.5
Iced, Caffe Mocha & Whip, Tall, Whole Milk, Starbucks*	1 Tall/335ml	248	14.1	74	2.1	8.4	4.2	0.4
Iced, Caramel Macchiato, Grande, Soy, Starbucks*	1 Grande/473ml	206	5.3	44	1.8	6.3	1.1	0.2
Iced, Caramel Macchiato, Tall, Soy, Starbucks*	1 Tall/335ml	152	4.2	45	1.8	6.6	1.2	0.0
Iced, Caramel Macchiato, Tall, Whole Milk, Starbucks*	1 Tall/335ml	191	7.5	57	2.0	7.2	2.2	0.0
Iced, Caramel Macchiato, Venti, Soy, Starbucks*	1 Venti/591ml	234	5.7	40	1.6	5.9	1.0	0.2
Iced, Caramel Macchiato, Venti, Whole Milk, Starbucks*	1 Venti/591ml	291	10.5	49	1.7	6.6	1.8	0.0
Iced, Grande, Starbucks*	1 Grande/473ml	4	0.1	1	0.1	0.0	0.0	0.0
Iced, Hazelnut Mocha, with Whip, Tall, Soy, Starbucks*	1 Tall/335ml	325	14.3	97	2.4	12.5	4.3	0.1
Iced, Latte, Vanilla, Grande, Skimmed Milk, Starbucks*	1 Grande/473ml	155	0.2	33	1.6	6.5	0.0	0.0
Iced, Latte, Vanilla, Grande, Soy, Starbucks*	1 Grande/473ml	168	3.2	36	1.3	5.7	0.7	0.2
Iced, Latte, Vanilla, Grande, Whole Milk, Starbucks*	1 Grande/473ml	207	6.5	44	1.5	6.3	1.4	0.0
Iced, Latte, Vanilla, Tall, Semi Skimmed Milk, Starbucks*	1 Tall/335ml	142	2.9	42	1.7	6.9	0.9	0.0
Iced, Latte, Vanilla, Tall, Skimmed Milk, Starbucks*	1 Serving/335ml	121	0.0	36	1.8	7.2	0.0	0.0
Iced, Latte, Vanilla, Tall, Soy, Starbucks*	1 Tall/335ml	128	2.5	38	1.5	6.0	0.7	0.2
Iced, Latte, Vanilla, Tall, Whole Milk, Starbucks*	1 Tall/335ml	158	5.2	47	1.6	6.6	1.5	0.0
Iced, Latte, Vanilla, Venti, S/Skimmed Milk, Starbucks*	1 Venti/591ml	218	4.4	37	1.4	6.1	0.7	0.0
Iced, Latte, Vanilla, Venti, Skimmed Milk, Starbucks*	1 Venti/591ml	182	0.2	31	1.4	6.3	0.0	0.0
Iced, Latte, Vanilla, Venti, Soy, Starbucks*	1 Venti/591ml	197	3.5	33	1.2	5.6	0.6	0.1
Iced, Latte, Vanilla, Venti, Whole Milk, Starbucks*	1 Venti/591ml	240	7.2	41	1.3	6.1	1.2	0.0
Iced, Tall, Starbucks*	1 Tall/335ml	3	0.1	1	0.1	0.0	0.0	0.0
Iced, Venti, Starbucks*	1 Venti/591ml	5	0.1	1	0.1	0.0	0.0	0.0
Mocha, Peppermint, Skimmed, Grande, Starbucks*	1 Grande/473ml	304	2.3	64	2.9	13.3	0.5	0.4
Mocha, Peppermint, Skimmed, Tall, Starbucks*	1 Tall/354ml	237	1.4	67	3.1	13.6	0.4	0.4
Mocha, Peppermint, Skimmed, Venti, Starbucks*	1 Venti/591ml	385	2.9	65	3.0	13.4	0.5	0.4
Mocha, Peppermint, Skimmed, Whip, Grde, Starbucks*	1 Grande/473ml	405	20.8	86	2.9	13.7	4.4	0.4
Mocha, Peppermint, Whole, Grande, Starbucks*	1 Grande/473ml	372	11.4	79	2.7	12.9	2.4	0.4
Mocha, Peppermint, Whole, Tall, Starbucks*	1 Tall/354ml	293	9.0	83	2.8	13.3	2.5	0.4
Mocha, Peppermint, Whole, Venti, Starbucks*	1 Venti/591ml	475	15.2	80	2.8	12.9	2.6	0.4
Mocha, Peppermint, Whole, Whip, Venti, Starbucks*	1 Venti/591ml	576	24.6	97	2.8	13.2	4.2	0.4
Vanilla Latte, Grande, Semi Skimmed Milk, Starbucks*	1 Grande/473ml	251	6.4	53	2.4	7.6	1.3	0.0
Vanilla Latte, Grande, Skimmed Milk, Starbucks*	1 Grande/473ml	199	0.3	42	2.5	7.8	0.1	0.0

	Measure INFO/WEIGHT	per Measure		Nutrition Values per 100g / 100ml				
		KCAL	FAT	KCAL	PROT	CARB	FAT	FIBRE
STARBUCKS								
COFFEE								
Vanilla Latte, Grande, Soy, Starbucks*	1 Grande/473ml	214	4.9	45	2.0	6.5	1.0	0.2
Vanilla Latte, Grande, Whole Milk, Starbucks*	1 Grande/473ml	284	10.6	60	2.4	7.6	2.2	0.0
Vanilla Latte, Short, Semi Skimmed Milk, Starbucks*	1 Short/236ml	127	3.3	54	2.5	7.6	1.4	0.0
Vanilla Latte, Short, Skimmed Milk, Starbucks*	1 Short/236ml	101	0.1	43	2.5	8.0	0.0	0.0
Vanilla Latte, Short, Soy, Starbucks*	1 Short/236ml	108	2.5	46	2.1	6.8	1.1	0.2
Vanilla Latte, Short, Whole Milk, Starbucks*	1 Short/236ml	144	5.4	61	2.4	7.6	2.3	0.0
Vanilla Latte, Tall, Semi Skimmed Milk, Starbucks*	1 Tall/335ml	195	5.2	58	2.7	8.1	1.5	0.0
Vanilla Latte, Tall, Skimmed Milk, Starbucks*	1 Tall/335ml	152	0.2	45	2.8	8.4	0.1	0.0
Vanilla Latte, Tall, Soy, Starbucks*	1 Tall/335ml	165	4.0	49	2.3	6.9	1.2	0.3
Vanilla Latte, Tall, Whole Milk, Starbucks*	1 Tall/335ml	221	8.6	66	2.7	8.1	2.6	0.0
Vanilla Latte, Venti, Semi Skimmed Milk, Starbucks*	1 Venti/591ml	321	8.5	54	2.5	7.8	1.4	0.0
Vanilla Latte, Venti, Skimmed Milk, Starbucks*	1 Venti/591ml	252	0.4	43	2.6	7.9	0.1	0.0
Vanilla Latte, Venti, Soy, Starbucks*	1 Venti/591ml	272	6.5	46	2.1	6.6	1.1	0.3
Vanilla Latte, Venti, Whole Milk, Starbucks*	1 Venti/591ml	364	14.0	62	2.5	7.6	2.4	0.0
COOKIES								
Chocolate, Chunk, Starbucks*	1 Cookie/90g	396	12.0	440	6.8	69.7	13.3	0.3
Fruit & Oat, Starbucks*	1 Cookie/80g	344	14.0	430	4.2	64.0	17.5	2.2
CORNFLAKE								
Chocolate, Belgian, Square, Starbucks*	1 Slice/62g	288	14.2	466	4.0	59.7	23.0	2.2
CREPE								
Ham, Mushroom & Tomato, Starbucks*	1 Pack/153g	148	4.7	97	4.3	14.0	3.1	1.0
CRISPS								
Strong Cheese & Onion, Starbucks*	1 Bag/50g	227	11.3	455	7.1	56.2	22.6	4.0
CROISSANT								
Almond, Starbucks*	1 Croissant/110g	465	24.1	423	7.0	48.2	21.9	2.2
Butter, Starbucks*	1 Croissant/70g	279	16.5	398	6.9	39.5	23.6	1.4
Cheese, & Ham, Starbucks*	1 Croissant/120g	378	21.0	315	13.8	25.2	17.5	0.9
Cheese & Mushroom, Starbucks*	1 Croissant/140g	427	27.3	305	9.2	22.6	19.5	1.1
Dry Cured Ham & Emmental, Starbucks*	1 Croissant/105g	333	19.2	317	13.0	26.9	18.3	1.0
CUPCAKES								
Banana & Chocolate Chip, Starbucks*	1 Cupcake/80g	342	14.9	428	4.7	57.8	18.6	0.5
Lemon, Sicilian, Starbucks*	1 Cupcake/80g	350	18.0	437	3.3	55.3	22.5	0.5
Strawberry, Starbucks*	1 Cupcake/83g	385	20.8	464	4.1	55.9	25.1	0.6
DOUGHNUT								
Chocolate & Custard, Mini, Starbucks*	1 Doughnut/25g	77	3.5	307	5.8	39.8	13.8	1.6
Classic Cake, Starbucks*	1 Doughnut/100g	449	24.1	449	3.6	54.5	24.1	1.0
Jam, Mini, Starbucks*	1 Doughnut/24g	77	2.7	323	6.2	49.6	11.1	1.4
DRIED FRUIT								
Starbucks*	1 Serving/30g	88	0.1	294	2.2	75.3	0.4	1.4
FLAPJACK								
Banana & Caramel, Starbucks*	1 Serving/70g	301	15.4	430	3.3	54.4	22.0	2.5
FRAPPUCCINO								
Caramel, Grande, Starbucks*	1 Grande/473ml	294	3.9	62	0.0	12.5	0.8	0.0
Caramel, Light, Grande, Starbucks*	1 Grande/473ml	158	1.6	33	1.3	6.3	0.3	0.5
Caramel, Light, Tall, Starbucks*	1 Tall/335ml	129	1.4	39	1.4	7.5	0.4	0.6
Caramel, Light, Venti, Starbucks*	1 Venti/591ml	192	1.7	32	1.2	6.4	0.3	0.5
Caramel, Tall, Starbucks*	1 Tall/354ml	228	3.1	64	0.0	12.7	0.9	0.0
Caramel, Venti, Starbucks*	1 Venti/591ml	370	4.7	63	0.0	12.7	0.8	0.0
Caramel, with Whip, Grande, Starbucks*	1 Grande/473ml	382	14.9	81	1.2	12.0	3.1	0.0
Caramel, with Whip, Tall, Starbucks*	1 Tall/335ml	302	11.0	90	1.3	13.7	3.3	0.0
Caramel, with Whip, Venti, Starbucks*	1 Venti/591ml	431	14.4	73	1.1	11.7	2.4	0.0
Caramel Cream, Grande, Starbucks*	1 Grande/473ml	351	16.0	74	1.0	10.1	3.4	0.0

STARBUCKS
FRAPPUCCINO

	Measure INFO/WEIGHT	per Measure KCAL	FAT	Nutrition Values per 100g / 100ml KCAL	PROT	CARB	FAT	FIBRE
Caramel Cream, Tall, Starbucks*	1 Tall/354ml	261	3.9	74	2.8	13.0	1.1	0.0
Caramel Cream, Venti, Starbucks*	1 Venti/591ml	409	6.0	69	2.6	12.3	1.0	0.0
Caramel Cream, with Whip, Grande, Starbucks*	1 Grande/473ml	431	14.2	91	2.6	13.5	3.0	0.0
Caramel Cream, with Whip, Tall, Starbucks*	1 Tall/254ml	329	10.4	130	3.6	19.7	4.1	0.0
Caramel Cream, with Whip, Venti, Starbucks*	1 Venti/591ml	489	13.6	83	2.4	13.0	2.3	0.0
Chocolate, Grande, Starbucks*	1 Grande/473ml	338	5.7	71	3.0	12.7	1.2	0.0
Chocolate, Tall, Starbucks*	1 Tall/354ml	260	4.5	73	3.0	13.0	1.3	0.0
Chocolate, with Whip, Grande, Starbucks*	1 Grande/473ml	469	17.9	99	3.0	13.1	3.8	0.1
Chocolate, with Whip, Tall, Starbucks*	1 Tall/354ml	354	13.2	100	3.0	13.6	3.7	0.2
Chocolate, with Whip, Venti, Starbucks*	1 Venti/591ml	544	19.3	92	2.8	13.0	3.3	0.2
Coffee, Grande, Starbucks*	1 Grande/473ml	239	3.1	51	1.1	10.1	0.7	0.0
Coffee, Light, Grande, Starbucks*	1 Grande/473ml	128	1.0	27	1.3	5.3	0.2	0.5
Coffee, Light, Tall, Starbucks*	1 Tall/335ml	91	0.7	27	1.3	5.4	0.2	0.5
Coffee, Light, Venti, Starbucks*	1 Venti/591ml	151	1.2	26	1.2	4.9	0.2	0.5
Coffee, Tall, Starbucks*	1 Tall/254ml	184	2.4	72	1.5	14.6	0.9	0.0
Coffee, Venti, Starbucks*	1 Venti/591ml	278	3.6	47	1.0	9.5	0.6	0.0
Cream, Caramel, with Whip, Tall, Starbucks*	1 Tall/335ml	329	10.4	98	2.7	14.9	3.1	0.0
Cream, Chocolate, with Whip, Grande, Starbucks*	1 Grande/473ml	425	14.2	90	2.7	13.5	3.0	0.1
Cream, Chocolate, with Whip, Tall, Starbucks*	1 Tall/335ml	322	10.4	96	2.9	14.6	3.1	0.2
Cream, Chocolate, with Whip, Venti, Starbucks*	1 Venti/591ml	480	14.1	81	2.5	13.0	2.4	0.2
Cream, Chocolate Chip, with Whip, Grande, Starbucks*	1 Grande/473ml	498	18.0	105	2.8	15.6	3.8	0.3
Cream, Chocolate Chip, with Whip, Tall, Starbucks*	1 Tall/335ml	368	12.9	110	3.0	16.7	3.8	0.4
Cream, Vanilla, with Whip, Grande, Starbucks*	1 Grande/473ml	431	14.2	91	2.6	13.5	3.0	0.0
Cream, Vanilla, with Whip, Tall, Starbucks*	1 Tall/335ml	310	9.8	93	2.7	14.0	2.9	0.0
Cream, Vanilla, with Whip, Venti, Starbucks*	1 Venti/591ml	470	13.0	80	2.3	12.7	2.2	0.0
Espresso, Grande, Starbucks*	1 Grande/473ml	209	2.7	44	1.0	8.9	0.6	0.0
Espresso, Tall, Starbucks*	1 Tall/335ml	146	1.9	44	1.0	8.7	0.6	0.0
Espresso, Venti, Starbucks*	1 Venti/591ml	243	3.1	41	0.9	8.1	0.5	0.0
Grande, Starbucks*	1 Grande/473ml	239	3.1	51	1.1	10.1	0.7	0.0
Java Chip, with Whip, Grande, Starbucks*	1 Grande/473ml	456	18.6	96	1.5	14.6	3.9	0.3
Mango Passion, Grande, Starbucks*	1 Grande/473ml	191	0.3	40	0.2	9.7	0.1	0.3
Mango Passion, Tall, Starbucks*	1 Tall/335ml	157	0.2	47	0.2	11.3	0.1	0.3
Mango Passion, Venti, Starbucks*	1 Venti/591ml	228	0.3	39	0.1	9.3	0.0	0.2
Mocha, Light, Grande, Starbucks*	1 Grande/473ml	144	1.4	30	1.3	6.1	0.3	0.6
Mocha, Light, Tall, Starbucks*	1 Tall/335ml	113	1.1	34	1.5	6.9	0.3	0.7
Mocha, Light, Venti, Starbucks*	1 Venti/591ml	184	2.0	31	1.3	6.3	0.3	0.6
Mocha, White Chocolate, Whip, Grande, Starbucks*	1 Grande/473ml	408	15.6	86	1.4	12.9	3.3	0.0
Mocha, White Chocolate, with Whip, Venti, Starbucks*	1 Venti/591ml	481	16.2	81	1.4	13.0	2.7	0.0
Mocha, with Whip, Grande, Starbucks*	1 Grande/473ml	378	14.8	80	1.3	12.0	3.1	0.1
Mocha, with Whip, Tall, Starbucks*	1 Tall/335ml	283	10.8	84	1.4	12.8	3.2	0.1
Mocha, with Whip, Venti, Starbucks*	1 Venti/591ml	428	14.9	72	1.3	11.7	2.5	0.1
Raspberry Tea, Grande, Starbucks*	1 Grande/473ml	200	0.2	42	0.1	11.0	0.0	0.2
Raspberry Tea, Tall, Starbucks*	1 Tall/354ml	144	0.1	41	0.1	10.4	0.0	0.2
Raspberry Tea, Venti, Starbucks*	1 Venti/591ml	261	0.2	44	0.1	11.3	0.0	0.2
Strawberries & Cream, Grande, Starbucks*	1 Grande/473ml	424	5.2	90	2.9	17.3	1.1	0.0
Strawberries & Cream, Tall, Starbucks*	1 Tall/354ml	299	3.6	84	2.7	16.4	1.0	0.0
Strawberries & Cream, Venti, Starbucks*	1 Venti/591ml	543	6.7	92	3.0	17.6	1.1	0.0
Strawberries & Cream, with Whip, Grande, Starbucks*	1 Grande/473ml	494	13.4	104	2.5	17.5	2.8	0.1
Strawberries & Cream, with Whip, Tall, Starbucks*	1 Tall/254ml	374	9.7	147	3.5	24.8	3.8	0.1
Strawberries & Cream, with Whip, Venti, Starbucks*	1 Venti/591ml	548	12.8	93	2.2	16.2	2.2	0.1
Tazo Chai, Tall, Starbucks*	1 Tall/354ml	294	3.8	83	2.9	15.8	1.1	0.0
Tazo Chai, with Whip, Grande, Starbucks*	1 Grande/473ml	536	17.3	113	2.9	16.9	3.7	0.0

STARBUCKS

INFO/WEIGHT		KCAL	FAT	KCAL	PROT	CARB	FAT	FIBRE
FRAPPUCCINO								
Tropical Citrus Tea, Tall, Starbucks*	1 Tall/354ml	128	0.2	36	0.3	9.0	0.1	0.3
Vanilla, with Whip, Grande, Starbucks*	1 Grande/473ml	364	14.2	77	1.2	11.4	3.0	0.0
Vanilla, with Whip, Tall, Starbucks*	1 Tall/254ml	284	10.4	112	1.7	17.3	4.1	0.9
FRUIT SALAD								
Starbucks*	1 Salad/182g	95	0.4	52	0.6	11.1	0.2	1.6
HOT CHOCOLATE								
Signature, with Whip, Grande, Soy, Starbucks*	1 Grande/473ml	515	29.8	109	3.0	11.8	6.3	1.6
Signature, with Whip, Grande, Whole Milk, Starbucks*	1 Grande/473ml	556	33.5	118	3.2	12.5	7.1	1.4
Signature, with Whip, Grde, Skimmed Milk, Starbucks*	1 Grande/473ml	505	27.0	107	3.3	12.5	5.7	1.4
Signature, with Whip, Short, Skimmed Milk, Starbucks*	1 Short/236ml	267	15.0	113	3.3	12.7	6.4	1.4
Signature, with Whip, Short, Soy, Starbucks*	1 Short/236ml	272	16.4	115	3.0	11.9	6.9	1.6
Signature, with Whip, Short, Whole Milk, Starbucks*	1 Short/236ml	293	18.1	124	3.2	12.7	7.7	1.4
Signature, with Whip, Tall, S/Skimmed Milk, Starbucks*	1 Tall/335ml	418	24.2	125	3.5	13.4	7.2	1.5
Signature, with Whip, Tall, Skimmed Milk, Starbucks*	1 Tall/335ml	393	21.3	117	3.5	13.7	6.4	1.5
Signature, with Whip, Tall, Soy, Starbucks*	1 Tall/335ml	401	23.5	120	3.2	12.8	7.0	1.7
Signature, with Whip, Tall, Whole Milk, Starbucks*	1 Tall/335ml	433	26.1	129	3.5	13.4	7.8	1.5
Signature, with Whip, Venti, S/Skimmed Milk, Starbucks*	1 Venti/591ml	665	37.2	113	3.3	12.7	6.3	1.4
Signature, with Whip, Venti, Skimmed Milk, Starbucks*	1 Venti/591ml	624	32.4	106	3.3	12.7	5.5	1.4
Signature, with Whip, Venti, Whole Milk, Starbucks*	1 Venti/591ml	690	40.4	117	3.2	12.5	6.8	1.4
Skimmed Milk, Grande, Starbucks*	1 Grande/473ml	261	2.4	55	3.3	10.6	0.5	0.4
Skimmed Milk, Tall, Starbucks*	1 Tall/354ml	209	1.5	59	3.5	11.3	0.4	0.4
Skimmed Milk, Venti, Starbucks*	1 Venti/591ml	340	2.9	58	3.3	11.2	0.5	0.4
White, Skimmed Milk, Grande, Starbucks*	1 Grande/442ml	361	16.6	82	3.8	13.9	3.8	0.0
White, Skimmed Milk, Tall, Starbucks*	1 Tall/354ml	301	3.9	85	4.1	14.4	1.1	0.0
White, Skimmed Milk, Venti, Starbucks*	1 Venti/591ml	493	7.1	83	4.0	14.2	1.2	0.0
White, Skimmed Milk, with Whip, Grande, Starbucks*	1 Grande/443ml	456	14.1	103	3.8	14.4	3.2	0.0
White, Skimmed Milk, with Whip, Tall, Starbucks*	1 Tall/354ml	381	11.9	108	4.1	14.7	3.4	0.0
White, Skimmed Milk, with Whip, Venti, Starbucks*	1 Venti/553ml	556	15.4	101	4.0	14.5	2.8	0.0
White, Whole Milk, Grande, Starbucks*	1 Grande/443ml	449	16.7	101	3.5	13.3	3.8	0.0
White, Whole Milk, Tall, Starbucks*	1 Tall/354ml	377	14.2	106	3.8	13.8	4.0	0.0
White, Whole Milk, Venti, Starbucks*	1 Venti/591ml	618	24.0	105	3.7	13.5	4.1	0.0
White, Whole Milk, with Whip, Grande, Starbucks*	1 Grande/443ml	543	25.5	123	3.5	13.7	5.7	0.0
White, Whole Milk, with Whip, Tall, Starbucks*	1 Tall/354ml	457	22.2	129	3.8	14.1	6.3	0.0
White, Whole Milk, with Whip, Venti, Starbucks*	1 Venti/553ml	673	31.2	122	3.7	13.9	5.6	0.0
Whole Milk, Grande, Starbucks*	1 Grande/473ml	347	14.1	73	3.0	9.9	3.0	0.4
Whole Milk, Tall, Starbucks*	1 Tall/354ml	277	10.7	78	3.1	10.7	3.0	0.4
Whole Milk, Venti, Starbucks*	1 Venti/591ml	448	17.6	76	3.0	10.7	3.0	0.4
Whole Milk, with Whip, Grande, Starbucks*	1 Grande/443ml	420	22.0	95	3.0	10.4	5.0	0.4
Whole Milk, with Whip, Tall, Starbucks*	1 Tall/354ml	357	18.7	101	3.1	11.0	5.3	0.4
Whole Milk, with Whip, Venti, Starbucks*	1 Venti/553ml	514	25.3	93	3.0	11.0	4.6	0.4
HOUMOUS								
with Tomato, Vegetables, Red Pepper, Starbucks*	1 Pack/218g	405	14.4	186	5.4	26.2	6.6	2.0
with Vegetable Sticks, Starbucks*	1 Pot/150g	96	3.9	64	2.9	7.3	2.6	4.5
JUICE								
Orange, Starbucks*	1 Bottle/250ml	112	0.2	45	0.8	11.4	0.1	0.3
MILK								
Steamed, Semi Skimmed, Grande, Starbucks*	1 Grande/473ml	203	8.0	43	2.8	4.0	1.7	0.0
Steamed, Semi Skimmed, Short, Starbucks*	1 Short/236ml	103	4.0	44	2.9	4.2	1.7	0.0
Steamed, Semi Skimmed, Venti, Starbucks*	1 Venti/591ml	258	10.2	44	2.9	4.1	1.7	0.0
Steamed, Skimmed, Grande, Starbucks*	1 Grande/473ml	257	0.6	54	5.4	7.9	0.1	0.0
Steamed, Skimmed, Tall, Starbucks*	1 Tall/254ml	114	0.3	45	4.4	6.4	0.1	0.0
Steamed, Skimmed, Venti, Starbucks*	1 Venti/591ml	175	0.4	30	2.9	4.4	0.1	0.0

STARBUCKS

	Measure INFO/WEIGHT	per Measure KCAL	FAT	Nutrition Values per 100g / 100ml KCAL	PROT	CARB	FAT	FIBRE
MILK								
Steamed, Soy, Grande, Starbucks*	1 Grande/473ml	157	6.1	33	2.3	2.7	1.3	0.3
Steamed, Soy, Short, Starbucks*	1 Short/236ml	80	3.1	34	2.4	2.5	1.3	0.0
Steamed, Soy, Tall, Starbucks*	1 Tall/254ml	120	4.7	47	3.3	3.9	1.8	0.5
Steamed, Whole, Grande, Starbucks*	1 Grande/473ml	244	24.6	52	5.2	7.1	5.2	0.0
Steamed, Whole, Short, Starbucks*	1 Short/236ml	123	6.7	52	2.8	3.8	2.8	0.0
Steamed, Whole, Tall, Starbucks*	1 Tall/254ml	187	10.1	74	3.9	5.5	4.0	0.0
MUFFIN								
Banana & Walnut, Starbucks*	1 Muffin/125g	469	25.1	375	5.7	42.9	20.1	4.2
Blueberry, Starbucks*	1 Muffin/125g	452	23.1	359	5.8	46.5	18.4	1.1
Raspberry, with White Chocolate Icing, Starbucks*	1 Muffin/121g	397	18.3	328	4.9	43.2	15.1	1.1
Skinny, Ginger Iced, Starbucks*	1 Muffin/140g	405	4.8	289	3.9	62.3	3.4	0.9
Skinny, Lemon & Poppy Seed, Iced, Starbucks*	1 Muffin/151g	424	6.3	281	4.3	60.4	4.2	4.2
Skinny Blueberry, Starbucks*	1 Muffin/145g	361	6.2	249	4.3	51.7	4.3	1.6
Skinny Peach & Raspberry, Starbucks*	1 Muffin/146g	344	4.2	235	5.7	45.1	2.9	3.0
Skinny Sunrise, Starbucks*	1 Muffin/131g	255	3.9	194	4.6	36.7	3.0	1.3
Sunrise, Starbucks*	1 Muffin/150g	592	34.6	395	5.5	40.8	23.1	1.9
PAIN AU CHOCOLAT								
Starbucks*	1 Pastry/70g	296	17.1	423	6.7	43.8	24.4	2.8
PAIN AU RAISIN								
Starbucks*	1 Pastry/120g	432	20.8	360	5.0	46.2	17.3	1.6
PANCAKES								
Buttermilk, Starbucks*	1 Serving/90g	227	2.4	252	4.6	51.9	2.7	1.2
PANINI								
Beef Pastrami & Roast Chicken, Starbucks*	1 Panini/220g	443	12.6	201	12.3	25.1	5.7	1.4
Cheese & Marmite, Starbucks*	1 Panini/130g	382	17.5	294	15.5	27.1	13.5	1.1
Chicken, Mediterranean, with Green Pesto, Starbucks*	1 Panini/224g	387	9.2	173	11.4	22.6	4.1	1.3
Chicken & Green Pesto, Starbucks*	1 Panini/203g	349	8.9	172	11.8	21.3	4.4	1.2
Chicken Pastrami, Starbucks*	1 Panini/205g	411	12.5	200	12.0	24.3	6.1	0.9
Croque Monsieur, Starbucks*	1 Panini/175g	410	16.6	234	13.2	23.8	9.5	0.9
Egg, Bacon & Mushroom, Breakfast, Starbucks*	1 Panini/153g	269	9.0	176	10.4	20.3	5.9	0.3
Egg Mayo, Breakfast, Starbucks*	1 Panini/146g	327	11.8	224	12.3	25.4	8.1	1.7
Falafel, Starbucks*	1 Panini/213g	362	7.0	170	6.4	28.5	3.3	2.4
Grilled Chicken Salsa, Lightly Spiced, Starbucks*	1 Panini/238g	385	8.1	162	7.9	25.0	3.4	2.0
Grilled Chicken Salsa, with Creme Fraiche, Starbucks*	1 Panini/180g	385	8.1	214	10.4	32.9	4.5	0.0
Ham, Cheese & Roasted Vegetable, Starbucks*	1 Panini/217g	388	8.0	179	11.0	25.4	3.7	1.4
Italian, Mozzarella & Slow Roast Tomato, Starbucks*	1 Panini/158g	419	19.4	265	12.1	26.5	12.3	1.6
Pesto Chicken, with Sunblush Tomato, Starbucks*	1 Panini/208g	399	10.0	192	13.1	24.1	4.8	3.0
Roast Chicken & Tomato, Starbucks*	1 Panini/207g	321	7.5	155	9.4	21.4	3.6	1.2
Roasted Vegetable & Taw Valley Cheddar, Starbucks*	1 Panini/226g	485	19.9	215	9.2	25.1	8.8	1.7
Roasted Vegetables & Cheese, Starbucks*	1 Panini/215g	542	32.5	252	8.7	20.6	15.1	0.0
Sausage, Egg & Baked Bean, Starbucks*	1 Panini/100g	395	9.8	395	16.9	59.8	9.8	1.5
Steak & Cheese, Starbucks*	1 Panini/204g	420	14.3	206	12.9	22.9	7.0	1.1
Tuna Melt & Mature Cheddar, Starbucks*	1 Panini/182g	459	20.9	252	14.6	22.6	11.5	1.3
SALAD								
Chicken, Roasted, Starbucks*	1 Pack/157g	165	10.2	105	7.1	5.1	6.5	1.2
Chicken Caesar, Starbucks*	1 Pack/233g	403	18.4	173	8.7	18.0	7.9	1.2
Mozzarella & Cherry Tomato, Starbucks*	1 Pack/172g	322	29.2	187	5.5	2.9	17.0	17.0
Pasta, Chicken & Red Pesto, Starbucks*	1 Pack/300g	390	13.2	130	7.1	15.3	4.4	1.2
Pasta, Salmon & Dill, Starbucks*	1 Pack/260g	614	34.8	236	7.8	21.0	13.4	1.0
Salmon Nicoise, Starbucks*	1 Pack/260g	291	18.2	112	6.9	7.2	7.0	1.0
Tuna, Minted Pea & Potato, Starbucks*	1 Pack/290g	276	12.8	95	5.4	8.5	4.4	2.2
Tuna & Bean Salad, Starbucks*	1 Pack/326g	254	3.6	78	7.1	9.9	1.1	2.5

STARBUCKS

INFO/WEIGHT	Measure	per Measure		Nutrition Values per 100g / 100ml				
		KCAL	FAT	KCAL	PROT	CARB	FAT	FIBRE
SALAD								
Tuna Nicoise, Starbucks*	1 Pack/184g	175	9.8	95	7.8	4.6	5.3	1.2
SANDWICH								
Atlantic Prawn, Starbucks*	1 Pack/185g	348	12.4	188	10.1	22.0	6.7	2.7
BLT, Starbucks*	1 Pack/181g	485	29.8	269	7.8	22.4	16.5	1.7
Cheddar, & Italian Style Roast Vegetables, Starbucks*	1 Pack/223g	553	30.6	248	5.3	25.8	13.7	0.0
Cheddar Cheese & Pickle, Starbucks*	1 Pack/190g	504	29.8	265	10.2	20.5	15.7	1.6
Cheese & Tomato, Apple Chutney, Starbucks*	1 Pack/200g	318	8.4	159	8.8	21.3	4.2	0.0
Chicken, & Bacon, Club, Starbucks*	1 Pack/252g	590	38.6	234	11.5	12.8	15.3	0.0
Chicken, Club, Starbucks*	1 Pack/206g	422	19.4	205	12.6	17.8	9.4	1.7
Chicken, in Lemon Pepper Dressing, Starbucks*	1 Pack/198g	307	6.9	155	11.8	19.4	3.5	1.6
Chicken, Lightly Spiced, Starbucks*	1 Pack/200g	286	4.8	143	11.2	18.2	2.4	0.0
Egg Mayonnaise, & Cress, Starbucks*	1 Pack/200g	410	20.4	205	10.5	17.4	10.2	1.9
Egg Mayonnaise, on Gluten Free Bread, Starbucks*	1 Pack/227g	340	11.6	150	6.2	20.3	5.1	2.9
Falafel & Houmous, in Flatbread, Starbucks*	1 Pack/250g	467	9.5	187	7.0	34.8	3.8	3.6
Free Range Egg Mayonnaise, Starbucks*	1 Pack/194g	372	15.1	192	10.4	20.0	7.8	2.0
Ham, & Tomato, Smoked, Starbucks*	1 Pack/206g	297	8.0	144	5.2	22.0	3.9	0.0
Ham, Yorkshire, Starbucks*	1 Pack/208g	374	11.0	180	10.0	23.0	5.3	2.3
Houmous, with Crunchy Vegetables, Starbucks*	1 Pack/219g	359	9.6	164	4.7	26.4	4.4	2.9
Prawn, Mayo, Starbucks*	1 Pack/183g	386	20.1	211	9.8	18.3	11.0	1.6
Salmon, Oak Smoked & Soft Cheese, Starbucks*	1 Pack/221g	523	24.1	236	9.6	12.6	10.9	1.9
Soft Cheese, & Tomato, Extra Light, Starbucks*	1 Pack/186g	283	5.0	152	8.0	24.0	2.7	3.1
Tuna, Mayonnaise, Starbucks*	1 Pack/184g	333	10.7	181	9.4	22.8	5.8	1.8
Turkey, & Salad, Smoked, Starbucks*	1 Pack/198g	303	4.8	153	10.8	22.3	2.4	1.5
Turkey, Pork & Herb, Starbucks*	1 Pack/198g	465	21.4	235	11.7	22.6	10.8	2.1
SCONE								
Berry, Starbucks*	1 Scone/143g	436	11.1	305	6.6	53.6	7.8	3.2
Blueberry, Starbucks*	1 Scone/128g	460	18.0	359	3.9	53.1	14.1	2.3
Extremely Fruity, Starbucks*	1 Scone/100g	325	8.5	325	5.7	57.1	8.5	2.3
Fruit, Starbucks*	1 Scone/75g	252	5.5	336	7.6	60.1	7.3	1.9
Plain, Starbucks*	1 Scone/75g	252	6.4	336	8.5	56.3	8.6	1.8
Raisin, Jumbo, Starbucks*	1 Scone/150g	564	22.2	376	5.9	54.9	14.8	2.1
Wheaten, Starbucks*	1 Scone/75g	197	4.7	262	8.6	43.3	6.2	2.7
SHORTBREAD								
Chocolate, Chunk, Fairtrade, Starbucks*	1 Bar/100g	508	26.8	508	7.6	59.3	26.8	1.0
Chocolate Caramel, Starbucks*	1 Bar/66g	357	20.7	541	4.2	59.9	31.4	0.8
SLICES								
Apricot, Pastry, Starbucks*	1 Pastry/115g	279	15.3	243	4.7	26.1	13.3	1.1
Belgian Chocolate & Orange, Swirl, Pastry, Starbucks*	1 Pastry/140g	525	18.5	375	7.5	57.4	13.2	2.6
Cheese, Savoury, Twist, Pastry, Starbucks*	1 Pastry/85g	370	20.0	435	13.5	42.3	23.5	1.8
Cinnamon Swirl, Pastry, Starbucks*	1 Pastry/140g	432	7.7	309	7.0	57.9	5.5	2.8
SYRUP								
Bar Mocha, 1 Pump, Starbucks*	1 Pump/17g	26	0.6	153	3.5	35.3	3.5	5.9
Flavoured, 1 Pump, Starbucks*	1 Pump/10g	20	0.0	200	0.0	50.0	0.0	0.0
Flavoured, Sugar Free, 1 Pump, Starbucks*	1 Pump/10g	0	0.0	0	0.0	0.0	0.0	0.0
Hazelnut Flavoured, Starbucks*	1 Pump/10g	20	0.0	200	0.0	50.0	0.0	0.0
TEA								
Brewed, Grande, Starbucks*	1 Grande/473ml	0	0.0	0	0.0	0.0	0.0	0.0
Brewed, Short, Starbucks*	1 Short/236ml	0	0.0	0	0.0	0.0	0.0	0.0
Brewed, Tall, Starbucks*	1 Tall/335ml	0	0.0	0	0.0	0.0	0.0	0.0
Brewed, Venti, Starbucks*	1 Venti/591ml	0	0.0	0	0.0	0.0	0.0	0.0
Chai, Black, No Sugar, Starbucks*	1 Serving/100ml	0	0.0	0	0.0	0.0	0.0	0.0
Chai, Latte, Tazo, Grande, Skimmed Milk, Starbucks*	1 Grande/473ml	204	0.2	43	1.6	9.3	0.0	0.0

STARBUCKS

	Measure INFO/WEIGHT	per Measure KCAL	per Measure FAT	Nutrition Values per 100g / 100ml KCAL	PROT	CARB	FAT	FIBRE
TEA								
Chai, Latte, Tazo, Grande, Soy, Starbucks*	1 Grande/473ml	213	3.2	45	1.3	8.7	0.7	0.2
Chai, Latte, Tazo, Grande, Whole Milk, Starbucks*	1 Grande/473ml	255	6.5	54	1.5	9.1	1.4	0.0
Chai, Latte, Tazo, Short, Skimmed Milk, Starbucks*	1 Short/236ml	103	0.1	44	1.6	9.3	0.0	0.0
Chai, Latte, Tazo, Short, Soy, Starbucks*	1 Short/236ml	108	1.6	46	1.4	8.5	0.7	0.2
Chai, Latte, Tazo, Short, Whole Milk, Starbucks*	1 Short/236ml	129	3.3	55	1.6	9.3	1.4	0.0
Chai, Latte, Tazo, Tall, Semi Skimmed Milk, Starbucks*	1 Tall/335ml	179	3.0	53	1.7	9.8	0.9	0.0
Chai, Latte, Tazo, Tall, Skimmed Milk, Starbucks*	1 Tall/335ml	154	0.2	46	1.7	9.8	0.1	0.0
Chai, Latte, Tazo, Tall, Soy, Starbucks*	1 Tall/335ml	162	2.4	48	1.4	9.2	0.7	0.2
Chai, Latte, Tazo, Tall, Whole Milk, Starbucks*	1 Tall/335ml	194	5.0	58	1.6	9.8	1.5	0.0
Chai, Latte, Tazo, Venti, Skimmed Milk, Starbucks*	1 Venti/591ml	256	0.3	43	1.6	9.5	0.0	0.0
Chai, Latte, Tazo, Venti, Soy, Starbucks*	1 Venti/591ml	268	4.0	45	1.3	8.6	0.7	0.2
Chai, Latte, Tazo, Venti, Whole Milk, Starbucks*	1 Venti/591ml	322	8.3	54	1.5	9.3	1.4	0.0
Iced, Chai, Latte, Tazo, Grande, Soy, Starbucks*	1 Grande/473ml	219	3.4	46	1.4	8.7	0.7	0.2
Iced, Chai, Latte, Tazo, Grande, Whole Milk, Starbucks*	1 Grande/473ml	259	6.9	55	1.5	9.3	1.5	0.0
Iced, Chai, Latte, Tazo, Tall, Semi Skimmed, Starbucks*	1 Tall/335ml	176	3.0	53	1.6	9.8	0.9	0.0
Iced, Chai, Latte, Tazo, Tall, Skimmed Milk, Starbucks*	1 Tall/335ml	152	0.2	45	1.6	9.8	0.1	0.0
Iced, Chai, Latte, Tazo, Tall, Soy, Starbucks*	1 Tall/335ml	162	2.4	48	1.4	9.2	0.7	0.2
Iced, Chai, Latte, Tazo, Venti, Soy, Starbucks*	1 Venti/591ml	256	3.5	43	1.2	8.5	0.6	0.2
Iced, Chai, Latte, Tazo, Venti, Whole Milk, Starbucks*	1 Venti/591ml	299	7.2	51	1.3	9.0	1.2	0.0
TOASTIE								
Ham & Cheese, Mini, Starbucks*	1 Pack/126g	327	11.1	260	13.3	31.7	8.8	1.8
TOPPING								
Caramel, Starbucks*	1 Serving/4g	15	0.6	375	0.0	50.0	15.0	0.0
Chocolate, Starbucks*	1 Serving/4g	6	0.1	150	2.5	25.0	2.5	2.5
Whipped Cream, Cold, Grande Beverage, Starbucks*	1 Serving/35g	114	11.2	326	1.7	8.6	32.0	0.0
Whipped Cream, Cold, Tall Beverage, Starbucks*	1 Serving/25g	81	8.0	324	1.6	8.0	32.0	0.0
Whipped Cream, Cold, Venti Beverage, Starbucks*	1 Serving/32g	104	10.2	325	1.9	9.4	31.9	0.0
Whipped Cream, Hot, Short Beverage, Starbucks*	1 Serving/16g	52	5.1	325	1.9	6.2	31.9	0.0
Whipped Cream, Hot, Tall Beverage, Starbucks*	1 Serving/19g	62	6.1	326	1.6	10.5	32.1	0.0
TZATZIKI								
with Vegetable Sticks, Starbucks*	1 Tub /140g	73	3.9	52	2.0	4.8	2.8	1.7
WAFFLES								
Caramel, Starbucks*	1 Waffle/30g	140	6.1	467	4.3	66.7	20.3	1.3
WRAP								
Chicken, Breast, in Honey Mustard, Starbucks*	1 Pack/200g	332	7.8	166	7.3	25.8	3.9	1.4
Chicken, Roasted, Starbucks*	1 Pack/197g	374	13.0	190	11.6	21.2	6.6	2.2
Chicken, with Lightly Spiced Salsa, Starbucks*	1 Pack/187g	320	8.2	171	10.4	22.5	4.4	1.6
Chicken with Salad, Starbucks*	1 Pack/223g	362	9.6	162	10.1	21.9	4.3	2.1
Emmental Cheese, & Roasted Aubergines, Starbucks*	1 Pack/225g	517	25.7	230	8.9	22.3	11.4	0.0
Greek Salad, Starbucks*	1 Pack/181g	265	7.3	146	6.1	21.5	4.0	2.0
Houmous & Falafel, Starbucks*	1 Wrap/213g	383	8.5	180	6.4	30.0	4.0	2.8
Houmous & Roasted Vegetable, Starbucks*	½ Pack/102g	205	6.9	200	6.2	29.2	6.7	3.5
Prawn Caesar, Starbucks*	1 Pack/173g	464	27.2	268	11.4	20.2	15.7	1.1
Roasted Chicken Salad, with Mange Tout, Starbucks*	1 Pack/184g	294	3.7	160	12.2	23.5	2.0	1.7
YOGHURT								
Blueberry, Starbucks*	1 Pot/130g	116	0.0	89	4.4	17.8	0.0	0.0
Blueberry with Mixed Seeds, Organic, Starbucks*	1 Pot/180g	194	6.5	108	3.6	15.1	3.6	0.6
Greek, with Crunchy Granola & Honey, Starbucks*	1 Pot/150g	267	15.0	178	1.7	20.5	10.0	1.1
Strawberry, Starbucks*	1 Pot/180g	176	6.5	98	3.6	12.4	3.6	1.7
Strawberry with Mixed Seeds, Organic, Starbucks*	1 Pot/180g	178	6.5	99	3.6	12.6	3.6	1.1

	Measure INFO/WEIGHT	per Measure KCAL	FAT	Nutrition Values per 100g / 100ml KCAL	PROT	CARB	FAT	FIBRE
SUBWAY								
BACON								
Bacon, 2 Strips, Subway*	1 Serving/9g	40	2.9	444	33.3	0.0	32.2	0.0
BREAD								
6" Hearty Italian, Subway*	1 Bread/79g	191	1.6	242	10.1	45.6	2.0	2.1
6" Honey Oat, Subway*	1 Bread/91g	228	2.4	251	9.9	44.0	2.6	3.0
6" Italian Herbs & Cheese, Subway*	1 Bread/86g	223	4.5	259	11.6	40.7	5.2	2.2
6" Italian White, Subway*	1 Bread/75g	180	1.4	240	9.3	45.3	1.9	1.6
6" Wheat, Subway*	1 Bread/80g	187	1.6	234	10.0	45.5	2.0	2.7
SUBWAY								
BREAD								
Wrap, Subway*	1 Wrap/101g	328	6.6	325	7.8	59.4	6.5	2.0
CHEESE								
American, Subway*	1 Serving/11g	40	3.6	364	18.2	0.0	32.7	0.0
Monterey Cheddar, Subway*	1 Serving/14g	55	4.4	393	25.0	2.1	31.4	0.0
COOKIES								
Chocolate Chip Cookie, Subway*	1 Cookie/45g	218	10.3	484	4.4	64.4	22.9	2.4
Chocolate Chunk Cookie, Subway*	1 Cookie/45g	224	11.7	498	4.4	62.2	26.0	2.0
Oatmeal Raisin Cookie, Subway*	1 Cookie/45g	190	8.8	422	4.4	55.6	19.6	4.2
Rainbow Cookie, Subway*	1 Cookie/45g	215	10.4	478	4.4	62.2	23.1	2.0
Sugar Cookie, Subway*	1 Cookie/45g	231	11.8	513	4.4	64.4	26.2	1.3
White Chip Mac Nut Cookie, Subway*	1 Cookie/45g	222	11.7	493	4.4	60.0	26.0	1.6
DOUGHNUTS								
Chocolate Donut, Subway*	1 Doughnut/55g	243	15.5	442	7.3	38.2	28.2	2.2
Sugared Donut, Subway*	1 Doughnut/49g	207	11.6	422	6.1	42.9	23.7	1.0
KIDS' PAK								
Ham, Subway*	1 Sub/147g	164	2.1	112	7.5	17.0	1.4	1.5
Turkey Breast, Subway*	1 Sub/156g	172	2.1	110	8.3	16.0	1.3	1.4
Veggie Delite, Subway*	1 Sub/118g	136	1.2	115	5.0	20.7	1.0	1.9
MEATBALLS								
Bowl of, Subway*	1 Bowl/206g	315	19.7	153	9.4	8.9	9.6	1.4
MUFFIN								
Blueberry Muffin, Subway*	1 Muffin/111g	352	20.6	317	4.5	36.0	18.6	2.7
Chocolate Chunk Muffin, Subway*	1 Muffin/111g	394	22.9	355	5.4	39.6	20.6	2.6
Double Chocolate Chunk Muffin, Subway*	1 Muffin/111g	389	22.0	350	5.4	40.5	19.8	2.8
SALADS								
Beef, Subway*	1 Serving/328g	118	2.4	36	4.9	1.8	0.7	1.2
Chicken Breast, Subway*	1 Serving/342g	143	3.2	42	6.1	2.0	0.9	1.2
Ham, Subway*	1 Serving/328g	108	2.9	33	4.0	2.1	0.9	1.2
Subway Club, Subway*	1 Serving/361g	147	3.4	41	6.1	1.9	0.9	1.1
Sweet Onion Teriyaki, Subway*	1 Serving/385g	201	3.4	52	5.4	5.2	0.9	1.1
Turkey Breast, Subway*	1 Serving/328g	105	2.4	32	4.3	1.8	0.7	1.2
Turkey Breast & Ham, Subway*	1 Serving/338g	115	2.9	34	4.4	2.1	0.9	1.2
Veggie Delite, Subway*	1 Serving/271g	52	1.0	19	1.1	2.2	0.4	1.5
SAUCE								
BBQ, Subway*	1 Serving/21g	40	0.1	190	0.9	45.7	0.5	0.5
Chipotle Southwest Sauce, Subway*	1 Serving/21g	88	9.0	419	0.0	9.5	42.9	0.9
Honey Mustard Sauce, Subway*	1 Serving/21g	32	0.2	152	0.0	33.3	0.9	0.5
Light Mayonnaise, Subway*	1 Serving/15g	56	6.0	373	0.0	6.7	40.0	0.0
Ranch Dressing, Subway*	1 Serving/21g	44	4.5	210	0.0	4.8	21.4	0.0
Sweet Onion Sauce, Subway*	1 Serving/21g	38	0.2	181	0.0	42.9	0.9	0.5
SNACKING								
Garden Side Salad, Subway*	1 Serving/135g	21	0.2	16	1.0	1.9	0.1	1.0
Melted Cheese Nachos, Subway*	1 Serving/126g	411	24.3	326	8.7	28.6	19.3	2.0

	Measure INFO/WEIGHT	per Measure		Nutrition Values per 100g / 100ml				
		KCAL	FAT	KCAL	PROT	CARB	FAT	FIBRE

SUBWAY

SOUPS

Beef Goulash, Subway*	1 Serving/250g	199	11.8	80	3.3	6.0	4.7	0.9
Carrot & Coriander, Subway*	1 Serving/250ml	81	1.8	32	0.9	5.6	0.7	1.1
Country Chicken & Vegetable, Subway*	1 Serving/250ml	168	11.0	67	2.7	4.2	4.4	0.2
Cream Of Chicken, Subway*	1 Serving/250ml	160	11.3	64	2.7	3.1	4.5	0.0
Cream Of Mushroom, Subway*	1 Serving/250ml	150	10.8	60	1.0	4.4	4.3	0.3
Highland Vegetable, Subway*	1 Serving/250ml	73	0.3	29	1.5	5.5	0.1	0.9
Leek & Potato, Subway*	1 Serving/250ml	124	3.0	50	1.7	8.0	1.2	1.1
Lentil & Bacon, Subway*	1 Serving/250ml	182	5.0	73	4.4	9.3	2.0	1.1
Minestrone, Subway*	1 Serving/250ml	81	3.3	32	0.7	4.4	1.3	0.7
Red Pepper & Tomato, Subway*	1 Serving/250ml	96	3.5	38	1.4	5.0	1.4	0.9
Thai Style Vegetable, Subway*	1 Serving/250ml	87	1.0	35	1.1	6.7	0.4	0.8
Tomato, Subway*	1 Serving/250ml	103	3.8	41	0.8	6.1	1.5	0.3
Wild Mushroom, Subway*	1 Serving/250ml	101	5.5	40	1.0	4.1	2.2	0.3

SUBS

Chicken & Bacon Ranch, Subway*	1 Sub/294g	496	20.1	169	12.6	13.3	6.8	1.1
Chicken Temptation, Subway*	1 Sub/249g	401	14.5	161	9.6	17.2	5.8	1.1
Chicken Tikka, Subway*	1 Sub/247g	366	10.8	148	11.3	15.4	4.4	1.3
Italian B.M.T, Subway*	1 Sub/239g	431	20.5	180	10.0	15.9	8.6	1.3
Meatball Marinara, Subway*	1 Sub/319g	511	20.9	160	8.5	17.2	6.5	1.9
Spicy Italian, Subway*	1 Sub/235g	506	28.9	215	10.2	15.7	12.3	1.4
Steak & Cheese, Subway*	1 Sub/247g	338	9.1	137	10.1	15.8	3.7	1.5
Subway Melt, Subway*	1 Sub/251g	352	10.3	140	10.8	15.1	4.1	1.3
Tuna, Subway*	1 Sub/247g	403	17.8	163	8.5	15.8	7.2	1.3
Veggie Patty, Subway*	1 Sub/261g	415	12.6	159	8.8	17.6	4.8	1.2

SUBS, BREAKFAST

Bacon, Subway*	1 Sub/98g	268	7.5	273	15.3	34.7	7.6	2.2
Bacon & Egg, Subway*	1 Sub/135g	337	13.6	250	12.6	25.9	10.1	1.7
Mega Breakfast, Subway*	1 Sub/211g	513	24.7	243	13.3	20.4	11.7	1.5
Sausage, Subway*	1 Sub/156g	364	12.7	233	12.8	26.9	8.1	1.9
Sausage & Egg, Subway*	1 Sub/202g	472	21.8	234	12.4	21.3	10.8	1.6

SUBS, LOW FAT

Beef, Subway*	1 Sub/221g	271	3.2	123	9.9	16.7	1.4	1.4
Chicken Breast, Subway*	1 Sub/235g	297	4.0	126	11.5	16.2	1.7	1.4
Ham, Subway*	1 Sub/221g	258	3.7	117	8.6	17.2	1.7	1.4
Subway Club, Subway*	1 Sub/254g	298	4.1	117	11.0	15.0	1.6	1.3
Sweet Onion Chicken Teriyaki, Subway*	1 Sub/278g	347	4.2	125	9.7	18.0	1.5	1.3
Turkey Breast, Subway*	1 Sub/221g	256	3.2	116	9.0	16.7	1.4	1.4
Turkey Breast & Ham, Subway*	1 Sub/230g	266	3.7	116	9.1	16.1	1.6	1.4
Veggie Delite, Subway*	1 Sub/164g	202	1.8	123	5.5	21.9	1.1	1.9

TOASTIE

Cheese, Subway*	1 Toastie/66g	200	9.5	303	16.2	26.5	14.4	0.9
Pepperoni Pizza, Subway*	1 Toastie/95g	241	12.7	254	12.3	21.7	13.4	0.9

THE REAL GREEK FOOD COMPANY LTD

COLD MEZE

Crudites, The Real Greek Food Company Ltd*	1 Serving/231g	37	0.4	16	0.6	3.1	0.2	1.6
Dolmades, The Real Greek Food Company Ltd*	1 Serving/131g	254	15.7	194	2.9	18.8	12.0	0.8
Flatbread, Greek, The Real Greek Food Company Ltd*	1 Serving/200g	615	15.7	307	6.6	52.6	7.8	7.4
Gigandes Plaki, The Real Greek Food Company Ltd*	1 Serving/210g	183	11.7	87	2.3	7.4	5.6	2.5
Htipiti, The Real Greek Food Company Ltd*	1 Serving/140g	305	24.8	218	8.0	7.8	17.7	3.5
Hummus, The Real Greek Food Company Ltd*	1 Serving/140g	298	19.1	213	7.6	15.6	13.6	5.2
Koliosalata, The Real Greek Food Company Ltd*	1 Serving/140g	506	47.8	361	12.1	1.6	34.1	0.3
Melitzanasalata, The Real Greek Food Company Ltd*	1 Serving/140g	236	21.8	168	1.2	7.1	15.5	3.2

	Measure INFO/WEIGHT	per Measure		Nutrition Values per 100g / 100ml				
		KCAL	FAT	KCAL	PROT	CARB	FAT	FIBRE
THE REAL GREEK FOOD COMPANY LTD								
COLD MEZE								
Revithia, The Real Greek Food Company Ltd*	1 Serving/160g	286	20.1	179	4.8	11.9	12.6	4.0
Salad, Tabouleh, The Real Greek Food Company Ltd*	1 Serving/165g	117	8.2	71	1.3	6.3	5.0	1.9
Taramasalata, The Real Greek Food Company Ltd*	1 Serving/140g	913	99.0	652	2.5	2.1	70.7	0.0
Tzatziki, The Real Greek Food Company Ltd*	1 Serving/140g	163	14.1	116	3.5	3.1	10.0	0.4
DESSERTS								
Loukoumia, The Real Greek Food Company Ltd*	1 Serving/66g	211	1.7	320	0.8	74.2	2.6	0.4
DIPS								
Aioli, Parsley, The Real Greek Food Company Ltd*	1 Serving/35g	176	18.8	504	2.3	2.3	53.8	0.6
Dip, Selection, The Real Greek Food Company Ltd*	1 Serving/140g	589	56.5	421	1.8	9.9	40.4	0.8
HOT MEZE								
Asparagus, Grilled, The Real Greek Food Company Ltd*	1 Serving/110g	140	9.8	127	3.3	9.3	8.9	2.3
Bifteki & Yoghurt, The Real Greek Food Company Ltd*	1 Serving/250g	252	60.3	101	21.6	3.7	24.2	0.0
Chicken, Skewer, The Real Greek Food Company Ltd*	1 Serving/144g	177	7.6	123	3.1	1.3	5.3	0.7
Fish, Cod, Salt, The Real Greek Food Company Ltd*	1 Serving/152g	346	1.5	227	21.1	34.2	1.0	0.6
Halloumi, Grilled, The Real Greek Food Company Ltd*	1 Serving/86g	151	11.8	175	10.3	74.5	13.7	0.9
Halloumi, Skewer, The Real Greek Food Company Ltd*	1 Serving/128g	118	8.5	92	6.8	49.7	6.6	0.5
Lamb, Cutlets, The Real Greek Food Company Ltd*	1 Serving/260g	881	79.1	339	16.3	0.0	30.4	0.0
Lamb, Kefte, The Real Greek Food Company Ltd*	1 Serving/216g	344	24.8	159	12.0	2.2	11.5	0.3
Lamb, Skewer, The Real Greek Food Company Ltd*	1 Serving/166g	255	18.8	154	11.8	1.1	11.3	0.6
Octopus, Grilled, The Real Greek Food Company Ltd*	1 Serving/128g	447	25.4	349	39.3	3.2	19.8	0.3
Pork, Skewer, The Real Greek Food Company Ltd*	1 Serving/165g	281	21.7	170	11.8	1.1	13.1	0.6
Potatoes, New, The Real Greek Food Company Ltd*	1 Serving/385g	293	5.2	76	1.7	15.2	1.3	1.4
Rice, Saffron, The Real Greek Food Company Ltd*	1 Serving/258g	406	2.8	157	3.2	32.2	1.1	0.3
Sardines, Grilled, The Real Greek Food Company Ltd*	1 Serving/360g	619	32.8	172	22.2	0.3	9.1	0.1
Tiropitakia, The Real Greek Food Company Ltd*	1 Serving/120g	416	21.2	344	10.0	37.3	17.5	1.3
KIDS MENU								
Chicken, Skewer, The Real Greek Food Company Ltd*	1 Skewer/72g	88	3.8	123	3.2	1.4	5.3	0.7
Lamb, Skewer, The Real Greek Food Company Ltd*	1 Skewer/82g	127	9.4	154	11.9	1.2	11.4	0.6
Pork Skewer, The Real Greek Food Company Ltd*	1 Skewer/82g	140	10.9	170	11.9	1.2	13.2	0.6
NIBBLES								
Nuts, Athenian, The Real Greek Food Company Ltd*	1 Serving/75g	479	45.4	638	17.7	6.1	60.5	9.2
Olives, The Real Greek Food Company Ltd*	1 Serving/110g	317	33.2	288	1.7	2.4	30.2	4.3
TOBY CARVERY								
BEEF								
Tewkesbury, Toby Carvery*	1 Serving/100g	176	5.6	176	31.4	0.1	5.6	0.0
DRESSING								
Sauce, Mint, Toby Carvery*	1 Serving/100g	67	0.1	67	1.1	15.6	0.1	0.0
Sauce, Parsley, Toby Carvery*	1 Serving/100g	42	1.3	42	1.6	5.9	1.3	0.0
GRAVY								
Beef, Toby Carvery*	1 Serving/100g	22	0.2	22	0.6	4.5	0.2	0.0
Caramelised Onion, Toby Carvery*	1 Serving/100g	80	0.8	80	1.7	16.4	0.8	0.0
Poultry, Toby Carvery*	1 Serving/100g	29	0.1	29	1.1	6.1	0.1	0.0
Vegetarian, Toby Carvery*	1 Serving/100g	18	0.1	18	1.2	3.2	0.1	0.0
PORK								
Horseshoe of, Toby Carvery*	1 Serving/100g	203	8.4	203	31.7	0.1	8.4	0.0
POTATOES								
Mashed, Toby Carvery*	1 Serving/100g	70	2.4	70	1.3	10.8	2.4	0.0
New, Toby Carvery*	1 Serving/100g	73	0.5	73	1.8	15.4	0.5	0.0
Roasted, Toby Carvery*	1 Serving/80g	137	3.7	171	2.7	28.9	4.6	0.0
TURKEY								
with Orange Glaze, Toby Carvery*	1 Serving/100g	145	1.8	145	32.0	0.1	1.8	0.0

	Measure INFO/WEIGHT	per Measure KCAL	FAT	Nutrition Values per 100g / 100ml KCAL	PROT	CARB	FAT	FIBRE

TOBY CARVERY

VEGETABLES

Broccoli, Toby Carvery*	1 Serving/100g	60	2.1	60	2.7	7.6	2.1	0.0
Cabbage, Toby Carvery*	1 Serving/80g	34	1.1	43	1.7	6.0	1.4	0.0
Carrots, Toby Carvery*	1 Serving/100g	46	1.1	46	1.1	3.0	1.1	0.0
Carrots, Toby Carvery*	1 Serving/100g	46	1.1	46	1.1	3.0	1.1	0.0
Leeks, Toby Carvery*	1 Serving/100g	32	0.1	32	0.8	7.1	0.1	0.0
Parsnips, Honey Glazed, Toby Carvery*	1 Serving/100g	148	3.2	148	1.7	28.1	3.2	0.0
Peas, Toby Carvery*	1 Serving/100g	107	1.8	107	6.2	16.6	1.8	0.0

YORKSHIRE PUDDING

New Muffin Style, Toby Carvery*	1 Serving/100g	331	11.7	331	15.3	41.0	11.7	0.0

WIMPY

BREAKFAST

Bacon & Egg Breakfast Roll, Wimpy*	1 Roll/194g	368	12.1	190	13.4	18.3	6.2	0.0
Bacon Breakfast Roll, Wimpy*	1 Roll/144g	278	5.1	193	13.3	24.7	3.5	0.0
Hashbrown, Wimpy*	1 Serving/424g	545	41.1	129	4.1	8.7	9.7	1.9
Sausage & Egg Breakfast Roll, Wimpy*	1 Roll/211g	527	28.4	250	11.8	20.3	13.5	0.0
Sausage Breakfast Roll, Wimpy*	1 Roll/161g	437	21.5	271	11.3	26.6	13.4	0.0
The Country Breakfast, Wimpy*	1 Serving/271g	392	23.1	145	9.4	6.9	8.5	1.7
The Great Wimpy Breakfast, Wimpy*	1 Serving/459g	910	53.6	198	10.7	12.7	11.7	1.2
Wimpy Club, Wimpy*	1 Serving/330g	767	38.6	232	14.7	18.2	11.7	0.8

BREAKFAST EXTRA

Toast with Jam, Wimpy*	1 Serving/89g	276	8.3	310	7.3	52.6	9.3	1.7

BURGERS

BBQ Burger, Wimpy*	1 Burger/236g	644	30.5	273	14.1	24.6	12.9	1.6
Bender in a Bun with Cheese, Wimpy*	1 Burger/170g	424	23.4	249	10.2	20.8	13.8	1.2
Chicken & Bacon Melt, Wimpy*	1 Burger/172g	443	20.2	258	12.6	25.4	11.7	0.0
Chicken Fillet, in a Bun, Savoury, Wimpy*	1 Burger/218g	356	13.8	163	10.4	16.1	6.3	1.1
Chicken Fillet, Wimpy*	1 Burger/327g	380	16.8	116	6.7	11.1	5.1	0.0
Chicken Fillet in a Bun, Hot & Spicy, Wimpy*	1 Burger/193g	398	18.5	206	10.6	19.1	9.6	1.8
Chicken in a Bun, Wimpy*	1 Burger/191g	449	21.4	235	10.4	22.7	11.2	1.3
Classic, Wimpy*	1 Burger/159g	337	15.1	212	12.4	19.9	9.5	0.0
Classic Bacon Cheeseburger, Wimpy*	1 Burger/192g	405	19.0	211	13.6	16.8	9.9	0.0
Classic Kingsize, Wimpy*	1 Burger/227g	551	31.1	243	16.2	14.2	13.7	0.0
Classic with Cheese, Wimpy*	1 Burger/175g	379	18.5	217	12.7	17.3	10.6	1.1
Halfpounder with Bacon & Cheese, Wimpy*	1 Burger/312g	892	50.5	286	19.2	15.5	16.2	0.8
Mega Burger, Wimpy*	1 Burger/206g	594	36.0	288	15.3	18.0	17.5	0.0
Quarterpounder, Wimpy*	1 Burger/200g	538	31.3	269	15.0	18.0	15.6	0.0
Quarterpounder with Bacon & Cheese, Wimpy*	1 Burger/237g	658	33.4	278	16.8	20.5	14.1	1.1
Quarterpounder with Cheese, Wimpy*	1 Burger/213g	578	34.6	271	15.1	17.2	16.2	0.0
Spicy Bean, Wimpy*	1 Burger/233g	611	29.4	262	5.9	30.5	12.6	2.7
Spicy Bean with Cheese, Wimpy*	1 Burger/245g	1459	98.3	596	24.2	35.5	40.1	2.7

CHICKEN

Chicken Chunks with Chips, Wimpy*	1 Serving/333g	779	46.8	234	8.3	19.0	14.0	1.5

CHOCOLATE

Crushed Flake for desserts, Wimpy*	1 Serving/20g	104	6.1	520	7.5	57.0	30.5	1.0

DESSERT

Brown Derby with Dairy Ice Cream, Wimpy*	1 Serving/180g	431	20.6	239	4.5	31.3	11.4	1.4
Brownie Sundae, Wimpy*	1 Sundae/252g	574	21.8	228	3.8	34.7	8.6	0.6
Cheese Cake, Wimpy*	1 Serving/144g	412	18.3	286	4.5	38.5	12.7	0.0
Chocolate Fudge Cake, Wimpy*	1 Serving/100g	371	12.4	371	4.7	60.2	12.4	0.0
Chocolate Waffle with Dairy Ice Cream, Wimpy*	1 Serving/178g	691	37.0	388	5.1	45.3	20.8	0.0
Chocolate Waffle with Squirty Cream, Wimpy*	1 Serving/158g	667	36.9	422	5.1	47.7	23.4	0.0
Dairy Ice Cream with Chocolate Sauce, Wimpy*	1 Serving/88g	200	8.1	227	3.4	32.5	9.2	0.0

	INFO/WEIGHT	KCAL	FAT	KCAL	PROT	CARB	FAT	FIBRE
WIMPY								
DESSERT								
Dairy Ice Cream with Strawberry Sauce, Wimpy*	1 Serving/88g	199	7.9	226	3.0	34.3	9.0	0.0
Deep Filled Apple Tart, Wimpy*	1 Serving/164g	339	10.2	207	1.7	36.2	6.2	0.0
Eskimo Waffle, Wimpy*	1 Serving/228g	694	30.2	304	4.6	42.7	13.2	1.3
Half Chocolate Waffle with Dairy Ice Cream, Wimpy*	1 Serving/116g	395	18.8	341	4.0	44.7	16.2	0.0
Ice Cream Sundae, Plain, Wimpy*	1 Sundae/170g	190	8.8	112	3.1	15.0	5.2	0.0
Mini Knickerbocker Glory with Dairy Ice Cream, Wimpy*	1 Serving/194g	190	8.5	98	1.6	13.2	4.4	0.0
Spotted Dick Pudding, Wimpy*	1 Serving/130g	400	16.5	308	4.1	44.2	12.7	0.0
Toffee Sundae, Wimpy*	1 Sundae/239g	537	23.6	225	3.8	30.8	9.9	0.8
Treacle Sponge Pudding, Wimpy*	1 Serving/130g	504	21.3	388	3.9	56.1	16.4	0.0
EXTRAS								
Bacon, Wimpy*	1 Serving/91g	267	22.0	294	24.2	0.0	24.2	0.0
Cheese, Slice, Wimpy*	1 Slice/12g	40	3.3	333	18.3	5.0	27.5	0.0
Chips Large Portion, Wimpy*	1 Portion/143g	333	17.1	233	3.0	30.4	12.0	3.0
Chips Standard Portion, Wimpy*	1 Portion/114g	267	13.7	234	3.0	30.5	12.0	3.0
Coleslaw, Wimpy*	1 Serving/50g	49	3.8	98	1.4	6.2	7.6	0.8
Egg, Wimpy*	1 Egg/50g	90	7.0	180	13.6	0.0	14.0	0.0
Hash Browns, Wimpy*	1 Serving/55g	93	7.8	169	2.2	19.6	14.2	1.8
Heinz Baked Beans, Wimpy*	1 Portion/110g	85	0.2	77	4.4	12.5	0.2	3.5
Mozzarella Meltz 3, Wimpy*	3 Meltz/79g	253	15.4	320	15.4	25.7	19.5	2.5
Mozzarella Meltz 6, Wimpy*	6 Meltz/157g	506	30.8	322	15.6	25.9	19.6	2.5
Onion Rings Large 12, Wimpy*	1 Portion/180g	401	23.2	223	3.2	23.6	12.9	0.0
Onion Rings Standard 6, Wimpy*	1 Portion/90g	201	11.6	223	3.2	23.6	12.9	3.0
Side Salad, Wimpy*	1 Portion/145g	44	0.3	30	1.4	6.1	0.2	0.8
FISH								
Haddock, Peas & Chips, Wimpy*	1 Serving/314g	674	37.9	215	6.6	21.2	12.1	2.4
Scampi & Chips with Peas, Wimpy*	1 Serving/303g	577	29.8	190	5.2	22.7	9.8	2.3
GRILL								
BBQ Rib Rack Platter, Wimpy*	1 Serving/439g	713	35.2	162	5.6	17.5	8.0	1.4
Classic Bacon Grill, Wimpy*	1 Serving/321g	722	45.3	225	11.5	14.0	14.1	0.0
Gourmet Chicken Platter, Wimpy*	1 Serving/392g	525	21.4	134	11.4	10.0	5.5	1.4
Sausage, Egg & Chips, Wimpy*	1 Serving/244g	597	38.8	245	9.0	17.4	15.9	1.7
Steak Platter, Wimpy*	1 Serving/424g	719	38.0	170	9.9	12.9	9.0	0.0
The International Grill, Wimpy*	1 Serving/416g	1010	71.3	243	13.9	9.9	17.1	0.9
Wimpy All Day Breakfast, Wimpy*	1 Serving/410g	731	39.7	178	8.3	14.5	9.7	0.0
ICE CREAMS								
Banana Longboat with Soft Ice Cream, Wimpy*	1 Serving/209g	260	6.0	124	2.3	23.9	2.9	0.0
Brown Derby with Dairy Ice Cream, Wimpy*	1 Serving/125g	397	19.7	318	5.6	38.9	15.8	0.0
Choc Nut Sundae, Wimpy*	1 Serving/83g	196	6.2	236	4.6	38.4	7.5	0.0
Fruit & Nut Sundae, Wimpy*	1 Serving/83g	138	5.8	166	4.2	23.3	7.0	0.0
Ice Cream Portion, Soft with Chocolate Sauce, Wimpy*	1 Serving/71g	137	3.2	193	2.8	36.1	4.5	0.0
Ice Cream Portion, Soft with Strawberry Sauce, Wimpy*	1 Serving/71g	137	3.0	193	2.4	38.3	4.2	0.0
Knickerbockerglory with Soft Ice Cream, Wimpy*	1 Serving/138g	196	6.0	142	2.7	24.7	4.3	0.0
Triple Strawberry Sundae with Soft Ice Cream, Wimpy*	1 Serving/170g	123	3.3	72	1.4	13.1	1.9	0.0
KIDS								
Cheese Toastie with Salad, Wimpy*	1 Serving/250g	367	8.8	147	5.9	24.2	3.5	1.2
Chicken Chunks Meal with Chips, Wimpy*	1 Serving/172g	440	26.1	256	8.4	22.1	15.2	1.8
Chicken Chunks Meal with Salad, Wimpy*	1 Serving/187g	265	16.8	142	6.8	8.4	9.0	0.7
Fish Bites Meal with Chips, Wimpy*	1 Serving/160g	380	20.9	237	6.7	24.7	13.1	2.1
Fish Bites Meal with Salad, Wimpy*	1 Serving/175g	205	11.6	117	5.2	9.8	6.6	0.9
Hamburger Meal with Chips, Wimpy*	1 Serving/184g	457	20.0	248	9.0	29.9	10.9	0.0
Hamburger Meal with Salad, Wimpy*	1 Serving/199g	283	10.7	142	7.5	16.4	5.4	0.0
Junior Cheeseburger Meal with Chips, Wimpy*	1 Serving/191g	497	23.5	260	10.0	27.7	12.3	2.1

	Measure INFO/WEIGHT	per Measure KCAL	FAT	Nutrition Values per 100g / 100ml KCAL	PROT	CARB	FAT	FIBRE

WIMPY

KIDS

	Measure/INFO/WEIGHT	KCAL	FAT	KCAL	PROT	CARB	FAT	FIBRE
Sausage Meal with Chips, Wimpy*	1 Serving/160g	428	27.7	267	8.9	19.9	17.3	1.9
Wimpy Hot Dog with Salad, Wimpy*	1 Serving/241g	425	21.1	176	7.0	17.3	8.8	0.0

MUFFIN

Giant Blueberry, Wimpy*	1 Muffin/108g	470	25.6	435	5.9	48.9	23.7	0.0

NUTS

Nibbed for desserts, Wimpy*	1 Serving/5g	32	2.8	640	26.0	6.0	56.0	12.0

PANINI

Cheese & Tomato, Wimpy*	1 Panini/225g	694	25.1	309	14.6	37.4	11.1	2.2
Cheese with Red Onion, Wimpy*	1 Panini/205g	673	22.8	329	14.6	42.7	11.1	1.9
Ham, Tomato & Cheese, Wimpy*	1 Panini/275g	1145	39.0	417	33.0	38.4	14.2	2.2
Ham & Cheese, Wimpy*	1 Panini/235g	944	33.3	402	32.0	35.7	14.2	1.4
Steak, Cheese & Onion, Wimpy*	1 Panini/305g	688	28.6	226	13.8	21.4	9.4	0.9

POTATO JACKET

Plain with Butter, Wimpy*	1 Serving/327g	453	7.6	139	3.5	27.7	2.3	2.4
with Baked Beans, Wimpy*	1 Serving/452g	549	7.9	121	3.4	23.5	1.7	2.7
with Beans & Cheese, Wimpy*	1 Serving/577g	1069	51.5	185	8.4	18.4	8.9	2.1
with Coleslaw, Wimpy*	1 Serving/452g	576	17.1	127	2.9	21.7	3.8	2.0
with Grated Cheese, Wimpy*	1 Serving/452g	973	51.2	215	9.6	20.0	11.3	1.7
with Tuna Mayo, Wimpy*	1 Serving/452g	764	34.2	169	5.9	20.6	7.6	1.7

RIBS

Pork Rib, Wimpy*	1 Rib/189g	463	22.4	245	13.0	21.6	11.9	0.0

ROLL

Bacon & Egg, in a Bun, Wimpy*	1 Roll/155g	702	41.7	453	29.6	22.6	26.9	1.4
Bacon in a Bun, Wimpy*	1 Roll/125g	341	16.1	273	16.0	22.6	12.9	1.4

SALAD

Fish, Wimpy*	1 Serving/356g	389	21.3	109	4.6	9.9	6.0	0.0
Gourmet Chicken, Wimpy*	1 Serving/358g	251	4.3	70	11.9	2.7	1.2	0.4
Hot & Spicy Chicken, Wimpy*	1 Serving/290g	283	15.2	98	6.1	6.7	5.2	0.9
Scampi, Wimpy*	1 Serving/356g	376	19.1	106	4.2	10.7	5.4	0.0
Steak, Wimpy*	1 Serving/355g	329	16.9	93	10.0	2.7	4.8	0.4

SAUCE

Chocolate for Sundae, Wimpy*	1 Serving/28g	80	0.4	286	1.4	66.1	1.4	1.1
Maple Flavoured Syrup for dessert, Wimpy*	1 Serving/28g	74	0.1	264	0.0	67.9	0.4	0.0
Strawberry for dessert, Wimpy*	1 Serving/28g	78	0.0	279	0.0	69.6	0.0	0.4

SWEETS

Mini Marshmallows for desserts, Wimpy*	1 Serving/10g	33	0.0	330	4.0	83.0	0.0	0.0
Mini Marshmallows for desserts, Wimpy*	1 Serving/10g	33	0.0	330	4.0	83.0	0.0	0.0

TEACAKE

Toasted with Butter, Wimpy*	1 Teacake/66g	227	2.3	344	1.7	10.4	3.4	0.4

VEGETARIAN

Lemon Pepper Quorn, Wimpy*	1 Serving/239g	586	26.5	245	8.0	29.2	11.1	0.0
Spicy Beanburger, Wimpy*	1 Serving/233g	593	29.2	255	5.4	30.8	12.5	0.0

WRAPID

WRAP

All Day Breakfast W22, Wrapid*	1 Wrap/223g	569	27.9	255	14.0	23.1	12.5	1.5
Breakfast Panini W35, Wrapid*	1 Wrap/181g	466	20.2	257	12.9	27.6	11.2	1.8
Chicken Fajita W18, Wrapid*	1 Wrap/226g	485	19.2	215	13.3	22.0	8.5	1.3
Chicken Tikka Balti W15, Wrapid*	1 Wrap/266g	476	13.7	179	8.5	24.4	5.2	1.5
Chicken Tikka Massala Pot WPOT004, Wrapid*	1 Pot/310g	487	14.7	157	5.4	20.8	4.7	1.2
Chilli Cheese Bean T8 & W46, Wrapid*	1 Wrap/189g	411	13.9	217	7.8	29.9	7.3	2.8
Chilli Con Carne & Rice W19, Wrapid*	1 Wrap/286g	505	13.9	176	3.9	28.8	4.8	1.2
Chilli Con Carne Pot WPOT001, Wrapid*	1 Wrap/310g	412	12.9	133	2.2	20.9	4.1	0.4

WRAPID

WRAP

	Measure INFO/WEIGHT	per Measure KCAL	FAT	Nutrition Values per 100g / 100ml KCAL	PROT	CARB	FAT	FIBRE
Croques Monsier, Ham & Cheese W30, Wrapid*	1 Wrap/231g	648	30.5	281	15.4	27.1	13.2	0.7
Fajita Chicken Panini W39, Wrapid*	1 Wrap/181g	336	8.4	186	10.0	25.5	4.6	1.6
Ham & Cheddar Panini W34, Wrapid*	1 Wrap/176g	501	21.4	284	13.1	30.9	12.2	1.5
Ham & Pineapple Pizza W28, Wrapid*	1 Wrap/270g	510	17.5	189	12.5	21.3	6.5	2.1
Margerita Panini W36, Wrapid*	1 Wrap/173g	441	18.7	255	11.6	28.6	10.8	2.2
Meat Balls Pasta Pot WPOT002, Wrapid*	1 Pot/291g	349	9.1	120	4.8	19.0	3.1	1.4
Mushroom, Cheese & Egg W20, Wrapid*	1 Wrap/210g	531	29.6	253	9.6	22.0	14.1	1.4
Pepperoni Pizza Panini W37, Wrapid*	1 Wrap/194g	570	30.7	294	13.9	25.0	15.8	1.8
Pepperoni Pizza W26, Wrapid*	1 Wrap/249g	688	36.8	276	16.5	21.2	14.8	2.3
Roast Vegetable Pasta Pot WPOT003, Wrapid*	1 Pot/311g	294	3.5	94	3.4	18.1	1.1	1.7
Roasted Peppers Pizza W27, Wrapid*	1 Wrap/261g	502	18.7	192	11.9	21.3	7.2	2.5
Steak & Mash, Wrapid*	1 Wrap/246g	424	9.7	172	6.6	26.2	4.0	1.0
Stir Fry Chicken with Noodles W23, Wrapid*	1 Wrap/251g	411	8.6	164	8.0	24.8	3.4	1.5
Tuna Melt Panini W33, Wrapid*	1 Wrap/178g	430	15.1	241	14.2	27.7	8.5	1.3
Tuna Melt W29, Wrapid*	1 Wrap/237g	538	21.3	227	16.3	21.2	9.0	1.3
Vegetable, Breakfast Panini W43, Wrapid*	1 Wrap/204g	366	11.0	180	7.0	25.8	5.4	1.8
Vegetable, Red Thai Panini W45, Wrapid*	1 Wrap/185g	360	12.8	194	6.8	30.1	6.9	2.1

Useful Resources

Weight Loss
Weight Loss Resources is home to the UK's largest calorie and nutrition database along with diaries, tools and expert advice for weight loss and health.
Tel: 01733 345592   Email: helpteam@weightlossresources.co.uk
Website: www.weightlossresources.co.uk

Exercise Equipment for Home
Diet and Fitness Resources has a range of equipment for exercise at home, from pedometers to treadmills and fitballs to weights. As well as diet tools such as food diaries, a weight loss kit and diet plates.
Tel: 01733 345592   Email: helpteam@dietandfitnessresources.co.uk
Website: www.dietandfitnessresources.co.uk

Dietary Advice
The British Dietetic Association has helpful food fact leaflets and information on how to contact a registered dietitian.
Tel: 0121 200 8080 Email: webmaster@bda.uk.com
Website: www.bda.uk.com

Healthy Eating
The British Nutrition Foundation has lots of in depth scientifically based nutritional information, knowledge and advice on healthy eating for all ages.
Tel: 0207 404 6504 Email: postbox@nutrition.org.uk
Website: www.nutrition.org.uk

Healthy Heart
The British Heart Foundation provides advice and information for all on all heart aspects from being healthy, to living with heart conditions, research and fundraising.
Tel: 0207 554 000   Email: via their website
Website: www.bhf.org.uk

Cancer Research
Cancer Research UK is the leading UK charity dedicated to research, education and fundraising for all forms of cancer.
Tel: 0207 242 0200 Email: via their website
Website: www.cancerresearchuk.org

Diabetes Advice
Diabetes UK is the leading charity working for people with diabetes. Their mission is to improve the lives of people with diabetes and to work towards a future without diabetes
Tel : 0845 120 2960 Email: info@diabetes.org.uk
Website: www.diabetes.org.uk

Beating Bowel Cancer
Beating Bowel Cancer is a leading UK charity for bowel cancer patients, working to raise awareness of symptoms, promote early diagnosis and encourage open access to treatment choice for those affected by bowel cancer.Tel: 08450 719301   Email: nurse@beatingbowelcancer.org
Website: http://www.beatingbowelcancer.org

Safety and Standards
The Food Standards Agency is an independent watchdog, set up to protect the public's health and consumer interests in relation to food.
Tel: 0207 276 8829 Email: helpline@foodstandards.gsi.gov.uk
Website: www.food.gov.uk

Feedback

If you have any comments or suggestions about The Calorie, Carb & Fat Bible, or would like further information on Weight Loss Resources, please call, email, or write to us:

Tel: 01733 345592
Email: helpteam@weightlossresources.co.uk
Address: Pat Wilson,
            Weight Loss Resources Ltd,
            29 Metro Centre,
            Woodston,
            Peterborough,
            PE2 7UH.

Reviews for The Calorie Carb & Fat Bible

'What a brilliant book. I know I'll be sinking my teeth into it.'
GMTV Nutritionist Amanda Ursell, BSc RD

'To help you make low-cal choices everyday, invest in a copy.'
ZEST magazine

'There is no doubt that the food listings are extremely helpful for anyone wishing to control their calorie intake in order to lose pounds or maintain a healthy weight.'
Women's Fitness magazine

'Useful if you don't want to exclude any overall food groups.'
Easy Living magazine

'Quite simply an astonishing achievement by the authors.'
Evening Post, Nottingham

'The book gives you all the basic information so you can work out your daily calorie needs.'
Woman magazine

'This is a welcome resource in view of the 'national epidemic of obesity.'

Bryony Philip, Bowel Cancer UK

'The authors seem to understand the problems of slimming.'

Dr John Campion

'Jam-packed with info on dieting, and full to bursting point with the calorie, carbohydrate and fat values of thousands of different foods, it's the perfect weight loss tool.'

Evening Express, Aberdeen

'Excellent resource tool - used by myself in my role as a Practice Nurse.'

Pam Boal, Sunderland

'I recently bought your book called the Calorie, Carb & Fat Bible and would love to tell you what a brilliant book it is. I have recently started a weight management programme and I honestly don't know where I'd be without your book. It has helped me a lot and given me some really good advice.'

Rachel Mitchell

About Weight Loss Resources

weightlossresources.co.uk

"What this does is put you in control with no guilt, no awful groups and no negativity! Fill in your food diary, get support on the boards and watch it fall off!"

LINDAB, Weight Loss Resources Member

How Does It Work?

Weight Loss Resources is home to the UK's biggest online calorie and nutrition database. You simply tap in your height, weight, age and basic activity level - set a weight loss goal, and the programme does all the necessary calculations.

What Does It Do?

The site enables you to keep a food diary which keeps running totals of calories, fat, fibre, carbs, proteins and portions of fruit and veg. You can also keep an exercise diary which adds the calories you use during exercise. At the end of a week, you update your weight and get reports and graphs on your progress.

How Will It Help?

You'll learn a great deal about how your eating and drinking habits affect your weight and how healthy they are. Using the diaries and other tools you'll be able to make changes that suit your tastes and your lifestyle. The result is weight loss totally tailored to your needs and preferences. A method you can stick with that will help you learn how to eat well for life!

Try It Free!

Go to **www.weightlossresources.co.uk** and take a completely free, no obligation, 24 hour trial. If you like what you see you can sign up for membership from £6.95 per month.